P9-CFQ-867

FOURTH EDITION

Neuroscience for the Study of Communicative Disorders

Subhash C. Bhatnagar, PhD, CCC-SLP

Neurolinguistics Laboratory
Speech Pathology and Audiology Department
Marquette University

Wolters Kluwer Health | Lippincott Williams & Wilkins

Philadelphia • Baltimore • New York • London
Buenos Aires • Hong Kong • Sydney • Tokyo

Senior Publisher: Julie Stegman
Product Manager: John Larkin
Marketing Director: Steven Rutberg
Designer: Joan Wendt
Compositor: SPi Global

Fourth Edition

351 West Camden Street
Baltimore, MD 21201

Two Commerce Square
2001 Market Street
Philadelphia, PA 19103

Printed in China

Library of Congress Cataloging-in-Publication Data
Bhatnagar, Subhash Chandra.
Neuroscience for the study of communicative disorders / Subhash C. Bhatnagar. —4th ed.
p. ; cm.
Includes bibliographical references and index.
ISBN 978-1-60913-871-4
I. Title.
[DNLM: 1. Central Nervous System—anatomy & histology. 2. Central Nervous System—physiology. 3. Communication Disorders—physiopathology. WL 300]
612.8—dc23

2011039961

To purchase additional copies of this book, call our customer service department at (800) 638-3030 or fax orders to (301) 223-2320. International customers should call (301) 223-2300.

Visit Lippincott Williams & Wilkins on the Internet: http://www.lww.com. Lippincott Williams & Wilkins customer service representatives are available from 8:30 am to 6:00 pm, EST.

9 8 7 6 5 4

The wealth of knowledge is the best of all possessions; it can neither be stolen, nor taken away by government, nor divided among brothers. It is never a burden to carry this wealth, which increases only by sharing and giving.

—A Sanskrit Saying

I dedicate this book to

My late father Shri Chiranji Lal Bhatnagar, who did everything possible, and more, to nurture and inspire

and

My late friend, Dr. Orlando J. Andy, who mentored me on cognitive aspects of neurosurgery.

Foreword

Once again, it is my deep pleasure to write the foreword for this latest edition of Subhash Bhatnagar's now classic text *Neuroscience for the Study of Communicative Disorders*. I have been honored to write the previous three forewords as well. It is enlightening to look back over those three earlier editions to note not only the increasing complexity of neuroscience as it is reflected therein but also to note the increasing sophistication, as well as the elegance with which Dr. Bhatnagar has made the subject, edition after edition, more accessible and user-friendly to students, teachers, and professionals who should keep it always near them as a fine reference work.

As neuroscience inevitably has advanced since the last edition 5 years ago, so has the technology of teaching. This volume takes advantage of these changes as well, with the addition of a Web site, PowerPoint outlines for instructional use, film clips, a structure mapping brain atlas, and much more.

Just as neuroscience and its study have advanced, so have the needs of students in Speech and Hearing Science. At its heart, I believe that neuroscience is the cornerstone of our profession and its clinical applications. Serious students can no longer slip by with a superficial knowledge or a modest appreciation of the role that neuroscience plays in their chosen profession. *Neuroscience for the Study of Communication* puts a sound foundation in that subject at their fingertips and provides their instructors with strong teaching tools to aid in the process.

Audrey L Holland, PhD
Regents' Professor Emerita
The University of Arizona
Tucson, Arizona

Preface

This genesis of this book is rooted in the growing recognition of the importance of neuroscience and its relationship with cognitive–communicative functions. This recognition has been furthered by the increasing emergence of a patient population with neurological conditions that includes roughly 50 million Americans, many with cognitive–communicative disorders (Castro et al., 2002), an area of primary concern to clinicians working in the field of human behavior.

FEATURES AND ORGANIZATION

The needs and challenges that provided the impetus for writing this book in the first place have not changed since its first edition went to print in 1995. This is now the fourth edition in this continuing endeavor, which was first envisioned by the late Dr. Orlando Andy and myself, to present the basics of neuroscience in a way that students could find both meaningful and interesting, while also giving academic faculty a tool for teaching the foundations and exploring the complexities of neuroscience. In order to make the study of neuroscience further accessible and user-friendly, and to promote an analytic approach to learning and critical thinking, the following improvements have been made in this print:

- A large part of the book has been rewritten so that the inherent, technical complexity of neuroscience is further simplified, in part, by focusing on the applications of theoretical and difficult concepts.
- Approximately 35% of the images have been modified to improve their effectiveness as a teaching and learning tool.
- Approximately 22 new MR and CT images (both normal and with pathologies) have been added to promote the application of learning to brain imaging.
- The text has been amended to include important clinical information in order to promote critical thinking, including
  - Approximately 60 boxes with clinical medical information
  - Approximately 10 more summarizing tables
  - Approximately 10 new, interactive problem-solving case studies
  - Neurogenic concepts related to human communication
- An updated discussion of cellular biology and neuroembryology is added.
- Additional clinical details about the embryonic synapse development and inherent cell loss (apoptosis) have been reexamined from a cognitive–communicative perspective.
- The section on neuroimaging has been rewritten, in conjunction with images, to address newer developments in the field of neuroimaging (functional MRI, diffusion-weighted MRI, perfusion-weighted MRI, diffusion tensor imaging, and MRI spectroscopy).
- The sections on respiratory control and consciousness have been rewritten to include newer concepts.
- The enhanced list of medical abbreviations has been categorized into practical categories, in order to increase its utility, such as assessment, body part, chemical, disease, hospital location, patient attribute, professional association, and treatment.
- The glossary has been enhanced and streamlined to make it a more effective quick-reference resource.

To assist instructors, each chapter has been reorganized to allow easy access to and retrieval of pertinent information. All of the chapters contain the following, uniform sections:

- Clinical considerations
  - Some have a section for lesion localizing rules and explanations.
- Problem-solving case studies
  - Inclusion of case study discussions at the end of the book
- Section or chapter summary
- Review questions (for classroom quizzes)
  - Inclusion of review question answers at the end of the book
  - The review questions and answers are written in such a way that they can be programmed on software like D2L that would allow immediate feedback to the students of their errors.

In addition, this edition has the following features:

- Fully outlined text in each section to facilitate reorganization for an individually tailored teaching.
  - This outline allows the instructors to reorganize the information to meet their specific teaching needs.
- Development of about 500 multiple choice and clinical case study questions with answers.
  - This resource with many images is available to the instructors on the book's Web site. Students have access to only questions.

- A Web site that contains a structure mapping brain atlas and movie clips to be used for additional study
- A reorganized structure that sequences the circulatory system before the chapters dedicated to sensorimotor physiology.
  - This reorganization, based on the feedback received from other teachers, will allow students to apply their knowledge of the vascular system to the sensorimotor brain.
- A developed PowerPoint outline of the book

These instructor and student ancillaries can be found at http://www.thepoint.lww.com/Bhatnagar4e

Despite these efforts to simply the book to increase its accessibility, the inherent complexity of neuroscience is maintained and appreciated in this book. It is my hope that these efforts at revision conform with Albert Einstein's famous aphorism: "Make everything as simple as possible, but not simpler."

Subhash C. Bhatnagar

Acknowledgments

At the outset, I wish to thank my many colleagues and students around the country, who have provided me with invaluable feedback about their experience with prior editions of this book. Their input has resulted in the addition of important information and improved the presentation of existing material, while keeping the study of neuroscience clear and accessible.

In preparing this edition of the book, I am grateful to many of my colleagues for their time, energy, and support. These colleagues, without whom this edition would not be possible, include Dr. Duane E. Haines, University of Mississippi Medical Center; Dr. Robin L. Curtis (retired), Medical College of Wisconsin; Dr. Alexandru Barboi, Medical College of Wisconsin; Dr. Lotfi Hacein-Bey, Radiological Associates of Sacramento Medical Group Inc; Dr. Satish Jain, Indian Epilepsy Center, New Delhi; Dr. Howard Kirshner, Vanderbilt College of Medicine; Dr. Madhuri Behari, All India Institute of Medical Sciences, New Delhi; Dr. William Mustain, University of Mississippi Medical Center, Milwaukee; Dr. Varun Saxena, Center for Neurological Disorders; Dr. Kunwar Bhatnagar, University of Louisville College of Medicine; Dr. Sanjeev Pradhan, University of Illinois Medical Center; Dr. Michelle Mynlieff, Marquette University; and Dr. Hugh Buckingham, Louisiana State University. I also thank Dr. Lotfi Hacein-Bey for jointly writing the 'Neuroradiology section'.

I also acknowledge the help that I received from Dr. Alexandru Barboi for jointly writing the clinical questions for 'ThePoint,' the website that accompanies this book.

Obviously this book would not have been possible without the support of many at Wolters Kluwer/Lippincott Williams and Wilkins. I express my thanks to Peter Sabatini and Julie Stegman (editors), Timothy Serpico (marketing manager), and John Larkin (product manager). I also thank Jennifer Clements for her hard work in preparing the artwork for the book.

I am especially grateful to Dr. Audrey L. Holland from the University of Arizona for agreeing to write the foreword of this edition, just as she has for the prior three editions of this book. It has been my honor to have her support and ongoing friendship from my days as a graduate student.

I also thank Ms. Martha Jerme, the health sciences librarian from Marquette University, for her invaluable assistance in ensuring all references in this edition are up-to-date.

I am indebted to my many students at Marquette University, whose comments and feedback over the years in the classroom have been both invaluable and encouraging. I am particularly thankful to three of my graduate students—Libby Kelley, Bridget Zmolek, and Amy Spilsky, each of whom has worked in my Neurolinguistics Lab and has diligently helped prepare many aspects of this edition. I also thank Kathryn Errek and Caitlin Fitzgerald for their help in preparing the PowerPoint for the book.

Finally, I thank Priti, my wife and my best friend. Without her understanding, support, and sacrifices, neither this edition nor any of the three that preceded it would have been possible. I also thank my children—Manav, Gaurav, and Kathryn—whose emotional support and encouragement underlies everything I do.

Contents

1

Essential Neurological Concepts and Principles

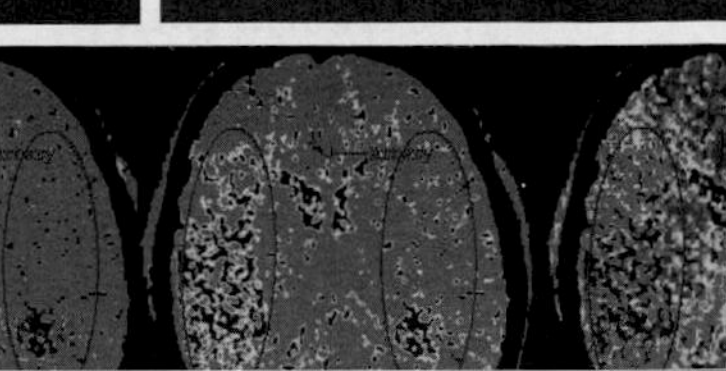

LEARNING OBJECTIVES

After studying this chapter, students should be able to:

- Describe the subject matter of neuroscience and speech–language–hearing pathology
- Discuss the relationship between neuroscience and speech–language–hearing pathology
- Explain the rationale for learning neuroscience
- Discuss the benefits of neuroscience training
- Describe the scope of the major branches of neuroscience
- Explain the components of a neurologic examination
- Describe common neurologic diseases that have clinical relevance to students of human behavior
- Explain the basic principles that govern human brain function
- Define technical terms used for directional reference, brain section planes, and anatomic structures
- Describe the major structures of the central nervous system and outline their functions
- Outline the classificatory components that categorize the nervous system functions
- Describe the architectural organization of the cerebral cortex
- Discuss Brodmann areas with respect to their use in neurolinguistics
- Display their familiarity with clinically established diagnostic signs
- Appreciate the rationale used for localizing lesions in the nervous system
- Appreciate the challenge posed by the solving of pertinent neurogenic problems

RELATIONSHIP BETWEEN NEUROSCIENCE AND SPEECH–LANGUAGE–HEARING PATHOLOGY

Speech–language–hearing pathology (SLP) and neuroscience are closely related disciplines. A well-developed and adequately connected neuronal organization of the brain serves as a prerequisite for the acquisition of language and other higher mental functions, whose normal use also reflects the brain's structural and functional integrity. This brain–behavior relationship was underscored over a century ago by the observations of the classical neurologists like Paul Broca (1861) and Carl Wernicke (1874) on the localization of specific expressive and receptive language functions in particular areas of the human brain. After examining a series of patients who could not speak, despite having no motor problems in their speech muscles and no difficulties understanding spoken language, Broca proposed in 1861 that speaking is controlled by the frontal lobe in the left hemisphere of the brain.

An examination of the brains of such patients during autopsy revealed a lesion in the lower posterior frontal region, a region now called the Broca area (see Fig. 2-5). Wernicke in 1874 described a different type of language disorder caused by reduced auditory comprehension instead of impaired expression. He related this aphasia type to a lesion in the left posterior temporal lobe (Fig. 9-10), a different area from the one described by Broca. These two observations of cortical functional specialization (different brain regions being associated with different functions) enhanced our knowledge of the brain–behavior relationship. In doing so, they established the groundwork for modern neurolinguistic studies, in which other language functions were assigned to different brain regions and their interactive connections. Language and speech disturbances have since become sensitive indicators of structural and physiologic impairment in the brain.

Key Terms :

Central nervous system
Cerebral cortex
Embryology
Neuroanatomy
Neurology
Neuropathology
Neurophysiology
Neuroradiology
Neurosurgery

Phylogenetically, the evolution of the brain is progressively linear, reaching its highest level in humans (*Homo sapiens*), in whom the brain is not just a scaled-up version of its primitive forms. Rather its advanced structural architecture reflects an enormously increased cellular complexity (in terms of cellular density and synaptic connectivity), and the brain regions associated with specific functions grow at different rates. Owing to this variable rate of cellular growth, the neocortex (six-layered cellular organization) occupies a large percentage of the **cerebral cortex**, which has a vast cytoarchitectural (cellular aggregates) complexity found only in the human brain. Thicker in appearance and highly laminated compared to other primates and comprising only 2% of the body weight, it is uniquely equipped to analyze and synthesize information in past, present, and future contexts. Through its biologic interaction with the environment, the human brain generates substrates for consciousness, cognition (attention, memory, and decision making), symbolic communication, learning, knowledge, personality, emotions, thoughts, creative ability, mental imagery, and skilled sensorimotor functions.

Domain of Neuroscience

The goal of neuroscience is to identify and explain the mechanisms the brain uses to acquire and regulate higher mental functions and to produce both basic and skilled actions. The biologic basis of such functions reflects an interface with both the cellular activities and the power of the mind, the seat of consciousness (Ward, 2010). The scope of neuroscience includes the study of the anatomic structures, cellular functions, and physiologic processes of the nervous system. Thus, neuroscience also makes it possible for clinicians to identify sites of structural and functional abnormalities in patients exhibiting altered mental and sensorimotor functions. Neuroscience is an important part of training in SLP and is indispensable for understanding the physiologic correlates and relationships among speech, language, gestures, and cognition. What raises the curiosity of students of human behaviors is the brain's relationship to the mind, the power it uses to create the representation of abstract attributes of thoughts, emotions, and cognition.

Domain of SLP

SLP deals with the normal mental processes and disorders (developmental and acquired) of human cognition and communication. Speech–language–hearing pathologists (SLPs) receive comprehensive training in normal development and in abnormal aspects of human communicative processes, including assessment and therapeutic management of such communication disorders. With an extensive background in the physiology and psychology of communication, they are also trained to undertake or assist in the neurolinguistic assessment of the behavioral effects of neurologic injuries and to pursue research in brain–behavior relationship issues.

Need for Training in Neuroscience

To understand the biological issues related to communicative disorders, one must have a functionally adequate background in neuroscience. Recent advances in medical care have generally increased longevity, prolonging the life span of many patients in the world. With an ever-increasing number of patients with cognitive and communicative disorders, resulting from head trauma, vascular accidents, embryologic malformations, degenerative conditions, tumors, epilepsy, and a variety of congenital and acquired organic disorders (Box 1-1), there is clearly a need for a comprehensive and effective rehabilitative intervention, which demands a broader training in SLP integrated with neuroscience as well as

BOX 1-1

Neurological Disorders in the United States

More than 20% (about 50 million people) of the U.S. population is estimated to have some form of chronic or acquired neurologic disorder; roughly 15 million of these individuals have either a developmental or an acquired communicative–cognitive disorder (Castro, 2002). Because of increasing longevity and a rapidly lowering average age for cerebral pathology, stroke not only constitutes the cause of >50% of cases of brain dysfunction but has become the leading cause of aphasia and the third leading cause of death and disability in adults. Stroke affects 600,000 to 700,000 people each year. Furthermore, as the number of people living into their 80s and beyond increases, so have the challenges and demands for supportive services. Speech-language-hearing-pathologists provide essential and valuable rehabilitative and supportive services for subjects with dementia and other communicative disorders.

other disciplines. The application of training in neuroscience is important in the diagnosis and treatment of communicative disorders across all ages and disorders. Training in neuroscience can be integrated throughout the speech–language–hearing curriculum. However, because of its complexity, neuroscience is best learned if it is studied as a separate course.

Nature of Training in Neuroscience

A well-trained professional in communicative disorders and human behavior must have a working knowledge of functional clinical neurology. Knowledge of how nerve cells communicate (how their axons serve as pathways for transmitting information to other cortical or subcortical regions, at what point they cross the midline, with what other pathways they travel, their cortical projections) provides a basis for understanding the neurologic correlates of higher mental functions and sensorimotor behaviors.

At times, some depth of discussion is unavoidable in learning neuroscience. However, students of behavioral science need not undergo the extensive training in neuroscience given to neurologists and neurosurgeons. Students of human behaviors only need basic familiarity with the functional and anatomic organization of the nervous system, including the cerebral cortex, the subcortical structures, and the spinal cord. It is a fallacy to assume that there is a simpler version of neuroscience related to hearing, speech, language, and mental functions. The fundamental sensorimotor rules that apply to locomotion also apply to complex skills in speaking. Similarly, the mental processes in the brain are also represented by their combined elementary operations.

Benefits of Training in Neuroscience

On a technical level, familiarity with the fundamentals of neuroscience does more than provide professionals in behavioral science with an understanding of the genesis of neurological conditions associated with communicative disorders. Training also enables these clinicians and researchers to appreciate the signs and symptoms associated with brain dysfunctions involving cortical and subcortical areas, to comprehend the principles of differential diagnosis, and to interpret neuroimaging. Such skills facilitate the recognition of clinically significant signs—covert and overt—and the detection of life-threatening conditions associated with a variety of pathologic processes. This training in neuroscience further facilitates a grasp of functional, structural, and neurolinguistic properties of the human brain, which helps us appreciate the rationale underlying neurologic management.

Students of communicative disorders and human behavior trained in neuroscience can provide a more effectively structured and realistic rehabilitation program for communication disorders. Their background in neuroscience makes them creative partners on a diagnostic team and helps forge a constructive working relationship with medical colleagues from a variety of disciplines (neurology, neurosurgery, radiology, pediatrics, and physiatry). Clinicians trained in neuroscience are able to appreciate the rationale of neurologic diagnoses, follow scientific literature, understand complex medical terminology, help solve neurologic problems, and promote neurolinguistic research; thus, they have a broad view of their profession.

SCOPE OF NEUROSCIENCE

Neurologic assessment and management involve many branches of neuroscience. A neurologic diagnosis means identifying clinical signs that characterize a particular disease and answering fundamental questions: What is the cause? Is it inflammatory, traumatic, genetic, psychological, or a combination? Which anatomic structures or pathways are involved? On what side (left or right) of the neuraxis is the lesion located? How best to optimize patient's functional skills? Knowledge of the anatomy of the nervous system is essential to diagnosing a neurologic problem, determining the cause, and localizing the lesion. The key for understanding the distribution and localization of deficits is knowledge of the neuroanatomic pathways in the nervous system, their cortical projections, sites of fiber crossing, and interactions with other functional systems. Relating the signs and symptoms with the site of the lesion helps the clinician to arrive at a diagnosis and recommendation for an optimal treatment. Access to family history provides information about the onset, susceptibility, genetic predisposition, and severity of the deficit. The most important branches of neuroscience are listed in Table 1-1.

Neurology

Neurology deals with diseases that disrupt the normal structural and physiologic properties of the nervous system. Neurologic disorders include the following: vascular disorders (thrombosis, embolism, hemorrhage); neoplastic conditions (benign or malignant tumor); cortical degenerative conditions (amyotrophic lateral sclerosis, Pick disease, Alzheimer disease); myeline degeneration (multiple sclerosis and Guillain–Barré syndrome); motor disorders (Parkinson disease and Huntington chorea); deficiency disorders (Wernicke–Korsakoff syndrome); bacterial and viral infections (meningitis and encephalitis); cellular toxicity; epileptic disorders; and traumatic brain injury. From the clinical history, the neurologist derives crucial information about the disease process and uses the data obtained from the clinical examination of sensory and motor (reflex quality and strength) functions and laboratory testing to diagnose and determine the site, nature, and cause of the pathology to recommend proper treatment. The reflex is measured on a scale of 1 to 5 (0 for absent

Table 1-1

Branches of Neuroscience

Branch	Domain
Neurology	Diagnosis and treatment of nervous system disorders
Neurosurgery	Surgical removal of dysfunctioning structures that impair the functions of the nervous system
Neuroanatomy	Study of structural framework of nervous system, consisting of nerve cells (neurons) and their tracts (fibers)
Neuroradiology	Imaging techniques for differentiating pathologic tissue of central nervous system; radiation therapy for nervous system tumors is a subspecialty
Neuroembryology	Study of embryologic origin and development of the nervous system
Neurophysiology	Study of chemical, electrical, and metabolic functions of nervous system
Neuropathology	Study of characteristics and origins of diseases and their effects on nervous system

reflex; 1 for reduced or hypoactive reflex; 2 for normal reflex; 3 for hyperactive reflex; 4 for clonus, contraction and relaxation of a muscle in rapid succession). The muscle strength is also graded on a scale of 1 to 5 (0/5 for no muscle movement; 1/5 for visible muscle movement, but not at the joint; 2/5 for movement at the joint but not against gravity; 3/5 for movement against gravity but not against added resistance; 4/5 for less than normal movement against resistance; 5/5 for normal muscle strength). The neurologist, with a keen interest in human behavior, also uses information from the assessment of higher mental functions in making the final diagnosis (Table 1-3) since the disordered processes of communication and cognition provide significant information about cortical integrity. SLPs play an important role in neurological diagnosis by undertaking a comprehensive assessment of higher mental functions (language, speech, memory, attention, and cognition). Two corollaries of cognitive neurology are closely related to SLP: cognitive neuropsychology and neurolinguistics. Cognitive neuropsychology uses brain-damaged patients to form the theories of normal cognition. Neurolinguistics, on the other hand, analyzes aphasic disorders to formulate hypotheses about the normal organization of language in the human brain.

Neurosurgery

Neurosurgery involves surgical intervention to treat a disease of the nervous system, which requires penetration of structures such as the skull, vertebral column, and meninges (brain and spinal cord coverings). Neurosurgical intervention is used for conditions such as removal of neoplastic (tumor) tissue; extraction of blood clots (hematoma); excision of vascular aneurysms; removal of carotid arterial plaque; blocking of vessel feeding to arteriovenous malformation; ablation of functionally impaired "convulsing" tissues (epileptogenic scars); placement of selective lesions in the thalamus (thalamotomy); placement of therapeutic brain stimulation electrodes in the basal ganglia, subthalamic nucleus, and mesothalamus (deep brain stimulation) for chronic pain and involuntary movements; and removal of herniated disks in the spine. Neurosurgery also involves intensive care management of patients neurologically ill from traumatic injury and other neurologic diseases. Pediatric neurosurgery has a special place in neurosurgery because of the high frequency of surgically amenable diseases that are diagnosed in infants and children. The removal of tissue, particularly from the vicinity of the sensorimotor and/or language cortex, involves mapping of cortex with language function in which an SLP can help with designing language tasks and executing intraoperative neurolinguistic testing (see Chapter 20).

Neuroanatomy

Neuroanatomy relates to the structural organization of the nervous system. It grossly and microscopically defines the structural elements of the nervous system, specifically neurons and their colonies, fiber tracts, nerves, ventricular structures, vascular networks, and supporting glial and meningeal tissues.

Neuroradiology

Neuroradiology enables the diagnosis of the **nervous system** abnormalities without intrusion into the cranial cavity and body tissues. It uses emission or transmission imaging to identify intact and pathologic structures of the nervous

Table 1-2

Major Brain Diseases

Disorder	Description
Cerebrovascular accident (stroke)	Sudden loss of sensorimotor, speech, and language functions caused by interrupted blood supply to the brain
Neoplasm	Damage caused by infiltration and invasion of normal structures by uncontrolled cell growth (benign or malignant) Clinically marked by progressive and diffuse symptoms
Demyelination	
Multiple sclerosis	Progressive autoimmune disease of myelin (oligodendroglia) degeneration in the CNS affecting nerve conduction speed Clinically marked by muscle weakness, sensation loss, and disequilibrium, incoordination, and speech disturbance, which come and go Guillain-Barré syndrome involves the body's own immune system attacking the axons and their coverings (Schwann) in the PNS
Degeneration	
Alzheimer disease	Progressive degenerative disease of the brain associated with dementia in elderly population Clinically marked by amnesia, personality changes and impaired cognition
Pick disease	Marked by the presence of abnormal substances (Pick bodies and Tau protein) in nerve cells of the frontal-temporal lobes. Clinically marked by behavioral and linguistic impairments
Amyotrophic lateral sclerosis	Degeneration of motor neuron in the brain and spinal cord Clinically marked by muscle weakness and spasticity
Motor disorders	
Huntington chorea	Degenerative brain disease of dominant inheritance appearing in the mid-30s Clinically characterized by personality deficit, dementia and chorea
Parkinson disease	Degenerative motor disease of the brain characterized by tremor, movement slowness, and reduced muscular strength affecting motor speech
Cerebral palsy	An encompassing term for developmental sensorimotor disorders in children with or without communicative and cognitive deficits Caused by lack of oxygen to the brain before, during, or immediately after birth
Deficiency disorders	Amnesia, confabulation, and psychosis (impaired reality awareness) caused by Thiamine deficiency due to chronic alcoholism (Wernicke-Korsakoff syndrome)
Bacterial and viral infections	Viral or bacterial inflammatory infection of CNS membrane (coverings); also called meningitis Marked with headache, fever, stiff neck, and long term cognitive impairments
Epilepsy	Impairment of sensory, motor, cognitive, and affective functions secondary to abnormal electrical activity in brain; also called seizures
Toxic and Metabolic Disorders	A cover term for any (internally generated or externally induced by drugs) condition with effects on brain's cellular functioning. Commonly associated with diabetes, abnormal liver functioning, drug intoxication, and anoxia.
Traumatic brain injury	Broken axons, ruptured arteries, and tissue damage secondary to an excessive bouncing around of the brain within the hard and edgy skull Clinically marked by coup (under the impact site) and contrecoup (opposite the impact site) injuries.

Table 1-3

Common Areas Included in a Neurologic Assessment

Motor Examination	Sensory Examination	Mental Functions
Reflexes	Reflexes	Language
Superficial and tendon	Testing of sensory functions	Auditory comprehension (commands and yes/no questions)
Testing of motor functions	Pain and temperature	Spontaneous speech (picture description and conversation)
Gait	Touch	Naming (common objects)
Muscle coordination	Nonlocalized touch	Repetition (digits, words, and clauses)
Involuntary movements	Two-point touch	Reading (written commands)
Muscle tone (resistance to passive limb manipulation)	Kinesthetic sensation	Writing (dictation and picture description)
Muscle strength	Proprioceptive sensation	Memory
Cranial nerve examination	Sensation of vibration	Short term (recall of two objects in 4 min)
Lens accommodation and pupil light reflex (CN II, CN III)	Stereognosis	Long term (past presidents)
Eye movements (CN III, CN IV, CN VI)	Graphesthesia	Nonverbal tasks
Facial movements	Cranial nerve examination	Copying (figures)
Jaw movement (CN V)	Smell (CN I)	Drawing (clock)
Facial strength, expression, and articulation (CN VII)	Vision (CN II)	Calculation (multiplication tables and basic subtraction)
Resonance, phonation, and speech (CN IX, CN X, CN XII)	Visual acuity	Abstraction (divergent/convergent thinking tasks)
Head rotation and shoulder elevation (CN XI)	Visual fields	
Tongue movement (CN XII)	Sensation from the face, mouth, nose, and eyes (CN V)	
Swallowing (CN IX, CN X)	Hearing and equilibrium (CN VIII)	

system in vivo. Some modern neuroradiologic techniques are **x-ray, angiography, computer tomography (CT), magnetic resonance imaging (MRI), single-photon emission computed tomography (SPECT), positron emission tomography (PET), and magnetoencephalography (MEG)** which maps brain activity by recording magnetic fields produced by electrical currents (see Chapter 20). Advances in neuroradiology have not only revolutionized the diagnosis of the diseased tissue but have also energized the study of the brain–behavior relationship as well as the interaction between brain structures and behavioral (psychiatric) disorders. Therapeutic radiation, a branch of radiology, is also used to treat various malignant body and brain tumors (with a γ-knife) and is often combined with drug treatment (chemotherapy) and tumor excision.

Neuroembryology

Neuroembryology deals with growth of the nervous system during the embryonic periods of development extending from conception to 7 weeks, by the end of which all brain structures have anatomically emerged and are in place. Usually, it is also used to cover all stages of the prenatal life. Teratology, a term related to embryology, is the study of fetal malformations, the most important of which, for our purposes, are cranial malformations, which have serious implications for the development of both higher mental functions and sensorimotor skills (see Chapter 4).

Neurophysiology

Neurophysiology focuses on the functional properties of the nervous system with respect to the structural, chemical, and electrical composition that is essential to living organisms.

Neuropathology

Neuropathology deals with the nature, cause, and diagnosis of diseased tissue in the brain and spinal cord, which functionally disrupts the nervous system. It identifies the cells affected by tumor, infarct, infection, and degeneration.

PRINCIPLES GOVERNING THE HUMAN BRAIN

Although the human brain has a complex anatomic organization, its basic functions are regulated by a few simple principles. Taken together, these simple principles account not only for complex anatomic organization but also for all the functional processes that govern brain functions. Eight common regulating principles of the human brain are given in Table 1-4.

Interconnectivity in the Brain

All functionally specific primary sensory and motor regions in the **cerebrum** are connected through association and commissural fibers. The cortical association areas are directly connected to each other, whereas the primary cortical areas are indirectly connected through the cortical association areas. The cortical association areas also serve as the hub through which the primary cortical areas are indirectly connected. The homologous areas of the two hemispheres are connected through the interhemispheric commissural fibers. This connective network allows constant interaction among the functional circuits within each hemisphere and between the two hemispheres of the brain; this integrated network also explains how a message from one source can trigger multiple integrated responses involving many brain regions and how messages from multiple sources are rapidly integrated for one appropriate response to a given stimuli.

Centrality of the Central Nervous System

The **central nervous system** (CNS) is responsible for integrating all incoming and outgoing information and for generating appropriate responses to the information received. The response can be integrated (mental functions), or volitional (internally generated), such as a spontaneous or reflexive (environmentally elicited) motor movement like the withdrawal of a limb.

Because of the centrality of decision making and the all-encompassing response, no two parts in the peripheral body can directly communicate with each other, regardless of the distance between them. Even the simplest form of communication between two adjacent body parts, such as the thumb and palm (as exemplified in the basic reflexes), is mediated through the CNS. The outgoing motor response is always different from the incoming sensory information as it contains a directive that was refined and synthesized with additional informative stimuli from other sources of the neuraxis. The ability to simultaneously analyze and synthesize multiple sources of information and to generate distinct responses best exemplifies the brain's centralized organization.

Table 1-4

Organizational Principles of the Brain

Organizational Principles of the Brain
Interconnectivity in the brain
Centrality of central nervous system
Hierarchy of neuraxial organization
Laterality of brain organization
Functional networking
Topographical representation
Plasticity in the brain
Culturally neutral brain

Hierarchy in Neuraxial Organization

The neuraxis of the CNS is hierarchically developed in complexity of functions. Lower levels of organization perform inherent specific functions that are modified to varying degrees of complexity by the axial segments above. The spinal cord, the lowest level of organization, serves simple sensorimotor functions in the form of reflexes that are partly influenced (inhibited or facilitated) by the upper axial levels. The complexity of information processing increases as the level of processing becomes more brain controlled. The cerebral cortex, organizationally the highest hierarchic level, is responsible for complex sensorimotor integration and higher mental functions (cognition, language, and speech). Functionally different neuronal structures and circuitries also exist in the brainstem and **diencephalon**, the intermediate level of organization. These structures consist of autonomic, chemical, and visceral systems, all of which contribute to the regulation of consciousness, blood pressure, respiration, sleep, temperature, endocrine levels, and neurotransmitter interactions. Together, these systems react to nonspecific stress and adverse bodily changes to maintain optimal homeostatic states. The intermediate level of organization, which may be considered the nonthinking part of the brain, is tightly integrated with the cerebral cortex, which serves the highest organization level of decision making.

Key Terms:

Bilateral	**Homunculus**
Contralateral	**Laterality**
Critical period	**Neuroplasticity**
Ipsilateral	**Planum temporale**

Laterality of Brain Organization

The three important aspects of brain organization are: (1) bilateral anatomic symmetry, (2) unilateral functional differences, and (3) contralateral sensorimotor control of the nervous system.

Bilateral Anatomic Symmetry

The two cerebral hemispheres are essentially identical in anatomy; they would be considered mirror images of each other if not for the **planum temporale** (Fig. 9-8). Sensorimotor cortices in both hemispheres are connected through the corpus callosum, the largest of the commissural fibers.

Unilateral Functional Differences

Immediately after birth, two cerebral hemispheres are functionally equipotential; each hemisphere has the functional capacity to develop all linguistic or nonlinguistic skills. However, after the first 2 years, each hemisphere acquires an advantage over the other for developing different specialized functions. For most people, right- or left-handed, the left hemisphere comes to dominate language, speech, and analytic processing (Box 1-2); whereas the right hemisphere develops a greater efficiency in emotions, musical skills, and paralinguistic functions such as metaphors and jokes. The right half of the brain is also involved with temporospatial attributes and regulating melodic feature attributes, such as stress, juncture, and intonation.

Mostly, lesions in the left hemisphere, irrespective of the handedness, affect language functions more than on the right side of the brain. Enlargement of the planum temporale in the left brain compared to the right has been associated with the laterality of language function (Fig. 9-8).

Contralateral Sensorimotor Control

A unique aspect of brain organization is that all sensory and motor fibers in the nervous system are contralaterally organized such that the descending and ascending fibers mediating sensorimotor functions cross (decussate) the body's midline. The left motor cortex controls movements in the right half of the body; the sensory information from the left half of the body projects to the right sensory cortex (Fig. 1-1). Most sensory and motor fibers cross the midline in the lower (caudal) medulla of the brainstem. Of course, there are exceptions to this rule; the fibers carrying bodily pain and temperature cross the midline at multiple points in the spinal cord (see Chapter 11); some pathways, such as those for hearing, cross and recross at numerous levels in the brainstem (see Chapter 9) and the visual pathway involves a complex pattern of fiber crossing (see Chapter 12).

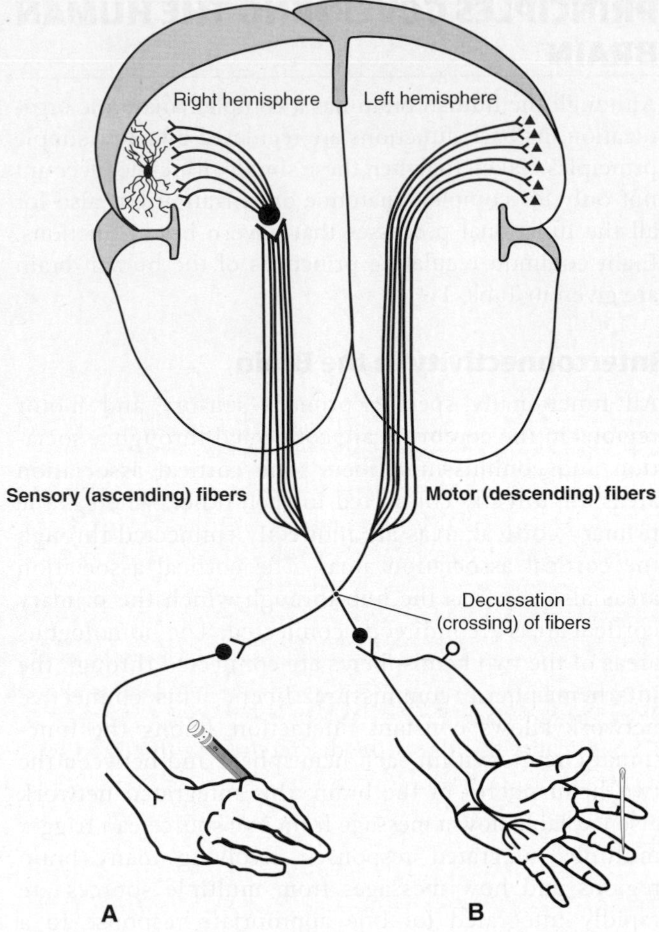

Figure 1-1 Contralateral brain organization. A. The decussation of the descending motor fibers before the synapse on the motor neurons. B. The ascending sensory fibers projecting to the contralateral somatosensory cortex after the midline crossing.

BOX 1-2

Wada Test

The Wada test, also referred to as "Sodium Amytal infusion," involves the intraarterial carotid injection of sodium amobarbital and is used for determining hemispheric dominance. The test involves the infusion of sodium amytal in the left and right integral carotid artery, which anesthetizes the brain for a period of 5 to 10 minutes. The neurolinguistic assumption is that if the drug is injected in the dominant hemisphere, it will result in aphasic symptoms, which helps identify the hemisphere dominant for language (see Chapter 20).

Functional Networking

The neuronal systems are functionally specialized. Sensory and motor systems possess specialized nerve cells that are separable and part of a selected network. These nerve cells incorporate specialized receptors and respond to functionally specific stimuli. The white matter in the brain is composed of many parallel pathways (tracts), each of which conducts different types of information. For example, sensory fibers exclusively carry sensations of pain, fine touch, and temperature; these fibers run parallel to one another and serve distinct functions that are determined by sensory receptor terminals in the peripheral body parts. The motor system also consists of several parallel but distinct pathways that transmit differentiated motor information to different limbs. For example, one path mediates skilled hand movements from the cortical and subcortical structures to the upper spinal cord, whereas the second transmits postural adjustment messages throughout the spinal cord and brainstem for trunk and limb movements. Another pathway contains short projections and controls speech and phonatory muscles in the face and neck through cranial nerves in the brainstem. The functional specificity of nerve cells and their projections accounts for their increased adaptability, processing speed, and the ability to make detailed and finer analysis of selected signals.

Topographical Representation

The topicality stands for the discreteness with which sensorimotor information is retained in the axonal pathways from the specialized peripheral receptors in the body to the brain. The spatial organization of neurons, tracts, and terminals reflects the spatial relationship of the body surface and functionally related muscle groups with the projected brain areas; this informational topicality also accounts for the somatosensory **homunculus**, an illustration of the human body superimposed on the brain (Fig. 2-6). For example, an orderly visual map is discretely projected to the visual cortex by way of the thalamus. This map is retained throughout the pathway to the visual cortex (Fig. 12-7). There is also continuity of representation; adjacent visual fields are represented in adjacent areas of the visual cortex. A similar relationship exists between a delineated area in the auditory cortex and the frequency-specific cells in the cochlea, called tonotopic representation.

Plasticity in the Brain

Plasticity or **neuroplasticity** is the brain's ability to change as a result of experience; the plasticity also includes the brain's ability to reorganize and gradually modify tissue functions when faced with pathologies. The inherent plasticity of brain cells permits the integration of specific cortical areas to serve additional functions and possibly to repair cortical circuitry in response to stroke, neoplasm, and degenerative changes in the brain. This adaptive property explains the reorganizational capacity of cellular functions.

Regeneration of nerves (sprouting) occurs to varying degrees in the nervous system. However, inflammatory responses, scar tissue, and protein expression interfere with but do not necessarily prevent the establishment of axonal reconnections in the CNS. The peripheral nervous system (PNS), with additional nerve trunk coverings (endoneurium, perineurium, and epineurium), has a greater opportunity for re-establishing connections (see Chapter 5).

The brain's ability to adapt to external and internal changes has important implications for learning; the functional plasticity in the brain's neuronal circuitry is greatest in the early years and substantially diminishes with age, but it never ends. Learning is better accomplished if one is given early experiences. Early exposure not only facilitates learning but also results in a finer and more efficient processing of information. Fine tuning of the internal system is best illustrated by the acquisition of a second language or a musical knowledge in the early years. Strongest support for a greater plasticity comes from the examples of brain injuries in early years. In such cases, the long-term effects of the injuries on language and cognition are not as dramatic and noticeable as they are in case of injuries in adult life; a provision for the better plasticity in younger age relates to the developing myelination and the ability to progressively establish new connections.

Accounting for the neuroplasticity, Gottlieb (1992) outlined two patterns of brain development: gene-governed predetermined and a probabilistic development. In the predetermined development, genes allocate specific functions to different areas of the brain and dictate what experiences these areas need. As part of the predetermined development, certain brain regions are committed to specific functions, the primary cortices (plural of cortex) are genetically programmed to serve sensation and movement, whereas the neurons in the association cortices are uncommitted at least at the time of birth. The brainstem possesses automatic control systems that are genetically acquired and cannot be modified. The functions involving the association cortical areas are programmed through experience, learning, and practice and are modifiable in the years to come. In a probabilistic development, the gene expression can be modified by experience and the internal and external environment. This view, representing the current neurolinguistic thinking, reinforces the brain's immense reorganizational ability that, to a certain extent, exists throughout the life. This not only underscores the importance of learning, but it also points to brain's ability to structurally change its circuitry through synaptic pruning, either by eliminating or recruiting synapses or by creating additional synapses. Neurons that are active together are more likely to be part of a coherent and integrated system.

Developing cellular density, establishing connectivity to target brain areas, and promoting synaptic patterns play an important role in the functional plasticity of the cerebral tissue. For the brain's functional reorganizational capacity, the **critical period** is another important concept; this is the period when an experience is most rewarding and effective in influencing the brain's potential. It is best illustrated by the axonal connectivity to the visual cortex as seen in the fetal period; structurally the axons carrying visual input from both eyes have equal access to the occipital visual cortex and equally compete for the available synaptic spaces. If for any reason, axons from one eye are not functional during this developmentally critical period, they lose the claim for synaptic spaces in the visual cortex. This allows for the axonal fibers from the good eye to become dominant and take initiative for controlling the available synaptic space in the brain, suggesting that it is not the experience alone, but rather the timing of the experience that regulates the potential for functional plasticity. The importance of the critical period has been widely discussed for facilitating the acquisition of language.

Substantial evidence has emerged to suggest that the brain's continued capacity to reorganize its synaptic connectivity underlies its plasticity. This capacity of tissue function reorganization continues throughout adult life. If a digit is amputated, for example, the projections from the digit to the cortex are lost and the target cortical area receives no sensory inputs. However, with functional reorganization, the tissue in the affected sensory cortex has been found to respond to stimuli from the intact digits adjacent to the amputated digit (Kingsley, 1999). Remapping of the functional brain has commonly been described in cases of phantom limbs (Ramachandran, 2001) with a substantial network remapping of the brain when the brain was deprived of input from the target limb. Similar observations of an ongoing tissue functional reorganization have been made during cortical stimulation in an adult brain. Within hours of the resectioning of a motor nerve, researchers observed the brain area that earlier controlled the muscles innervated by the sectioned nerve now regulated a different group of muscles (Donoghue and Sanes, 1988). What happens to the brains of congenitally blind individuals? Touch appears to be processed in the visual cortex of early Braille readers (Sadato et al., 1996); no such activation of the visual cortex was found in late-blind and sighted individuals. There is ample evidence to suggest that the cortical representation of the activated sensory sites increases during an attended behavior (Jenkins et al., 1990). MRI-based investigation has revealed an increased neural density in the cortex resulting in the brain subsequent to a constant and patterned mental activity (Draganski et al., 2004) underscoring the hope for therapy-assisted recovery in patients with stroke. Cochlear implant has been documented with reversal of atrophic changes in the central auditory mechanism (Guiraud et al., 2007).

An issue that is closely related to the plasticity in the brain of patients with strokes and other brain pathologies is the protection of injured or dying neurons.

Culturally Neutral Brain

In spite of the complex architectural organization, multiple interconnected pathways, and functionally independent specialized areas, the brain's basic functioning is straightforward. Its operations are not governed by any personal characteristics of gender, color, or cultural variations. The brain's functioning is unaffected by normal variations in size, shape, or weight. Its power is judged by the efficiency with which it remembers, processes information, generates responses, attends to tasks, plans, programs, makes decisions, and projects information.

ORIENTATION TO TECHNICAL TERMINOLOGY

A set of descriptive terms is used in neuroscience to indicate direction and position of structures with respect to their relative orientation within the brain. Special terminology is also used for visually delineating anatomic structures according to the various planes of brain sections.

Key Terms :

Caudal	**Forebrain**	**Ventral**
Dorsal	**Rostral**	

Directional Brain Orientation

To understand the directional orientation of the human nervous system, it is important to consider first the brain of a mammal such as a dog, which, because of its quadrupedal posture, is organized in a straight (anteroposterior) line in the horizontal plane of the body. The term **rostral** refers to a location toward the nose; **caudal** is the location toward the tail; **dorsal** refers to a location toward the back, and **ventral** is the location toward the abdomen (Fig. 1-2).

This directional terminology is slightly different in humans. During phylogenetic development, the longitudinal CNS bends just above the brainstem. This cephalic flexure results in the spinal cord and brainstem developing vertically and the **forebrain** developing horizontally (Fig. 1-2). Therefore, in humans, the CNS (brain and spinal cord) is organized along two different axes: horizontal (brain) and vertical (spinal cord).

Because of this difference in axial orientation, the terms used for describing the locational orientaion of structures in the CNS vary (Fig. 1-2; Table 1-5). For the forebrain above the cephalic flexure (bend), rostral refers to locations toward the nose and caudal refers to locations toward the back of the brain, whereas dorsal refers to the top of the brain and ventral refers to the lower brain toward the jaw (Fig. 1-2*B*). The directions of these terms below the cephalic flexure (neuraxial bend) change and are similar to the ones used for lower vertebrates (Fig. 1-2*A*). For the spinal cord and brainstem, rostral refers to locations toward the brain, caudal points to the coccyx (a bone at the end of the spinal column) of the spinal cord, dorsal refers to locations toward the back of the body, and ventral refers to locations toward the abdomen (Fig. 1-2*D*).

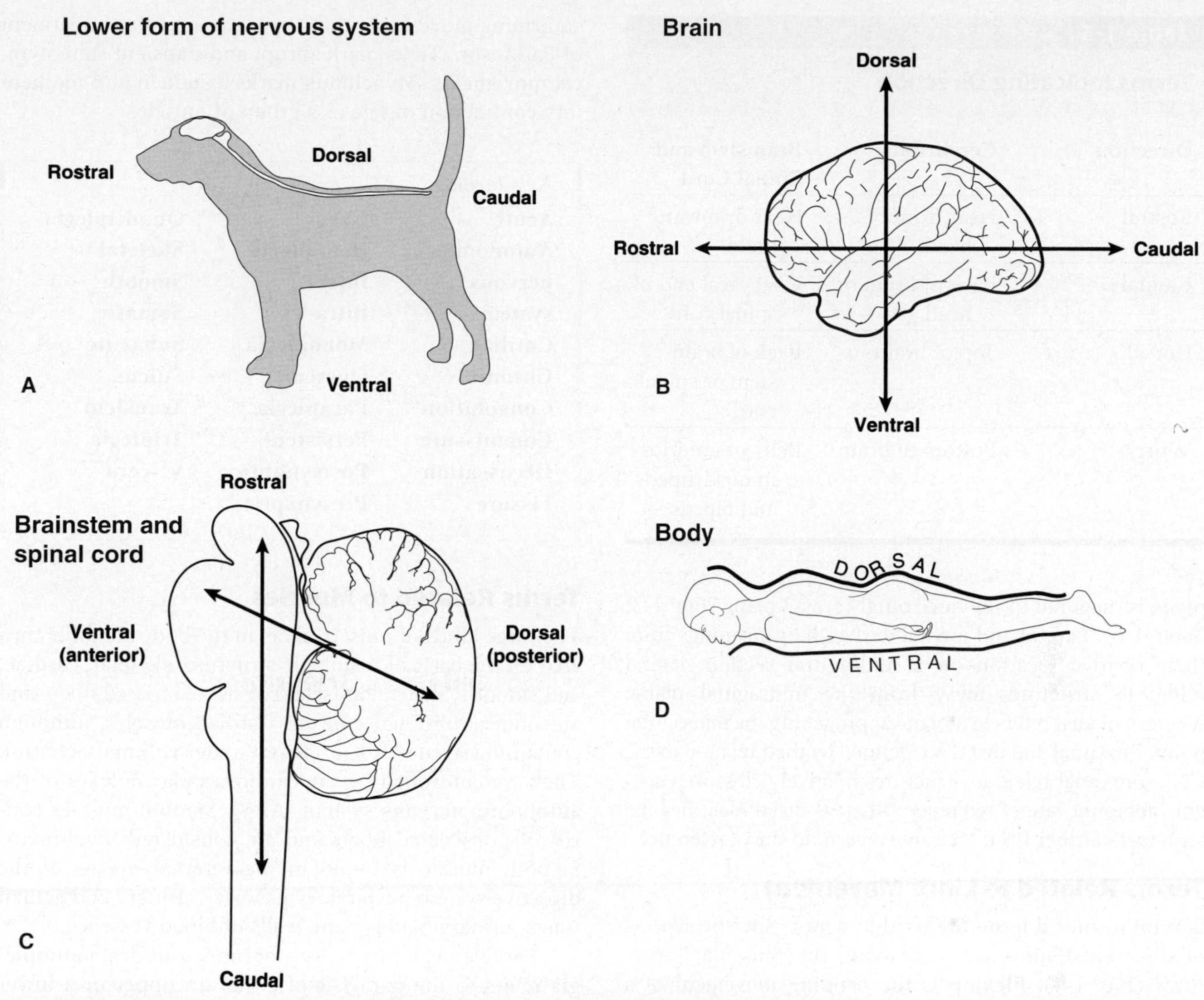

Figure 1-2 Nervous system axes and directional terms. A. The nervous system organization in primates along a straight line. B. The organization of the human nervous system develops along horizontal and vertical axes. The directional terms used for the brainstem (C) and spinal cord (D) are similar to those for lower vertebrates.

Key Terms:

Abduction	**Dystonia**	**Proximal**
Adduction	**Extension**	**Sagittal**
Akinesia	**Flexion**	**Supination**
Bradykinesia	**Lateral**	**Transverse**
Coronal	**Midsagittal**	**Tremor**
Distal	**Myoclonus**	
Dyskinesia	**Pronation**	

Planes of Brain Section

Not all cortical structures are on the brain's surface. Some can be examined only after sectioning the brain, which may be cut into three primary planes: **sagittal**, **coronal** and **horizontal** (Fig. 1-3). The sagittal plane, named after the sagittal suture in the skull, is a vertical cut that passes longitudinally and divides the brain into left and right portions. A sagittal section at the center separates the brain into two equal halves and is called the **midsagittal**. A coronal plane, a vertical section made perpendicular to the sagittal section, divides the brain into front and back parts. A horizontal plane, a cut perpendicular to both coronal and sagittal planes, divides the brain into upper and lower parts. A cross-section of the spinal cord at a right angle to its longitudinal axis divides the cord into upper and lower portions (Fig. 1-3*D*; Table 1-6).

There are three additional orienting terms regarding brain planes: **transverse**, **lateral**, and **medial**. A transverse plane is a crosscut at a right angle to the longitudinal axis on a bend. Because of the curvature of the brainstem, this

Table 1-5

Terms Indicating Direction

Direction	Cerebrum	Brainstem and Spinal Cord
Rostral	Near front of head	Near or toward brain
Caudal	Back of brain or head	Coccygeal end of spinal cord
Dorsal	Top of brain	Back of brain-stem or spinal cord
Ventral	Bottom of brain	Belly or anterior in quadrupeds and bipeds

plane is diagonal to the horizontal (cross) plane (Fig. 1-3; Table 1-6). Lateral and medial derive their meanings from their relative location on a midsagittal section: lateral refers to structures away from the midsagittal plane, whereas medial refers to a plane approaching the midsagittal point. **Proximal** and **distal** are defined by their relation to the CNS. Proximal refers to structures relatively close to a specific anatomic site of reference, whereas distal identifies the structures farther from the same anatomic site of reference.

Terms Related to Limb Movement

Several technical terms are used to denote specific aspects of directional movement involving the muscular structures (Fig. 1-4). **Flexion** is the bending movement of a limb.**Extension** involves the straightening movement of a limb. In **abduction**, a limb is moved away from the central axis of the body, whereas in **adduction** a limb is moved toward the central axis of the body. **Pronation** is the movement that turns the palm downward (or lying on the belly) and **supination** is the action that turns the palm upward (lying on the back).

The following terms are used for describing movements that are associated with brain pathology, mostly affecting basal ganglia structures. **Tremor** is a repetitive movement secondary to alternate contraction of opposing muscles. Two major types of tremors are **resting** and **action**. Resting tremor, associated with Parkinson disease, is prominent when the body is at rest against gravity. Action tremor, on the other hand, is associated with cerebellar pathology and it is apparent only during voluntary muscle contractions. **Akinesia** represents a lack of voluntary motor activity, whereas a slowness of movement is known as **bradykinesia**. **Dystonia** refers to any atypical posture with abnormally sustained muscle contraction. **Dyskinesia** stands for any involuntary and abnormal movement but it is specially used to mark the restless and squirming movements that appear as a result of treatment of Parkinson. **Ticks** mark abrupt and transient stereotypical movements. **Myoclonus** marks a sudden and momentary contraction of one or a group of muscles.

Key Terms:

Acute	**Gyrus**	**Quadriplegia**
Autonomic nervous system	**Hemiplegia**	**Skeletal**
Cardiac	**Inter-**	**Smooth**
Chronic	**Intra-**	**Somatic**
Convolution	**Monoplegia**	**Subacute**
Commissure	**Opercular**	**Sulcus**
Decussation	**Paraplegia**	**Transient**
Fissure	**Persistent**	**Triplegia**
	Postsynaptic	**Viscera**
	Presynaptic	

Terms Related to Muscles

The three kinds of muscle fibers in the body are differentiated on the basis of histologic structure: **skeletal, cardiac**, and **smooth**. Skeletal muscles consist of striated fibers and are under volitional control. Cardiac muscles, although containing striated fibers, are not under voluntary control. They are controlled by the cardiovascular reflexes of the **autonomic nervous system** (ANS). Smooth muscles consist of nonstriated fibers and are considered involuntary. Smooth muscle is found in the internal organs of the digestive system, respiratory passages, urinary and genital tracts, urinary bladder, and walls of blood vessels.

Paralysis can involve one or more muscles: **monoplegia** refers to the paralysis of either an upper or a lower limb, whereas **hemiplegia** is used for the paralysis of both the upper and the lower limbs on one side. **Triplegia** is used to describe the paralysis of three limbs (both extremities on one side and one on the other side) and **quadriplegia** refers to a paralysis pattern involving all four limbs. **Paraplegia** refers to the paralysis of both lower limbs.

Terms Related to Neuroanatomical Structures

The bony cavity of the skull restricts the expansion of the cortical mantle containing nerve cells; consequently, the human cortex is highly convoluted, giving the brain a folded appearance (Fig. 2-3). The crest of every fold is called a **gyrus** (pl. gyri) or **convolution**. The groove or valley separating adjacent gyri is called the **sulcus** (pl. sulci) or **fissure** (in case of greater depth). **Opercular** refers to the margins of the cerebral convolutions serving as a cover. For example, the margins of the operculum of three lobes cover the **insular cortex** (Fig. 2-13). A **commissure** is a band of fibers connecting part of the brain or spinal cord on one side with the same structures on the opposite side of the midline.

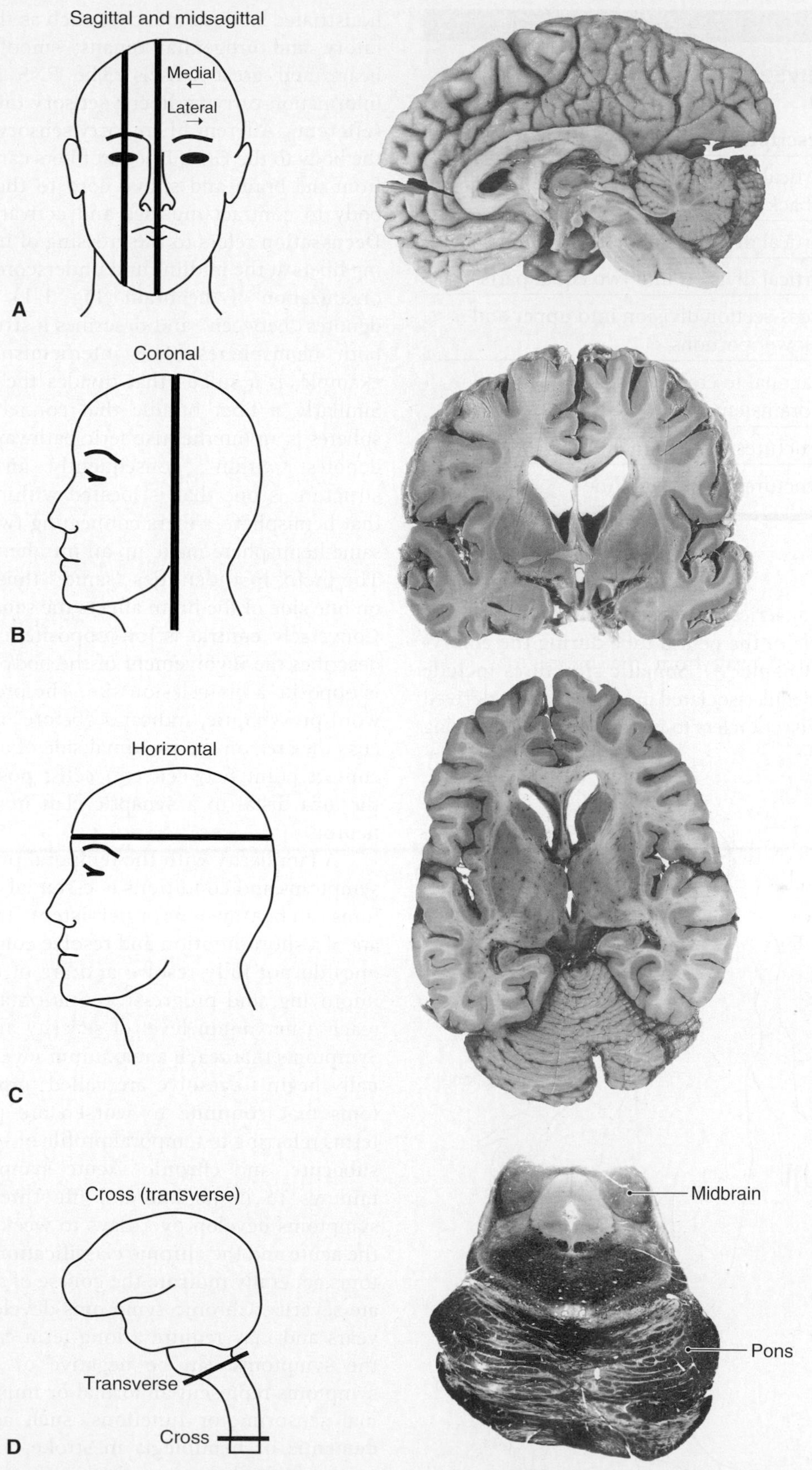

Figure 1-3 The four common planes/cuts of the brain with corresponding brain sections: (A), sagittal, (B) coronal, (C) horizontal, and (D) transverse.

Table 1-6

Terms for Brain Sections

Section	Description
Coronal	Vertical section into front (rostral) and back (caudal)
Sagittal	Vertical division into left and right
Midsagittal	Vertical division into two equal parts
Horizontal	Cross-section division into upper and lower portions
Transverse	Diagonal to cross-plane at curving brainstem
Lateral	Structures away from midline
Medial	Structures toward midline

Somites are a series of mesodermal tissue blocks found on each side of the neural tube during the embryonic period (see Chapter 4). **Somatic** structures include most axial skeletal and associated muscles that are derived from the somite. **Viscera** refers to internal organs containing nonstriated smooth muscles, such as the digestive, respiratory, and urogenital organs; smooth glands; spleen; heart; and great vessels. The PNS has two types of information-carrying fibers: **sensory (afferent)** and **motor (efferent)**. Afferent fibers carry sensory information from the body to the CNS. Efferent fibers carry motor impulses from the brain and spinal cord to the periphery of the body to contract muscles and activate gland secretion. **Decussation** refers to the crossing of incoming or outgoing fibers at the midline and underscores the contralateral organization of the brain (Fig. 1-1). The prefix **inter-** denotes "between" and describes a structure common to both hemispheres. The interhemispheric fissure, for example, is a sulcus that divides the two hemispheres. Similarly, a fiber bundle that connects the two hemispheres is an interhemispheric pathway. The prefix **intra-** denotes "within"; consequently, an intrahemispheric structure is one that is located within the substance of that hemisphere. Fibers connecting two areas within the same hemisphere make up an intrahemispheric pathway. The prefix **ipsi**-identifies "same," thus **ipsilateral** lesion on one side of the brain affects the same side of the body. Conversely, **contra-** is for "opposite," thus **contralateral** describes the involvement of the body on the side which is opposite a brain lesion site. The prefix **pre-**, as in the word **presynaptic**, indicates "before" and is used to discuss the area on the proximal side of a synaptic cleft, the contact point between two cells; **postsynaptic** denotes the area distal to a synaptic cleft involving the second neuron.

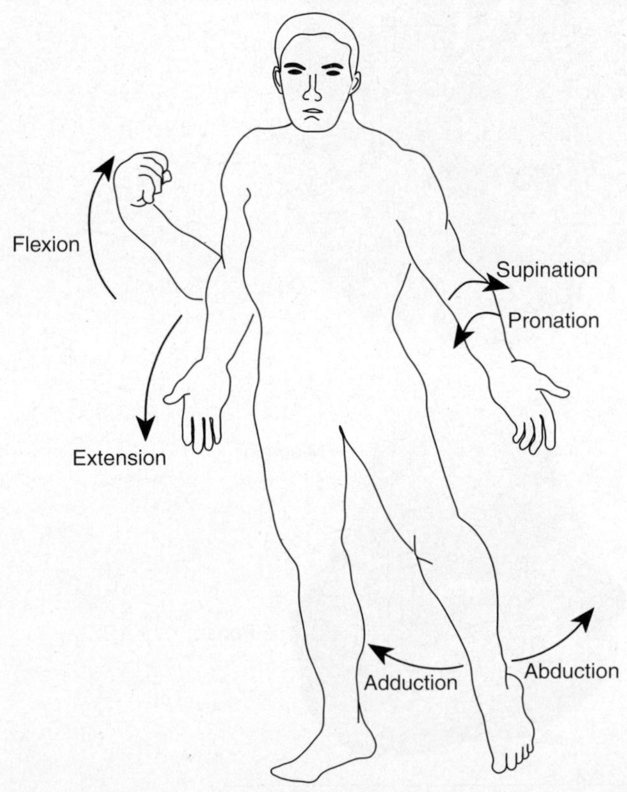

Figure 1-4 An illustration of terms related to limb movements.

A familiarity with the temporal profile of neurologic symptoms and conditions is essential. Neurologic symptoms can be **transient** or **persistent**. Transient symptoms are of a short duration and resolve completely; persistent ones do not fully resolve and are of three types: static, improving, and progressive. Static/stationary symptoms reach a maximum level of severity and do not change. Symptoms that reach a maximum severity and then gradually begin to resolve are called improving and symptoms that continue to worsen are progressive. Other terms referring to temporal profile of symptoms are **acute subacute**, and **chronic**. Acute symptoms evolve over minutes to hours and are life threatening. Subacute symptoms develop over days to weeks and fall between the acute and the chronic classifications. Subacute symptoms generally indicate the course of a disease of moderate severity. Chronic symptoms develop over months to years and may require a long-term care. Diagnostically, the symptoms can be negative or positive. Negative symptoms represent abnormal or impaired states of normal sensorimotor functions, such as memory loss in dementia or hemiplegia in stroke. The positive symptoms are the behaviors that confirm the presence of a disease process, such as pin-rolling tremor (for Parkinson disease) and hallucination of a specific smell (temporal seizures).

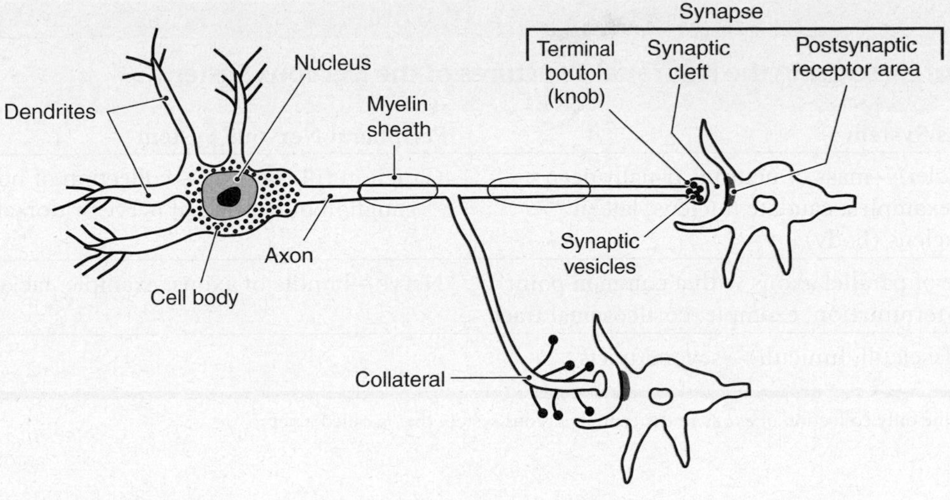

Figure 1-5 A typical nerve cell with its major structures.

Key Terms:

Appendicular	**Colliculus**	**Gray matter**
Axial	**Dendrite**	**Nerve**
Axon	**Fasciculus**	**Soma**
Brachium	**Ganglion**	**Synapse**
Cerebellum	**Glial cells**	**White matter**

Terms Related to the Neuronal Structures

The brain, by a conservative estimate, consists of 15 to 20 billion nerve cells (neurons) and their axonal processes; two-thirds of the neurons are hidden within sulci. **Gray matter** refers to the gross appearance of the cells in the brain, which consists of nerve cells, supporting glia cells, and many unmyelinated fibers. Representing only 10% of the brain cells, the neurons are concentrated in the cerebral cortex as layers and in the subcortex as nuclei. The cells appear gray in the absence of myelin; thus they are also called gray matter. **White matter** is made of nerve fibers that form tracts and carry information from one brain site to another. It is white because of the white appearance of the myelin lipid (fat-like) substance surrounding many of the axons.

As the basic building block of the brain, the neuron is responsible for generating, receiving, transmitting, and synthesizing electrical/chemical impulses. The cellular activity of the primary cells is responsible for generating the nerve impulses that underlie all sensorimotor and higher mental functions. **Glial cells** support nerve cell function by providing structural support and insulating framework around the nerve cells, by contributing to the neuronal metabolism, by regulating the ionic balance in the extracellular fluid of the CNS, and by participating in the repair of damaged nerve cells. A typical neuron, enclosed by a continuous plasma membrane, consists of a cell body, dendrites, and an axon (Fig. 1-5).The cell body, also called **soma** (pl. somata) or perikaryon (pl. perikarya), contains the cytoplasm with standard but important cellular organelles, which are needed for cellular metabolism and keep the cell alive and functional. Also contained in the cytoplasm is a **nucleus**, which contains ladder-like micromolecules of DNA with genetic blueprint and is responsible for vital cellular activities. Dendrites, highly specialized processes that look like trees, receive neural signals (synaptic activity) from other neurons through contacts (synapses).

Generation and Transmission of Action Potential

The axon, arising from an elevation of the cell body (called **axon hillock**), transmits neural messages (action potentials) away from the soma to axonal terminals where they make contact with other neurons through synapses (contacts). **Synaptic terminals** (terminal boutons, knobs, or buttons) are the end portions of the axon and contain many vesicles that store and release neurotransmitters between the end of the axon and the surface of the next nerve cell. This narrow space between two cells is the **synaptic cleft**. Once a neuron is adequately stimulated, the resulting action potential (neural impulse) travels along the axon, and the terminal boutons (knobs) release the neurotransmitters to activate the receptor site of the next or target nerve cell. The **synapse** includes the boutons, synaptic cleft, and receptor sites of the next nerve cell. A neuron that ends at the synapse is a presynaptic nerve cell. A neuron that receives an impulse from a presynaptic neuron is a postsynaptic neuron.

Cellular Connectivity

The most intriguing aspect of the brain's cellular organization for students of human behavior is the mechanism that, during the embryonic period, guides the connectivity of axons to the predetermined target areas. What makes the early developing axons the path-finding fibers, and how do their growth cones actively or passively spot the target cell surfaces for connectivity? Since not all axons are properly connected and not all the synaptic connections

Table 1-7

Terms Used for Describing the Neuronal Structures of the Nervous System

Central Nervous System	Peripheral Nervous System
Nucleus (pl. nuclei)—mass of neurons usually deep in the brain; examples: caudate nucleus, lateral geniculate nucleus (body)	Ganglion (pl. ganglia)—collection of neurons; example: ganglion of trigeminal nerve or dorsal root
Tract—a bundle of parallel axons with a common point of origin and termination; example: corticospinal tract	Nerve—bundle of axons; example: facial nerve[a]
Fasciculus (pl. fasciculi, funiculi)—several tracts	

[a]The optic nerve is the only collection of axons in the central nervous system that is called a nerve.

survive, trophic factors play an important role in the survival of neurons and their synapses. In general, an overabundance of neurons is produced during normal development and >50% of neurons in some areas die a programmed death during development (apoptosis); most of these cells die because of their inability to establish synaptic connections or because they develop weak connections. See Chapter 5 for a detailed discussion.

Terminology of the Central and Peripheral Nervous Systems

A well-defined collection of nerve cells in the CNS is called a nucleus or cell column; a similar collection of nerve cells in the PNS is called a **ganglion** (Table 1-7). A sensory ganglion contains cell bodies of the sensory nerves; there are no synapses around cell bodies. A motor ganglion of the ANS contains cell bodies of fibers that supply the smooth muscles and glands.

Nerve fibers transmit information. A collection of nerve fibers that share a common origin as well as termination is called a **tract** or **fasciculus** in the CNS. Another name for a bundle of connecting pathways is **brachium**, which specifically connects the **cerebellum** to the brainstem. **Stria** is used to denote a band of fibers that may differ in color and/or texture. **Colliculus** refers to a small prominence of nervous system tissue.

A bundle of fibers in the PNS is called a **nerve** or nerve trunk (Table 1-7). Axial structures are differentiated from the appendicular structures. **Axial** refers to the central part of the body and is made up of the head and trunk. **Appendicular** relates to the limbs, which are attached to the axial structures.

Key Terms:

Brainstem
Cerebellum
Cerebrum
Hypothalamus
Medulla
Midbrain
Pons
Spinal roots
Thalamus

STRUCTURES OF THE CNS

The human nervous system is divided into the CNS and PNS. The CNS consists of the brain and the spinal cord. The brain consists of three major structures: **cerebrum**, **brainstem** (**midbrain**, **pons**, and **medulla**), and **cerebellum** (Fig. 1-6; Table 1-8). Each of these structures serves some common and some specific functions. The cerebrum consists of two hemispheres; each hemisphere contains the cerebral cortex and diencephalon (**thalamus** and **hypothalamus**).

With over 15 to 20 billion neurons, the cerebrum is a vital aspect of cortical thalamic circuits that enables higher symbolic functions required of all vertebrates, and of special importance for humans as it regulates language, thinking, reasoning, memory, personality, emotion, and attention. Each cerebral hemisphere also houses the limbic lobe and the basal ganglia. The limbic lobe, made up of an array of subcortical brain structures and their connections, regulates motivational and emotional states and reflexes that ensure survival of the species. The basal ganglia serve as an auxiliary motor system and play an important role in maintaining muscle tone and in regulating motor activities by modifying the information received from the motor cortex and returning it to the motor cortex. The basal ganglia have also been connected with the regulation of symbolic and cognitive functions (Bhatnagar and Mandybur, 2006; see Chapter 15).

The thalamus is a collection of subcortical nuclei, which are an essential part of the thalamus–cerebral cortex–thalamic circuit, the basic functional circuitry of the forebrain. Integrated closely with the cerebral hemispheres in sensorimotor functions, the thalamic nuclei control circuit activity by evaluating incoming sensory signals before directing them to the functionally specific cortex. The hypothalamus is involved with endocrinic (hormonal) and autonomic functions. It serves as the central site of hormonal secretion and the central structure for the control of various metabolic activities, such as water balance, sugar and fat metabolism, body-rhythm control, and body temperature.

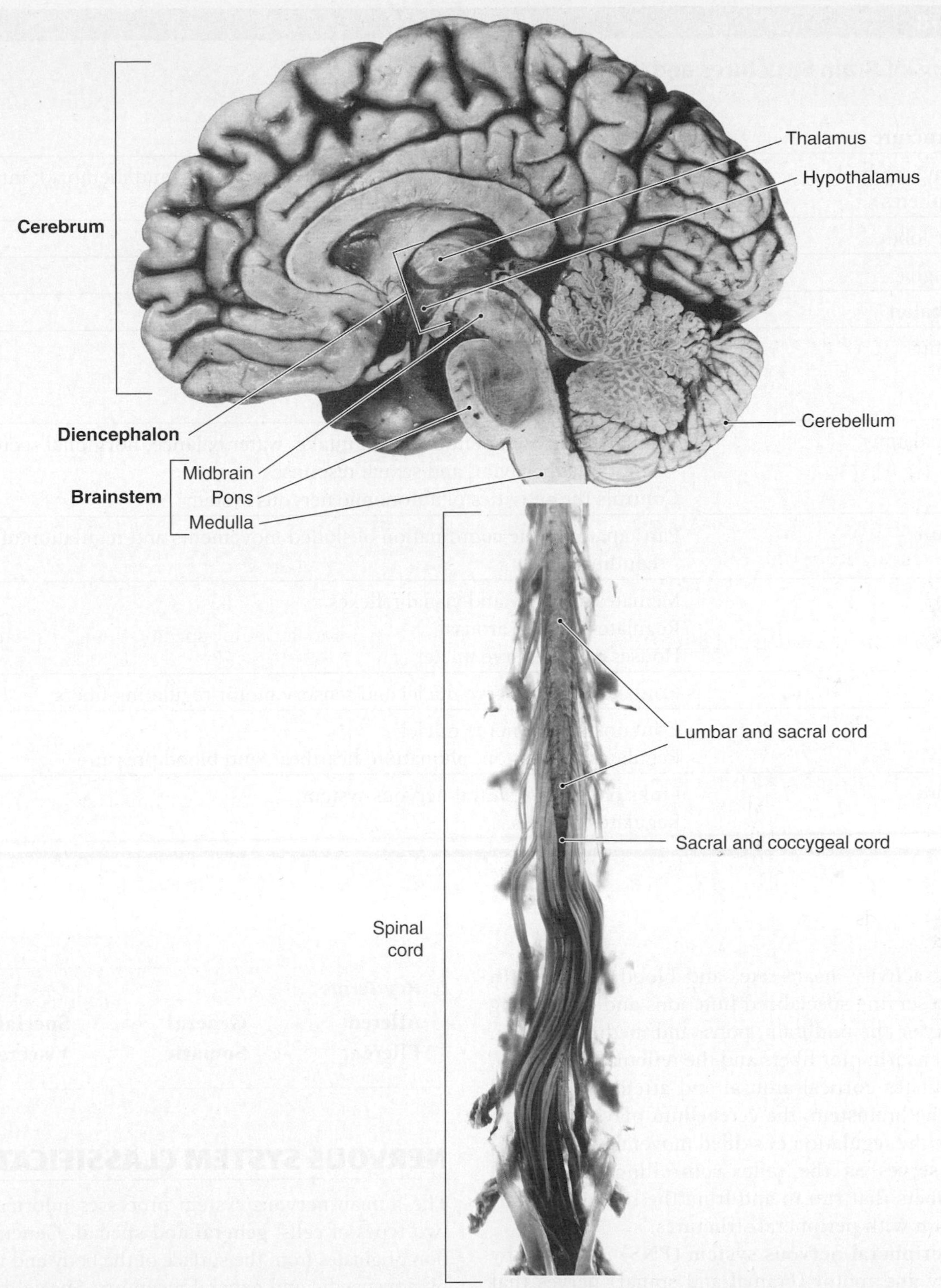

Figure 1-6 The major anatomical structures of the central nervous system: the cerebrum, brainstem, and spinal cord.

The brainstem consists of the midbrain, pons, and medulla. Besides linking the brainstem and lower neuraxial structures with the brain, the midbrain also controls pupil size, auditory reflexes, and reflexive eye movements in response to external stimuli. The pons contains a specialized center that controls the rhythm of respiration; it also regulates facial movements and sensation through cranial nerves. The medulla controls

Table 1-8

Functions of Brain Structures and the Spinal Cord

Brain Structure	Functions
Cerebrum (cerebral hemispheres)	Serves higher mental functions (cognition, language, and memory); integrates sensorimotor functions and perceptual experiences
Limbic lobe	Regulates motivational and emotional states
Basal ganglia	Regulates motor movements and muscle tone
Diencephalon	
Thalamus	Channels sensorimotor information to cortex Participates in cortex-mediated functions Regulates crude awareness of sensation
Hypothalamus	Regulates body temperature, food intake, water balance, hormonal secretions, emotional behavior, and sexual responses Controls the activities of autonomic nervous system
Cerebellum	Participates in the coordination of skilled movements and regulation of equilibrium
Midbrain	Mediates auditory and visual reflexes Regulates cortical arousal Houses cranial nerve nuclei
Pons	Contains cranial nerve nuclei and sensory motor-regulating fibers
Medulla	Contains cranial nerve nuclei Regulates respiration, phonation, heartbeat, and blood pressure
Spinal cord	Links body with central nervous system Regulates reflexes

respiratory activity, heart rate, and blood pressure. In addition to serving specialized functions and controlling cranial nerves, the midbrain, pons, and medulla contain common sensorimotor fibers and the reticular formation, which regulates cortical arousal and attention. Located dorsal to the brainstem, the cerebellum plays an important role in the regulation of skilled movements. The spinal cord serves as the reflex-controlling center and contains fibers that run to and from the brain, connecting the brain with peripheral structures.

The **peripheral nervous system (PNS)** is formed by the sensory and motor (cranial and spinal) nerves that connect the CNS with the peripheral structures. Conveying pain, touch, and temperature information, the sensory fibers enter the spinal cord via the dorsal spinal roots. The motor fibers that innervate muscles and glands exit through the ventral spinal roots. The ANS, as an independent entity, uses the components of both the CNS and PNS and controls the activities of the cardiac muscles, smooth muscles of the internal organs, and glandular secretion.

Key Terms :

Afferent	**General**	**Special**
Efferent	**Somatic**	**Visceral**

NERVOUS SYSTEM CLASSIFICATION

The human nervous system processes information using two types of cells: **general** and **special**. General information originates from the surface of the body and is processed by nonspecific and general receptors. Special information is mediated by the specialized receptors to specialized functionally committed cells in the nervous system. Pain and temperature are examples of general information, whereas vision, smell, taste, and audition are examples of special information. Each information type (general and special) is involved with body structures that are either **somatic** or **visceral**. Somatic refers to striated skeletal muscles that are embryologically derived from somites. Visceral nonstriated muscles are concerned with vegetative tasks and relate to the internal vital body organs involved in the respiratory, vascular, and digestive systems controlled by the ANS. Thus, general and special information is divided into somatic and visceral subtypes, both of which are further divided based on the efferent (motor) and afferent (sensory) fibers. The only exception to this classification is the absence of a special somatic efferent system. Therefore, the functional classification of the CNS consists of seven components and is important for understanding all sensory and motor functioning of spinal and cranial nerves (Table 1-9).

Key Terms:

Anatomic orientation	**Isocortex**
Archicortex	**Lenticular**
Babinski sign	**Neocortex**
Brodmann area	**Paleocortex**
Chorea	**Peduncle**
Clinical orientation	**Pyramidal layer**
Cytoarchitecture	**Rigidity**
Granular layer	**Spasticity**
Hippocampus	**Ventricles**

CELLULAR CORTEX

Neuron Types

There are three major types of cells in the cortex: **pyramidal**, **granular/satellite**, and **interneurons**. The pyramidal cells, the most common of these, are found in all cortical layers except the first (the molecular) layer. They are the only cells with outgoing axons that project to the adjacent association cortex and also connect with subcortical structures, spinal cord, and basal ganglia nuclei. The largest of the pyramidal cells (giant cells of Betz) are mostly present in the primary motor cortex. The nonpyramidal (Stellate and interneurons) cells serve as the only local circuit, and their axons mostly project to the association cortices and do not leave the immediate regions of the cell body. Interneurons serve as the association cells contributing to the facilitation or inhibition of the local circuitry.

Layered Cerebral Cortex

The human brain contains a 3- to 5-mm thick layer of neurons (gray matter) covering the entire surface of the cerebral hemispheres. Arranged in six horizontal layers, the cerebral cortex is highly developed in *Homo sapiens*. Histologically, the six-layered cortex, **isocortex** or **neocortex**, is essential for serving higher mental (cognition and language) and sensorimotor functions. Two regions of the brain, however, have fewer than six layers: **archicortex**, **cerebellum**, and **paleocortex**. The archicortex contains three cellular layers and includes structures like hippocampus, amygdala, and septum which are important in memory consolidation and instinctual reflexes that are essential for survival. Containing three to five layers, the paleocortex includes the structures like olfactory–sensory–cortex and periamygdaloid cortex that serve emotional behavior.

Each of the neocortical layers is classified by its neuronal density and architecture (morphology of the cellular composition) as seen under light microscopy: molecular

Table 1-9

Functional Components of the Nervous System

General				Special			
Somatic		Visceral		Somatic		Visceral	
Efferent (GSE)	Afferent (GSA)	Efferent (GVE)	Afferent (GVA)	Efferent (SSE)	Afferent (SSA)	Efferent (SVE)	Afferent (SVA)
Activates muscles derived from somites, including skeletal, extraocular, and glossal (tongue) muscles	Mediates sensory innervation from somatic muscles, skin, ligaments, and joints	Projects to muscles of visceral organs, including pupillary constriction, gland secretion, and regulation of heart and tracheal muscles	Mediates sensory innervation from visceral organs, including larynx, pharynx, and abdomen	Does not exist	Mediates special sensations of vision from retina and of audition and equilibrium from inner ear	Projects to muscles of face, palate, mouth, pharynx, and larynx; does not include eye and tongue muscles	Mediates visceral sensations of taste from tongue and of olfaction from nose

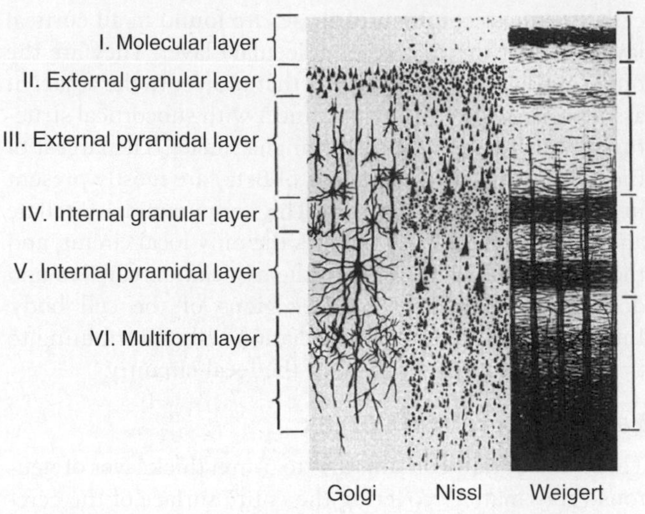

Figure 1-7 Six cellular layers of the neocortex, the most evolved type of cerebral cortex.

layer, external granular layer, external pyramidal layer, internal granular layer, internal pyramidal layer, and multiform layer (Fig. 1-7; Table 1-10). Each layer functions as a functional module, processing input and giving rise to outgoing axons. Some axons project to other cortical areas, and others form the descending tracts. These layers of the cerebral cortex starting from external to internal are numbered from one to six.

The presence of six cortical layers is not uniform in the entire cerebral cortex. The cellular composition variations depend on the function. For example, in the motor cortex, the layers three and five are dominated by large pyramidal cells with outgoing axons. In contrast to the motor region, the primary sensory cortex has distinctive layer of two and four that are dominated by the presence of stellate cells. Their projections are limited to the association cortex. This brain region is also called the granular cortex as opposed to nongranular motor cortex.

Brodmann Areas

Different cortical regions contain varied configurations (thickness and cellular morphology) at different cellular layers, which reflect the specialized functions served by each brain area. This variable cellular architecture of the six cortical layers was the basis for Brodmann's discovery of various distinct functional areas in the brain (Brodmann, 1909). His cytoarchitectural map is the most frequently used brain map in neurologic and neurolinguistic literature; it divides the brain into approximately 47 regions and serves as a standard for referring to specific brain areas by number (Fig. 1-8). For example, Brodmann area 4 is the primary motor cortex, which contains large pyramidal cells (Betz cells) in the leg and foot cortical areas. Sensory cortical areas have more densely packed granular cells and only a few pyramidal cells. Primary sensory areas include the somatosensory cortex in the postcentral gyrus (Brodmann areas 3, 1, 2), the primary visual cortex (Brodmann area 17), and the primary auditory cortex, or gyri of Heschl (Brodmann areas 41 and 42, in the superior temporal gyrus).

Tertiary areas of the temporal, parietal, and prefrontal cortex are called association areas of the brain. The association areas are concerned mostly with the processing of cross-modality input from other cortical areas and integrating and elaborating complex functions. Familiarity with the commonly used Brodmann areas is necessary for working in medical SLP (Table 1-11).

Table 1-10

Six-layered Cerebral Gray Matter

Cellular Layer	Cellular Characteristics
Layer I: molecular	Terminal dendrites and axons from cortical neurons that run parallel to the surface of the brain and communicate with neighboring cortical areas
Layer II: external granular	Small granular cells, interneurons, and some small pyramidal cells that receive inputs from other cortical regions
Layer III: external pyramidal	Small- to medium-sized pyramidal neurons with projections to neighboring ipsilateral and contralateral cerebral cortex and basal ganglia
Layer IV: internal granular	Granular interneurons that receive input from thalamus and other subcortical nuclei. They form a thick layer in somatosensory, visual, auditory, and vestibular cortex
Layer V: internal pyramidal	Large pyramidal neurons (Betz cells of the primary motor cortex) that project to subcortical sites, such as brainstem, cerebellum, and spinal cord
Layer VI: multiform	Multiform layer with some neuronal projections to basal ganglia and remaining projections to superficial cellular layers within same cortical area

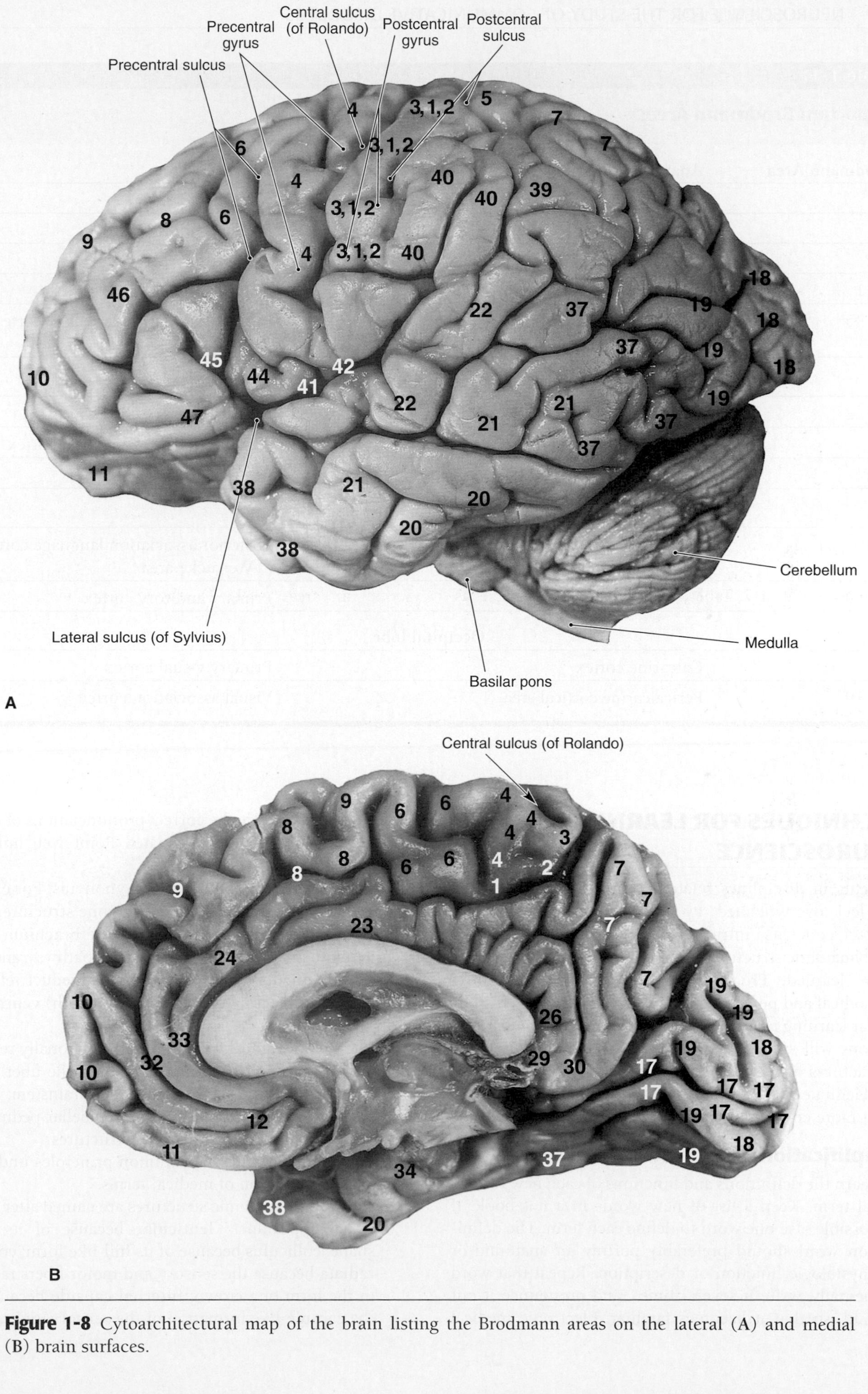

Central sulcus (of Rolando)
Precentral gyrus
Postcentral gyrus
Postcentral sulcus
Precentral sulcus
Cerebellum
Medulla
Lateral sulcus (of Sylvius)
Basilar pons

A

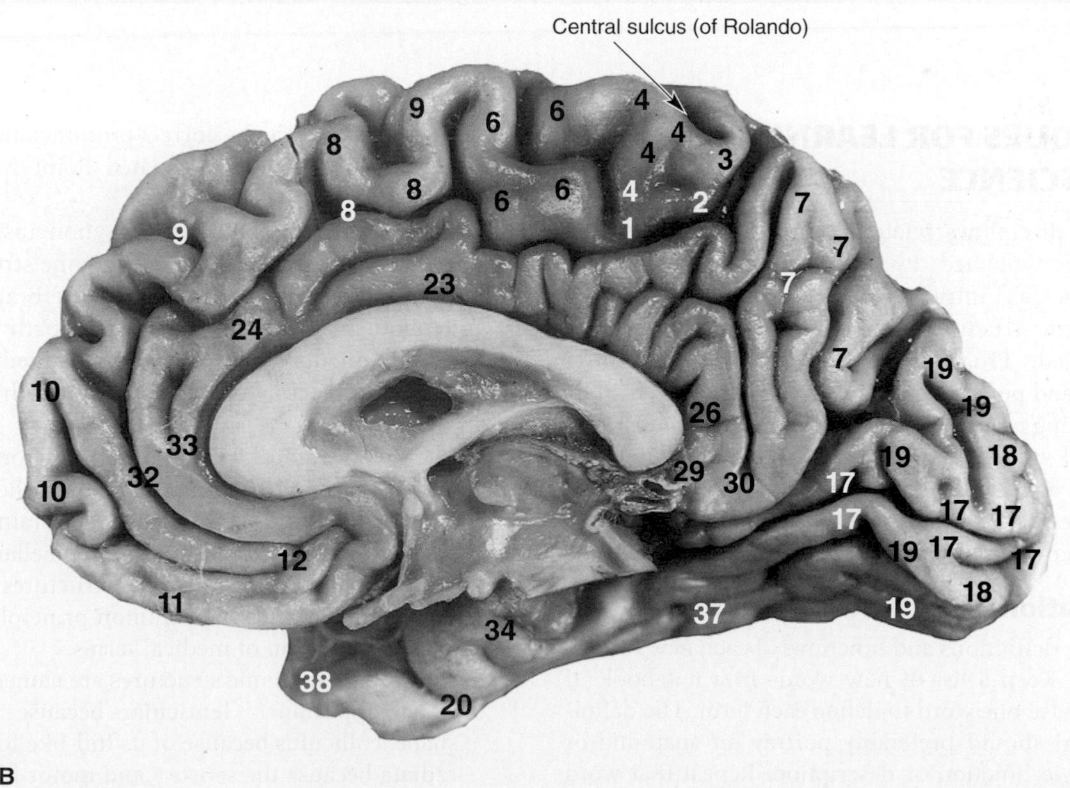

Figure 1-8 Cytoarchitectural map of the brain listing the Brodmann areas on the lateral (A) and medial (B) brain surfaces.

Table 1-11

Important Brodmann Areas

Brodmann Area	Anatomic Location	Function
	Frontal lobe	
4	Precentral gyrus	Primary motor cortex
6, 8	Anterior to precentral gyrus	Premotor cortex
9–11	Prefrontal region	Cognitive association cortex
44, 45	Inferior frontal lobule	Frontal association language cortex; Broca area
	Parietal lobe	
3, 1, 2	Postcentral gyrus	Primary sensory cortex
5, 7	Posterior to postcentral gyrus	Somatosensory association cortex
39	Angular gyrus	Reading and writing
	Temporal lobe	
22	Subtemporal and posterior temporal gyrus and planum temporale	Posterior association language cortex; Wernicke area
41, 42	Gyri of Heschl	Primary auditory cortex
	Occipital lobe	
17	Calcarine cortex	Primary visual cortex
18, 19	Pericalcarine cortical area	Visual association cortex

TECHNIQUES FOR LEARNING NEUROSCIENCE

Students in disciplines related to human behavior need not feel overwhelmed by the technical terminology, abstract concepts, intricate connections, multiplicity of neuroanatomic structures, or amount of technical material to be learned. Progressively adding knowledge in a methodical and persistent fashion is the best proven strategy for learning neuroscience. The following practical suggestions will simplify the technical terminology and the abstractness of the material presented. These suggestions will facilitate the learning process while making the time spent more enjoyable (Table 1-12).

Simplification of Technical Terminology

1. Learn the definitions and functions of each new technical term. Keep a list of new words in a notebook. If possible, use one word to define each term. The definition word should preferably portray an anatomic or physiologic function or description. Repeat that word mentally, write it several times, and pronounce it out loud, so that it becomes familiar. Electronic medical dictionaries provide the correct pronunciations of medical words (check the associated Point web link for access).
2. Relate each technical word to its synonyms. For example, fissure and sulcus refer to the same structure. The **superior cerebellar peduncle** and the **brachium conjunctivum** refer to the same cerebellar pathway, and the **cerebral aqueduct**, iter, and sylvian aqueduct refer to the canal connecting two (**third and fourth**) **ventricles** in the brain.
3. Relate each technical term to other functionally related terms. For example, **peduncle** refers to the fiber bundles connecting the cerebellum to the brainstem; thus, the superior, middle, and inferior cerebellar peduncles are functionally related anatomic structures.
4. Become familiar with the common principles underlying the formulation of medical terms.
   - Some neuroanatomic structures are named after their visual appearance: **lenticular** because of its lens shape; colliculus because of its hill-like form; **corona radiata** because the sensory and motor fibers radiate in the form of a crown; **internal capsule** because of the capsule-like formation of the sensory and motor

Table 1-12

Strategies for Overcoming the Complexity of Neuroscience

Relate each structure to its definition and function
Be familiar with the synonyms for each structure
Relate each term with other functionally related terms
Be familiar with the idiosyncratic patterns for coining technical terms based on the following: • Visual appearance • Researcher's name • Anatomic projection • Roots in Greek and Latin
Undertake a visual approach to neuroanatomy: • Learn the shape, size, location, and function of each structure • Orient each structure in relation to its adjoining structures
Apply clinical orientation to anatomic structures
Find a functional context for neurologic concepts and structures
Discover the meaning and purpose of each new concept by solving clinical problems
Be familiar with the rules of lesion localization

fibers deep in the brain; **amygdaloid nucleus** because of its almond shape; and **hippocampus** because of its seahorse shape in a sagittal or horizontal section.

- Some terms are eponyms, named after pioneer researchers—for example, circle of Willis, Babinski reflex, Brodmann area, Huntington chorea, foramen of Monro, Sylvian fissure, fissure of Rolando, Parkinson disease, and Broca area.
- Names of pathways are established according to sites of fiber origin and termination. The corticospinal tract, for instance, originates in the motor cortex and terminates in the spinal cord. The corticobulbar tract originates in the motor cortex and terminates in the bulbar area (medulla and adjacent brainstem areas). The reticulospinal system extends from the reticular formation of the brainstem to its termination in the spinal cord. Although the names of fiber tracts primarily emphasize the points of origin and termination, they sometimes include unnamed brain structures along the entire length of the tract.
- Most neurology terms are derived from Greek or Latin. Familiarity with lexical roots and derivational morphology can simplify learning. Some examples follow.
  - **Ataxia: a-** means "without," and the Greek root taxis means "order"; thus, ataxia is loss of motor coordination. (See Appendix B on the Point web site for common lexical roots.)
  - **Chorea:** the Greek root choros means "dance"; thus, chorea is a dance-like (involuntary) movement.
  - **Lemniscus:** the Greek root lemniskos means "a fillet or ribbon"; thus, lemniscus refers to a ribbon form collection (bundle) of nerve fibers in the CNS.
  - **Brachium:** the Greek root brachios means "arm" (arm-like fiber bundle), as in **brachium conjunctivus**, the crossing fibers of the cerebellum.
- Many medical terms derived from Greek or Latin roots have a combining form of the word that is different from its root form. For example, the combining form of the Greek root skleros (hard) is scler-, as in sclerosis; the combining form of Greek root soma (body) is somat-, as in somatic; the combining form of Greek root stethos (chest) is stetho-, as in stethoscope (see Appendix B on the Point web site for a list of such combining forms).

Visual Approach to Learning

The human nervous system is complex, but it is organized logically. Most concepts can be understood and remembered after the learner has acquired the basics in neuroscience. Some concepts and facts, however, must be familiarized with and repeated until they become incorporated in a readily available knowledge bank. Neuroanatomy is best learned by persistent repetition and visual orientation. Neuroanatomic structures are not abstract entities; they are real, occupy space, and serve specific functions. All brain structures are anatomically and physiologically integrated to form a whole entity with one purpose—preservation of the species. The visual learning of anatomic structures (with reference to shape, size, texture, function, and location in the nervous system and relationship to bordering structures) is the most successful tool. No other effective way has been found. Consequently, developing a visual memory by correlating written descriptions of cortical and subcortical structures with their anatomic illustrations and figures has been found to be invaluable. As a student learns more, s/he should become better equipped to solve clinical problems, a highly valued and most stimulating skill. Thus, some practical suggestions for learning the concepts and functions of neuroscience follow:

1. Take a visual approach to learning brain structures in the context of their locations. Each external and internal neuroanatomic structure is visually distinct. Visual familiarity with a structure as it appears in space facilitates learning neuroanatomy and reduces the fear of learning. For example, widely dispersed sensory and motor fibers are responsible in part for the bulging appearance of the pons; the four adjacent egg-shaped structures located dorsally in the midbrain are the **corpora quadrigemina** (four bodies) with a role in visual and auditory reflexes, and the slit cleavage between two football-shaped thalami is the **third ventricle**. The fillet-shaped fibers at the midbrain (**pes pedunculi** or **crus cerebri**) contain the sensory (**medial lemniscus**) and the motor fibers.
2. Familiarity with adjacent structures and landmarks helps form a three-dimensional image that further facilitates learning. For example, it is easier to remember the location of various cortical and subcortical structures if they are visualized in relation to the **ventricular system**. Another important anatomic landmark is the differing shapes of the sensorimotor fibers throughout the neuraxis (see Fig. 3-1).

Clinical Orientation to Neuroscience

There are two types of orientations involved in learning in neuroanatomy: **anatomic orientation** and **clinical orientation**. Structural neuroscience is learned with an anatomic orientation where in diagrams, the left brain structures are on the left side and right brain structures are on the right. This is identical to the left and right of the clinician. In this orientation, the posteriorly (dorsal) located structures are at the top of figures, whereas the anterior (ventral) structures are located at the bottom in the figures.

In clinical orientation, the patient lies on his/her back (supine) and the clinician looks at the patient from a pedal view, as if facing the patient's feet (Dougherty et al., 2003). This makes the patient's right and left, respectively, the physician's left and right (Fig. 1-9*A*); this reverse anatomic representation also applies to the brainstem and spinal cord anatomy (Fig. 1-9*B*). Clinical orientation not only facilitates reading radiological images, such as MRI (Figs. 1-10–1-13) and CT (Figs. 1-14–1-16) but also enhances the ability of students of human behavior to use neuroradiologic studies in the management of neurologic patients

Functional Context for Learning

Every structure in the nervous system has a purpose and is part of an integrated functional system, with ascending and/or descending projections. Determining how each newly introduced structure fits into the broader organization of the brain is a meaningful learning activity. To what other structure is it functionally and/or anatomically related? For instance, the **medial lemniscus** refers to the brainstem location of the fibers that conduct sensory information from the peripheral body parts to the thalamus, whereas the **lateral lemniscus** refers to brainstem location of the fibers that conduct auditory impulses to the thalamus. The **superior colliculi** are concerned with visual reflexes, whereas the adjacently located **inferior colliculi** are the auditory-relay structures in the midbrain. Together, they regulate bodily reflexes in response to visual and auditory stimuli.

Deductive Reasoning and Problem Solving

The most important aspect of training in neuroscience is to learn to narrow down choices of possible lesion sites or localize a lesion in the nervous system using a multistep, clinical problem-solving approach (Box 1-3). The process of localizing a lesion involves finding the limits of affected limbs and point of breakdown in the neural circuitry by examining both the spared and the disrupted functions. Basic knowledge of coexisting anatomic structures and axonal pathways with respect to their origin, termination, and crossing (decussation) helps determine how a patient with a lesion on a specific site is likely to exhibit a combination of symptoms on the body—ipsilateral or contralateral to the lesion site. For example, oculomotor nerve (cranial nerve III) palsy on the left side and hemiparesis on the right side of the body (alternating ophthalmic-hemiplegia) are most likely to result from a midbrain lesion in the left pes pedunculi (crus cerebri). A lesion affecting the oculomotor nerve (with already crossed fibers) in the brainstem produces paralysis of the eye muscles on the same side (ipsilateral), but the paralysis of the limbs is contralateral because of the involvement of the corticospinal tract, which has not yet crossed in the medulla. Furthermore, loss of sensation (of pain and temperature) and paralysis in a single limb implies a lesion either in the spinal roots or nerves or in the brain. This is because these are the only two neuraxial locations in which the sensory and motor fibers from the implicated limb are together. The bilateral presence of paralysis and sensory loss below a certain level on the trunk while they are spared above suggests a complete spinal cord cut; a spinal disorder is likely to interrupt the fibers below the lesion while sparing those above.

Neurological Indicators

Reported symptoms of abnormality and confirmed clinical signs play an important role in the ultimate diagnosis of

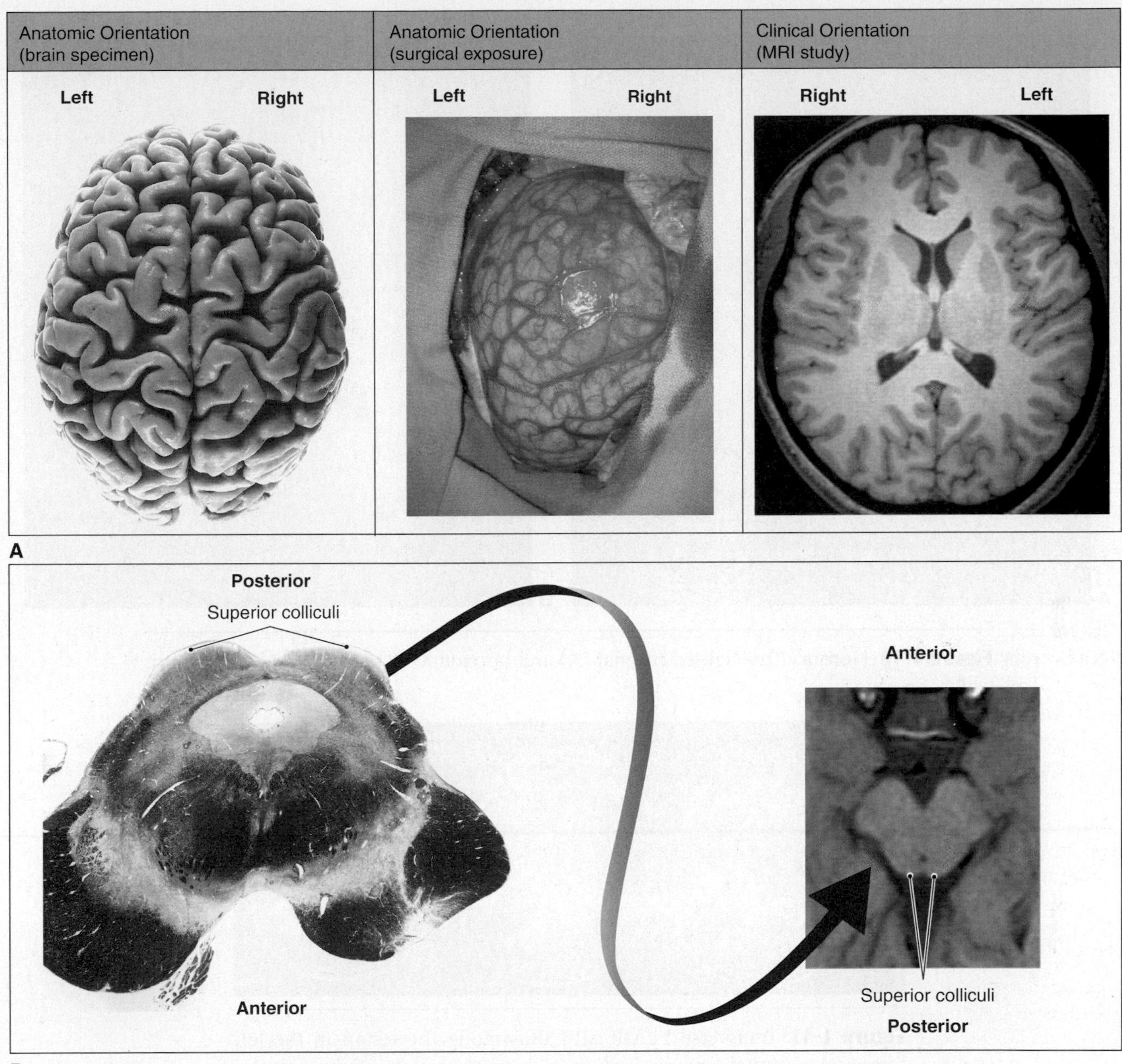

Figure 1-9 Reverse relationship between the anatomic and clinical orientations. A. Cerebral hemispheres. B. Midbrain.

the nervous system disease. Their presence, if occurring with other clinically established signs, is of importance in clinical neurology as it helps move in the direction of right diagnosis decision making. A familiarity with common behavioral abnormalities and diseases also enhances the clinical skills of students of communicative disorders as it guides their decision-making rationale about a proper diagnosis and effective treatment as well as the optimal timing of the treatment. A lack of this understanding about the disease process can limit the applications of the clinical skills as best pointed out by Dr. Arnold Aronson commenting on his first-day experience as an SLP at the Mayo Clinic: "Now, 20,000 neurologic patients later, I have come to appreciate the importance of a solid background in medical neuroscience in preparation for the practice and teaching of speech, language and audiologic disorders from neurologic diseases" (1990, pp IX).

A recently developed condition is clinically more significant than a chronic one. Reduced strength, muscle tone, and reflexes are likely to result from a lesion in the PNS or one involving the lower (spinal or cranial) motor neurons. On the other hand, increased muscle tone and

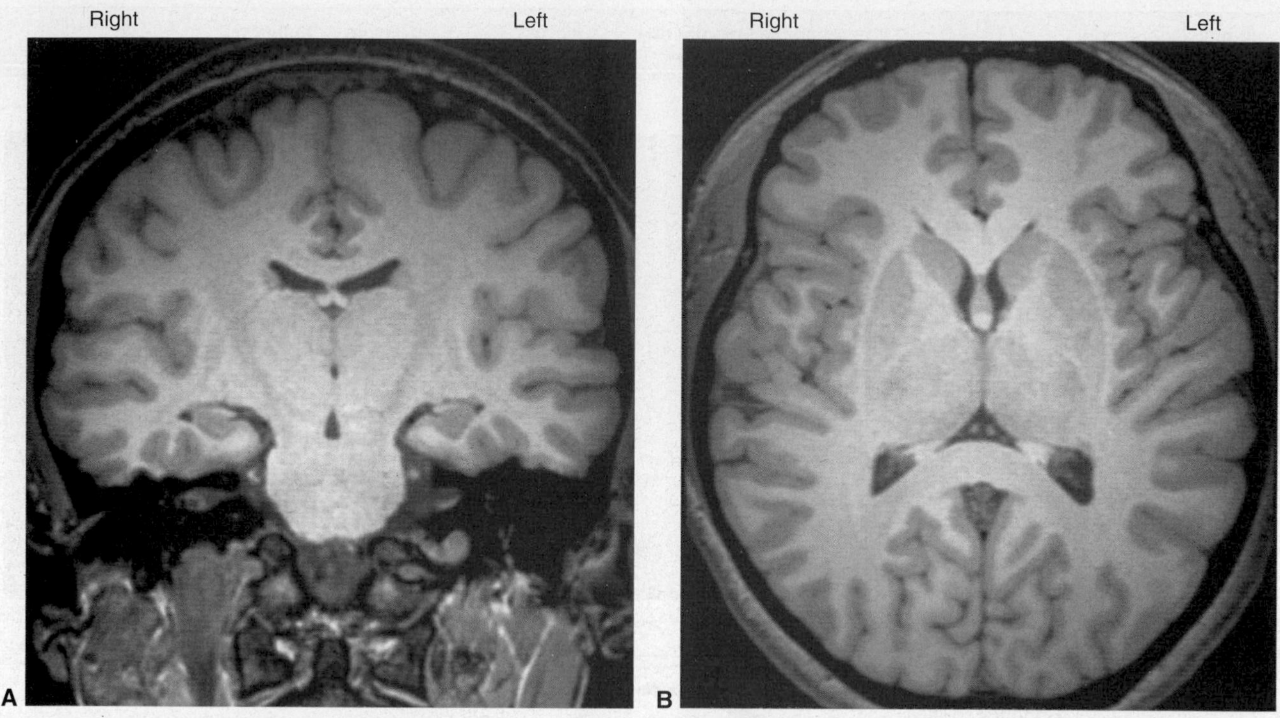

Figure 1-10 Normal T1-weighted coronal (A) and horizontal (B) MR images of the brain.

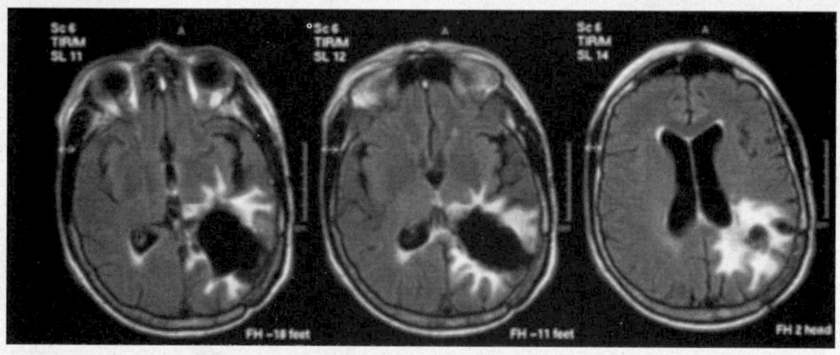

Figure 1-11 Transverse FLAIR MRI illustrating the lesion in the left temporal–occipital area including a large resection cavity from a surgery.

hyperactive reflexes are the indicators of lesions involving the upper motor neurons in the forebrain and/or their long descending fibers. Decerebrate posture provides significant clinical information. Marked by extended legs and internally rotated arms, this posture results from a lesion in the midbrain (below the red nucleus). Sudden emergence of focal symptoms is often an indicator of a cerebrovascular accident, while gradually emerging symptoms point in the direction of a progressive lesion like neoplasm or a degenerative condition. The best indicator of a healthy muscle is its natural tone; that is, the natural resistance experienced by the examiner during a passive limb movement. Muscle tone changes also help differentiate central and peripheral lesion. **Spasticity** refers to an increased muscle tone and is best illustrated by a "clasp-knife pattern," where there is resistance to flexion but gives way abruptly to allow further easy movement. Its presence is clinically associated with the lesion involving the upper motor neurons in the brain; this spasticity also co-occurs with **Babinski sign** (see Chapter 16). Other increased muscle tone abnormality is **rigidity**, which is marked by the constant resistance present throughout the passive limb movement (lead-pipe rigidity); it implies an extrapyramidal lesion involving basal ganglia structures (see Chapter 15). Parkinson patients show a different pattern of rigidity called "cog-wheel" where because of tremor the muscle responds with jerks (ratchety feeling) to a constant limb bending. Muscle atrophy and fasciculation

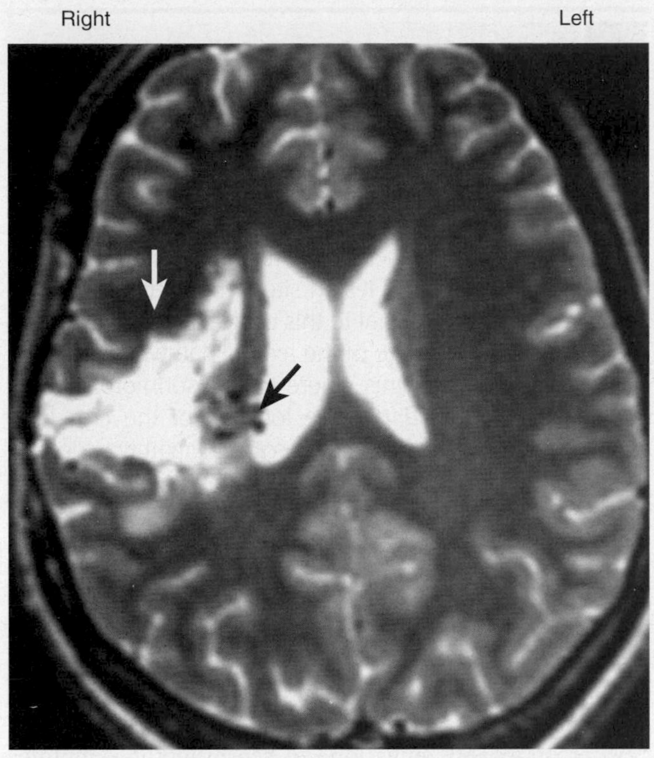

Figure 1-12 T2 axial MRI illustrating a small residual arteriovenous malformation (AVM) in a right periventricular area (*black arrow*) and a large hemorrhagic lesion (*white arrow*).

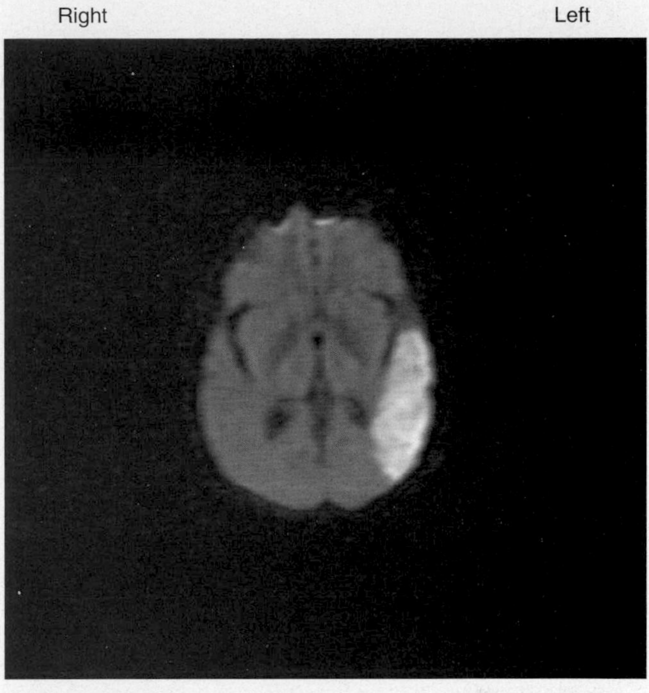

Figure 1-13 An acute infarct in the left temporal lobe on a diffusion-weighted MR image.

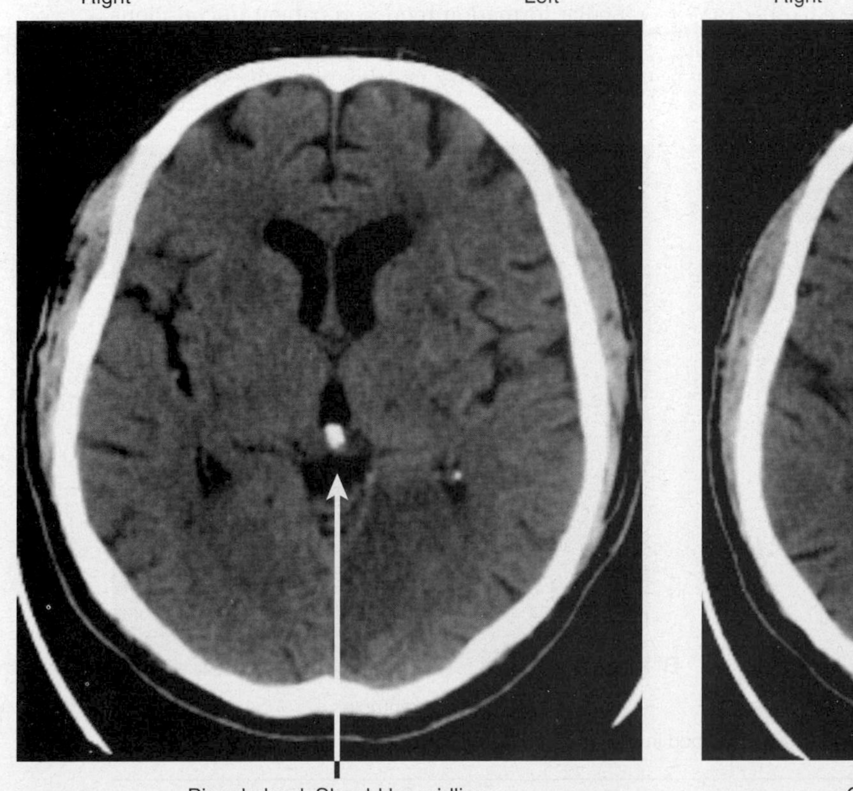

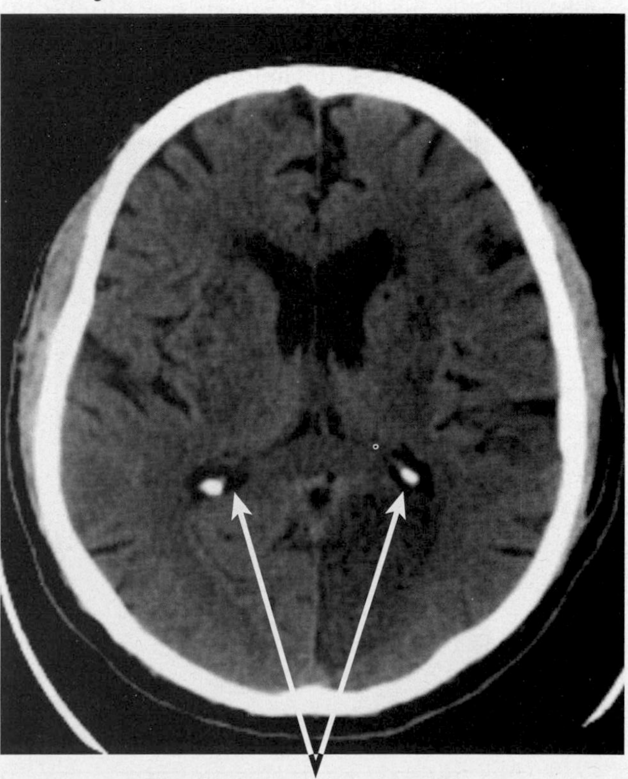

Figure 1-14 Two axial CT scans with normal calcified landmarks of pituitary gland and choroid plexus in the posterior horns of the lateral ventricle.

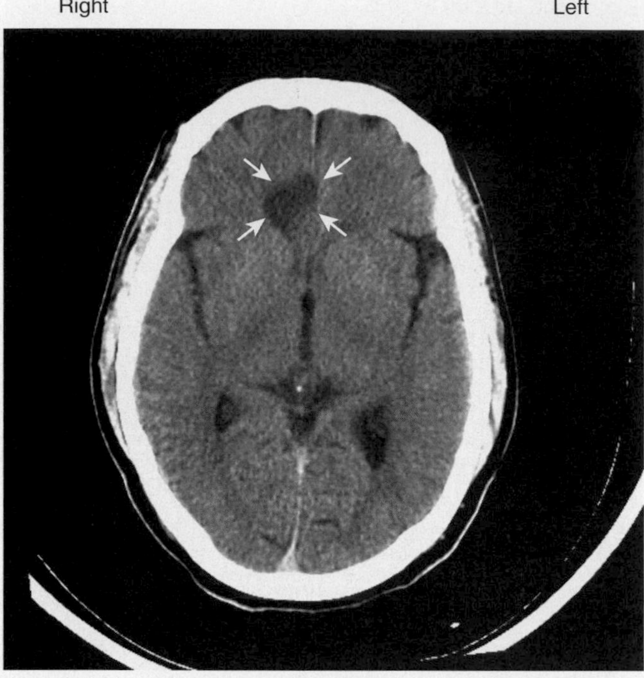

Figure 1-15 A CT image of an infarct (**white arrows**) in the parafalcine region of the right frontal lobe in patient who developed neurogenic stuttering.

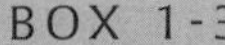

BOX 1-3

Clinical Problem Solving

Lesion localization, crucial for differential diagnosis, is the foundation for learning clinical neurology. Perhaps the most challenging aspect of learning neuroscience is relating symptoms with their underlying lesion sites. The anatomic information that is vital to this clinical problem solving is the knowledge of the axonal pathways and the anatomical points where the sensorimotor fibers cross the midline. The location of the crossing points for the information-carrying pathway determines if the symptoms of brain injuries will manifest ipsilateral or contralateral to the lesion site.

(twitching of a group of muscle fibers) are usually seen in patients with the diseases of lower motor neurons or peripheral lesions involving the muscle (see Chapter 13). Permanently dilated or constricted pupils are indicative of autonomic abnormalities. In clinical terms, the presence of a "Kayser–Fleischer ring" (pigmented ring encircling the cornea) indicates the **Wilson disease**, a disorder of copper metabolism, characterized by basal ganglia degeneration with subsequent speech and cognitive impairments. The "exacerbation and remission" of sensorimotor symptoms are considered an indicator of multiple sclerosis, the most common demyelinating disease of the CNS. Maintaining consciousness requires the integrity of both hemispheres and the brainstem reticular formation. A massive and diffuse injury affecting both hemispheres or the brainstem reticular formation renders a patient unconscious.

Further, any limb asymmetry is a confirmed sign of an abnormality in the nervous system. Students of

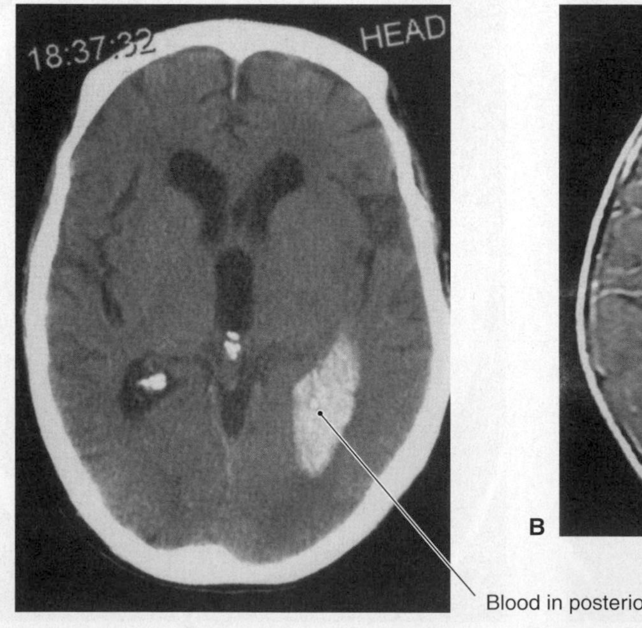

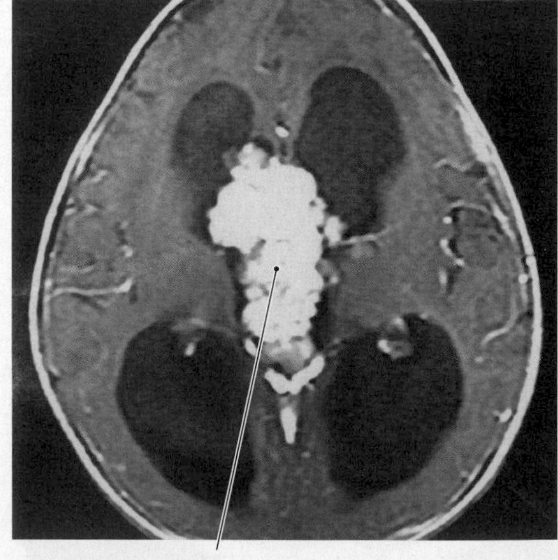

Figure 1-16 A CT image of blood presence in the posterior horn of the lateral ventricle (**A**) and a large tumor in the third ventricle (**B**).

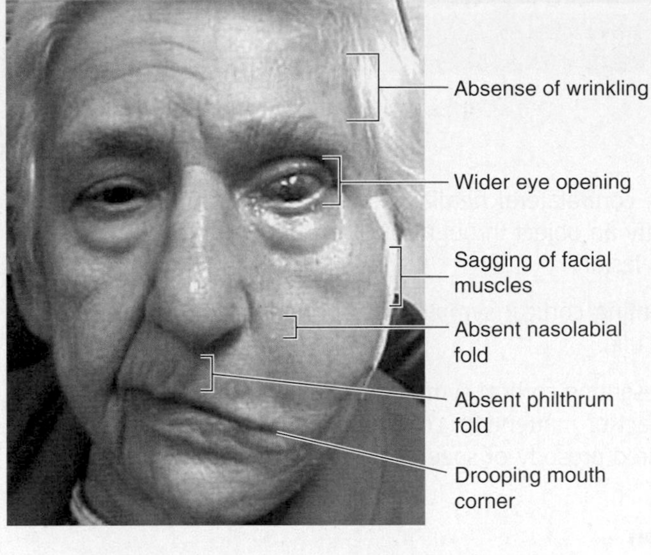

Figure 1-17 Facial asymmetry (Bell palsy).

communicative disorders must be sensitive to the asymmetry of face and oral structures which is in direct response to cranial nerve dysfunctions. Six altered facial locations contribute to facial asymmetry: forehead (absent wrinkling), eye (droopy eyelid and wider eye opening), facial contour (sagging face muscles), labial curve (loss of nasolabial fold) upper lip (loss of philtrum fold), and mouth (drooping mouth corner) (Fig. 1-17).

Gradually expanding on such an analytical approach by adding more and more clinically confirmed facts can make learning neuroscience enjoyable and help you realize clinical potential possible from the application of your neuroscience knowledge.

Lesion Localization

Lesion localization is crucial to differential diagnosis in neurology and is perhaps the most challenging aspect of learning neuroscience. Most of the systems in the brain are considered to be vertically organized systems that connect the CNS to the peripheral body region. Each abnormal sign in a patient presumably reflects a breakdown at a point in the linear (ascending or descending) pathway. If the implicated linear fibers mediating sensory and motor information intersect, a lesion involving this single point, understandably, will impair both sensory and motor functions. However, the intersection of these fibers at two different anatomic sites would indicate two possible potential lesion sites. In this case, one will have to attend to other co-occurring symptoms in order to determine which of these lesion sites could more plausibly be implicated. Localizing a lesion becomes complex in cases with multiple clinical symptoms that involve numerous pathways and multiple points of their intersections. Lesion localization in such patients requires a systematic analysis of symptoms, use of problem-solving skills, in-depth understanding of neuroanatomy, and a specialized professional training; only neurologists are able to complete the diagnosis.

Nevertheless, a set of simple clinical rules can account for many common neurological signs and explain many pertinent neurologic conditions since some neurologic signs point to specific lesions and their sites (Box 1-4; Table 1-13). For example, a pathologic involvement of the sensorimotor cortex leads to impairment in the deliberate and voluntary control of movements. Basal ganglia lesions lead to increased muscle tone, resulting in stiff muscles and involuntary movements like tremors and chorea. Cerebellar lesions affect the ability to balance and are characterized by

Table 1-13

Lesion-Localizing Signs

Clinical Symptoms	Implicated Lesion Sites
Reduced (deep tendon) reflex	Lower motor neuron syndrome: impaired muscle stretch afferents involving motor nuclei (brainstem or spinal corda and their axons in the peripheral pathway)
Flaccid tone (loss of muscle resistance to passive stretching)	Lower motor neuron syndrome: injury to motor nuclei in the brainstem or spinal cord
Babinski sign (extension of great toe and abduction of other toes)	Upper motor neuron syndrome: damage to the motor neurons in the motor cortex or interruption in the descending fibers
Hyperactive (brisk) reflex	Upper motor neuron syndrome: damage to the motor neurons in the motor cortex or interruption in the descending fibers Diffuse massive cortical, subcortical, or brainstem dysfunction or bilateral affection of the ascending reticular projections

BOX 1-4

Ten Rules That Assist in Localizing a Lesion

Rule 1: Symptoms Suggesting a Cortical Lesion

- **Presenting symptoms:** Contralateral hemiplegia; contralateral hemianesthesia of face, trunk, and upper extremity; and cortical sensory loss (failure to identify an object through touch or to identify a letter or word written on the surface of the skin) suggest a cortical lesion.
- **Dominant hemisphere:** In addition to the presenting cortical symptoms, a dominant hemisphere lesion results in aphasia, apraxia, finger agnosia, and acalculia.
- **Nondominant hemisphere:** In addition to the presenting cortical symptoms, an injury in the nondominant (right) hemisphere can also result in left-sided neglect or inattention, constructional and/or dressing deficits (apraxia), spatial and temporal disorientation, impaired prosody of speech, and impaired ability to recognize faces.

Rule 2: Symptoms Suggesting a Subcortical Lesion

- **Presenting symptoms:** Contralateral hemiplegia and diminution or loss of pain and temperature equally for the face, arms, and legs, but with no loss of higher mental functions, is associated with a subcortical (internal capsule) lesion. Emergence of involuntary movements suggests a basal ganglia involvement.

Rule 3: Symptoms Suggesting a Disorder in Vascular System

- **Presenting symptoms:** Sudden development of contralateral paralysis of the lower face, arm, and upper extremity (more than the leg), with accompanying sensory loss, results from an occlusion (thrombosis or embolism) of the middle cerebral artery. Additional symptoms may include the ones discussed under rule 1. (An abrupt onset of symptoms usually indicates vascular disease, whereas a gradual progression of symptoms indicates a mass lesion.)
- **Presenting symptoms:** Toe, foot, and leg paralysis as well as sensory loss and mental impairments (distractibility, indecisiveness, and lack of spontaneity) are associated with ischemia owing to embolism or thrombosis in the anterior cerebral artery distribution.
- **Presenting symptoms:** Homonymous hemianopsia (blindness in contralateral eye) and memory impairment are associated with posterior cerebral artery involvement. Visual agnosia, if present, involves a bilateral involvement of this artery.

Rule 4: Symptoms Suggesting a Central Gray Matter Spinal Lesion

- **Presenting symptoms:** Bilateral loss of pain and temperature sensation with a preserved sense of touch in the same limbs (usually the two upper limbs) implies a lesion (e.g., cavitation or syringomyelia) in the spinal central gray.

Rule 5: Symptoms Suggesting a Visual Pathway Lesion

- **Presenting symptoms:** Blindness in one eye suggests an optic nerve lesion anterior to the optic chiasm.
- **Presenting symptoms:** Bitemporal hemianopsia (the patient does not see things laterally in the visual fields) results from an optic chiasm lesion compressing or interrupting the crossing fibers from the nasal retina of each eye.
- **Presenting symptoms:** Homonymous hemianopsia is associated with a lesion in the optic tract fibers anywhere between the optic chiasm and the occipital lobe.
- **Presenting symptoms:** Alexia (failure to comprehend written word) and homonymous hemianopsia, along with spared macular vision, are associated with a lesion of the primary visual cortex (area 17) and visual association cortex (areas 18 and 19). Visual agnosia is associated with bilateral occipital lesions.

Rule 6: Symptoms Suggesting a Complete Spinal Cord Transection

- **Presenting symptoms:** Paralysis and sensory loss bilaterally below the level of the lesion with spared functions above indicates a complete spinal cord transection injury.

BOX 1-4 *(Continued)*

Rule 7: Symptoms Suggesting a Spinal Hemisection Lesion

- **Presenting symptoms:** Ipsilateral loss of proprioception and vibratory sensation, ipsilateral loss of skilled motor activity due to paralysis, and contralateral loss of pain and temperature sensation below the level of the lesion indicate a spinal hemisection (Brown–Séquard syndrome).

Rule 8: Symptoms Suggesting a Peripheral or Central Lesion

- **Presenting symptoms:** Paralysis and sensory (pain and temperature) loss involving the same single limb suggests either a lesion in the peripheral nerve or a large lesion in the sensory cortex.

Rule 9: Symptoms Suggesting an Upper or Lower Motor Neuron Lesion

- **Presenting symptoms:** Increased reflexes, hemiplegia, and spastic muscle tone in a symptomatic (sensorimotor) limb indicate upper motor neuron lesions. Reduced reflexes, muscle atrophy, and weakness in the same symptomatic limb imply peripheral or lower motor neuron lesions.

Rule 10: Symptoms Suggesting a Brainstem Lesion

- **Presenting symptoms:** Motor and sensory losses of the extremities on one side with contralateral cranial nerve signs imply a brainstem lesion. An altered level of consciousness is also associated with such a lesion. An extension of this rule is that lesions lower than the mid-pons will not impair the function of the facial muscles.

wide-based and unsteady (ataxic) gait, clumsy and inaccurate movements with a tendency to fall on the affected side. Additional symptoms associated with cerebellar pathology are tremor during action and inaccurate (dysmetria) and irregular (asynergia) movements. Common rules that assist in localizing a lesion are presented in Box 1-4.

These rules will become meaningful as students become more familiar with neuroanatomy and sensorimotor pathways. An understanding of the lesion-localizing rules facilitates the grasp of the rationale for using selected tasks and activities when examining a patient with left or right hemiplegia. For example, establishing a left cortical lesion in a patient with right hemiplegia requires that the patient be tested for aphasia (naming, verbal output, reading, and writing); the differential paralytic involvement of face, arm, and leg; right-sided cortical sensory loss; and homonymous hemianopsia. To determine a lesion in the right (nondominant) hemisphere, testing should include the assessment of inattention to the left body space, left sensorimotor involvement, spatial orientation, constructional and/or dressing activities, and speech prosody and denial of disease. Determining a subcortical lesion requires that the patient be tested for contralateral hemiplegia and equal sensorimotor involvement of face, arm, and leg; dystonic postures; and reduced pain threshold. To confirm a brainstem lesion, one must test the patient for alternating hemiplegia, which is characterized by ipsilateral cranial nerve symptoms (left ear hearing loss, left tongue deviation, left facial weakness, swallowing, and dysarthria) and crossed hemiplegia. Establishing a spinal cord lesion requires that the patient be examined for muscle tone, reflex quality, paralysis, and sensory loss.

CLINICAL CORRELATES

CASE STUDIES FOR PROBLEM SOLVING

CASE ONE (1-1)

A 25-year-old speech–language–hearing pathologist (SLP) on the first day of her medical placement received a case study with the following magnetic resonance imaging (MRI) study and a report identifying it as a glioblastoma involving the right frontal cortex. Because the lesion was clearly located on the left side of the image, the SLP thought the report localizing the tumor in the right hemisphere was in error.

Question: How can you explain the confusion in reading the MRI?

Case (1-1) Discussion: See discussion of case studies

(continued)

CASE STUDIES FOR PROBLEM SOLVING

CASE TWO (1-2)

On his first day of work at a hospital, a 28-year-old SLP met a neurologist who informally began discussing an interesting 20-year-old patient she had just seen. This patient had no apparent cognitive or communicative problem but presented with a history of big appetite, excessive perspiration, irregular sleep–wake cycle, and altered sexual behavior, with no libido. The neurologist noted that this was a classical case of a lesion in the lower diencephalon.

Question: How can you explain these symptoms in relation to the lesion site?

Case (1-2) Discussion: See discussion of case studies

CASE THREE (1-3)

A rookie SLP read the report of a patient with impaired speech, language, cognitive, and sensorimotor functions subsequent to a traumatic brain injury caused by an automobile accident. The neurologic report identified multiple sites with laceration and contusing tissues—most important, those involving Brodmann areas 4, 3, 1, 2, 10, 11, and 38.

Question: What sensorimotor and behavioral symptoms are you likely to see in this patient?

Case (1-3) Discussion: See discussion of case studies

CASE FOUR (1-4)

A beginning SLP went to a grand-round discussion, which focused on a patient who had profound aphasic symptoms disproportionate to the extent of the lesion displayed on a coronal MRI study. The SLP was asked what she could tell about this patient's language dysfunctions. The SLP said that she wanted to see a different view of the brain before commenting.

Question: Which view of the brain would give the SLP a better clinical picture?

Case (1-4) Discussion: See discussion of case studies

CASE FIVE (1-5)

An SLP attended the grand rounds in the neurology department where a 75-year-old man was being discussed. This man with a slow and progressive history of cognitive impairment had recently suffered a stroke. MRI revealed this to be a brainstem injury, which resulted in impaired sensorimotor functions and unintelligible speech. Additional clinical symptoms included:

- Ptosis (paralysis of eye lid on the left)
- Dilated left pupil with no response to light
- A laterally deviated left eye
- Left-sided limb incoordination
- Right-sided spastic paralysis

Answering questions from the floor, the presenter stated that a physical therapy consultation was sought for the patient but there was nothing that required an SLP consultation and then he looked toward the SLP.

Question: What do you think about this statement? Do you think that there is some missing information about this patient?

Case 1-5 Discussion: See discussion of case studies

SUMMARY

Neuroscience and communicative disorders are two closely related disciplines. Basic understanding of neuroscience is essential for a comprehensive training in SLP. This knowledge provides students with a broad framework for diagnosing communication disorders and for providing effective remediation. Such a background also helps students of communicative disorders become creative partners in a team approach to managing a patient's clinical condition, and nurturing good working relationships with colleagues in the medical and paramedical professions.

In spite of the difficulty in learning neuroscience, there are ways to overcome its technical complexity. A familiarity with brain–behavior governing rules, basic neuroanatomical structures, clinical–neurological concepts, technical word-formation rules, neuronal functions, and diagnostic tools is prerequisite for learning neuroscience; this knowledge is needed for solving clinical neurological problems, the most satisfying part of learning neuroscience. Familiarity with technical terms and approaches that emphasize persistent repetition, visual orientation, and deductive reasoning can make learning neuroscience easier and challenging. Further, a visual familiarity with the graphic details presented in Chapters 2 and 3 will help develop the foundation for understanding the functional and structural organization of the nervous system.

REVIEW QUESTIONS

1. Complete the following statements using the appropriate technical terms:
   - A. A left hemispheric lesion results in __________ hemiplegia and __________ hemianesthesia.
   - B. In __________ __________, the patient faces the clinician so that the patient's left and right corresponds to clinicians' right and left.
   - C. Brain's inherent capacity to reorganize when faced with injuries is known as __________.
   - D. The __________ of sensory and motor fibers accounts for the contralaterality of sensorimotor organization in the brain.
   - E. Clinical symptoms are __________ if they appear on the side of the body which is identical to the lesion side.
   - F. The __________ __________ refers to the discreteness with which sensorimotor information is retained in the axonal pathways from the specialized peripheral receptors in the body to the brain.
   - G. __________ refers to a hypertonic state of muscle which is marked by increased tone.
   - H. As an example of muscle tone abnormality, _______ refers to a constant resistance that is present throughout a passive limb movement.
   - I. The central part of the body which is made up of the head and trunk is known as the __________ region. __________, on the other hand, relates to the limbs, which are attached to the central body region.
   - J. The __________ consists of three structures: midbrain, pons, and medulla.
   - K. Cerebral hemispheres, limbic lobe, and basal ganglia are derived from the __________, which itself relates to the __________.
   - L. __________ is a collection of nerve fibers that have a common origin and termination.

2. Match each of the following functional categories with its examples.

A. general somatic afferent (GSA)	a. pain and temperature
B. special somatic afferent (SSA)	b. autonomic nervous system activity
C. general visceral afferent (GVA)	c. limb movement involving skeletal muscles
D. special visceral afferent (SVA)	d. audition
E. general somatic efferent (GSE)	e. organ content
F. general visceral efferent (GVE)	f. taste and smell
G. special visceral efferent (SVE)	g. articulation, phonation, facial expression, and swallowing

3. Match the following lexical roots with their meanings. (see Appendix C for help)

A. Kinesis	a. paralysis
B. Opsis	b. old
C. Phagein	c. tongue
D. Plege	d. eat
E. Prattein/praxis	e. vision
F. Presbys	f. movement
G. Taxis	g. order
H. Gloss	h. act or action

4. Match the Brodmann area numbers for the following cortical regions.

A. Primary motor cortex	a. 41, 42
B. Primary somatosensory area	b. 3, 1, 2
C. Primary visual cortex	c. 4
D. Primary auditory cortex	d. 17

5. Provide the directional terms above and below the neuroaxial bend on the figures below:

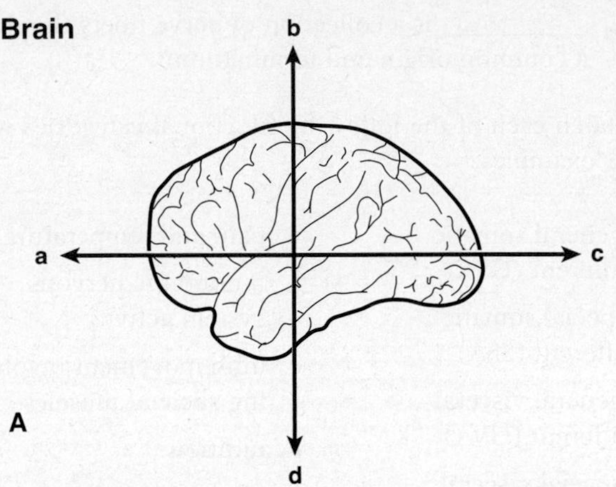

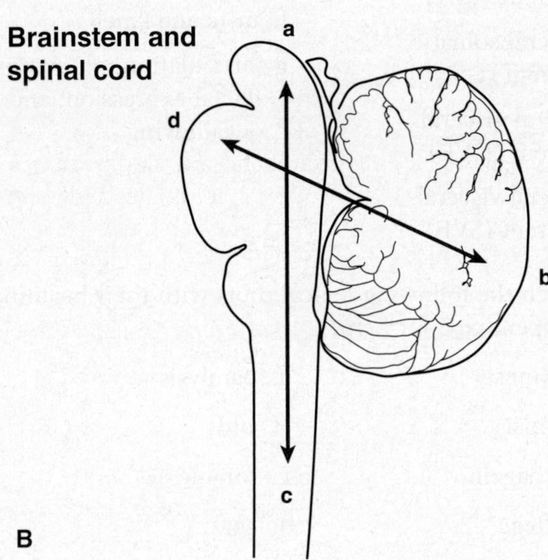

A. Above the neuroaxial bend (the brain):

a.
b.
c.
d.

B. Below the neuraxial bend (the brainstem and spinal cord):

a.
b.
c.
d.

6. Match each of the branches of neuroscience with its associated definition.

A. Neurology	a. nervous system and its diseases
B. Neurosurgery	b. structure and anatomy of the CNS
C. Neuroanatomy	c. imaging of brain structures in vivo
D. Neuroradiology	d. development of the CNS
E. Neuroembryology	e. chemical/physical processes of the CNS
F. Neurophysiology	f. pathologic changes in the CNS
G. Neuropathology	g. surgical removal of pathologic tissue from the nervous system

7. Match the following neurological conditions with the associated statement.

A. Huntington disease	a. a degenerative disease of the aging brain associated with dementia
B. Cerebral palsy	b. a motor disorder caused by damage to the brain pre, post, or during birth
C. Parkinson disease	c. an abnormality in the brain's electrical activity
D. Alzheimer	d. a progressive and hereditary brain disease leading to chorea and dementia
E. Stroke	e. a progressive demyelinating disease of the CNS
F. Epilepsy	f. a loss of function due to the interruption of blood circulation in the brain
G. Multiple sclerosis	g. a progressive disease of the brain characterized by tremor, reduced strength, and slow movements

8. Provide two examples of reorganization in the adult brain as a reflection of cerebral plasticity:
9. List six reasons why training in neuroscience helps you become a better SLP clinician:
10. How does a stroke (cerebral vascular accident) affect cortical functions?
11. How does familiarity with clinical orientation help reading brain images?
12. Name the principles that regulate brain functions dealing with connectivity, decision making, dominance, reorganization, and discreteness of sensorimotor representation.
13. Name the three major structures of the brain.
14. Name the brain region that contains the six-layered cortex and list its function.
15. Name the three major areas covered in a neurological examination.

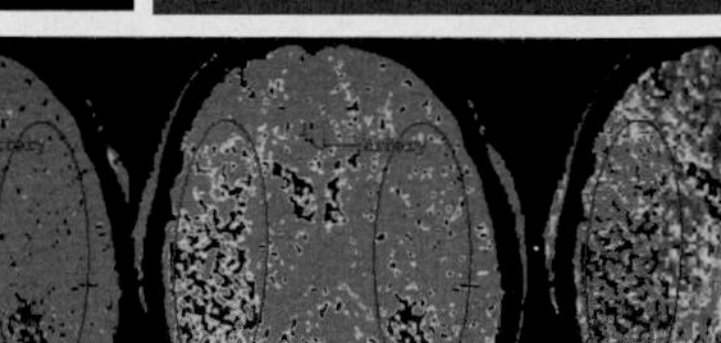

2 Gross Anatomy of the Central Nervous System

LEARNING OBJECTIVES

After studying this chapter, students should be able to:

- Differentiate between the central and peripheral nervous systems
- Describe the functions of the major structures of the central and peripheral nervous systems
- List principal embryonic divisions of the brain and gross anatomic structures related to each division
- Identify the internal structures of the cerebral cortex, thalamus, midbrain, pons, and medulla and describe their functions
- Identify the gross anatomic structures of the spinal cord and explain their functions
- Discuss the structural and functional importance of the brainstem reticular formation
- Discuss parts and functions of the ventricular cavities
- Describe the meninges, their locations, and their functions
- Differentiate the various medullary fibers and appreciate the structural complexity and functional connectivity of the brain structures
- List the cranial nerves, cite their anatomic locations, and describe their major sensory and motor functions
- Discuss the anatomy and functions of the autonomic nervous system

The human nervous system can best be described as a cellular system specialized for rapid intercellular communication by means of the electrical and chemical energy distributed throughout the body, which it uses to respond to static or dynamic changes in the internal and external environment as they impinge on the body. With the endocrine system, it is able to reach target cells in all organs by long axons with multiple branches. Cellular communication along an axon involves rapid electrochemical changes in the cell membranes (action potential). The axonal branches terminate in close contact with the target cells, so the diffusion of the chemical messenger to the receptors of the target cell is precise, rapid, and localized.

Through rapid communication, complex integrative functions, and massive data storage, the network of neurons in the brain and spinal cord provides the mechanism of function for the nervous system, which has four categories of function: sensor, effector, integrator, and regulator. As the sensor, it receives all environmental and bodily generated changes and stores it. As the effector, it initiates and controls all body movements. As the integrator, it analyzes and combines information received from all sources and modalities. As the regulator, it maintains the homeostatic state for the optimum control of peak body performance and repair.

Key Terms :

Autonomic nervous system
Cerebrospinal fluid (CSF)
Diencephalon
Meninges
Mesencephalon
Metencephalon
Midbrain
Myelencephalon
Parasympathetic nervous system
Pons
Prosencephalon
Rhombencephalon
Somatic nervous system
Spinal nerves
Sympathetic nervous system
Telencephalon

CENTRAL AND PERIPHERAL NERVOUS SYSTEMS

Anatomically, the nervous system consists of two major parts: the central nervous system (CNS) and the peripheral nervous system (PNS). The CNS consists of the brain and spinal cord (Fig. 2-1*A*). The brain is responsible for initiating, controlling, and regulating all sensorimotor and cognitive (mental) functions that generate and regulate human

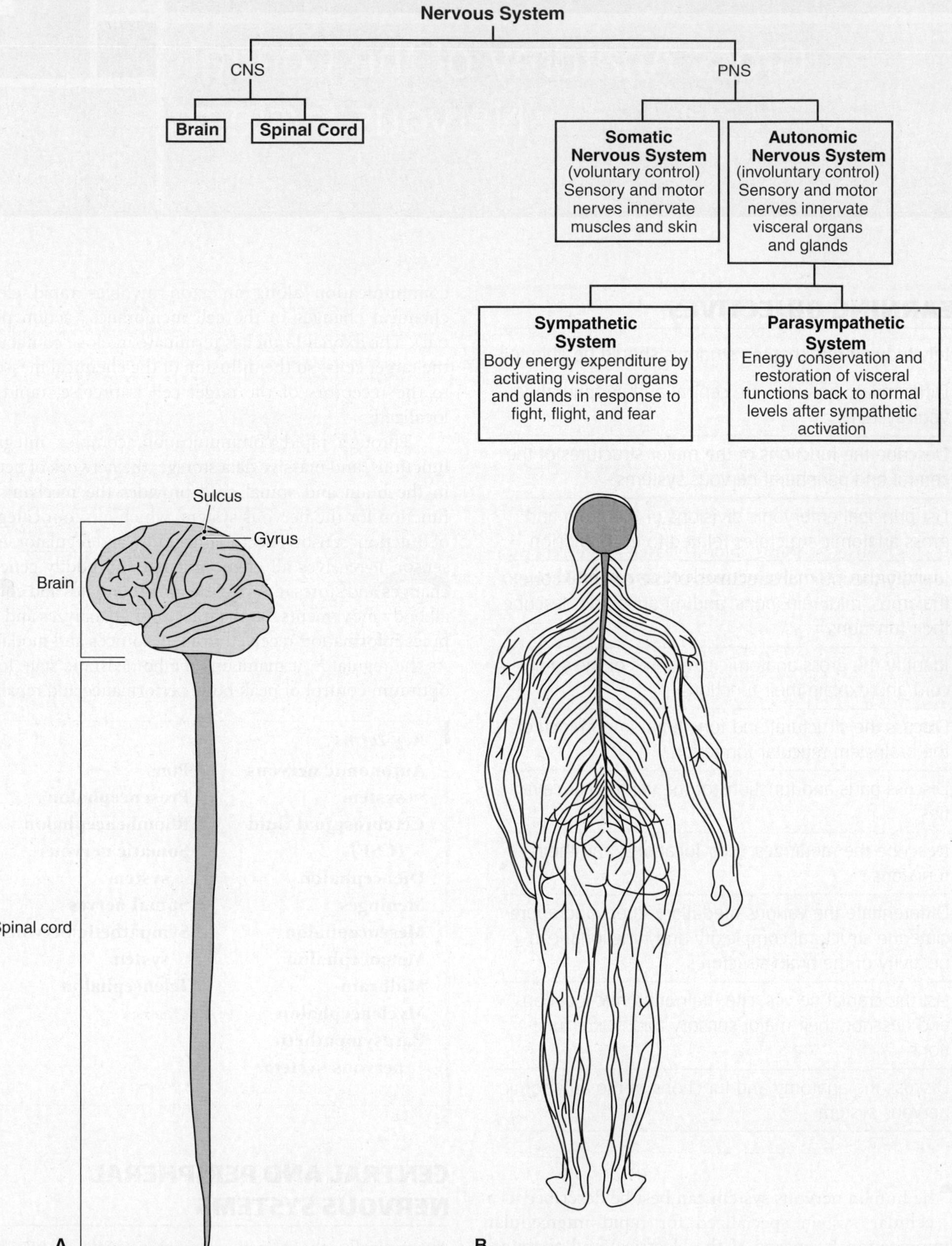

Figure 2-1 The human nervous system. A. The central nervous system: brain and spinal cord. B. The peripheral nervous system: cranial nerves and spinal nerves.

behavior. The spinal cord is primarily a wired-cable structure in the CNS that transmits motor commands to various body parts, which interact with the environment. Also, the sensory information that is collected from the peripheral body parts and the environment is transmitted to the brain via the spinal cord. Some sensory input is processed locally in the spinal cord and regulates peripheral reflexive motor activity.

The CNS is protected by a bony shell. The brain is encased in a tough bony skull, and the spinal cord is similarly protected by the vertebral column, which consists of a series of bones and cartilaginous washer-like structures; the washers buffer body movements to bear weight. The CNS is encased in three membranous coverings, known as the **meninges** and visualized as three diapers. Between the two inner diapers, there is the **cerebrospinal fluid (CSF)**, which serves both as a protective mechanical buffer and as a chemical mediator for metabolic functions. The meninges also provide the supporting framework for the CNS vessels that carry blood to and from the heart.

The PNS consists of sensory and motor nerves that are connected to the spinal cord (**spinal nerves**) and the brainstem (**cranial nerves [CNs]**). These nerves extend to the organs, muscles, joints, blood vessels, and skin surface, forming an extensive network of fine wires throughout the body (Fig. 2-1*B*). The PNS consists of two major systems: the **somatic nervous system** and the **autonomic nervous system** (ANS). Each of these systems consists of two subsystems: sensory (**afferent**) and motor (**efferent**) fibers. The afferent fibers consist of nerves and cells that transmit sensory information to the CNS from receptors in the skin, muscles, and visceral organs. The efferent fibers transmit commands from the CNS to activate the muscles and glands located throughout the body.

The **somatic** afferents and efferents mediate the skeletal muscle reflexes. **Visceral sensory** inputs of the ANS communicate with **visceral motor** outputs to activate the visceral organ reflexes and glands. The ANS regulates the activity of organs, such as the salivary glands, heart, lung, blood vessels, stomach, intestines, kidneys, and bladder.

The ANS (also called the visceral, involuntary, autonomic, and vegetative system) uses both CNS and PNS components and is made up of two functionally different divisions: the **sympathetic nervous system** and the **parasympathetic nervous system**. Functionally both of these systems produce opposite effects when innervating the same organ. For example, the sympathetic system spends energy (catabolic) and prepares for fight and flight. The parasympathetic system conserves energy (anabolic) and is dominant during relaxation or sleep (see the end of this chapter and Chapter 18).

PRIMARY DIVISIONS OF THE BRAIN

Familiarity with the three major **vesicles** of the embryonic brain facilitates understanding of the development of the human brain and its structures. The 4- to 5-week embryonic brain is well developed in terms of its structures. It has three vesicles: **prosencephalon** (forebrain), **mesencephalon** (midbrain), and **rhombencephalon** (hindbrain). These vesicles are demarcated by three brain **flexures** (bends): **midbrain**, **pontine**, and **cervical** (Fig. 2-2). The midbrain flexure (also called the cephalic) demarcates the midbrain region in the brainstem. The cervical flexure is at the junction of the hindbrain and the spinal cord. An unequal development of the hindbrain produces the pontine flexure, which causes the thinning of the hindbrain roof.

The prosencephalon develops into the **telencephalon** and **diencephalon**. The **cerebral hemispheres**, **limbic lobe**, and **basal ganglia** are the principal derivatives of the telencephalon, whereas the **thalamus** and **hypothalamus** are derived from the diencephalon. The

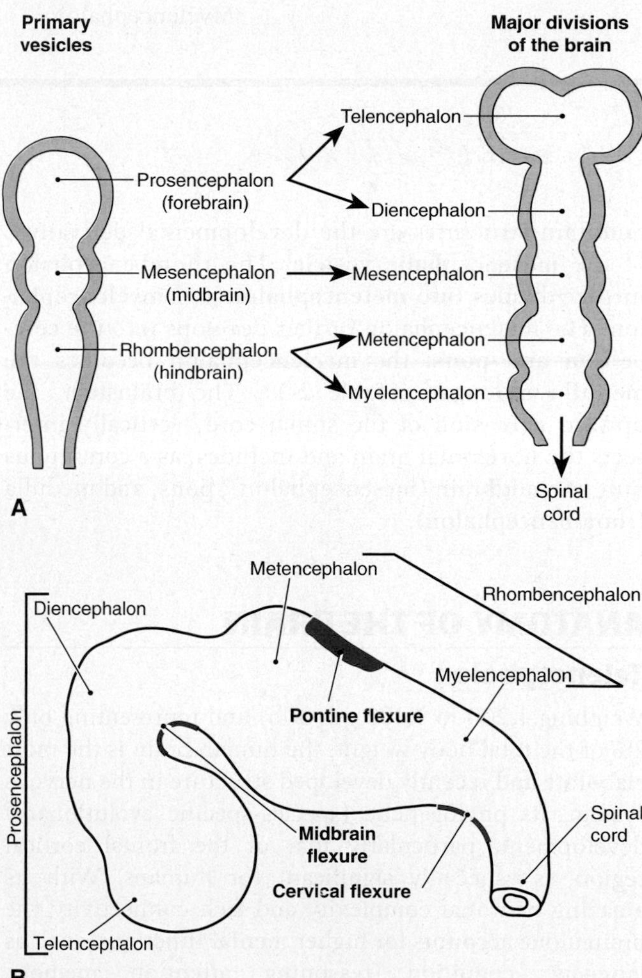

Figure 2-2 A. Three embryonic primary vesicles (**left**) and secondary vesicles and derived structures (**right**). B. Lateral view of the vesicles and the dividing three flexures in the developing brain at end of the embryonic week 5.

Table 2-1

Adult Brain Structures Derived from Embryonic Vesicles

Embryonic Brain Vesicles	Major Divisions of the Brain	Gross Anatomic Structures
Prosencephalon (forebrain)	Telencephalon	Cerebral cortex (frontal, parietal, occipital, temporal cortices), basal ganglia (caudate nucleus, putamen, globus pallidus), and limbic system (cingulate, hippocampus, amygdala) Lateral ventricles
	Diencephalon	Thalamus and hypothalamus Third ventricle
Mesencephalon (midbrain)	Mesencephalon	Midbrain structures (red nucleus substantia nigra, corporal quadrigemina) Cerebral aqueduct
Rhombencephalon (hindbrain)	Metencephalon	Pons and cerebellum Fourth ventricle
	Myelencephalon	Medulla oblongata No ventricle

midbrain structures are the developmental derivatives of the **mesencephalic vesicle**. The rhombencephalon further divides into **metencephalon** and **myelencephalon**. The metencephalon further develops into the **cerebellum** and **pons**; the myelencephalon becomes the **medulla oblongata** (Table 2-1). The brainstem, the upward extension of the spinal cord, vertically intersects the horizontal brain and includes, as a contiguous unit, the midbrain (mesencephalon), pons, and medulla (rhombencephalon).

Key Terms:

Agnosia	**Lateral (Sylvian) fissure**
Association visual cortex	**Occipital**
Astereognosis	**Papez circuit**
Broca area	**Postcentral gyrus**
Dominant and nondominant hemispheres	**Parietal**
Fissure of Rolando	**Precentral gyrus**
Insular	**Precentral sulcus**
Interhemispheric/ longitudinal fissure	**Prefrontal cortex**
	Premotor cortex
	Primary motor cortex
	Primary sensory cortex
	Wernicke area

ANATOMY OF THE BRAIN

Telencephalon

Weighing 1,200 to 1,400 g (~3 lb) and representing only 2% of the total body weight, the human brain is the most elaborate and recently developed structure in the nervous system. Its phylogenetic (species-specific evolutionary) development, particularly that of the frontal cortical region, is especially significant for humans. With its amazing neuronal complexity and rich connectivity, the brain alone accounts for higher mental functions, such as language; cognition (reasoning, attention, memory, temporospatial orientation, judgment, and reflective thinking); emotion and personality; imagination; and consciousness. These functions are integrated by the combined activities of the well-connected cerebral hemispheres and diencephalon.

Cerebral Hemispheres

The **cerebrum** consists of the cerebral hemispheres, which make up the largest part of the brain (Fig. 2-3). Composed of a 3.5-mm-thick layer of neurons, the cerebral cortex is the convoluted surface of the brain; it overlies the internal white matter and more deeply located basal ganglia. The convolutions form ridges and valleys (grooves): the cortical ridges are called **gyri** and the valleys are called **fissures** or **sulci** (Fig. 2-3). The convolutions allow for the accommodation of a large cellular volume within a limited cranial space.

The cerebral hemispheres are separated along the midline by the **longitudinal fissure**, also called the

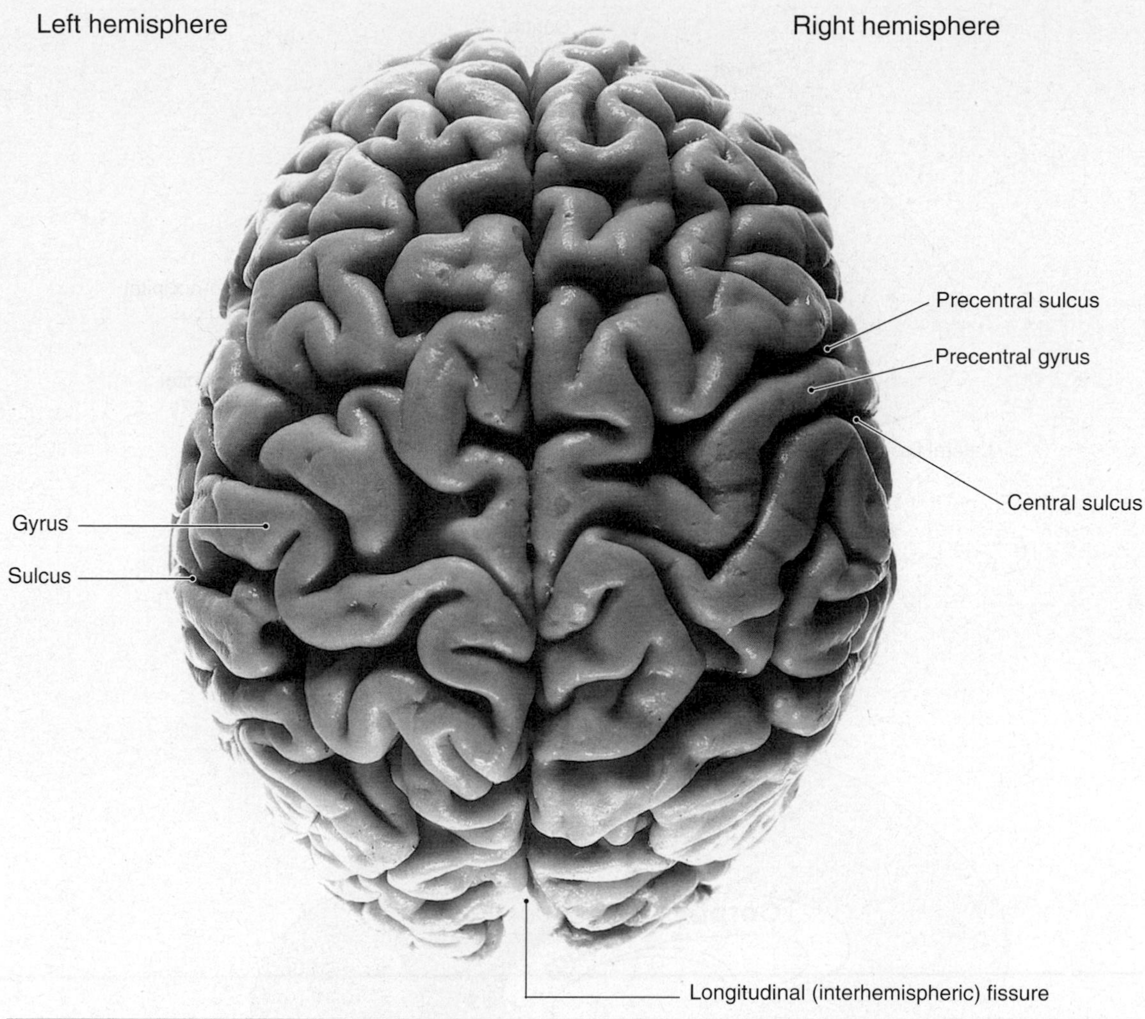

Figure 2-3 Dorsal view of the human brain with the cerebral hemispheres, major sulci, and gyri.

interhemispheric fissure (Fig. 2-3). The paired cerebral hemispheres are essentially mirror images, containing similar centers for processing sensory and motor functions. Besides controlling the sensorimotor functions in the opposite side of the body (Fig. 1-1), each hemisphere possesses specialized skills. For example, the left (dominant) hemisphere is superior in processing language, speech, calculation, and verbal memory, whereas the right (nondominant) hemisphere is better equipped to process and regulate pragmatic skills and visual and spatial concepts. Visual and spatial concepts refer to a series of cognitive processes that we use in recognizing visual objects, designing objects, orienting ourselves within the framework of time and space, and perceiving and expressing music and emotions.

Each cerebral hemisphere consists of five lobes: four primary (**frontal**, **parietal**, **occipital**, **temporal**) and one secondary (**insular**). The primary lobes are named after the overlying bones of the skull (Fig. 2-4). Considered a secondary lobe, the insular lobe (not a universally accepted nomenclature) is a small cortical island hidden in the depths of the sulcus, covered by the overgrown opercular regions of the frontal, parietal, and temporal folds of the cortex (Fig. 2-13). The primary lobes are divided by various sulci; the boundaries of these lobes, although well marked, are arbitrary, especially in the temporal, parietal, and occipital areas. The sulci and gyri markings of the brain are highly variable, particularly on the medial and basal surfaces of the brain. Consequently, maps of the hemispheric lobe boundaries serve as only rough frames of reference.

Cortical Surfaces

Dorsolateral Surface

Some sulci and gyri serve as important landmarks for dividing the hemisphere into lobes. Three major sulci are present on the dorsolateral surface of the brain: **central sulcus (fissure of Rolando)**, **lateral fissure (sylvian**

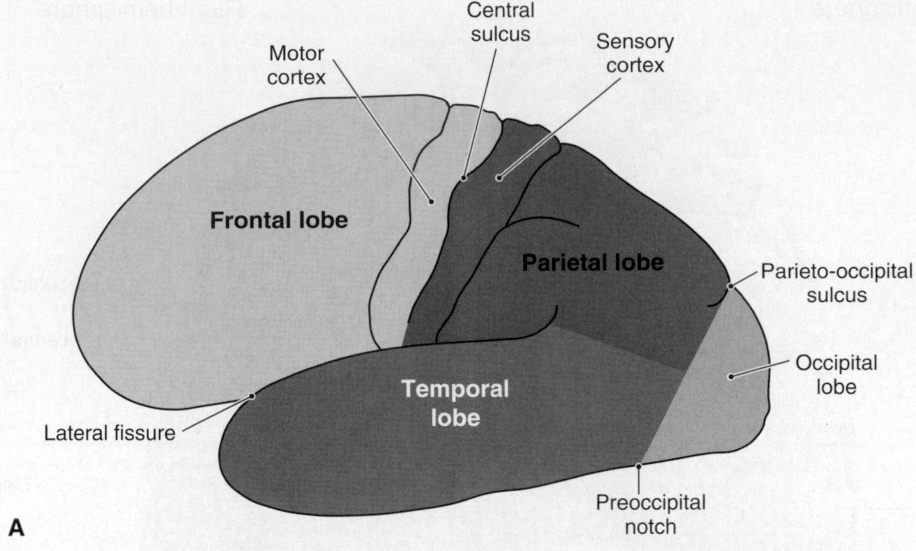

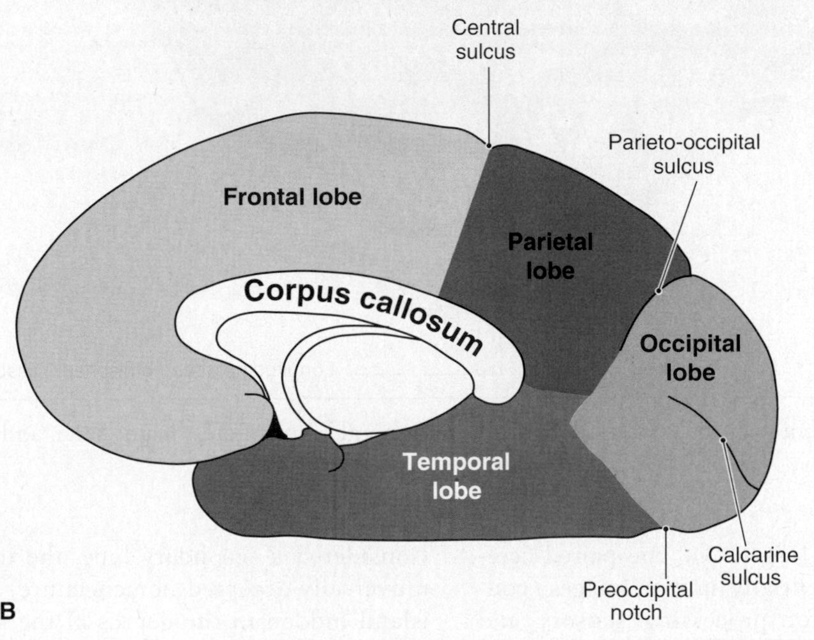

Figure 2-4 Lateral (A) and medial (B) views of the primary hemispheric lobes.

fissure), and **parieto-occipital sulcus** (Figs. 2-4 and 2-5). The central sulcus begins at the top of the brain, extends along the dorsolateral surface in a downward and rostral (anterior) direction, and ends at the lateral fissure. The central sulcus is about 2 cm deep, a depth that marks the boundary between the frontal and the parietal lobes. It also separates the **primary motor cortex** from the **primary sensory cortex**. The lateral fissure, which is the most constant feature of the dorsolateral surface of the brain, begins rostrally below the frontal pole and extends posteriorly up toward the inferior parietal lobe. Anteriorly, the lateral fissure separates the frontal and temporal lobes; posteriorly, it extends partially between the parietal and the temporal lobes. The parieto-occipital sulcus, a vertically oriented deep fissure on the lateral and medial surfaces of the cerebral cortex, separates the parietal lobe from the occipital lobe (Figs. 2-4 and 2-5).

Frontal Lobe

The frontal lobe is rostral to the central sulcus and dorsal to the lateral fissure. As the largest lobe, it occupies about one-third of the hemisphere and contains four important gyri: the vertical **precentral gyrus** and three horizontal gyri. The precentral gyrus lies rostral to the central sulcus;

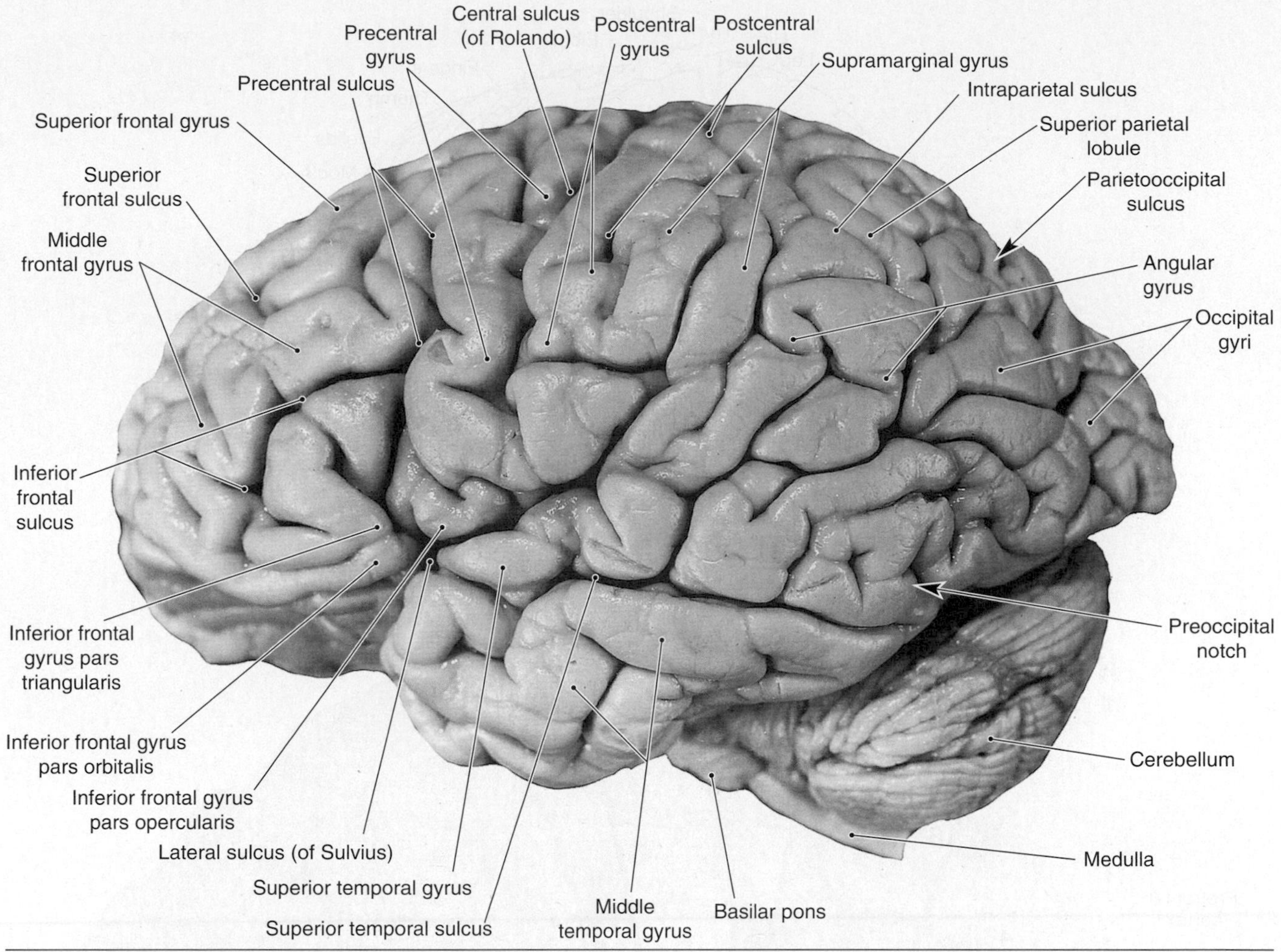

Figure 2-5 Lateral view of the major sulci and gyri of the left cerebral hemisphere.

its anterior boundary is marked by the **precentral sulcus**, which runs parallel to the central sulcus. The precentral gyrus, the site of the primary motor cortex (Brodmann area 4), contains the representation of the human body (homunculus) and regulates the fine and graded movements of the arms, legs, and face (Fig. 2-6); the disproportionate representation of various body portions in the homunculus is based on their role in skilled movements. Bioelectrical activity of nerve cells in this area is responsible for activating and controlling motor acts on the **contralateral** half of the body.

The area immediately rostral to the precentral sulcus is the **premotor cortex** (Figs. 2-5 and 2-6*B*; Brodmann area 6), which is involved with complex and skilled movements and regulates the responsiveness of the primary motor cortex. There are specific areas within the premotor cortex for controlling speech, hand, and finger movements and eye–head coordination. The remaining anterior portion of the frontal lobe is the **prefrontal cortex** (Brodmann areas 10–12). Aside from contributing to personality and mood, the prefrontal cortex is also involved with the regulation of cognitive functions such as reasoning, abstract thinking, self-monitoring, decision making, planning, and the control of executive decisions and pragmatic behaviors. There are three large horizontal gyri in the frontal lobe: superior (first), middle (second), and inferior (third) frontal gyri (Fig. 2-5). The inferior frontal gyrus in the dominant hemisphere constitutes the **anterior language cortex**, or **Broca area** (Brodmann areas 44 and 45). Broca area is located in front of the area of the primary motor cortex (Brodmann area 4), which controls jaw, lip, tongue, and vocal cord movement (Box 2-1).

Clinical Information

Patients with a lesion of the lateral dorsal region of the prefrontal cortex exhibit difficulty with planning, thinking, reasoning, and performing executive functions. Such subjects often appear normal but display difficulty in solving problems and planning the number and order of steps involved in task execution. Patients with orbital prefrontal region pathology exhibit personality disorders, emotional disinhibition, and abnormal impulsive social behaviors. A

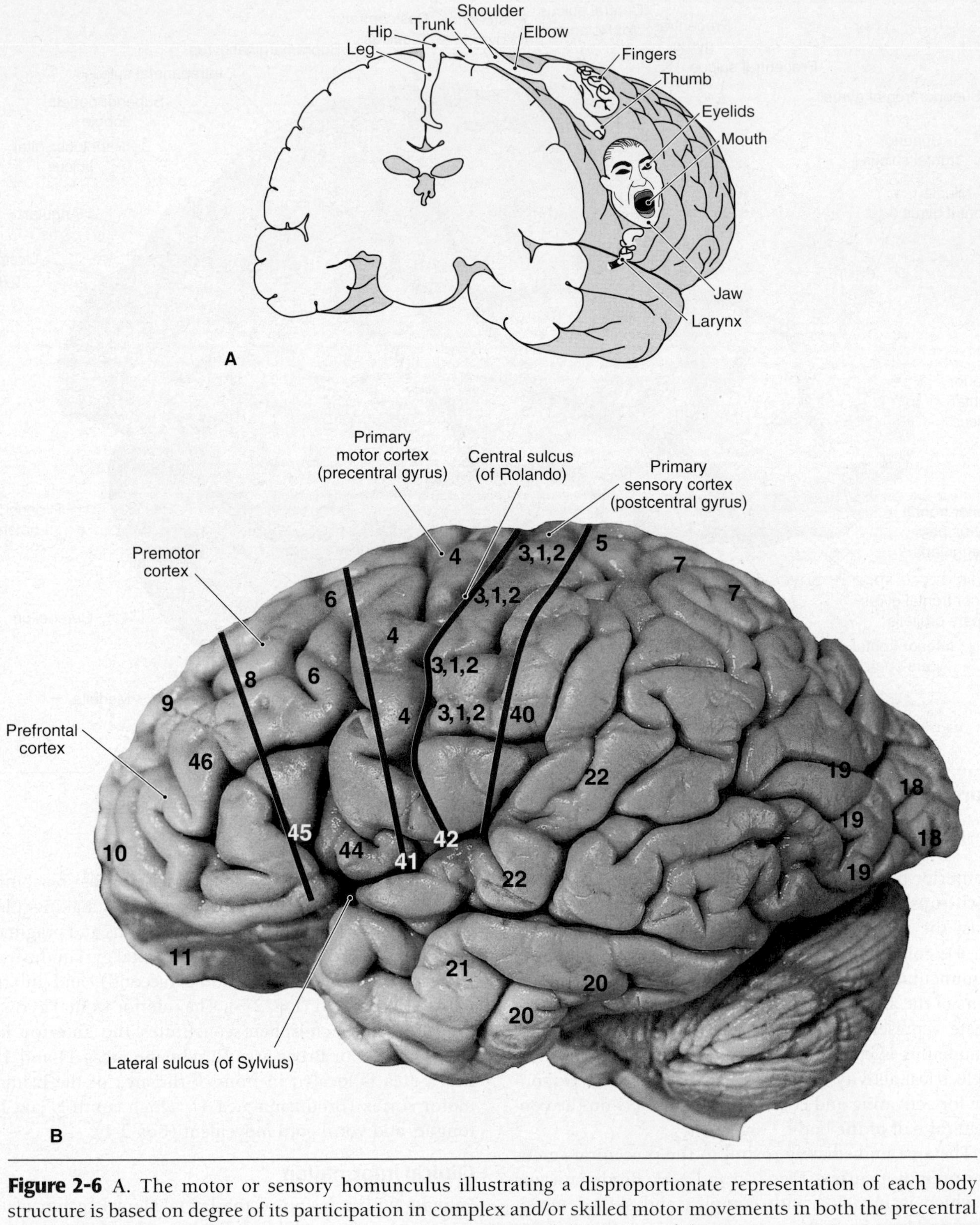

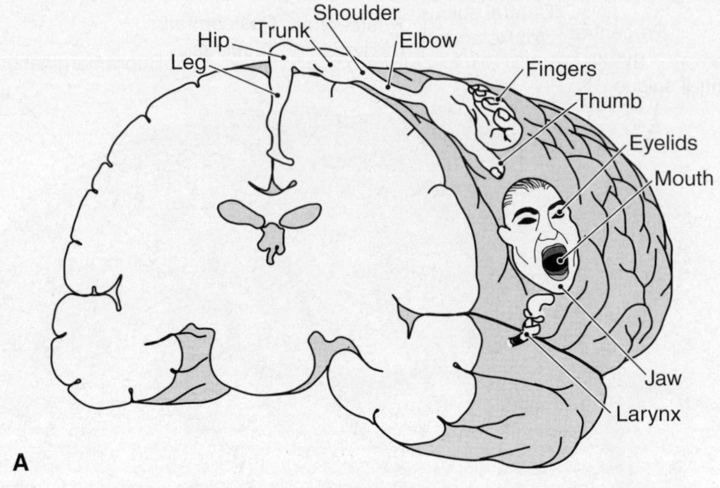

Figure 2-6 A. The motor or sensory homunculus illustrating a disproportionate representation of each body structure is based on degree of its participation in complex and/or skilled motor movements in both the precentral gyrus (motor cortex) and the postcentral gyrus (sensory cortex). B. A view of the primary motor, premotor, prefrontal, and primary sensory cortices and central sulcus is depicted on the lateral surface of brain with Brodmann areas marked.

BOX 2-1

Broca area

The inferior frontal gyrus consists of three sections: pars opercularis, pars triangularis, and pars orbitalis. The opercular and triangular portions of the gyrus in the dominant hemisphere constitute the Broca area (anterior language cortex corresponding to Brodmann areas 44–45). The Broca area is important for verbal expression and is connected with the posterior language cortex (Wernicke area) through the fibers of the arcuate fasciculus. The Wernicke area, which is located in the posterior temporal and inferior parietal region, is responsible for the comprehension of spoken and written language.

lesion of the medial prefrontal region affects the regulation of attention and motivation and the responsiveness to external cognitive stimuli. Such patients may appear abulic (reduced speech movements and emotional reaction), apathetic, and incognizant of their surroundings. Commonly seen in cases of traumatic brain injury, patients are usually apathetic, procrastinators, indecisive, or confused. They appear unaware of social expectations and the consequences of their actions, and they are unable to monitor and regulate their behavior (Table 2-2).

This symptomatology of the prefrontal lobe syndrome was best illustrated by the century-old case of an industrial worker named Phineas Gage in 1823. In an accident, a railway spike passed through his cheek and into the orbitofrontal region of the brain. He survived for many years with the spike protruding from his skull. However, his personality and social attitudes radically changed, and he became impulsive, rude, erratic, and unpredictable.

Parietal Lobe

The **parietal lobe** is between the frontal and the occipital lobes and above the temporal lobe. The central sulcus marks the anterior boundary of the parietal lobe. An arbitrary line from the **ramus** of the parieto-occipital sulcus extending to the preoccipital notch marks its posterior boundary (Figs. 2-4 and 2-5). The inferior boundary of the parietal lobe is represented by a line drawn from the posterior ramus of the lateral fissure to the middle of the line connecting the preoccipital notch to the parieto-occipital sulcus.

The parietal lobe is concerned with spatial orientation, cross-modality integration, memory, recognition and

Table 2-2

Clinical Symptoms and Associated Lesion Sites

Anatomic Structure	Associated Symptoms
Frontal lobe	Contralateral paralysis; impaired cognition (reasoning, self-monitoring, attention, abstraction, and problem solving); decreased spontaneity; impaired judgment; reduced concentration; apathy; inappropriate/uninhibited social behavior; and expressive (left hemisphere) aphasia
Parietal lobe	Contralateral hemisensory loss, impaired tactile discrimination, tactile agnosia, inattention, constructional and visual-spatial deficits, anosognosia (denial of impaired functioning), and aphasia (left parietal lobe involvement)
Occipital lobe	Blindness or scotoma in the opposite visual field, impaired recognition, visual agnosia, alexia, and impaired recognition of colors
Temporal lobe	Contralateral homonymous hemianopsia, receptive aphasia (Wernicke area in the left lobe), memory disturbance, and Klüver–Bucy syndrome (bilateral temporal lobes)
Thalamus	Altered regulation of cortical functions and contralateral unpleasant or painful sensation
Hypothalamus	Impaired autonomic functions; disturbance in the regulation of temperature, salt, water metabolism, and the sleep–wake cycle; hormonal disorders; altered sexual functioning
Basal ganglia	Reduced (hypokinesia) movement, involuntary movement, and abnormal posture
Brainstem	Altered consciousness, vertigo, nystagmus (involuntary rhythmic ocular movement), cranial nerve dysfunctions, and crossed (alternating) sensorimotor deficits
Cerebellum	Reduced single or multiple limb coordination and synergy as well as impaired balance
Spinal cord	Reduced reflexive movement as well as limb paralysis and sensory loss

expression of emotions and prosodies, and cognition as well as the perceptual interpretation and elaboration of somatic sensation. The **postcentral gyrus** (Brodmann areas 3, 1, and 2) is the **primary sensory cortex**, in which all modalities of bodily experienced (somatic) sensation are perceived; these sensations are recognized as awareness in the parietal sensory association cortex, probably Brodmann areas 5 and 7 (see Fig. 2-5*B*; Fig. 1-8). The sensory representation of the entire body, like the motor representation in the precentral gyrus, is disproportionately perceived, beginning with the face and head in the lower third of the postcentral gyrus and the trunk, hands, arms, and legs in the upper portion of the gyrus (Fig. 2-6). The oblique intraparietal sulcus divides the remaining parietal lobe into the superior and the inferior parietal lobules (Fig. 2-5). The analysis and integration of sensory information in the superior parietal lobule contributes to complex perceptual experiences.

Clinical Information

A lesion in this parietal area results in contralateral sensory loss including perceptual–conceptual disorders of tactile recognition, constructional skills, spatial orientation, and memory (Table 2-2). A lesion involving a large part of the somesthetic association cortex also causes both tactile **agnosia** and **astereognosis**, which are closely related. The most extreme form of astereognosis is cortical neglect in which the patient ignores existence of one side of the body, and/or corresponding visual fields. Lesions affecting the **angular** (Brodmann area 39) and **supramarginal** (Brodmann area 40) **gyri** in the inferior parietal lobule of the dominant hemisphere result in disorders of reading (alexia), writing (agraphia), calculation (acalculia), and language (aphasia). Pathology in the inferior parietal lobule of the nondominant hemisphere affects body schema and spatial attention and results in neglect of the contralateral half of the body.

Occipital Lobe

Only a small portion of the occipital lobe lies on the lateral surface (Figs. 2-4 and 2-5); it is more fully developed along the medial surface of the hemisphere. Containing the primary (Brodmann area 17) and secondary (Brodmann area 18) visual cortical areas, the anterior boundary of the occipital lobe is marked by an imaginary line extending from the ramus of the parieto-occipital sulcus to the preoccipital notch. (See the clinical characteristics under the midsagittal surface.)

Temporal Lobe

The temporal lobe, which serves audition, memory, thought elaboration, comprehension of spoken and written language, and olfaction, is located ventral to the frontal and parietal lobes (Figs. 2-4 and 2-5). The lateral fissure and an arbitrary line extending from its posterior ramus toward the occipital pole mark the dorsal limit of the temporal lobe and separate it from the frontal and parietal lobes. The ventral continuation of the imaginary line connecting the parieto-occipital fissure to the preoccipital notch separates the temporal lobe from the occipital lobe.

The lateral surface of the temporal lobe contains three prominent gyri: **superior**, **middle**, and **inferior** (also called the first, second, and third) **temporal gyri**. The superior temporal gyrus and sulcus run parallel to the lateral fissure and posteriorly turn upward in the parietal lobe, where they are bordered on the parietal side by the angular gyrus. The dorsal surface of the superior temporal gyrus, the area hidden by the opercular portions of the frontal, parietal, and temporal lobes, dips into the **insular cortex** and houses a few short, oblique convolutions, the **Heschl gyri**. These gyri form the **primary auditory cortex**, which is buried within the lateral sulcus in front of the insular cortex. It receives projections from both ears (Fig. 9-10).

Clinical Information

A lesion of the primary auditory cortex (Brodmann areas 41-42) causes merely a partial binaural attenuation in the hearing sensitivity, but it significantly affects the auditory perceptual function and the skills for phonemic discrimination. A pathology involving the language association cortex in the dominant (usually left) hemisphere (**Wernicke area**; Brodmann area 22) results in receptive aphasia, which is marked by impaired comprehension of spoken and written language and word-finding deficit. A lesion in the association cortex on the nondominant (usually right) side of the brain primarily affects the ability to process nonverbal material, such as music and environmental sounds.

Ventral Surface

The ventral (inferior) surface of the brain displays structures of the frontal, temporal, and occipital lobes (Figs. 2-7 and 2-8); no parietal structure is visible. The two most visible structures are the orbital portion of the frontal lobe and the basal portion of the temporo-occipital lobes. The orbital frontal region is known to serve emotions, personality, and inhibition. It also includes the olfactory region. The interhemispheric fissure extends to the ventral surface separating the orbital portions of both frontal lobes. The **olfactory bulb** and **tract**, located in the olfactory sulcus, serve the sense of smell. The **gyrus rectus** is medial to the olfactory structures, and the area lateral to it is occupied by many small orbital gyri.

The posterior structures in the temporal and occipital lobes are the inferior temporal gyrus, occipitotemporal **(fusiform) gyrus**, **lingual gyrus**, **collateral sulcus**, **parahippocampal gyrus**, and **uncus**. The inferior temporal gyrus is partially on the lateral and partially on the ventral surfaces of the temporal lobe. The hippocampus, a structure identified with the encoding of short-term memory, is beneath the parahippocampal gyrus and can be seen after removal of this gyrus (Fig. 3-30). The hippocampal gyrus is posteriorly connected

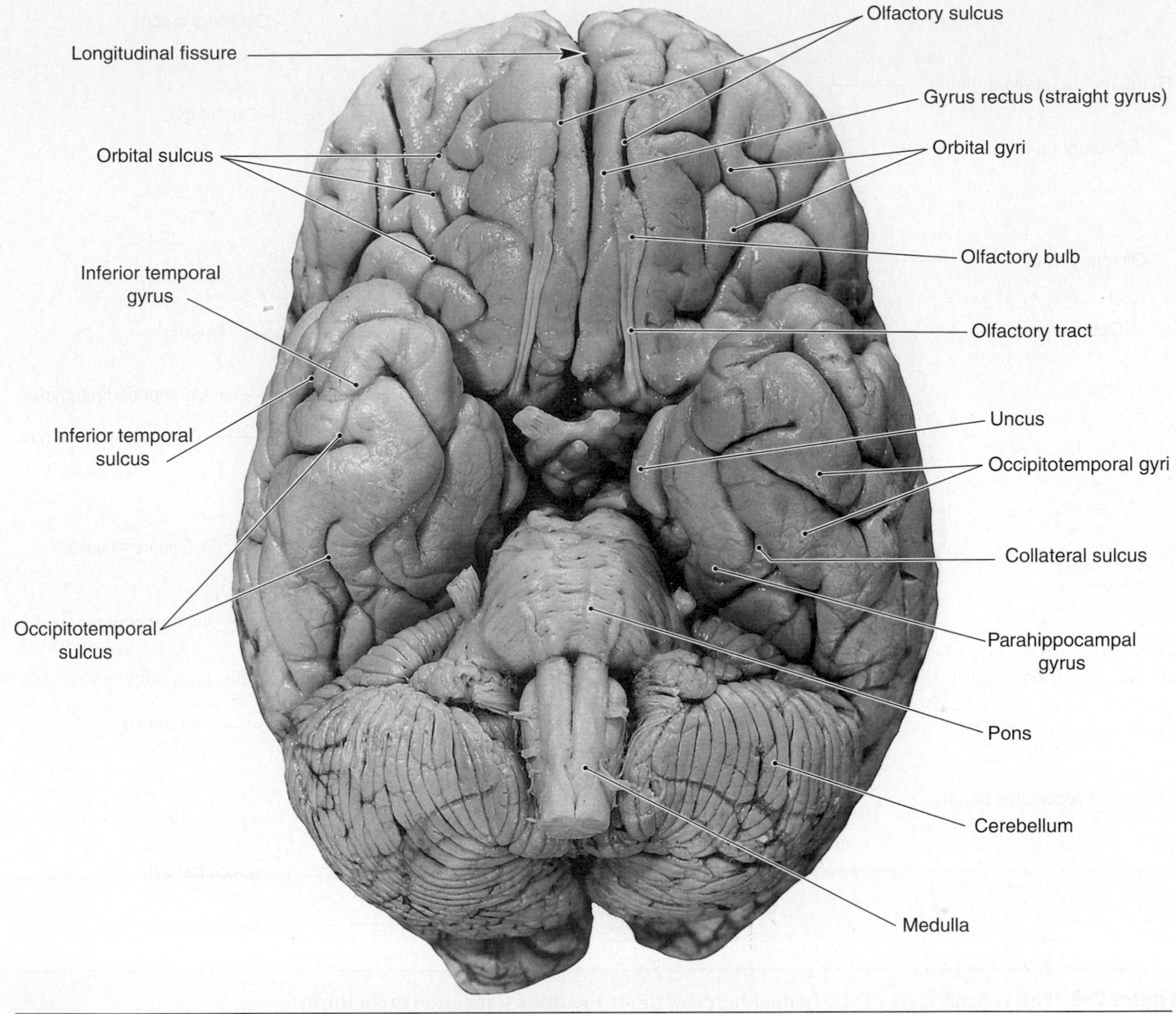

Figure 2-7 The ventral view of the important sulci and gyri.

to the **cingulate gyrus** by a narrow isthmus beneath the **splenium** (posterior part) of the **corpus callosum** (Figs. 2-10 and 2-14). Collectively, the parahippocampal gyrus, isthmus, and cingulate gyrus are the components of the **limbic lobe**. The collateral sulcus marks the lateral limit of the parahippocampal and lingual gyri and separates these from the medially located occipitotemporal gyrus (Figs. 2-7 and 2-8).

Clinical Information

A pathologic involvement of the orbitofrontal region is associated with emotional disturbance, detached personality, and behavioral disinhibition. The occipital-temporal gyrus, also known as the fusiform gyrus, is part of the visual association cortex; electrical stimulation in this region not only evokes various hallucinations but memories needed for the recognition of objects. A lesion in the fusiform gyrus leads to failure of object recognition, which results in visual agnosia (a higher-order visual impairment) and prosopagnosia (impaired recognition of previous known faces).

Midsagittal Surface

Cortical structures on the medial surface of both hemispheres are best examined after both hemispheres are separated by sectioning the fibers of the corpus callosum (Figs. 2-9–2-11). Although portions of all four lobes are seen on the midsagittal surface, their sulci and gyri—except for the cingulate and parahippocampal gyri—do not present consistent lobar boundaries.

Frontal Lobe

A line drawn from the notch of the central sulcus to the cingulate sulcus marks the caudal boundary of the frontal lobe (Fig. 2-4). A portion of the frontal lobe on the medial

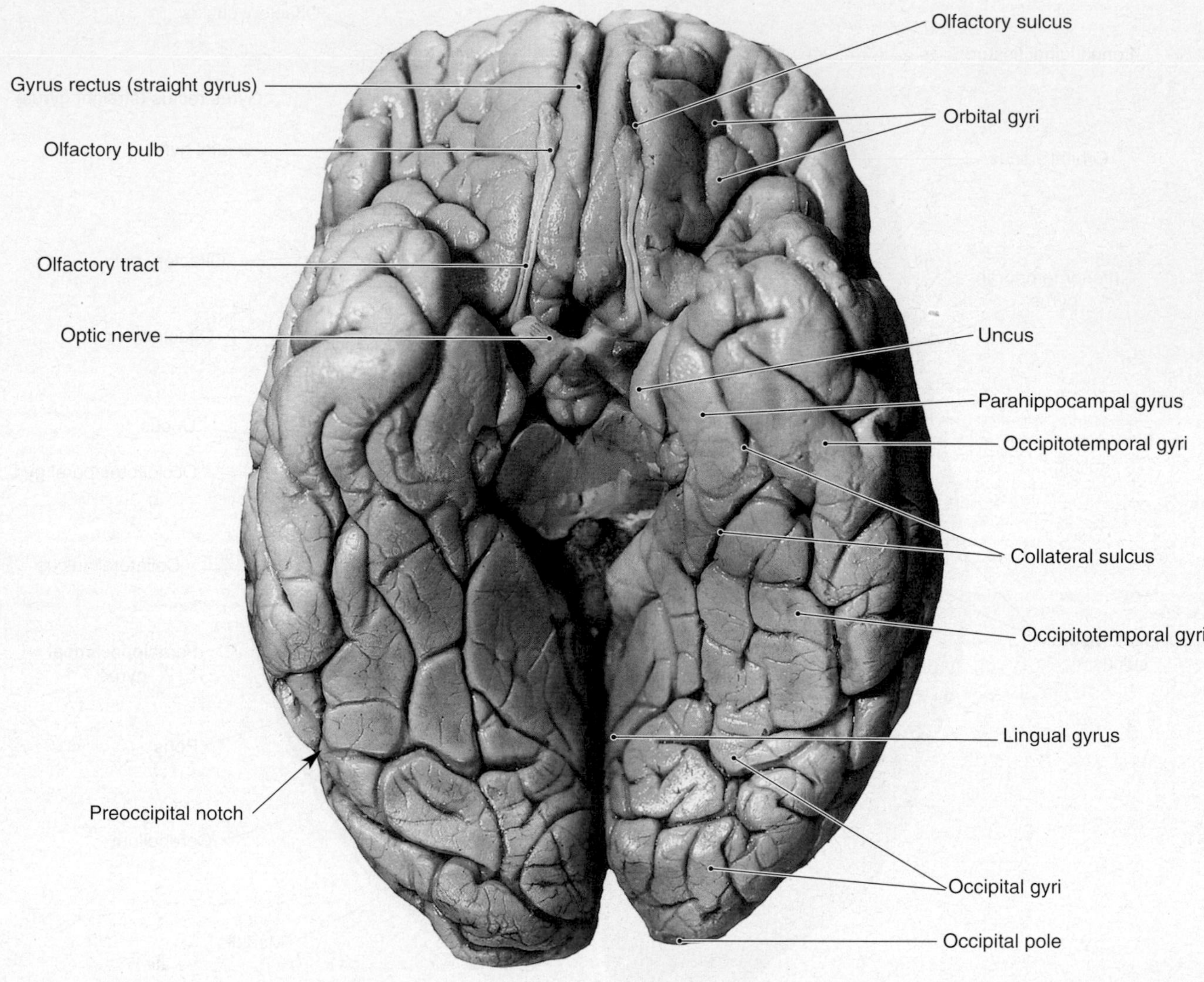

Figure 2-8 The ventral view of the hemispheres without the brainstem and cerebellum.

surface is part of the superior frontal gyrus extending from the dorsolateral surface.

Parietal Lobe

Portions of the parietal lobe on the midsagittal surface extend from the superior parietal lobule of the lateral surface (Fig. 2-4). A line drawn from the notch of the central sulcus to the cingulate sulcus also demarcates the rostral boundary of the medial parietal lobe. The posterior boundary of the medial parietal lobe is marked by the parieto-occipital sulcus on the medial and the lateral surfaces. The precentral and postcentral gyri from the lateral surface continue midsagittally and constitute the **paracentral lobule**, an area notched by the central sulcus (Fig. 2-10).

Occipital Lobe

The portion of the occipital lobe located on the medial surface is larger than the portion on the lateral surface. A line extending from the parieto-occipital sulcus to the preoccipital notch separates the occipital lobe from the parietal and the temporal lobes (Fig. 2-4). The occipital lobe has two important structures on the medial surface: **calcarine sulcus** and lingual gyrus (Fig. 2-10). The calcarine sulcus divides the **primary visual cortex** (Brodmann area 17) into the upper and lower operculum, which in turn are surrounded by the **association visual cortex** (Brodmann areas 18 and 19) which is involved with the elaboration, recognition, and appreciation of visual stimuli. There are spatial patterns of representation in the primary visual cortex; the upper calcarine operculum receives information from the lower quadrants of the visual field, and the lower calcarine operculum receives visual impulses from the upper quadrants of the visual field.

Clinical Information

A destructive lesion in the primary visual cortex causes blindness (homonomous hemianopsia) in the opposite

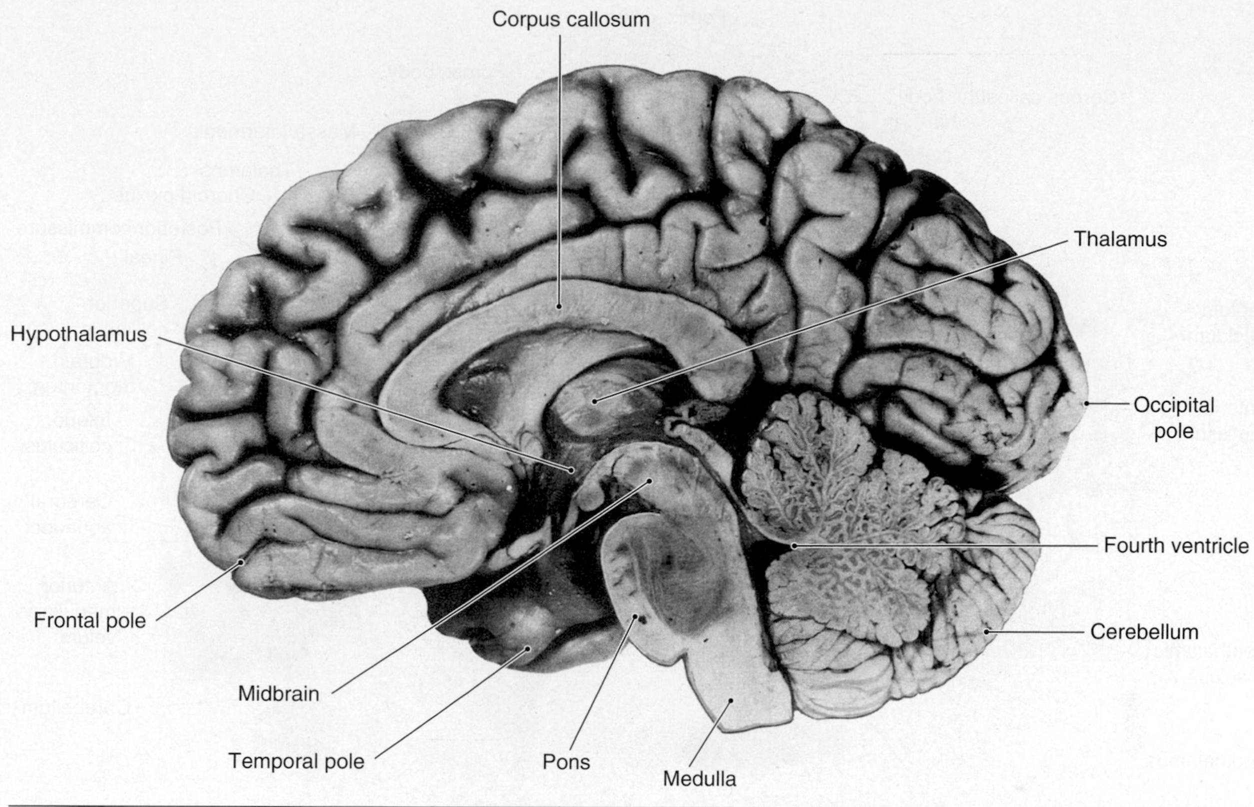

Figure 2-9 Midsagittal section of the brain with the brainstem structures in place. Detailed topography illustrated in Figure 2-11.

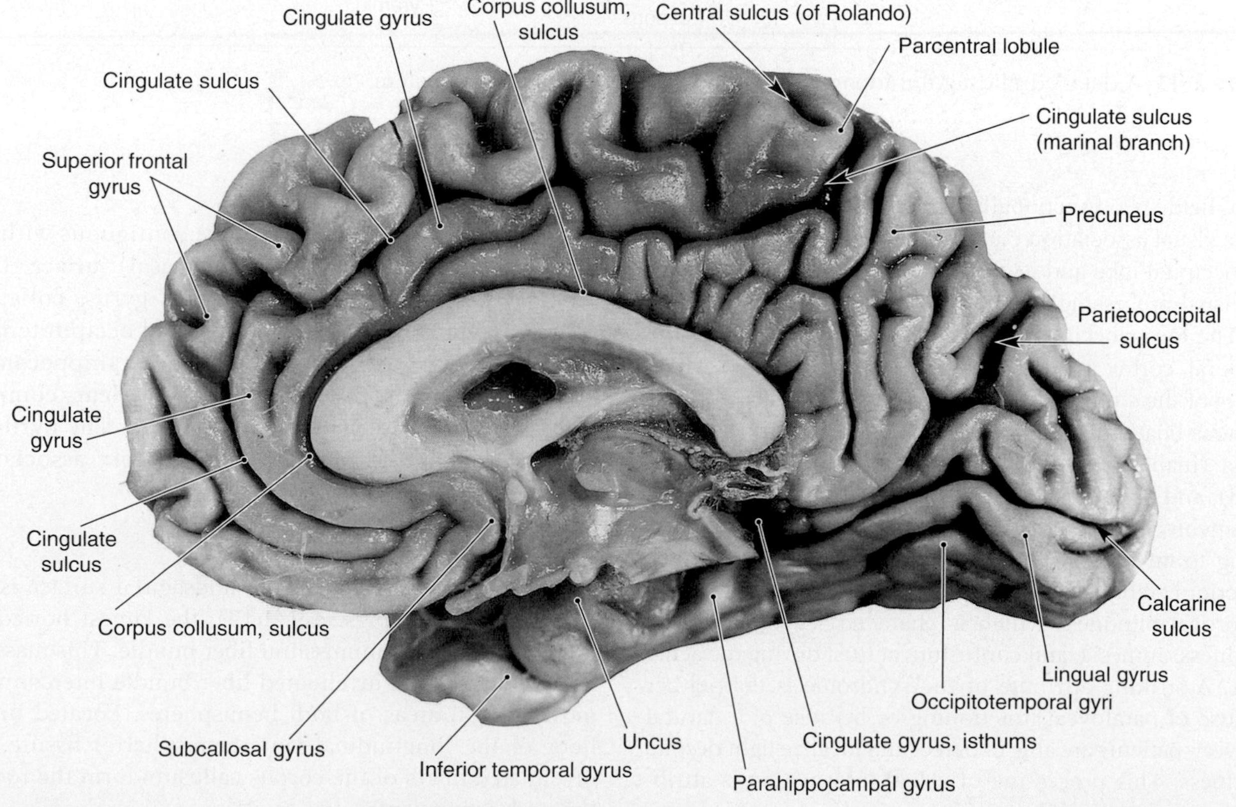

Figure 2-10 Midsagittal view of the structures in the right cerebral hemisphere without the brainstem and cerebellum.

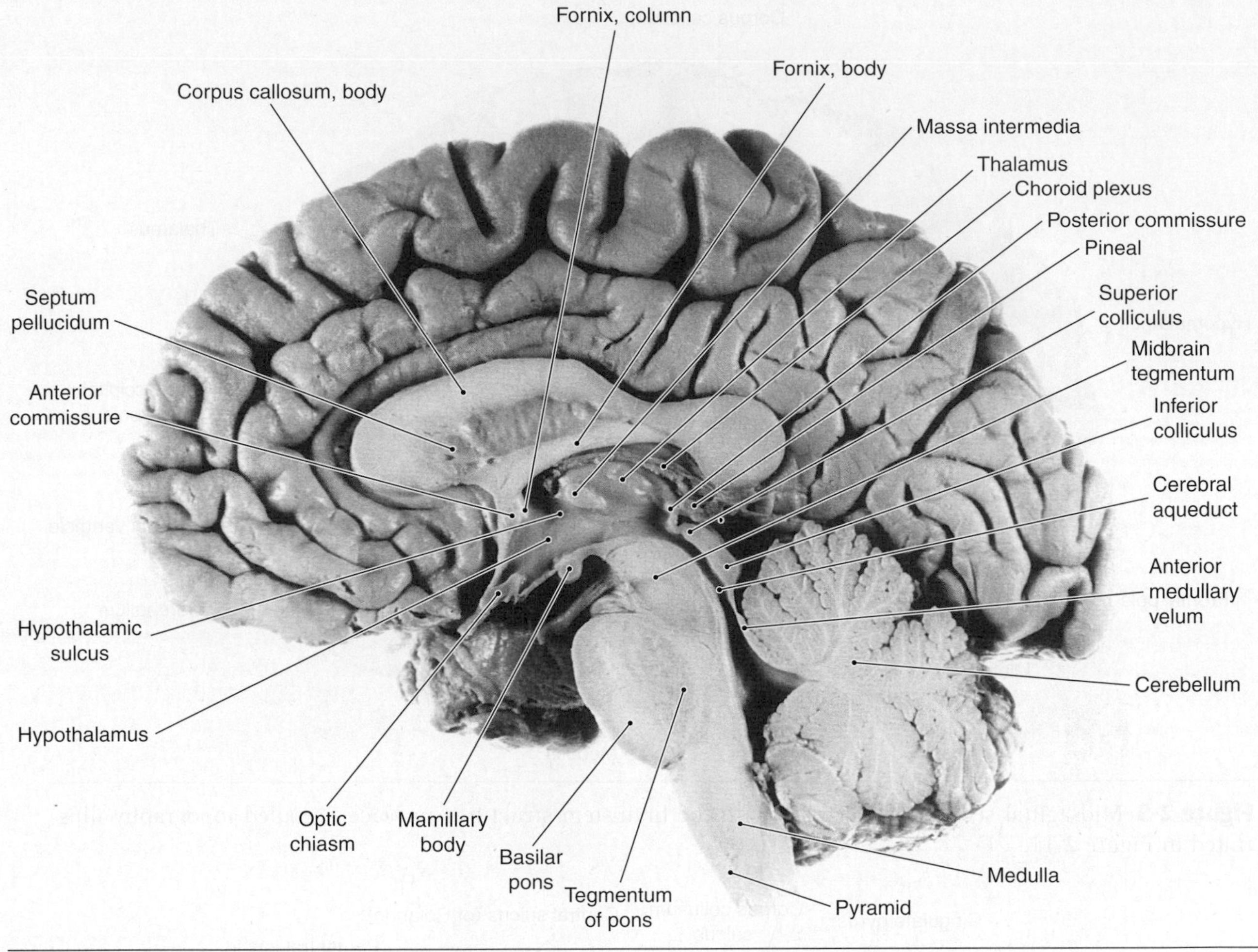

Figure 2-11 A detailed midsagittal topography of the diencephalon and brainstem.

visual field. Two functionally distinct regions are identified in the visual association cortex: where and what. The superior occipital lobe and its parietal projections contribute to the visual processing "where" attributes of the visual stimuli. The lower occipital region with its projections to the temporal cortex participates in determining the "what" nature of the stimuli. A lesion involving the visual association area bilaterally results in visual agnosia, color agnosia, alexia (inability to comprehend the meaning of written word), and impaired visual memories (Table 2-2). A bilateral involvement of the primary visual cortices—usually owing to an ischemic stroke involving the basilar artery, posterior cerebral arteries, or the calcarine arteries—results in cortical blindness which is characterized by complete blindness, amnesia, and confusion, at least during the acute stage. A striking attribute of the syndrome is that, either because of parafoveal functioning or because of a natural recovery, patients are able to detect and localize light despite blindness. This processing of visual information is attributed to a subcortical integration of visual information.

Temporal Lobe

The medial temporal structures are contiguous with the ones that are visible on the ventral (basal) surface. They include the **uncus**, parahippocampal gyrus, collateral sulcus, isthmus of cingulate gyrus, and occipitotemporal gyrus (Fig. 2-10). The uncus and parahippocampal gyrus along with the **amygdaloid nuclear complex** form the **pyriform (pear-shaped) cortex**. The pyriform cortex includes the higher-order olfactory association cortex.

Additional Structures

Among other structures on the midsagittal surface is the corpus callosum (Figs. 2-9–2-12), the largest horizontal interhemispheric commissural fiber bundle. This massive, half moon–shaped myelinated fiber bundle interconnects most cortical areas of both hemispheres. Located in the floor of the longitudinal (interhemispheric) fissure, the myelinated fibers of the corpus callosum form the roof of the underlying ventricular cavities.

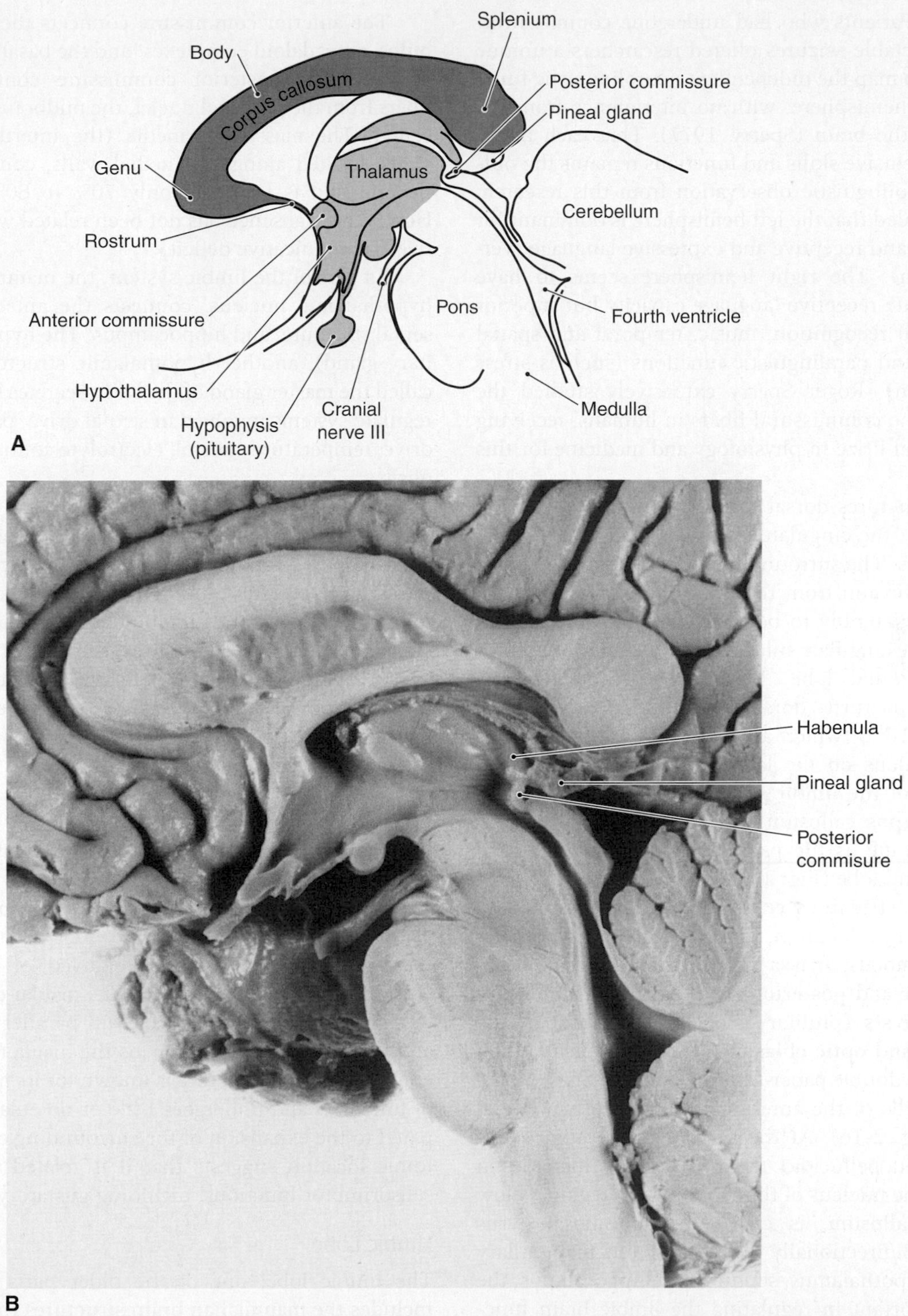

Figure 2-12 Midsagittal view of the corpus callosum, its major parts (A) and other structures (B): brainstem and diencephalon.

The corpus callosum consists of the following four parts, from its rostral to its caudal extent: rostrum, the most anterior portion; genu, the anterior bend; body, the large portion caudal to the genu; and splenium, the posterior most region (Fig. 2-12). Memories, experiences, and actions of both hemispheres are shared and integrated by way of the corpus callosum.

A complete sectioning of the corpus callosum (commissurotomy) makes both hemispheres independent and incapable of communicating with each other or sharing information. Patients who had undergone commissurotomy for intractable seizures offered researchers a unique opportunity to map the independent neurolinguistic functions of each hemisphere, with no interference from the other half of the brain (Sperry, 1977). That each hemisphere has exclusive skills and functions remains the outstanding neurolinguistic observation from this research. Findings revealed that the left hemisphere is dominant for analytic skills and receptive and expressive language (verbal expression). The right hemisphere seems to have merely adequate receptive language capacity but superior skills for facial recognition, music, temporal and spatial information, and paralinguistic functions (such as stress and intonation). Roger Sperry extensively studied the functions of the commissural fibers in humans, receiving the 1981 Nobel Prize in physiology and medicine for this work.

Major structures dorsal to the callosal fibers are the callosal sulcus, the cingulate gyrus, and the sulcus of the cingulate gyrus. The surrounding callosal sulcus separates the corpus callosum from the overlying cingulate gyrus, curving ventrolaterally to become the sulcus of the hippocampus. The cingulate sulcus marks the inferior boundary of the frontal lobe. Running rostrocaudally, the cingulate sulcus turns dorsally to become its marginal branch (Fig. 2-10), which ascends and continues as the postcentral sulcus on the lateral surface. The cingulate gyrus, a part of the **limbic** or **visceral–emotional brain**, circles the corpus callosum and posteriorly curves ventrally to continue as the parahippocampal gyrus in the medial temporal lobe (Fig. 2-10).

Important structures ventral to the corpus callosum are the **septum pellucidum**, **fornix**, thalamus, hypothalamus and its sulcus, **massa intermedia** (thalamic adhesion), **anterior** and **posterior commissures**, **mammillary body**, **hypophysis** (pituitary gland), **subcallosal gyrus**, **pineal body**, and **optic chiasm**. The septum pellucidum, consisting of a double paper-thin set of membranes, marks the medial walls of the anterior horns of the two lateral ventricles (Fig. 2-16). At the base of the septum pellucidum (pl. septa pellucida), the medial cortex increases in thickness as the nucleus of the septum. This region, below the corpus callosum, is called the subcallosal gyrus (Fig. 2-14). Bidirectionally connecting the mammillary body of the hypothalamus, septum, and hippocampus, the fornix is important in regulating the limbic brain functions of emotions and memory. Forming the basic forebrain circuit, the thalamus is important in sensorimotor integration and speech–language–hearing functions. The hypothalamus, ventral to the thalamus, controls endocrine and autonomic functions. Specifically, it controls food and water intake, sexual behavior, and body temperature, important for preserving the survival capabilities of the organism. The boundary between the thalamus and the hypothalamus is identified by the hypothalamic sulcus, an indentation along the medial wall (Fig. 2-11).

The anterior commissure connects the two olfactory bulbs, amygdaloid complexes, and the basal temporal pole cortices. The posterior commissure contains crossing fibers from the pretectal nuclei, the midbrain's visual reflex center. The massa intermedia (the interthalamic adhesion), located along the medial walls, connects the two thalami and is found in only 70% to 80% of humans. However, its absence has not been related with any cognitive-communicative deficit.

As part of the limbic system, the mammillary body, a hypothalamic nucleus, connects the anterior thalamus, septal structure, and hippocampus. The hypophysis (pituitary gland), another hypothalamic structure commonly called the master gland of the body, secretes hormones that regulate systems involved in sexual drive, pain, emotional drive, temperature control, electrolyte control, and metabolism.

The subcallosal gyrus, also known as the paraolfactory area, is a part of the limbic lobe. The pineal body is a cone-shaped structure at the level of the posterior commissure. It secretes important neurotransmitters (serotonin, melatonin, and norepinephrine) that regulate the circadian rhythm and control the sexual reproduction cycles. The optic chiasm is the site at which optic fibers from the medial retina of each eye cross the midline, join the uncrossed fibers of the lateral retina, and continue to the opposite hemisphere.

Insular Lobe

The **insular cortex** (**isle of Reil**) is concealed within the depths of the lateral fissure by the overgrowth of the opercula of the frontal, parietal, and temporal lobes (Fig. 2-13). The structures of this secondary lobe are exposed when these opercular tissues are removed or spread apart. Outlined by the circular sulcus, the insular cortex consists of short and long gyri, which run parallel to each other and the limen insula that opens the insula toward the lateral fissure. This structure is known for its nonelaboration of functions and undergoes little or no enlargement compared to the expansion of the surrounding cortex. Its anatomic location suggests that it is related to limbic and sensorimotor functions, including gustatory functions.

Limbic Lobe

The limbic lobe, one of the older parts of the brain, includes the mammalian brain structures that form a ring around the medial-most margins of the frontal, parietal, and temporal lobes (Fig. 2-14). The limbic lobe consists of the cingulate gyrus, hippocampal formation, parahippocampal gyrus, uncus, and subcallosal gyrus. All of these structures, through their connections with diencephalic and brainstem nuclei, provide the emotional drive to visceral and vegetative functions, which are fundamental to survival; these include instinctual reflexes and drives (fleeing, feeding, fighting, and mating behaviors), aggression, anxiety, and fear. The limbic circuit begins with

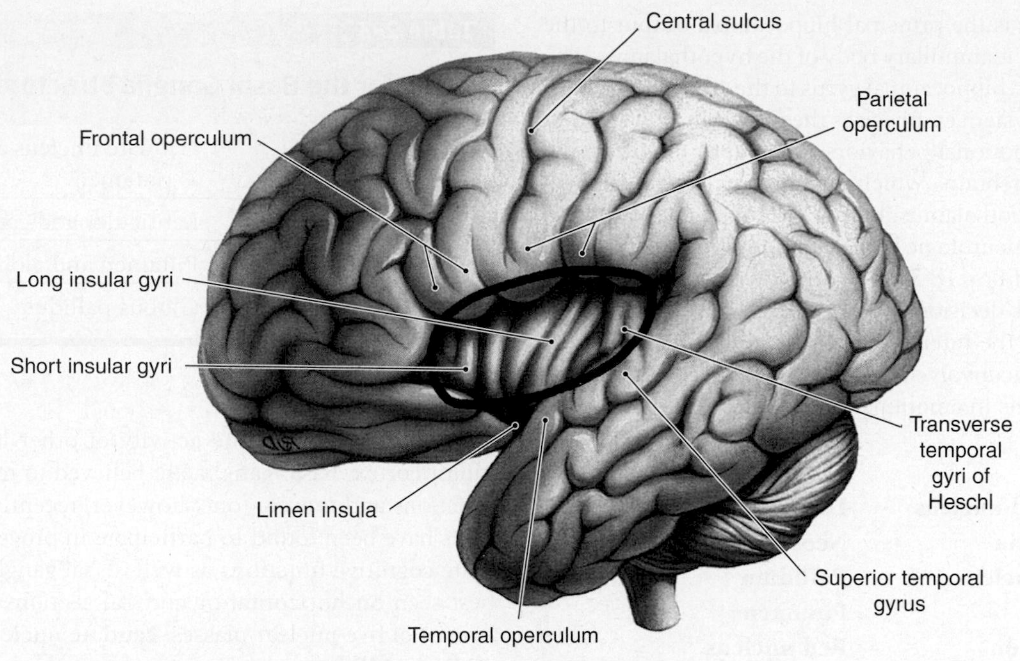

Figure 2-13 Lateral view of the left cerebral hemisphere with both lateral fissure banks separated to reveal the insular cortex.

hippocampal projections via the fornix to the hypothalamic mammillary bodies, which use the **mammillothalamic tract** for projecting to the cingulate gyrus by way of the anterior thalamic nucleus; the cingulate gyrus completes the circuit by projecting back to the parahippocampal gyrus (see Chapters 6 and 18).

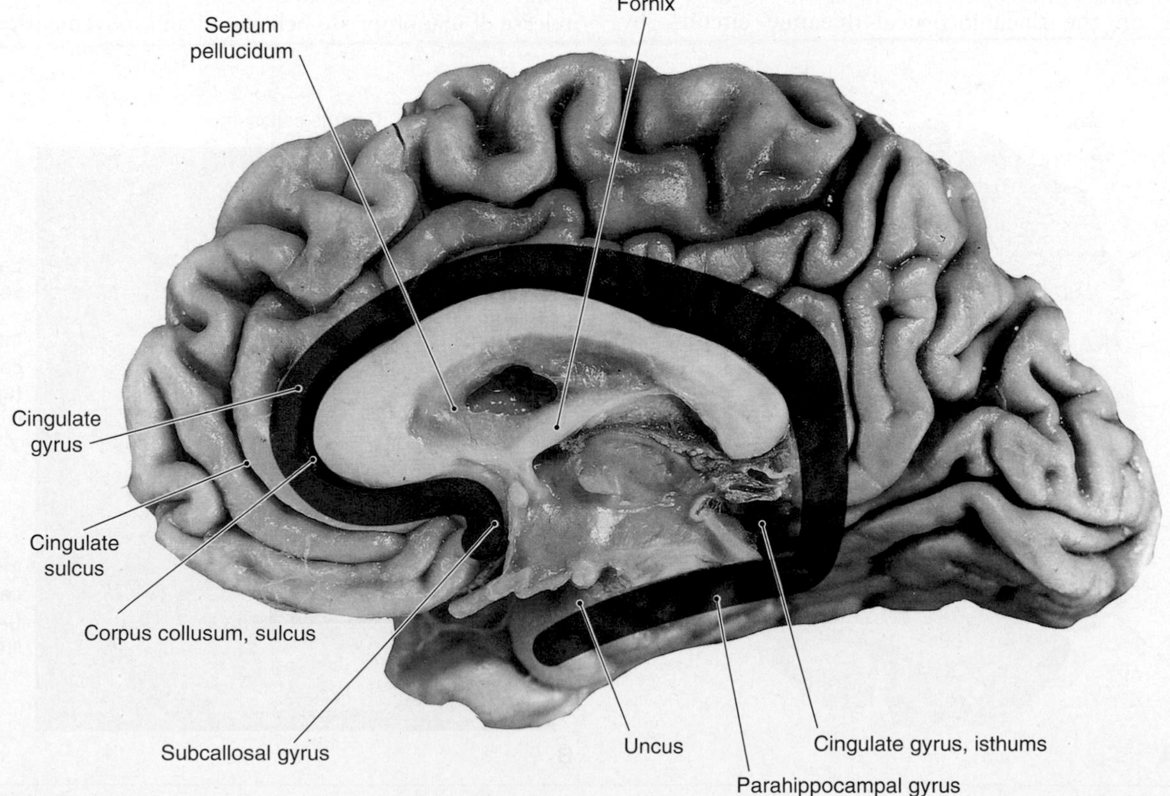

Figure 2-14 Midsagittal view of the limbic structures: cingulate gyrus, parahippocampal gyrus, and uncus.

The fornix is the principal hippocampal output to the septum and the mammillary body of the hypothalamus. The proximity of the hippocampal gyrus to the amygdala, uncus, and olfactory system emphasizes the importance of smell in visceral and emotional behaviors. The **Papez circuit** in the mammalian forebrain, which involves neuronal connections of the hypothalamus, limbic system, and thalamus, is considered the neurologic base of emotional expression (see Chapter 18 and Box 18-3). The limbic system also governs our values and decisions about perceptions and feelings, which regulate the intensity and strength of the emotional drive. Pathologic involvement of the Papez circuit produces profound deficits in emotional behavior.

Key Terms:

Amygdaloid nucleus	**Lenticular nucleus**
Basal ganglia	**Neostriatum**
Caudate nucleus	**Pallidum**
Claustrum	**Putamen**
Diencephalon	**Red nucleus**
Globus pallidus	**Striatum**
Interventricular foramen	**Substantia nigra**

Basal Ganglia

Formed by a series of complex neuronal circuits, the basal ganglia regulates cortical output processing, which impinges on the thalamocortical–thalamic circuits, by slowing or inhibiting the activity of other loops and the motor cortex. Basal ganglia are believed to regulate motor functions and muscle tone; however, recently these structures have been found to participate in processes that regulate cognitive functions as well. Basal ganglia structures, best seen on horizontal or coronal sections of the brain, consist of five nuclear masses: **caudate nucleus, putamen, globus pallidus, claustrum**, and amygdaloid nucleus (Figs. 2-15–2-17). Various anatomic terms are used for grouping the basal ganglia nuclei (Table 2-3): **Neostriatum** for the histologically identical nuclei of the caudate nucleus and putamen, **corpus striatum** for lenticular and caudate nuclei, **lenticular nucleus** for the putamen and globus pallidus, and **pallidum** for globus pallidus.

Damage to the basal ganglia circuitry by physical injury or by the loss of one of the neurotransmitters results in the release of inappropriate behavioral and movement patterns

Table 2-3

Terms for the Basal Ganglia Structures

Neostriatum or striatum	Caudate nucleus and putamen
Corpus striatum	Lenticular and caudate nuclei
Lenticular nucleus	Putamen and globus pallidus
Pallidum	Globus pallidus

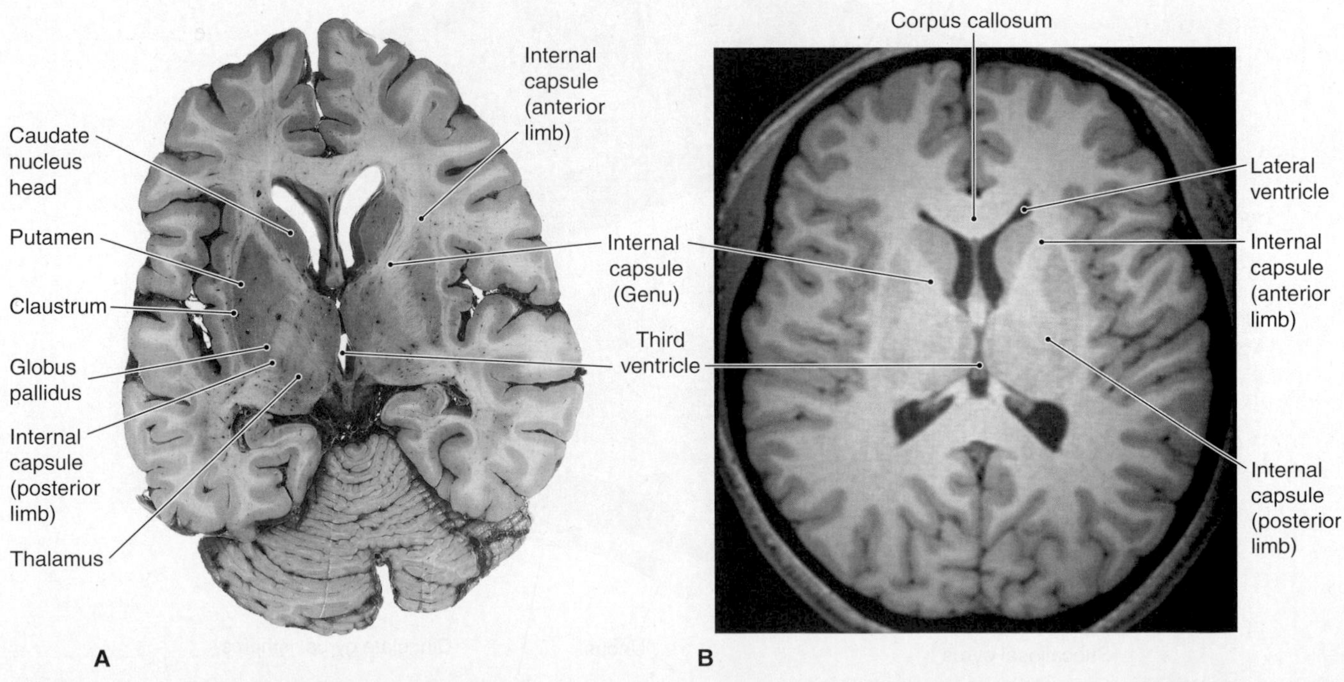

Figure 2-15 Horizontal section (A) and the corresponding MRI (B) showing the subcortical basal ganglia structures in relation to the internal capsule and its parts.

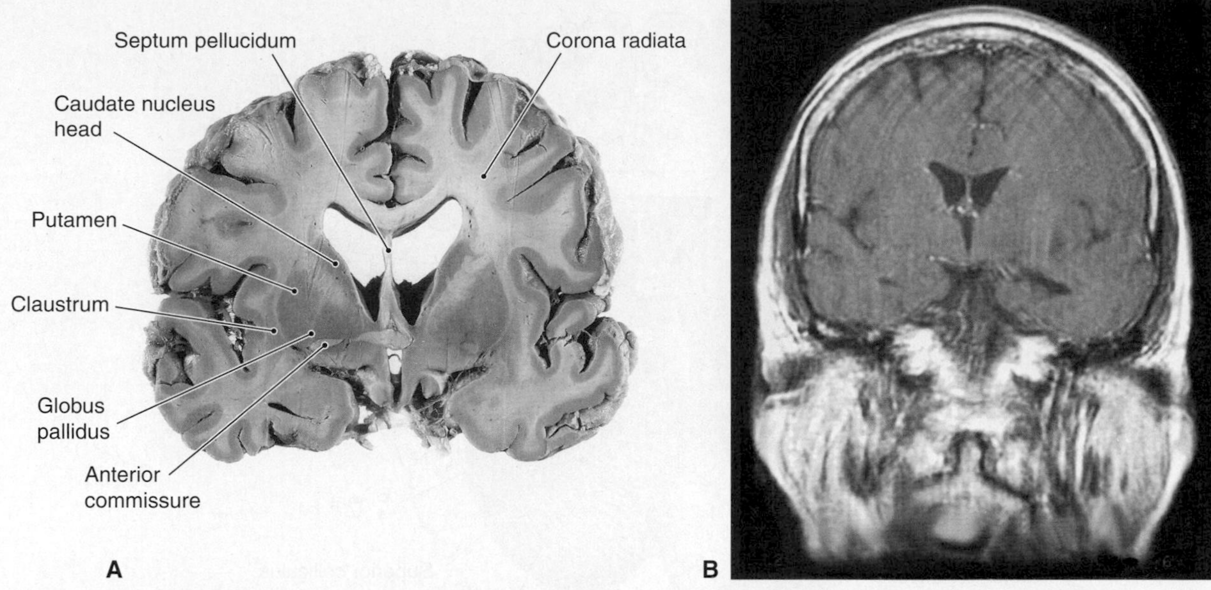

Figure 2-16 Rostral surface of a coronal brain section (A) and the corresponding MRI (B) showing the basal ganglia nuclei and other subcortical structures.

because of the disinhibition. These released and abnormal patterns are seen in patients with Parkinson disease, Huntington disease, Tourette syndrome, Wilson disease, and Sydenham chorea (see Chapter 15). Basal ganglia lesions do not cause paralysis. Rather, they produce involuntary movements, such as the tremor, chorea, ticks, and ballism.

Caudate Nucleus

The caudate nucleus is a large C-shaped structure. It has a massive pear-shaped head and a long curved tail. Rostrally, the head of the caudate forms the lateral wall of the anterior horn of the lateral ventricle into which it bulges. The tail of the caudate extends caudally (posteriorly) from the head, curves around the ventricular trigone to enter the inferior horn, and ends at the level of the amygdala in the temporal lobe (Figs. 2-16, 2-17, and 3-30).

Putamen

The putamen, a half moon–shaped basal ganglia nucleus, lies within the subcortical white core of the brain. It is located caudal lateral to the caudate and lateral to the globus pallidus. Lateral to the putamen is the **external capsule**, a long and slender fiber bundle. Other structures lateral to the putamen are the claustrum and **extreme capsule**, lying over the insular cortex (Figs. 2-15 and 2-16).

Globus Pallidus

The wedge-shaped globus pallidus is medial to the putamen (Figs. 2-15 and 2-16). It consists of medial and lateral components. The globus pallidus is ventrally bordered by the optic tract fibers and amygdala and medially by the posterior limb of **internal capsule**.

Claustrum

The claustrum is a slender mass of gray matter buried in the white matter between the insular cortex and the lateral margin of the lenticular nucleus (Figs. 2-15 and 2-16). It is connected with sensory cortical areas and contributes to visceral functions and sensory integration.

Amygdaloid Nucleus

The amygdaloid nucleus is a small round nucleus that lies in the rostral-medial temporal lobe at the end of the temporal horn and is contiguous to the tail end of the caudate

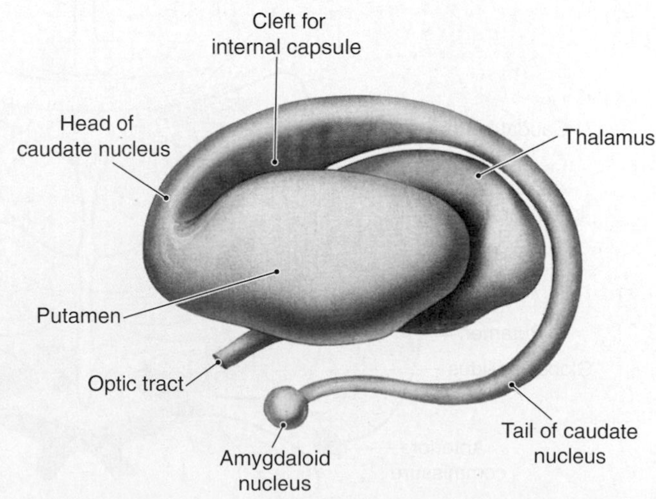

Figure 2-17 An anatomical orientation to the isolated striatum: the caudate and putamen merging, the tail of the caudate nucleus, and the amygdaloid nucleus.

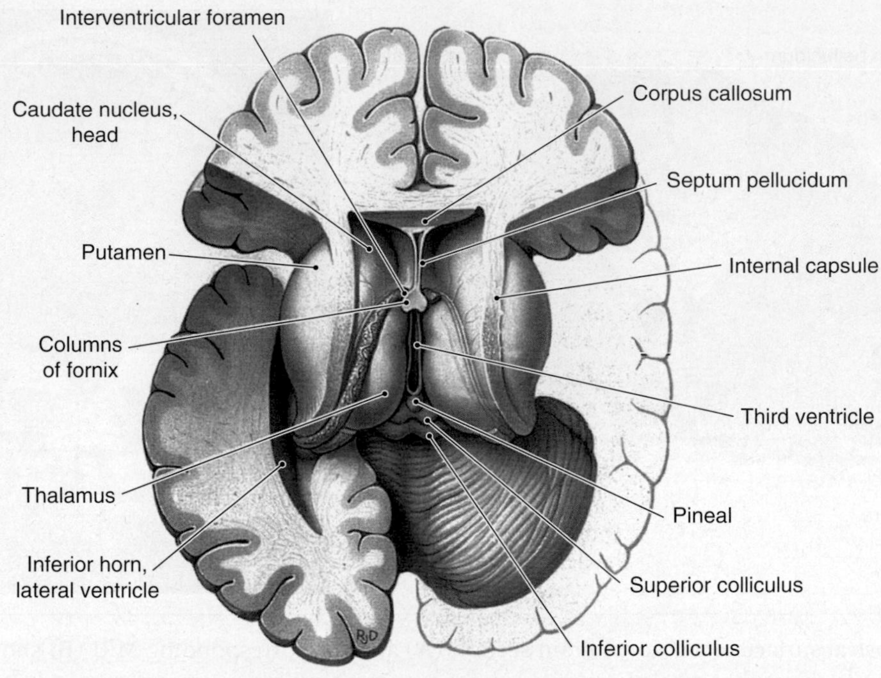

Figure 2-18 A horizontally dissected brain with the thalamus, striatum (caudate and putamen), internal capsule, and cavity of the lateral ventricle.

nucleus (Figs. 2-17 and 3-30). Although anatomically included in the basal ganglia, the amygdaloid nucleus is related functionally to the limbic system.

The **substantia nigra, red nucleus**, and **subthalamic nucleus** are additional important subcortical nuclei that participate in motor activity (Figs. 2-19 and 2-24). Although functionally related, these are not true basal ganglia structures. The structural and functional details of these structures are discussed in Chapter 15.

Diencephalon

The diencephalon includes the subcortical nuclear masses that form the central core of the brain. The thalamus and hypothalamus are the two major substructures of the diencephalon and can be seen on sagittal and coronal sections of the brain (Figs. 2-11, 2-18, and 2-19). The diencephalon is divided in half by a vertical slit of the third ventricle that demarcates the medial limit of the diencephalon.

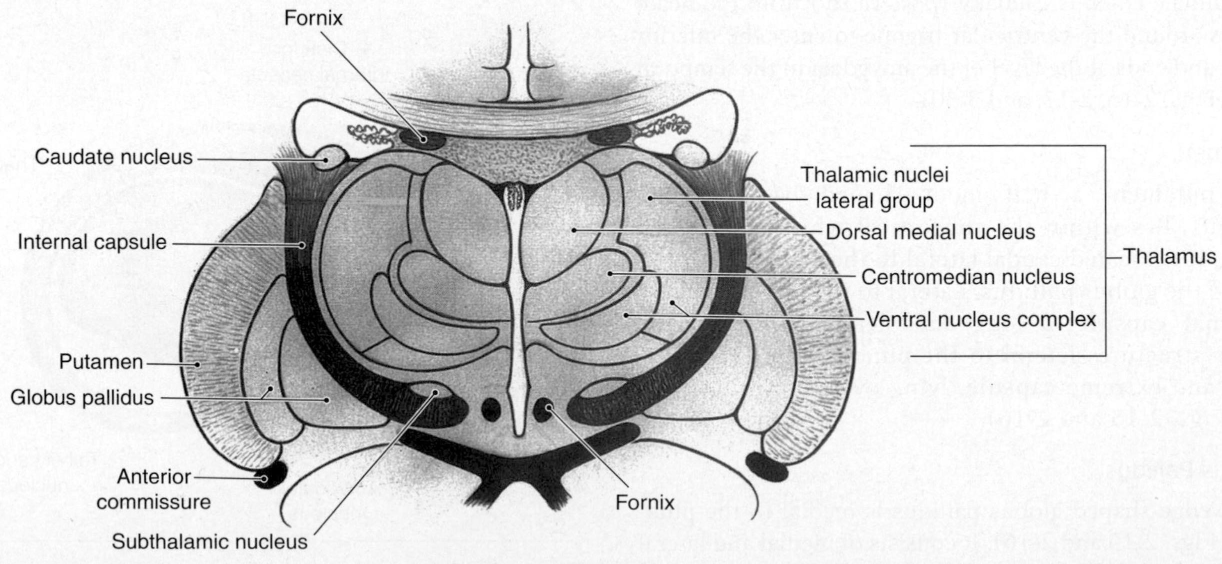

Figure 2-19 A coronal brain section through the diencephalon marked with the presence of the thalamus, hypothalamus, third ventricle, internal capsule, striatum, corpus callosum, and fornix.

The interventricular foramen, bilaterally located at the rostral end of the third ventricle, marks the rostral limit of the diencephalon (Fig. 2-18). The caudal boundary of the diencephalon is contiguous with the rostral end of the midbrain, and its dorsal boundary is delineated by the lateral ventricles. Laterally, the diencephalon extends to the internal capsule (Fig. 2-15).

Thalamus

The thalamus, an oval nuclear mass, is above the hypothalamus in the floor of the lateral ventricle. The interventricular foramen and the posterior commissure, respectively, mark the anterior and posterior limits of the thalamus (Fig. 2-11). The third ventricle delineates the medial border, and the internal capsule delineates the lateral border (Figs. 2-15, 2-18, and 2-19). Both thalami are bridged by a loose fibrous tissue, the massa intermedia (thalamic adhesion), that crosses the midline through the third ventricle (Fig. 2-11).

The thalamus is made up of numerous small specific and nonspecific nuclei, each serving definite functions and projecting to different parts of the brain. A major function of the thalamus is to relay sensorimotor information to the cortex. Research evidence from patients with thalamic infarcts and thalamotomy (surgically induced lesion of the thalamus for treatment of intractable pain and motor disorders) suggests that the thalamus also contributes to cortically mediated speech and language functions. Vascular or neoplastic thalamic lesions cause impaired contralateral somatic (bodily experienced) sensation, as well as a burning sensation, and low threshold for pain (Table 2-2). The anatomy and function of the thalamus are discussed in Chapter 6.

Hypothalamus

The hypothalamic sulcus separates the hypothalamus from the dorsally located thalamus (Figs. 2-11 and 2-19). The optic chiasm and anterior commissure mark the anterior limit, and the mammillary body marks the caudal limit of the hypothalamus (Fig. 2-11). Consisting of many nuclei, the hypothalamus communicates with the brain, brainstem, and spinal cord by neural and hormonal efferents. The hypothalamus uses overlapping neuronal circuitry to serve four primary functions: autonomic, endocrinic, regulatory, and drive and emotion. With efferent projections to the brainstem and spinal cord, it controls the ANS and its functions. By releasing various hormones directly into the blood system, it regulates all endocrinic functions of the body. Major regulatory functions of the hypothalamus include maintaining body temperature, blood volume, food and water intake, body mass, reproduction, and the regulation of circadian rhythms. With projections to the limbic system, the hypothalamus contributes to drives and emotions. The structures and functions of the hypothalamus are discussed in Chapter 18. Hypothalamic pathology results in impaired control of body temperature regulation, food and water intake, salt metabolism, sleep–wake cycles, and endocrine functions (Table 2-2).

Key Terms:

Brachium pontis	**Medial lemniscus**
Brachium conjunctivum	**Pes pedunculi**
Cerebellar peduncle	**Pyramidal tract**
Corpora quadrigemina	**Restiform body**
Dura mater	**Reticular formation**
Flocculus	**Superior Colliculus**
Foramen magnum	**Trigeminal nerve**
Fourth ventricle	**Vagus nerve**
Glossopharyngeal nerve	**Pyramid**
Hypoglossal nerve	**Reticular formation**
Inferior Colliculus	**Tegmentum**
Inferior olivary nucleus	**Tectum**

Brainstem

The brainstem is a short extension of the brain that connects the diencephalon to the spinal cord (Figs. 2-20–2-22). It consists of the midbrain, pons, and medulla oblongata, but it does not include the cerebellum. Integrating and coordinating both centrally and peripherally acquired information, the brainstem monitors all brain outputs. It possesses automatic control systems that are genetically acquired. This is opposite of the cortical functions, which are programmed through daily experience and learning. Brainstem syndrome includes impaired ocular control, altered consciousness, and sensorimotor deficit of the opposite half of the body (Table 2-2).

The entire ventral surface of the brainstem can be seen in Figure 2-20. The dorsal and lateral surfaces are exposed only after the overlying cerebellar tissues are removed (Figs. 2-21 and 2-22). Located on the ventral surface of the midbrain is the **pes pedunculi** (crus cerebri) which contains sensorimotor fibers and is situated on each side of the midline peduncular groove. Caudal to the peduncular groove and pes pedunculi is the large protruding body of the pons. Attached to the pons below is the medulla, the cone-shaped caudal portion of the brainstem, which becomes contiguous with the spinal cord at the level of the **foramen magnum** (Fig. 2-31).

The superior surface of the brainstem is seen after the cerebellum is removed (Fig. 2-21). The structures on the brainstem's dorsal surface are the **corpora quadrigemina** (**superior** and **inferior colliculi**), the floor of the **fourth ventricle**, and three **cerebellar peduncles**. The fourth ventricle floor contains many CN nuclei. The **fasciculus gracilis** and **fasciculus cuneatus** are the most evident structures of the dorsal medulla. These structures mediate fine discriminative touch from the body (see Chapter 11). Figure 2-22 provides a lateral view of the entire brainstem and its gross anatomic structures.

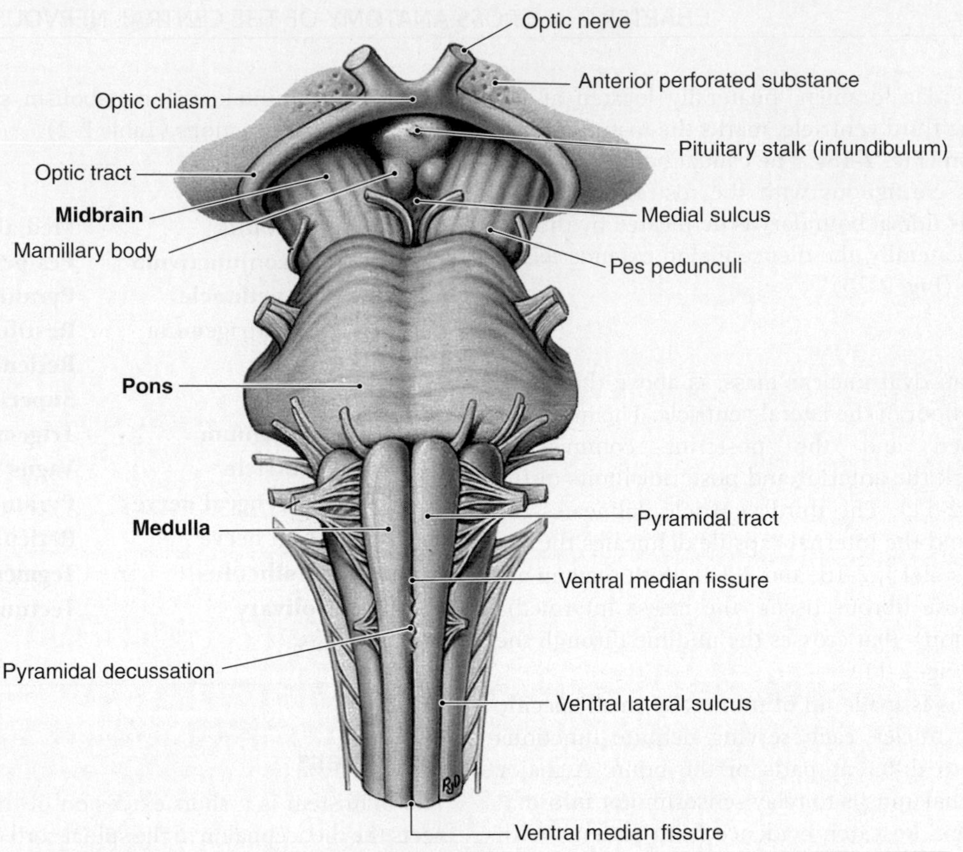

Figure 2-20 The ventral brainstem view with the midbrain, pons, and medulla as well as several cranial nerve rootlets.

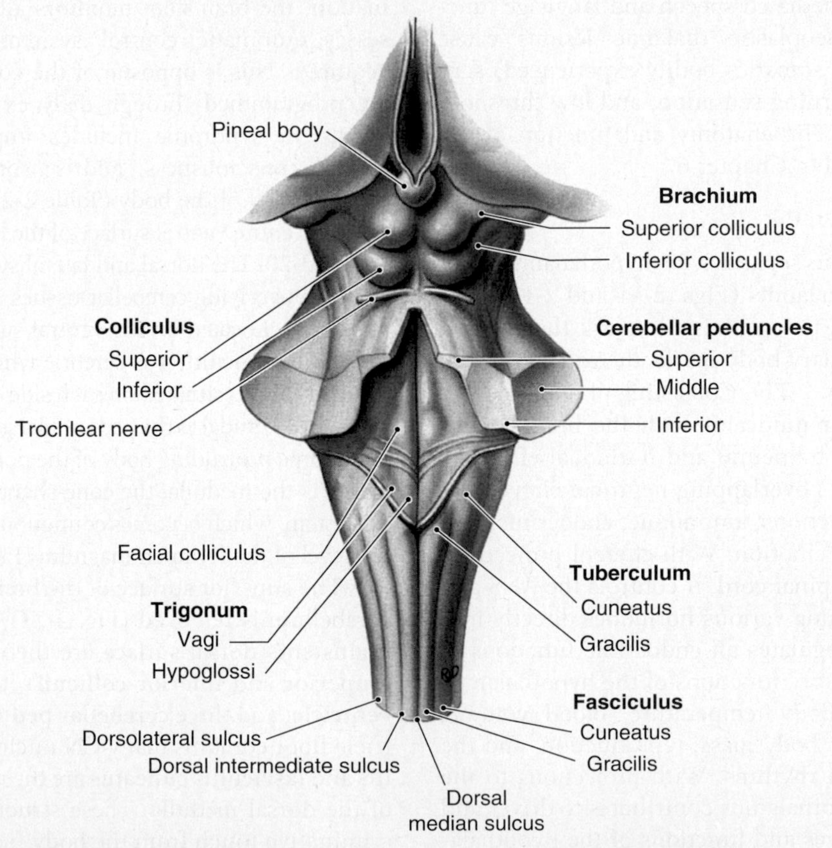

Figure 2-21 Dorsal view of the brainstem with the exposed cavity of the fourth ventricle after the removal of the overlying cerebellum.

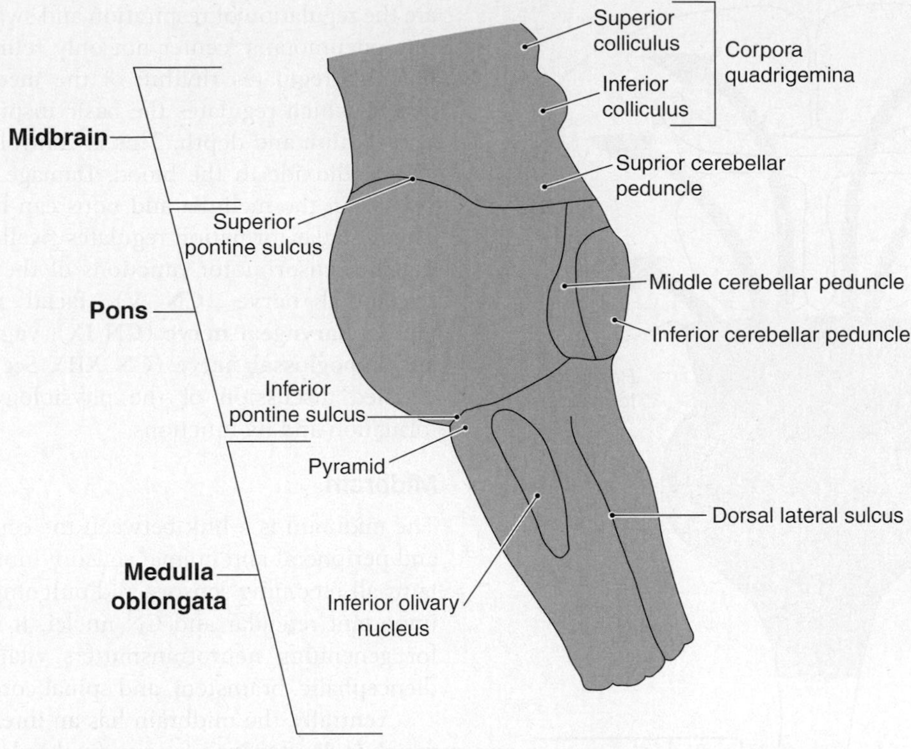

Figure 2-22 Lateral view of the brainstem and the cerebellar peduncle locations.

Internally, the brainstem consists of **cranial nerve nuclei, longitudinal fiber tracts**, and the **reticular formation**. The reticular formation collectively represents groups of diffusely located specialized nerve cells that are entangled in a network of fibers, which are interconnected with parallel- and serial-running neuronal circuits (Box 2-2). Composing most of the brainstem, the divergent circuitry of the reticular formation is functionally wired to nuclei in the thalamus and spinal cord (Fig. 2-23). By virtue of their central locations, the reticular neuronal circuits inhibit, facilitate, modify, and regulate all cortical functions. The reticular formation integrates all sensorimotor stimuli with internally generated thoughts, emotions, and cognition. It is also responsible for maintaining the homeostatic state of the brain, which is essential for regulating visceral, sensorimotor, and neuroendocrine activities, including blood pressure and movement.

The complex multisynaptic ascending projections of the reticular formation to the brain, thalamus, hypothalamus, and basal ganglia form the reticular activating system (RAS), which has a controlling influence on the levels of cortical arousal and consciousness. A lesion of the RAS leads to altered states of arousal, such as drowsiness, stupor, or prolonged unconsciousness (comatose). The level of alertness is correlated with the electroencephalic activity of the brain.

Besides alertness, two functions of the reticular formation that are closely related to communicative disorders

BOX 2-2

Brainstem Reticular Formation

The brainstem reticular formation plays an important role in regulating cortically mediated functions. With its diffuse and interactive circuitry, it not only modifies all the cortically generated functions, such as language, thinking and reasoning, but it also integrates all sensorimotor stimuli with internally generated thoughts, emotions, and cognition. Being responsible for maintaining the homeostasis (equilibrium state) of the brain, it has a role in maintaining visceral, sensorimotor, and neuroendocrine activities. By controlling the consciousness and arousal (cortical activating system), it also regulates the quality of language, memory, and thoughts. During sleep, the specialized reticular nuclei repair the body's metabolic systems and reawaken the brain after energy is replenished. Two other functions of the reticular formation, closely related to communicative disorders, are the regulation of respiration and swallowing (which involve the pontine pneumotaxic center) and the regulation of the multiple cranial nerves (see Chapter 18).

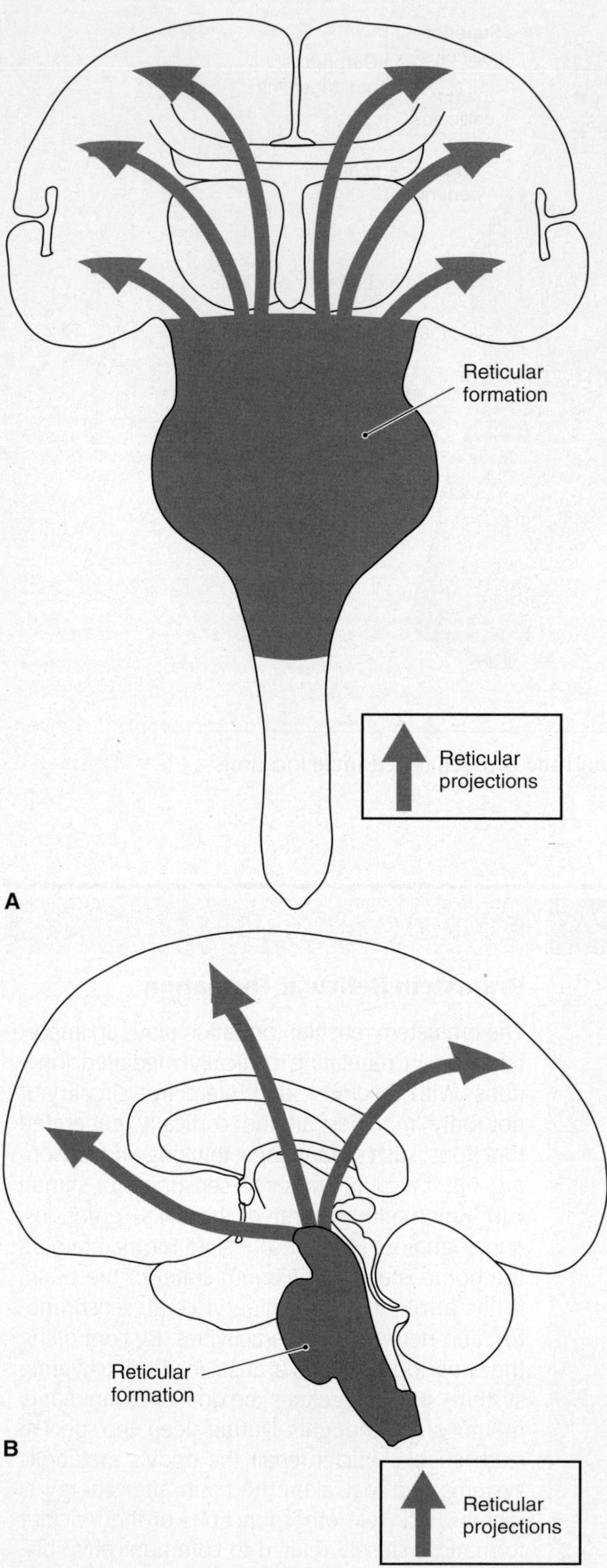

Figure 2-23 Frontal (A) and lateral (B) views of the brainstem reticular formation.

are the regulation of respiration and swallowing. The pontine pneumotaxic center not only refines the respiration but also regulates rhythm of the medullary respiratory center, which regulates the basic inspiration and expiration rhythm and depth. This is controlled by the level of carbon dioxide in the blood. Damage to the respiratory centers in the medulla and pons can be life-threatening. The reticular formation regulates swallowing by integrating the sensorimotor functions of the CNs that include **trigeminal nerve** (CN V), **facial nerve** (CN VII), **glossopharyngeal nerve** (CN IX), **vagus nerve** (CN X), and **hypoglossal nerve** (CN XII). See Chapter 18 for a detailed discussion of the physiology of the reticular formation and its functions.

Midbrain

The midbrain is a link between the cerebral hemispheres and peripheral and cranial sensory input systems. It contains all incoming sensory and outgoing motor fibers and important reticular and CN nuclei. It is also responsible for generating neurotransmitters vital to telencephalic, diencephalic, brainstem, and spinal cord functions.

Ventrally, the midbrain has an interpeduncular fossa, which is divided by a longitudinal indentation (peduncular groove). The elevation on each side is formed by the pes pedunculi tracts of pyramidal motor fibers (Fig. 2-20). Dorsally, the midbrain has four rounded elevations (corpora quadrigemina), which are located just beneath the overlapping pineal gland of the thalamus (Fig. 2-11) and form the roof (**tectum**) of the midbrain (Fig. 2-21). The two upper rounded elevations are the superior colliculi, which participate in reflexive control of eye movements, visual reflexes, and coordination of vestibular generated head and eye movements. The two lower rounded elevations are the inferior colliculi, which mediate the transmission of auditory impulses from the ear to the thalamus and auditory cortex. The inferior colliculi also mediate reflexes triggered by auditory stimuli (Box 2-3).

Lateral to the corpora quadrigemina are swellings of the two brachia (sing. brachium). Fibers of the **brachium** of the **superior colliculus** connect the superior colliculi with the visual relay nucleus of the thalamus, and fibers of the **brachium** of the **inferior colliculus** connect the inferior colliculi with the auditory relay nucleus of the thalamus.

Internally, the midbrain contains many important nuclei and bundles of sensory and motor fibers (Fig. 2-24). There are three subdivisions in the midbrain: **tectum** (roof), **tegmentum**, and **basis pedunculi**. The tectum is located dorsal to the cerebral aqueduct, a small tubular connection between the third and the fourth ventricles. The tectum has an important role in the survival of the organism because it provides the organism with a three-dimensional orientation map. This map guides eye movements and head and body turning in response to bright light and directional sounds. The tectum also mediates

BOX 2-3

The Midbrain

The midbrain has four rounded elevations (corpora quadrigemina), which form the roof (**tectum**) of the midbrain. The upper two rounded elevations are the superior colliculi, which participate in reflexive control of eye movements, visual reflexes, and coordination of vestibular-generated head and eye movements. The lower two rounded elevations are the inferior colliculi, which mediate the transmission of auditory impulses from the ear to the thalamus and auditory cortex. The inferior colliculi also mediate reflexes triggered by auditory stimuli. The superior colliculi have an important role in the survival of the organism. Together with auditory cortex and visual tract, the superior colliculi provide a three-dimensional map of an organism's stimulus-generated external world. The complex multisensory integrated circuit of the superior colliculi receives tactile and proprioceptive information and projects to the ipsilateral motor nuclei of the brainstem and to all contralateral spinal levels. This complex circuitry makes it possible for the organism to rapidly adjust limb, head, and eye movements to a sudden stimulus (startle) or stumbling (equilibrium reflex). We consider most of these behaviors, automatic.

visual reflexes, such as pupil constriction and lens accommodation. The tegmentum region of the midbrain contains numerous scattered nuclei, such as the red nucleus, CN nuclei, and reticular central gray region. The basis pedunculi is ventral to the tegmentum; it consists of the pes pedunculi (crus cerebri), a group of cortical pyramidal tract fibers, which terminate in the brainstem, spinal cord, and the substantia nigra. The substantia nigra contains a group of nuclei that produce dopamine, an inhibitory basal ganglia neurotransmitter; degeneration of these dopamine-secreting cells leads to Parkinson disease.

Pons

The pons, a metencephalic structure, is separated from the midbrain by the superior pontine sulcus and from the medulla by the inferior pontine sulcus (Fig. 2-22). The ventral pontine surface is convex both longitudinally and horizontally, whereas dorsally the pontine structures are hidden by the overlying cerebellum (Fig. 2-12). The pons contains all descending motor fibers and ascending sensory fibers, numerous cranial nuclei, the reticular formation, and transverse fibers that form the **middle cerebellar peduncle**, which attaches the cerebellum to the brainstem. The rhomboid fourth ventricle is dorsal to the pons and is visible after removal of the overlying cerebellum. The ventricular floor is broad in the middle and narrows toward its caudal end. The floor is divided in half by the dorsal median sulcus, and it contains important CN nuclei (Fig. 2-21). Along the medial eminence of the ventricular floor is a small round protrusion, the facial colliculus, formed by the facial nerve (CN VII) fibers.

Internally, the pons consists of two parts: the **pontine tegmentum** and the **basis pontis**, which is also called the base of the pons (Fig. 2-25). The tegmentum of the pons contains ascending and descending fibers and numerous diffusely scattered pontine reticular nuclei. The fibers of the **medial lemniscus** are responsible for mediating fine discriminative touch in the body. The basis pontis contains the cortical descending fiber tracts, pontine nuclei, and pontocerebellar fibers. The base of the pons also contains descending corticospinal fibers, which form the medullary pyramids in the medulla and continue in the spinal cord.

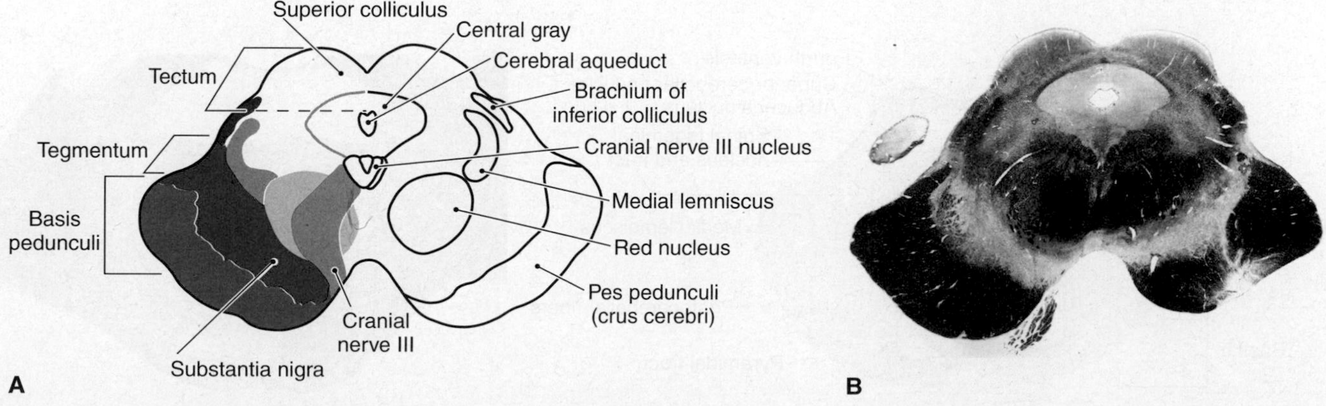

Figure 2-24 A. A view of the internal midbrain anatomy on a transverse section. Also marked are the locations of the tectum (superior and inferior colliculi), cerebral aqueduct, and the tegmentum. B. The corresponding transverse section of the midbrain.

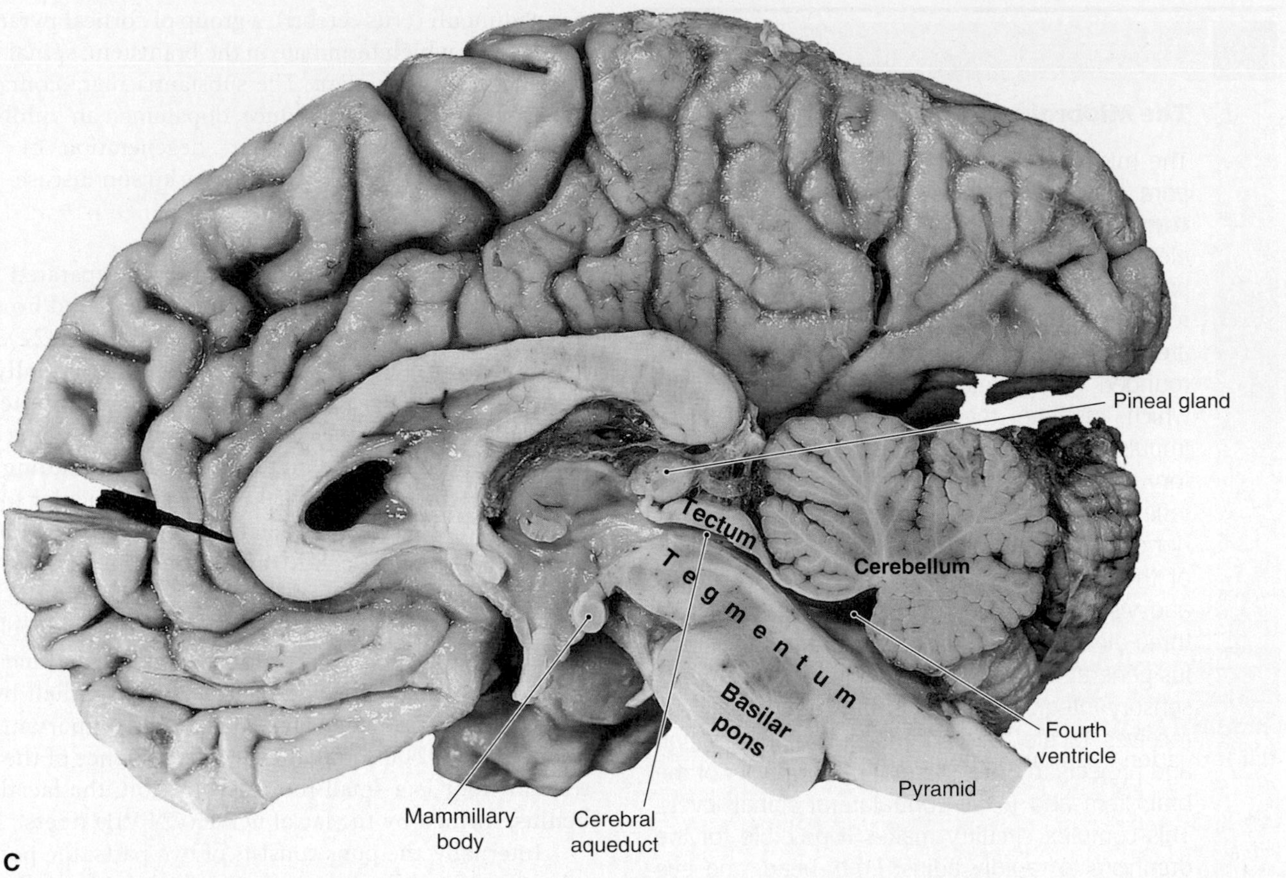

Figure 2-24 (*Continued*) C. Sagittal view of the brainstem.

Medulla Oblongata

The medulla oblongata is the most caudal part of the brainstem (Fig. 2-20 and 2-22). It contains all the motor fibers that descend to the spinal cord and all the sensory fibers that carry sensory information from the body to the more rostral brain areas. Major surface structures of the medulla are the ventral median sulcus, **pyramidal tract**, **inferior olivary nucleus**, and dorsal tubercula (gracile fasciculus and cuneate fasciculus).

The ventral median fissure divides the medulla in half. Parallel to the ventral median fissure is the ventrolateral sulcus. Between both these sulci is the pyramidal tract, which carries motor information from the motor cortex to the spinal cord for activation of skeletal muscles.

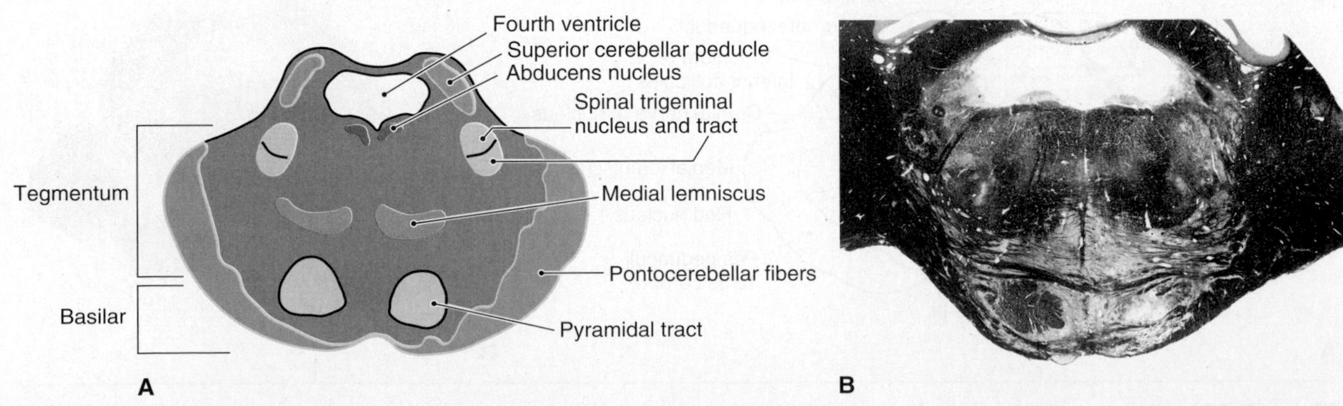

Figure 2-25 A. Internal; anatomy of the mid-pons on a transverse section marked with the tegmentum and basilar pons. B. Corresponding transverse section of the pons.

The descending fibers of the pyramidal pathway decussate at the level of the caudal medulla. After the motor fibers cross the midline, they form the **lateral corticospinal tract**, a motor pathway of the spinal cord.

The **dorsal median sulcus** divides the dorsal surface of the medulla in half; the caudal floor of the fourth ventricle forms a trigonum, which contains the hypoglossal and vagus nuclear complexes (Fig. 2-21). Located between the dorsolateral sulcus and the dorsal median sulcus are two sensory pathways, the gracile fasciculus and cuneate fasciculus, that carry fine discriminatory sensory information from the body to the medulla and then to the thalamus. On the lateral medullary surface is an oval protrusion produced by the underlying enlarged inferior olivary nucleus. Fibers from the inferior olivary nucleus project to the cerebellum by way of the **inferior cerebellar peduncle**.

Internally, the medulla consists of two parts: the tegmentum and **pyramid** (Fig. 2-26). The tegmental area contains several nuclei, the reticular formation, medial lemniscus fibers, and fibers projecting to the cerebellum. Numerous CN nuclei are anchored and interconnected through the reticular bed that extends up and down the brainstem tegmentum. Some nuclei of the medullary reticular formation form three vital reflex centers. The **cardiac center** regulates the rate and strength of heartbeat; the **vasomotor center** monitors and alters the diameter of the blood vessels and the **respiratory center**, in conjunction with the pontine pneumotaxic center, controls the rhythm and rate of breathing. Consequently, injuries to the medulla that damage those centers may be fatal. The pyramid contains the descending motor fibers that are ventral in the medulla and cross the midline in the caudal medulla.

Cerebellum

The cerebellum is dorsal to the pons and medulla (Figs. 2-9, 2-11, and 2-12). It is separated from the cerebral hemispheres above by a **meningeal layer** of **dura mater** and from the brainstem by the fourth ventricle.

This three layered structure contributes to the maintenance of equilibrium and coordination of skilled motor activity by modifying cortical motor functions, but, like basal ganglia structures, it does not initiate motor activity. Through direct and indirect projections to the motor cortex, basal ganglia, and spinal cord, the three layered cerebellum coordinates and modifies the tone, speed, and range of muscular excursions in the execution of motor functions. For example, it adjusts the strength needed to lift 10 lb versus 200 lb, and it ensures smooth movement. The cerebellar projections to the vestibular system make crucial contributions to the equilibrium-maintaining mechanism. A lesion in the cerebellum leads to tremor, paucity of movement, ataxia (muscular incoordination), and impaired equilibrium, mostly ipsilaterally.

The cerebellum has a highly distinctive appearance; its surface consists of a large number of transverse thin sulci formed by narrow rows of tightly packed gyri called folia. The wedge-shaped cerebellum is divided into the cerebellar hemispheres (Fig. 2-27). The structures in the midline portion of the cerebellum are grouped into the vermis (Fig. 2-28). Each cerebellar hemisphere is divided into three lobes: **anterior**, **posterior**, and **flocculonodular** (Fig. 2-28). The portion of the cerebellum rostral to the primary fissure is the anterior lobe. The posterior lobe lies between the primary fissure and the posterolateral fissure. The flocculonodular lobe, the oldest part of the cerebellum, is on the inferior surface; it consists of the **nodulus** and the paired **flocculi** which are two vermal structures (Fig. 2-29).

A midsagittal section of the vermis reveals its central structures and provides a better view of the overall internal anatomy of the cerebellum. The nodulus portion of the flocculonodular lobe is medial; the remaining part of this older lobe, the paired **flocculi**, is ventrolateral on the inferior surface of the cerebellum (Fig. 2-29). Both the **flocculus** and the nodulus are involved in coordinating movements with equilibrium (vestibular system activation) while throwing a ball.

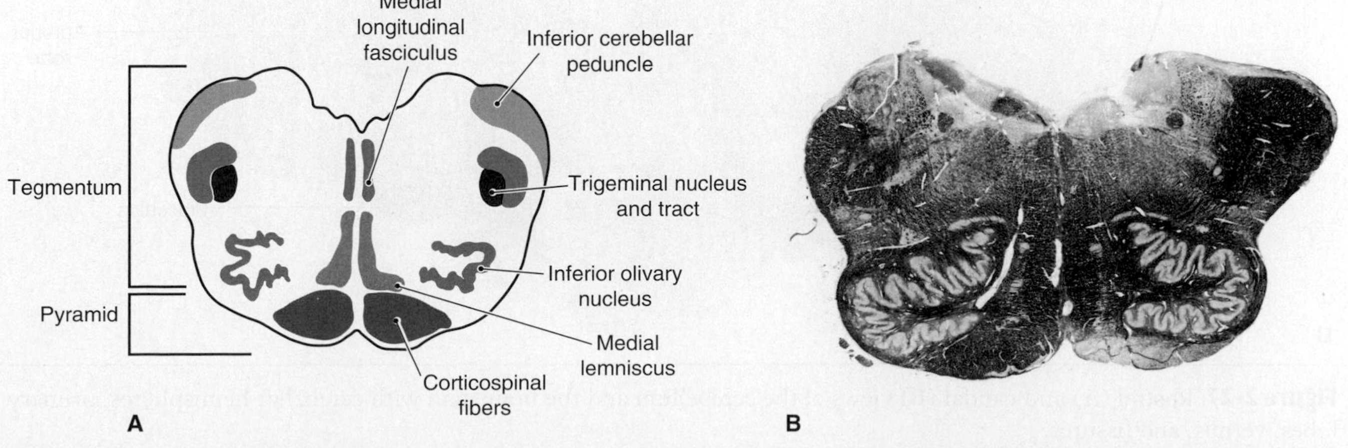

Figure 2-26 A. Internal anatomy of the medulla on a transverse section containing the tegmentum and pyramid. B. Corresponding transverse section of the medulla.

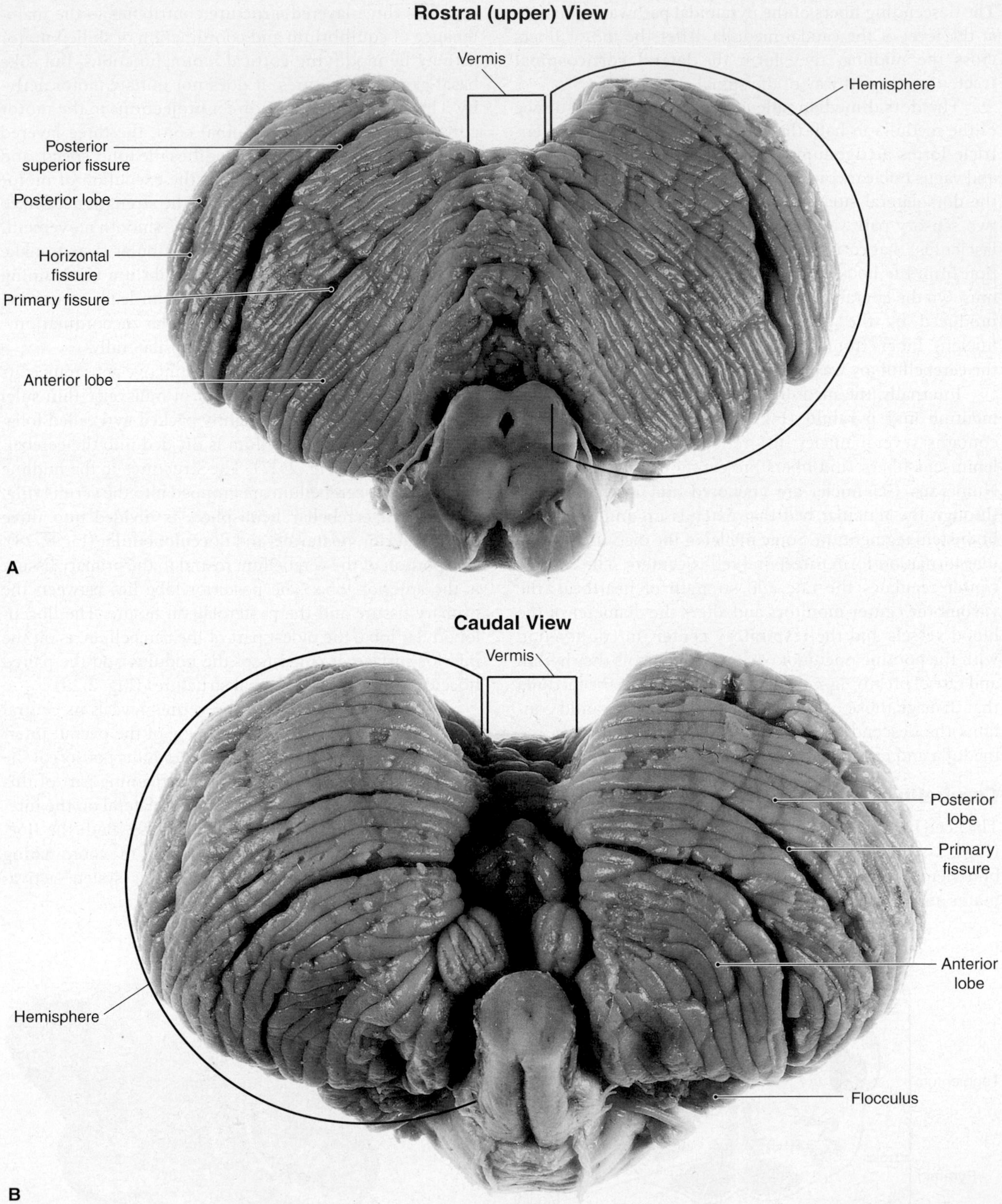

Figure 2-27 Rostral (A) and caudal (B) views of the cerebellum and the brainstem with cerebellar hemispheres, primary lobes, vermis, and fissures.

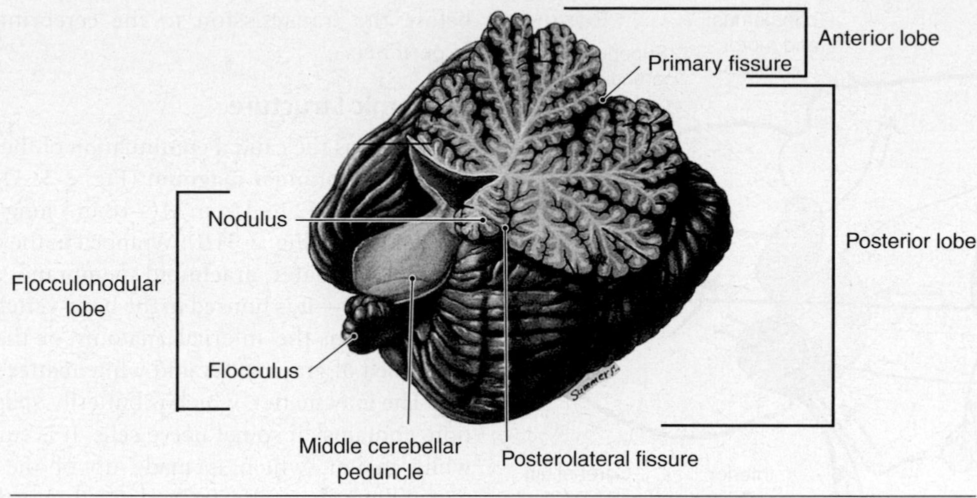

Figure 2-28 An exposed view of the cerebellar vermis on a sagittal surface.

Structurally, the cerebellar lobes consist of a surface area of gray matter and a medullary core of white matter. Within the core of the white matter are important intrinsic cerebellar nuclei that participate in the analysis and synthesis of sensorimotor information and project motor-modulating impulses to all motor control centers.

Cerebellar Peduncles

The cerebellum is connected to the brainstem through three fiber bundles called the **superior (brachium conjunctivum)**, **middle (brachium pontis)**, and **inferior (restiform body) cerebellar peduncles**. The lateral inferior surface of the cerebellum reveals the connections of the peduncles to the brainstem (Figs. 2-29 and 2-30). The superior peduncle is stem shaped. Located ventrally, the middle and inferior peduncles appear as a bulging, thick semicircular collar attached to the pontine ventrolateral brainstem.

Input to the Cerebellum

The cerebellum receives its input information from two sources. Afferents from the motor cortex by way of the pons enter through fibers of the middle cerebellar peduncle. Fibers of the inferior cerebellar peduncle transmit proprioceptive afferent information from the trunk and limbs and the vestibular information to the cerebellum (Fig. 2-30). The cerebellar cortex near the midline (vermis), which receives all the input, plays an important role in the integration of vestibular data with the ongoing movement mechanism.

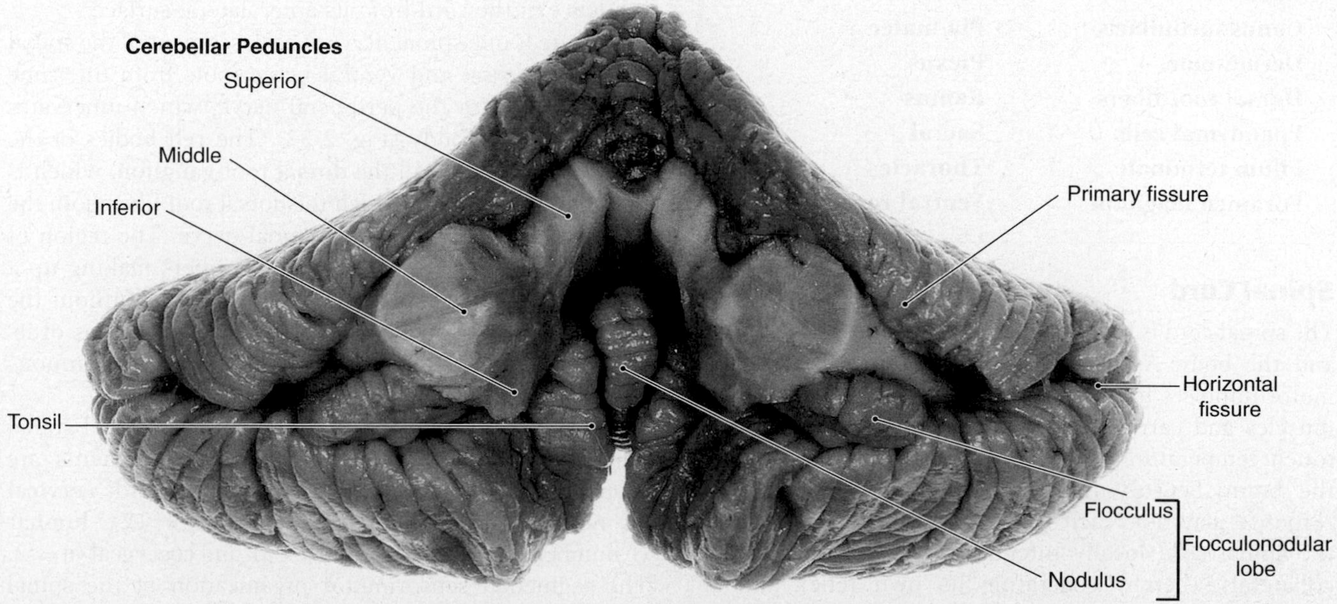

Figure 2-29 Inferior view of the cerebellum, cerebellar peduncles, and vermal structures.

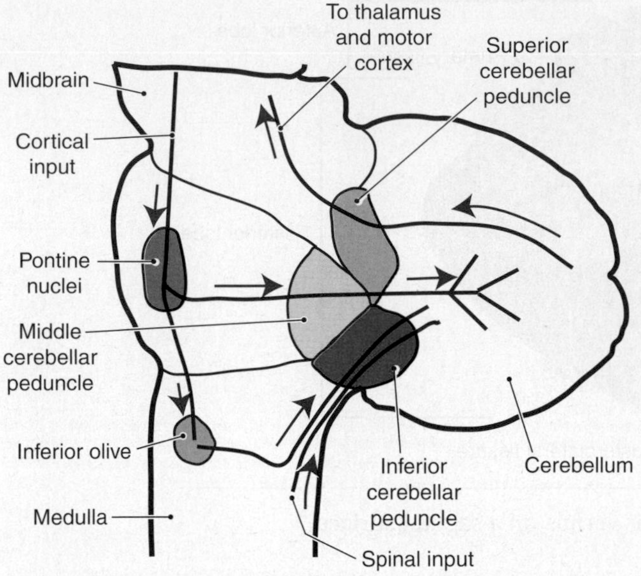

Figure 2-30 A diagrammatic illustration of the lateral brainstem and the three connecting cerebellar peduncles.

Output from the Cerebellum

After analyzing and synthesizing the received sensorimotor information, the cerebellum projects its corrective feedback predominantly to the opposite motor context, through the superior cerebellar peduncle (Fig. 2-30).

Key Terms:

Arachnoid membrane	**Foramen of Luschka**
Brachial	**Foramen of Magendie**
Cauda equina	**Hydrocephalus**
Cervical	**Lumbar**
Coccyx	**Myotome**
Conus medullaris	**Pia mater**
Dermatome	**Plexus**
Dorsal root fibers	**Ramus**
Ependymal cells	**Sacral**
Filum terminale	**Thoracic**
Foramen magnum	**Ventral root fiber**

Spinal Cord

The spinal cord is the transmission link between the brain and the body. As a bidirectional pathway, it transmits motor impulses from the brain to the visceral organs and muscles and carries sensory information, such as pain, touch, temperature, and proprioception, from the body to the brain. Sensory input that requires an immediate response may not reach the level of awareness. Instead, the spinal cord locally integrates such information via collaterals, thereby generating its own reflex and an immediate response to environmental changes. Even the reflexes that involve multiple synapses are well under way before the transmission to the cerebrum can result in experience.

Anatomic Structure

Beginning as the caudal continuation of the medulla oblongata at the **foramen magnum** (Fig. 2-31*A*), the cylindrical spinal cord is 42 to 45 cm (16–18 in.) long with a diameter of about 1 cm (Fig. 2-31*B*). Wrapped in the three **meningeal layers—pia mater, arachnoid membrane**, and **dura mater** (Fig. 2-32*B*)—it is housed in the bony vertebral column. On cross section, the internal anatomy of the spinal cord is composed of gray matter and white matter (Fig. 2-32*A*).

The gray matter, which is butterfly-shaped in cross section, contains all spinal nerve cells. It is surrounded by the white matter, which is made up of the ascending and descending fibers arbitrarily divided into three myelinated funiculi (fasciculi): dorsal, lateral, and ventral. The gray matter consists of two **dorsal horns** and two **ventral horns**. The dorsal horns contain the nerve cells that receive sensory information from the body through the **dorsal root fibers**. The ventral horns contain motor nerve cells whose axons leave the cord through the anterior roots to activate visceral and skeletal muscles and glands. In addition, the ventral horns contain many interneurons that communicate with each other and the **lower motor neurons (LMNs)** of synergistic motor units and agonistic and antagonistic muscles, producing coordinated movements of limbs. After exiting through the **intervertebral foramina**, the fibers of the dorsal and ventral roots join to form the spinal nerves (Fig. 2-32). In the center of the spinal cord is the small opening of the **central canal**, an invisible duct containing CSF that extends from the fourth ventricle to the conus medullaris.

The spinal cord has a series of nerve roots attached to it (Fig. 2-32). A continuous series of dorsal rootlets enters the cord on its posterolateral surface. Similarly, a series of rootlets exit the cord from its anterolateral surface.

There is one spinal nerve at each segment of the spinal cord. The dorsal and ventral nerve roots from the same side join to form the peripheral nerve, which innervates that side of the body (Fig. 2-32). The cell bodies of the dorsal root fibers form the **dorsal root ganglion**, which is proximal to the site at which the dorsal root fibers join the **ventral root fibers** to form a spinal nerve. The region of the spinal cord that gives rise to the fibers making up a spinal nerve is called a spinal cord segment. Without the rootlet fibers, the spinal cord would show no signs of its segmental nature; rather it would appear as a continuous column of gray and white matter.

There are 31 segments in the spinal cord and 31 spinal nerves on each side (Fig. 2-33). These segments are grouped into five divisions of the spinal cord: **cervical** (*C* number = 8), **thoracic** (*T* number = 12), **lumbar** (*L* number= 5), **sacral** (*S* number = 5), and **coccygeal** (*n* = 1). The segmental sensorimotor organization of the spinal cord is reflected by the peripheral overlapping of sensory and motor innervations for body parts and areas. The area

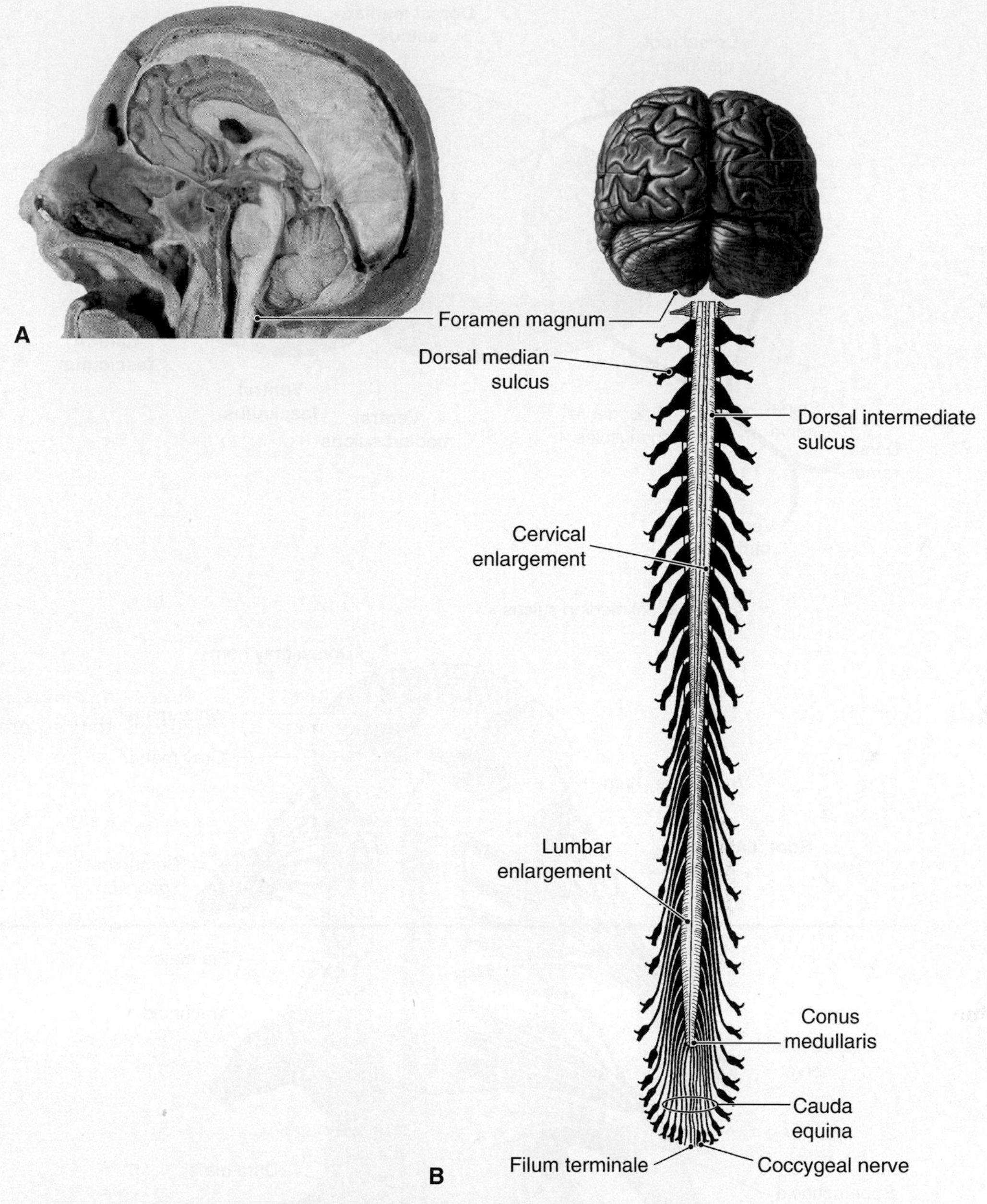

Figure 2-31 A. Sagittal view of the foramen magnum. B. Posterior view of the spinal cord with a series of dorsal root ganglia and spinal nerves.

of the body innervated by the neurons in a single dorsal root ganglion is a **dermatome**. The entire body is divided into numerous dermatomes. The muscles or a part of muscles, innervated by all the axons exiting the cord via a single ventral root, is called a **myotome**. Familiarity with a dermatome–myotome chart and the corresponding spinal segments can aid in making clinical diagnoses of sensorimotor disorders (Fig. 2-34; Table 2-4; Box 2-4).

In earthworms and fish, the body area (dermatome) related to each spinal segment is not only equal in width to the spinal cord but is also parallel to the spinal segment. The segmental organization of spinal innervation did not change during phylogenetic development. What has changed is the level of the innervated area that used to be parallel to the cord. In humans, before approximately the fourth fetal month, the cord segments have the same location as the corresponding segments of the vertebral column. In later months, however, the bony column grows faster than the cord. Consequently, the lumbar and sacral nerve roots descend below the level of the **conus medullaris** and form the **cauda equina** (Fig. 2-33). The nerves from the caudal segments of the spinal cord continue to exit from the same intervertebral foramina as they did in earlier; however, the nerves progressively stretch and

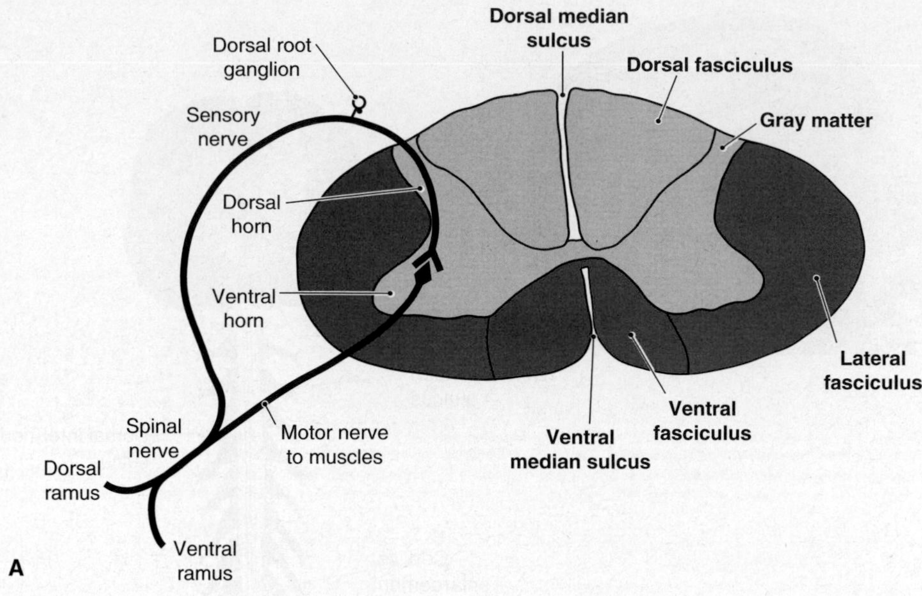

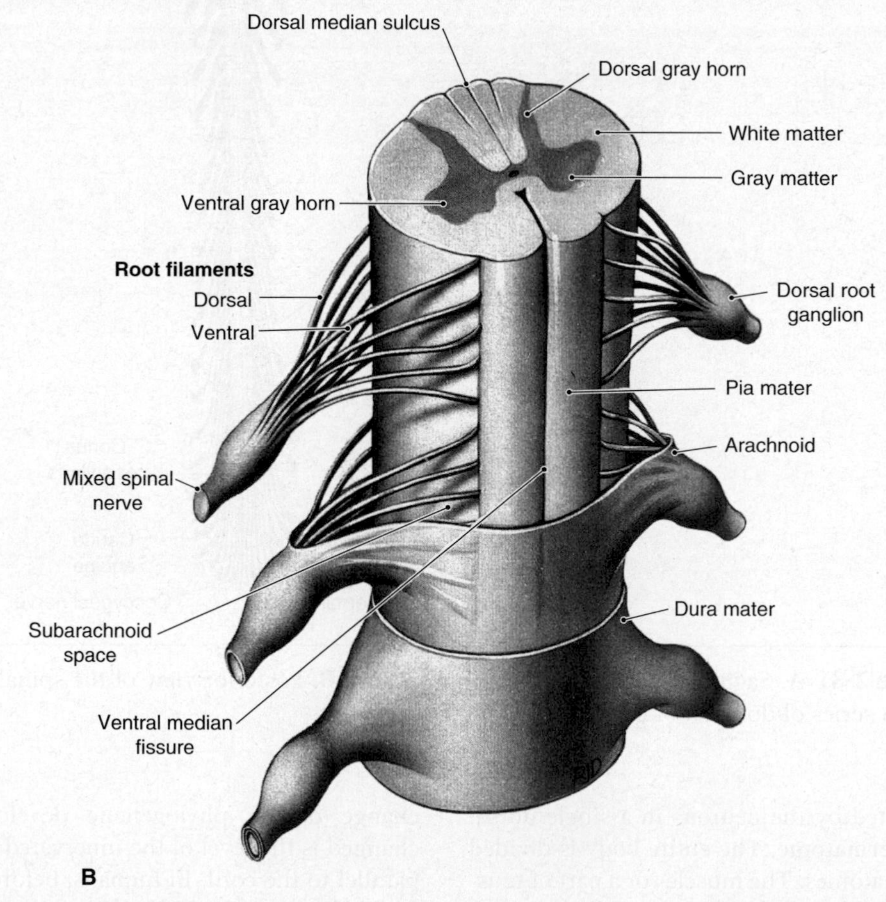

Figure 2-32 A. View of the internal spinal topography on a cross section. B. The structures of the spinal cord with the fibers of the dorsal and ventral roots, dorsal root ganglion, spinal nerves, meninges, and subarachnoid space.

appear as a bundle of roots descending in the fluid-filled spinal canal before exiting the spinal column. The **filum terminale** is the fibrous extension from the cord that is attached to the **coccyx** (Fig. 2-33).

Networking of Spinal Nerves

The 31 pairs of spinal nerves, named after the regions from which they arise, are formed by the merging of the dorsal (sensory) and ventral (motor) roots of the spinal cord.

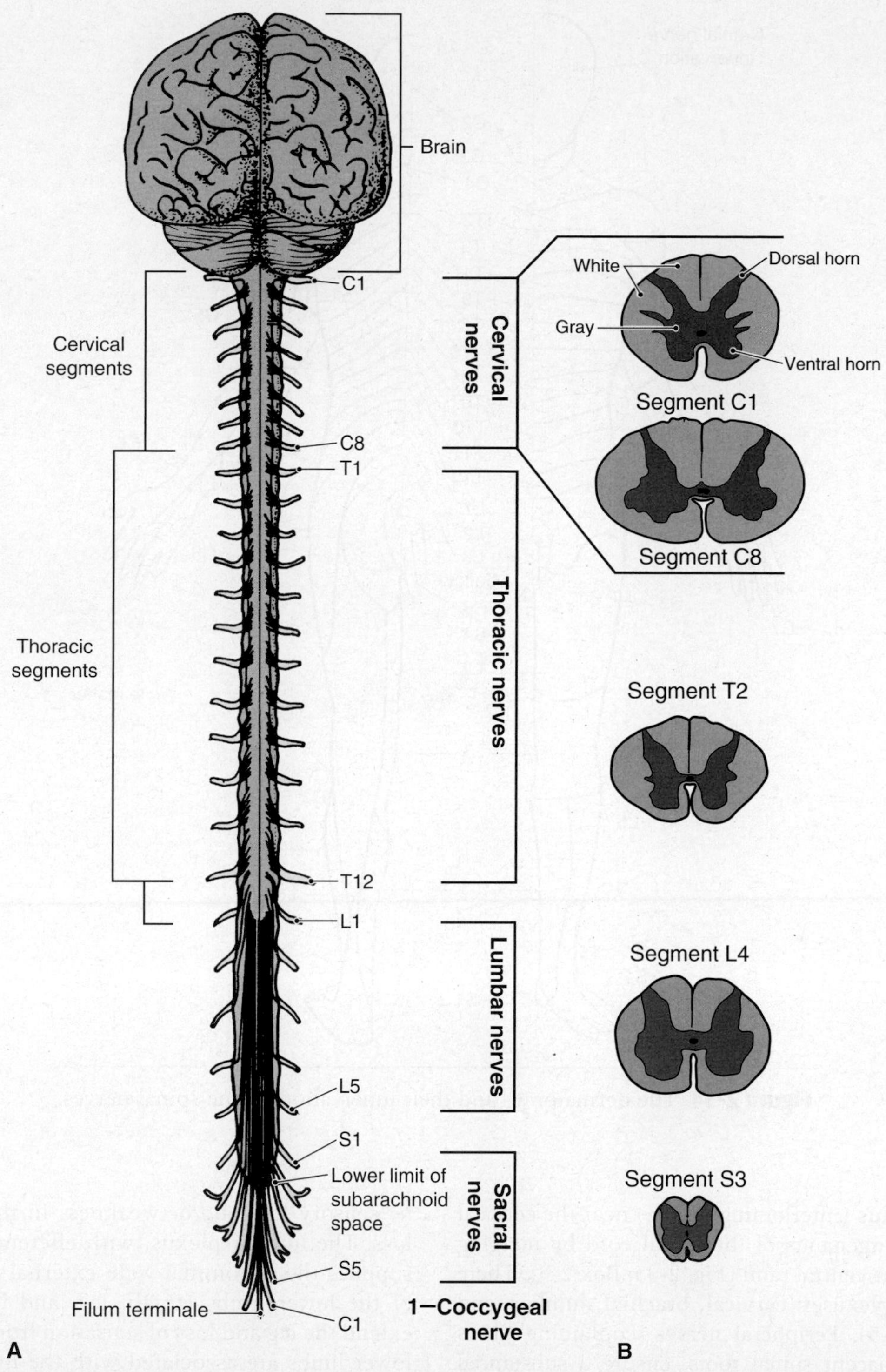

Figure 2-33 A. The spinal nerve positions in relation to the vertebrae. B. Cross sections of the spinal cord with varying sizes and shapes of the gray matter at different spinal levels.

After traveling a centimeter, each nerve divides into two rami: **dorsal** and **ventral**. Each **ramus**, like a spinal nerve, contains both sensory and motor fibers. Thus a lesion of a ramus or spinal nerve results in paralysis and loss of sensation (pain and touch) for a specific limb. The dorsal rami serve the sensorimotor functions of the posterior trunk (skin and dorsal back muscles). The ventral rami, which contain a greater number of fibers, innervate a larger area of the body. Other than those originating from T1 to T12, ventral rami do not go directly to body structures. Rather

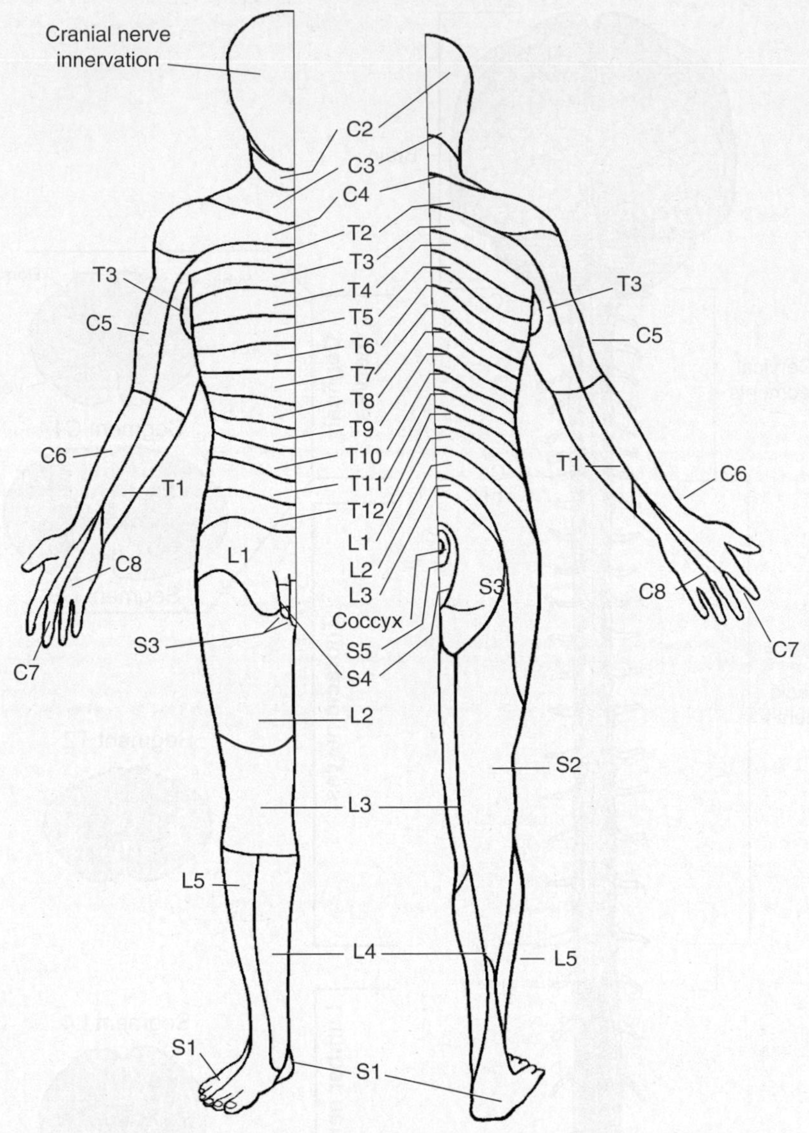

Figure 2-34 The dermatomes and their innervation by the spinal nerves.

they form a **plexus** (interjoining nerves) near the cervical and lumbar enlargements of the spinal cord by merging with the adjacent ventral rami (Fig. 2-35; Box 2-5). There are four major plexuses: **cervical**, **brachial**, **lumbar**, and **sacral** (Table 2-5). Peripheral nerves, containing fibers from several adjacent spinal roots, ensure a substantial overlap in the sensorimotor innervations to the skin and muscles.

The cervical plexus, formed primarily by the projections from C1 to C4, supplies the muscles and skin of the head, neck, and part of the shoulders and most importantly the diaphragm (the primary muscle of inhalation). Its pathology results in cervical pain and respiratory palsy. The brachial plexus, with efferents from C5 to C8, provides the nerve supply for the shoulders and upper limbs. Its pathologic involvement is characterized by sensory loss and/or weakness in the arm and reflex loss. The lumbar plexus, with efferents from L1 to L4, supplies the abdominal wall, external genitals, and part of the lower limbs (thigh, leg, and foot). Inability to extend the leg and loss of sensation from the genitals and lower limbs are associated with the involvement of the lumbar plexus. The sacral plexus, with spinal efferents from L4 to S4, supplies the buttocks, perineum, and lower limbs. Foot-drop and pain extending down from the buttocks to the leg indicates involvement of the sacral plexus.

Neuritis (nerve inflammation) marks the common pathologic condition involving peripheral (spinal or cranial) nerves; it is marked by inflammation of one (mononeuropathy) or more (polyneuropathy) nerves from either structural irritation or inflammation (Box 2-6).

Table 2-4

Major Spinal Roots and Their Distribution

Roots	Myotomal Activity	Dermatomal Distribution
C5	Shoulder abduction	Shoulder, lateral
C5–C6	Forearm flexion	Biceps
C6	Elbow supination/pronation	Thumb
C7	Finger extension; forearm extension at elbow	Third finger
C8–T1	Digital abduction and adduction (check the patient's ability to move fingers apart and together against resistance)	Finger, ring
T4		Nipple
T10	Umbilical contraction	Umbilicus
L2–L4	Knee extension, hip flexion, and adduction	Anterior-medial thigh and medial leg below the knee
L5	Ankle and great toe dorsiflexion (check the patient's ability to walk on heels)	Foot, dorsal
S1	Ankle plantar flexion (check the patient's ability to walk on tiptoes)	Sole of foot, lateral

Spinal Regulation of Muscles for Respiration

Understanding the spinal control of the muscles of respiration is an important aspect of training for students in communicative disorders (Table 2-6). In addition to being vital for survival, respiration, with its patterned cycle of inhalation and exhalation, also regulates our speaking and speech intelligibility (see Chapters 13 and 18).

BOX 2-4

Peripheral Spinal Distribution

Familiarity with dermatome (with projections from the dorsal root ganglion) and myotome (motor fibers that pass through the ventral root) charts and the corresponding body regions aids in making clinical diagnoses of sensorimotor disorders. It also helps explain instances of visceral pain from internal organs that are masked. There is some overlap between neighboring dermatomes that makes their boundary limits somewhat less clear. Nonetheless, this also provides some safety by reducing the area of anesthesia following the involvement of one dorsal root or dorsal root ganglion Likewise, multiple segment innervation of many muscles reduces the functional damage should a ventral root be lost. For students in human behaviors, the myotomes responsible for innervating respiratory muscles are important. Their pathology causes serious respiratory problems, particularly if the muscles of inhalation are affected.

VENTRICLES

The primary function of the ventricular cavities in the brain is to circulate the CSF, which is secreted by the **choroid plexus** in the **ventricular cavities**. Circulating around the CNS, the CSF forms a spongy cushion to protect the brain and spinal cord from excessive accelerating and decelerating head movements.

There are four interconnected ventricles within the brain (Figs. 2-36 and 2-37): two lateral ventricles (one in each hemisphere; the first and second ventricles), the third ventricle, and the fourth ventricle. Both lateral ventricles are connected by way of the interventricular foramen to the midline third ventricle. The third ventricle is connected to the fourth ventricle in the brainstem through the cerebral aqueduct. The inner wall of these interconnected ventricular cavities is lined with a layer of **ependymal cells**; these glial cells, in part, prevent diffusion of substances from the CSF into the brain. A common pathologic condition associated with CSF circulation is **hydrocephalus**.

Lateral Ventricles

The lateral ventricles are C-shaped structures that form an arch (Fig. 2-36). Each lateral ventricle consists of the central part, or body, and three extensions: **anterior**, **posterior** (occipital), and **inferior** (temporal) **horns**. The roof of the body of the lateral ventricle is formed by the fibers of the

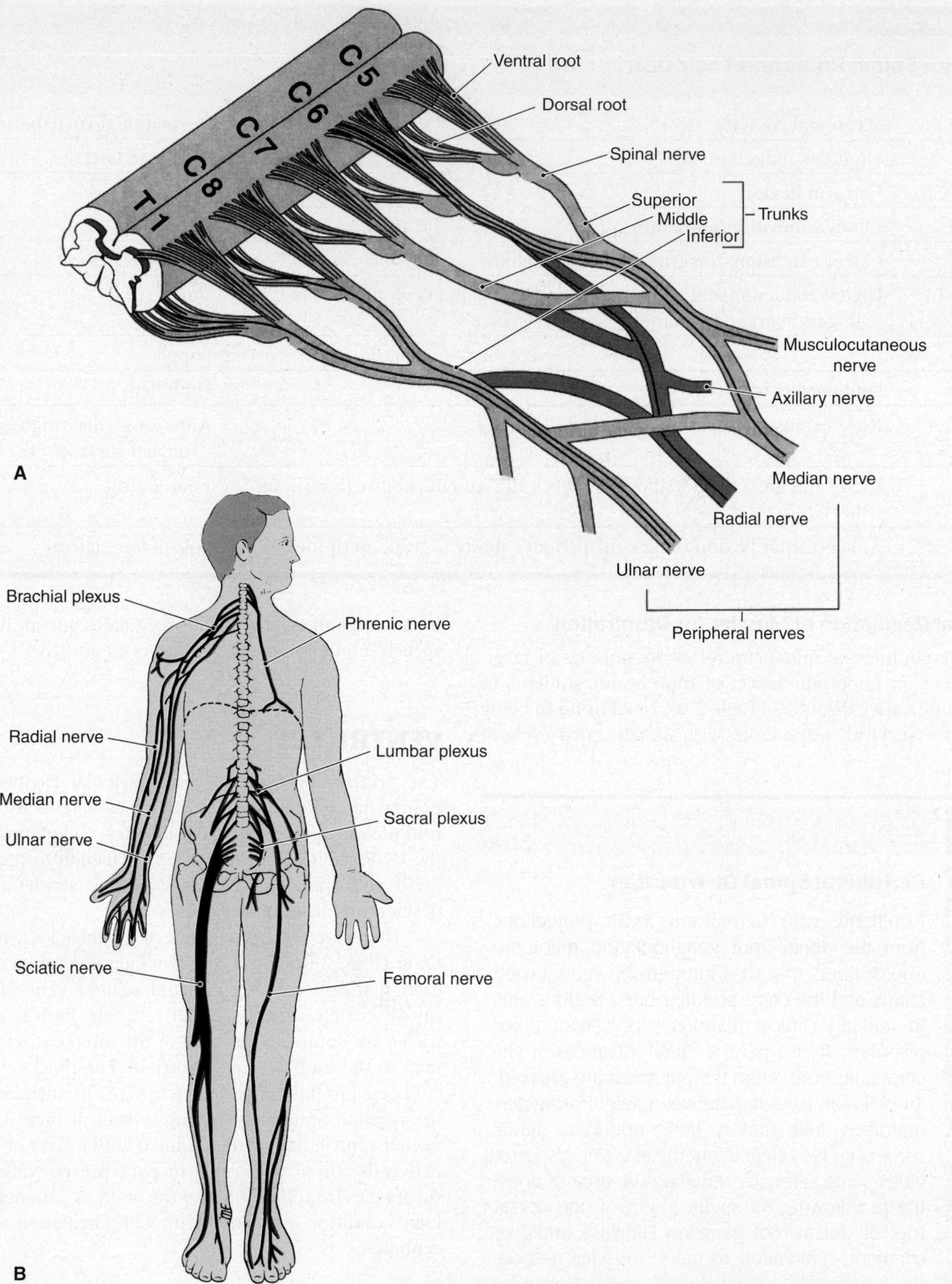

Figure 2-35 A diagrammatic view of plexus formation (A) and major spinal plexuses (B).

Table 2-5

Nerve Plexus and Motor Functions

Plexus and Origin	Nerves	Served Body Areas	Clinical Characteristics
Cervical (C1–C5)	Phrenic	Diaphragm; muscles of shoulder and neck	Respiratory paralysis
Brachial (C5–C8, T1)	Radial	Triceps and extensors of arm	Wrist-drop and inability to extend hand at wrist
	Median	Flexors of forearm	Inability to pick up objects; failure to abduct thumb and index finger; neuropathy associated with carpal tunnel syndrome
	Ulnar	Wrist muscles	Inability to spread fingers
Lumbar (T12, L1–L4)	Femoral	Lower abdomen, buttocks, and anterior thigh	Inability to extend leg and flex hip
Sacral (L4–L5, S1–S4)	Sciatic	Lower trunk and posterior surface of thigh and leg	Inability to the extend hip and flex knee
	Peroneal	Foot and lateral leg	Foot-drop and inability to dorsiflex foot

corpus callosum. The superior surface of the thalamus constitutes the floor of the lateral ventricle. The body of the lateral ventricle extends from the interventricular foramen (of Monro) to an imprecisely defined point near the splenium of the corpus callosum. The arch-shaped body of the lateral ventricle enlarges near the **collateral trigone** area, the broader portion in the posterior floor of the lateral ventricle. At this point, the ventricular body diverges into the posterior and inferior horns. The anterior horn is the extension of the lateral ventricle in the frontal lobe rostral to the interventricular foramen. The membranous thin part of the septum pellucidum forms the medial wall of the anterior ventricular horns (Figs. 2-11 and 2-16). The posterior horn, shaped like an elongated slender finger, is the caudal extension of the ventricle from the

BOX 2-5

Spinal Plexus

Spinal nerves, other than those originating from T1 to T12 ventral rami, do not go directly to body structures. Rather, they form a plexus (interjoining nerves) near the cervical and lumbar enlargements of the spinal cord by merging with the adjacent ventral rami. There are four major plexuses: cervical, brachial, lumbar, and sacral. The peripheral nerves, containing fibers from several adjacent spinal roots, ensure a substantial overlap in the sensorimotor innervations to the skin and muscles. For students in human behaviors, the cervical plexus is clinically important as it supplies the diaphragm (the primary muscle of inhalation). An injury affecting the diaphragm results in respiratory palsy; such patients, if not provided with mechanical respiration, can die.

BOX 2-6

Peripheral Neuropathy

Peripheral neuropathy involves structural damage to the peripheral nerves, which can result in a generalized loss of sensory and motor functions in the area supplied by the nerve. Involvement of an isolated nerve (focal neuropathy) may result in difficulty using the hands owing to nerve compression after a sustained use of limbs (seen in construction workers) and a limited movement of the wrist after the use of a computer mouse for a sustained period (carpal tunnel syndrome involving median mononeuropathy at the wrist). The loss of motor control in the leg after sitting a long time in the same position is another example of a focal neuropathy involving the sciatic nerve, by which walking and standing become difficult as a result of the numbness. Nutritional deficits, alcoholism, diabetes, tumors, and autoimmune diseases are common causes of neuropathy which affects one or multiple nerves.

Table 2-6

Spinal Control of the Muscles of Respiration

Spinal Roots	Muscles	Functions
C3–C5	Diaphragm	Contracts to increase thoracic diameter for inspiration
T1–T12	External intercostals	Contract to raise ribs for inspiration
T1–T12	Internal intercostals	Assist in rib depression for forced expiration
T6–T12	Abdominal muscles Rectus abdominus Internal oblique External oblique Transversus abdominus	Increase intrathoracic pressure for forced expiration

trigone area into the occipital lobe. The inferior horn is the curved inferior extension of the lateral ventricle from the trigone area into the temporal lobe. Some important anatomic structures in the floor of the inferior horn are the hippocampus, amygdala, tail of the caudate nucleus, and crus (leg) of the fornix.

Third Ventricle

The third ventricle is a narrow vertical space between the two thalami and is rostrally connected to the lateral ventricles through the interventricular foramen of Monro (Fig. 2-36). The hypothalamic nuclei form the floor of the third ventricle (Fig. 2-19). Caudally in the midbrain, the cavity of the third ventricle narrows to become the cerebral aqueduct, which connects the third and fourth ventricles (Fig. 2-11).

The cerebral aqueduct is an important reference point for the transition between the dorsal and the ventral midbrain areas. The area dorsal to the cerebral aqueduct, the tectum, includes the corpora quadrigemina in addition to the tectal nuclei. The midbrain region ventral to the cerebral aqueduct is the tegmentum, which contains important structures, such as the red nucleus and reticular formation nuclei.

Fourth Ventricle

The tegmentum of the pons and medulla constitute the triangular floor of the fourth ventricle; the cerebellum forms its roof. The rhomboid floor of the fourth ventricle can be seen completely after removal of the cerebellum (Figs. 2-9 and 2-21). Beneath the floor of the ventricle are the nuclei of CN V–CN XII. At the widest portion of the fourth ventricle, there are three openings: two lateral apertures (**foramina of Luschka**) and one medial aperture (**foramen of Magendie**) (Fig. 2-36). Through these three openings, the CSF gains access to the subarachnoid space surrounding the CNS (see Chapter 8).

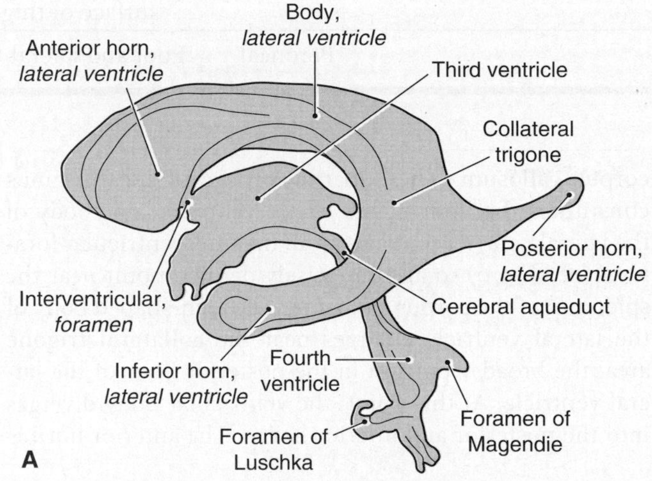

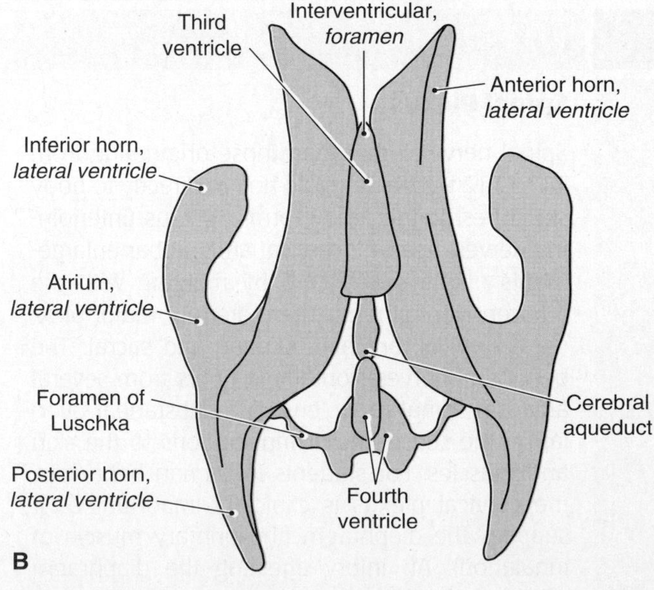

Figure 2-36 Lateral (A) and dorsal (B) views of the ventricular system.

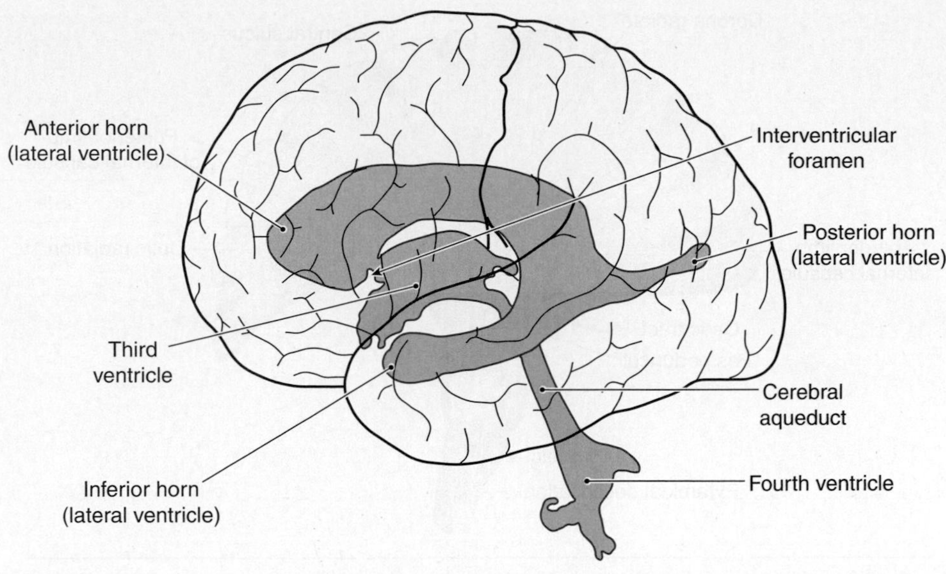

Figure 2-37 Lateral view showing the relation of the ventricular cavity within the brain.

Key Terms:	
Arcuate fasciculus	**Cingulum**
Association fibers	**Disconnection syndrome**
Commissural fibers	**Projection fibers**
Corona radiata	**Uncinate fasiculus**

CORTICAL WHITE MATTER

Besides containing the cellular laminae (gray matter) and ventricular cavities, each cerebral hemisphere includes a large volume of fibers (white matter). The myelinated fibers form the medullary core of the brain and account for all **inter-** (between hemispheres) and **intrahemispheric** (within a hemisphere) axonal connectivity. The comprehensive and well-organized connectivity through these fibers accounts for the efficiency with which external information is quickly analyzed, synthesized, and transferred from one modality to another and adequate responses are formulated and executed promptly with the left, right, or both limbs. These interconnecting fibers keep all brain areas informed of information processed, decisions made, steps undertaken, and actions performed. The medullary core in the brain consists of three types of fibers: **projection, association,** and **commissural**.

Projection Fibers

While carrying sensory and motor information, the projection fibers travel vertically to connect the cortex with the brainstem and spinal cord structures. These fibers project through the **corona radiata** and coalesce as a large fiber bundle in the **internal capsule** (Figs. 2-16 and 2-38). The internal capsule, a subcortical band of fibers, contains all ascending (projecting to the cerebral cortex) and descending (projecting downward from the telencephalon) fibers as they pass between the basal ganglia and the thalamus. Appearing as a left-facing V-shaped structure, the internal capsule can be seen on a coronal or horizontal section; it consists of an **anterior limb, genu,** and **posterior limb** (Figs. 2-15, 2-16, and 2-38). The anterior limb contains corticothalamic and thalamocortical fibers, which connect the thalamic nuclei with the frontal cortex and limbic-cingulate gyrus. Also located here are the corticopontine fibers that mediate frontal projections. The genu of the internal capsule is the site for the corticobulbar fibers that descend to innervate the CN nuclei and play an important role in motor speech processes. The posterior limb is much larger and is known to contain the corticospinal fibers that project to the spinal motor neurons.

The motor fibers of the corticospinal (pyramidal) tract primarily originate from the precentral gyrus and descend through the corona radiata, internal capsule between the basal ganglia and the thalamus, and pes pedunculi in the midbrain (Fig. 2-38). They form the pyramid in the medulla before crossing the midline and entering the spinal cord. The **sensory projection fibers** collect cutaneous and proprioceptive sensation from the skin and joints and project to the CNS. These sensory fibers enter the spinal cord, ascend through the brainstem and internal capsule, and then fan out through the corona radiata and project to the primary sensory cortex in the parietal lobe. Interruption of the projection fibers results in sensorimotor syndromes.

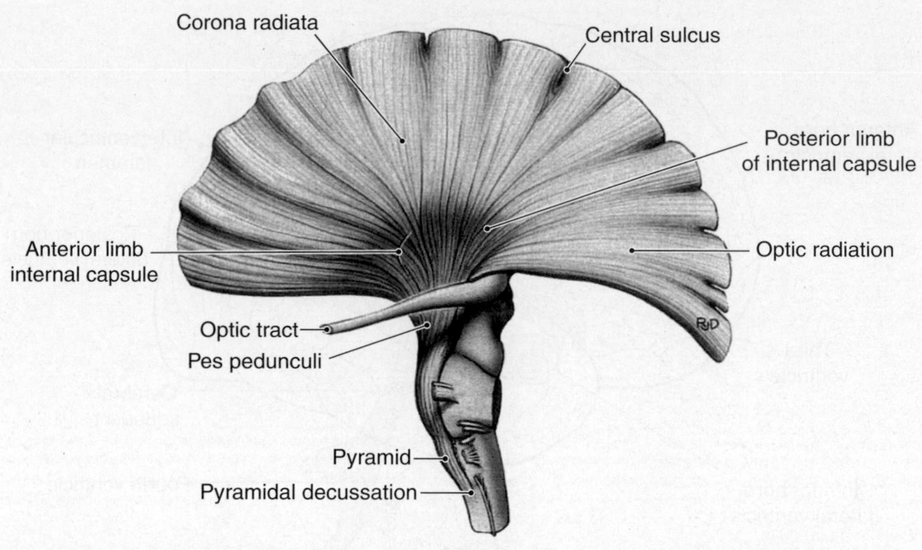

Figure 2-38 Continuity of the longitudinally arranged projection fibers from the cortex through the corona radiata, internal capsule, and midbrain pedunculi to the pyramids in the medulla.

Association Fibers

Association fibers, the most numerous of the three types of fibers, are confined within the hemisphere. Some of the association fibers are short and connect adjacent gyri, whereas some are long and connect distant cortical areas. Functionally, they share the same goal, which is to provide efficient bidirectional channels for communication among cortical areas within each hemisphere. They are also important in refined and integrated behavioral responses. Lesions involving these pathways result in disconnections between two areas within a hemisphere. Selective involvement of one or more of these pathways may result in a peculiar symptom complex, such as conduction aphasia as an example of the **disconnection syndrome** (Box 2-7).

Short association fibers are U-shaped arcuate fibers that bend sharply around a sulcus and connect two adjacent gyri. The important long association fiber bundles are the following: **superior longitudinal fasciculus, cingulum, inferior longitudinal fasciculus**, and **uncinate fasciculus**. The general location of these pathways is best seen on a coronal section of the brain (Fig. 2-39).

The superior longitudinal fasciculus, also known as the **arcuate fasciculus**, lies anteroposterior above the insular cortex. This associational fasciculus connects the frontal lobe with the occipital lobe. Many of its fibers diverge from the parietal lobe, curve around as the arcuate fasciculus, and project to the temporal lobe (Fig. 2-40). This fasciculus is an important communication link among the frontal, parietal, occipital, and temporal lobes. The curved arcuate fibers of the fasciculus are known to connect the classical Wernicke area (posterior language cortex) in the temporal lobe with Broca area (anterior language cortex) in the frontal lobe. This pathway is significant in the normal acquisition of language functions, auditory–verbal (repetition) memory, and propositional communication.

The inferior longitudinal fasciculus is a well-defined compressed bundle of fibers beneath the sylvian fissure and the insular cortex. It connects the temporal and occipital lobes. Its fibers travel anteroposteriorly from the occipital to the temporal lobe. Traveling in close proximity of the inferior longitudinal fasciculus are the short fibers of the uncinate fasciculus (Fig. 2-40*A*); these fibers connect the orbital frontal gyri with the rostral region (superior and middle gyri) of the temporal lobe.

The cingulum, a C-shaped association fiber bundle, is beneath the cingulate gyrus, which lies above the corpus callosum. The cingulum is an association fiber bundle of the limbic lobe connecting the medial, frontal, and parietal cortices with the temporal cortex. Its fibers originate in the subcallosal area beneath the genu of the corpus callosum, circle around the corpus callosum within the cingulate gyrus, and terminate in the parahippocampal gyrus of the medial temporal lobe (Fig. 2-40*B*).

Commissural Fibers

Commissural fibers in the brain run horizontally and connect the corresponding cortical areas in both cerebral hemispheres. Most neocortical commissural fibers are included in the corpus callosum, and the remainder of the fibers constitutes the anterior commissure. The corpus callosum, the largest commissural bundle of fibers, is a thick plate of 300 to 400 million fibers (Figs. 2-15, 2-16, and 2-41). The fibers of the corpus callosum connect the corresponding cortical areas in both hemispheres, except for the primary

BOX 2-7

Disconnection Syndromes

In a disconnection syndrome, two major functional centers are disconnected from each other rather than damaged directly (see association fibers under "Medullary Centers" in the "Brain" in this chapter; also see Chapter 19 and the "Diffusion Tensor Imaging" in Chapter 20). This syndrome makes reference both to anatomy and to function. The symptomatology of the functional disconnection is different from the symptomatology that arises from disruption to one or another of the functional centers, themselves. It is important to know what clinically and linguistically happens when there is a disconnection syndrome or if the lesion is confined to either of the language centers where the functions are represented. The general understanding about the disconnection syndrome is that the functions themselves are not disturbed, but rather the functions of each disconnected center cannot "communicate" with each other. Sigmund Freud was the first to distinguish "center" lesions from "disconnecting" lesions, while other 19th-century medical thinkers used the metaphor of the "telephone line," whereby the lines could be damaged, leaving the functional machinery of the individual telephones intact.

Disconnecting lesions can sever long intrahemispheric association fibers, or they can disturb different amounts of the interhemispheric commissural fibers. A great portion of the corpus callosum may be sectioned by a surgical procedure referred to as a "commissurotomy" to alleviate mostly intractable epilepsy. Lesser parts of the corpus callosum may be damaged by lesions disconnecting the right hemisphere sensorimotor systems from the left hemisphere systems. In the clinic, when a verbal command is given to "move your left hand," the response is often disrupted, because the movement centers and the language comprehension centers are disconnected. Damage in the left frontal lobe in zones where colossal fibers from the right hemisphere are extending to the left will often cause a "left-handed" apraxia, because as a result the right motor strip will be disconnected from the stored movement formulae in the left posterior areas. This is commonly referred to as a "sympathetic apraxia." In addition, lesions may disconnect the undamaged visual centers of the right hemisphere from the left hemisphere language systems that convert visual letter representations into "graphemic/phonemic" verbal codes for reading comprehension. In this case, there is a disconnecting lesion in the splenium of the posterior portion of the callosum and another that disconnects left occipital regions from the more rostral language zones in the left. The patient with this disconnection syndrome, startlingly, cannot read, but can write (called "alexia without agraphia"). Moreover, the well-known breakdown in repeating "heard words" has been classified as a disconnection phenomenon that does not involve damage to acoustic perceptual or motor planning centers, but rather to the smooth connective integration of these two functions. Again, emanating from the telephone metaphor, this syndrome has been classically referred to as "conduction aphasia" (see Chapter 19). The disconnected association fiber tract in this syndrome is usually the superior longitudinal fasciculus, often referred to as the "arcuate fasciculus." A newly emerged clinical concept related to the connectionist model is 'hodology',' which is concerned with a neuroanatomical focus upon the connectionist- tissue in the nervous system, (Catani, 2007). The awareness of hodology' is increasing in cognitive-communicative disorders since SLP professionals in medical settings will often be asked for cognitive interpretations of diffusion tensor images from fMRI measurements and relate them to various kinds of "disconnection" syndromes they will see, diagnose, and treat.

centers for motor, sensory, auditory, and visual functions. The primary centers in both hemispheres are connected to each other only through the association cortical areas, which in turn are interconnected through the callosal fibers.

The corpus callosum contains four parts: rostrum, genu, body, and splenium (Figs. 2-12 and 2-41). The fibers in the genu and rostrum of the corpus callosum interconnect the anterior and orbital regions of the frontal lobes. The fibers from the posterior frontal lobes and the parietal lobes pass through the body of the corpus callosum. The fibers forming the splenium originate from the occipital and temporal lobes. Because the corpus callosum is shorter than the hemispheres from front to back, its fiber radiations extend anteriorly and posteriorly to the frontal and occipital poles.

The fibers of the corpus callosum allow each hemisphere to access the memory traces, experiences, and unique learning abilities of the contralateral hemisphere. This close interaction underlying normal behavior is best illustrated by the studies conducted on patients who had undergone commissurotomy, described earlier in this chapter, which produced the so-called split brain paradigm. Surgical sectioning of the callosal fibers, undertaken as a medical treatment for epilepsy, rendered the cerebral hemispheres functionally independent.

The smaller **anterior commissure**, a second commissural bundle, contains crossing fibers other than the neocortical ones (Figs. 2-11 and 2-16). Originating from the ventral temporal lobe cortices, the anterior commissure interconnects two amygdaloid complexes and both olfactory systems.

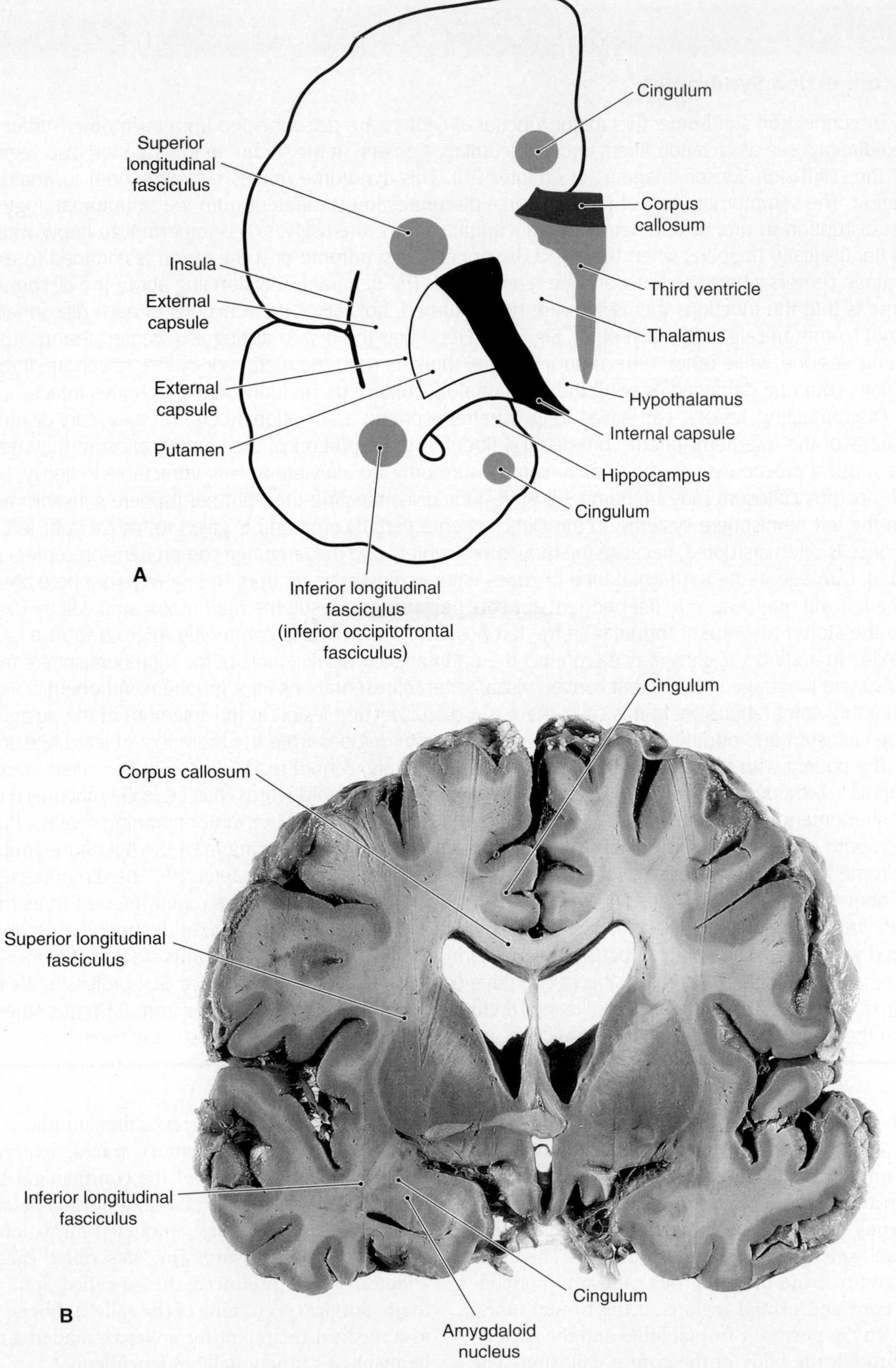

Figure 2-39 Locations of the major intrahemispheric association pathways: in a diagrammatic view (A) on a coronal section of the brain (B).

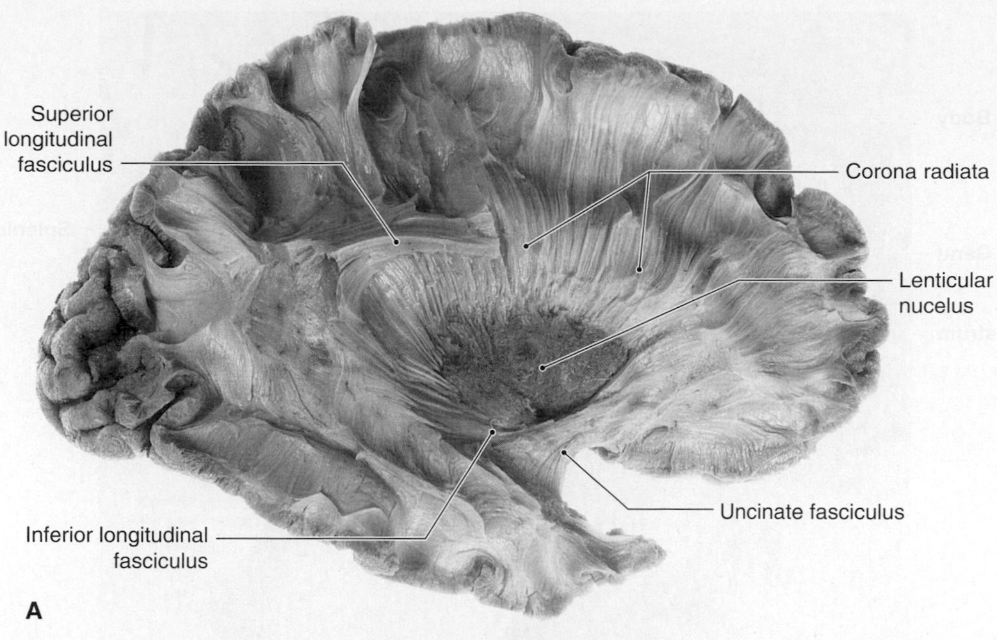

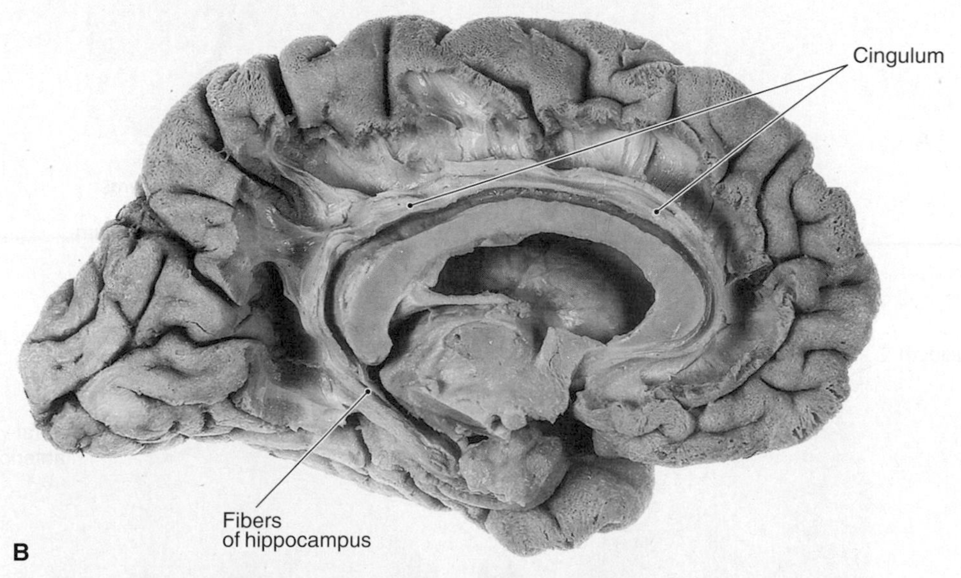

Figure 2-40 Dissected views of the long intrahemispheric association fibers: **A.** Superior and inferior longitudinal and uncinate fasciculi; **B.** The cingulate fasciculus.

Key Terms :

Epidural space	**Subarachnoid space**	**Tentorial notch**
Falx cerebri	**Subdural space**	
Meninges	**Tentorium cerebelli**	
Septum pellucidum		

MENINGES OF THE BRAIN

The soft and gelatinous nature of the CNS makes the brain and spinal cord susceptible to traumatic injuries. The structures that provide the basic protections to the CNS include the three meningeal layers: the cushioning CSF, the bony wall of the skull, and the vertebral column. The meninges consist of three concentric fibrous tissue membranes that encase the CNS: dura mater, arachnoid

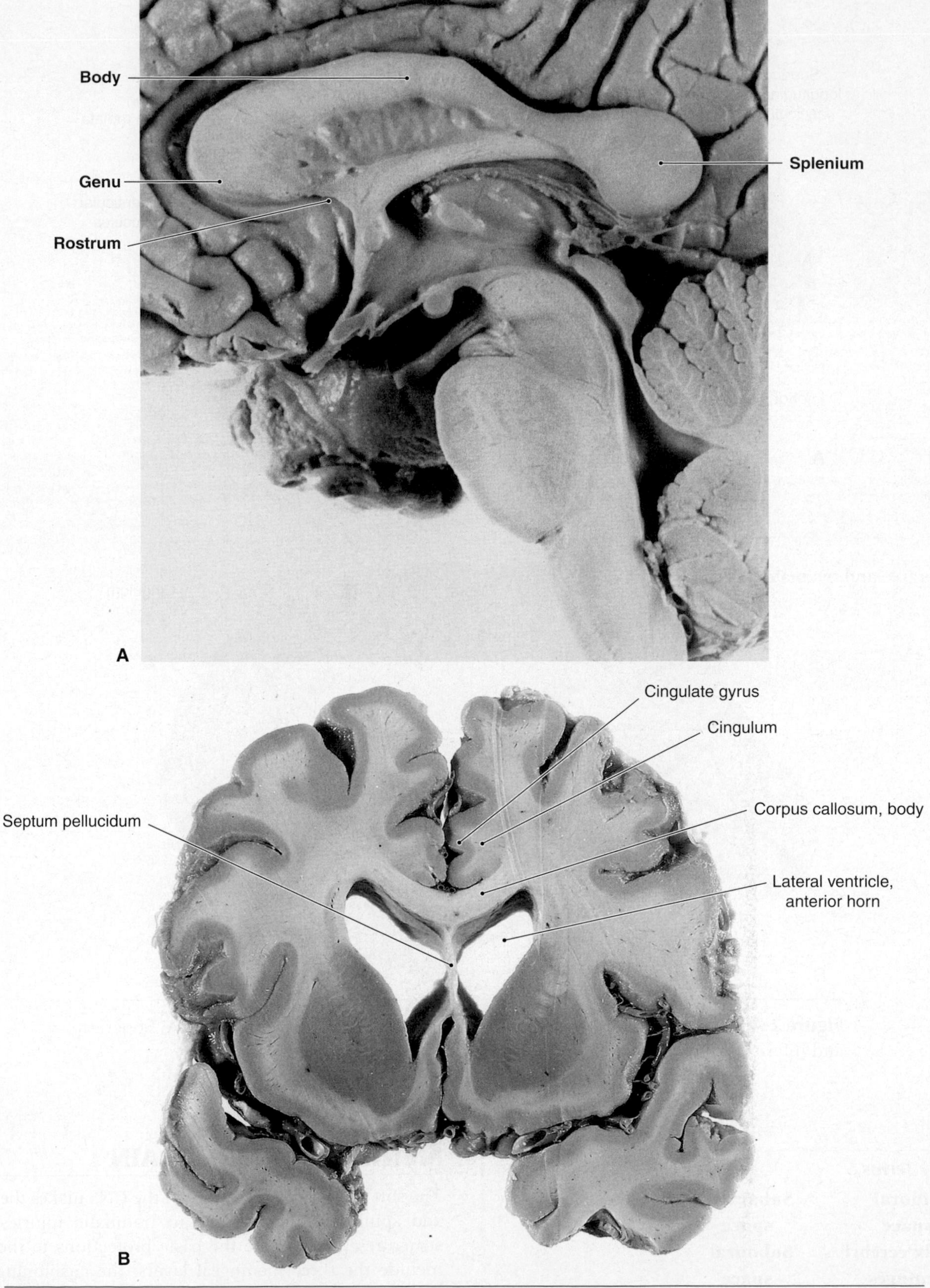

Figure 2-41 A. Midsagittal view of the corpus callosum. B. Coronal view of the corpus callosum and its radiating fibers.

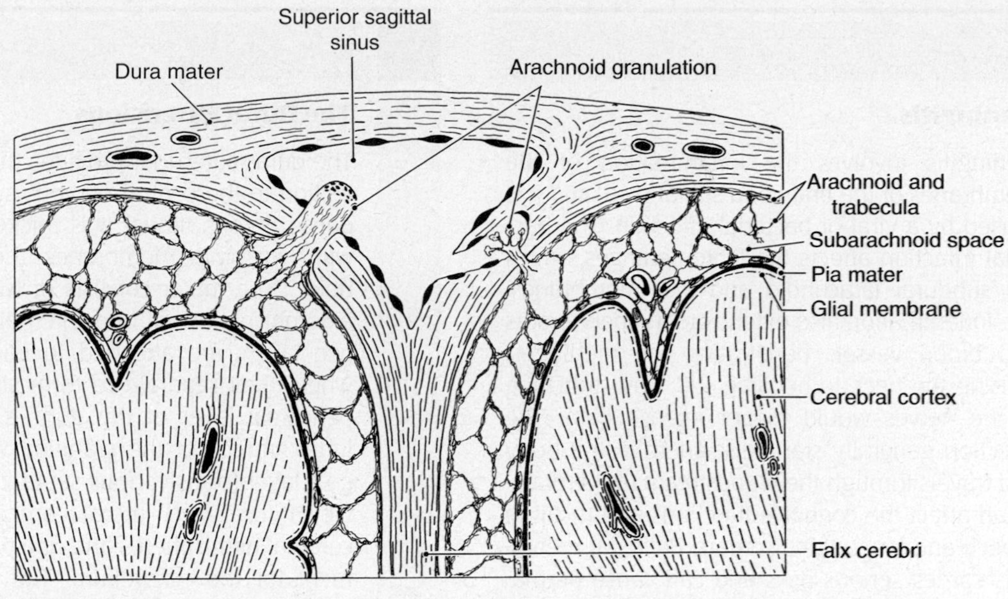

Figure 2-42 Diagrammatic illustration of the three meninges on a coronal section.

membrane, and pia mater (Fig. 2-42; Table 2-7). A pathologic condition associated with membranes of the CNS is viral or bacterial meningitis, which is associated with meningeal inflammation (Box 2-8).

Dura Mater

The dura mater, the gray outermost membrane, consists of dense, fibrous connective tissue and provides the maximum meningeal protection to the CNS. It is thicker and tougher than the pia and arachnoid membranes. The dura is attached to the inner surface of the skull and overlies the underlying arachnoid. There are two potential (not real) spaces around the cranial dura: **epidural** and **subdural**. The potential spaces are apparent only subsequent to pathologies. Epidural refers to the space between the dura mater and the bone; subdural is the space between the dura mater and the arachnoid. Both of these are the sites of vascular hemorrhages. Dura mater consists of two fibrous layers: external **periosteal** and internal **meningeal** (Box 2-9). The two layers are attached to each other, except where they separate to form sinuses that carry the blood from veins and absorb the circulated CSF (Fig. 2-43). The outer periosteal layer of the dura mater is attached to the inner surface of the cranium, and its meningeal layer forms various septa (dural extensions), which form

Table 2-7

Cerebral Versus Spinal Meninges

Cerebral Meninges	Spinal Meninges
Dura	
Adheres to inner skull; composed of two fused (periosteal and meningeal) layers that split to form sinuses	Composed of only meningeal layer; separates from vertebrae by epidural (potential) space
Arachnoid	
Attaches to dura in living condition (no subdural space); subarachnoid space with several cisterns	Attaches to dura in living condition (no subdural space); subarachnoid space with sacral cistern
Pia	
Adheres to the surface of brain, with extension within depth of sulci; follows vessels as they pierce cerebral cortex	Adheres to the surface of cord; specializations in the form of denticulate ligaments and filum terminale that attach to dural sac

BOX 2-8

Meningitis

Meningitis involves the inflammation of the membranes of the brain and spinal cord, and it is caused by a viral or bacterial infection. The bacterial infection affects the leptomeninges, which are subdural (arachnoid and pia) membranes. The inflammation also extends to the nerve roots and blood vessels penetrating the meninges, causing the neck to become stiff; any stretching of the nerves would trigger intense pain. The infection generally starts elsewhere in the body and travels through the bloodstream to the brain. It can affect the cognitive functions and result in speech and language disorders. Bacterial meningitis carries serious risks and can cause permanent brain damage and death. Group B streptococcus (in newborns), pneumococcus, Haemophilus influenzae type B, and meningococcus are common bacteria associated with meningitis. Viral meningitis is considered to have less serious consequences and its symptoms resolve on their own.

BOX 2-9

The Dural Extensions

The dura mater that provides the maximum protection to the central nervous system consists of dense fibrous tissue. It is thicker in comparison with two other membranes, the pia and arachnoid. Dura mater consists of two fibrous layers: external periosteal and internal meningeal. The two layers are attached to each other, except where they separate to form sinuses. The outer periosteal layer of the dura is attached to the inner surface of the cranium, while the meningeal layer forms various septa (dural extensions), which form two lateral compartments for the cerebral hemispheres and one posterior compartment for the cerebellum. The terms related to dural extensions (falx cerebri, tentorium cerebelli, and falx cerebelli) can be confusing but they are related structures.

two lateral compartments for the cerebral hemispheres and one posterior compartment for the cerebellum (Fig. 2-44).

Falx Cerebri

The **falx cerebri**, a dural extension, is named for its sickle shape and is the largest dural reflection. It extends longitudinally in the interhemispheric fissure and forms a vertical partition in the cranial cavity between the cerebral hemispheres (Fig. 2-44). Anteriorly, this dural reflection is attached to the crista galli of the ethmoid bone in the inner cranium; posteriorly, it extends to the internal occipital protuberance and the **tentorium cerebelli**, another dural reflection. At the dorsal edge of the interhemispheric fissure, the falx cerebri forms the cavity for the **superior sagittal sinus**. Within this fissure and above the corpus callosum, the **inferior sagittal sinus** is located along the free inferior margin of the falx cerebri.

Tentorium Cerebelli

The tentorium cerebelli, a dural extension, arises from the petrous portion of the temporal bone. Its attachments to the falx cerebri along the midline pull it up, creating a tent-like structure over the posterior fossa, which houses the cerebellum (Fig. 2-44). Its margins are between the cerebellum and the basal surface of the temporal and occipital lobes, so that the occipital lobes lie over it and the cerebellum is below it. Anteriorly, the free borders of the tentorium cerebelli constitute the opening named the tentorial incisure, or **tentorial notch**. The brainstem descends through the free borders of tentorial notch toward the foramen magnum. The space above the tentorium, the supratentorial space, contains the cerebral cortex. The space below the tentorium, the infratentorial space, contains the cerebellum and brainstem (Fig. 2-45).The supra and infratentorial spaces have clinical implications in traumatic brain injuries: increased intracranial pressure mostly due to cerebral edema, tumor, or subdural hematoma involving stretched veins results into an uncal (temporal) herniation through the notch in to the infratentorial space. Similarly, any increased cranial pressure in the infratentorial space results in the extension of the cerebellum (tonsillar) through the foramina Magnum. Both herniations critically affect sensorimotor skills and consciousness (Fig. 2-31*A*; Box 2-10).

Falx Cerebelli

The falx cerebelli is a small triangular vertical extension from the tentorium cerebelli that separates the cerebellar hemispheres (Figs. 2-44 and 2-45).

Arachnoid Membrane

The arachnoid membrane is a thin, nonvascular membrane between the internal pia mater and the external dura mater. It does not adhere to the cortical surface like the pia

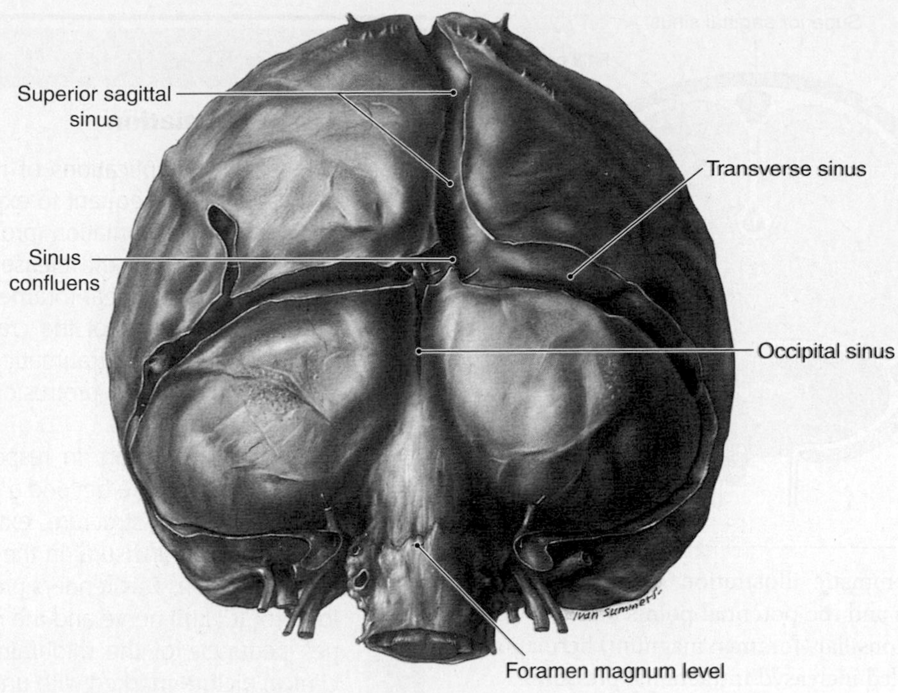

Figure 2-43 The dura surrounding the brain. The removed periosteal layer of the dura exposes the prominent dural sinuses.

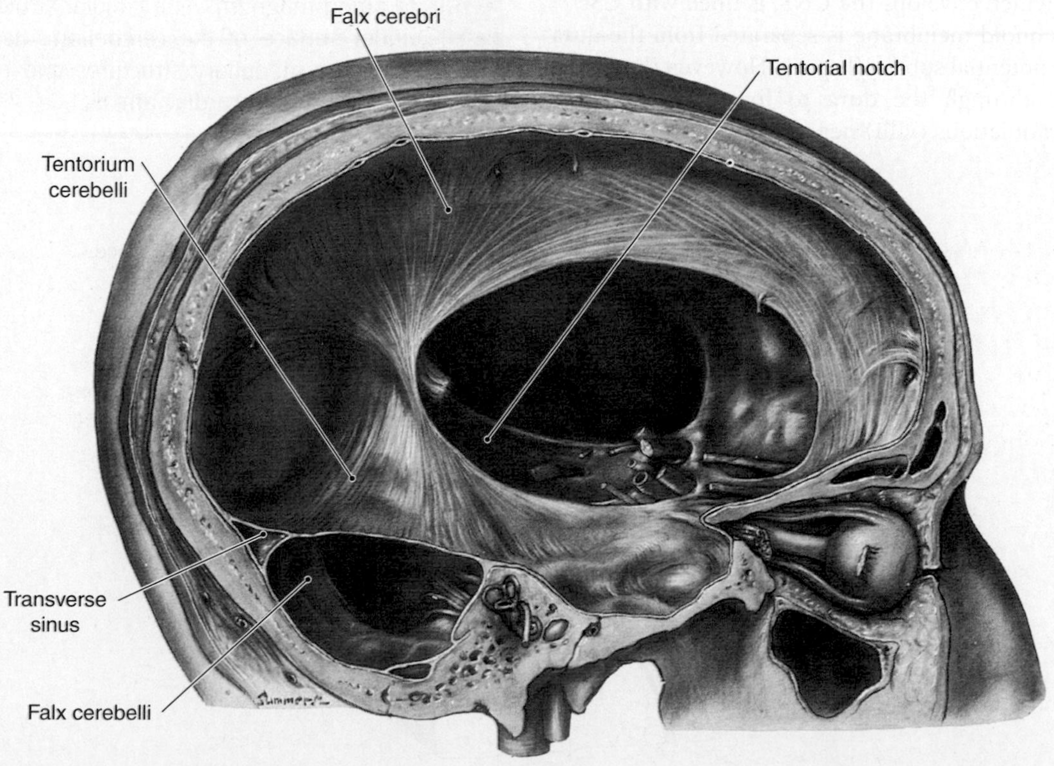

Figure 2-44 Midsagittal section of the brain with the dural extensions (falx cerebri, falx cerebelli, and tentorium cerebelli).

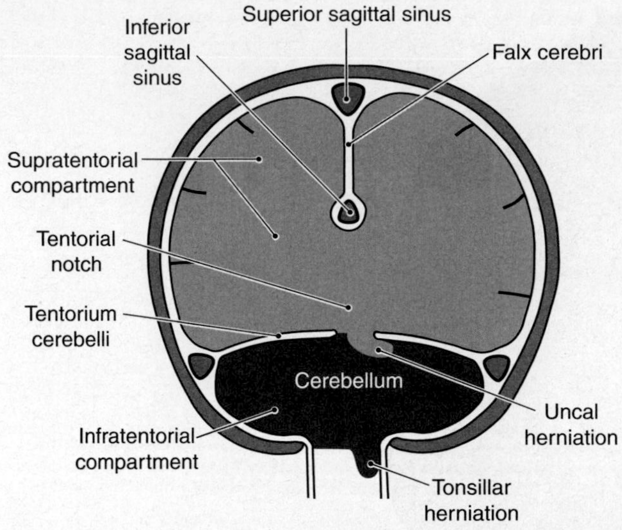

Figure 2-45 Diagrammatic illustration of the supra and infratentorial spaces and the potential points of uncal (tentorial incisure) and tonsillar (foramen magnum) herniations in case of uncontrolled increased intracranial pressure.

mater (Figs. 2-42 and 2-46) but bridges the cortical surface and the pia mater. The space between the pia and the arachnoid is traversed by the arachnoid **trabeculae**, which consist of fibrous and elastic connective tissue. Located between the arachnoid and the pia mater, the **subarachnoid space**, which envelops the CNS, is filled with CSF.

The arachnoid membrane is separated from the dura mater by the potential subdural space. However, the arachnoid pushes through the dura to form flower-shaped arachnoid granulations (villi) near the vertex of the brain.

BOX 2-10

Tissue Herniation

One of the complications of increased intracranial pressure subsequent to expanding lesions in the brain is the herniation (protrusion) of cortical tissue through the soft release points (openings) that involve meningeal foramen and are located in the lower region of the cranium. Commonly seen in subjects with traumatic brain injuries, two major cortical tissue protrusions are uncus and the cerebellar tonsils.

Uncal Herniation. In response to increased intracranial pressure beyond a point, the uncus, a medial temporal structure, extends through the tentorial notch (incisura) in the infratentorial cavity of the brain. This renders pressure on the oculomotor (CN III) nerve and the motor fibers in the pes peduncle of the midbrain and results in a clinical picture marked with unilateral or bilateral pupil dilations, lateral deviation of the affected eye, and weakness on the contralateral side of the body. A large or bilateral supratentorial lesion may give rise to decorticate rigidity (flexed upper extremities and extended lower extremities).

Cerebellar (tonsillar) Herniation. This involves the extension of the cerebellar tonsil through the foramen magnum. As a circular structure on the under surface of the cerebellum, its protrusion damages medullary structures and can lead to respiratory and cardiac arrests.

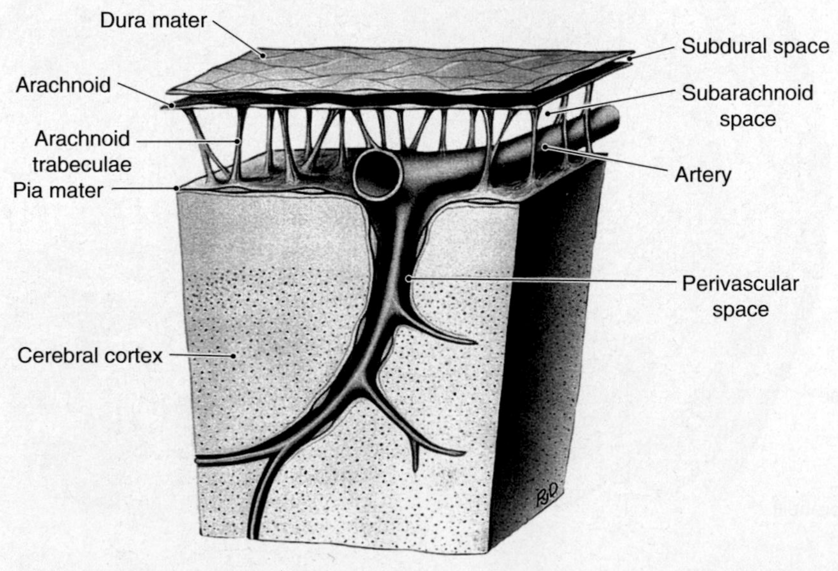

Figure 2-46 Diagrammatic illustration of the meninges of the brain in relation to the subarachnoid and perivascular space.

The arachnoid granulations, through which CSF drains into the vascular system, are predominantly located around the superior sagittal sinus on the dorsal surface of the brain.

Pia Mater

The pia mater, a thin, transparent, collagenous (connective tissue) membrane, is closely attached to the surface of the brain (Fig. 2-42). It adheres to the entire surface of the brain and thus follows the contours of the gyri and the sulci (Fig. 2-46). The pia mater also surrounds the blood vessels and forms the perivascular space. Both the pia and arachnoid membranes are relatively delicate, and together they are called the leptomeninges; they are most involved in cases of meningitis.

MENINGES OF THE SPINAL CORD

Spinal Dura Mater

As a part of the CNS, the spinal cord is equally protected by the three meningeal membranes, the CSF, and the bony vertebral column (Figs. 2-32 and 2-47). However, the spinal dura mater is a single-layer meningeal membrane; it lacks the cranial periosteal layer (Table 2-7). The spinal dura looks like a loose tube pierced by the spinal nerve roots. It is rostrally attached to the foramen magnum (Fig. 2-31), the opening in the occipital bone through which the spinal cord passes. The spinal dura is separated from the wall of spinal canal by an extradural space and extends in a sac formation to the S2 vertebral level, at which point it merges with the filum terminale to form the coccygeal ligament, a thin fibrous cord (Figs. 2-47 and 2-48). Anesthetic agents are injected into the epidural space to block nerve transmission of pain in the lower body.

Spinal Arachnoid Membrane

The arachnoid covering for the spinal cord begins at the foramen magnum and extends to the cauda equina. The subarachnoid space around the cord is filled with CSF. The arachnoid also invests the tubular projections of the spinal nerve roots from the cord to their foramina of exit. At the lumbar level of the spinal column, with the diminished cord size, the subarachnoid space extends into the **lumbar cistern**. With no cord structure present, the lumbar level is the best site for the **lumbar puncture** (spinal tap).

Spinal Pia Mater

The pia, the innermost protective layer, surrounds and tightly adheres to the spinal cord. The fibers of the dorsal and ventral spinal roots pierce the pia membrane. The cord suspended within the dural tube is not free; it is attached to the surrounding dura mater by a series of denticulate ligaments on both sides. These fibrous ligaments originate from the pia mater at the lateral surface

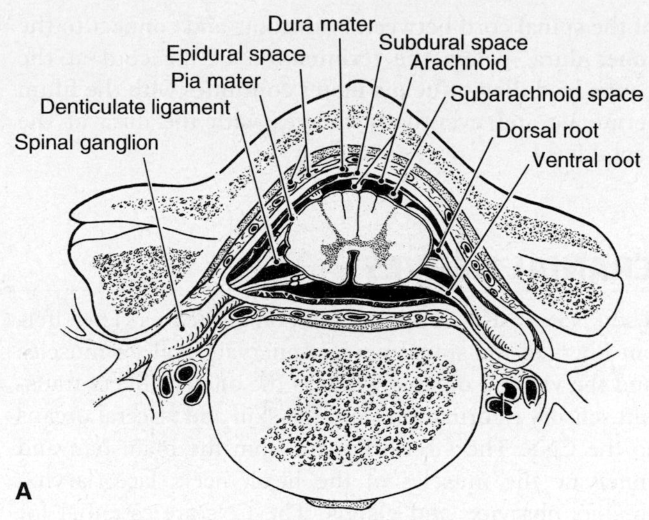

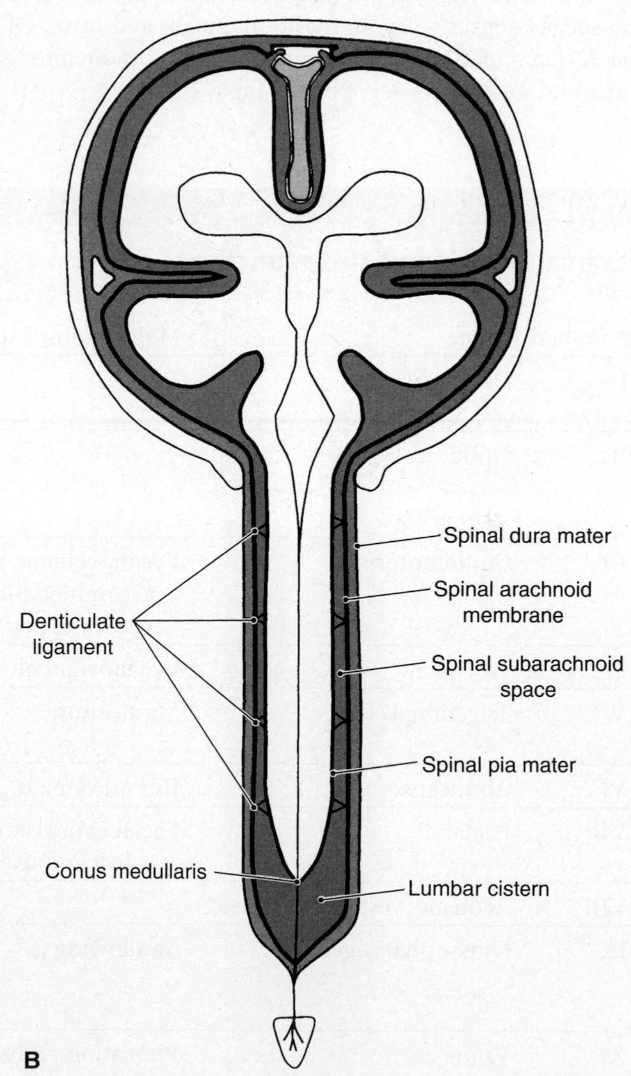

Figure 2-47 A. Cross section of the spinal cord and its meningeal coverings. B. The relationship of the meningeal membranes to the brain and spinal cord.

of the spinal cord between both roots and connect to the inner dura. Below the termination of the cord at the conus medullaris, the pia mater continues with the filum terminale and eventually merges with the dura at the sacral level.

CRANIAL NERVES

The PNS consists of **spinal** and **cranial nerves**. The efferent fibers of the spinal nerves innervate skeletal muscles and the visceral organs, whereas the afferent fibers transmit sensory information from the skin and visceral organs to the CNS. The CNs originate from the brainstem and innervate the muscles of the head, neck, face, larynx, tongue, pharynx, and glands. The CNs are essential for speech, resonance, and phonation. In addition, they serve the special senses—vision, audition, smell, and taste. Of the 12 pairs of CNs, some serve either sensory or motor functions, and others serve both (Table 2-8).

Nomenclature

CNs are both numbered and named. The Roman numerals (CN I–CN XII) indicate the sequence in which the CNs exit and/or enter the brain. The names contain information describing some or all the functional characteristics of the nerves (Table 2-8). A series of acronyms (listing the first letter) can be used to learn the names of the CNs, such as OOO for olfactory, optic, and oculomotor nerves.

Another method of learning the names and order of the CNs is the following commonly used acrostic: **O**n (olfactory) **o**ld (optic) **O**lympus' (oculomotor) **t**opmost (trochlear) **t**op (trigeminal), **a** (abducens) **F**inn (facial) **a**nd (acoustic; vestibulocochlear) **G**erman (glossopharyngeal) **v**iewed (vagus) **a** (accessory) **h**op (hypoglossal).

Functions

CNs exit and/or enter the CNS at various points. Consequently, they have also been categorized in relation to their anatomic location in the CNS (Table 2-9). The first two (olfactory and optic) CNs are related to the cerebral

Table 2-8

Cranial Nerves and Their Functions

Number	Name	Major Motor Function	Major Sensory Function
I	Olfactory		Smell: sends information from nasal mucosa to olfactory bulb
II	Optic		Vision: sends messages from retina to visual cortex (vision) and superior colliculus (reflexes)
III	Oculomotor	Eye movement; regulation of pupil; accommodation of lens for near vision; upper lid elevation	
IV	Trochlear	Eye movement	
V	Trigeminal	Mastication	Sensation: face, orbit, and oral structures
VI	Abducens	Eye movement	
VII	Facial	Facial expression; secretion of saliva and tears	Taste: anterior two-thirds of tongue
VIII	Acoustic; vestibulocochlear		Equilibrium and audition
IX	Glossopharyngeal	Swallowing	Taste: posterior third of tongue; visceral sensation from palate and oral pharynx
X	Vagus	Phonation and swallowing	Sensation: pharyngeal cavity, thoracic and abdominal organs
XI	Accessory	Head movement and shoulder elevation	
XII	Hypoglossal	Tongue movement	

Table 2-9

Location-Based Classification of the Cranial Nerves

Location	Cranial Nerves
Prosencephalon (forebrain)	
Telencephalon	I (olfactory)
Diencephalon	II (optic)
Mesencephalon (midbrain)	III (oculomotor) IV (trochlear)
Rhombencephalon (hindbrain)	
Metencephalon (pons)	V (trigeminal) VI (abducens) VII (facial) VIII (acoustic; vestibulocochlear)
Myelencephalon (medulla oblongata)	IX (glossopharyngeal) X (vagus) XI (spinal accessory) XII (hypoglossal)

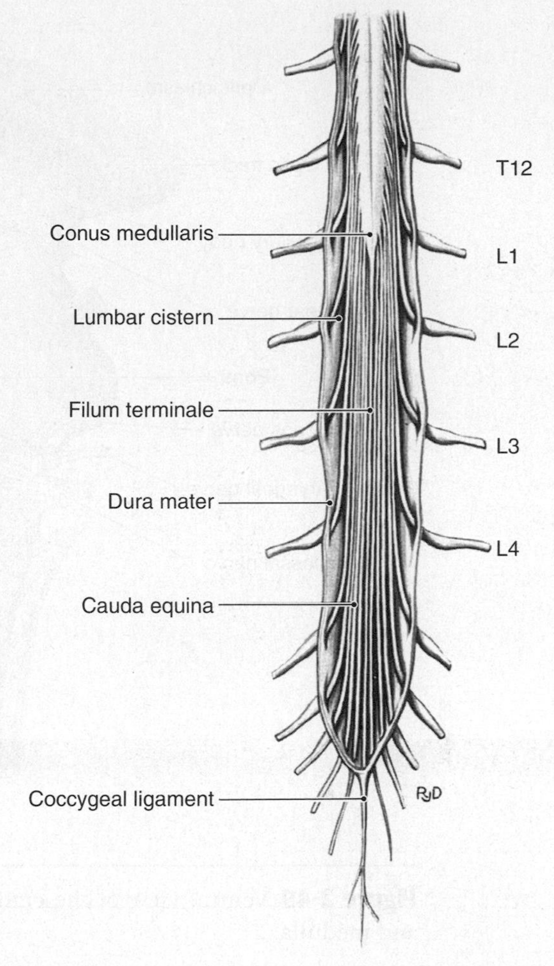

Figure 2-48 Posterior view of the lumbosacral cord, conus medullaris, and lumbar cistern.

cortex; the remaining ten nerves originate from the brainstem. CNs are best seen on the ventral or lateral surface of the brainstem (Fig. 2-51).

The **olfactory nerve** (**CN I**), a sensory nerve, is responsible for the perception of smell. It originates from the receptor cells in the mucosa of the nasal cavity and synapses in the olfactory bulbs on the orbital surface of the frontal lobe. The axons from the bulb travel in the olfactory tract and terminate in the cortical olfactory area (pyriform cortex) of the medial temporal lobe (Figs. 2-7 and 2-8). An interruption of olfactory fibers impairs the sense of smell.

The **optic nerve** (**CN II**) is a brain tract concerned with visual sensation. Optic nerves originate from the retina in both eyes and unite at the optic chiasm at the base of the brain. The crossed and uncrossed optic fibers continue in the optic tract and, via the thalamus, project information from each eye to the visual cortex in the occipital lobes (Figs. 2-7, 2-8, and 2-50). Injury to any part of the visual pathway results in a selective visual field loss (scotoma).

The **oculomotor nerve** (**CN III**), a motor nerve, controls four of the six muscles responsible for moving the eyeball. It emerges from the ventral surface of the midbrain medial to the pes pedunculi (Fig. 2-49). Complete interruption of the oculomotor nerve results in ptosis of the eyelid, dilation of the pupil, and an abducted (laterally deviated) position of the eye. The oculomotor nerve also innervates the **levator palpebrae**, which raises the upper eyelid. Interruption of the nerve to this muscle causes ptosis through the loss of this function.

The **trochlear nerve** (**CN IV**), a motor nerve, controls one of the muscles responsible for eye movement. The trochlear nerve exits from the brainstem below the inferior colliculus (Fig. 2-51). It is the only motor nerve to exit the brainstem from the dorsal surface. A trochlear lesion or injury is associated with impaired downward gaze.

The **trigeminal nerve** (**CN V**) and the next three nerves (CN VI–CN VIII) originate in the tegmentum of the pons. The trigeminal is a functionally mixed nerve with both sensory and motor functions. Primarily, it is a sensory nerve for the face, head, and oral structures and a motor nerve for jaw movements. It is a large nerve in the pons, and its sensory and motor roots leave the brainstem from the ventrolateral surface of the pons (Fig. 2-49 and 2-51). Loss of trigeminal function is associated with facial sensory loss and paralysis of the jaw.

The **abducens nerve** (**CN VI**), a motor nerve, controls the lateral rectus muscle, which turns the eyeball away from the nose. Fibers of the abducens nerve originate in the tegmentum of the pons and emerge ventrally from the junction of the pons and the medulla oblongata

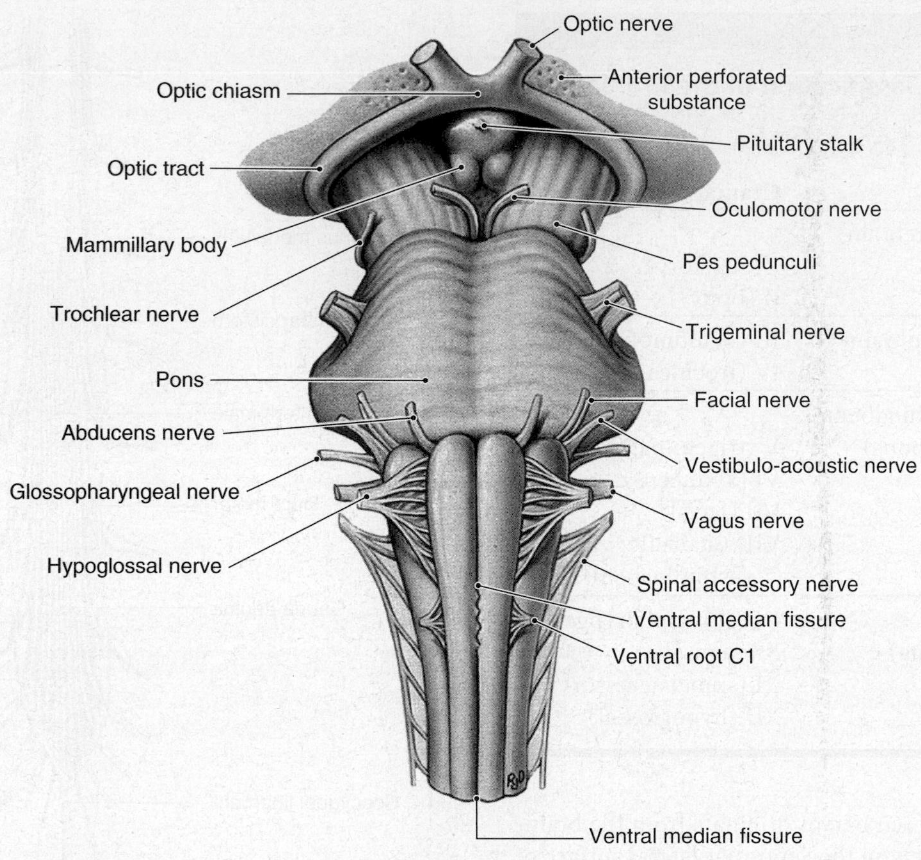

Figure 2-49 Ventral view of the cranial nerves exiting from the midbrain, pons, and medulla.

(Fig. 2-49 and 2-51). Interruption of this nerve results in partial ocular paralysis with a medially fixed eye.

The **facial nerve** (**CN VII**) is primarily a motor nerve, but it also has some sensory functions. As the name implies, this nerve controls all muscles of facial expression. It also serves the sense of taste from the anterior two-thirds of the tongue. Fibers of this nerve exit from the ventrolateral surface of the pons at its border with the medulla (Figs. 2-49 and 2-51). A facial nerve lesion results in facial paralysis and loss of taste sensation.

The **vestibulocochlear**, or **acoustic, nerve** (**CN VIII**), is a sensory nerve with, as its name implies, two divisions: **vestibular** and **acoustic**. The vestibular division is concerned with the position of the head in space; the acoustic portion is concerned with hearing.

This is a large nerve: its rootlets are lateral to the roots of the facial nerve, and its fibers enter the brainstem at the ventrolateral surface of the pons at its junction with the medulla. As such, the vestibulocochlear nerve's location is the landmark of the pontomedullary junction (Figs. 2-49 and 2-51). Interruption of the vestibulocochlear nerve is associated with impaired hearing and equilibrium disorders.

The **glossopharyngeal nerve** (**CN IX**) originates in the medulla oblongata (Figs. 2-49 and 2-51). It serves both sensory and motor functions: its sensory function is to process the sensation of touch and taste from the posterior third of the tongue and oral pharynx; its motor function is to contribute to the process of swallowing. Its fibers leave the medulla just below the acoustic nerve from the lateral surface. A glossopharyngeal lesion results in the loss of taste sensation from the posterior third of the tongue and mild dysphagia (swallowing disorder).

The **vagus nerve** (**CN X**), the largest CN, has a wide distribution of its fibers. Its fibers leave the brainstem from the lateral medulla just below the point of exit for the glossopharyngeal nerve (Figs. 2-49 and 2-51). Although the vagus is primarily a sensory nerve, it has a motor component, which activates the muscles of the pharynx, larynx, and soft palate. Vagus nerve pathology results in decreased sensation from and activation of visceral organs and paralysis of the larynx and pharynx.

The **spinal accessory nerve** (**CN XI**), a motor nerve, innervates muscles for controlling head movement. The spinal roots exit from the four cervical segments and contribute to the innervation of neck and shoulder muscles. A spinal accessory nerve injury causes restricted neck movement and weakness of the shoulder.

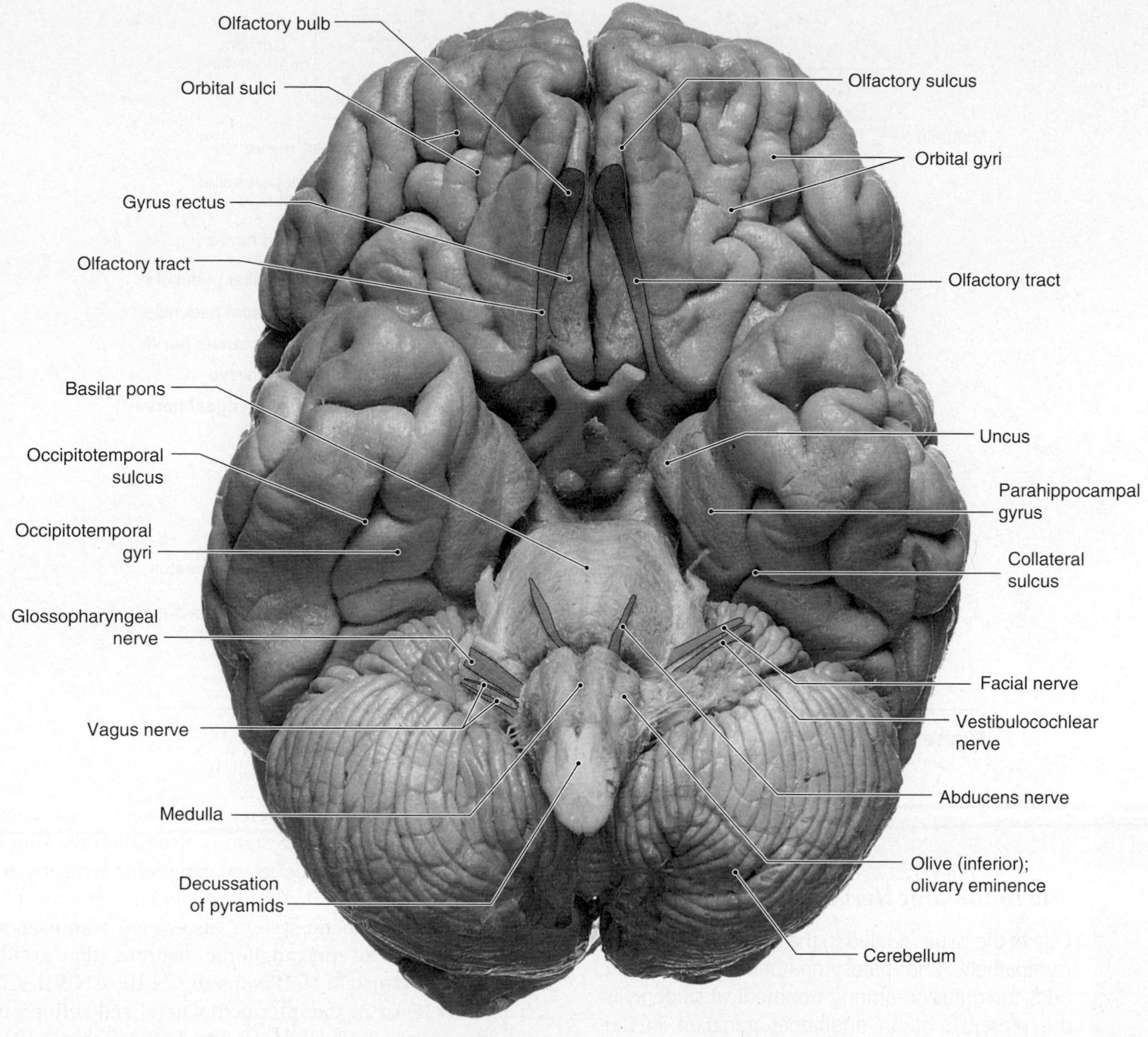

Figure 2-50 Ventral view of the cerebral hemispheres, brainstem, and cerebellum with exposed cranial nerves.

The **hypoglossal nerve** (CN XII) is a motor nerve, innervating the muscles of tongue. The nucleus is in the medulla, and its fibers exit the medulla just lateral to the pyramid (formed by axons of the corticospinal tract) in the medulla (Figs. 2-49 and 2-51). The branches of this nerve innervate all intrinsic and some extrinsic muscles of the tongue. A pathologic condition of the hypoglossal nerve results in paralysis of half of the tongue.

Key Terms :

Parasympathetic system	**Preganglion**
Postganglion	**Sympathetic system**

AUTONOMIC NERVOUS SYSTEM

The ANS, an autonomous and self-monitoring system, is regulated by the hypothalamus in the CNS. The ANS consists of sensory and motor components (Box 2-11). It receives a constant flow of sensation (general visceral afferents) from the visceral organs, the detectors of carbon dioxide levels in the blood, and from the stretching of internal organs or blood vessels. It controls the motor activity of smooth and cardiac muscles, such as the lungs, kidney, urogenital area, gastrointestinal tract, blood vessel walls, eyes, and heart. The ANS also regulates the secretion of the glands that produce salivation, sweating, and lacrimation (tears) as well as the gastric, intestinal, and pancreatic glands.

The motor component of the ANS consists of the **sympathetic** and **parasympathetic systems**. There are

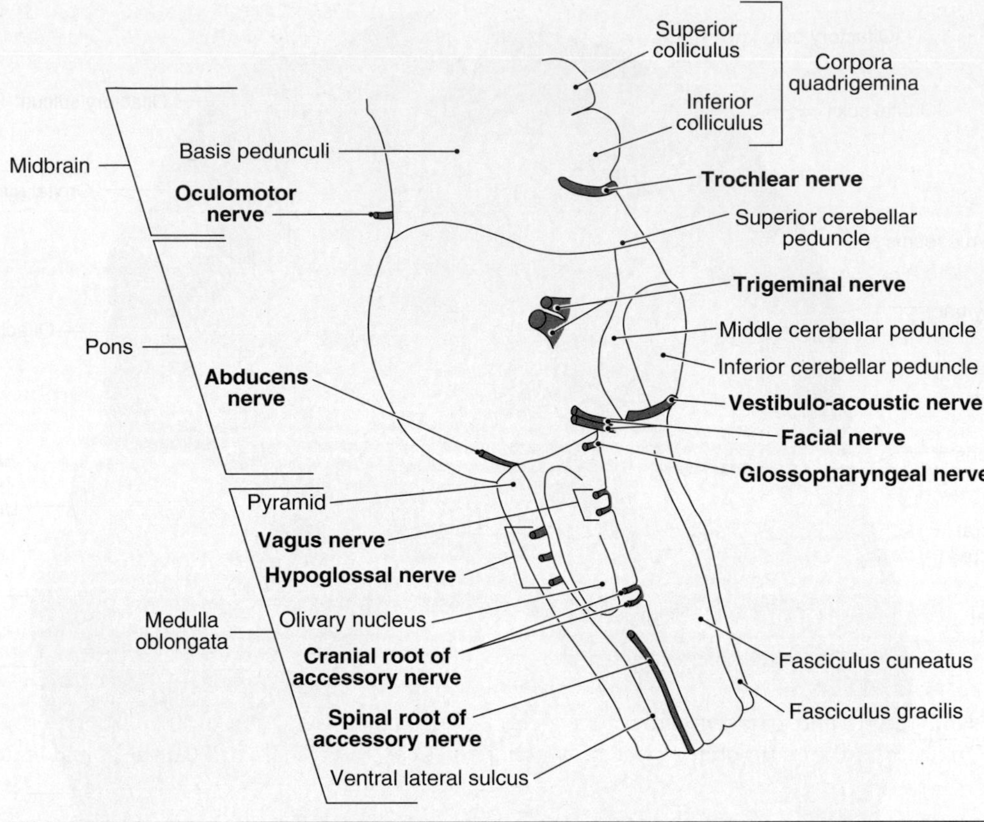

Figure 2-51 Lateral view of the brainstem with cranial nerve roots.

BOX 2-11

The Autonomic Nervous System

One of the issues related to the autonomic nervous (sympathetic and parasympathetic) system that adds to confusion among nonmedical students is the presence of an additional ganglion in the peripheral nervous system. This additional ganglion, not included in the somatic efferent system, is part of the circuitry used for controlling the autonomic activities of limbs and trunk. Its presence gives rise to two additional terms: preganglionic and postganglionic. The fibers from the CNS projecting to this peripheral ganglion are preganglionic axons, and the fibers from this ganglion to the target organs are postganglionic. The sympathetic and parasympathetic systems also differ in terms of the location of this peripheral ganglion, which is next to the spinal cord (in the spinal chain) in the case of the sympathetic system but is closer to the target organ in the parasympathetic system. The sympathetic fibers innervate sweat glands, smooth muscles of blood vessels of skin and vessels of the central nervous system. The parasympathetic efferents influence the glands, smooth muscles of the eye, trachea, lungs, and esophagus.

anatomic and functional differences between these components. The sympathetic system is also called the **thoracolumbar division** because its preganglionic neurons are present in the lateral cell column of spinal segments T1–L2. The parasympathetic system, also called **craniosacral system**, consists of preganglionic neurons that reside either in the brainstem (for axons to CN III, CN VII, CN IX, and CN X) or in the intermediolateral cell column of spinal segments S2–S4 (Figs. 18-2 and 18-4; Table 2-10).

Sympathetic ganglia (clusters of nerve cells) usually innervate many organs, whereas parasympathetic ganglia innervate a single organ. Together the sympathetic and parasympathetic systems monitor, regulate, and sustain optimum visceral functions essential to survival. They function by exerting a dual innervation on the visceral organs and glands; both systems serve the same visceral organs but produce opposite effects. For example, the sympathetic system spends energy (catabolic) and prepares for fight and flight. In so doing, it constricts the blood vessels of the skin, visceral organs, and bronchial passages; induces perspiration; dilates pupils; and mobilizes glucose (see Chapter 18). The parasympathetic system conserves energy; dominant during relaxation or sleep, it constricts the pupils, decreases body metabolism, and lowers the heart rate (see Chapter 18). This is possible because of the involvement of different neurotransmitters.

Functionally, the sympathetic system spends energy by stimulating the organs and preparing for fight and

Table 2-10

Subdivisions of the Autonomic Nervous System

Division	Nuclei Location	Function
Sympathetic system	Thoracolumbar	Expending energy in flight, fright, or fight conditions
Parasympathetic system	Craniosacral	Restoring energy

flight. In doing so, it induces perspiration; dilates the pupils; accelerates heart rate; and mobilizes glucose by dilating the blood vessels in skeletal muscles, cardiac muscles, and the branchial passage.

Most of the visceral organs are under dual innervation by efferent fibers of the sympathetic and parasympathetic systems. Some internal organs, however, are innervated by only one system. The structures under only sympathetic innervation are the sweat glands, pili erector muscles (attached to the hair follicles), kidneys, and most blood vessels. The lacrimal gland, on the other hand, receives only parasympathetic innervation.

The ANS (sympathetic and parasympathetic) system structurally differs from the somatic motor system, which is used for activating the limbs and trunk (Fig. 2-52). In the somatic motor system, the motor nuclei are in the spinal cord, and their axons (spinal nerves) extend to skeletal (striated) muscles. The ANS uses an additional ganglion in the PNS, which is a cause of confusion for students of human behavior as it introduces two additional words: **preganglionic** and **postganglionic**. The fibers from the CNS projecting to this ganglion are preganglionic axons, and the fibers from this ganglion to the target organs are postganglionic. Preganglionic fibers are mostly myelinated; the postganglionic fibers, on the other hand, are largely unmyelinated, and thus the conduction of impulses in them is slow, ranging from 1 to 2 m per second. The sympathetic and parasympathetic systems also differ in terms of the location of this peripheral ganglion, which is next to the spinal cord (in the spinal chain) in the case of the sympathetic system but closer to the target organ in the parasympathetic system (Figs. 18-2 and 18-4).

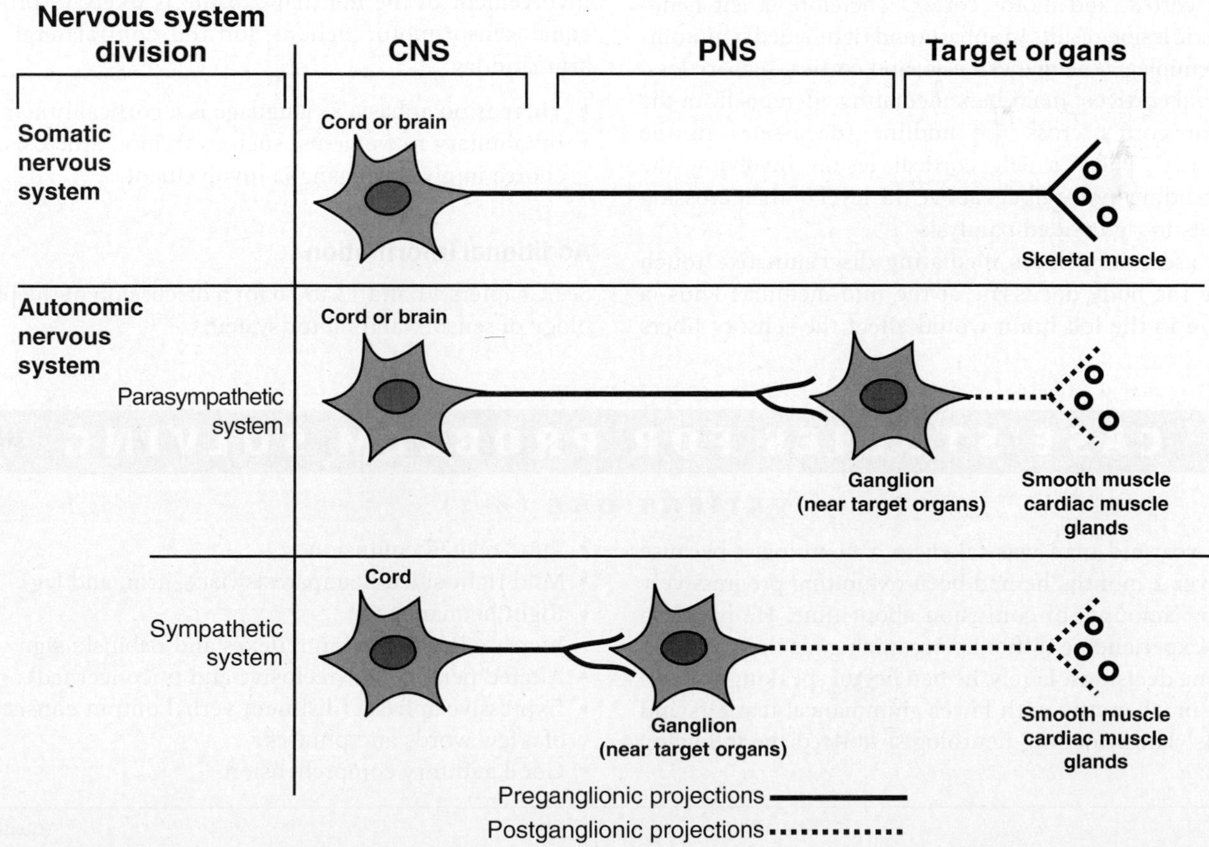

Figure 2-52 Diagrammatic illustration of the projectional difference between the somatic and the autonomic nervous systems.

CLINICAL CORRELATES

Lesion Localization

Rule 1: Symptoms Suggesting a Cortical Lesion

Dominant Hemisphere

Contralateral hemiplegia, contralateral hemianesthesia of face, trunk, upper, and lower extremity, and cortical sensory loss (failure to identify an object through touch or to identify a letter or word written on the surface of the skin) suggest a cortical lesion.

Dominant Hemisphere

In addition to presenting cortical symptoms, a dominant hemispheric lesion results in aphasia, apraxia, finger agnosia, and acalculia.

Nondominant Hemisphere

In addition to presenting cortical symptoms, an injury in the nondominant (right) hemisphere also results in left-sided neglect or inattention, constructional and/or dressing deficits (apraxia), spatial and temporal disorientation, impaired prosody in speech, and impaired ability to recognize faces.

Rationale

- The cerebrum contains the language cortex, somatosensory cortex, and motor cortex. Therefore, a left hemispheric lesion results in aphasia and right-sided symptoms of hemiplegia, hemianesthesia, and cortical sensory loss.
- Lateral corticospinal fibers mediating efferents from the motor cortex cross the midline (decussate) in the medulla. Thus, a left cortical lesion involving the descending motor fibers above the level of their crossing results in right-sided paralysis.
- The ascending fibers mediating discriminative touch from the body decussate at the mid-medulla. Thus, a lesion in the left brain would affect the sensory fibers originating from the right half of the body and result in sensory loss (anesthesia) in the right side of the body.
- The right (nondominant) hemisphere regulates visuospatial orientation, emotional and prosodic function, attention, and sensorimotor control for the left half of the body. Thus, visual-spatial functions would be affected by a right cortical lesion.

Additional Information

See Chapter 7 for the vascular system, Chapter 11 for somatic sensation, Chapters 13 to 16 for the physiology of motor systems, and Chapter 19 for neurolinguistic properties of the brain and higher mental functions.

Rule 2: Symptoms Suggesting a Subcortical Lesion

Presenting Symptoms

Contralateral hemiplegia and diminution or loss of pain and temperature equally for the face, arms, and legs, but with no loss of higher mental functions, are associated with a subcortical (internal capsule) lesion. Emergence of involuntary movements suggests a basal ganglia lesion.

Rationale

All of the descending motor fibers and ascending sensory fibers pass through the internal capsule. Thus, any involvement of the internal capsule is likely to produce equal sensorimotor deficits for the contralateral face, arm, and leg.

- There is no aphasia as language is a cortical function.
- Involuntary movements, such as tremor, athetosis, and chorea imply basal ganglia involvement.

Additional Information

See Chapters 11 and 13 to 16 for a discussion of the physiology of sensory and motor systems.

CASE STUDIES FOR PROBLEM SOLVING

PATIENT ONE (2-1)

A 52-year-old man was taken to a neurologist because for over 2 months he had been exhibiting progressively greater amounts of confusion about time. He had also been experiencing difficulty organizing his thoughts and making decisions. Lately, he had begun speaking a somewhat incoherently with fewer grammatical markers and words. The attending neurologist noticed the following signs:

- Time-related confusion
- Mild right-sided hemiparesis (face, arm, and leg)
- Right hemianopsia
- Increased deep tendon reflexes and Babinski sign
- Altered personality (reclusive and unconcerned)
- Expressive aphasia (disfluent verbal output consisting of a few words and phrases)
- Good auditory comprehension

(Continued)

CASE ONE (2-1) *(CONTINUED)*

The physician suspected a brain tumor (neoplastic growth). MRI studies revealed a left cortical neoplastic mass bordering the frontoparietotemporal region. The patient was referred for biopsy; surgical removal of the tumor, if possible; and then radiation treatment, if needed.

Question: How can you relate these clinical signs to the structures involved? What made the neurologist rule out a stroke during the examination?

Case (2-1) Discussion: See discussion of case studies.

PATIENT TWO (2-2)

The family of a 75-year-old man with progressive difficulty with language and bladder control took him to the family physician. Suspecting a case of a tumor, he ordered an MRI investigation and speech language pathologist (SLP) consult. MRI studies revealed two tumors: first involving the tempora parietal regions in the left brain and second involving the cauda equina region of the spinal cord.

The patient had difficulty in urinary retention and fecal continence which was clear during his SLP evaluation which indicated markedly confused and incohesive language with moderate memory problems.

Question: How can you relate these social symptoms to his lower spinal tumor?

Case 2-2 Discussion: See discussion of case studies.

PATIENT THREE (2-3)

A 30-year-old man who had a history of being social, detail oriented, and focused had gradually changed, becoming depressed, indifferent, and socially detached. For the past 2 to 3 months, he did not want to work and spent time sitting, staring, and procrastinating. He was seen by a neurologist who noted the following:

- Indifferent attitude and little desire to do anything
- Easily distractable
- Socially inappropriate use of language
- Impaired sense of smell
- Nose picking in public
- Paucity of verbalization
- A brain MRI study revealed a tumor in the anterior cranial fossa bilaterally affecting the frontal lobes.

Question: Can you relate these symptoms to the associated region of the brain?

Case (2-3) Discussion: See discussion of case studies.

PATIENT FOUR (2-4)

A husband and wife speech language pathologist team participated in a cognitive experiment in which they were examined with functional brain MRI studies. Both were horrified to see that one had a structure bridging the space in the third ventricle, but the other did not. Each attributed this as the cause of the other's weird personality and psychosomatic discomforts.

Question: Can you identify the structure that crosses through the third ventricle to connect both thalami?

Case (2-4) Discussion: See discussion of case studies.

PATIENT FIVE (2-5)

A 60-year-old woman developed severe dysarthria after undergoing carotid endarterectomy. This is a surgical procedure used to clean the atherosclerotic plaque from the right internal carotid artery, a major artery that supplies blood to the brain. The surgeon assured the patient that the symptoms would resolve soon and she could expect a full recovery. The consulting SLP noted the woman exhibited the following:

- Paresis involving the right half of the face
- Paralysis of the right half of the tongue
- Unintelligible speech owing to slurred speech
- Slow articulatory movements
- Distorted consonants and vowel prolongation
- Aphonia, diplophonia, and breathiness
- Difficulty swallowing
- Good auditory comprehension and no signs of aphasia

Question: Can you discuss the cranial nerves that were affected in this patient?

Case (2-5) Discussion: See discussion of case studies.

(Continued)

CASE SIX (2-6)

A 55-year-old man, who initially complained of a constant headache, had gradually developed poor balance and lacked concentration. He was seen by a neurologist who noted the following:

- Difficulty walking, with small shuffled steps
- Slow thinking and inattentiveness, which caused loss of immediate memory
- No signs of motor weakness or sensory loss
- Bladder incontinence
- The brain MRI study revealed two large lateral ventricles, a wide third ventricle, and a normal size fourth ventricle.

Question: Can you identify the foramen that was blocked in this case?

- Foramen of Magendie
- Foramen of Luschka
- Interventricular foramen
- Cerebral aqueduct
- Foramina of Magendie and Luschka

Case (2-6) **Discussion:** See discussion of case studies.

CASE SEVEN (2-7)

A 75-year-old right-handed man, who was diagnosed with stroke and aphasia, was seen by a SLP, who noted the following:

- Fluently spoken and well-articulated speech
- Speech consisting of meaningless strings of words
- Poor repetitions
- Impaired comprehension for both spoken and written language
- Moderate anomia
- Optimistic attitude

The MRI study revealed a large ischemic stroke in the left inferior parietal lobule involving Brodmann areas 22, 39, and 40.

Question: Can you identify the type of aphasia and the lesion site?

- Transcortical aphasia related to a lesion in the pars triangularis region
- Conduction aphasia related to a postcentral gyrus lesion
- Wernicke aphasia related to a lesion affecting the posterosuperior temporal, angular, and supramarginal gyri
- Visual agnosia related to a lesion in the anterior temporal gyrus
- Anomic aphasia related to a prefrontal lesion

Case (2-7) **Discussion:** See discussion of case studies.

SUMMARY

The human nervous system, which consists of the CNS (brain and spinal cord) and PNS (spinal and CNs), is the generator of the electrical and chemical energy that controls body parts and their functions. The brain is responsible for initiating, controlling, and regulating all sensorimotor and cognitive (mental) functions. The spinal cord carries sensory and motor commands, both somatic and visceral, to and from body parts that interact with the environment. The bony shell of the skull; the vertebral column; and the dural, arachnoid, and pial layers of the meninges protect the CNS. CSF in the subarachnoid space also helps protect the brain and spinal cord by serving as a mechanical buffer. Embryologically, the brain is derived from three vesicles: prosencephalon, mesencephalon, and rhombencephalon. The cerebral hemispheres, basal ganglia, limbic lobe, thalamus, hypothalamus, and lateral and third ventricles are derived from the prosencephalon. The mesencephalon develops into the midbrain and cerebral aqueduct, whereas the rhombencephalon gives rise to the pons, cerebellum, medulla oblongata, and fourth ventricle. Each of these structures serves a specific sensorimotor or regulating function. The PNS, which includes spinal and cranial nerves, extends to organs, muscles, joints, blood vessels, and skin surfaces, forming an extensive network of cables and fine wires throughout the body. The PNS consists of the somatic and autonomic nervous systems. The somatic motor and sensory nerves innervate skeletal muscles, whereas the autonomic sensory and motor nerves innervate the visceral organs and glands. CNs regulate the sensory and motor functions of the face and head.

REVIEW QUESTIONS

1. Complete the following statements using the appropriate technical terms:

   A. Comprised of caudate nucleus, putamen, globus pallidus, claustrum, and amygdaloid nucleus, the __________ are known to regulate cortically generated motor functions.

   B. Consisting of cranial nerve (CN) nuclei, longitudinal fiber tracts, and the reticular formation, the __________ connects the forebrain to the spinal cord.

   C. The brainstem exits the cranium through the __________ and connects with the spinal cord.

   D. The __________ represents the spinal nerve roots that arise from the lumbosacral region and pass through the lumbar cistern before exiting the vertebral canal

   E. The lower terminal point of the spinal cord is referred to as the __________.

   F. Bordering medially the inferior horns of the lateral ventricles, the limbic structure of __________ is thought to be related to memory functions.

   G. As the controller of the autonomic nervous system, the __________ also regulates endocrinic functions and maintains body temperature, blood volume, food and water intake, body mass, reproduction, and the regulation of circadian rhythms.

   H. The brain system that regulates emotional drive to visceral and vegetative functions such as instinctual reflexes, aggression, anxiety, and fear is the __________

   I. The meninges that protect the central nervous system (CNS) consist of three layers of concentric fibrous tissue that include the __________, __________, and __________.

   J. Also referred to as the craniosacral system, the __________ functions to conserve energy and regulates optimum visceral functions essential to survival.

   K. A __________ is a network of interconnected nerves that originate from multiple segments of the __________.

   L. Also referred to as the thoracolumbar division of the autonomic nervous system, the __________ functions to expend energy in flight, fright, or fight conditions.

   M. Besides providing the organism with a three-dimensional orientation map which guides eye movements and head and body turning in response to bright light and directional sounds, the __________ also mediates visual reflexes.

   N. The free borders of the __________ form an opening called the __________ through which the brainstem exits the posterior cranial fossa.

   O. __________ axonal fibers carry sensory impulses toward the CNS while the __________ fibers carry the commands away from the CNS.

   P. The corpora quadrigemina that consist of the __________ and __________ serve as the reflex centers for vision and audition.

   Q. The __________ is the bundle of fibers that connects the cerebellum with the brainstem.

2. Match each of the following structures with the associated vesicle.

A. pes pedunculi	a. telencephalon
B. limbic system	b. diencephalon
C. fourth ventricle	c. mesencephalon
D. basal ganglia	d. metencephalon
E. thalamus	e. myelencephalon
F. substantia nigra	
G. medulla	
H. pons	
I. cerebellum	

3. Match each of the following cortical structures to the lobes in which they are located.

A. supramarginal gyrus	a. frontal
B. angular gyrus	b. parietal
C. calcarine sulcus	c. temporal
D. olfactory sulcus	d. occipital
E. uncus	
F. parahippocampal gyrus	
G. premotor cortex	
H. amyglala	
I. precentral gyrus	
J. postcentral gyrus	

4. Match each of the following cortical structures to the associated cortical surface.

A. central sulcus	a. dorsal lateral
B. lateral sulcus	b. ventral
C. supramarginal gyrus	c. midsagittal
D. angular gyrus	
E. calcarine sulcus	
F. olfactory sulcus	
G. parahippocampal gyrus	
H. collateral sulcus	

I. orbital cortex

J. olfactory nerve

K. cingulate gyrus

L. corpus callosum

5. Match the major divisions of the brain with the corresponding ventricular spaces.

A. telencephalon	a. cerebral aqueduct
B. diencephalon	b. fourth ventricle
C. midbrain	c. lateral ventricles
D. metencephalon	d. third ventricle

6. List the number of spinal nerves that exit from the following spinal regions:

A. cervical

B. thoracic

C. lumbar

D. sacral

7. List the cranial nerves by name and in the order they exit the brainstem:

8. Match each of the following pathologies to the associated statement.

A. lesion in area 17 on the left	a. incomprehension of spoken language
B. lesion in area 41 on the left	b. right hemianopsia
C. lesion in area 22 on the left	c. loss of executive function
D. prefrontal lobe white matter lesion	d. auditory imperceptibility
E. cutting the corpus callosum	e. separation of hemispheres

9. Match each of the dysfunctions to the associated lesion site.

A. hemiplegia	a postcentral gyrus
B. hemianesthesia	b. cerebellum
C. impaired motivation and emotion	c. ventricles and cerebrospinal fluid
D. involuntary movements	d. precentral gyrus
E. hydrocephalus	e. hypothalamus
F. hormonal disorder	f. limbic lobe
G. meningitis	g. arachnoid–pia membranes
H. incoordination	h. basal ganglia

10. Why should speech language pathologists be concerned about traumatic injuries at the cervical spinal cord?

11. List two common herniations that occur after increased intracranial pressure in the brain.

12. Which system is responsible for expending energy in flight, fight, and fright conditions? Which system helps to restore energy when threats are gone?

13. List the primary and secondary brain vesicles along with their brain derivatives.

14. Name the three meninges in the order from external to inward.

15. Name the three types of fiber bundles in the brain.

16. List three extensions of the meningeal layer of the dura mater.

17. Name the location of the reticular cortical arousal system.

18. Name the parts of the corpus callosum.

3

Internal Anatomy of the Central Nervous System

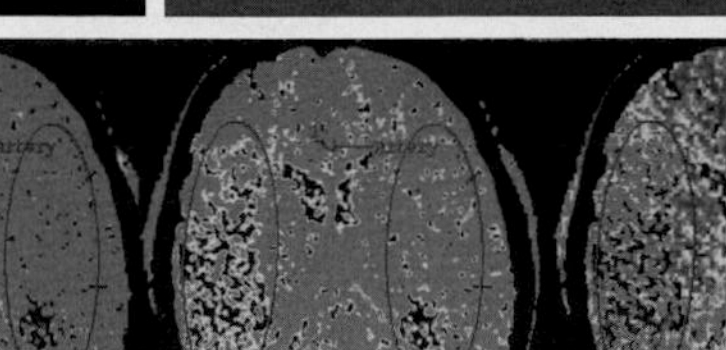

LEARNING OBJECTIVES

After studying this chapter, students should be able to:

- Identify the varying shapes of corticospinal fibers at different neuraxial levels
- Recognize the varying ventricular cavity shapes at various neuraxial levels
- Recognize major internal structures of the spinal cord and describe their functions
- Identify major structures of the medulla and explain their functions
- Recognize functionally pertinent structures of the internal pons and describe their functions
- Identify major structures of the midbrain and discuss their functions
- Recognize major structures of the forebrain (diencephalon, basal ganglia, and limbic structures) and relate to their functions
- Follow the continuation of major anatomic structures in sequential sections of the brain
- Identify major forebrain structure brain slices and match to their locations on the corresponding MR images

The major neuroanatomical (cortical, subcortical, meninges, ventricles, and axonal pathways) structures and their functions have been discussed in Chapter 2. The next step is to use specific and easily identified anatomic structures as signposts for developing an orientation to the internal anatomy of the brain in relation to the locations of surrounding structures. An understanding of the internal brain anatomy is the most significant part of training in clinical neuroscience, and this knowledge is essential not only for solving clinical problems but also for reading brain images and deriving neurolinguistic implications. Exposure to the internal brain structures often is neglected in teaching neuroscience to students of communicative disorders; however, this limits the students' learning potential and their ability to apply their knowledge to clinical problem solving. Internal anatomy is best learned by repeated exposure to the serial sections of the spinal cord, brainstem, and forebrain. In this chapter, the spinal cord, and brainstem are examined via stained sections, and the forebrain is studied on unstained coronal and horizontal sections of the brain.

As per the rule of topographical representation (see Chapter 1), nuclear structures and fiber tracts related to different functional systems exist side by side in the central nervous system. Since disease processes in the brain rarely strike only selective structures or pathways, a series of related and unrelated clinical signs are seen after a brain injury. A thorough knowledge of the internal brain structures—including their location, proximity, shape and size—makes it easier both to understand their functional significance for the syndrome composition and to explain why multiple clinical signs may develop from a single lesion site (Box 3-1).

BOX 3-1

Exposure to Internal Anatomy of the Forebrain

Learning internal brain anatomy is a significant part of the training in functional neuroscience. This knowledge of the locations of the major axonal pathways, anatomical structures, and their structural and functional connectivity is essential not only for appreciating the rationale for co-occurring symptoms but also for solving clinical problems. This also helps in reading brain images and deriving neurolinguistic implications of lesion and lesion sites. A lack of familiarity with the internal brain structures limits learning potential of the students of communicative disorders and restricts their ability to apply the knowledge to clinical thinking.

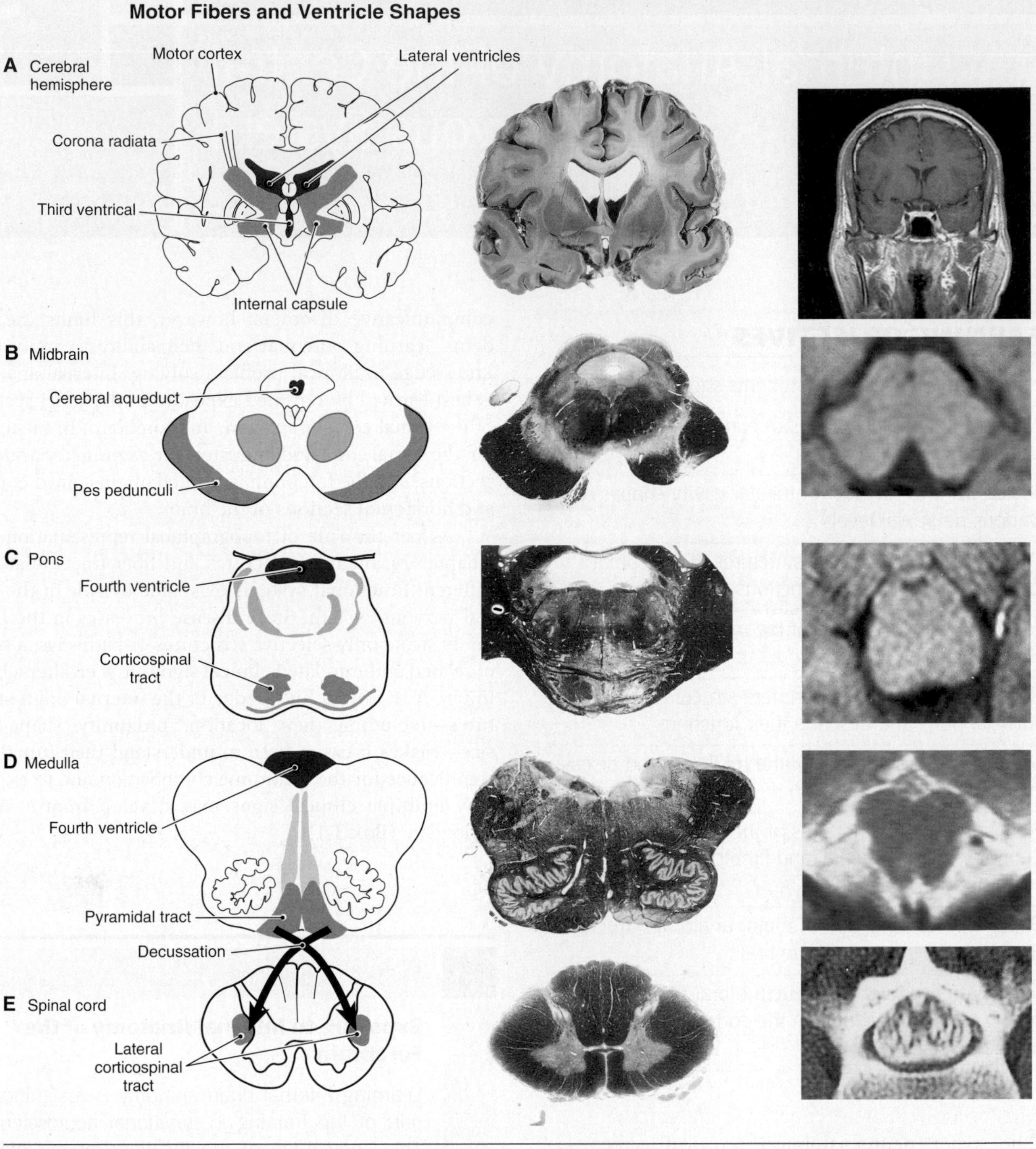

Motor Fibers and Ventricle Shapes

A Cerebral hemisphere
Motor cortex
Lateral ventricles
Corona radiata
Third ventrical
Internal capsule

B Midbrain
Cerebral aqueduct
Pes pedunculi

C Pons
Fourth ventricle
Corticospinal tract

D Medulla
Fourth ventricle
Pyramidal tract
Decussation

E Spinal cord
Lateral corticospinal tract

Figure 3-1 A–E. The shapes of the corticospinal fibers and the ventricular cavities at various neuroaxial levels.

ANATOMICAL LANDMARKS

Two distinct anatomic landmarks used for visual orientation to the internal anatomy of the brain are the shapes of the descending corticospinal fibers and the ventricular cavities (Fig. 3-1). Both are present throughout the brain, although their shape and size vary as one progresses from the forebrain (telencephalon) to the caudal brainstem. A familiarity with the progressively changing shapes and sizes of these structures is essential for identifying not only the various brain levels that they represent but also the coexisting structures on these levels.

Shapes of Corticospinal Fibers

Immediately after their origin in the sensorimotor cortex, the descending corticospinal fibers fan down through the corona radiata (see Figs. 2-16 and 2-38) to enter the wedge-shaped internal capsule at the diencephalic level (Fig. 3-1*A*; see Figs. 2-15 and 2-16). Along the ventral surface of the midbrain, they form the pes pedunculi (crus cerebri), a bilaterally compact fillet-shaped mass of fibers well visible on a cross section (Fig. 3-1*B*; see Fig. 2-24). The fibers of the corticospinal tract later disperse among the scattered pontine nuclei and appear as many irregular round axonal masses scattered throughout the basal pons (Fig. 3-1*C*; see Fig. 2-25). The corticospinal tract fibers recombine when entering the medulla and form a pyramid, which is best viewed in microscopic cross section of the caudal brainstem (Fig. 3-1*D*; see Fig. 2-26). The term pyramid gave origin to the term pyramidal tract, which is synonymous with the corticospinal tract. Pyramidal fibers cross the midline at the caudal medulla; after crossing, they enter the **lateral funiculus** of the spinal cord and are known as the lateral corticospinal tract (Fig. 3-1*E*).

Shape of the Ventricular Cavities

The lateral and third ventricles together are butterfly shaped in a cross section of the rostral brain (Fig. 3-1*A*; see Fig. 2-16). The two lateral ventricles are the wings, and the medially located narrow slit of the third ventricle serves as the body. The cerebral aqueduct of Sylvius is the small tube-shaped midbrain canal (Fig. 3-1*B*; see Fig. 2-24) that connects the third and fourth ventricles. The fourth ventricle overlies the pons (Fig. 3-1*D*; see Fig. 2-9); it tapers to end in the rostral medulla (Fig. 3-1*E*).

Important internal anatomic landmarks of the CNS have been serially examined starting caudally. The spinal cord is examined in cross section. The midbrain, pons, and medulla are reviewed in transverse section. The forebrain structures (cerebral cortex, diencephalon, and basal ganglia) are studied in both coronal and horizontal sections.

SPINAL CORD IN CROSS SECTIONS

The internal anatomy of the spinal cord is studied in four sections; a representative section is taken from each of the following anatomic sections beginning caudally: sacral, lumbar, thoracic, and cervical. The internal anatomic pattern of the spinal cord remains the same throughout its extent from sacral to cervical regions. The central region (gray matter) of the cord, made up of cell bodies, is shaped like a butterfly and appears gray in freshly cut sections. The outer part of the cord, which looks like the rim of a wheel, consists of ascending and descending fiber tracts (white matter) and surrounds the butterfly-shaped central gray matter. The fiber tracts form functionally related longitudinal funiculi, which are demarcated by longitudinal grooves and spinal nerve attachments along the surface of the spinal cord.

The only change that occurs in the internal spinal anatomy throughout its axis is the ratio of white to gray matter at each of the four spinal levels. In the transition from the sacral to cervical region, this ratio gradually increases as new fibers are added to the afferent tracts. Additional changes relate to the shape of the gray matter; the spinal cord enlarges in the cervical and lumbar regions because of the relatively large nerve supply needed for the sensory and motor functions of the upper and lower extremities (see Fig. 2-33). The important internal spinal structures include the sensory and motor nuclei and various ascending and descending tracts (Table 3-1; Box 3-2).

Sacral Section

The sacral structures of the spinal cord are seen in Figure 3-2. This level of the cord, which is small in diameter, contains a thin mantle of white matter and a larger gray region with bulky ventral and dorsal horns. The **dorsal lemniscal column** consists of the ascending fibers of the **fasciculus gracilis**, which carry information concerning discriminative touch, pressure, and limb position from the lower half of the body. The fasciculus gracilis contains sensory fibers that enter the cord from the sacral to midthoracic level. The lateral column of the white matter at this level contains the lateral corticospinal tract and fibers of the **anterolateral**

Table 3-1

Anatomic Structures of the Spinal Cord
Dorsal median sulcus
Ventral median sulcus
Dorsal intermediate sulcus
Gray matter Dorsal horns Ventral horns
White matter Dorsal fasciculus Lateral fasciculus Anterior fasciculus
Dorsal root
Ventral root
Sensory nuclei in gray column
Motor nuclei in gray column
Fasciculus gracilis and cuneatus
Spinothalamic (lateral and anterior) tracts
Spinocerebellar (dorsal and ventral) tracts

BOX 3-2

Clinical Spinal Syndromes

The anatomic pattern of the spinal cord remains the same throughout from sacral to cervical regions. However, the ratio of the white to gray matter changes at each of the spinal levels proceeding from sacral to cervical, since new fibers are added to the afferent and efferent tracts.

Depending on the extent of the spinal lesion, vascular spinal pathology can affect the dorsal column fibers, corticospinal tract, and the fibers of the anterolateral system. A spinal syndrome includes limb paralysis, loss of pain and temperature, and the loss of discriminative (proprioception and kinesthetic) awareness below the lesion site. Two frequent conditions associated with spinal cord are: Brown–Sequard syndrome and syringomyelia.

Brown–Sequard syndrome, often caused by traumatic injury, affects half of the cord and results in ipsilateral paralysis and loss of discriminative sensation, and contralateral loss of pain and temperature (see Chapter 11).

The spinal central canal is formed by the embryologic tube closing. There are different consequences if the cavity within the neural tube remains large (syringomyelia), which can be localized to a few segments. In syringomyelia, a congenital condition, the enlarged cavity interferes with the normal crossing of pain and temperature fibers through the ventral white commissure on the path to the contralateral half of the brain. A bilateral loss of pain and temperature occurs for the involved segments. The pain and temperature fibers that have crossed the midline below are usually preserved. The cavitation, if large, can also affect the development of the ventral horn motor neurons causing a bilateral limb weakness.

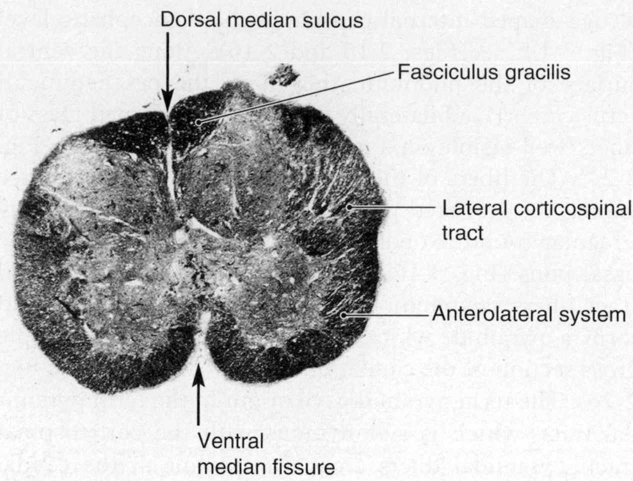

Figure 3-2 Cross section of the spinal cord at the sacral level.

system. The lateral corticospinal tract transmits commands from the motor cortex via the **lower motor neurons** to the muscles. The anterolateral system of fibers consists of the anterior and lateral spinothalamic tracts, which mediate sensations of diffuse touch, pain, and temperature.

The large ventral horns are the sites of motor nuclei. The dorsal horns contain the sensory nuclei, which include the **substantia gelatinosa** and **nucleus proprius** (see Chapter 11); these nuclei are present throughout the spinal cord and receive input predominantly from spinal sensory nerves. Other sensory spinal cells include the **nucleus dorsalis of Clarke**. Many dorsal horn cells give rise to fibers of the spinocerebellar (unconscious proprioception) and anterolateral system (pain and temperature).

Lumbar Section

Present in Figure 3-3 is the anatomic views of the spinal lumbar (L4) structures. The gray matter at this level contains larger dorsal and ventral horns in relation to the surrounding white matter. Located lateral to the dorsal median sulcus, the dorsal lemniscal column continues to exclusively represent fibers of the fasciculus gracilis, which mediates fine discriminative touch-related information to the brain. This level also contains the lateral corticospinal tract and the anterolateral system, consisting of the spinothalamic and spinocerebellar tracts. (The spinocerebellar tract is not identified in Fig. 3-3.) The dorsal horns contain the sensory nuclei and the ventral horns contain the motor nuclei. Also present in this cross section are the dorsal and ventral root fibers.

Thoracic Section

The anatomic view of the spinal thoracic structures (T4) is shown in Figure 3-4. This spinal level is characterized by the reduced gray matter size and the enlarged share of the white matter. Compared to the previously discussed sections, the dorsal and ventral horns are smaller and tapered. The dorsal lemniscal column at this level is larger because of additional sensory fibers entering from the higher body levels. The additional sensory fibers form the fasciculus cuneatus, which ascend lateral to the fasciculus gracilis in the dorsal columns of the cord. The fasciculus cuneatus fibers carry the sensations of fine

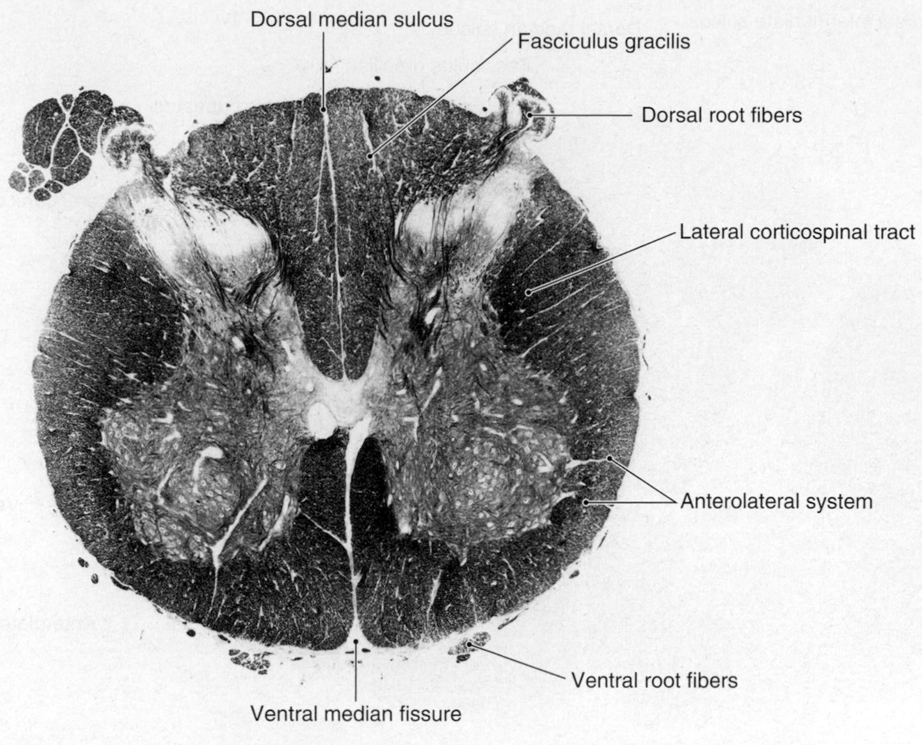

Figure 3-3 Cross section of the spinal cord at the L4 level.

discriminative touch, pressure, and limb position from the upper body; its fibers enter the spinal cord at the midthoracic through cervical levels. With emergence of the fasciculus cuneatus, the dorsal intermediate sulcus is visible as it separates the medially located fasciculus gracilis from the laterally located fibers of the fasciculus cuneatus. The lateral corticospinal tract is larger here than at lower levels, although it retains the same relative lateral location. Mediating sensations of diffuse touch, pain, and temperature, the fibers of the spinothalamic

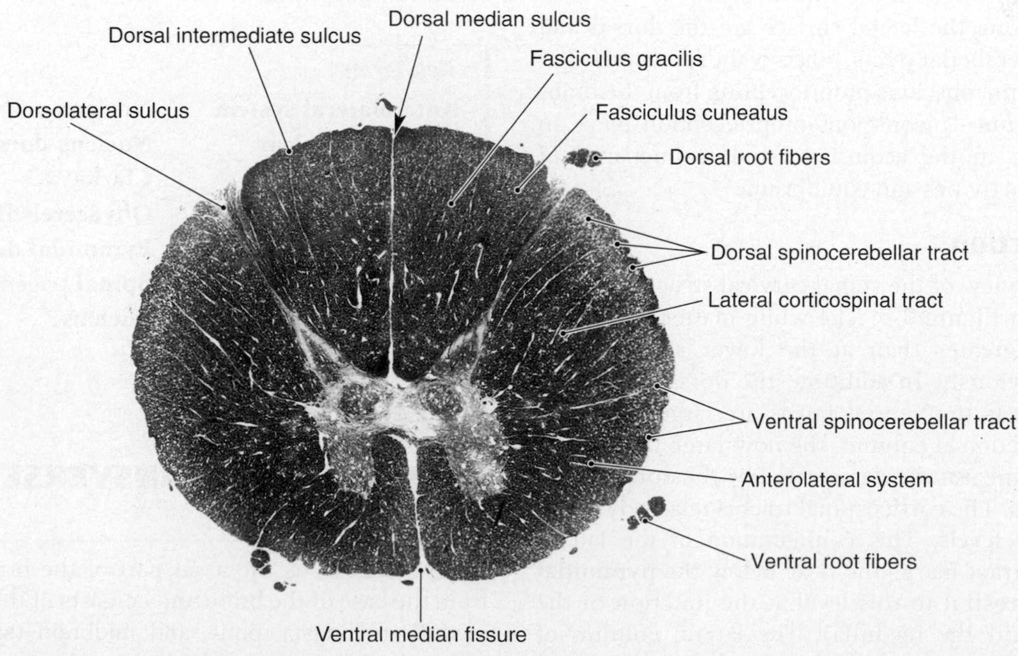

Figure 3-4 Cross section of the spinal cord at the T4 level.

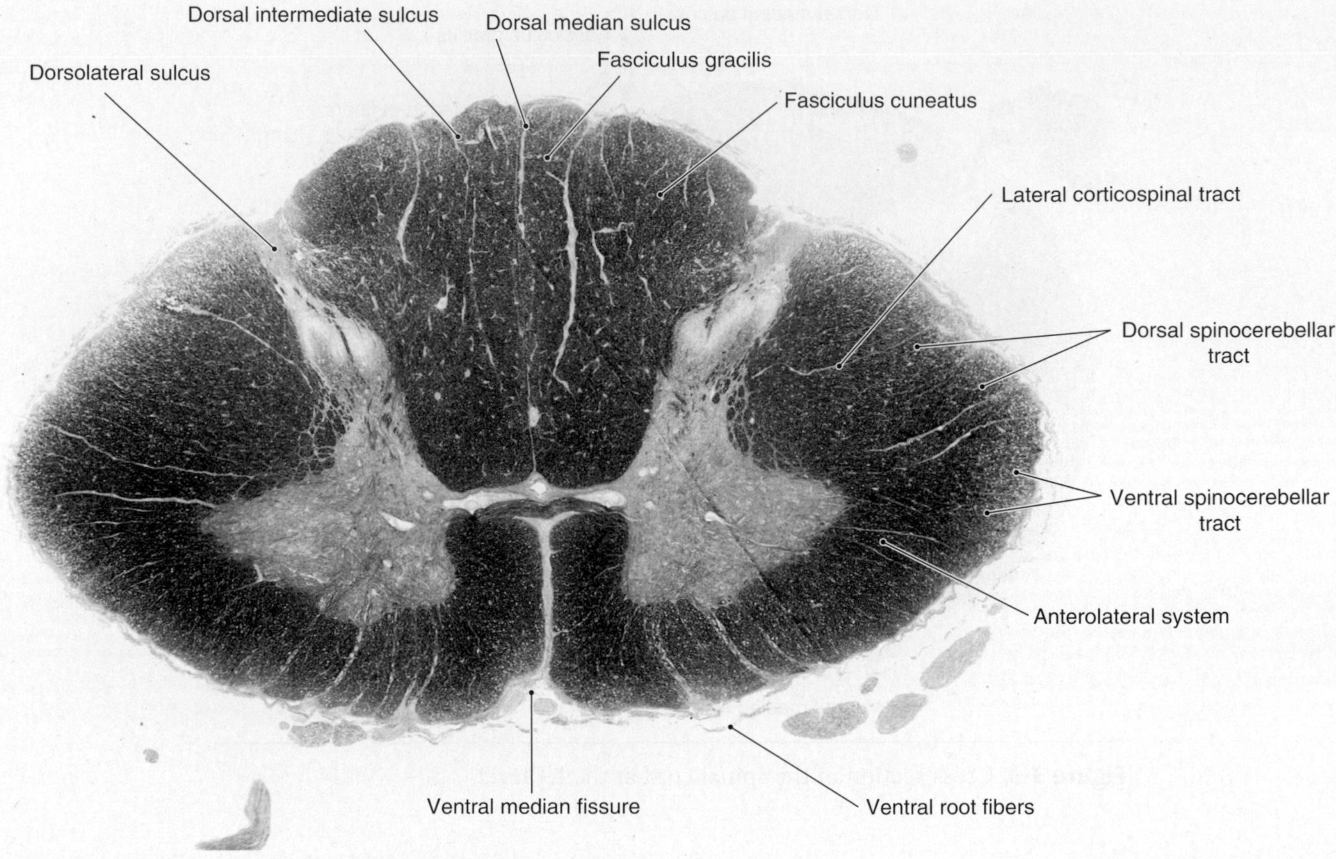

Figure 3-5 Cross section of the spinal cord at the C7 level.

tracts (anterolateral system) continue to occupy the same general space throughout the spinal cord.

Present along the lateral surface are the **dorsal and ventral spinocerebellar tracts**. Fibers of the spinocerebellar tracts mediate unconscious proprioception from the limbs to the cerebellum. Unconscious proprioception plays an important role in the acquisition and maintenance of skilled motor activities and equilibrium.

Cervical Section

The anatomic view of the spinal cervical structures (C7) is displayed in Figure 3-5. The white matter volume at this level is greater than at the lower spinal levels discussed previously. In addition, the dorsal horns are slender, whereas the ventral horns are large and wing shaped. In the dorsal column, the now-large fasciculi of gracilis and cuneatus are demarcated by the dorsal intermediate sulcus. The corticospinal tract is relatively larger than at lower levels. This configuration of the lateral corticospinal tract marks the level below the **pyramidal decussation** (rostral to this level at the junction of the spinal cord and the medulla). The lateral column of fibers continues to contain the spinothalamic and spinocerebellar pathways.

Key Terms:

Anterolateral system	**Nucleus ambiguous**
Cochlear nuclear complex	**Nucleus dorsalis of Clarke**
Dorsal lemniscal column	**Olivocerebellar fibers**
Dorsal and ventral spinocerebellar tracts	**Pyramidal decussation**
Fasciculus gracilis	**Spinal trigeminal nucleus**

BRAINSTEM IN TRANSVERSE SECTIONS

The brainstem, as the axial part of the brain, protrudes from the base of the brain and consists of three structures: medulla oblongata, pons, and midbrain (see Fig. 2-22).

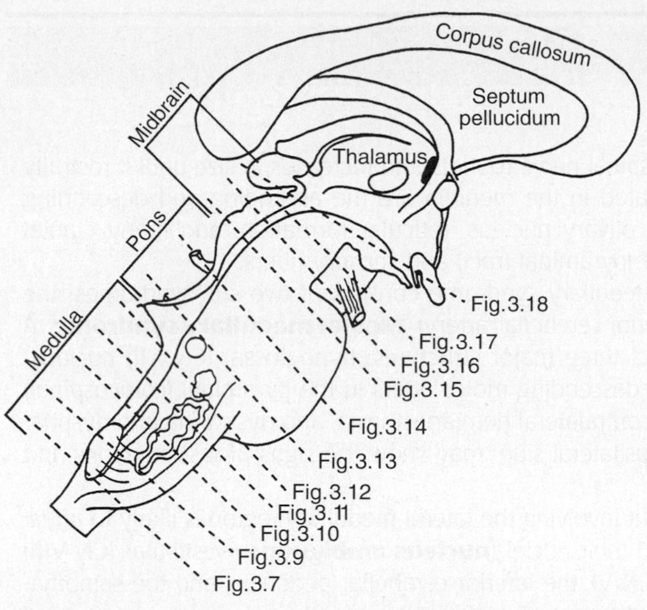

Figure 3-6 Location of the transverse sections of the brainstem shown in the specified figures.

Table 3-2

Anatomic Structures of the Medulla

Anatomic Structures of the Medulla
Caudal (low) medulla
Pyramid
Decussation of pyramidal fibers
Fasciculus gracilis and cuneatus
Nucleus gracilis and cuneatus
Spinal trigeminal nucleus and tract
Middle medulla
Fasciculus gracilis and cuneatus
Nucleus gracilis and cuneatus
Inferior cerebellar peduncle (restiform body)
Sensory decussation
Internal arcuate fibers
Medial lemniscus
Principal inferior olivary nucleus
Pyramid
Spinal trigeminal nucleus and tract
Rostral (high) medulla
Principal inferior olivary nucleus
Inferior cerebellar peduncle
Cochlear nuclear complex
Vestibular nuclear complex
Medial lemniscus
Pyramid
Spinal trigeminal nucleus and tract

Besides containing all ascending (sensory) and descending (motor) fiber tracts, the brainstem includes a large group of nuclei that relate to the sensorimotor functions of the cranial nerves, serve various vital visceral (cardiac and respiratory) functions, and mediate the special senses and reflexive functions. The transverse sections of the brainstem discussed here are indicated in Figure 3-6.

Medulla Oblongata

The medulla oblongata, the most caudal portion of the brainstem, begins above the rootlets of the first cervical spinal nerve and gradually increases in size until it merges rostrally with the pons. Important structures in the medulla are the corticospinal fibers (pyramidal tract), dorsal lemniscal column (fasciculus gracilis and fasciculus cuneatus), medial lemniscus, inferior cerebellar peduncle, principal (inferior) olivary nucleus, reticular formation, and many cranial nerve nuclei (Table 3-2; Box 3-3). The medulla is also the site for the decussation (crossing) of sensory and motor fibers which accounts for the contralateral organization of the brain.

Caudal (Lower) Medulla

The transverse section in Figure 3-7 is the most caudal view of the brainstem, where the medulla merges with the spinal cord at the foramen magnum (see Fig. 2-31*A*). Four important structures in the dorsal medulla are the nucleus gracilis, fasciculus gracilis, nucleus cuneatus, and fasciculus cuneatus.

The ascending fibers of the fasciculus gracilis synapse on the cells of the nucleus gracilis, and those of the fasciculus cuneatus synapse on the cells of the nucleus cuneatus. In the lower center of this medullary section, the fibers of the pyramidal tract cross the midline and move to a lateral position to form the lateral corticospinal tract in the spinal column (Fig. 3-5). This crossing of the corticospinal fibers accounts for the motor cortex of one side of the brain controlling the opposite side of the body. Lateral to the fasciculus cuneatus is the massive formation of the **spinal trigeminal nucleus** and its (**spinal trigeminal**) **tract**.

The spinal trigeminal tract consists of the fibers of the trigeminal (CN V) nerve, which mediates pain, touch, and temperature in the face. Fibers of this tract enter the brainstem, descend ipsilaterally in the medulla, and terminate in the spinal trigeminal nucleus. Secondary fibers from the spinal trigeminal nucleus cross the midline and ascend to the thalamus, from which impulses are relayed to the primary sensory cortex in the parietal lobe (see Chapter 11).

BOX 3-3

Clinical Medullary Syndromes

The medulla oblongata begins above the first cervical spinal nerve rootlets and increases in size until it rostrally merges with the lower pons. Important structures located in the medulla are the ascending and descending fibers, inferior cerebellar peduncle, principal (inferior) olivary nucleus, reticular formation, and many cranial nerve nuclei. It is also the site for the crossing of motor (pyramidal tract) and sensory fibers.

Receiving blood from two different sources, the medullary syndrome consists of two sub-syndromes: the medial (anterior spinal artery) and lateral (posterior inferior cerebellar artery). **Medial medullary syndrome**: A vascular involvement of the medial medulla can affect three major structures: hypoglossal (CN XII) nucleus/nerve, sensory fibers of the medial lemniscus, and the descending motor fibers in the pyramidal (corticospinal) tract. Clinical deficits include contralateral hemiplegia, contralateral hemianesthesia, and dysarthria and dysphagia. The tongue, which on protrusion deviates to the ipsilateral side, may show the signs of fasciculations and atrophy.

Lateral medullary syndrome: A vascular accident involving the lateral medullary region is likely to affect vagus (CN X) and glossopharyngeal (CN IX) nerves and their nuclei (**nucleus ambiguous**), vestibular (CN VIII) nerve and nuclei, spinal trigeminal tract and nucleus (CN V), the inferior cerebellar peduncle, and the spinothalamic tract. Clinical deficits include the loss of pain and temperature from the ipsilateral face, dysphagia, and dysarthria because of the paralysis of pharyngeal, laryngeal, and soft palate muscles, tendency to fall to the ipsilateral side, vertigo, ataxia in ipsilateral upper and lower limbs, and contralateral loss of pain and temperature.

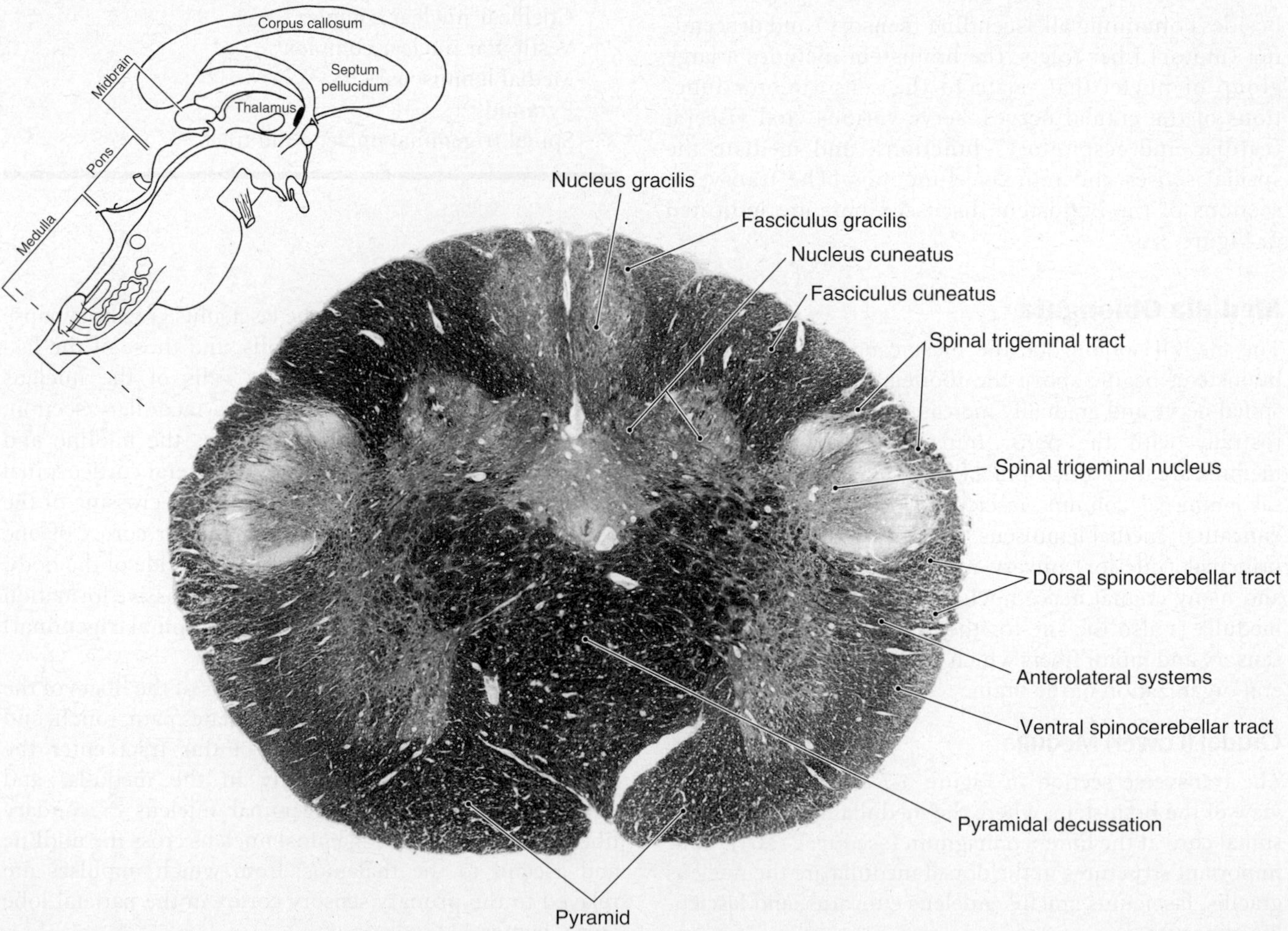

Figure 3-7 Transverse section of the medulla through the pyramidal decussation.

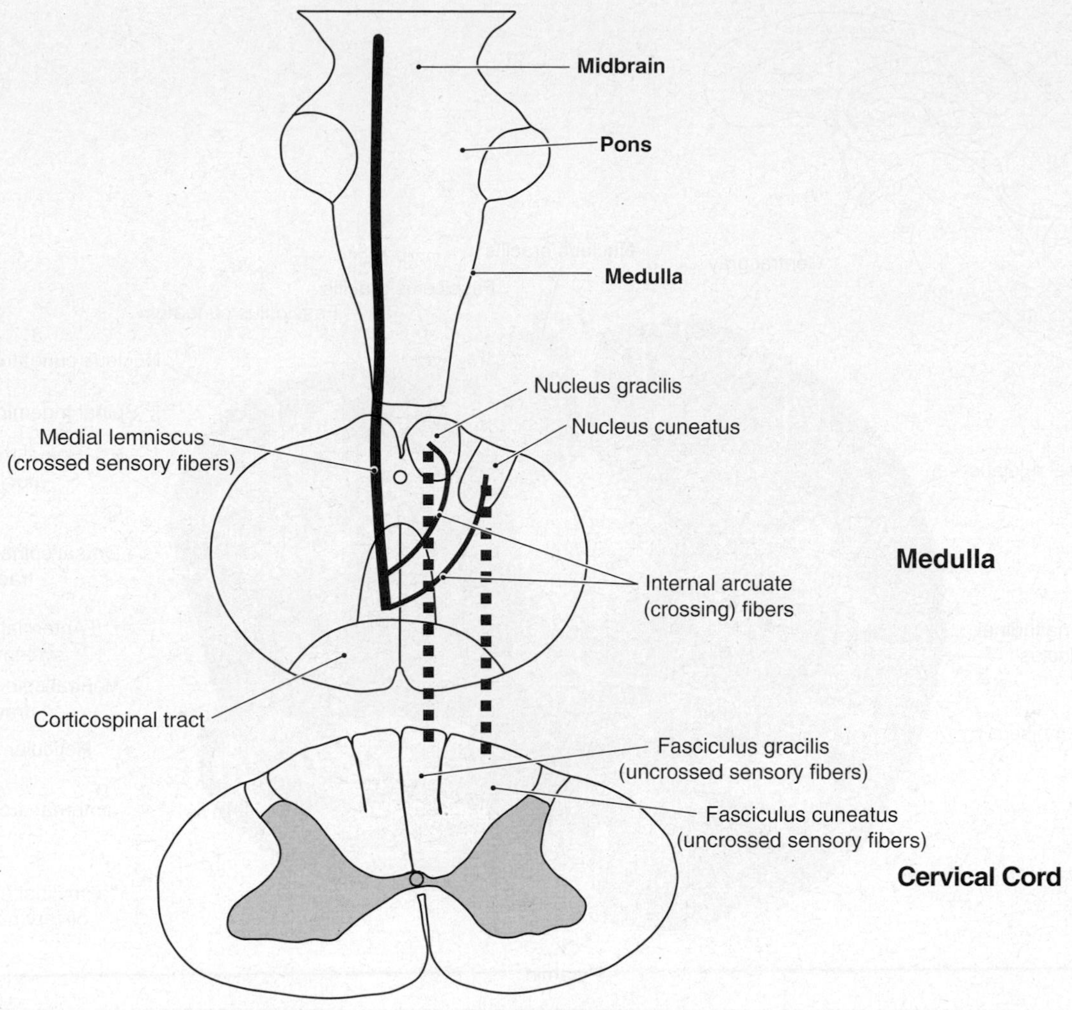

Figure 3-8 Crossing of the dorsal lemniscal fibers in the caudal medulla.

Medial to the trigeminal tract and nucleus are diffusely located cellular and fibrous components of the reticular formation. Extending throughout the brainstem, the reticular formation is responsible for the regulation of cortical arousal and consciousness (see Fig. 2-23). The reticular formation also integrates all sensorimotor stimuli with internally generated thoughts, emotions, and cognition. It also maintains the homeostatic state of the brain, which is essential for regulating visceral (cardiovascular), sensorimotor (respiration), and neuroendocrine activities such as blood pressure and movement.

A discussion of the events related to the crossed and uncrossed sensory fibers is important for an orientation to the course of the dorsal column fibers (Fig. 3-8). The fasciculi of gracilis and cuneatus are the first-order sensory fibers; their sensory neurons are in the spinal dorsal root ganglion. Fibers of these two fasciculi enter the spinal cord and ascend on the same side in the dorsal lemniscal column and synapse on their respective nuclei in the medulla. These nuclei project secondary fibers across the midline as the **internal arcuate fibers**, which form the medial lemniscus and travel upward to relay information related to fine discriminative touch (deep touch, two-point touch, stereognosis, and proprioception) to the thalamus. The thalamocortical projections transmit the sensory information to the primary sensory cortex (Brodmann areas 3, 1, 2). Thus, three different terms (dorsal lemniscal column, internal arcuate fibers, and medial lemniscus) relate to the very fibers that mediate the same sensory information received from the fasciculi of gracilis and cuneatus, which transmit sensation from the lower and the upper body, respectively.

The transverse section in Figure 3-9 provides a better view of the crossing internal arcuate fibers that arise from the gracilis and cuneatus. The gracile and cuneate nuclei reach their largest size at this level. The internal arcuate fibers from those nuclei cross the midline to form the medial lemniscus and then travel rostrally to the thalamus. At the medullary level, this decussation thus allows for the transmission of tactile and discriminative sensation from

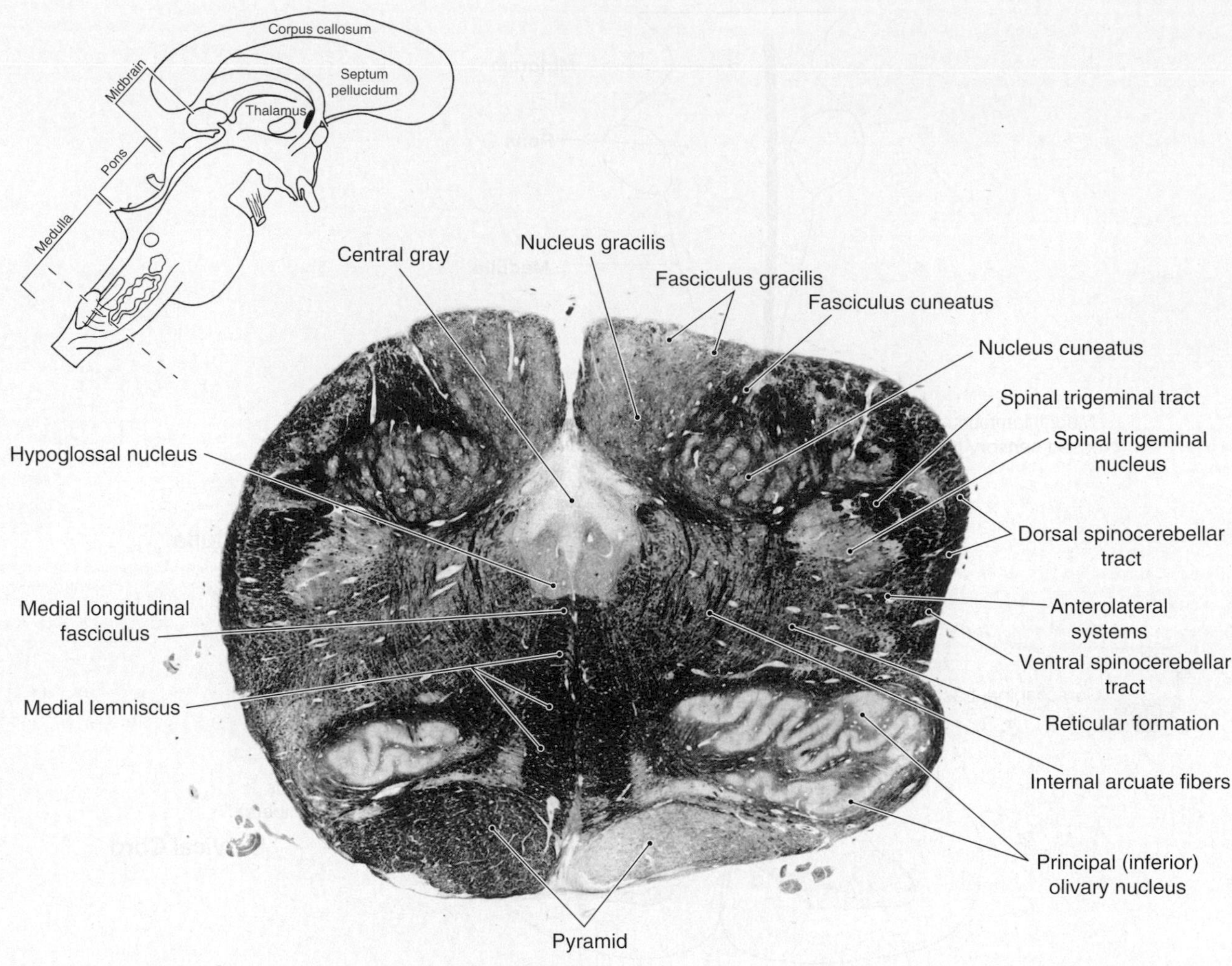

Figure 3-9 Transverse section of the medulla through the dorsal column (gracilis and cuneatus) nuclei, caudal portions of hypoglossal nucleus, caudal end of inferior olivary nucleus, and middle portions of the sensory decussation.

one side of the body to the opposite half of the brain. The pyramids in the ventromedial medulla appear as a compact bundle of fibers just rostral to the level at which they decussate. The decussations of the sensory internal arcuate fibers and motor pyramidal fibers are two landmarks of the caudal medulla.

The core of the reticular formation in the central third of the medulla is continuous with the lower levels. It is a net-like arrangement of cell bodies and interwoven projections that interact with virtually all sensorimotor systems and regulate brain functioning (see Fig. 2-23). The central gray matter is the midbrain reticular–limbic area, which regulates somatic and visceral functions. Beneath the central gray is the nucleus of the hypoglossal nerve (CN XII). It controls all intrinsic and most extrinsic tongue muscles and is an important nerve for speech production and swallowing.

The structure below the hypoglossal nucleus is the medial longitudinal fasciculus. This fiber bundle receives visual and vestibular projections and is located longitudinally from the cervical cord to the brainstem. It interconnects the motor nuclei of four cranial nerves (oculomotor [CN III], trochlear [CN IV], abducens [CN VI], and spinal accessory [CN XI]) and regulates head–eye coordination. The principal (inferior) olivary nucleus, also seen in this area, relays spinal and brainstem afferents to the cerebellum. Some of the previously described structures like the pyramidal tract, medial lemniscus, and inferior olivary nucleus also remain present in this section of the brainstem.

Middle Medulla

Present in the Figure 3-10 are the structures of the middle third of the medulla. The rostral portion of the hypoglossal nucleus is larger here than in the lower medulla. Located above the pyramidal tract, the principal (inferior) olivary nucleus occupies a major portion of the lower half of the medulla. The principal olivary nucleus, a wrinkled and saggy structure, is an important relay center for motor and proprioceptive information to the cerebellum. This nucleus

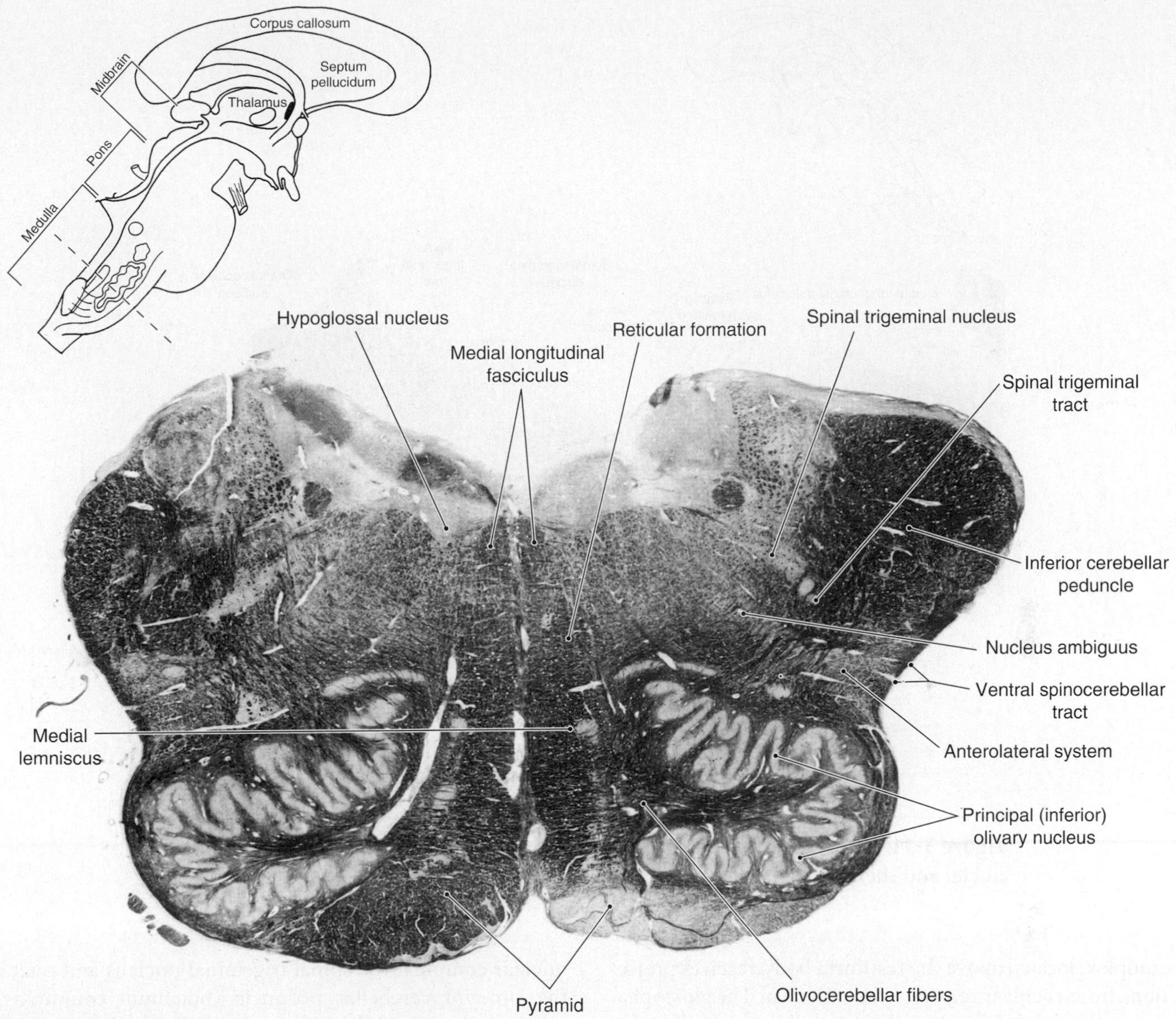

Figure 3-10 Transverse section of the medulla through the rostral portions of the hypoglossal nucleus and middle portions of the principal (inferior) olivary nucleus.

receives input related to pain, touch, and position of the limbs from the spinal cord (**spino-olivary**) and reticular formation (**reticulo-olivary**). The **olivocerebellar fibers** cross the midline and project to the opposite cerebellar hemisphere through the inferior cerebellar peduncle (**restiform body**). The inferior cerebellar peduncle appears along the lateral–dorsal surface of the upper half of the medulla. It is one of the three peduncles that connect the brainstem to the cerebellum (see Figs. 2-29 and 2-30).

The cranial nerve nuclei, which are related to the glossopharyngeal (CN IX) and vagus (CN X) nerves, are found in the region between the inferior cerebellar peduncle and the reticular formation. One of the important nuclei at this level is the **nucleus ambiguus**, the motor nucleus of the glossopharyngeal (CN IX) and vagus (CN X) nerves; it regulates phonation and swallowing functions by controlling the muscles of the soft palate, pharynx, larynx, and upper esophagus. The nuclei of the reticular formation are scattered and occupy a larger core area in the center of the medulla.

Rostral (High) Medulla

Located in the transverse section through the rostral third of the medulla (Fig. 3-11) are the inferior cerebellar peduncle and the principal (inferior) olivary nucleus, larger than they were in Figure 3-10. Among the newly appearing structures are the **cochlear nuclear complex** and glossopharyngeal (CN IX) nerve. The cochlear (CN VIII) nuclear

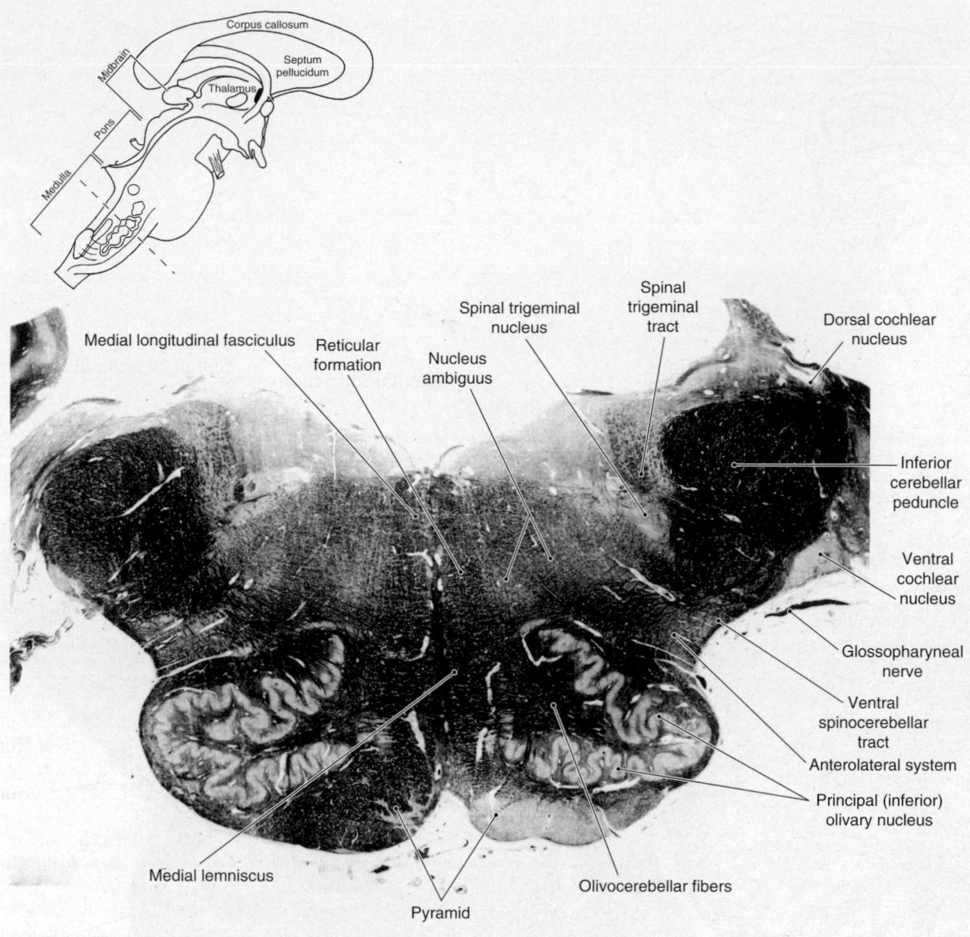

Figure 3-11 Transverse section of the medulla through the dorsal and ventral cochlear nuclei and the root of the glossopharyngeal nerve.

complex, located above the restiform body, receives projections from cochlear region of the inner ear. The glossopharyngeal nerve mediates taste and contributes to swallowing.

The compact pyramidal motor fibers are in the ventral medulla. The principal (inferior) olivary nucleus is present in its fully developed form. The medial lemniscus (mediating fine and discriminative touch) and the medial longitudinal fasciculus (interconnecting the motor nuclei of the ocular cranial nerves with vestibular input) are present along the midline in the medulla dorsal to the pyramids. The spinal trigeminal nucleus and its tract can also be seen in this section. The reticular formation occupies a large core in the middle third of the medulla, spanning the area dorsal to the principal (inferior) olivary nucleus.

Pons

The major pontine structures are the corticospinal fibers interspersed within diffused **pontine nuclei**, the crown-shaped cavity of the fourth ventricle, the massive middle cerebellar peduncle (brachium pontis), the medial lemniscus, the **crossing pontocerebellar fibers**, the **trigeminal nuclear complex**, the spinal trigeminal nucleus and tract, the superior cerebellar peduncle (brachium conjunctivum), remnants of the inferior cerebellar peduncle, and many cranial nerve structures (Table 3-3; Box 3-4).

Lower Pons

The transitional anatomic structures between the medulla and pons are presented in Figure 3-12. The enlarged fourth ventricle and diffuse pontine nuclei represent the pons, whereas the pyramid characterizes the medulla. The superior cerebellar peduncle forms part of the lateral roof of the fourth ventricle. The convex anterior medullary velum, in the dorsal area of this section, forms the roof of the fourth ventricle. The ventral teardrop-shaped pyramid does not hug the ventromedial area here, as it does in the lower medullary levels.

The cochlear nucleus, seen in Figure 3-11, is not present anymore. Appearing beneath the floor of the fourth ventricle, the **vestibular nuclear complex** receives projections from the semicircular canals in the inner ear and plays a role in equilibrium and head–eye coordination (see Chapter 10).

Table 3-3

Anatomic Structures of the Pons

Lower Pons	Middle Pons
Full-size crown-shaped fourth ventricle	Middle cerebellar peduncle
Diffuse pyramidal fibers piercing basal pons	Trigeminal nuclear complex
Remnants of inferior cerebellar peduncle	Pontine nuclei
Facial nucleus and nerve	Superior cerebellar peduncle (brachium conjunctivum)
Middle cerebellar peduncle (brachium pontis)	Fourth ventricle cavity
Medial lemniscus (marking upper limit of basal pons)	Anterior medullary velum
Spinal trigeminal nucleus and tract	Medial lemniscus Diffuse corticospinal fibers

The fibers of the **vestibular branch** of the vestibulocochlear nerve (CN VIII) exit laterally from the pontomedullary junction along the ventral surface of the middle and inferior cerebellar peduncles. The structures beneath the vestibular complex are the spinal trigeminal tract and spinal trigeminal nucleus.

BOX 3-4

Clinical Pontine Syndromes

The vascular support to the pons is through the paramedian branches of the basilar artery (see Chapter 7), which supply the medial pontine region that contains the corticospinal tract, medial lemniscus, and abducens nerve/nucleus. The lateral pons, supplied by the longer branches of the basilar, contains the middle cerebellar peduncles, vestibular-cochlear (CN VIII) nerve/nuclei, and facial (CN VII) nerve/nucleus. Clinical deficits include various combinations of disorders depending on the artery affected. Commonly occurring deficits include contralateral hemiplegia (involving both the upper and lower extremities), contralateral losses of discriminative (position and vibratory sensation) touch, medially deviated eye (the paralysis of the ipsilateral lateral rectus muscle), diplopia (double vision) on gaze toward the side of lesion (involving the abducens nerve), unsteady gait, ipsilateral facial palsy, vertigo, nausea, and deafness in the ipsilateral ear. Involvement of cranial nerve symptoms on ipsilateral side and contralateral limb paralysis presents an important clinical concept of alternating hemiplegia (see Chapter 16).

The spinal tract fibers of the trigeminal nerve descend ipsilaterally to synapse in the trigeminal nucleus, which relays somatosensory sensation from the face through its fiber tracts. After crossing, the trigeminal spinal tract fibers join the medial lemniscus to terminate in the thalamus. The nucleus of the facial nerve (CN VII) is visible in the pontine tegmentum. The facial nerve (CN VII) innervates the muscles of facial expression and not only controls smiling, frowning, and laughing but also assists in speaking. Fibers of the facial nerve (CN VII) exit laterally from the pontomedullary junction (see Figs. 2-49–2-51).

The massive body of the middle cerebellar peduncle, by far the largest of the cerebellar peduncles, is located laterally in this section. Its fibers connect the pons with the cerebellum and mediate information from the motor cortex to the contralateral cerebellar hemisphere. The fibers located medial to the middle cerebellar peduncle belong to the inferior cerebellar peduncle, which carry vestibular and spinal proprioceptive afferents to the cerebellum. Also emerging are the crescent-shaped fibers of the superior cerebella peduncle, which are more prominent at the higher pontine levels.

Middle Pons

The transverse section of the middle pons shown in Figure 3-13 is at the level of the trigeminal (CN V) nerve (the principal sensory nerve for the face) as it exits laterally through the middle cerebellar peduncle. The most characteristic features of the pons are the interspersed **corticospinal–corticopontine fibers** and the crown-shaped lumen of the fourth ventricle. Fibers of all three cerebellar peduncles are present laterally in this section, although the inferior cerebellar and superior cerebellar peduncles are relatively small.

Scattered pontine nuclei receive massive input from the ipsilateral primary motor and sensory cortices and

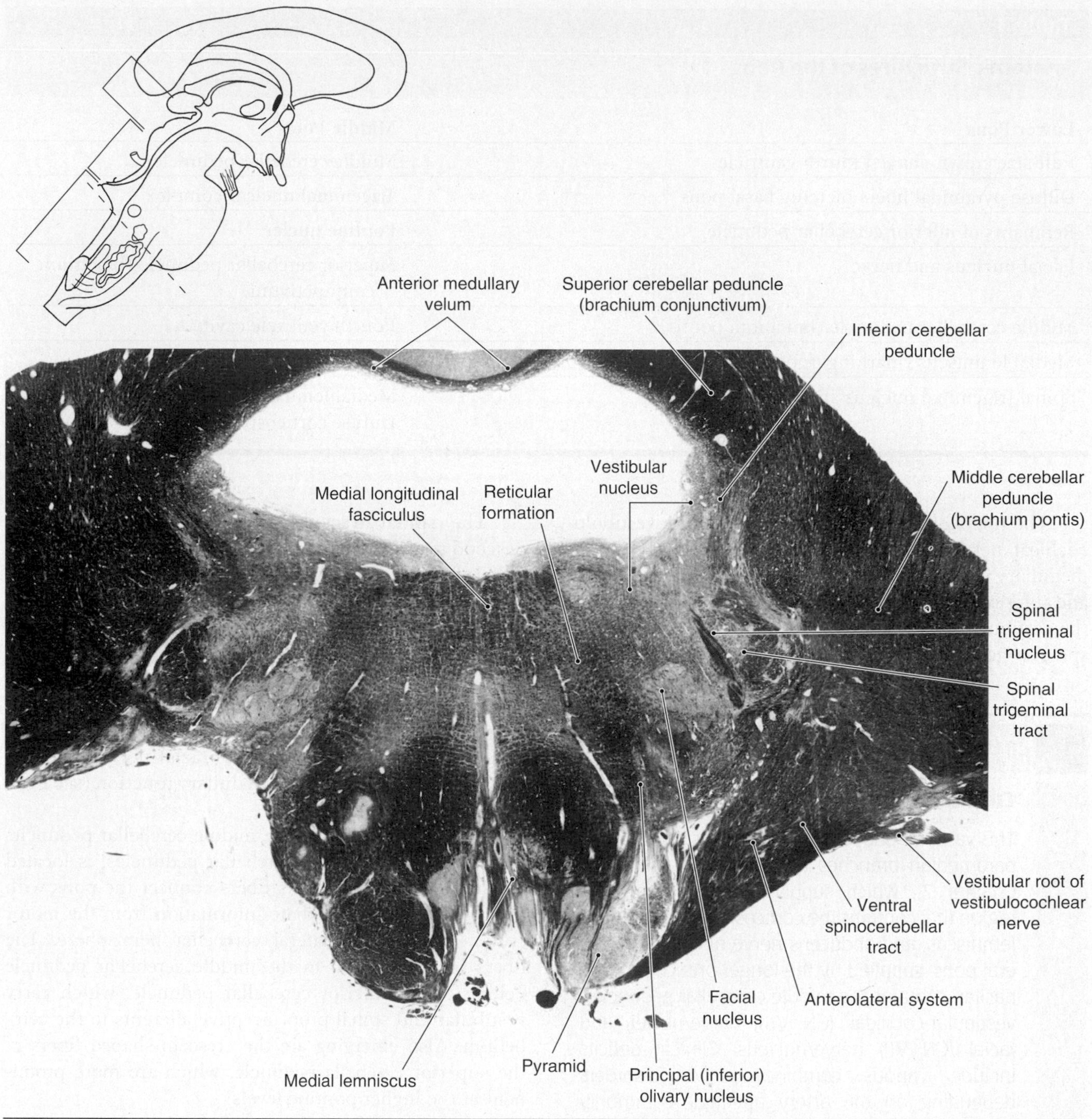

Figure 3-12 Transverse section of the pontomedullary junction through the rostral pole of the inferior olivary nucleus and facial nucleus.

cross the midline to project to the **pontocerebellar fibers** to the contralateral cerebellar hemisphere. Thus, they mediate information from the opposite primary motor, sensory, and visual cortices and are concerned with limb movement during skilled acts. Laterally, the crescent-shaped superior cerebellar peduncle provides cerebellar feedback to the primary motor cortex via the **red nucleus**. Located ventrolaterally are fibers of the **lateral lemniscus**, which carry auditory information from both the ears to the cortex (see Chapter 9).

This pontine section also demonstrates spatial relationships among the facial nucleus, facial nerve, abducens nucleus, and abducens nerve. The internal genu refers to fibers of the facial (CN VII) nerve as they curve over the nucleus of the abducens (CN VI) nerve just below the floor of the fourth ventricle (see Figs. 15-3 and 15-4).

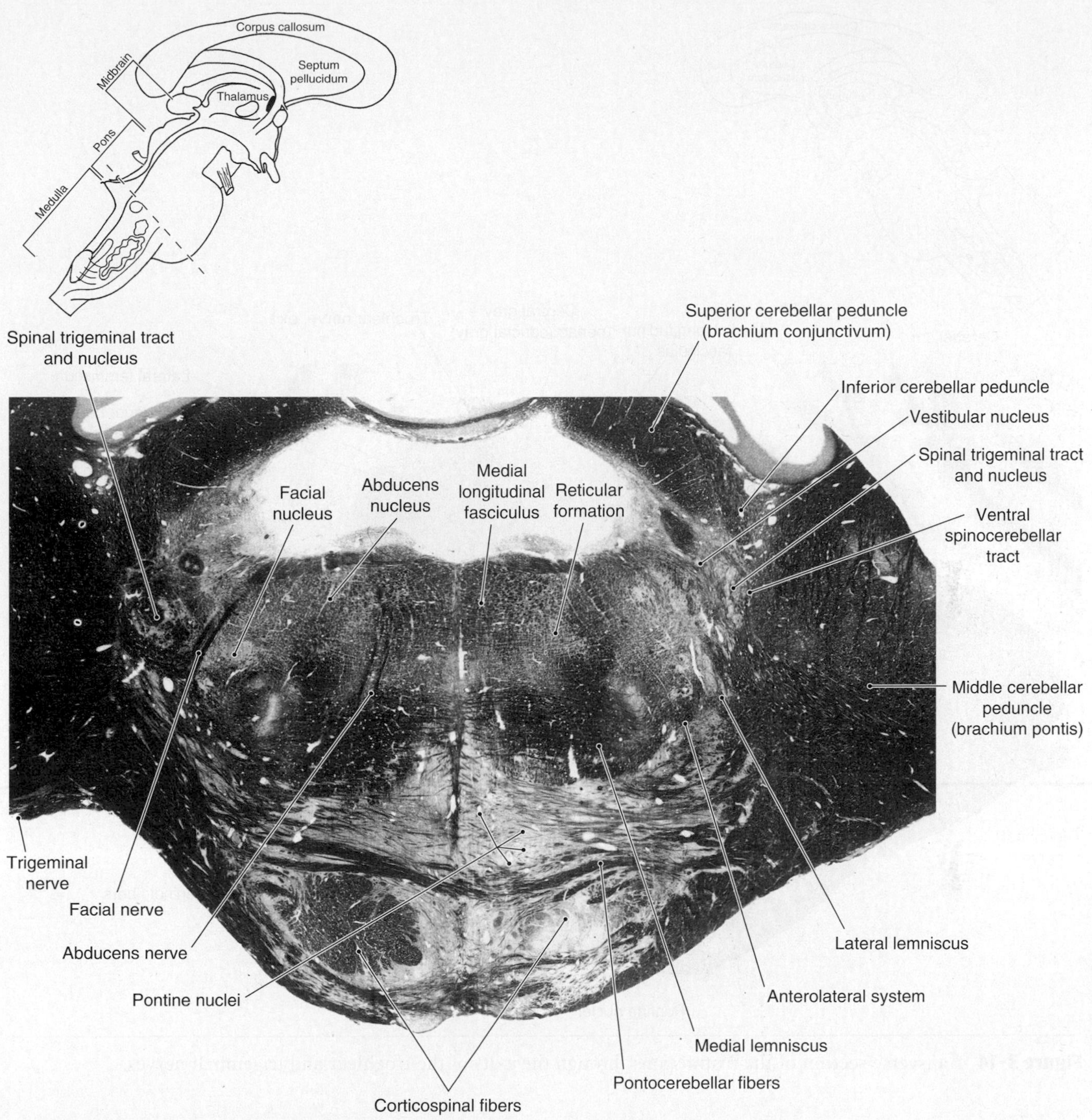

Figure 3-13 Transverse section of the pons through the rostral pole of the facial nucleus and internal genu of the facial nerve.

Key Terms:

Edinger–Westphal nucleus	**Neostriatum**
Hemiballism	**Parkinson disease**
Medial geniculate body	**Tectobulbar tract**
	Tectospinal tract
	Trochlear nerve root

Pons–Midbrain Junction

The section shown in Figure 3-14 is located at the transition between the rostral pons and the midbrain. This transition is marked by a reduction in the size of the fourth ventricle. The ventricular floor is formed by the enlarged central gray of the reticular formation, which contains important somatic and visceral nuclei. Located dorsally in this section is the **trochlear nerve root**, which is one of

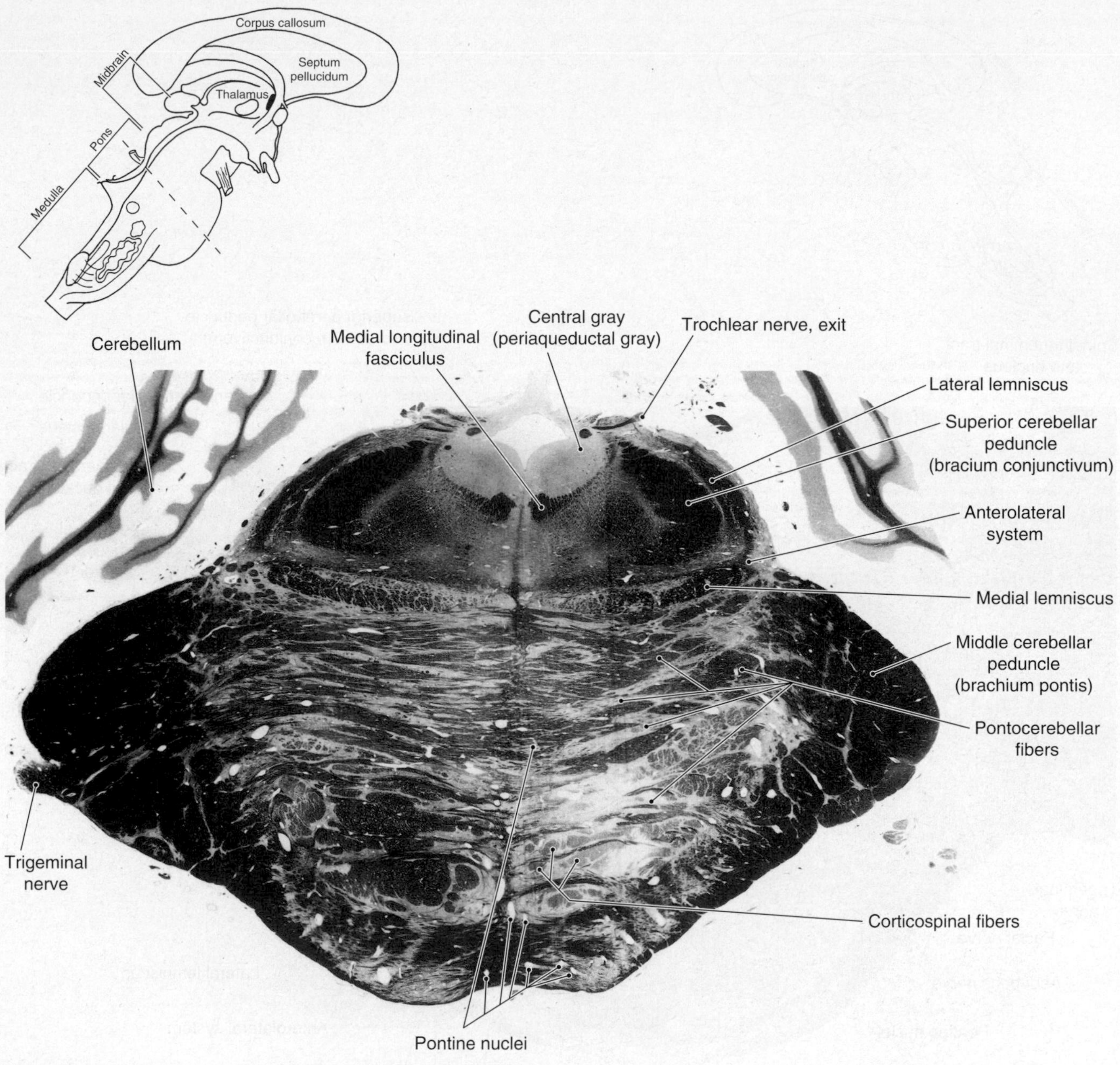

Figure 3-14 Transverse section of the rostral pons through the exits of the trochlear and trigeminal nerves.

three cranial nerves (the other two are oculomotor [CN III] and abducens [CN VI]) responsible for innervating the eye and is the only motor nerve that exits dorsally. The medial longitudinal fasciculus is buried within the central gray substance of the reticular formation. The massive cerebellum is dorsal to the ventricular cavity.

Ventral to the reticular central gray are fibers of the superior cerebellar peduncle, which occupy the outer third of the tegmentum and decussate at a higher level in the midbrain (Fig. 3-15). These fibers originate in the deep cerebellar nuclei and provide feedback to the opposite thalamic and cortical centers. Lateral to the fibers of the superior cerebellar peduncle are the lateral lemniscus fibers, which relay information from both the ears to the midbrain structures. The ventral region in this section contains diffuse pontine nuclei and a massive amount of crossing pontocerebellar fibers that make up the large middle cerebellar peduncles; also seen here are the scattered corticospinal tract fibers on each side of the midline. Located laterally is the root of the trigeminal nerve (CN V).

Midbrain

The midbrain consists of the tectum, tegmentum, and basis pedunculi (see Fig. 2-24). The tectum consists of the

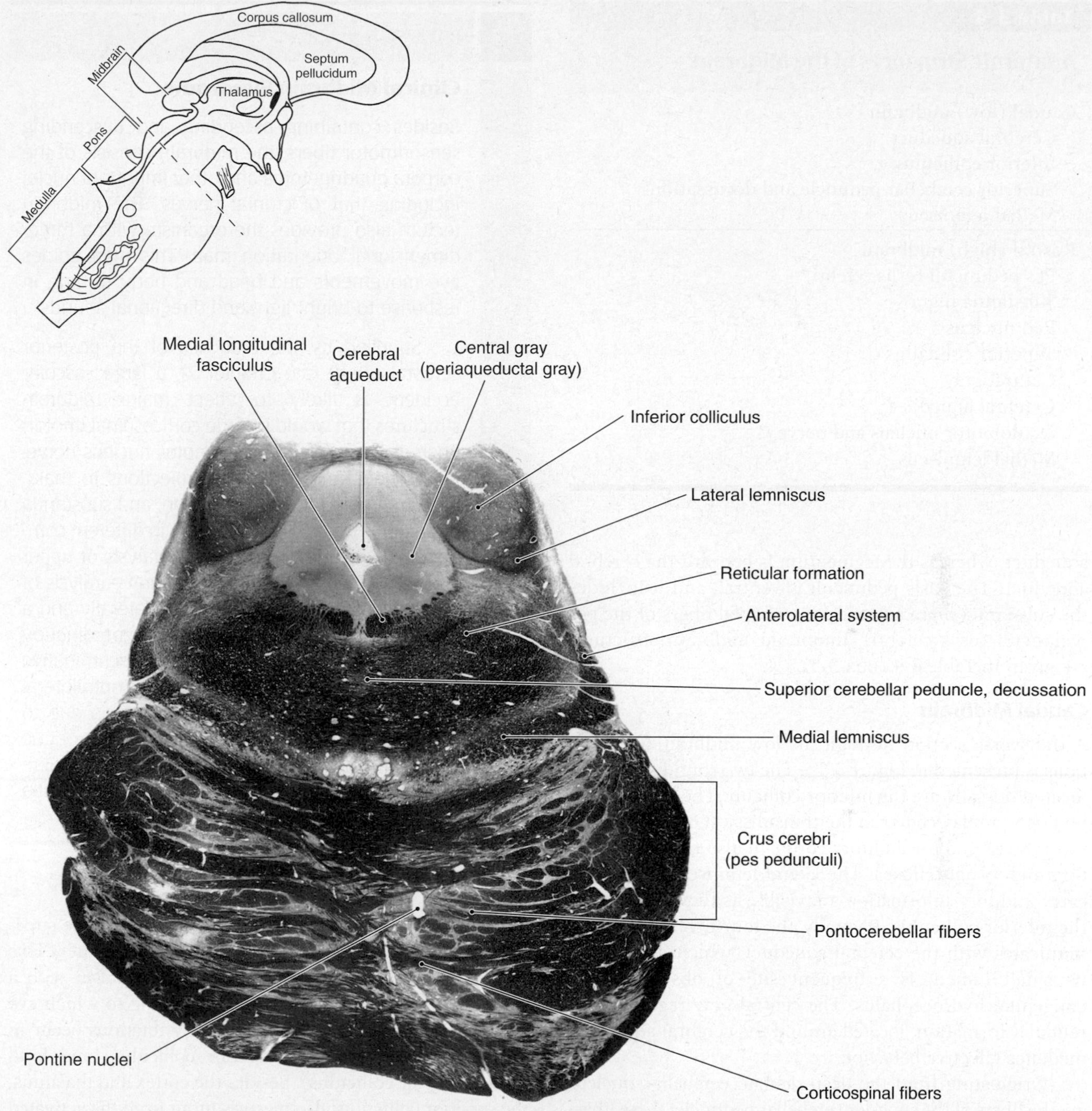

Figure 3-15 Transverse section of the pons–midbrain junction through the inferior colliculus, caudal portions of the decussation of the superior cerebellar peduncle, and rostral parts of the basilar pons.

corpora quadrigemina, which refers to four egg-shaped structures (see Figs. 2-21 and 2-22). The upper two nuclei are the superior colliculi and the lower two nuclei are the inferior colliculi. Below the midbrain tectal structure is the cerebral aqueduct, a narrow canal that connects the third and fourth ventricles.

The tegmentum is an elongated mass of nuclei and white matter in the center of the brainstem that includes decussation of the superior cerebellar peduncle, reticular formation, and red nucleus. The tectum and tegmentum are distinguishable by their locations with respect to the cerebral aqueduct. The tectum is dorsal to the cerebral

Table 3-4

Anatomic Structures of the Midbrain

Caudal (low) midbrain
Cerebral aqueduct
Inferior colliculus
Superior cerebellar peduncle and decussation
Medial lemniscus
Rostral (high) midbrain
Pes pedunculi (crus cerebri)
Substantia nigra
Red nucleus
Superior colliculus
Central gray
Cerebral aqueduct
Oculomotor nucleus and nerve
Medial lemniscus

aqueduct, whereas the tegmentum is beneath the cerebral aqueduct. The basis pedunculi is ventral, and it includes the substantia nigra and the wing-shaped fibers of the pes pedunculi (crus cerebri). Important midbrain structures are given in Table 3-4 (Box 3-5).

Caudal Midbrain

A transverse section through the low midbrain and high pons is presented in Figure 3-15. The two round structures located dorsally are the inferior colliculi. The inferior colliculus is a relay center in the transmission of information from the ears to the auditory cortex; it also regulates auditory and visual reflexes. The lateral lemniscus fibers that carry auditory information are visible as they merge with the inferior colliculus. Rostrally, the fourth ventricle communicates with the cerebral aqueduct, which, because of its small lumen, is a frequent site of obstruction in congenital hydrocephalus. The central gray region of the reticular formation, located around the cerebral aqueduct, mediates affective behavior.

Originating from the deep dentate cerebellar nucleus are the fibers of the superior cerebellar peduncle; these fibers course ventromedially below the aqueduct to cross the midline before going to the thalamus and cortex. This decussation of the superior cerebellar peduncle fibers accounts for the cerebellar projections to the contralateral motor cortex. Also present is the emerging pes pedunculi. The medial lemniscus, medial longitudinal fasciculus, lateral lemniscus, pontine nuclei, pontocerebellar fibers, and corticospinal fibers, identified earlier, are also present in this section.

Rostral Midbrain

The slightly oblique section shown in Figure 3-16 reveals the anatomic characteristics of the high midbrain. The tectum consists of two dorsally located round structures, the superior colliculi, which serve as the visual reflex center. This with other tectal structures provides the organism with a three-dimensional orientation map according to which eye movements and/or head turns and body rotations occur in response to bright lights (superior colliculus) and loud noises (inferior colliculus). Besides the cortex and thalamus, the superior colliculus also receives input from the activated spatial points in the retina. Ascending auditory signals also send collaterals into the inferior colliculus for similar spatial orientation processing.

Tectobulbar and **tectospinal** projections to the spinal cord and brainstem motor nuclei result in the appropriate turning of the eyes, head, and body toward the sound source. These startle reflexes are quite rapid, occurring before the cerebral cortex becomes aware of them. The superior colliculus and the adjacent pretectal area mediate reflexes involving intrinsic eye muscles; they also regulate pupil constriction (light reflex) and lens accommodation for near vision (see Chapter 12).

BOX 3-5

Clinical Midbrain Syndrome

Besides containing ascending and descending sensorimotor fibers, the midbrain consists of the corpora quadrigemina and other important nuclei including that of cranial nerves. The midbrain tectum also provides the organism with a three-dimensional orientation map. This map guides eye movements and head and body turning in response to bright light and directional sounds.

Supplied by the branches of the posterior cerebral artery (see Chapter 7), a large vascular accident is likely to affect major midbrain structures that would include corticospinal (motor) fibers in crus cerebri, oculomotor nucleus/nerve, red nucleus and cerebellar projections to thalamus, midbrain reticular formation, and substantia nigra. A midbrain syndrome may in different combinations include contralateral paralysis of upper limb, lower limb and trunk, ipsilateral paralysis of eye movement with the eye fixed laterally and a dilated pupil, contralateral limb incoordination (ataxia), and loss of contralateral discriminative touch. Additional symptoms include contralateral facial, pharyngeal, and tongue paralysis due to the affection of the corticobulbar fibers; tongue deviation contralaterally on protrusion; contralateral paralysis of lower face; akinesia (of substantia nigra); and frequent altered consciousness.

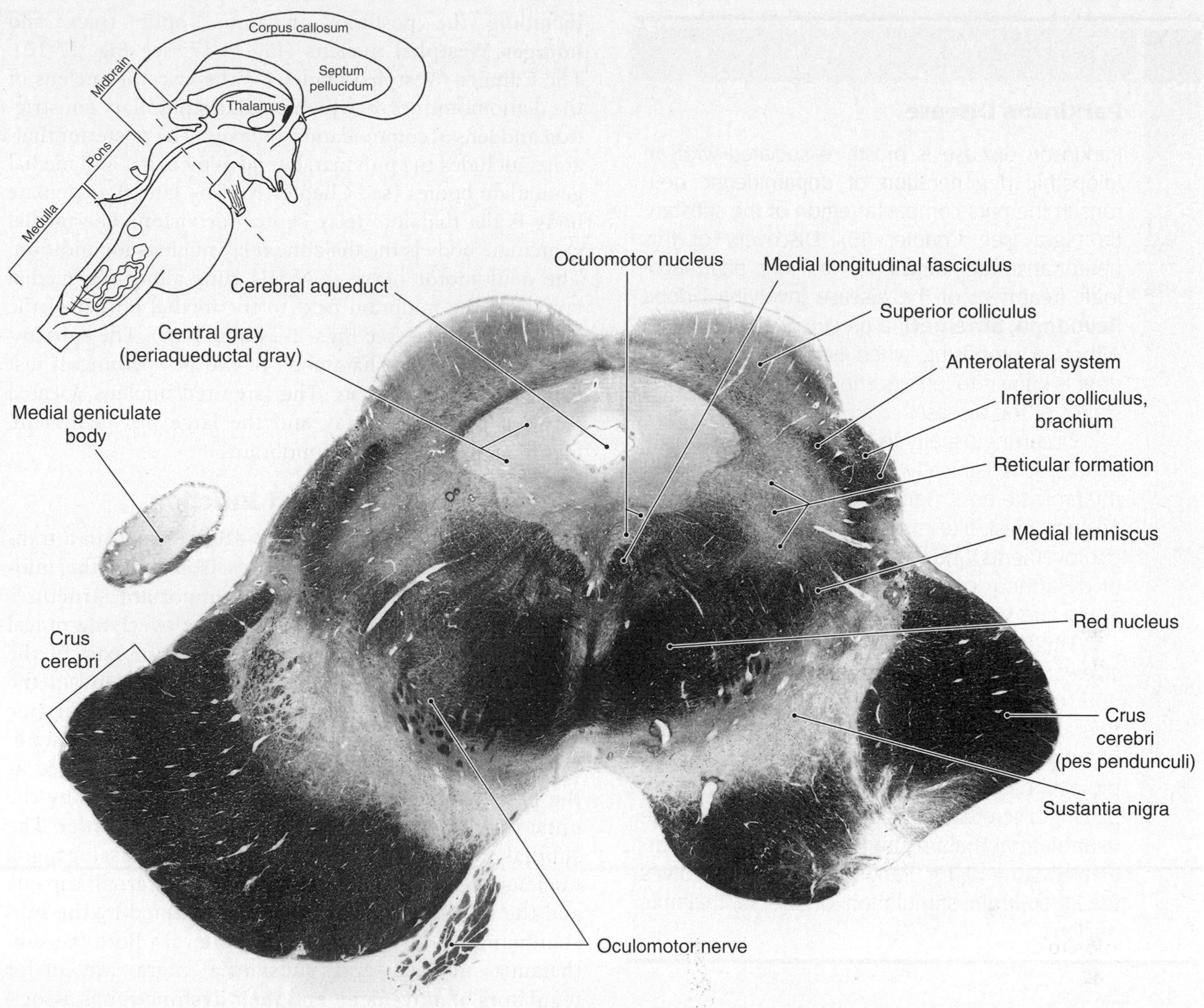

Figure 3-16 Transverse section of the midbrain through the superior colliculus, caudal parts of the oculomotor nucleus, and red nucleus.

The superior colliculi look similar to the inferior colliculi, but can be differentiated by comparison to their co-occurring structures. When seen on a cross section or transverse section, the decussation of the superior cerebellar peduncle fibers is the important landmark for identifying the inferior colliculus. The presence of the red nucleus and the substantia nigra characterizes the level of the superior colliculus.

Lateral to the superior colliculus is the brachium of the inferior colliculus, which carries auditory information from the inferior colliculus to the **medial geniculate body**, the thalamic relay nucleus for audition to the brain. The round nucleus in the midbrain tegmentum is the red nucleus, which has two important functions. First, it receives the cerebellar projections through the crossed superior cerebellar peduncle fibers and sends cerebellar feedback to the thalamus and motor cortex. Second, it transmits descending motor information to the spinal and cranial motor nuclei and regulates muscle tone.

Located below the red nucleus is the substantia nigra, an important nucleus in the extrapyramidal circuitry. Cells of the substantia nigra secrete **dopamine**, an inhibitory basal ganglia neurotransmitter; the nigrostriatal fibers project dopamine from the substantia nigra to the caudate nucleus of the **neostriatum**, another important nucleus in the extrapyramidal circuitry. The degeneration of the dopamine-producing cells in substantia nigra is associated with **Parkinson disease**, a slow progressive degenerative condition characterized by resting tremor, expressionless

BOX 3-6

Parkinson Disease

Parkinson disease is mostly associated with an idiopathic degeneration of dopaminergic neurons in the pars compacta region of the substantia nigra (see Chapter 15). Discovery of this neurotransmitter deficiency led to a pharmacologic treatment of the disease involving L-dopa (**levodopa, Sinemet**), a precursor of dopamine. Although promising when first introduced; this drug is known to lose its effectiveness in the later stages of the disease.

Occurring usually in late years of life, mostly in 60s, it is clinically characterized by bilateral rhythmic tremors, rigidity of movement, stooped posture, mask-like expressionless face, slowness of movements, and unintelligible speech because of dysarthria; cognitive symptoms may emerge in the late stages of the disease.

The lack of adequate treatment for progressive Parkinson disease led to a surgical intervention (stereotaxic neurosurgery) involving the neural circuitry of the basal ganglia. It was used to interrupt the basal ganglia circuitry and its projections to the motor cortex originally by placing discrete lesions in the pallidum or in the ventrolateral thalamic nucleus. More recent surgical treatment for Parkinson disease involves the deep-brain stimulation of the subthalamic nucleus.

(mask-like) face, muscular rigidity, flexed posture, slow movements, and moderate to severe progressive dysarthria (Box 3-6; see Chapter 15).

Ventrally located in this section are the wing-shaped large bundle fibers of the pes pedunculi (crus cerebri), which indicate the midbrain location of the descending corticospinal and corticobulbar fibers. In the floor of the central gray is the oculomotor nerve (CN III) nucleus, one of the three cranial nerves responsible for eye movements. Fibers of the oculomotor nerve (CN III) exit in the interpeduncular fossa (see Fig. 2-50). Located below the oculomotor nucleus is the medial longitudinal fasciculus, an important fiber bundle that interconnects three cranial nerves (oculomotor [CN III], trochlear [CN IV], and abducens [CN VI]) with the vestibular system. It not only regulates synergetic conjugate eye movement but it also coordinates head and eye movements.

High Rostral Midbrain

A transverse section through the rostral midbrain contains structures that are not present at lower levels, including the posterior thalamus, optic tract, and **Edinger–Westphal nucleus** (Fig. 3-17; see Fig. 17-10). The Edinger–Westphal nucleus is the visceral nucleus of the oculomotor nerve, which mediates pupillary constriction and lens accommodation reflexes. The posterior thalamus includes the pulvinar, lateral geniculate, and medial geniculate bodies (see Chapter 6). The lateral geniculate body is the thalamic relay center for vision. The medial geniculate body is the thalamic relay nucleus for audition. The oculomotor nerve (CN III) runs along the medial border of the midbrain next to the medial border of the large red nucleus (see Figs. 2-24 and 3-16). The substantia nigra sits in the hammock of the pes pedunculi just beneath the red nucleus. The large red nucleus, located between the central gray and the large pes pedunculi, identifies this level of the midbrain.

Midbrain–Diencephalon Junction

The oblique section in Figure 3-18 is located in a transitional area, revealing structures from both the midbrain and the diencephalon. The important structures are the posterior commissure with the overlying pineal gland in the dorsal midline; the posterior part of the thalamus, the pulvinar nucleus; the rostral end of the red nucleus flanked laterally by the medial lemniscus; and the large diagonal internal capsule–pes pedunculi. Fibers of the internal capsule, which were identified as the pes pedunculi below this level, are hugged by the optic tract that runs along its ventrolateral border. The subthalamic nucleus, a very important basal ganglia nucleus, is sandwiched between the internal capsule and the red nucleus; this area was occupied by the substantia nigra at the caudal midbrain levels. Both the subthalamic nucleus and substantia nigra are major regulators of movement, and their dysfunction is associated with movement disorders.

The pineal gland, an endocrine organ, is located dorsally and is important in the body's diurnal (repeating once each 24 hours) rhythm. Inhibition of its secretion has also been associated with the onset of puberty. This calcified structure serves as a landmark for reading the neurological images. The posterior commissure is considered to connect the two superior colliculi. The posterior thalamus includes the pulvinar, lateral, and medial geniculate bodies (see Chapter 6). The lateral geniculate body is the thalamic relay center for vision. The medial geniculate body is the thalamic relay center for audition. The pulvinar, the most caudal part of the thalamus, is reciprocally connected with the parietotemporal association cortex. Its association with speech and language functions is discussed in neurosurgical literature (see Chapter 6).

The dysfunction of the subthalamic nucleus, an important extrapyramidal structure, results in **hemiballism**, a neurologic condition characterized by an abrupt onset of violent and flinging movements.

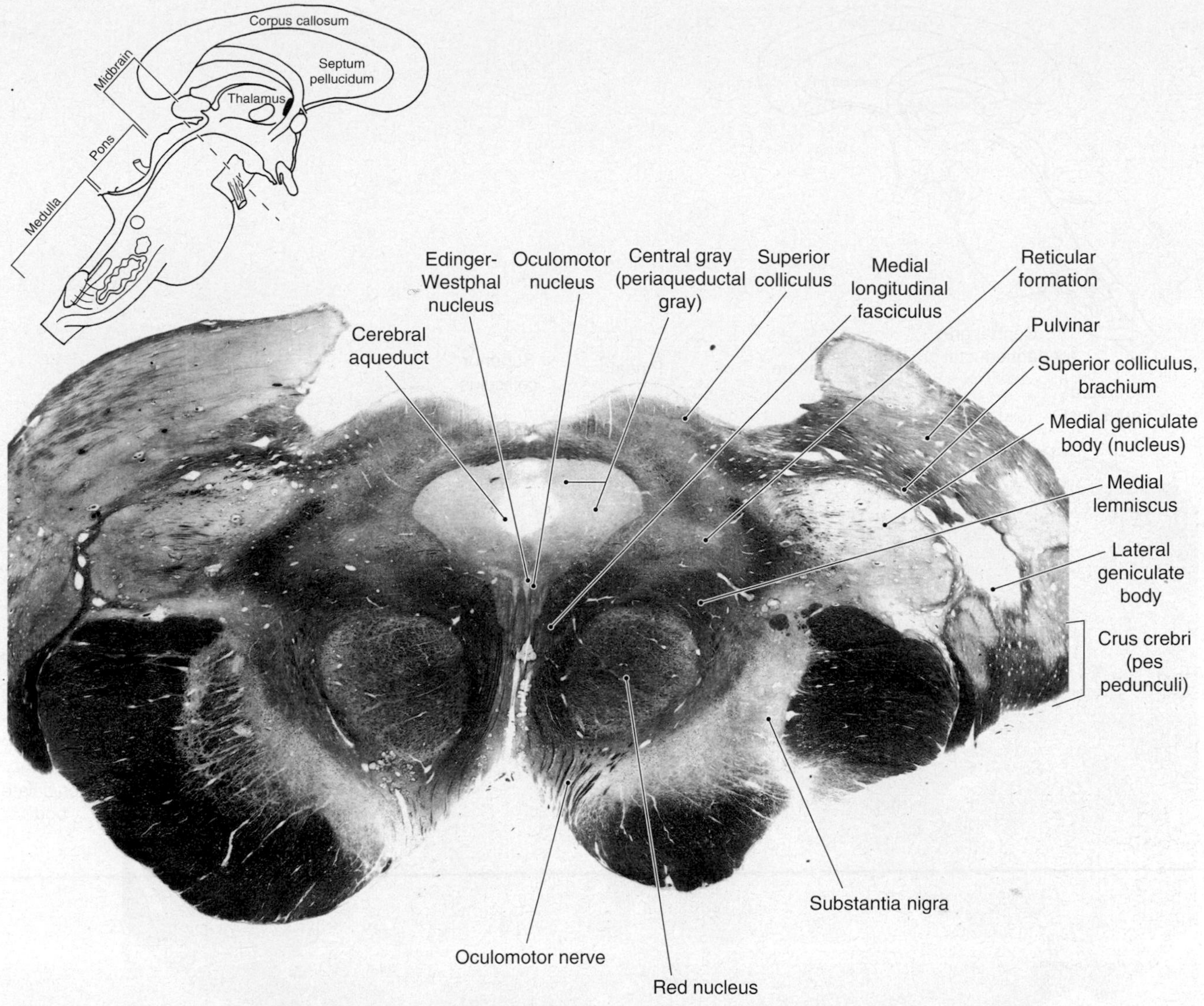

Figure 3-17 Transverse section of the midbrain through the superior colliculus and rostral portions of the oculomotor nucleus.

FOREBRAIN IN CORONAL SECTIONS

Learning the forebrain internal anatomy entails orientation to the subcortical structures: basal ganglia (caudate nucleus, putamen, globus pallidus, and functionally related subthalamic nucleus), diencephalon (thalamus and hypothalamus), ventricular cavity (lateral and third ventricles), and limbic structures (amygdala, fornix, hippocampal formation, and cingulate gyrus). Other important structures are the corpus callosum, optic chiasm, insular cortex (isle of Reil), septum pellucidum, anterior commissure, internal capsule, external capsule, extreme capsule, and claustrum (Table 3-5; Box 3-7). A familiarity with the internal forebrain anatomy is a prerequisite for training in neuroscience, since it promotes the ability to read neurological images of the brain, contributes to neurological clinical problem solving, and helps explain the pathophysiology of degenerative brain etiologies associated with higher mental dysfunctions; it also explains the reasons for the multiplicity of clinical signs that can occur even after a focal lesion. Since the neuroanatomical structures in the brain are in fixed positions, a review of their relative locations on a horizontal section would facilitate the orientation to them on subsequent coronal serial sections of the brain (Figs. 3-19 and 3-20).

Located rostrally in a horizontal section of the brain are the frontal lobes on each side of the midline corpus (genu) callosum (Fig. 3-19); for a better orientation, also see Figure 2-41. The fibers of the corpus callosum connect the homologous cortical areas in both hemispheres by corticocortical fibers. The septum pellucidum is in the midline extending from the ventral surface of the corpus callosum and ending along the anterior limits of the thalamus. On each side of the septum pellucidum are the anterior horns of the lateral

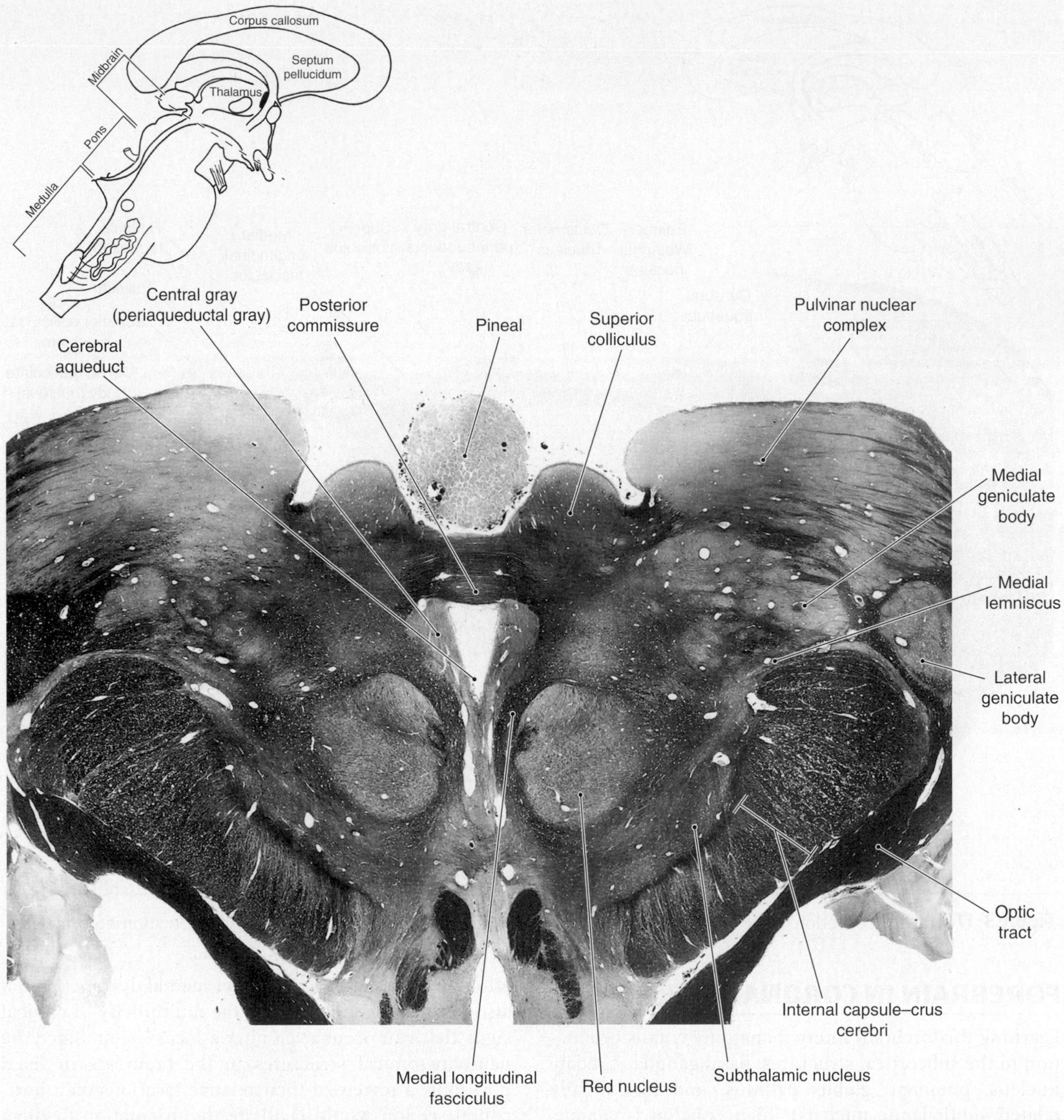

Figure 3-18 Oblique section through the midbrain–diencephalon junction.

ventricle (Figs. 2-15 and 3-19). The septal nuclei are located at the base of the anterior ventricular horns. With connections to the limbic (hippocampal formation and amygdala), hypothalamic (mammillary) structures, and hippocampus, the septal nuclei are known to play a role in autonomic (reproductive) behaviors and memory regulation. The third ventricle is in the midline between two the thalami. Each lateral ventricle communicates with the midline third ventricle through the **interventricular foramen of Monro** (see Figs. 2-18 and

Table 3-5

Anatomic Structures of the Forebrain

Posterior thalamus	
Pineal gland	Lateral geniculate body
Corpus callosum, splenium	Medial geniculate body
Pulvinar of thalamus	Internal capsule merging in crus cerebri/pes pedunculi
Cerebral aqueduct	
Midthalamus	
Corpus callosum, body	Third ventricle
Fornix	Hypothalamus
Subthalamic nucleus	Diminishing globus pallidus and putamen
Lateral ventricle	
Anterior thalamus	
Anterior commissure	Internal capsule, genu
Caudate	Corpus callosum, body
Putamen	External capsule
Globus pallidus	Extreme capsule
Third ventricle	Septum pellucidum
Hypothalamus	Claustrum
Anterior internal capsule	
Corpus callosum, body	Septum pellucidum
Head of the caudate nucleus	Internal capsule, anterior limb
Putamen	External capsule
Lateral ventricle, anterior horn	Claustrum
	Extreme capsule

3-19). The interventricular foramen is located at the junction of the septum and thalamus on each side of the midline.

The two large nuclear masses projecting into the lateral ventricles are the heads of the caudate nuclei, which are important contributors to motor functions. Caudal to the caudate nuclei are the two thalami on each side of the third ventricle. The junctional area between the caudate and the thalamus is indented by the genu of the internal capsule, which connects the anterior limb of the capsule to its posterior limb. The anterior limb is associated predominantly with fronto-pontine and anterior thalamic radiation fibers; the posterior limb is associated with the ascending (sensory) and descending (motor) cortical projections.

The bend of the internal capsule is produced in part by the lenticular nucleus (putamen and globus pallidus). These two nuclei contribute to motor control and, in conjunction with the caudate nucleus, constitute the basal ganglia. Just lateral to the putamen is the claustrum, a thin, wavy line of cells that possesses two-way projections predominantly with the sensory cortical areas of the brain. The insular cortex, concerned with visceral functions, overlies the claustrum and lenticular nucleus.

The caudal end of the third ventricle is identified by the posterior commissure and the pineal gland in the midline. This level is the transitional area between the posterior thalamus and the midbrain. More caudally, the cerebellum is in the midline between the occipital lobes. The cerebellum overlies the fourth ventricle and is attached to the brainstem by the cerebellar peduncles. The next six figures are used to illustrate the forebrain anatomy on sequentially related coronal section (Fig. 3-20). Corresponding MR images are included so that students can efficiently read brain images by relating their acquired knowledge of internal brain anatomy to the very structures as they appear in the images.

Coronal Section through the Posterior Thalamus

The distinction between white and gray matter with sulci and gyri markings is vividly present on the fist coronal section of the brain (Fig. 3-21). The large fissure in the middle separating the hemispheres is the **interhemispheric longitudinal fissure**. The body of the corpus callosum forms the roof of the lateral ventricles. The splenium of the corpus callosum, not present on this cut, connects both occipital lobes.

BOX 3-7

Clinical Forebrain Syndrome

The forebrain serves all higher mental functions, including consciousness, cognition, symbolic communication, knowledge, imagination, creativity, and skilled sensorimotor skills. Vascular accidents are the primary causes of forebrain dysfunction and include aphasia, agnosia, apraxia, dysarthria, visual special deficits, altered consciousness, and sensorimotor deficits. With vascular supply to brain through three different (anterior, middle, and posterior) cerebral arteries, most of the vascular cortical symptoms are focal, depending on the cortical artery that was involved (see Chapter 7). In general, left brain lesions result in language deficits which involve alexia, aphasia, verbal apraxia, acalculia, and aphasia. The right nondominant cortical lesions mostly lead to the deficits related to visual-spatial processing, musical appreciation, comprehension and expression of prosody, processing of paralinguistic (joke, humor, metaphor, and idiom) skills, and attention. Irrespective of the hemisphere involved, cortical vascular lesions also affect sensorimotor fibers and result in contralateral paralysis and loss of discriminative touch, pain, and temperature.

The large cavities in this section are the bodies of the lateral ventricles; the small cavities in the temporal lobe mark the inferior horns of the lateral ventricles. Located in the floor of the lateral ventricle is the fornix, a bundle of fibers that serve as a two-way connection between the mammillary body of the hypothalamus and hippocampus (see Chapter 19). Forming the medial wall of the inferior horn of the lateral ventricles is the hippocampal formation, which is thought to serve memory functions by consolidating new information. Its involvement is most marked in degenerative diseases of the brain that are associated with higher mental function disorders.

The thalamic nucleus in this caudal section is the pulvinar, the most posterior nucleus of the thalamus, which is connected reciprocally to the parietal association cortex and participates in language functions (see Chapter 6). Ventral to the pulvinar are the geniculate (medial and lateral) bodies, which serve as thalamic relay centers. The medial geniculate body mediates auditory information from the ears to the primary auditory cortices in the transverse **gyri of Heschl** (Brodmann area 41). The lateral geniculate body transmits visual information from homonymous halves of the retinas to the primary visual cortex in the occipital lobe (Brodmann area 17).

Dorsal to the inferior horn and lateral to the thalamus is the posterior limb of the internal capsule, which contains the ascending (sensory) and descending (motor) fibers. In the middle of this section, the following brainstem structures can be seen: cerebral aqueduct, decussation of the superior cerebellar peduncle, basal pons, and the pretectal structure. The pretectal area regulates visual reflexes (see Chapters 12 and 17).

Coronal Section through the Midthalamus

The section of the brain shown in Figure 3-22 retains most of the structures previously identified at the posterior thalamic level and a few newly visible structures. Emerging bilaterally from the walls of the lateral ventricle is the larger body of the caudate nucleus. The caudate nucleus, with its long tail, is a C-shaped structure in sagittal views of the brain (see Fig. 2-17); it can be seen in many sequential coronal sections of the brain. The caudate is an important nucleus, contributing to motor activity; it may have a role in cognitive processing. Its pathologic involvement of this structure is associated with Huntington chorea, a neurodegenerative disease characterized by dysarthria, chorea, personality changes, and dementia. (Box 3-8). This genetically transmitted condition is characterized by dominant inheritance with complete penetrance and onset in the third or fourth decade of life.

Forming the floor of the lateral ventricles in this section are the large gray masses of the thalamus. Both thalami are connected through the **massa intermedia**, a thalamic loose fibrous tissue. In the midline between the two lateral ventricles is the septum pellucidum. Through the base of the septum courses the fornix, an important C-shaped limbic structure that connects the mammillary bodies of the hypothalamus to the hippocampus and septum and is involved in autonomic functions. Located lateral to the internal capsule, the lenticular nucleus consists of the globus pallidus and putamen. The globus pallidus and putamen are parts of the basal ganglia and are important in regulating motor functions and muscle tone (see Chapter 17).

The external capsule is a thin band of fibers lateral to the lenticular nucleus. Lateral to the external capsule is the claustrum, a thin layer of gray matter. The thin bundle of fibers lateral to the claustrum is the extreme capsule. The most lateral structure in this section is the insular cortex. The vertical slit in the center is the third ventricle, formed by the medial walls of each thalamus. In the center of the section, the remaining brainstem structures include the crus cerebri (pes pedunculi), basilar pons, red nucleus, and substantia nigra.

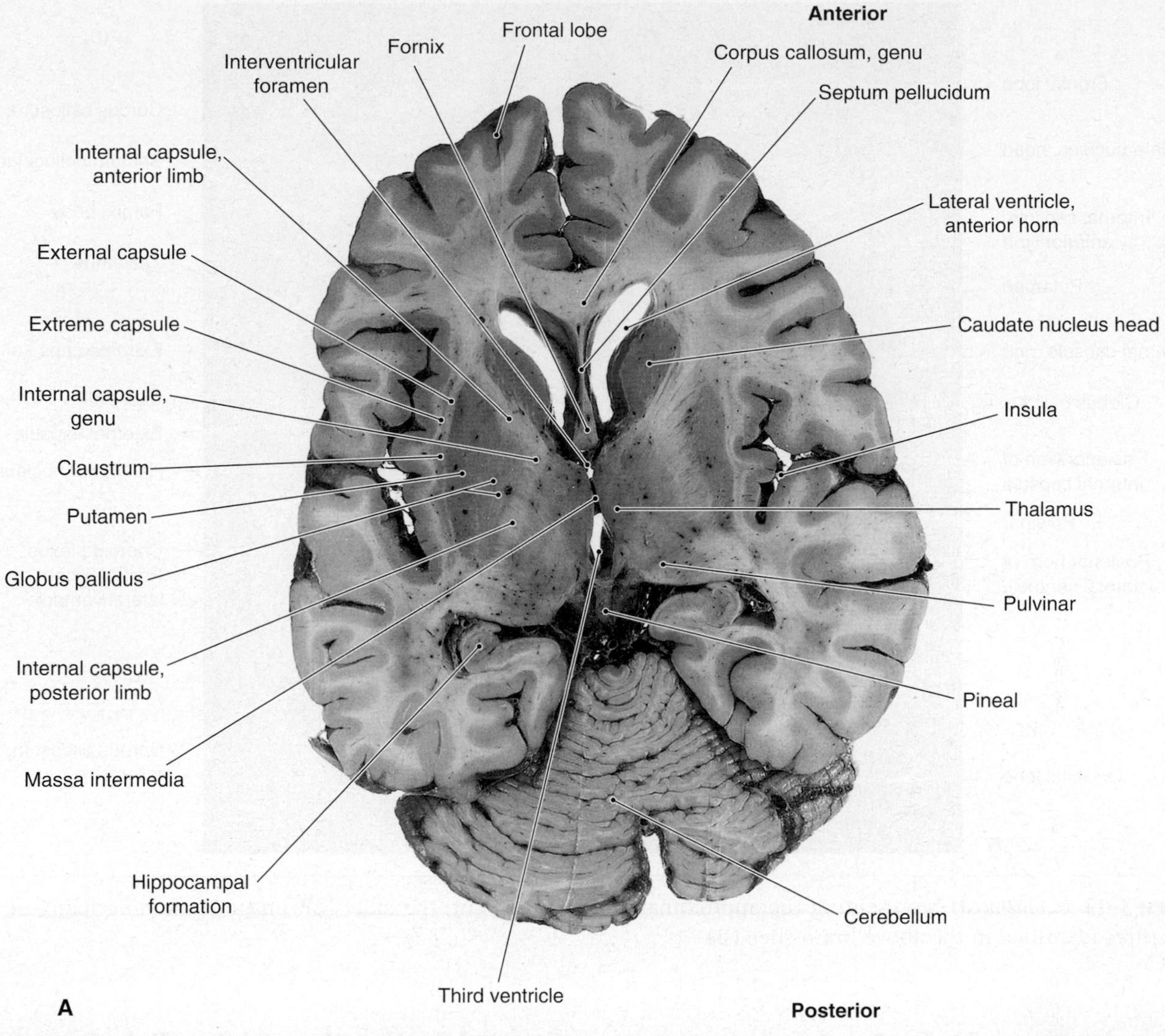

Figure 3-19 Dorsal view of a horizontal section through the interventricular foramina, third ventricle, and pulvinar (A);

Coronal Section through the Anterior Thalamus

The general orientation of the forebrain anatomy in a coronal section through the anterior thalamus is similar to that of the previous section, although the one shown in Figure 3-23 is more rostral at the anterior thalamic nucleus level. The rough, saggy, and worm-shaped structure in the lateral ventricles is the choroid plexus, which secretes cerebrospinal fluid. Forming the floor of the lateral ventricle is the anterior nucleus, the most rostral nucleus of the thalamus. This nucleus receives afferents (mammillothalamic tract) from the mammillary bodies of the hypothalamus and projects to the cingulate gyrus of the limbic lobe. Along the lateral wall of the lateral ventricles is the caudate nucleus, a C-shaped structure. This section of the forebrain is unique because it simultaneously reveals the dorsal component (body of the caudate nucleus in the lateral ventricle) and ventral component (tail of the caudate nucleus in the lateral wall of the temporal horn).

Medial to the internal capsule is the biconvex-shaped subthalamic nucleus, an important nucleus in the basal ganglia circuitry. It receives afferents from the lateral segment of the globus pallidus and projects to both of the pallidal segments as well as to the pars reticulata region of the **substantia nigra**. Subthalamic pathology results in hemiballism, a condition of involuntary movement marked by the onset of violent and flinging movements.

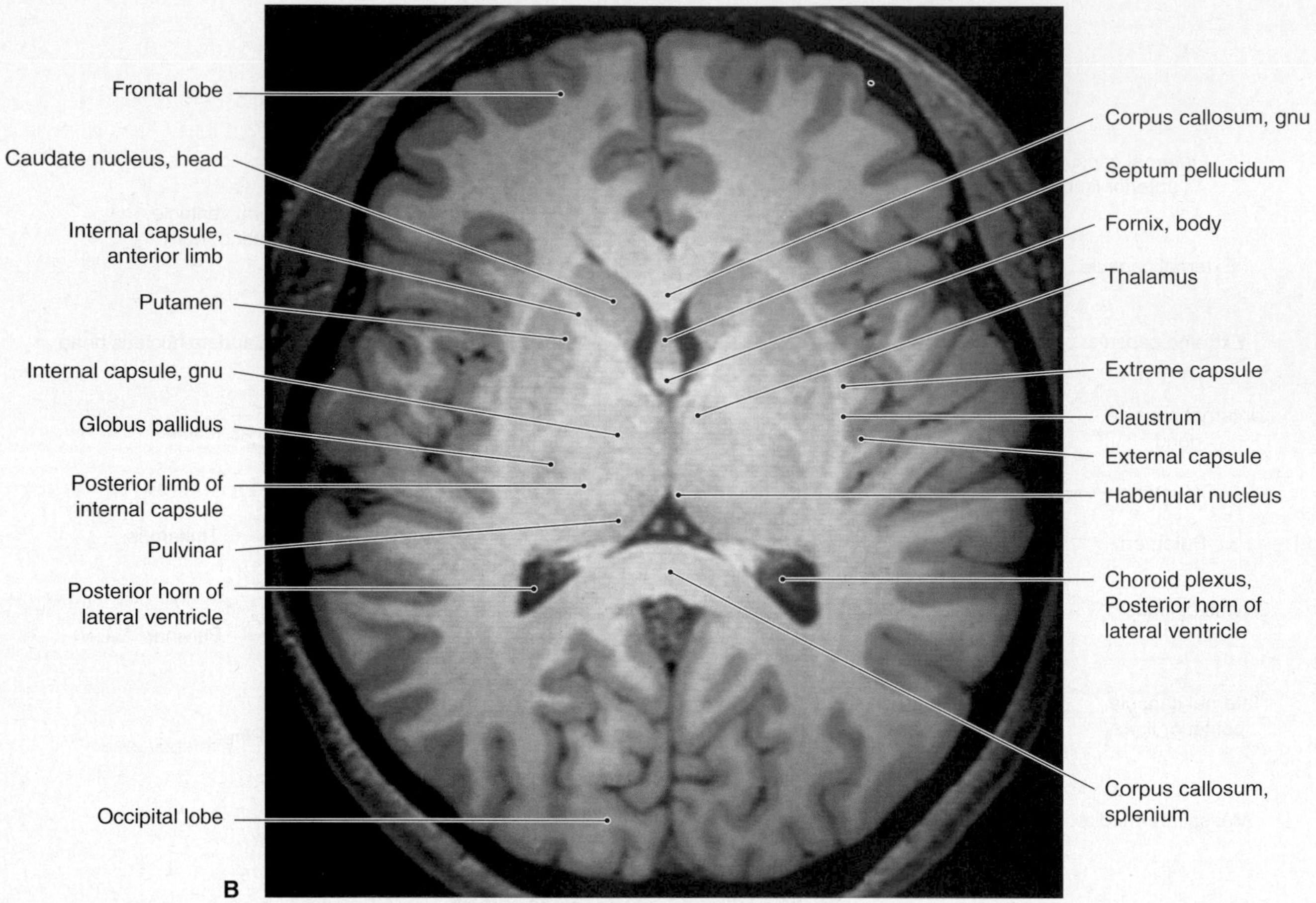

Frontal lobe
Caudate nucleus, head
Internal capsule, anterior limb
Putamen
Internal capsule, gnu
Globus pallidus
Posterior limb of internal capsule
Pulvinar
Posterior horn of lateral ventricle
Occipital lobe
Corpus callosum, gnu
Septum pellucidum
Fornix, body
Thalamus
Extreme capsule
Claustrum
External capsule
Habenular nucleus
Choroid plexus, Posterior horn of lateral ventricle
Corpus callosum, splenium
B

Figure 3-19 (*Continued*) representing the approximate plane of the cut, the axial MR image containing many of the structures identified in the above brain slice (B).

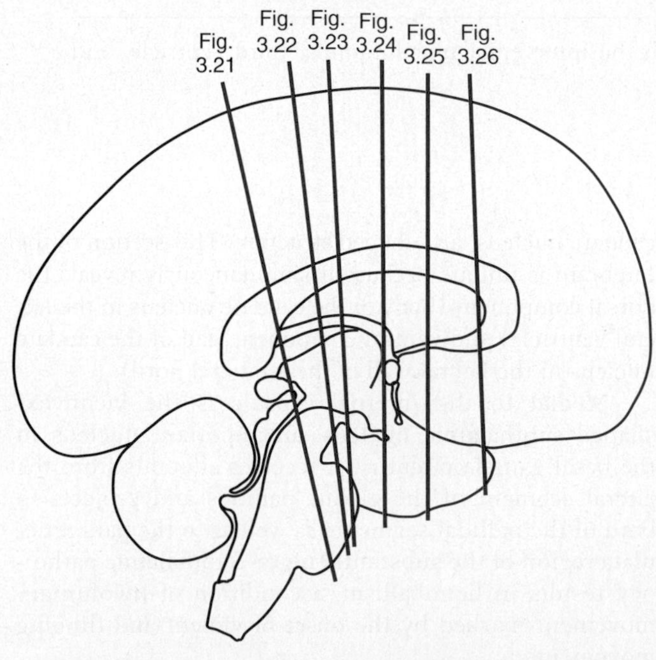

Figure 3-20 Midsagittal view identifying the locations of the coronal brain sections shown in the indicated figures.

Coronal Section through the Anterior Commissure

A coronal section of the forebrain through the anterior commissure and the anterior limb of the internal capsule provides a more rostral view of the forebrain structures (Fig. 3-24). The head of the caudate nucleus emerges as a larger structure at this point in the ventricular cavity than at the more caudal levels. There is a clear view of the anterior commissure and its crossing. The anterior commissure is a small forebrain fiber bundle that contains bidirectional olfactory fibers and connects the temporal cortices.

The septum, which anteriorly separates the lateral ventricles, is centrally located in the section. Many hippocampal projections through the fornix terminate in the septum verum nuclei, which are part of the limbic system. Forming the lateral walls of the third ventricle below the level of the anterior commissure is the hypothalamus. Two important structures of the hypothalamus, not seen in this section, are the mammillary body and pituitary gland. Hypothalamic nuclei produce neurosecretions that are important in controlling water balance, sugar and fat metabolism, body temperature, and

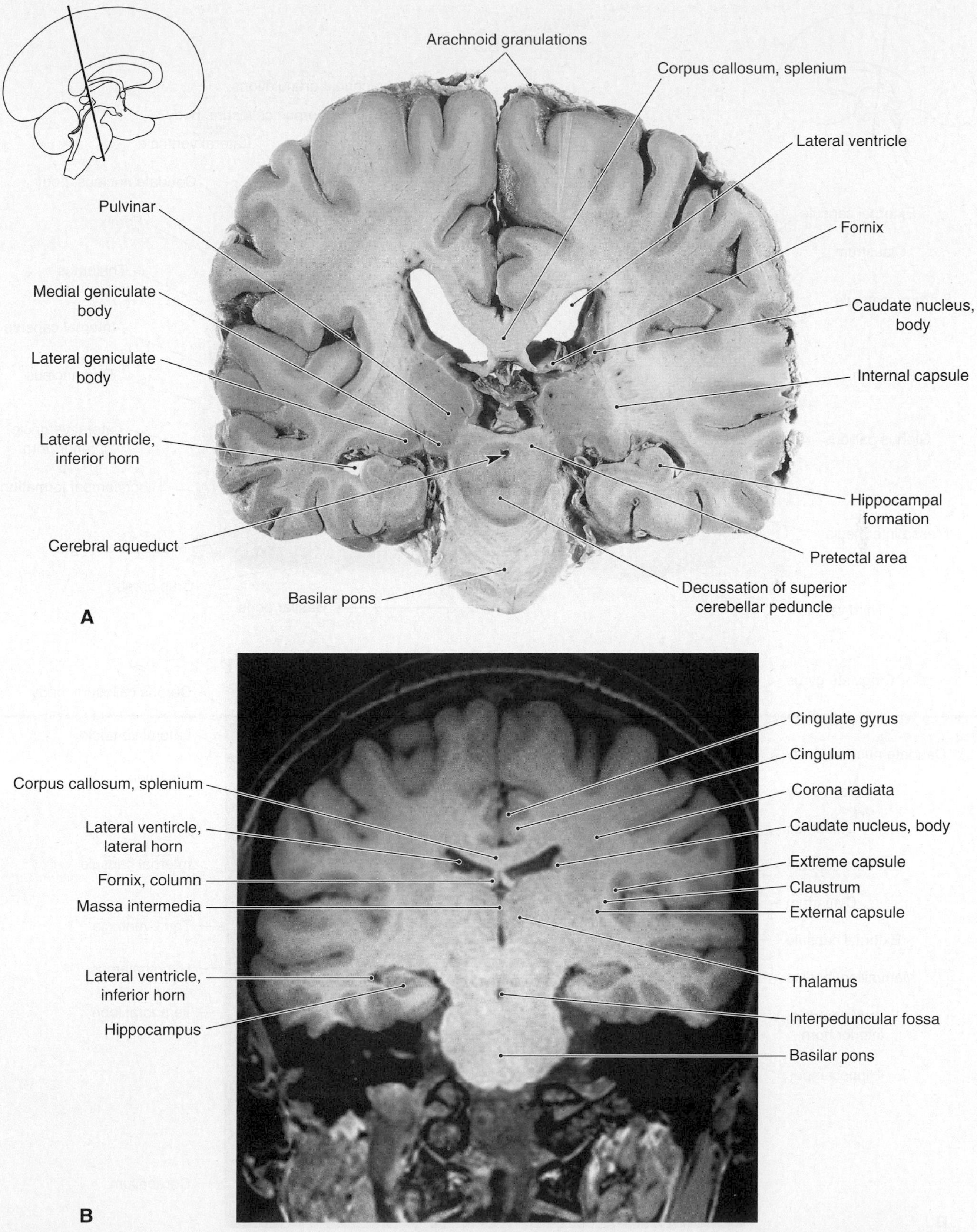

Figure 3-21 Caudal surface of a coronal section through the posterior thalamus (A); coronal MR image (B) approximately at the same plane illustrating many of the structures identified in the brain slice.

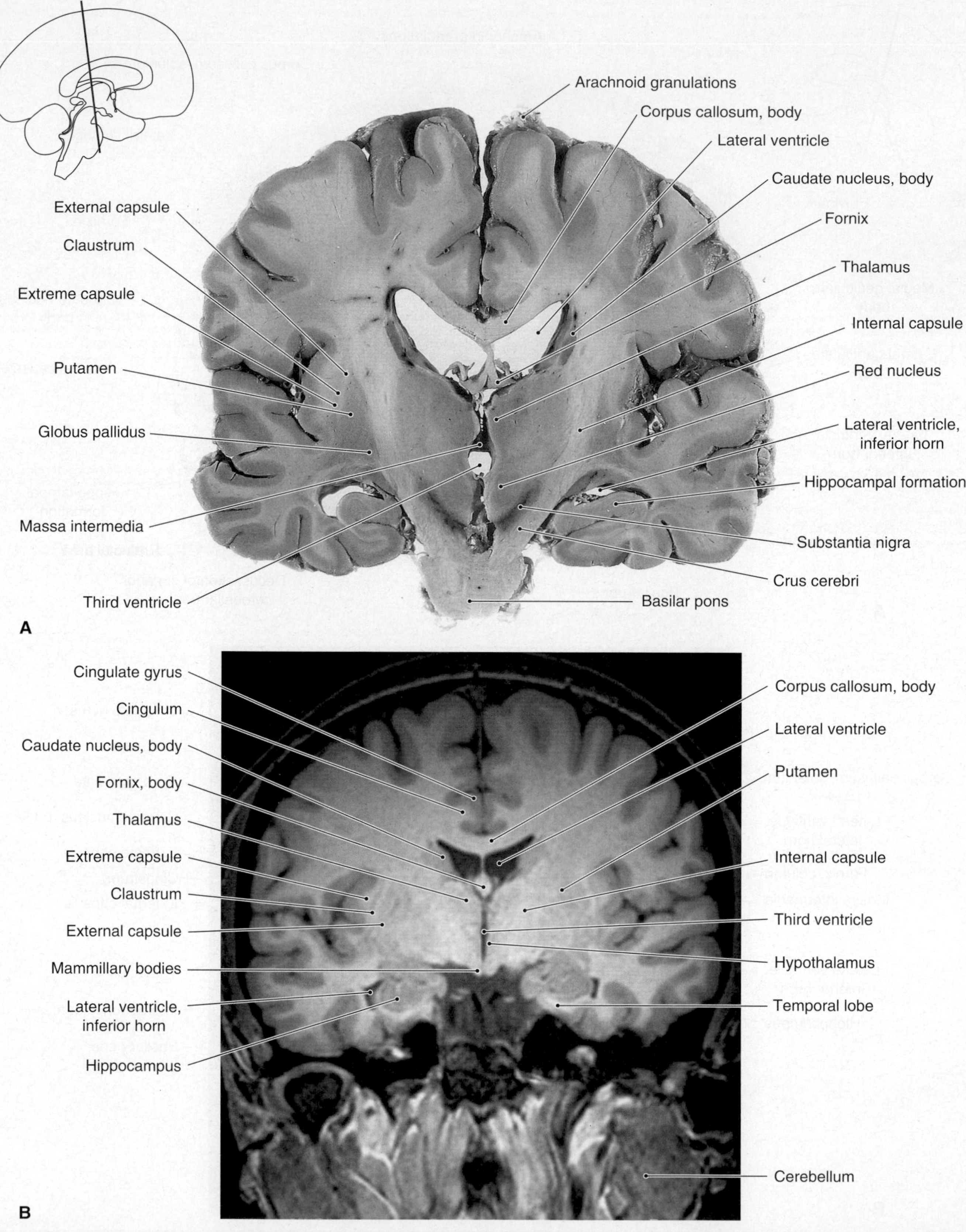

Figure 3-22 Caudal surface of a coronal section (A) through the medial thalamus and massa intermedia; coronal MR image (B) approximately at the same plane illustrating many of the structures identified in the brain slice.

BOX 3-8

Huntington Chorea

Huntington chorea, a progressive neurodegenerative disease of dominant autosomal inheritance, is associated with complete gene penetration with an onset in the fourth or fifth decade of life. The mutation, a repeat of the Huntington gene locus, has been mapped to chromosome 4p. The disease causes cellular death in the caudate nucleus, putamen, and cerebral cortex. Clinically, it is characterized by choreic movements of the upper and lower limbs, altered personality, dysarthria, and dementia. There is no medical treatment for preventing the degenerative process in Huntington chorea; however, dopamine receptor blockers have been used to control the choreic movements. Speech–language pathologists are involved with the management of this syndrome because of the presence of dysarthria and dementia.

hormone production. The hypothalamus is also the regulator of the autonomic (sympathetic and parasympathetic) nervous system.

The amygdaloid nucleus is seen here at the level at which the tail of the caudate nucleus terminates (see Fig. 2-17). The amygdala, a massive round structure in the medial temporal lobe, is generally responsible for activating emotional behavior. Pathology of the amygdaloid nucleus has been known to lead to aggression and other abnormal behavior, such as hypersexuality; surgical removal of amygdala in animals has caused aggressive animals to become docile and hyposexual.

The following previously identified structures are also present in this section and remain unchanged in basic configuration: corpus callosum, septum pellucidum, fornix, caudate nucleus, putamen, globus pallidus, internal capsule, external capsule, claustrum, extreme capsule, and insular cortex.

Coronal Section through the Caudate Head

A coronal section of the forebrain at the rostral region of the basal ganglia reveals the large head of the caudate nucleus, the anterior horn of the lateral ventricles, and the anterior limb of the internal capsule (Fig. 3-25). At this level of the brain, the thalamus and globus pallidus are no longer present (Fig. 3-19). The massive caudate nucleus head forms the ventrolateral wall of the lateral ventricle at the level of the anterior horn. Laterally, the ventral component of the caudate nucleus merges with the putamen to form the corpus striatum.

The portion of the internal capsule at this level is the anterior limb, which courses between the bodies of the caudate and putamen. In the middle, forming the medial ventricular wall is the septum pellucidum, which is attached to the medial basal forebrain area. The cingulate gyrus, a limbic structure involved with emotional drive and anxiety, is dorsal to the body of the corpus callosum. The cingulum, a bundle of mediofrontal parietal cingulate association fibers, is beneath the cingulate gyrus. Also visible is the septum pellucidum with its underlying nucleus, a limbic structure related to visceral functions, reward, and gratification.

The cortical regions rostral to this level undergo only a few changes. The ventricular cavity rostrally ends at the genu of the corpus callosum (see Fig. 2-12). Anterior to the corpus callosum is the massive accumulation of white matter that consists of callosal radiations and corona radiata. These changes can be seen in Figure 3-26.

Coronal Section through the Anterior Horn

A coronal section of the forebrain at the genu of the corpus callosum reveals the end of the lateral ventricle (anterior horn) and the rostral striatum (caudate head and putamen) (Fig. 3-26). Other previously identified rostral structures seen here include the septum, internal and external capsules, claustrum, cingulate gyrus, and cingulum.

FOREBRAIN IN HORIZONTAL SECTIONS

A review of the forebrain anatomy on horizontal sections contributes to the visual orientation of the internal anatomy of the brain and helps consolidate previous learning. In Figures 3-27 to 3-30, the human brain has been dissected horizontally to provide a three-dimensional view of the corpus callosum, ventricular cavity, thalamus, and basal ganglia structures.

Further, the removal of a 1-cm-thick layer of the cerebral cortex exposes the underlying brain structures (Fig. 3-27). The residual indentation of the interhemispheric longitudinal fissure is evident in the middle, including the central sulcus; other sulci and gyri are seen in the periphery of this section. Each hemisphere contains a **semiovale center**, a massive accumulation of white matter that contains the blended association, commissural, and projection fibers above the internal capsule level. The sensorimotor fibers form the corona radiata, in which the descending motor fibers fan down toward the internal capsule and

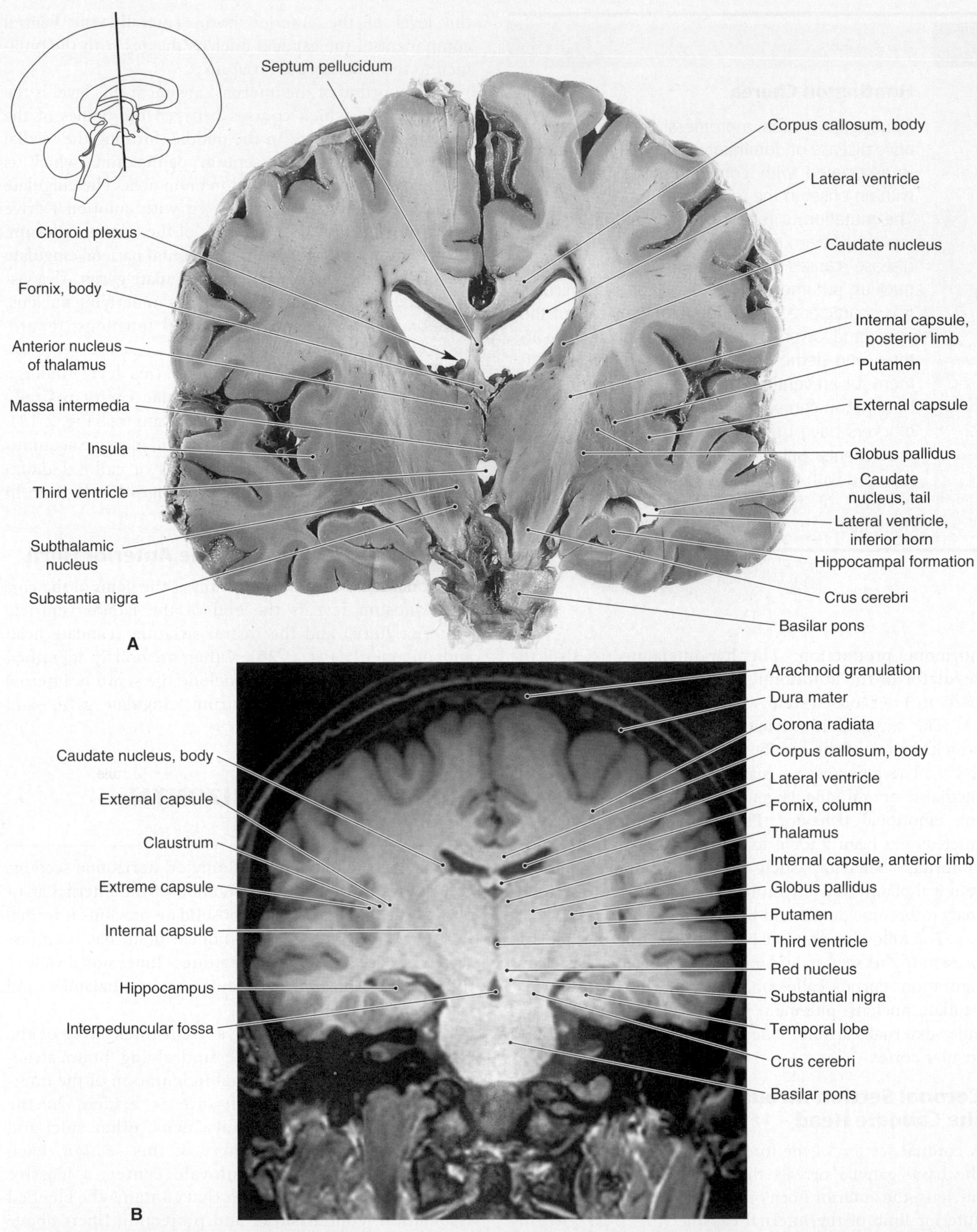

Figure 3-23 Rostral surface of a coronal section (A) through the rostral thalamus, massa intermedia, and subthalamic nucleus; coronal MR image (B) approximately at the same plane illustrating many of the structures identified in the brain slice.

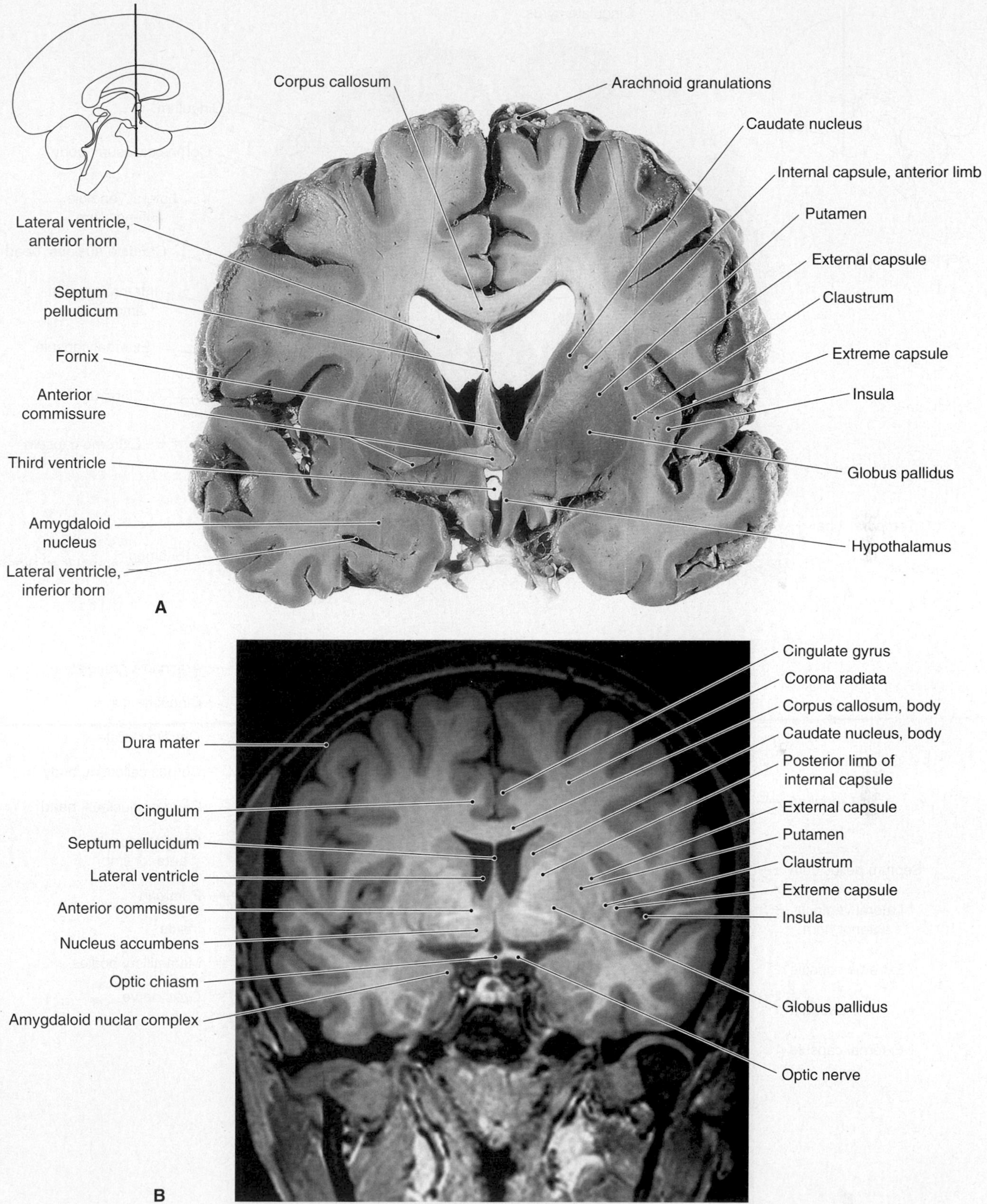

Figure 3-24 Rostral surface of a coronal section (A) through the level of the anterior commissure rostral to the genu of the internal capsule; coronal MR image (B) approximately at the same plane illustrating many of the structures identified in the brain slice.

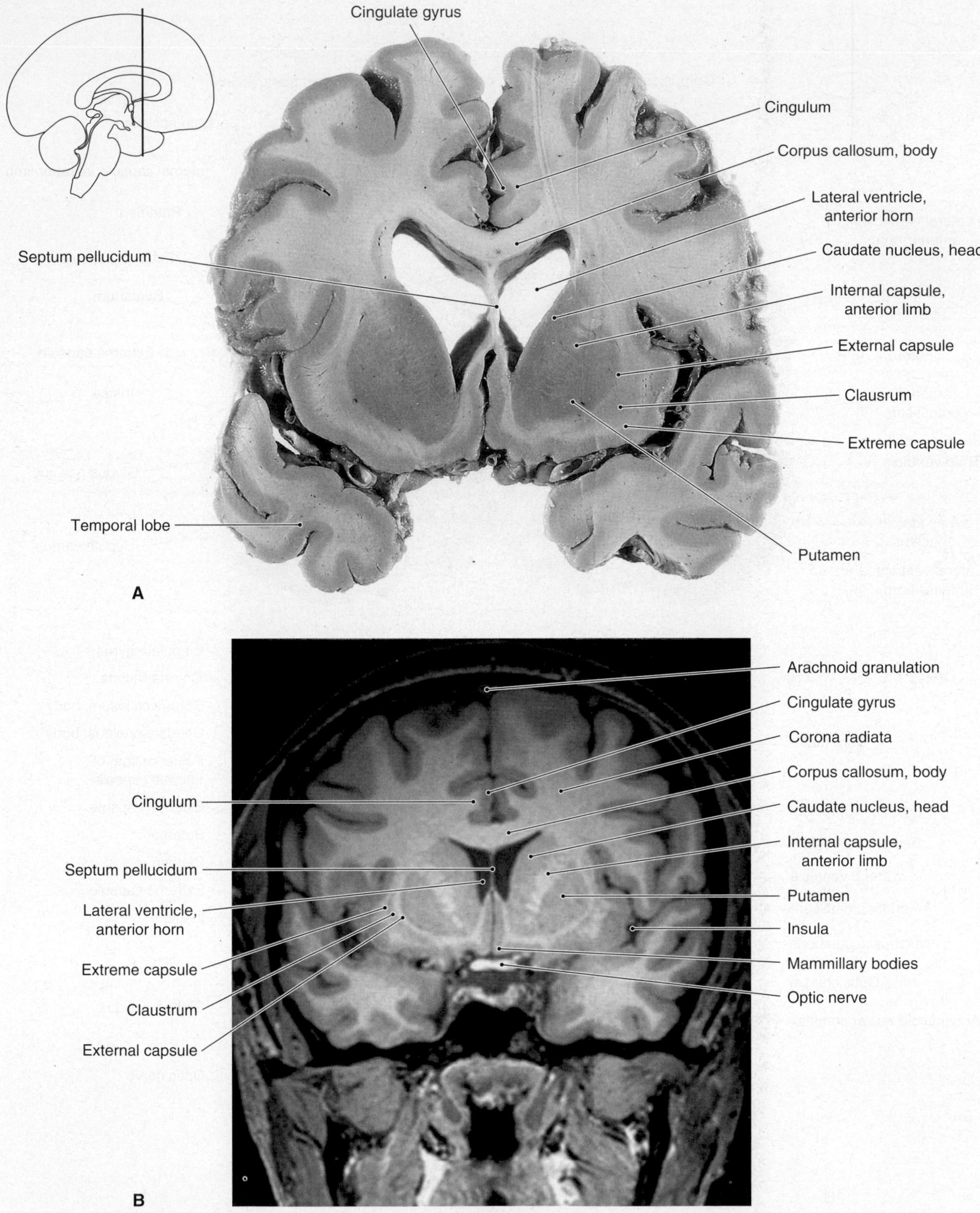

Figure 3-25 Caudal surface of a coronal section (A) through the head of the caudate nucleus; coronal MR image (B) approximately at the same plane illustrating many of the structures identified in the brain slice.

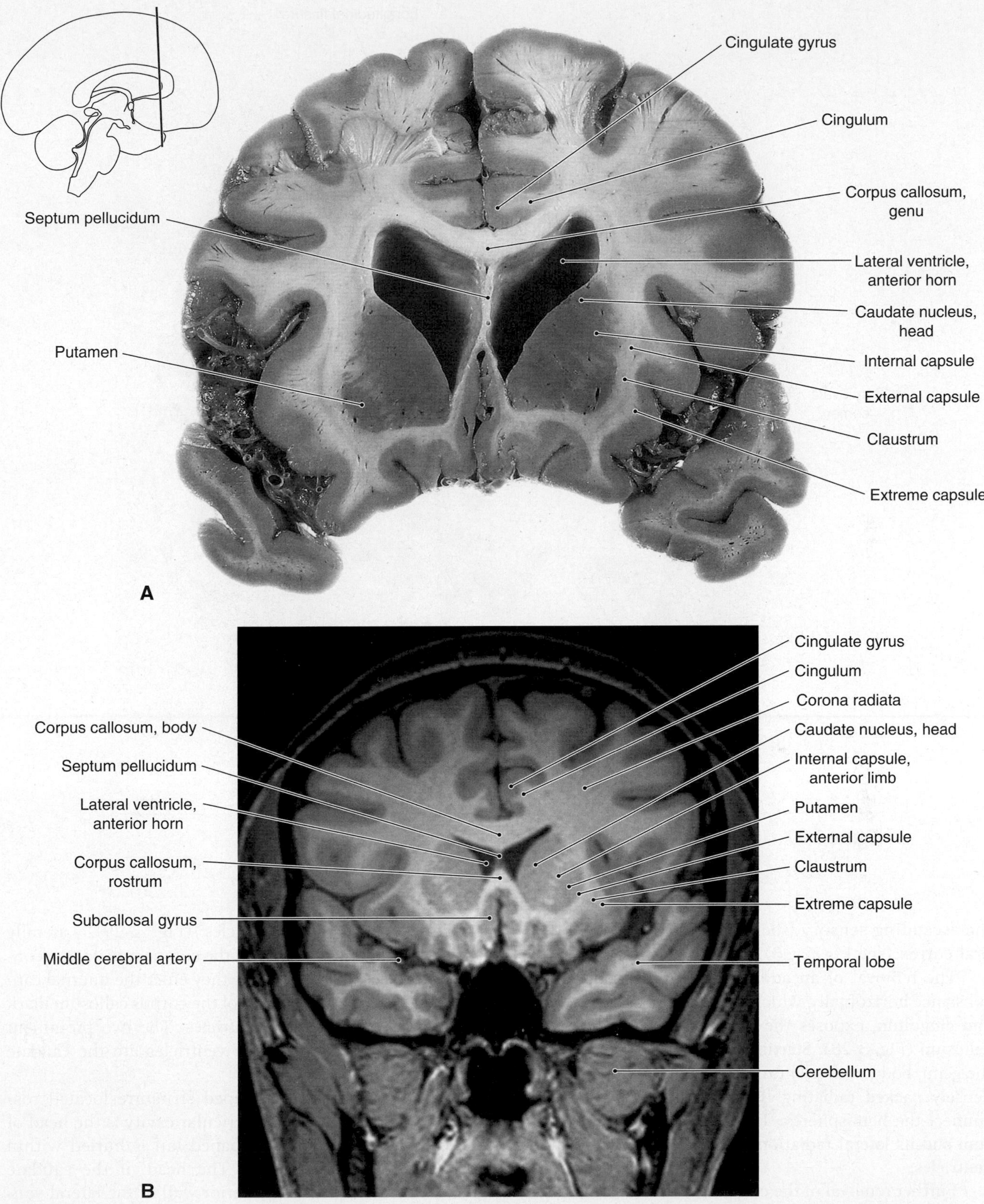

Figure 3-26 Caudal surface of a coronal section (A) just caudal to the genu of the corpus callosum and the rostral end of the anterior horns; coronal MR image (B) approximately at the same plane illustrating many of the structures identified in the above brain slice.

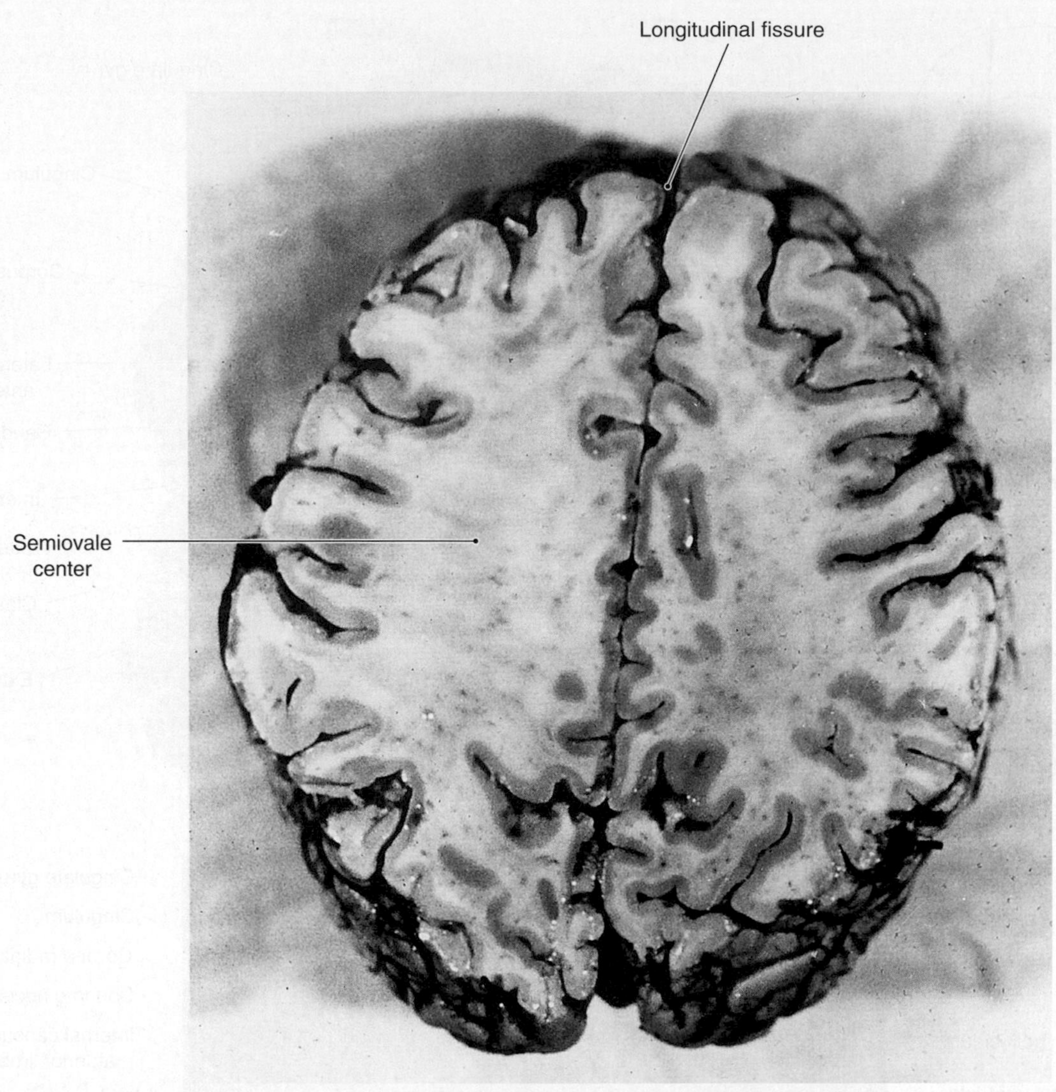

Figure 3-27 Horizontal section of the brain above the corpus callosum.

the ascending sensory fibers fan out to reach the cerebral cortex (see Fig. 2-38).

The removal of an additional 1 to 2 cm of cortical substance horizontally, which includes the cingulate gyrus and cingulum, exposes the dorsal surface of the corpus callosum (Fig. 3-28). Starting rostrally in this section are the genu, body, and splenium of the corpus callosum. The densely packed radiating fibers of the corpus callosum connect the hemispheres. The body of the corpus callosum and its lateral radiations form the roof of the lateral ventricles.

Further removal of the corpus callosum and its radiating cortical fibers reveals the large underlying subcortical structures and lateral ventricles (Fig. 3-29). Laterally located are the fibers that form the corona radiata, the condensed projection fibers before they enter the internal capsule. The spaces on both sides of the corpus callosum mark the cavities of the lateral ventricles. The two prominent structures in the floor of the ventricles are the caudate nucleus and the thalamus.

The massive balloon-shaped structure located rostrally and laterally in the ventricular cavity is the head of the caudate nucleus; its C-shaped tail is buried within the adjoining white matter. The head of the caudate nucleus forms the lateral anterior wall of the lateral ventricles. The thalamus, the largest diencephalic structure,

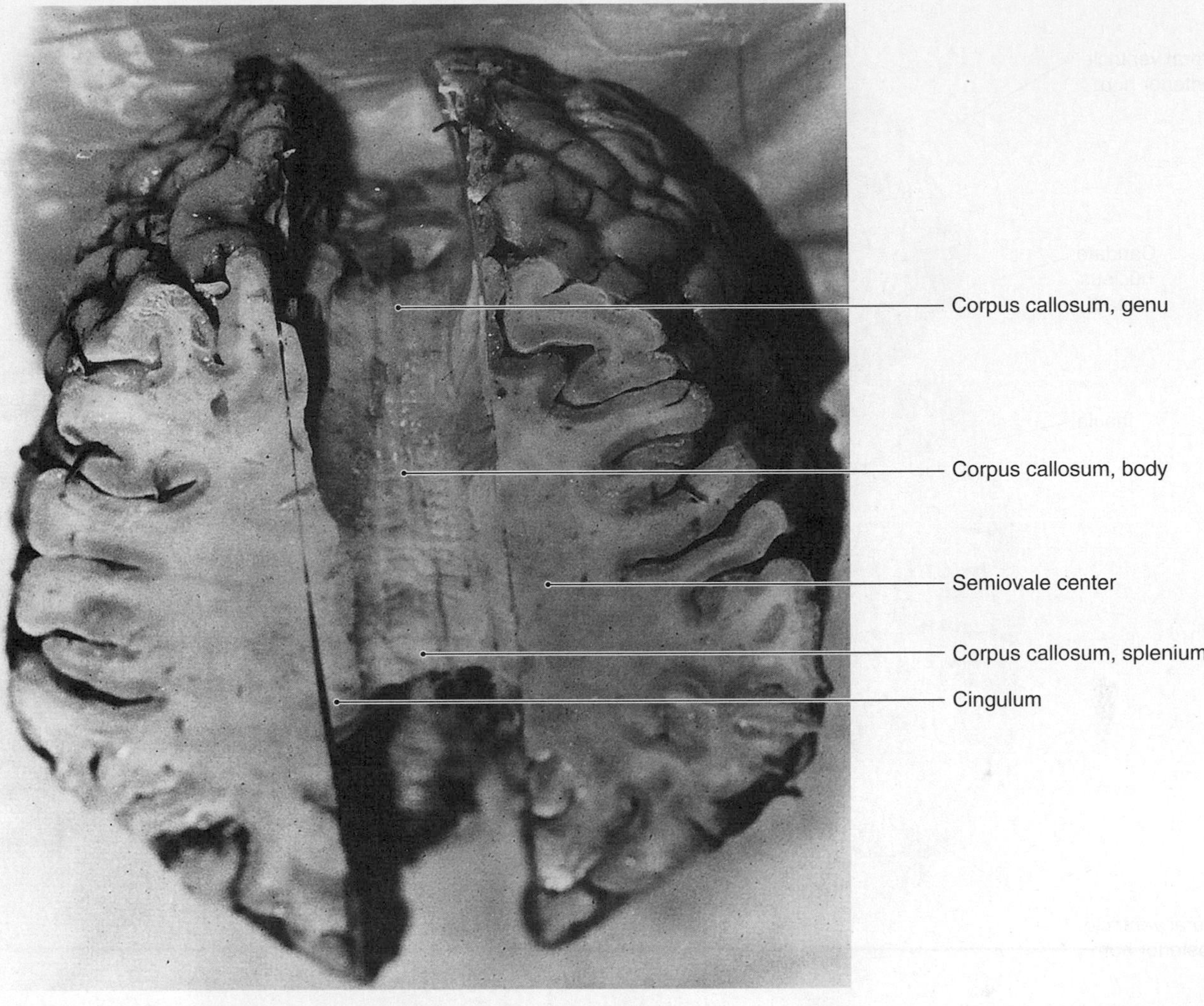

Figure 3-28 Horizontal section exposing the corpus callosum.

is located posteriorly in the floor of the ventricular cavity; caudate is clinically connected to the basal ganglia circuitry and Huntington chorea. Removal of parietal and occipital tissues has also exposed the caudal portion of the lateral ventricles, particularly the posterior horns in the occipital lobe regions. The remaining genu, body, and splenium portions of the corpus callosum are identified easily above the lateral ventricles. Also present is the point at which the tail of the caudate nucleus enters the temporal lobe.

Further removal of the overlying white medullary substance, caudate nucleus, and thalamus by sectioning rostral to the genu of the corpus callosum exposes the cavity of the lateral ventricles and the surrounding subcortical structures (Fig. 3-30). The exposed inner temporal lobe contains the slender temporal horns of the lateral ventricles. The hippocampus, amygdala, and uncus are located medially in the inferior horn. The hippocampus forms the medial wall of the temporal horns. It receives direct projections from the fornix and indirect projections from the cingulum via the parahippocampal gyrus and is associated with Alzheimer disease (Box 3-9).

Anterior to the tip of the hippocampus is the amygdaloid nucleus, an important limbic structure with a protruding cortical component called the uncus. With a complete removal of the callosal fibers, the floor of the lateral ventricles becomes fully visible. The septum is seen rostrally, separating the anterior horns of the lateral ventricles. The structure at the base of the septum is the fornix column. Also present are the head of the caudate nucleus, the medial dorsal thalamus, and the third ventricle.

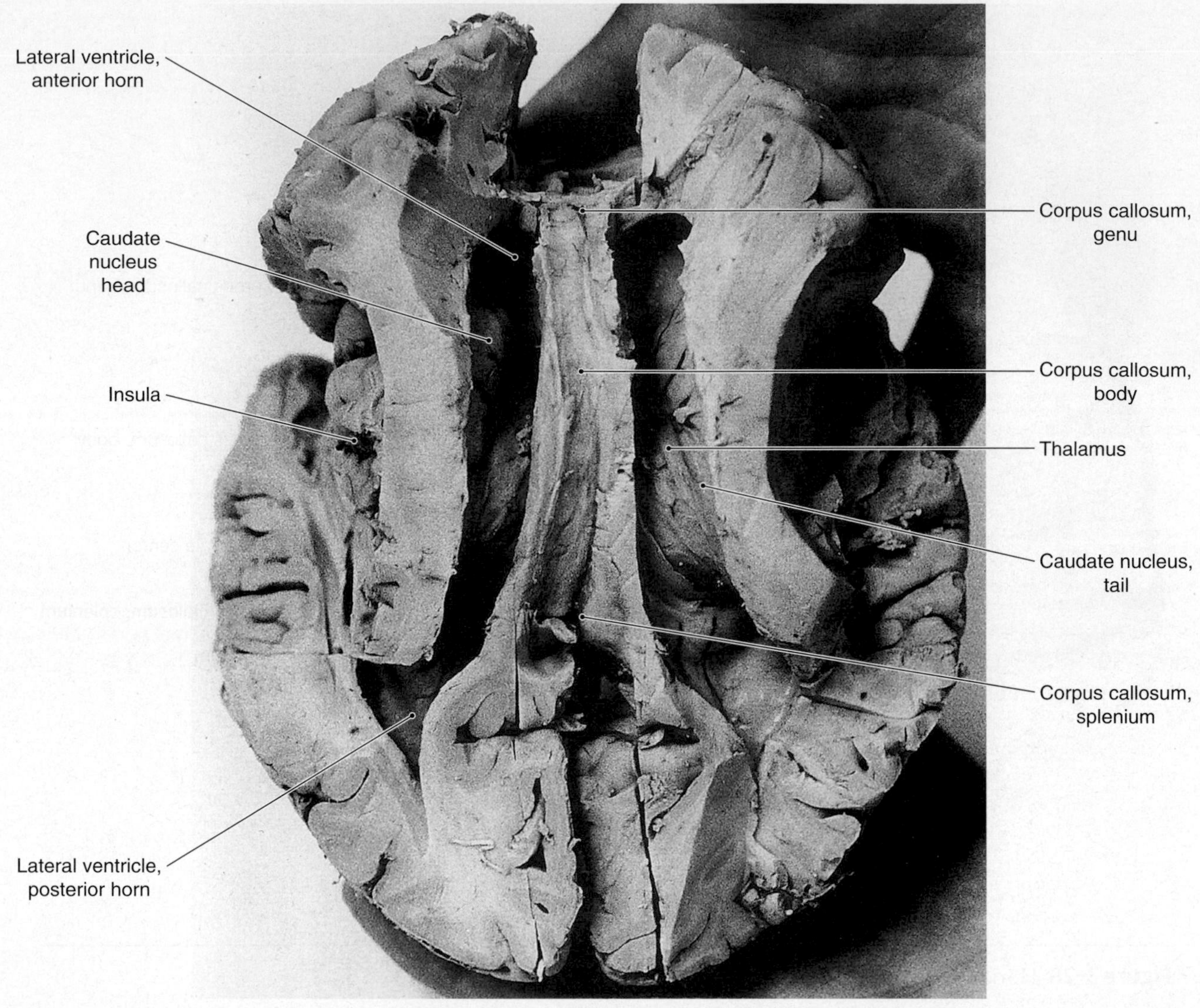

Figure 3-29 Horizontal section exposing the ventricles and basal ganglia.

BOX 3-9

Degenerative Brain Diseases: Alzheimer and Pick

With increased life expectancies, many disabling brain degenerative diseases, which cause behavioral and cognitive deficits in the elderly population, have become more apparent. Most common among these diseases are Alzheimer and Pick disease.

Alzheimer disease, a slowly progressive condition, results from the cellular degeneration in the brain that leads to the formations of the senile plaques in the gray matter and neurofibrillary tangles (strands of coarse and twisted intracytoplasmic fibers) in the neurons of the regions of the associational cerebral cortex, hippocampus, and the cholinergic neurons in the nucleus basalis of Meynert. The pathology of Alzheimer disease can be difficult to separate from that of normal aging of the brain since nearly 50% of people >80 years meet the clinical criteria for dementia. The cellular loss begins behaviorally with memory loss and gradually results in profound problems with thinking and behavior, and eventually the patient is incapable of caring for his or her self and requires 24-hour care.

Pick disease, a less common condition associated with dementia, results from a slow shrinking of brain cells in the temporal and frontal lobular regions. It also involves excessive build-up of protein, called Tau, in the cortical cells which forms the pick bodies. Besides cognitive impairments, patients also exhibit personality changes and a disinterest in communicating. Such patients often are initially considered depressed and suffering from mental illnesses.

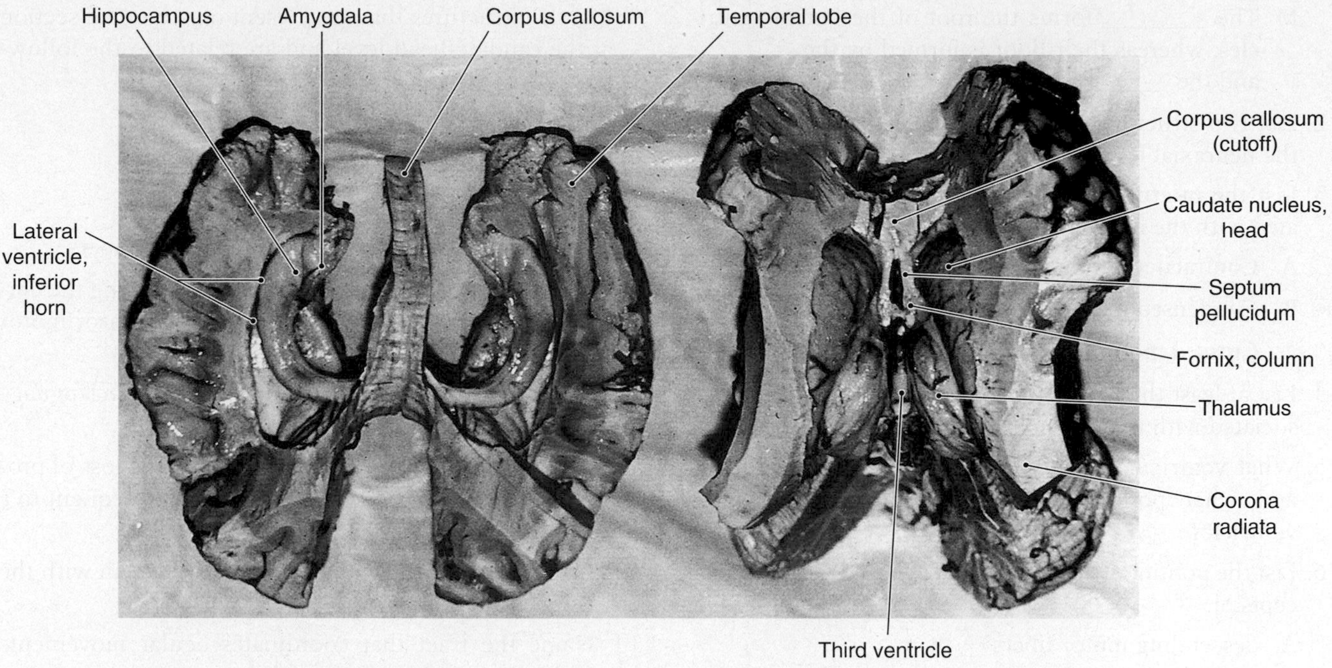

Figure 3-30 Horizontal section in which sectioning of the corpus callosum from the adjacent cortical structure exposes the hippocampus, ventricular cavity, and basal ganglia structure.

SUMMARY

Knowledge of the internal brain anatomy is the most important part of training in neuroscience and is essential for solving clinical problems and reading neuro images. It is learned best by repeated study of the internal structures on serial sections of the spinal cord, brainstem, and forebrain and by relating the structures to their functions. Visual orientation to the structures and functional knowledge of the internal anatomy are essential because they form the basis for the overall understanding of brain structures and their relation to clinical symptoms. Brainstem anatomy is dissected on cross sections, while the forebrain anatomy is examined on sequential coronal and horizontal sections of the brain.

REVIEW QUESTIONS

1. Complete the following statements using the appropriate technical terms:

   A. The ________ connects the third and fourth ventricles.

   B. The ________ in the midbrain is concerned with the transmission of auditory signals to the medial geniculate body of the ________

   C. The ________ of the thalamus relays visual information to the cortex.

   D. The ________ plays an important role in coordinated conjugate eye movements by integrating vestibular projections with ocular cranial nerve nuclei.

   E. The ________ of motor fibers in the caudal most medulla accounts for contralateral motor organization in the brain.

   F. The midbrain cell cluster in the ________ relays cerebellar output to the motor cortex as well as the spinal cord.

   G. The dopaminergic nuclei, with inhibitory projections to the caudate and putamen, are located in the ________. Degeneration of these inhibitory nuclei is associated with ________.

   H. The ________, a basal ganglia nucleus located between the internal capsule and the substantia nigra, is involved with hemiballism.

   I. The ________, a midbrain structure, regulates visual reflexes such as ocular accommodation and coordinated head and eye movements.

   J. Located above the internal capsule, fanned sensorimotor fibers are known as the ________.

   K. The ________ provides a two-way connection between the hypothalamic mammillary bodies and hippocampus.

   L. The ________, containing the sensory fibers that mediate proprioception and discriminative touch, projects to the ________ sensory cortex.

M. The ________ forms the roof of the lateral ventricles, whereas their floor is formed by the ________ and the ________.

2. List two structures whose varying shapes help identify the neuraxial levels in the brain.

3. List the internal medullary constructs that are associated with the following concepts:
   A. Contralateral motor organization
   B. Condensed motor fibers
   C. Crossed motor fibers

4. List at least three structures in the medulla that are associated with the transmission of somatic sensation.

5. What ventricular cavity is located dorsal to the pons and what pontine region is located beneath this ventricle?

6. List the pontine structures that are related with the concepts of
   A. descending motor fibers
   B. somatic sensation
   C. projections to the cerebellum
   D. auditory transmission

7. What structure differentiates the tectal and tegmental regions in the midbrain?

8. Name the internal structures of the midbrain that are associated with the clinical concepts of
   A. dopamine-secreting cells
   B. mediation of visual reflexes
   C. relay nuclei for the auditory information
   D. cerebellar projections to the motor cortex

9. List the structures that are present on a coronal section at the caudate-head level and are related to the following constructs:
   A. Interhemispheric fibers
   B. Separation of the lateral ventricles
   C. Huntington chorea
   D. Concentrated descending sensorimotor fibers.

10. A lesion in the right caudal medulla involving the corticospinal fibers is likely to result in a sensorimotor loss on what half of the body?

11. Will a lesion at internal capsule level result in language disorders? Why or why not?

12. What half of the body is involved with the loss of proprioception and discriminative touch subsequent to a cervical spinal lesion?

13. List three fiber tracts that connect brainstem with the cerebellum.

14. Name the tract that coordinates ocular movements and integrates it with vestibular input.

15. A lesion in the right medulla involving the medial lemniscus fibers is likely to result in a loss of discriminative touch on what half of the body?

16. What are the three parts of the internal capsule?

17. Order the structures starting medial to laterally from the third ventricle: thalamus, claustrum, external capsule, globus pallidus, internal capsule, and insula.

4

Development of the Nervous System*

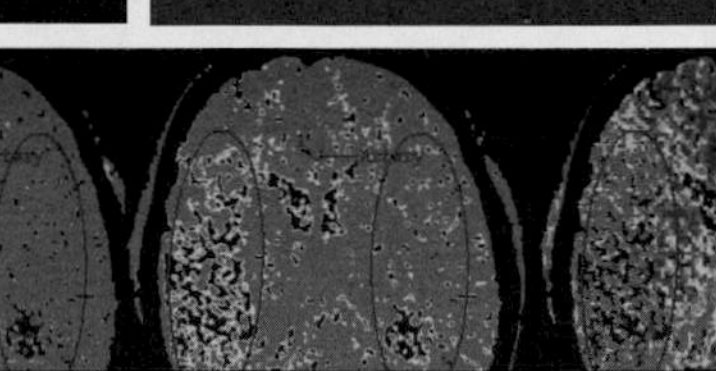

LEARNING OBJECTIVES

After studying this chapter, students should be able to:

- Define basic embryologic terms
- Describe the basic process involved with the development of sperm and ovum
- Discuss the development of the human from single cell to the adult form
- Discuss the differences between oogenesis and spermatogenesis
- Explain why the mother's lifestyle is vital for normal embryologic development
- Explain human development during the first 3 weeks
- Discuss the development of the central and peripheral nervous systems
- List the major brain structures that are derived from the three primary brain vesicles
- Discuss the critical periods of susceptibility to teratogenesis for the central nervous system
- Explain the developmental cerebrospinal malformations

Key Terms:

Autosome	**Gamete**	**Meiosis**
Chromatin	**Gametogenesis**	**Mitosis**
Diploid	**Gene**	**Spermatogenesis**
Genome	**Haploid**	

HUMAN CHROMOSOMES, GENES, AND CELL DIVISION

Human somatic cells are **diploid**, or contain 2*n* chromosomes—that is, 46 chromosomes: 44 **autosomes** and 2 **sex chromosomes** (written as either 46, XY for the male, or 46, XX for the female as per international code). The **haploid** normal **gamete**, or sex cell, contains *n* chromosomes—that is, 23 chromosomes: either 23, Y or 23, X. It is only the male gamete that has either an X or a Y chromosome (Box 4-1). (The division of the primary **spermatocyte** into four spermatids—two 23, X and two 23, Y.)

Abnormalities in Chromosome Number

The term **euploid** refers to any exact multiple of *n* chromosomes, such as **triploid** (23 × 3) or **tetraploid** (23 × 4). **Aneuploid** is the term used for any chromosome number that is not euploid (e.g., when an extra chromosome is present, as in trisomy of chromosomes 13 (Patau syndrome), 18 (Edwards syndrome), or 21(Down syndrome) or when one chromosome is missing, as in monosomy). Such abnormalities in chromosome number originate during **gametogenesis**. Some of these abnormalities are listed in Table 4-1.

Genes and Genome

The diploid human **genome** is made up of 6 to 7 billion base pairs of **deoxyribonucleic acid (DNA)** arranged linearly on the autosomal and sex chromosomes. Molecularly defined, a **gene** is the sequence of chromosomal DNA required for a functional product—a polypeptide or ribonucleic acid molecule—to be produced. The human genome consists of

BOX 4-1

Chromosomal Composition

Human somatic cells are **diploid** and contain 2*n* chromosomes: 44 autosomes and 2 sex chromosomes. This composition is based on the gender. It is 46, XY for the male or 46, XX for the female. In the cellular division (gametogenesis), a missing chromosome changes the number of chromosomes and causes a trisomy to occur. Three common chromosomal trisomies involve either chromosome 13, or 18, or 21; each trisomy involves symbolic and cognitive dysfunctions.

* This chapter is written by K.P. Bhatnagar, PhD, University of Louisville School of Medicine, Louisville, KY.

Table 4-1

Trisomies of the Autosomal and Sex Chromosomes

Condition	Incidence	Characteristics
	Autosomal chromosomes	
Trisomy 13[a]	1 in 25,000 births	Mental retardation; severe central nervous system malformations; bilateral cleft lip and palate; polydactyly; malformed ears
Trisomy 18[a]	1 in 8,000 births	Mental retardation; growth retardation; low-set, malformed ears
Trisomy 21 (Down syndrome)	1 in 800 births	Mental retardation; flat nasal bridge; upward or slant to palpebral fissures; protruding tongue; simian crease (a single transverse palmar crease)
	Sex chromosomes	
45, X (Turner syndrome); monosomy	1 in 8,000 births	Short neck; gonadal dysgenesis (faulty development); puffiness and swelling of feet
47, XXX	1 in 960 female births	15%–25% are mentally retarded
47, XXY (Klinefelter syndrome)	1 in 1,080 male births	Small testes; disproportionately longer lower limbs; impaired intelligence; 40% of males with abnormally developed mammary glands
47, XYY	1 in 1,080 male births	Tall; exhibit aggressive behavior

[a]Rarely survive beyond 6 months after birth.
Data from Moore KL, Persaud, TVN. *The Developing Human: Clinically Oriented Embryology*. 8th ed. Philadelphia: Saunders, 2007.

31,778 known genes and gene predictions that encode a similar number of proteins. The total number of human genes is still in question and is subject to change as research continues (Lander et al., 2001).

Except for the small mitochondrial chromosome, each chromosome is made up of a single continuous DNA double helix, or DNA molecule. DNA molecules have been estimated to range in size from about 50 million base pairs for the smallest (chromosome 21) to 250 million base pairs for the largest (chromosome 1). The DNA molecule appears along with **histones** (chromosomal proteins) and other proteins. The combined DNA and protein complex is called the **chromatin**.

Cell Division

Cell division is indispensable for living organisms. Whereas embryonic cells and some adult cells divide by **mitosis** (equal division), sex cells, or gametes, are formed by a special type of cell division called **meiosis**. Meiosis is the reduction division that occurs during gametogenesis. In meiosis, the chromosome number is reduced to half the usual number, ensuring the constancy of chromosome number from generation to generation. Maternal and paternal chromosomes are independently assorted and crossed over, which shuffles the genes and recombines genetic material, creating a unique genome.

Mitosis (equal division) has four phases: **prophase**, **metaphase**, **anaphase**, and **telophase**. During prophase, the chromosomes appear within the nucleus and double longitudinally (fold in half), forming two **chromatids** united at a **centromere** (Fig. 4-1). During **prometaphase**, the nuclear envelope breaks down, and kinetochore fibers form. The chromosomes then arrange themselves on the equatorial plate, or metaphase plate. The chromosomes move apart during anaphase and reach the spindle poles during telophase. The division of the cytoplasm takes place and leads to the formation of two sibling cells. The increase in cell numbers and, consequently, the growth of tissue lead to development and maturation. Details of mitosis are readily available in human biology textbooks.

EARLY HUMAN DEVELOPMENT

Even though human development is a continuous process, its origin is found in gametogenesis, or the formation of the male and female gametes, the spermatozoa and the ova, respectively. With the union of a spermatozoon and an ovum (secondary oocyte), fertilization is complete. The large cell that results is called a **zygote**. The zygote undergoes repeated divisions, giving rise to the multicellular human form.

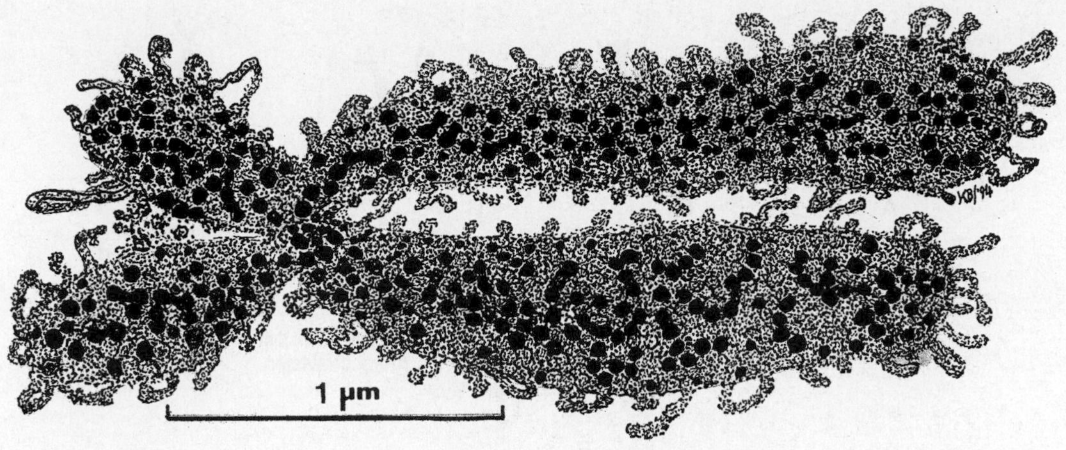

Figure 4-1 An unsanctioned human chromosome 12 from a dividing cell as seen by electron microscopy. The chromosome is divided in half along its length (into two chromatids) except at the centromere. This chromosome contains about 4 cm of deoxyribonucleic acid double helix per chromatid. (Some of the looping and coiling that allows all the DNA to be contained in a chromosome 3 μm long is visible.) (40,200×), (Modified from Fig. 1-21 in Kelly DE, Wood RL, Enders AC. Baily's Text book of Microscopic Anatomy. Baltimore, MD: Williams & Wilkins, 1984).

Gametogenesis

The formation of **germ cells** called gametes (**spermatozoa** and **ova**) involves the halving of chromosomes (i.e., haploid cells are created from diploid cells) and an alteration in cell shape. The reduction of chromosome number, from 46, XY for males and 46, XX for females to 23, Y (spermatozoa) or 23, X (ovum and spermatozoa), occurs during a unique process of cell division called meiosis (Figs. 4-2 and 4-3). This is in contrast to mitosis, in which the new cells remain diploid.

During gametogenesis, two meiotic divisions occur, one after the other. During the first meiotic division, the homologous chromosomes (one from each parent) in the primary spermatocyte or oocyte pair during prophase (Fig. 4-2*A*). They separate during anaphase, with each chromosome going to one of the poles of the cell (Fig. 4-2*E*). Therefore, at the end of this process, each of the two resulting cells (the secondary spermatocyte or oocyte) contains half of the original number of chromosomes (Fig. 4-2*G*). This **disjunction** of homologous chromosomes enables the separation of the **allelic genes** during meiosis. Without an interphase (break in the process of cell division), the second meiotic division follows. Each chromosome, consisting of two **chromatids**, divides; the chromatids are drawn to opposite poles of the cell during division (Fig. 4-2*F*, *G*). The haploid number of chromosomes in the resulting daughter cells is maintained. Meiosis ensures that the number of chromosomes in the next generation remains the same and that chromosomes are recombined to create a mix of genetic material from each parent (Box 4-2).

Nondisjunction is one cause of abnormal gametes that are able to develop into a fetus. The resulting newborns tend to display congenital malformations. During gametogenesis, each primary spermatocyte gives rise to four spermatozoa. However, each primary oocyte develops into only one mature ovum and three nonfunctional **polar bodies**, which soon degenerate.

In the human male, spermatogonia lie dormant in the testes from the fetal period through puberty. **Spermatogenesis** begins at puberty and continues through life. In males, the BMP8B gene (bone morphogenetic protein 8B or osteogenic protein 2), the DAZ1 gene (deleted in azoospermia 1), and paternal effect genes influence gametogenesis. In the human female, however, oogenesis begins before birth. All oogonia, possibly as many as two million, develop into primary oocytes before birth and are retained as primordial follicles. These begin the first meiotic division before birth. However, prophase is not complete until after puberty, at which time no more than 40,000 primary oocytes can be seen. Of these, it is estimated that only about 400 become secondary oocytes and are expelled one at a time on a monthly cycle (Moore and Persaud, 2007). Thus the entire reproductive period of a human female can be considered to last only about 400 months, or 33 years, from about age 12 to about age 45. A small number of the expelled ova never reach the status of secondary oocytes (Box 4-3).

Fertilization and the First Week of Development

Once spermatozoa and the secondary oocyte are united, human development begins. Only one spermatozoon can gain entry through the thick **zona pellucida** surrounding the secondary oocyte. Binding of spermatozoon to zona pellucida is brought about by the proteins **zona pellucida 3**

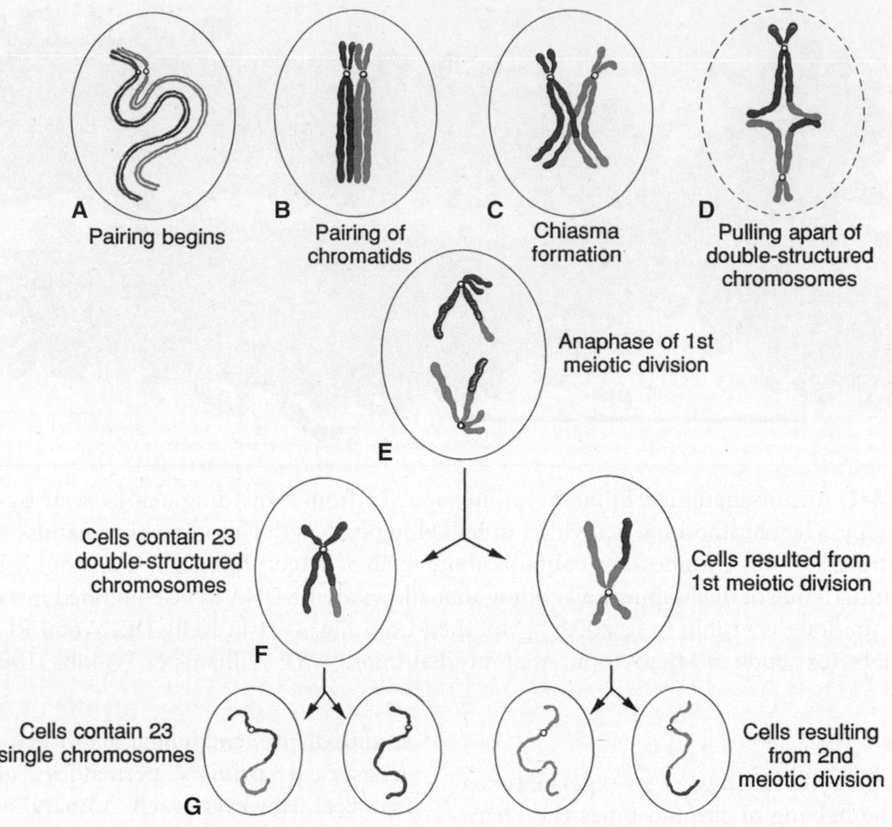

Figure 4-2 First and second meiotic divisions with crossover. A. Homologous chromosomes approach each other. B. The homologous chromosomes pair, each member of the pair consists of two chromatids. C. The intimately paired homologous chromosomes interchange chromatid fragments (crossover). Note the chiasma. D. The double-structured chromosomes pull apart. E. Anaphase of the first meiotic division. F, G. During the second meiotic division, the double-structured chromosomes split at the centromere. At the completion of division, the chromosomes in each of the four daughter cells are different from each other.

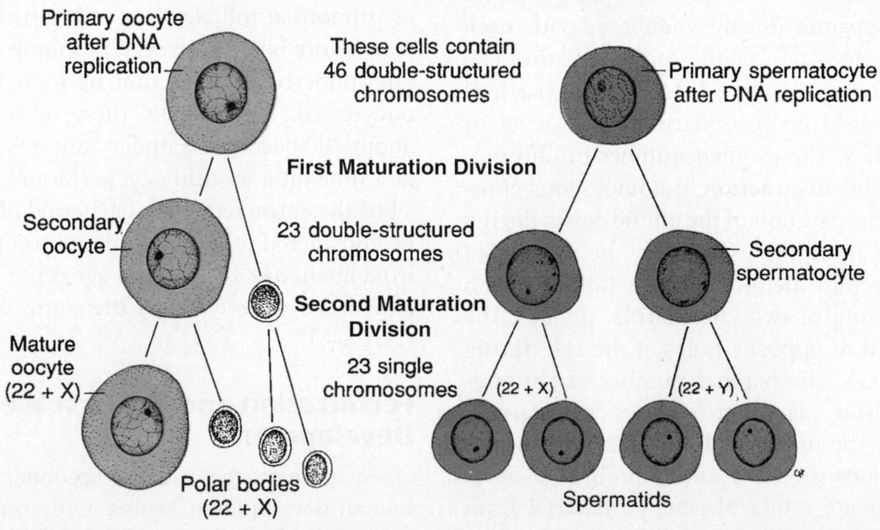

Figure 4-3 Reduction in the number of chromosomes during the maturation divisions. Female germ cell (left). Male germ cell (right).

BOX 4-2

Importance of Cellular Division

A meiotic division of the cell ensures that the number of chromosomes from one generation to the next remains the same and that the recombination of chromosomes creates a mix of genetic blueprint from each parent. An error in recombination causes an abnormal gamete to form, which leads to congenital malformations.

BOX 4-3

Male and Female Gametogenesis

There is a difference between the development of spermatogonia and oogonia. Spermatogenesis for a male begins at puberty and continues through life. However, in the human female, oogenesis starts before birth with the beginning of the first meiotic division, but its prophase is not completed until after puberty. This long period of development for oogonia makes the female ova highly susceptible to internal and external toxicity, which has implications for cognitive and linguistic deficits.

(ZP3), the zona pellucida-binding **protein sp56**, **zona receptor kinase (ZRK)**, and **galactosyl transferase**. At the time of contact between the two gametes, the secondary oocyte completes the second meiotic division and becomes a mature ovum. Its nucleus becomes the female pronucleus. The head of the spermatozoon forms the male pronucleus. With the fusion of these pronuclei, a zygote is formed.

Within 24 hours of ovulation, fertilization is complete, the diploid number of chromosomes is restored, and sex and species variation are determined. The zygote then begins to divide slowly by mitotic division. Mitosis-promoting factor, cyclins, and cdc-25 phosphatase participate in the cleavage. The new cells, called **blastomeres**, gradually become smaller, because they remain confined within the zona pellucida. After the two-, three-, and four-cell stages, the ball of 12 to 16 blastomeres (embryonic cells) is called a **morula** (Fig. 4-4).

This stage, about 3 days after fertilization, occurs when the morula enters the uterus. The morula develops a central cavity—the **blastocyst cavity**—that gets larger as more uterine fluid gains access to it. Cells are now clustered into an outer ring-like cell mass (**trophoblast**) and a group of cell clusters, or the inner cell mass (**embryoblast**) (Fig. 4-5). The blastocyst formation plays a role in the adhesion molecules, including cadherin. The blastocyst remains free in the uterine cavity for about 2 days, during which time the zona pellucida gradually degenerates, allowing the blastocyst to grow in all directions. About 6 days after fertilization, the blastocyst attaches to the **uterine endometrium** at the embryonic pole, most frequently on the upper part of the posterior fundic wall near the midsagittal plane. The first week of human development begins with fertilization and ends with the blastocyst superficially implanted in the uterine lining (endometrium) (Box 4-4).

Second Week of Development

In week 2, the blastocyst becomes completely implanted, and the **bilaminar embryo** develops. Other structures that develop during this period are **cytotrophoblast** and **syncytiotrophoblast** (both differentiated from the trophoblast), **amniotic cavity, amnion, chorion, primary** and **secondary yolk sacs, connecting stalk, chorionic cavity** or **extraembryonic coelom, extraembryonic mesoderm**, and the two components of the bilaminar embryo (the **epiblast** and the **hypoblast**). Another important structure that emerges during this time is the **prechordal plate**, a thickened

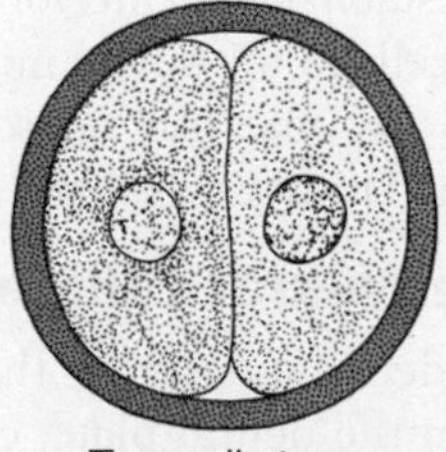

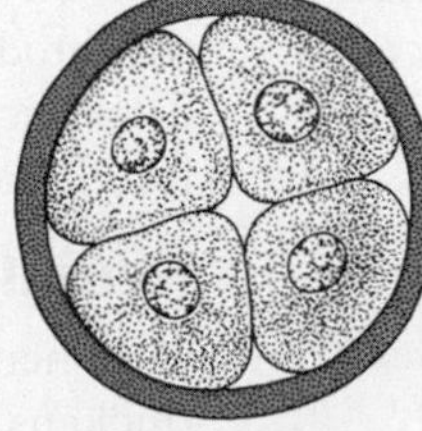

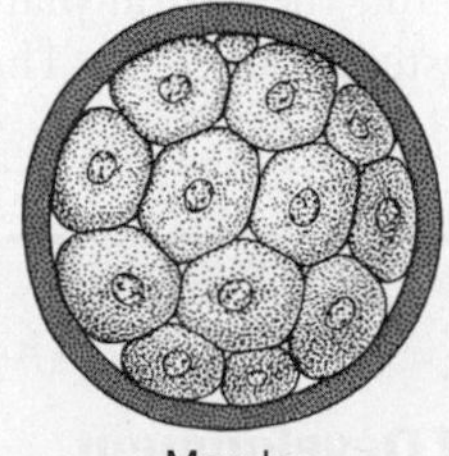

Figure 4-4 Development of the zygote from the two-cell stage to the late morula stage. The two-cell stage is reached approximately 30 hours after fertilization; the four-cell stage at approximately 40 hours; the 12- and 16-cell stages at approximately 3 days; and the late morula stage at approximately 4 days.

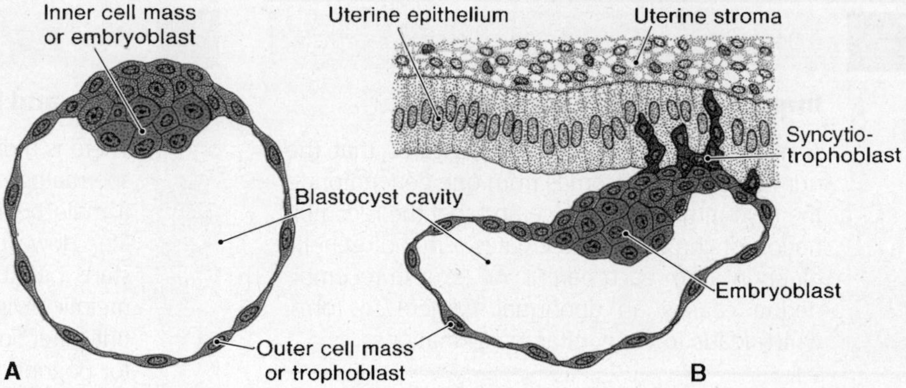

Figure 4-5 A. A section through a human blastocyst recovered from the uterine cavity at approximately 4.5 days. B. A section of a blastocyst at day 9 of development. The human blastocyst likely begins to penetrate the uterine mucosa by day 5 or 6.

cranial region of both the hypoblast and epiblast that is the site of the future mouth (Fig. 4-6; Box 4-5).

Key Terms:

Alar plate	**Neural tube**
Basal plate	**Neurulation**
Neural crest	**Notochord**
Neural plate	

Third Week of Development

The third week of gestation generally coincides with the week after the first missed menstrual period—that is, the fifth week after the onset of the last normal menstrual period. The embryo becomes **trilaminar**; the three germ layers are **ectoderm**, **mesoderm**, and **endoderm** (Fig. 4-7). A caudal midline thickening on the dorsal embryonic disc forms. Through this **primitive streak**, epiblastic cells move between the epiblast and the hypoblast, ultimately giving rise to the mesoderm and the endoderm. The rest of the epiblastic cells become ectoderm.

The **notochord** is the first skeletal structure that develops; it is retained in the adult intervertebral discs as the **nucleus pulposus** (Fig. 4-8). Mesodermal masses arrange themselves segmentally into paired **somites**, which give rise to muscles and other tissues (Fig. 4-9). The **allantois** appears, and the **neural plate**, the forerunner of the nervous system, develops. The **neural crest** separates as the **neural tube** closes and gives rise to numerous components of the peripheral nervous system (PNS). Any disturbance in the development of the neural plate results in severe abnormalities of the nervous system. The intraembryonic coelom, the primitive placenta, and the cardiovascular system—including the plasma and blood cells—also develop in week 3. Of the 8 weeks of embryonic development, week 3 can be considered the most significant because of the definitive beginnings of numerous structures (Box 4-6).

BOX 4-4

First Week of Development

The first week of human development begins with fertilization (with the restoration of the diploid number of chromosomes) and ends with the superficial implantation of the blastocyst in the uterine lining (endometrium) of the uterus.

THE CENTRAL NERVOUS SYSTEM

Development of the brain and spinal cord begins early in week 3 of gestation under the inductive influence of the notochord and the paraxial mesoderm adjacent to it. **Neurulation** is one of several important processes that begin during the trilaminar stage of human development and is complete by the end of week 4. The entire trilaminar stage is completed in week 3.

As the embryo enters week 3, epiblastic cells give rise to endoderm and mesoderm through the region of the primitive streak. The remaining epiblastic cells are now called ectodermal cells. The hypoblast moves to form the secondary yolk sac. Thus in the third week of gestation, the three primary germ layers (ectoderm, mesoderm, and endoderm) are established. Anterior to the primitive streak, the ectodermal cells in the dorsal midline of the embryonic disc thicken to become the neuroectodermal layer, the forerunner of the entire central and PNSs (Box 4-7).

Neural Plate, Neural Tube, and Neural Crest

The neuroectoderm overlying the midline notochord thickens to form the neural plate, cranial to the primitive knot. The neural plate later extends caudally with the receding primitive streak. On day 18, the neural plate invaginates along the midline to form a neural groove flanked by neural folds on either side (Fig. 4-8). At this time, some neuroectodermal cells on the crest of each neural fold are identifiable. These cells first fuse and later

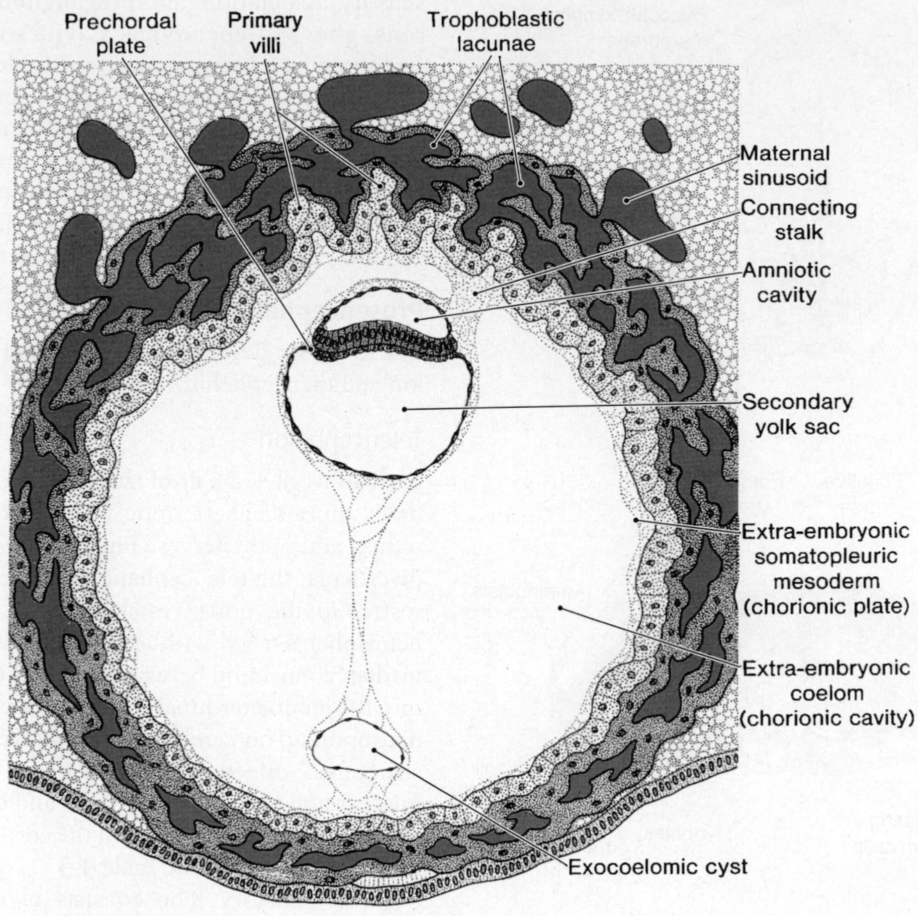

Figure 4-6 A 13-day-old human blastocyst is completely embedded in the endometrium. The dark region between the amniotic cavity and the secondary yolk sac is the bilaminar germ disc.

split; after the split, they lie on the right and left sides of the neural tube when it closes on approximately day 22. The neural tube develops into the brain and the spinal cord, and the segmentally arranged neural crest tissue develops into the **cranial** and **spinal ganglia, nerve sheaths, postganglionic autonomic nerves**, and other structures (Figs. 4-8, 4-9, and 4-10). The neural tube soon separates from the adjacent ectoderm and differentiates into a **posterior (dorsal) alar lamina** or **alar plate** and an **anterior (ventral) basal lamina** or **basal plate**. These two

BOX 4-5

Second Week of Development

The second week of development marks the formation of a bilaminar (epiblast and hypoblast) embryo that gets fully implanted in the uterine lining (endometrium) of the uterus.

regions are separated by a groove, the **sulcus limitans**, midway on the inner surface of the lateral walls of the neural tube. The gap over the neural tube is bridged dorsally by ectoderm that will give rise to skin.

Brain

Early in week 4 (days 22–23), the rostral two-thirds of the neural tube represents the future brain, and the caudal third represents the future spinal cord. The fusion of the neural folds occurs irregularly. The resulting neural tube is at first open at both the cranial and the caudal ends (Fig. 4-11). The rostral opening (anterior neuropore) closes on day 25. The caudal opening (posterior neuropore) closes 2 days later. In the brain, the anterior-most closure of the anterior neuropore is represented by the **lamina terminalis**. Closure of the posterior neuropore must be sought within the filum terminale. As the neural folds fuse dorsocranially and the rostral neuropore closes, three primary brain **vesicles** form. The brain proper develops from the following vesicles, which are formed during week 4: prosencephalon, or

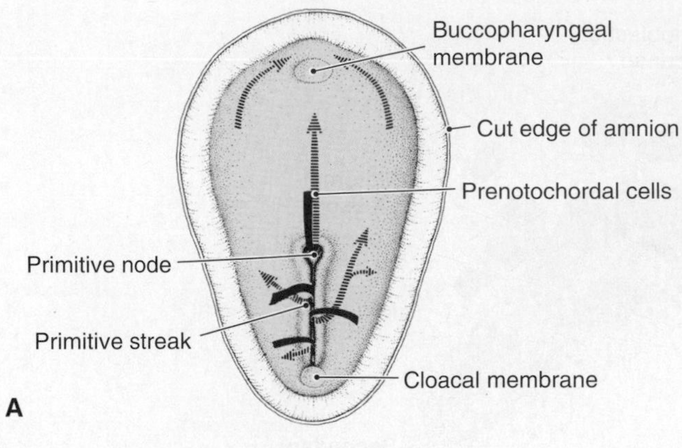

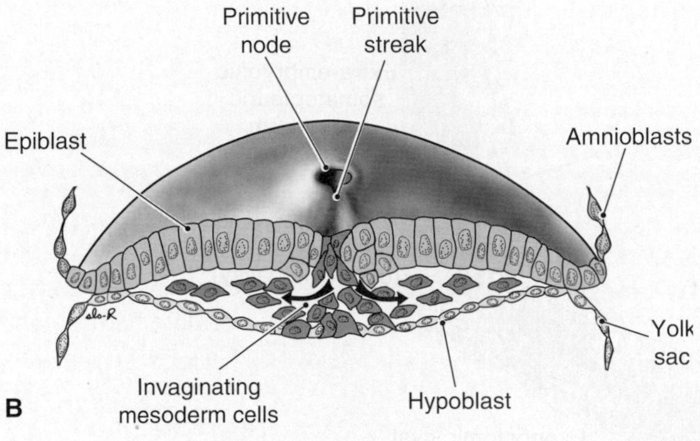

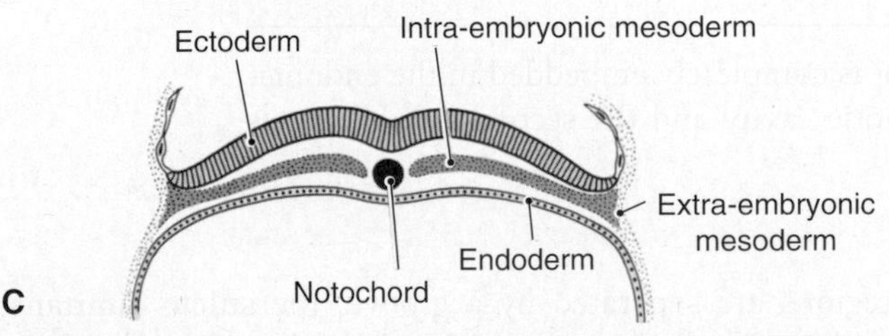

Figure 4-7 A. The germ disc of a 16-day-old embryo from the dorsal aspect indicating the movement of the surface epiblastic cells (*solid lines*) through the primitive streak and the subsequent cellular migration between the hypoblast and the epiblast (*broken lines*). **B.** A cross section through the cranial primitive streak showing the invaginating epiblastic cells. **C.** Cross section of the three primary germ layers: ectoderm, mesoderm, and endoderm.

forebrain; mesencephalon, or midbrain; and rhombencephalon, or hindbrain (Figs. 4-12–4-14). A week later, the prosencephalon develops into two secondary vesicles, the telencephalon and the diencephalon. Likewise, the rhombencephalon develops into the metencephalon and myelencephalon. The mesencephalon does not divide. The brain is now represented by five secondary brain vesicles, each with its own epithelial lining of neuroectoderm that gives rise to motor, sensory, association, and **preganglionic autonomic neurons**, glia, and **ependyma**. Cavities in each vesicle differentiate into brain ventricles (Table 4-2).

Three **brain flexures**, or bends, develop with the rapid growth and folding of the brain. The **midbrain** and **cervical flexures** develop ventrally in the midbrain region and at the junction of the hindbrain and spinal cord. The **pontine flexure** develops dorsally between these two flexures, thinning the roof of the hindbrain (see Fig. 2-2*B*).

Prosencephalon (Forebrain)

The forebrain develops into two subdivisions: telencephalon and diencephalon.

Telencephalon

Early in week 4, a pair of lateral outgrowths from the forebrain appears. These optic vesicles are the primordia for retinas and optic nerves (Fig. 4-12). Soon another pair of diverticula, the telencephalic vesicles, appears dorsal and rostral to the optic vesicles. These grow into cerebral hemispheres, each with anteriorly a lateral ventricle. The median connection between the cerebral vesicles develops into the lamina terminalis, the site of closure of the **rostral neuropore**. The cerebral vesicles give rise to three main structures: **olfactory lobe, corpus striatum (caudate nucleus** and **lentiform nucleus**), and **cerebral cortex**. The timeline for the maturation of the cortical areas, tracts, and myelination is given in Table 4-3.

The olfactory lobe consists of the **olfactory bulb, olfactory tract, anterior perforated substance**, and certain other structures collectively known as the **pyriform lobe** (see Chapters 17 and 18). The olfactory parts of the brain constitute the rhinencephalon (see Chapter 15). An accessory olfactory (vomeronasal) system complex develops in the human embryo but degenerates in the fetal stage (Bhatnagar and Smith, 2001).

The entire forebrain is considered to be an alar lamina derivative. The cerebral cortex in early development consists of three concentric zones: a germinal zone surrounding the lateral ventricles; an intermediate zone, which becomes the white matter; and an outer cortical zone, which develops into the six-layered (gray matter) neocortex/isocortex. The olfactory cortex, the hippocampal formation, and the dentate gyrus constitute the allocortex, because these do not have six layers.

The cerebral hemispheres are smooth (lissencephalic) up to about 20 weeks of gestation. By week 24, various sulci and gyri gradually appear. At birth, all topographical features of the adult brain are present. The various lobes (frontal, parietal, occipital, temporal, and insular) become clearly identifiable during the third trimester. Commissures connecting the right and left hemispheres develop. The principal ones are the **anterior commissure, commissure of the fornix, corpus callosum, habenular commissure**, and **posterior commissure**. The latter two develop in relation to the **pineal body**.

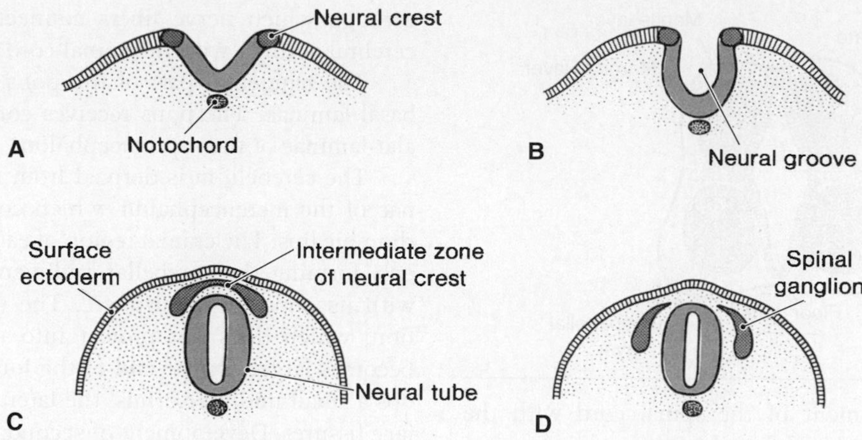

Figure 4-8 Transverse sections through successively older embryos showing the formation of the neural crest (A), neural groove (B), and neural tube (C). The cells of the neural crest, initially forming an intermediate zone between the neural tube and the surface ectoderm, develop into the spinal and cranial sensory ganglia (D) and other structures.

Diencephalon

The caudal forebrain develops into the diencephalon. Its cavity is the **third ventricle**, to which small contributions are added from the telencephalic cavities. The **epithalamus, thalamus, metathalamus, hypothalamus**, and **subthalamus** develop in the lateral walls of the third ventricle. The epithalamus differentiates into the pineal body, **habenular trigone, stria medullaris, tenia thalami**, and posterior commissure. The posterior commissure separates the diencephalon from the mesencephalon. The thalamus is a large structure. Its rapid development reduces the third ventricle to a narrow cavity. In about 70% of humans, the two thalami fuse and form the short bridge-like massa intermedia. The medial and lateral geniculate bodies constitute the metathalamus. The hypothalamus develops into the inferior lateral wall and floor of the third ventricle. The optic chiasm, infundibulum, tuber cinereum, mammillary bodies, and neurohypophysis are grossly identifiable hypothalamic structures. The subthalamus is small and lies between the thalamus and the tegmentum.

The **pituitary gland**, or **hypophysis** of hypothalamus, develops during weeks 4 and 5 of gestation. An ectodermal diverticulum grows dorsally from the roof of the mouth cavity and comes into close contact with the ventral diencephalic diverticulum, the infundibulum. These two diverticula develop into the anterior lobe/**adenohypophysis** (which consists of the **pars distalis, pars tuberalis**, and **pars intermedia**) and the posterior lobe/ **neurohypophysis** (which consists of the **pars nervosa, infundibular stem**, and **median eminence**), respectively.

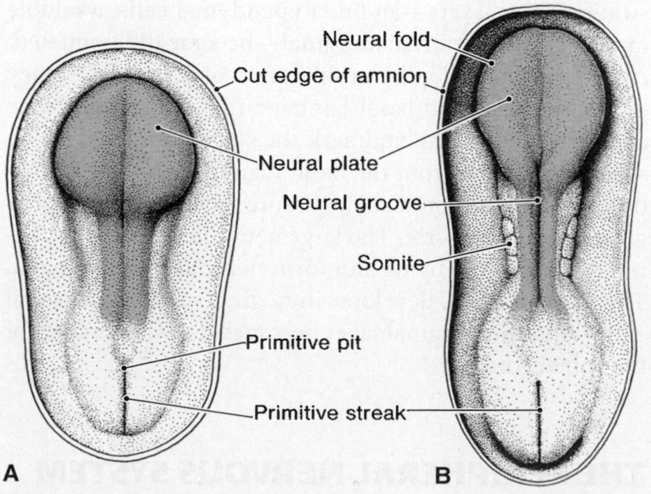

Mesencephalon (Midbrain)

The midbrain is the least modified subdivision. The **superior** and **inferior colliculi** form in its roof, or **tectum**. The

Figure 4-9 A. Dorsal view of a late presomite embryo (~18 days). The amnion has been removed, and the neural plate is clearly visible. B. Dorsal view at approximately 20 days. Note the somites, neural groove, and neural folds.

BOX 4-6

Third Week of Development

The third week of development coincides with the week after the first missed menstrual period. A trilaminar embryo results. A primitive streak appears along with the notocord, somites, and the neural crest.

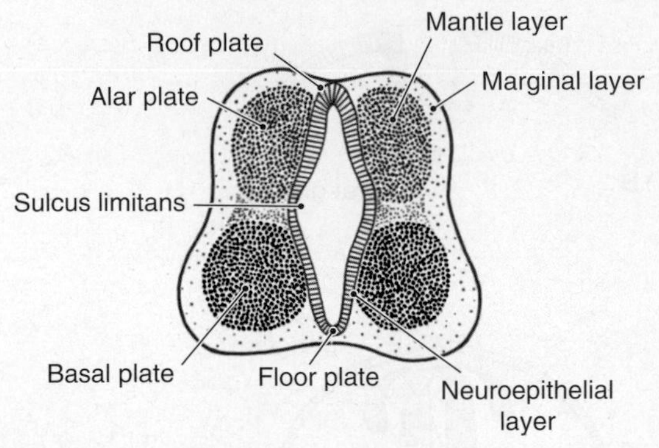

Figure 4-10 Development of the spinal cord with the formation of the ventral and dorsal roots.

superior colliculi relay visual impulses. The inferior colliculi relay auditory impulses. The basal laminae become the **tegmentum**, which includes **red nuclei, substantia nigra, reticular nuclei**, and nuclei of **oculomotor nerve** (cranial nerve [CN] III) and **trochlear nerve** (CN IV). The substantia nigra and **cerebral peduncles** develop anteriorly.

Rhombencephalon (Hindbrain)

The hindbrain develops into the metencephalon (pons and cerebellum) and the myelencephalon (**medulla oblongata**), whereas its cavity develops into the fourth ventricle and **central canal**, which continues into the spinal cord.

Metencephalon

The pons develops in the anterior region of the metencephalon. It is the region of the brainstem (which also includes the medulla oblongata and mesencephalon) through which nerve fibers connect the cerebellar and cerebral cortices with the spinal cord.

The tegmental part of the pons is derived from the basal laminae. The pons receives contributions from the alar laminae of the myelencephalon.

The cerebellum is derived from the dorsal alar laminae of the metencephalon, which comes together as the rhombic lips. The cranial region of each rhombic lip thickens, forming the cerebellar rudiment, which later fuses with its opposite hemisphere. The extraventricular portion, which does not project into the fourth ventricle, becomes larger. By the end of the fourth month, it develops a small midline vermis, the lateral lobes, and the surface fissures. Development of secondary fissures gives rise to the characteristic folia of the cerebellum.

Myelencephalon

The medulla oblongata develops from the most caudal brain region, the myelencephalon. It is continuous with the brainstem superiorly and the spinal cord inferiorly. Here, the **sulcus limitans** divides the alar lamina and the basal lamina in such a manner that the alar region lies lateral to the basal lamina. The bilaminar roof plate in the region of the fourth ventricle consists of an outer thin layer of pia mater and an inner layer of ependymal cells. Together, these two layers constitute the tela choroidea, which projects into the fourth ventricle (and into other ventricles in a similar manner) as the choroid plexus. Two lateral apertures (**foramina of Luschka**) and a median aperture (**foramen of Magendie**) connect the fourth ventricle and the entire ventricular system, including the spinal central canal, with the cerebellomedullary cistern.

BOX 4-7

Neural Concepts

The neural tube that gives rise to the central nervous system develops from the neuroectoderm; the neuroectoderm arises from a specialized region of the embryonic ectoderm.

Formation of the neural tube (neurulation) occurs along the dorsal midline of the embryo. As the neural plate begins to fold inward, it forms neural grooves. Increased cellular growth at the lateral margin of the plate makes the neural folds thicker and causes them to merge so that the neural tube is formed. The anterior and posterior neuropores (openings) close in timely manner. The rostral opening (anterior neuropore) closes on day 25. The caudal, or posterior, neuropore closes 2 days later on day 27. Failure of this closing causes serious birth defects.

Spinal Cord

As the neural tube begins to close, its walls thicken and stratify. Three layers—an inner **ependymal cells**, a middle **mantle**, and an external **marginal**—become differentiated. As the layers develop by proliferation of neuroblasts, they give rise to alar and basal laminae; roof and floor plates; and a morphological landmark the sulcus limitans, which separates the alar from the basal regions. With the formation of the anterior median fissure, the central canal is greatly reduced in size. The large neuroblasts near the central canal rapidly divide and form neurons and neuroglia. The mantle layer develops into gray matter (neuronal zone), and the marginal layer becomes the white matter of the spinal cord.

THE PERIPHERAL NERVOUS SYSTEM

Normal Development

The PNS is composed of ganglia and projections of the cranial, spinal, and the autonomic nervous system. The **suprarenal gland medulla**, which is derived from the postganglionic

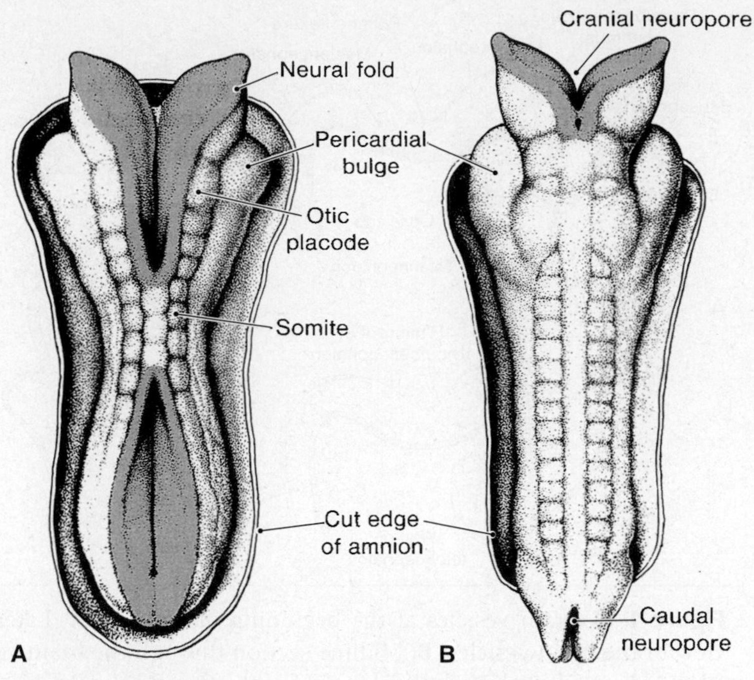

Figure 4-11 A. Dorsal view of a human embryo at approximately day 22. Seven distinct somites are visible on each side of the neural tube. B. Dorsal view of a human embryo at approximately day 23. The central canal is in communication with the amniotic cavity through the open cranial and caudal neuropores.

sympathetic neurons, also falls in this category. Of the 12 pairs of cranial nerves, 4—oculomotor (CN III), facial (CN VII), glossopharyngeal (CN IX), and vagus (CN X)—belong to the cranial parasympathetic system. Likewise, the S2, S3, and S4 spinal nerves form the components of the sacral parasympathetic system (see Chapter 18).

The motor nuclei for all cranial and spinal nerves, and all preganglionic neurons for the autonomic nervous system, are derived from the neural tube. Therefore, the PNS as a whole is derived from the neural tube. Both are within the brain and the spinal cord. Therefore, axons of all such neurons, even though they collectively

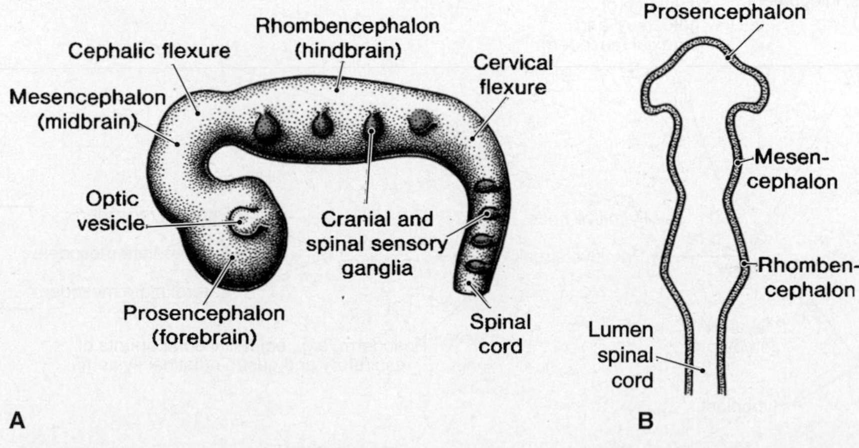

Figure 4-12 A. Lateral view of the brain vesicles and part of the spinal cord in a 4-week-old embryo. Note the sensory ganglia formed by the neural crest on each side of the rhombencephalon and spinal cord. B. Lumina of the three brain vesicles and spinal cord.

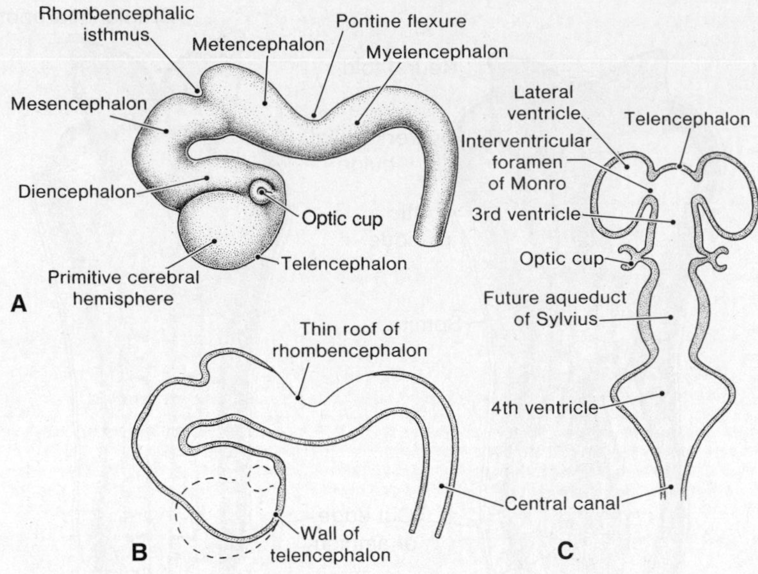

Figure 4-13 Brain vesicles at the beginning of week 6. A. Lateral view of the brain vesicles. B. Midline section through the brain vesicles and spinal cord. Note the thin roof of the rhombencephalon. C. The lumina of the spinal cord and brain vesicles.

Brain, spinal cord, and nuclei within

Neural tube

Neural crest

Cranial ganglia
Spinal ganglia
Autonomic ganglia
Sheaths of nerves
Suprarenal medulla
Pigment cells
Leptomeninges
Branchial cartilages
Head mesenchyme
Parafollicular (C) cells of thyroid gland

Neuroectoderm

Ectoderm (under inductive influence of notochord and paraxial mesoderm)

Ectoderm (epidermis, integument, enamel)

Notochord

Chordamesoderm

Fetal membranes, placenta, and umbilical cord, in part

Primitive node

Paraxial mesoderm

Epiblast

Primitive streak

Embryonic mesoderm

Intermediate mesodem

E.g., muscle, bone, cartilage, blood, kidney

Lateral plate mesoderm

Trophoblast

Bilayered embryo

Inner cell mass

Endoderm, e.g., epithelial components of respiratory and gastrointestinal systems

Morula

Hypoblast

Secondary yolk sac

Zygote

Ovum

Spermatozoon

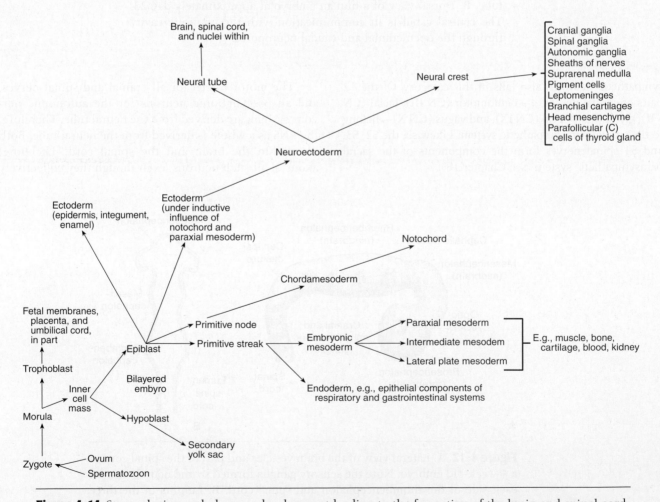

Figure 4-14 Stages during early human development leading to the formation of the brain and spinal cord.

Table 4-2

Development of the Human Brain[a]

Week 3	Week 4	Week 5	Cavity	Weeks 6–12 Alar Lamina	Basal Lamina
Neural tube	Prosencephalon[b]	Telencephalon	Lateral ventricles and choroid plexus; rostral 3rd ventricle	Cerebral hemispheres, cortex, and corpus striatum	None
		Diencephalon	Caudal part of the 3rd ventricle and choroid plexus	Thalamus, hypothalamus, and epithalamus, including pineal body	None
	Mesencephalon	Mesencephalon	Cerebral aqueduct	Tectum: superior and inferior colliculi	Cerebral peduncles and tegmentum
	Rhombencephalon	Isthmus rhombencephali	Rostral part of 4th ventricle	Superior cerebellar peduncles	None
		Metencephalon	Middle part of 4th ventricle	Cerebellum, middle cerebellar peduncles, and sensory nuclei of cranial nerves V and VIII (in part)	Pons
		Myelencephalon	Posterior part of 4th ventricle and choroid plexus	Inferior cerebellar peduncles and sensory relay nuclei of cranial nerves VII, IX, and X (in part)	Medulla oblongata

[a]See also Figures 4-11 and 4-12.
[b]"Many embryologists consider that the prosencephalon is formed of alar laminae alone." (Hamilton WJ, Mossman, HW. Hamilton, Boyd, and Mossman's Human Embryology: Prenatal development of form and function. 4th ed. Cambridge: Helfer, 1972.)

form peripheral nerves, are derived from the **central nervous system (CNS)**. The spinal or dorsal root ganglia, sensory ganglia of the cranial nerves, all autonomic ganglia, and postganglionic autonomic neurons are derived from the neural crest in a similar manner from tissue that separated from the closing neural tube. The suprarenal medulla, the **mucosal** and **submucosal enteric ganglia**, the **capsular cells** that enclose the sensory nerve bodies, and the myelin-producing **Schwann cells** also develop from the neural crest. Some cranial ganglia—glossopharyngeal (CN IX) and vagus (CN X)—and the first-order olfactory and accessory olfactory (vomeronasal) neurons arise not from the neural tube but from the surface ectoderm—that is, they are placodal in origin.

Key Terms :

Anencephaly	**Microcephaly**
Cranium bifidum	**Myelinogenesis**
Embryogenesis	**Synaptogenesis**
Holoprosencephaly	**Spina bifida**
Hydrocephalus	**Teratogenesis**

CLINICAL CORRELATES

Abnormal Development of the CNS

The brain and spinal cord, with the exception of the cerebellum, reach the full complement of neurons by week 25

Table 4-3

Gradients of Maturation for Cortical Areas and Myelination of Tracts

Period	Maturation for Cortical Areas and Myelination
8th week of gestation to birth	Cerebral cortex is established from deeper layers toward the surface Neuroepithelial cells in ventricular zone, which cease to divide, are postmitotic; these are guided by glial cells toward cortex
4th month to 2–3 years after birth	Process of myelination is related to functional maturation of neuronal interconnections Myelination starts at soma and proceeds distally Tracts concerned with tasks necessary for life are myelinated first In spinal cord: myelination starts in cervical region and proceeds caudally Anterior root motor fibers are myelinated first; then posterior root sensory fibers Ascending spinal tracts start myelination in the fetal 6th month, followed by descending tracts Pyramidal tract fibers are fully myelinated about 2 y after birth
6th fetal month to before birth	Myelination of cranial nerves takes place (optic nerve myelinated before birth) Nuclear groups develop in their own time, but not simultaneously
Newborn to adult	Synaptic density per neuron at time of birth begins to decline gradually By puberty, the number of synapses is drastically reduced Formation of new synapses is closely related to learning

Data from Brodal P. The Central Nervous System: Structure and Function. 3rd Ed. New York: Oxford University Press, 2010.

of gestation. After this point and well into the postnatal years, glial cells develop and multiply, various neuronal processes develop, and **synaptogenesis** occurs. Glial cells proliferate from midgestation to the end of the second year of life and beyond. **Myelinogenesis** begins at the end of the first trimester (month 3 of gestation) and extends to age 4. In **embryogenesis**, the timing of an insult is more detrimental than the nature of the insult in causing cerebrospinal malformations; hence **teratogenesis** is a time-specific but insult-nonspecific phenomenon (Table 4-4). Of patients with cerebrospinal disorders admitted to hospitals, some 90% relate to neural tube closure, notably spina bifida cystica and anencephaly. Table 4-5 summarizes the critical periods and relative vulnerability of the neural regions to insult leading to specific defects (Box 4-8).

Anencephaly

Defective fusion of the neural tube anteriorly results in **anencephaly**, in which the cranial vault is congenitally absent. Cerebral hemispheres are either missing or reduced and attached to the base of the skull. This abnormality has an incidence of 1 in 1,000 deliveries and occurs more commonly in females. Indications of the defects include absence of the optic nerves, although the eyes appear normal, and exposure or herniation of cerebral tissue (Fig. 4-15). Folic acid with a multivitamin preparation taken by the mother even before conception has been used to prevent such a defect. Anencephaly is incompatible with extrauterine existence; survival in many cases lasts between 3 and 48 h after birth.

Cranium Bifidum

Cranium bifidum is a condition in which bone fusion is prevented in the posterior midline of the skull. As a result, the brain or spinal cord protrudes through the opening.

Spina Bifida

When a fusion failure of the dorsal part of the neural tube, similar to cranium bifidum, occurs in the vertebral column, it is called **spina bifida**. Spina bifida can be classified into several subtypes, based on severity and tissue involvement. In **spina bifida cystica**, the posterior vertebral arches fail to fuse, and meninges herniate, but neural tissues do not; lumbar or lumbosacral defects are common. In **spina bifida occulta**, the skin of the back is epithelialized and always shows a surface marking in the form of a dimple, a dermal sinus, or a hairy region. Several skin, spinal cord, and bone deformities of this kind can be revealed through radiograms.

The caudal displacement of cerebellar tissue through the foramen magnum is called **Arnold–Chiari malformation**. It occurs with every case of spina bifida cystica. Two abnormalities commonly associated with syndrome are

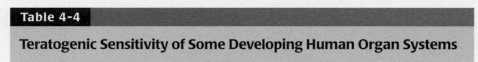

Table 4-4

Teratogenic Sensitivity of Some Developing Human Organ Systems

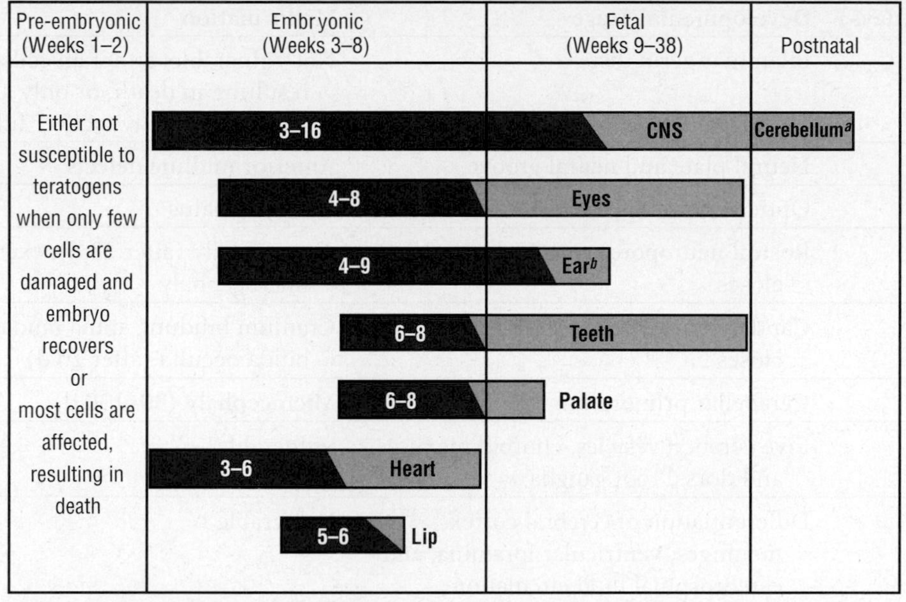

[a]DNA synthesis has been reported to occur in the cerebellar granular layer during the first few years of life; antiviral therapy in infants may cause extensive damage to the developing cerebellar neurons (Langman J, Shimada M, Rodier P. Floxuridine and its influence on postnatal cerebellar development. Pediatr Res 1972;6:758–764.). Other brain regions in infants are also known to continue mitotic division of neurons postnatally.
[b]Week 16.
CNS, central nervous system; *dark red*, major congenital defect; *light red*, minor defect or functional malformation.

BOX 4-8

Abnormal Development of the Brain

In embryogenesis, the timing of an insult is more detrimental than the nature of the insult in causing cerebrospinal malformations; hence teratogenesis is time specific but insult nonspecific. Of pediatric patients with cerebrospinal disorders admitted to hospitals, some 90% have malformations that relate to neural tube closure, notably spina bifida cystica (most common congenital defect in the United States) and anencephaly. About 40% of the infant deaths during the first year are related to central nervous system malformations.

Reportedly, the women taking anticonvulsant drugs are at three to four times more risk for carrying a congenitally malformed baby. Sodium valproate has been associated with spina bifida. While genetic predisposition is well established, there is evidence to suggest that there is a higher prevalence of congenital neurological conditions in children born to diabetic mothers (Castro et al., 2002).

hydrocephalus and syringomyelia. This tissue protrusion results in cerebellar and medullary symptoms.

Hydrocephalus

Hydrocephalus is characterized by an enlarged head, a prominent forehead, brain atrophy, mental deficiency, and convulsions. Cerebral ventricles enlarge because of excessive production of cerebrospinal fluid and/or obstruction of the cerebrospinal fluid drainage pathways. Hydrocephalus is caused by the obstruction of cerebrospinal fluid circulation. The ventricles are enlarged and the cerebral mantle is thin. Neurologic findings are abnormal.

Microcephaly

Microcephaly is an uncommon condition in which the brain, and **calvaria** (skull cap), and face are small. Because the brain is underdeveloped, infants with this condition are mentally retarded. Environmental disturbances, genetic abnormalities, and ionizing radiation during the critical period of CNS development have been implicated as the primary causes of the defect.

Holoprosencephaly

The incomplete development of midline structures as well as fused eyes, single nasal chamber, a single ventricle

Table 4-5

Critical Periods of Development of the Human Central Nervous System (CNS)

Gestational Age (days)	Developmental Stage	Malformation
14	Bilaminar germ disc	Not vulnerable; either all cells are damaged, resulting in death, or only a few cells are affected and may recover fully
18	Neural plate and neural groove	Anterior midline defects
22	Optic vesicles	Hydrocephalus
25	Rostral neuropore (anterior neuropore) closes	Anencephaly (after 23 d), exencephaly, and microcephaly
27	Caudal neuropore (posterior neuropore) closes	Cranium bifidum, spina bifida cystica, and spina bifida occulta (after 26 d)
32	Cerebellar primordium	Microcephaly (30–130 d)
33–35	Five cerebral vesicles, choroid plexuses, and dorsal root ganglia	Vulnerable
56	Differentiation of cerebral cortex, meninges, ventricular foramina, and cerebrospinal fluid circulation	Vulnerable
70–100	Corpus callosum	Vulnerable
140–175	Neuronal proliferation in the CNS (except cerebellum) fully completed	Defects of cellular circuitry and myelin
175 d to 4 y of life	Neuronal migration, glia, and myelin formation and synaptic connections	Vulnerable

instead of lateral ventricles, olfactory bulbs and tracts, and carpus callosum are hypoplastic or absent The brain and face are highly malformed.

Lissencephaly

Lissencephaly is defined as gross neural defect where sulci and gyri do not develop and thus the brain appears smooth surfaced.

Additional Abnormalities

Other less common structural abnormalities of the nervous system are craniorachischisis, encephalocele, meningocele, cyclopia, and agenesis of the cortex, corpus callosum, and cerebellum.

Developmental Disabilities

Commonly known developmental disabilities are **mental retardation, Down syndrome, fragile X syndrome, Williams syndrome**, childhood **autism**, and **attention deficit hyperactivity disorder** (ADHD). In general, children with the developmental disorders tend not to develop normal cognition skills and emotional/social maturity. Besides, these children are also at risk of ADHD, epilepsy, and behavioral abnormalities.

Mental Retardation

Mental retardation is a disability characterized by significant limitations both in intellectual functioning and in adaptive behaviors (Luckasson, et al. 2002). This disability originates before age 16 and affects one's ability to conceptualize age-appropriate cognitive, linguistic, and social skills. Its causes can include idiopathic factors, genetic conditions, and congenital disorders including maternal Rubella, cytomegalovirus, and toxoplasmosis infection. The genetic causes include chromosomal abnormalities (Down, Williams, and Patau syndromes) or gene mutations. The most common preventable cause of mental retardation in present time is maternal alcohol abuse. Gestational weeks 3 to 16 is the period of greatest teratogenic sensitivity for fetal brain damage (Table 4-5). Cell depletion in the cerebral cortex results in severe mental retardation and social/communicative disorders.

Down Syndrome

Marked by a range of cognitive abnormalities, Down syndrome results from a translocation of chromosome 21. The affected individual has three copies of this chromosome; this condition is also known as trisomy 21. Its clinical findings include mental retardation, retarded growth, flat

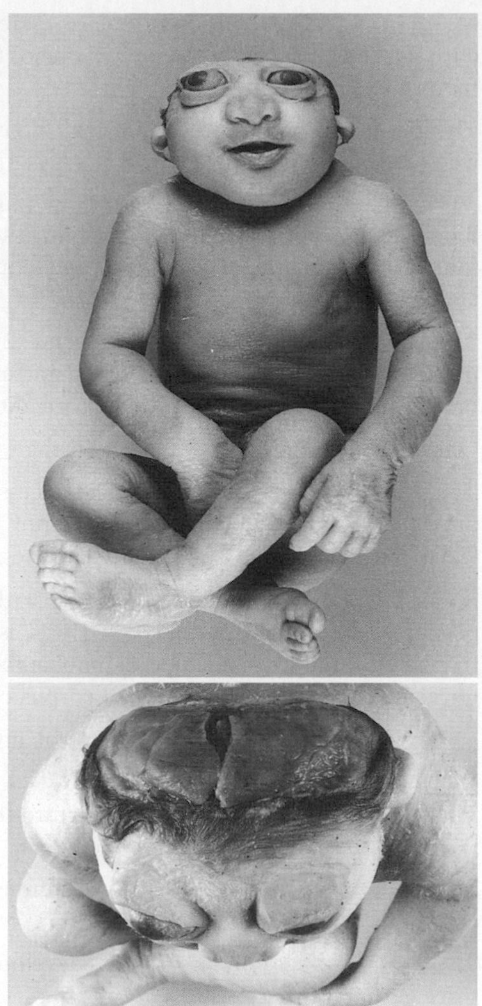

Figure 4-15 Newborn female with anecephaly. Front view showing the large eyes and absence of the cranial vault (upper figure). Dorsal view showing the exposed poorly formed brain.

face with short nose, low-set ears, thickened tongue, broad hands and feet, and stubby fingers (Table 4-1).

Fragile X Syndrome

Fragile X syndrome is one of the most common causes of mental retardation. Affected individuals have a fragile site near the end of the long arm of the X chromosome, which looks almost as if it were a detached segment. Special culture conditions are required for demonstration. It has a frequency of 1 in 1,500 male births and may account for the excess of males in the mentally retarded population.

Williams Syndrome

Williams syndrome, another genetic cause of mental retardation, is characterized by distinct facial features of a small upturned nose and long ridges of philtrum and a high level of empathy (overly friendly). Most subjects develop a sensorineural hearing loss by the age 30. Additional symptoms are delayed development, learning disorders, high anxiety, attention deficit disorder, and phobia to loud sounds. This is a contiguous gene deletion syndrome with occurrence of 1 in 8,000 births.

Childhood Autism

Autism is a mental-social disorder of unknown cause characterized by abnormal development of brain circuitry that is essential for integrating social interaction and communicative skills. Affected individuals have limited interests and keep busy by being involved with only a few selected items. Their lifelong disability diminishes their social–emotional–communicative capacities and hinders their linguistic interaction with other people. They also lack the skills that are needed for imaginative play. Many of the affected children later display impaired cognitive and language skills; many are hyperactive and exhibit a slow development of somatosensory functions.

An autism-related neurological condition is Asperger syndrome, named after an Austrian pediatrician Hans Asperger. Currently considered within the autistic spectrum, the distinctive behavioral disorders that he documented were apathy, lack of eye contact, clumsy movements, stereotyped behavior or language use, obsessive interests, and impaired ability to socially interact.

Early intervention using controlled social and linguistic stimulation has been found to make significant improvement in the functional skills of these patients.

Attention Deficit Hyperactivity Disorder

ADHD, one of the most common developmental disabilities, has serious implications for cognitive development, social interaction, and educational performance. The origins of ADHD are mostly unknown. The condition is characterized by persistent inattention, chronic hyperactivity, and impulsivity. Early diagnosis of children with ADHD is important because it saves them, along with parents and teachers, from frustration, anger, and anxiety. It also helps in providing them with systematic treatment to promote their cognitive and linguistic functions.

Abnormal Development of the PNS

Abnormal development of the PNS cannot ordinarily be distinguished from the developing central nervous structures. Anencephalic fetuses lack optic nerves, but the eyes, although large, appear normal. Another example of such a disorder is congenital **aganglionic megacolon (Hirschsprung disease)**. In this condition, the colon is greatly dilated because of lack of muscular tone and contractile activity of the bowel segment, which causes fecal retention. This is because the postganglionic parasympathetic neurons are congenitally decreased in the myenteric plexus, which is located in the distal segment of the large intestine. The innervation of the muscle layers is defective even when ganglionic neurons are present. Generally, only the rectum and sigmoid colon are affected, but occasionally more proximal parts of the colon are affected as well.

SUMMARY

There are 46 human somatic chromosomes. Human sex cells divide by meiosis. Further division occurs through mitosis. Human development begins with the union of a spermatozoon with a secondary oocyte. During week 1 of development, a zygote forms and divides into blastomeres that pass through the two-, three-, and four-cell stages. In the 12- to 16-cell stages, on about day 6, the morula becomes the blastocyst and attaches to the endometrium. During week 2, trophoblast differentiation and formation of the amnion and chorion, the two yolk sacs, and the two germ layers (epiblast and hypoblast layers) occur. In week 3, the mesoderm and endoderm form from the epiblast through the primitive streak, and the ectoderm differentiates. Somites and the neural tube develop at this time. The five brain vesicles appear early in week 4 and gradually differentiate into corresponding brain structures and ventricles. Sulci and gyri appear in approximately week 24. Abnormal development of the CNS causes deficits such as anencephaly, cranium bifidum, spina bifida, hydrocephaly, and microcephaly. The PNS is derived from a specialized portion of the neural tube, the neural crest. The nervous system continues to develop for many years after birth.

REVIEW QUESTIONS

1. Complete the following statements using the appropriate technical terms:

   A. The haploid normal gamete, or sex cell, contains 23________: either 23, Y or 23, X. It is only the ________gamete that has either an X or a Y________.

   B. ________ represents the normal separation of pairs of chromosomes.

   C. The ________ refers to the developing human organism from conception until the end of the eighth week, whereas the developmental period from 2 months to the birth is the ________ stage.

   D. ________ refers to the formation of the male and female gametes, the spermatozoa and the ova, respectively.

   E. Sex cells or gametes are formed by a type of cell division called ________, which is characterized by reduction of chromosomes to half the usual number.

   F. The other type of cellular division is________ in which the daughter cell contains the number of chromosomes that is ________ to the mother cell.

   G. ________ ________ is the neuroectodermal region of the early embryo's dorsal surface that later develops into the nervous system.

   H. ________ refers to a failure of one or more pairs of chromosomes to separate, which is one of the common causes of abnormal________.

   I. The disturbed growth process in malformed babies is ________.

   J. ________ ________ ________ ________ is a common cause of developmental disability with profound implications for cognitive and educational abilities.

   K. A ________ involving the chromosome 21 results in________ ________, which is characterized by mental retardation and physical abnormalities.

   L. One of the original two germ layers is the ________.

   M. ________ ________ is an X-linked recessive syndrome characterized by mental retardation, atypical facial appearance, and abnormally large testicles.

   N. As an embryonic forebrain syndrome with poorly developed midline structures, ________ is characterized by fused eyes, a single nasal chamber, a single ventricle, and underdeveloped corpus callosum.

   O. ________ refers to the development of myelin before and after the birth.

   P. The ________ ________ is the structure that gives rise to the peripheral nervous system.

   Q. The ________ ________ is the forerunner of the central nervous system (CNS).

   R. ________ ________ refers to the development of three germ layers.

   S. ________ involves the presence of an extra chromosome.

   T. The anterior and posterior pores of the ________ ________, respectively, close on the 25th and 27th day; otherwise, serious birth defects result.

   U. Except for some later developing cells in the cerebellum and possibly in hippocampus, the full complement of neurons is in place by week ________ ________ ________, and no cells develop after the________.

2. By which gestation week does the human embryo has three primary brain vesicles?
3. True or false? Normally developing humans have 46 somatic chromosomes.
4. True or false? There are 24 types of human chromosomes; 22 autosomes, and one X and one Y chromosome.
5. Name the structure that is the forerunner of the nervous system.
6. True or false? The neural tube develops into the brain and the spinal cord.

7. Name the duration, in which the CNS is most susceptible to major congenital defects.
8. Match the following disorders with their associated statements.

A. anencephaly	a. failure of the brain to form two hemispheres
B. holoprosencephaly	b. developmental failure of the gyri/sulci formation
C. lissencephaly	c. miniature brain and small skull cap with normal face size
D. microcephaly	d. congenital absence of the cranial vault with missing or reduced forebrain
E. Arnold–Chiari syndrome	e. cerebellar protrusion into the vertebral foramen

9. List three common trisomies naming the involved chromosome number.
10. List four common forebrain malformations.
11. List two structural malformations that are associated with the Arnold–Chiari malformation.
12. Name the single most important difference between oogenesis and spermatogenesis.
13. List four common developmental disorders.
14. What percent of infant deaths occurring during the first year of life are related to CNS malformations?

5 Nerve Cell Physiology

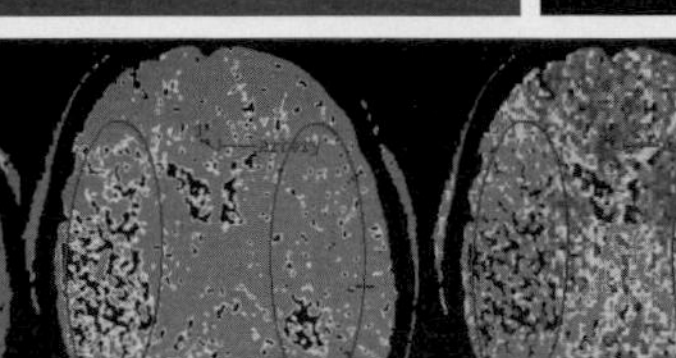

LEARNING OBJECTIVES

After studying this chapter, students should be able to:

- Explain the major parts of a nerve cell and outline their functions
- Describe the types and functions of glial cells
- Explain the mechanisms involved with the synapse establishment and neuronal pruning during embryogenesis
- Discuss cognitive and linguistic implications of errors in neuronal pruning and synaptic development
- Explain the process of action potential generation conduction and outline the ways in which extracellular (Na^+) and intracellular (K^+) chemical properties alter the cell membrane potential
- Explain the role of myelin in the nervous system and the effect of demyelination on impulse transmission
- Outline the nerve cell responses to injuries in the nervous system
- Explain differences in the regenerative processes between the central and peripheral nervous systems
- Outline the tumor types in the brain and their graded classification abnormalities

The **nerve cell** is the basic functional unit in the central nervous system (CNS). Each nerve cell participates in activities that are vital to the life of the cell and the organism. Each cell uses identical mechanisms to synthesize protein, thereby using and transforming energy. More than 15 to 20 billion nerve cells in the human brain generate **nerve impulses** and are the means of communication within the nervous system and between the nervous system and body parts. The CNS consists of two primary types of cells: nerve cells (**neurons**) and **neuroglia** (or simply **glia**) **cells**. Through excitatory and inhibitory impulses, nerve cells in the CNS drive the power of mind by regulating higher mental (attention, problem solving, memory, thinking, reasoning, calculation, and language) and sensorimotor activities. Neuroglial cells support and protect nerve cells; they also actively participate in tissue repair in response to brain injury and disease.

NEURON

A nerve cell consists of three primary elements: **cell body** (soma), **dendrites**, and **axon** (Fig. 5-1*A*). Cells receive impulses primarily via the dendrites and secondarily through the soma and the initial segment of the axons. Cells conduct nerve impulses through their axonal fibers, which travel various distances and **synapse** on the receptive ends of other nerve cells and target organs. Whether the effect is excitatory or inhibitory on the target cell depends on the identity of the neurotransmitter released by the neuron. Nerve cells are highly specialized in responding to excitatory and inhibitory neurotransmitters. Factors that add to the operational complexity of nerve cells are the various ways in which the cell bodies are interconnected and respond to electrochemical signals.

Key Terms :

Cell body	**Dendrites**
Cytoplasm	**Nissl bodies**
Axon	**Synapse**

Nerve Cell Structure

Cell Body

The cell body of a neuron consists of two major components, a **nucleus** and **cytoplasm**, both of which work closely to maintain the viability of the entire organ. Cytoplasm consists of protein molecules and an aqueous (watery) substance enclosed within the cell membrane. The cytoplasmic material of the cell contains many microscopic subcellular units called **organelles** (Fig. 5-1*B*), which include **mitochondria, ribosomes, lysosomes, rough** and **smooth endoplasmic reticulum** (ER), and the **Golgi apparatus**. The primary function of these organelles and associated structures is to metabolize protein essential for the maintenance

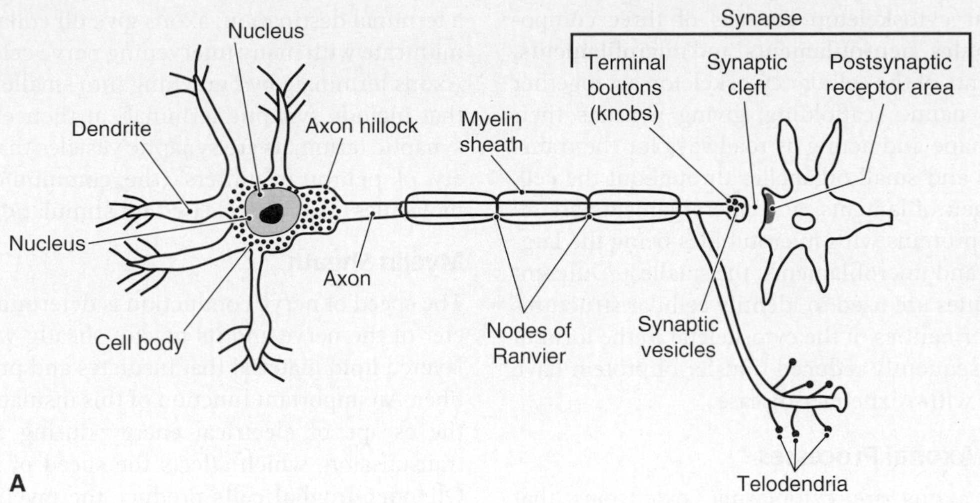

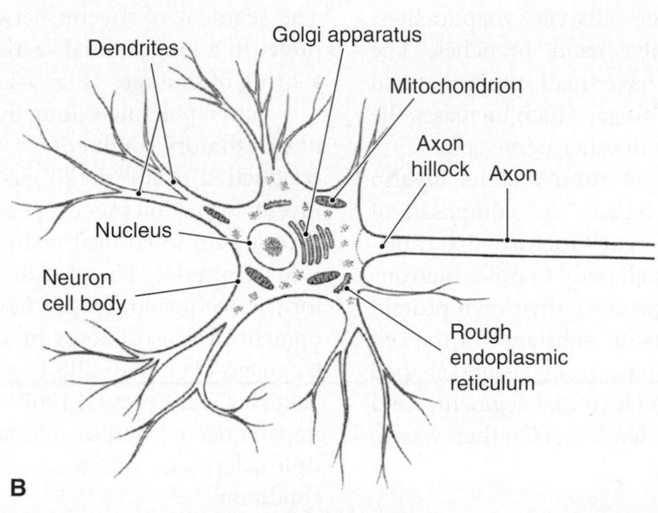

Figure 5-1 A. A nerve cell and its major parts: body, dendrites, and axon. B. Soma organelles, the most important of which are neurofibrils, mitochondria, rough endoplasmic reticulum, and Golgi apparatus.

and growth of the cell body and its processes and to add to the capability of the organ. Nerve cells have a high metabolic activity that depends on the availability of **glucose**. Cells manufacture their own proteins, which are transported throughout the cell via a network of **cylindrical microtubules**. This transport can occur both from the cell body to axons and dendrites (anterograde) and from the axonal processes back to the cell body (retrograde).The nucleus contains **deoxyribonucleic acid** (**DNA**), macromolecules with genetic information that determines the characteristics of specific cell types. The transformation and replication of DNA through cell division make up the mechanism for genetic inheritance (see Chapter 4 for gametogenesis). Visible within the nucleus is the **nucleolus**, which contains RNA and is the site of the assembly of ribosomes.

The ribosomes are transported out of the nucleolus into the cytoplasm, where they play a key role in protein synthesis. Proteins destined to be free in the cytoplasm are synthesized by free ribosomes, whereas all other proteins (membrane bound or within organelles) are synthesized by ribosomes attached to the rough ER. Compared to other cell types, neurons contain a large amount of rough ER as well as free ribosomes for protein production, which are viewed as Nissl bodies (or substance) when stained with basic dyes (such as methylene blue) for histology (study of the minute structure of cells and its functions). Further processing of proteins occurs in the smooth ER and Golgi apparatus. Mitochondria, scattered throughout the cell body, contain **enzymes** involved with cellular metabolic energy. Lysosomes contain the enzymes that participate in intracellular digestion.

The cellular cytoskeleton consists of three components: **microtubules, neurofilaments**, and **microfilaments**. These components of the cellular cytoskeleton act together to provide a dynamic scaffolding, giving neurons their characteristic shape and acting as roadways for the transport of proteins and small organelles throughout the cell. Microtubules, neurofilaments, and microfilaments are all long strands of proteins with microtubules being the largest of the three, and microfilaments, the smallest. Different staining techniques are used to identify cellular structures (Box 5-1). Abnormalities of the cytoskeletal in the form of tangles and subsequently reduced transfer of protein have been associated with Alzheimer disease.

Dendritic and Axonal Processes

Dendrites and axons are cytoplasmic extensions that extend from the cell body and mediate nerve impulses. Dendrites are afferent (receptive), transmitting information to the cell body from other cells via synaptic sites. They tend to be short and have many branches. The branching dendrites sometimes have small spines that add to their arborization (sub-branching), which increases the surface available for synapses with other nerve cells.

The **nerve fiber** refers to an axon and its **myelin sheath** covering (see below). Nerves are composed of many nerve fibers. Axons are efferent structures that transmit information away from the cell body to other neurons or target organs. Axons do not produce their own protein and thus depend on the cytoplasmic substance of the cell body for survival. Axons originate from a cone-shaped region of the cell, the **axon hillock** (initial segment), and extend longer distances than do dendrites. On their way to a terminal destination, axons give off collaterals that communicate with many intervening nerve cells along the way. Axons terminate by branching into smaller multiple fibers that include synaptic terminals at their ends. Within the synaptic terminals are synaptic vesicles that contain a variety of neurotransmitters (the communicating chemical molecules) that are released on stimulation of the cell.

BOX 5-1

Cellular Staining Techniques

The gray matter in the cerebral cortex consists of cell bodies of various sizes and shapes that are intermixed with myelinated or unmyelinated fibers. Various staining methods are used to identify the cell bodies and their parts. Two staining methods that are commonly mentioned are Nissl and Golgi. Nissl stain because of ionic attraction binds to the rough endoplasmic reticulum, and, thus helps identify the cell body; however, the Nissl technique does not identify axonal and dendritic processes. For identifying axonal process, the Golgi method is used; the Golgi stain binds to the lipoprotein in myelin sheath of the axons and dendrites. This staining technique helps visualize the axonal pathways fibers such as corticospinal and corticobulbar fibers.

Myelin Sheath

The speed of nerve conduction is determined by the diameter of the nerve and its myelin sheath, which is a multilayered lipid material that insulates and protects the nerve fiber. An important function of this insulation is to prevent the escape of electrical energy during action potential transmission, which affects the speed of nerve impulses. **Oligodendroglial cells** produce the myelin sheath in the CNS. The myelin sheath is formed in small segments that are interrupted by intervals called the **nodes of Ranvier**. The segment of myelin between two nodes is the **internode**. In a longitudinal section, the nerve fiber looks like a string of sausages (Fig. 5-1*A*).

Action potentials jump from one node of Ranvier to the next (**saltatory conduction**), which facilitates rapid impulse conduction of up to 120 m/s (typical rate = 10 m/s). The myelin formation process begins during the fetal period and it continues to cortical maturity and beyond to adulthood (see Chapter 4). The growth rate and time span for myelin formation (myelogenesis) have implications for the development of sensorimotor functions, learning, and speech–language–cognitive skills (Lecours, 1975; Lenneberg, 1967; Yakovlev and Lecours, 1967). Damaged myelin in the CNS impairs nerve impulse conduction, a deficit found in **multiple sclerosis**, a progressive and autoimmune degenerative condition.

In the peripheral nervous system (PNS), the myelin sheath is produced by the **Schwann cells**, which are located along the axons. One characteristic of myelin formation in the PNS is that each Schwann cell is associated with only one axon, whereas one oligodendroglial cell contributes to the myelination of a group of adjacent axons in the CNS.

Synapse

The synapse is the space between the presynaptic terminal and the postsynaptic cell and includes three parts: **presynaptic terminal, synaptic cleft**, and **postsynaptic cell**. Structurally, the presynaptic terminal may be a clearly defined bouton, or it may occur merely where there is close opposition of the membrane of two cells. The synaptic terminals contain vesicles filled with neurotransmitters that mediate communication between cells. The membrane of the postsynaptic cell contains receptor proteins, the sites for binding the neurotransmitter molecules (Box 5-2).

Nerve impulses do not actually cross chemical synapse. Communication at the synapse occurs through a neurotransmitter released from the terminals. The

BOX 5-2

Receptors

Consisting of protein molecules and located on cellular surface, the receptor sites play an important role in regulating cellular activity. With selective affinity, a receptor binds to a drug, antigen, or neurotransmitter. By responding to acetylcholine, the receptors contribute to the activation of muscle movement. In autoimmune diseases, the antibodies block the receptors and make the neurotransmitter with affinity ineffective. This is true of myasthenia gravis in which the blocked receptors in the postsynaptic membrane contribute to the underactivity of acetylcholine causing weakness and muscle fatigue. This concept also has therapeutic implications in neuropharmacological treatment, where drugs are used to regulate the cellular functioning through influencing the receptor activities.

presynaptic cell is stimulated to release its neurotransmitter by an action potential that travels down the axon. The depolarization, caused by an action potential traveling down the axon to the terminal, causes the vesicles at the axon terminals to release stored neurotransmitters into the cleft area. Activation of the postsynaptic receptors can have many effects, such as **depolarizing** the postsynaptic membrane, **hyperpolarizing** the postsynaptic membrane, and activating various second messenger pathways, depending on the neurotransmitter and receptor type involved in the synapse (Box 5-2). If a depolarization of the postsynaptic membrane is large enough to cause the membrane potential to reach threshold, the cell will fire an action potential that will move up the dendrite to the cell body. (See "Nerve Impulse" later in this chapter.) Axons usually synapse with dendrites (**axodendritic synapse**) but may synapse with axons (**axoaxonic synapse**) or directly on cell bodies (**axosomatic synapse**).

A second type of synapse in the nervous system is an electrical synapse. Electrical synapses are present where extremely fast communication must occur between cells (such as in vision or hearing) or where synchronization of the excitation of cells is necessary (e.g., in the heart). With an electrical synapse, both surfaces are in close proximity containing large channels embedded in the membranes. Small molecules such as ions can flow directly from one cell to the next, allowing for very rapid changes in membrane potential to be transmitted from one cell to the next without the use of extracellular chemical signaling molecules.

Nerve Cell Types

The ability of a cell to process specialized information depends not only on how it is connected with other cells but also on its shape, size, and structural configuration. Accordingly, this structural diversity serves as the basis for nerve cell classification. Nerve cells are classified according to the number of receptive processes coming out of their bodies and by the length of their axons. Both dendritic and axonal processes add to a cell's ability to respond differentially to various types of sensorimotor information.

Based on the number of processes arising from the cell body, nerve cells are either **multipolar**, **bipolar**, or **unipolar** (Fig. 5-2). Multipolar cells have many dendrites and one axon. Differing in size and shape, the cells make numerous synaptic contacts with other cells. Most cells in the CNS are multipolar. Spinal **interneurons** and cerebellar **Purkinje cells** are the best examples of the multipolar type. Bipolar cells have two processes (dendrite and axon), one extending from each pole of the body. These are found in retina and inner ear. Unipolar cells are T shaped, with one process extending from the body and dividing into an axon and dendrite away from the cell body. Cells in the spinal dorsal roots, for example, are unipolar.

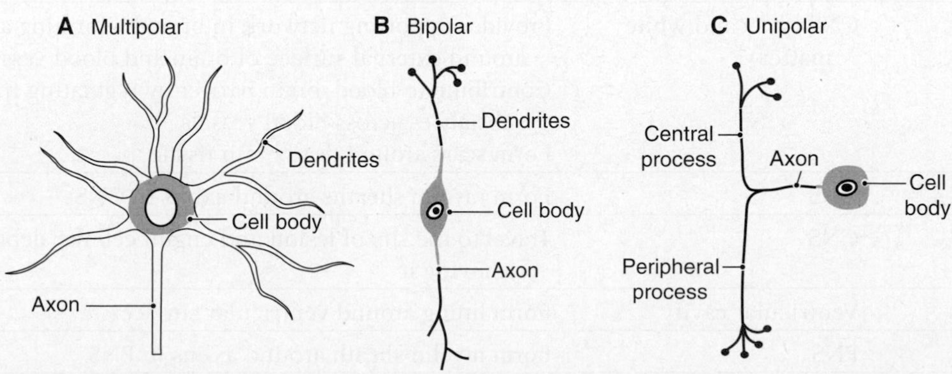

Figure 5-2 Nerve cell types based on their processes: (A) multipolar, (B) bipolar, (C) unipolar.

An alternative classification of neurons is based on axon length. **Golgi type I** cells have a long axon, ranging from inches to feet; many form the sensory or motor tracts connecting cells across long distances. **Golgi type II** cells, such as the interneurons that connect with other adjacent cells, have a short axonal process.

> ***Key Terms:***
> **Microglia cells** | **Oligodendroglia cells**
> **Astrocyte cells** | **Schwann cells**

Neuroglial Cells

Located in the gray and white matter of the brain, the neuroglia cells support and protect the nerve cells (Table 5-1). There are 40 to 50 times as many glial cells as nerve cells. The glial cells are small and do not participate in the generation and transmission of nerve impulses. There are four types of glial cells in the CNS: **astrocytes, oligodendroglia, ependymal**, and **microglia** (Fig. 5-3). Glial cells of the PNS are Schwann cells and **satellite cells**. Schwann cells may be capable of acting as **fibroblasts** (connective tissue), while the satellites are only supportive.

Located predominantly in the CNS white matter, the astrocytes function as connective tissue and provide skeletal support for the brain cells and their processes. In the gray matter, the astrocytes protect the brain by forming **external** and **internal limiting** membranes. By contacting capillary surfaces with their end feet and by forming tight junctions, astrocytes contribute to the **blood–brain barrier** (the selective **permeability** of capillaries and arteries that restricts the movement of harmful substances from the blood to the brain; see Chapter 7). Astrocytes also regulate the extracellular concentration of ions and, in some instances, can degrade released neurotransmitters. After an injury to the brain, the astrocytes and microglial cells proliferate and migrate to the lesion site. Microglia phagocytose (engulf and digest) cellular debris, leaving a cavity. In the case of a large lesion, astrocytes seal the cavity, forming a **cyst**. In the case of a limited-size lesion, astrocytes fill the space with a glial scar.

Oligodendroglia cells form and maintain the myelin sheath in the CNS. Each of the processes that radiate from the oligodendrocyte contributes to forming myelin. Thus, each oligodendrocyte may supply myelin for 25 or more axons. The sheath of myelin insulates the axons and speeds up action potential conduction. The myelin that covers PNS fibers is formed by Schwann cells, which are derived from the neural crest.

Ependymal cells line the inner surface of the **ventricles**. In conjunction with the astrocytes, the ependymal cells form the internal limiting membrane. The **choroid plexus**, which secretes cerebrospinal fluid (CSF) in the ventricular cavity, consists of a vascular membrane surrounded by an epithelial layer of ependymal cells. Microglial cells do not perform day-to-day functions in the nervous system but are called on during injury. In response to injury, the microglia, as scavengers of the CNS, proliferate and migrate to the injury site. Once at the site, they transform into **macrophages** that phagocytose dead tissue debris and pathogens.

> ***Key Terms:***
> **Endoneurium** | **Perineurium**
> **Epineurium**

Table 5-1

Neuroglia and Their Functions

Glia Cells	Locations	Functions
Astrocytes	CNS (gray and white matter)	Provide supporting network in brain by forming a complete lining around external surface of brain and blood vessels in CNS Contribute to blood–brain barrier by regulating transmission of substances across blood vessels Form scars around dead brain tissue
Oligodendrocytes	CNS	Form myelin sheaths around axons in CNS
Microglia	CNS	Travel to the site of lesion and engulf cellular debris before removing it
Ependymal cells	Ventricular cavity	Form lining around ventricular surface
Schwann cells	PNS	Form myelin sheath around axons in PNS
		Constitute fibrous connective tissue around fibers in PNS

CNS, central nervous system; PNS, peripheral nervous system.

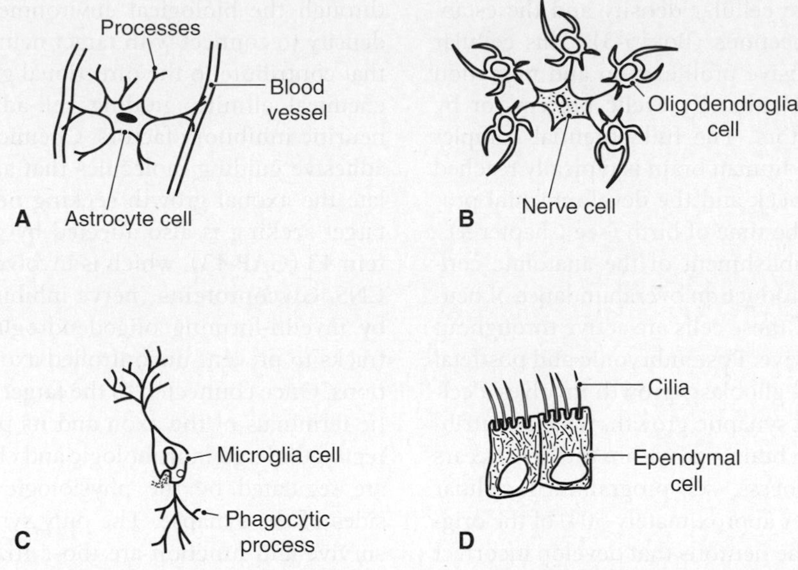

Figure 5-3 Glia cells. A. Astrocyte. B. Oligodendroglia. C. Microglia. D. Ependyma.

CENTRAL AND PERIPHERAL NERVOUS SYSTEMS

The two important cytologic differences between the CNS and the PNS are the different myelin-forming cells and the presence in the PNS of **endoneurium**, a fibrous connective tissue covering for axons. Schwann cells myelinate the fibers in a jelly-roll manner. One Schwann cell forms myelin exclusively for one internode of a peripheral nerve fiber, whereas one oligodendrocyte myelinates many axons in the CNS. Myelin formation by these two types of cells is otherwise similar.

The composition of nerve fibers differs between the CNS and PNS. Peripheral nerve fiber bundles are held together by connective tissues, such as the collagen fibers of the fibroblasts and other cells that form the **endoneurial membrane** (Fig. 5-4). This covering surrounds each peripheral nerve individually. This fibrous connective tissue (endoneurial membrane) is not known to exist in the CNS and may be related to the lack of regenerative growth in the CNS.

NEURONAL PRUNING AND SYNAPSE ESTABLISHMENT

The human brain's ability to serve cognitive–linguistic–speech functions relates to its unique neuronal growth pattern during its embryonic period, which reflects a balanced

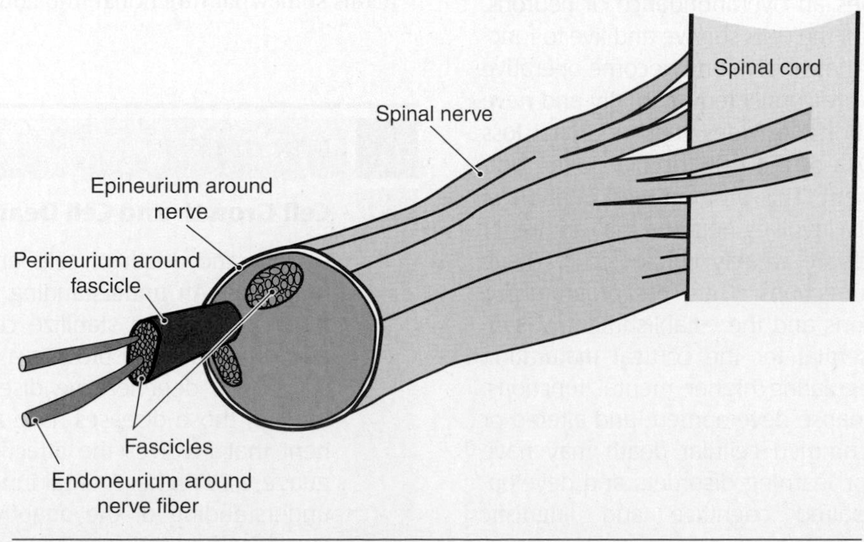

Figure 5-4 Peripheral nerve components.

development between the cellular density and the establishment of axonal connections (Box 5-3). This cellular growth involves an extensive proliferation and migration of cells that is regulated either by cyclic proteins or by trophic (nutritional) factors. The full potential complement of nerve cells in the human brain is typically reached by the 25th gestational week and the developmental process is virtually over by the time of birth (see Chapter 4).

Embryogenesis (establishment of the anatomic configuration) is known to produce an overabundance of neurons in the brain; most of these cells are active throughout life, but some do not survive. Postembryonic and postfetal neuronal (neuroblast and glioblast) growth involves a cellular reduction and rapid synaptic growth, which contributes to a 350% increase in brain size within the first 2 years of life. As an active process, self-programmed cellular death (apoptosis) involves approximately 50% of the original cells and applies to the neurons that develop incorrect or transient synaptic connections to the target areas, as well as to the neurons that are unable to develop these connections.

During the development of the brain, there are specific mechanisms that guide the ways cells are connected through traveling axons in the brain. Once a neuron has migrated and is established in its final destination, it extends an axon with **growth cones** (path finders) containing sensory or motor inclination. These growth cones navigate the directional axonal paths by finding ways through the biological environment of enormous cellar density to connect with target neurons. Additional factors that contribute to the directional growth of axons include chemical affinity, guiding cell-adhesive molecules, and neuritic inhibitory factors. Chemical factors, such as cell-adhesive guiding molecules that attract axons, also regulate the axonal growth seeking neuronal targets. Axonal target seeking is also affected by **growth-associated protein 43 (GAP-43)**, which is involved with repairing of the CNS. **Glycoproteins** (nerve inhibitory factors), produced by myelin-forming oligodendroglia cells, serve as train tracks to prevent uncontrolled axonal growth in all directions. Once connected to the target neurons, the presynaptic terminals of the axon and its postsynaptic (receptive) region undergo morphologic and chemical changes, which are regulated by the physiologic compatibility of both sides of the synapse. The only synaptic connections that survive and function are those that meet the criterion of biocompatibility on both sides.

This results in the retention of only a few synapses out of many competing connections. This networking stabilization is the basis for the formation of a mature axonal pathway, whose function is reinforced by experience on its each repeated activation.

Repeated activation influences the brain's organization and contributes to its astonishingly creative capacity for serving a variety of cognitive behaviors and allocating functions to different regions. The repeated use of this specialized network is of immense value in language acquisition and the development of musical skills. Some of these mechanisms are: retention of particular connections through use and function, removal of redundant and incompatible connections, and reduction of neurons through the process of programmed cell death during the critical period of the first 5 years of age (Box 5-4). Cerebral plasticity and the brain's ability to re-establish functional communication are most visible in the early years of life; however, cerebral plasticity remains somewhat functional into adult life.

BOX 5-3

Neuronal Pruning and Synapse Establishment

Cellular growth during the embryonic and fetal periods involves an overabundance of neurons. However, not all the cells survive and live to function. The cells that survive and become operative are those that are connected optimally and have assigned functions. A widespread neuronal loss involving >50% of the cells occurs during normal development. This programmed attrition of neurons largely involves neurons that are either not connected, are weakly connected, or have redundant connections. Thus, the programmed death of neurons and the establishment of synapses are essential for the cortical maturation needed for regulating higher mental functions. Attenuated synapse development and altered or reduced programmed cellular death may have implications for learning disorders and developmentally impaired cognitive and linguistic functions.

BOX 5-4

Cell Growth and Cell Death

Growth and death of cells are highly regulated processes. An understanding of these processes that regulate and stabilize cellular connectivity and cell death will provide a better understanding of the degenerative diseases of the brain; most of those diseases have a cognitive component that involves the affection of speech, language, and higher mental functions. Much of the understanding of the adaptive processes must await the future research.

Knowledge of the physiologic processes involved in nervous system development and the identification of factors that can either stop, slow down, or interrupt programmed cell death will help researchers evaluate the natural restitution process seen in most brain-damaged patients. Research is under way to find methods of stopping, or slowing the rate of, cellular death in the brains of stroke patients by administering nerve growth proteins and incorporating the brain's own trophic factors.

Key Terms:

Action potentials	**Excitatory postsynaptic potentials**
Depolarization	**Inhibitory postsynaptic potentials (IPSP)**
Polarization	
Hyperpolarization	
Nerve impulse	

NERVE IMPULSE

Nerve cells communicate with one another through impulses that represent all neuronal activity. Nerve impulses have a chemical component that underlies the electric potential of the cells (Fig. 5-5). The excitability of nerve cells depends on the ion channels in the neuronal membrane. An action potential results from charged particles (ions) moving through the cell membranes. Nerve impulses activate the release of a neurotransmitter in a presynaptic neuron. The transmitter often causes the adjacent postsynaptic receptors to open the ionic channels (either directly or indirectly through second messengers). By selectively opening or closing ion channels, the released neurotransmitter controls the excitability as well as inhibition of the interconnecting neuron.

A cell is in a **resting state** when it is not excited and not conducting an impulse. In the resting state, there is a specific level of **membrane potential** in which the distribution of positive and negative ions on each side of the membrane is unequal (polarized). Consequently, there is a difference between electrical charges on the inner and outer sides of the cell membrane (Fig. 5-5*A*). The specific resting membrane potential depends on the cell type but is typically between –50 and –70 mV in relation to the outside of the cell. The membrane potential is maintained by an unequal distribution of positively charged **sodium (Na)** and **potassium (K)** ions and negatively charged **chloride** (Cl) ions and proteins across the membrane. The concentration of negative ions is slightly higher inside the cell, and the concentration of positive ions is slightly higher outside the cell. Although the unequal distribution of positive and negative ions is small, it is large enough to generate potentials on an mV scale.

Even during a resting state, when the nerve cell is not conducting an impulse, some ions constantly pass through

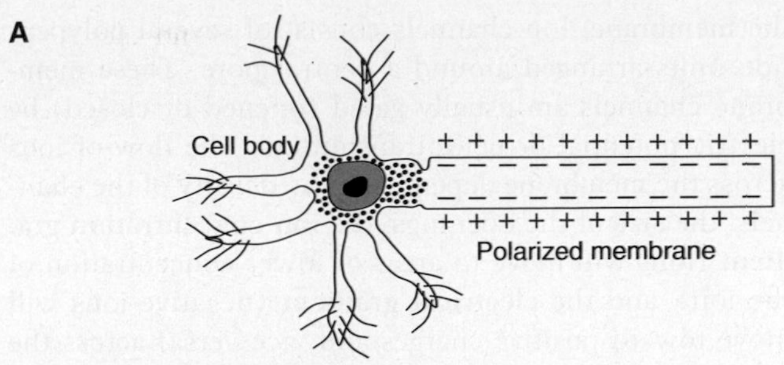

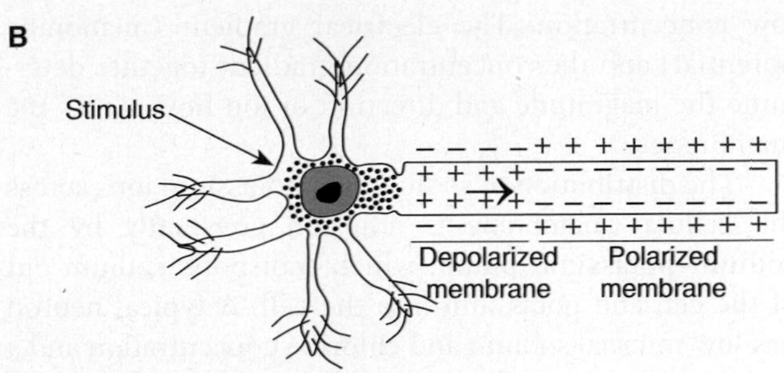

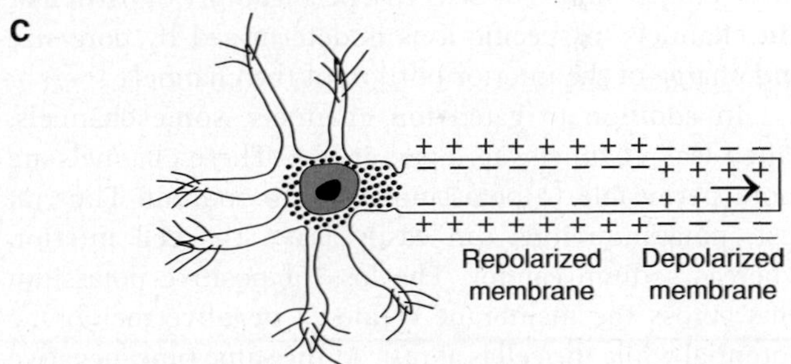

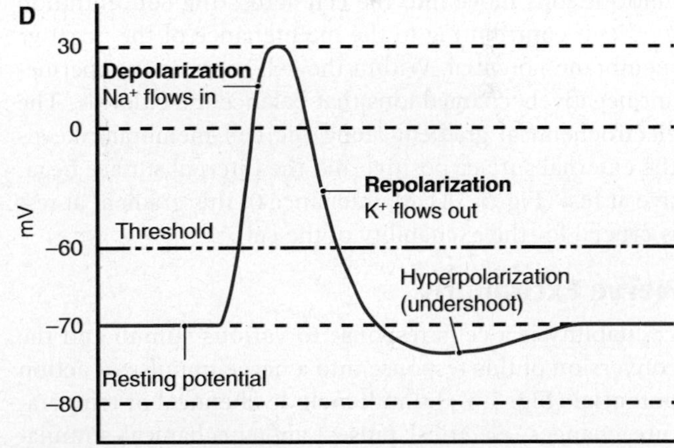

Figure 5-5 Action potential. A. The resting potential with a polarized membrane. B. The generation of the action potential with a depolarized membrane. C. The conduction of the action potential along the membrane. D. Recorded changes in the membrane potentials, threshold excitatory postsynaptic potentials, and inhibitory postsynaptic potential.

the membrane. Ion channels consist of several polypeptide units arranged around a central pore. These membrane channels are usually gated (opened or closed) by electric potential or neurotransmitters. The flow of ions across the membrane depends on the density of the channels, the size of the openings, the **ion concentration gradient** (ions will move to areas of lower concentration of the ion), and the **electrical gradient** (negative ions will move toward positive charges and vice versa) across the membrane. The steeper the gradient concentration across the membrane, the greater the flow of ions from high to low concentration. The electrical gradient (membrane potential) and the concentration gradient together determine the magnitude and direction of ion flow across the membrane.

The distribution of sodium and potassium ions across the cellular membrane is adjusted constantly by the **sodium–potassium pump**, which transports sodium out of the cell and potassium into the cell. A typical neuron has low internal sodium and chloride concentration and a high internal potassium concentration relative to the extracellular fluid. The selective permeability of particular ion channels to specific ions is determined by pore size and charge of the interior portion of the channel.

In addition to gated ion channels, some channels, called leak channels, are open at rest. These channels are more permeable to potassium than to sodium. Thus, at rest, potassium ions can easily leave the cell interior, whereas sodium cannot. The loss of positive potassium ions across the membrane creates a negative membrane potential while the cell is at rest. At the same time, negative chloride ions move into the cell across the concentration gradient, contributing to the maintenance of the negative membrane potential. Within the cell there are nonpermeant negatively charged ions that balance the chloride. The electrochemical gradient along the cell membrane keeps the external surface positive and the internal surface negative at rest (Fig. 5-5*A*). Maintenance of this gradient at rest is crucial for the excitability of the cell.

Nerve Excitability

Excitability is a cell's response to various stimuli and the conversion of this response into a nerve impulse or **action potential** (Fig. 5-5). Stimuli include chemical or temperature changes, electrical pulses, and mechanical stimulation. All these stimuli are converted to changes in the membrane potential of the cell. When the neuron becomes **hyperpolarized** (the cell interior becomes more negative), it is less capable of triggering a large spike, called an action potential. An action potential is triggered when the change is in the other direction of less negativity (**depolarization**) and the cell reaches threshold. Neurotransmitters released by the presynaptic cell cause one of two graded (of different magnitudes) electrical responses. If the postsynaptic cell demonstrates **hyperpolarization** in response to the neurotransmitter, it is called an **inhibitory postsynaptic potential** (**IPSP**). An IPSP will take the membrane potential further away from the action potential threshold so that the cell becomes less likely to fire an action potential in response to other stimuli. If the neurotransmitter causes a depolarization of the membrane potential, it is called an **excitatory postsynaptic potentials** (**EPSP**). If the EPSP is of sufficient magnitude, the cell will reach threshold for firing an action potential.

The threshold for triggering an action potential varies from cell to cell but is typically 5 to 10 mV depolarized from the resting membrane potential. The depolarization of a cell membrane opens specific voltage-gated ion channels, allowing ions to flow in and out of the cell. Initially, sodium flows quickly into the cell, causing a large depolarization, to potentials >0 mV. These sodium channels close rapidly, allowing a return to the resting membrane potential. The **repolarization** of the cell is aided by the opening of voltage-gated potassium channels that allow more potassium to flow down the concentration gradient. The membrane potential can become slightly more hyperpolarized than the original resting membrane potential (undershoot). As the cell becomes hyperpolarized, the potassium channels also close, so that the cell can reestablish its membrane potential. All this occurs in a matter of milliseconds; hence relatively few ions flow across the membrane. In this way, the concentration gradient is not disturbed during the brief action potential, and the electrical chemical gradient that established the membrane potential in the first place remains intact.

For a period following the action potential, the cell is incapable of producing a second action potential. This is called the **absolute refractive period**. Unlike the graded IPSPs and EPSPs, action potentials are all-or-nothing responses. If the cell reaches threshold, it will always fire an action potential, and the action potential will have the same shape and magnitude every time it occurs.

Not all stimuli are strong enough to cause the cell to reach threshold for firing an action potential. However, if many stimuli with subthreshold strength occur at about the same time (or in series), or in the same place, an action potential can be initiated.

Action Potential Conduction

An action potential is passively conducted a short distance in the axon by sodium entering the cell membrane. The interior of the axon becomes more positive than the adjacent neighboring area (Fig. 5-5*B*). This gradually changes the membrane potential in the neighboring area, and the action potential continues to allow positively charged ions to enter the cell membrane as it moves distally along the axon (Fig. 5-5*C*). Action potential conduction in a myelinated axon is the same as in an unmyelinated axon, except the action potential conduction in the myelinated axon is faster as the action potential jumps from one node of Ranvier to the other (saltatory conduction). Conduction velocities depend on the diameter of the axon; the largest diameter axons have the greatest conduction velocity. Large axons are typically myelinated for efficient conduction and have velocities of 72 to 120 m per second and diameters of 12 to 20 μm. In contrast, small-diameter axons (0.2–1.5 μm) are unmyelinated and have conduction velocities of 0.4 to 2 m per second.

Key Terms :

Axonal reaction	**Chromatolysis**
Macrophage	**Wallerian degeneration**

NEURONAL RESPONSES TO BRAIN INJURIES

Nerve cells in the human brain are less capable of further cell division and regeneration than other cell types. Limited cellular regeneration restricts the recovery of sensorimotor functions and higher mental functions including that of language after lesions in the brain. The nerve cell synapses serve as good points of reference for discovering the effects of cellular injuries because, in addition to conducting an impulse, the cells transmit nutritive (trophic) substances between neurons. Trophic factors are crucial for normal cell maintenance on both sides of the synapse. A neuron may degenerate if either the presynaptic or the postsynaptic terminal degenerates. Axotomy affects not only the directly injured neuron but also postsynaptic neurons and neurons that innervate the injured neuron. The severity of the effect on other neurons depends on the extent to which each of the other neurons interacts with the surrounding noninjured neurons.

Understanding the physiologic events that cells undergo after injuries explains the processes of spontaneous recovery after trauma and vascular accident. The two types of degenerative changes that follow axonal sectioning are the **axonal (retrograde) reaction** and **Wallerian (anterograde) degeneration** (Fig. 5-6*A*; Table 5-2). During **axonal reactions**, retrograde degenerative changes occur in the cell body in response to sectioning the axon (axotomy). This is secondary to the interruption of trophic factors that flow from the axon to the cell body and to the reprogramming of the cell body in the face of metabolic changes. Axonal injury extends from the site of injury to the cell body. In **Wallerian degeneration**, the degenerative changes occur in the axon region detached from the cell body. The axonal segment still attached to the cell body is the **proximal segment**, and the detached axonal segment is the **distal segment** (Fig. 5-6*C*).

Axonal Reaction

Nerve cells undergo a series of changes in response to an injury (Fig. 5-6*B*, Table 5-3). The microscopic structures

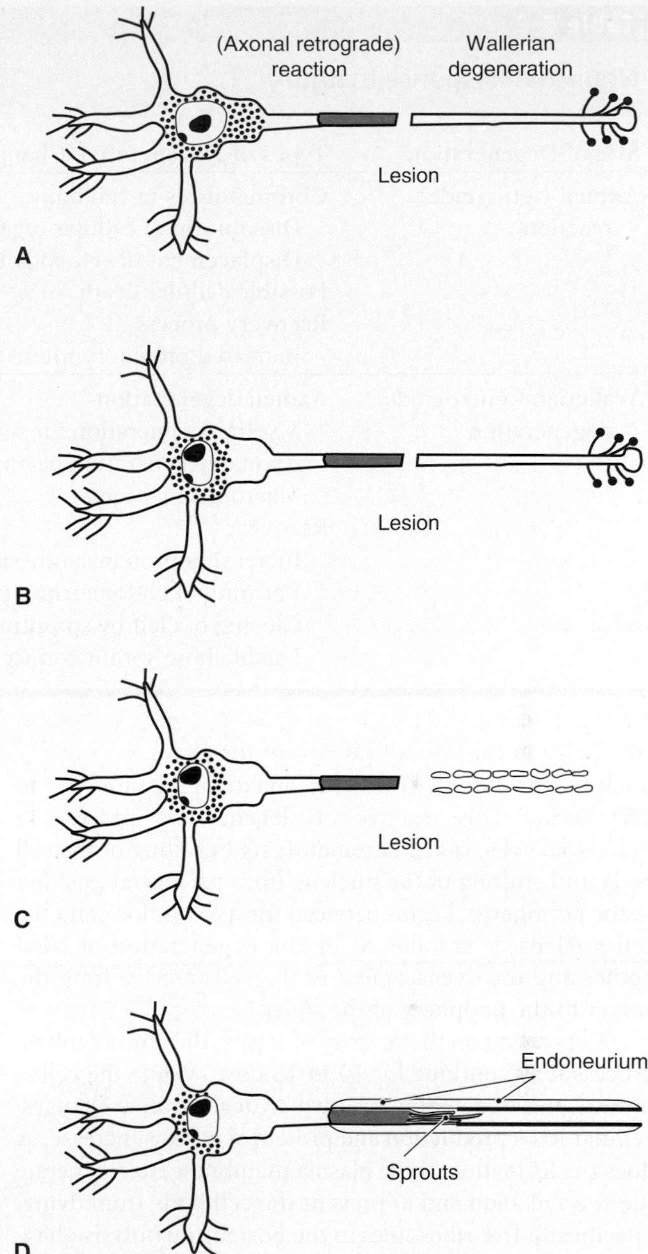

Figure 5-6 The neuronal response to injury (here, a severed axon) and the recovery process in the peripheral nervous system. A. Types of neuronal responses to injury. B. Axonal (retrograde) reaction. C. Wallerian degeneration. D. Peripheral nerve regeneration.

(organelles) of the soma undergo structural-degenerative alterations that are evident within 24 to 48 hours after injury. The first cytologic signs of changes in the cell body are swelling of the organelles and dissolution of coarse clumps of **Nissl bodies** into fine granules. Cellular edema, caused by an altered blood–brain barrier, obliterates structural details of the gray and white matter and triggers

Table 5-2

Neuronal Response to Injury

Site of Degeneration	Types of Degenerative Changes
Axonal (retrograde) reaction	Chromatolysis in cell body Dissolution of cellular organelles Displacement of cell body to periphery Possible cellular death Recovery process Increased protein synthesis to regenerate severed axon and prevent cell body from dying
Wallerian (anterograde) degeneration	Axonal degeneration Myelin degeneration for sectioned axon Axonal degeneration beginning with its distal end Macrophagic process Recovery Increasing protein synthesis to promote recovery Forming of endoneurium tube by Schwann cells Closing of cleft by sprouting of cut ends of axons Establishing sprout connections between both axonal ends

nuclear shrinking. Edema is maximal within 90 to 100 hours. This reactive or degenerative process in individual cells, called **chromatolysis** (swelling of the cell body and shifting of the nucleus from its central position to the periphery), begins between the axon hillock and the cell nucleus. It is followed by the degeneration of Nissl bodies and the displacement of the cell nucleus from the center to the periphery of the soma.

Depending on the severity of injury, the chromatolytic process may continue for 10 to 18 days. While the cell is injured and undergoing reactive or degenerative changes, cellular RNA production and protein synthesis increase, as does the formation of the plasma membrane, to regenerate the severed axon and to prevent the cell body from dying. Specifically, free ribosomes in the postchromatolysis phase synthesize increased structural proteins that are needed for restoring cellular structure and rebuilding Nissl bodies and cellular fibers. If the connection of the severed axon is properly restored, the chromatolysis process ends, and the cell may return to its normal appearance with some function. Some cells, if not seriously damaged, may respond to the natural recovery process and survive the injury. In such cases, all cell body organelles resume their normal appearance, and the nucleus again assumes a central location. However, this restoration may take months. Cells that are severely injured do not survive. They shrink and assume irregular shapes because of the degenerated organelles. They gradually atrophy and leave only debris.

Cellular swelling, if not medically treated, can lead to death of the cell by elevating intracranial pressure. By the end of a week, swelling may begin to go down, but necrotic tissues are invaded by a considerable number of new capillaries (hyperplasia) and a proliferation of macrophages (astrocytes and microglia). The period after the first week is marked by liquefaction of necrotic tissue and **phagocytosis**,

Table 5-3

Sequence of Pathologic Features in the Necrotic Process

Time	Pathologic Changes
1 d	No visible sign of tissue death
2–4 d	Elimination of structural details between gray and white matter owing to cellular edema and shrinking of cells
4+ d	Maximum swelling in necrotic tissues owing to impaired blood–brain barrier Infiltration of infection-fighting blood monocytes
1 wk	Attenuation of swelling and astrocytic and capillary proliferation (hyperplasia and hypertrophy)
1 wk to 3 mo	Liquefaction of necrotic tissues and their phagocytosis by macrophagic microglial cells
3–6+ mo	Formation of a cystic cavity Scar formation if small infarct

in which lipid-laden macrophagic microglia cells engulf and remove the dead tissue. Phagocytosis may take 3 or more months, depending on the size of the lesion. In the case of a large lesion, tissue removal is likely to leave a cavity filled with some macrophagic cells and fluid (CSF); the cavity area is outlined by a sheet of astrocytes. The presence of such a cystic cavity in the brain of a stroke patient has made some pessimistic about the benefits of rehabilitative efforts. However, the recovery process is highly dynamic and presumably involves multiple steps, most importantly the potential development of alternate networks and functional reallocation and reorganization.

Wallerian Degeneration

Survival of the axon depends on cytoplasmic flow from the cell body. Survival of the axon depends on metabolic activity, trophic substance, and cytoplasmic flow from the cell body. The Wallerian reaction (Fig. 5-6*C*) refers to the degeneration of the axonal part that is separated from its cell body. The distal portion of the sectioned axon swells and begins to degenerate within 12 to 20 hours. Axons degenerate before the myelin sheath, and, within 2 to 3 days, the connected muscles become denervated. Within 7 days, the axon and its myelin are broken into small pieces, which gradually disintegrate, setting the stage for the macrophagic action of microglia cells. Phagocytosis begins in 7 days and is complete in 3 to 6 months (Table 5-3).

Neuroglial Responses

Neuroglial cells react to cellular injuries and brain tissue necrosis by multiplying in number (**hyperplasia**) and by increasing their size (**hypertrophy**). The infection-fighting **neutrophils** (scavenger white blood cells) arrive at the lesion site within a few days of an injury. This is followed by the migration of microglia and the proliferation of the astrocytes and other macrophages in the region of the dying cells. The breakdown of the blood–brain barrier allows monocytes (phagocytic white blood cells) to invade brain tissues. In the case of a small lesion, the astrocytes form a glial scar, called replacement **gliosis**. In large lesions, they outline the fluid-filled space, forming a **cystic cavity**.

Microglias are the primary scavengers of the nervous system. In case of inflammation or injury, they rapidly proliferate and migrate toward dead tissue within 24 hours. Their function is to phagocytose the cellular debris. Normally, microglia cells are small, but they become large after phagocytizing dead cells; their cytoplasm becomes less dense and their nucleus more prominent. Within 1 week, they look like typical macrophages, with pale cytoplasm. As the macrophages ingest the debris of myelin, cells, and lipid droplets, the nucleus is pushed to the side. The phagocytic cells dominate the injury site from the first week, and it may take several months or even years to remove the debris of dead brain tissue (Table 5-3).

In addition, the proliferation and migration of glial cells displace presynaptic and postsynaptic terminals and cell bodies of axotomized neurons, thus impairing transmission between neurons. After normal input to the cell body is removed, new synaptic trigger zones may develop on its dendritic aspect and begin to excite the cell.

Axonal Regeneration in the PNS

The regeneration of fibers in the PNS has been confirmed clinically (Fig. 5-6*D*). The sectioned nerve endings proximal to the cell body begin regenerating within 3 to 4 days. This regeneration cannot occur unless the proximal and distal ends of the severed nerve are cleaned and attached. The Schwann cells and fibroblasts contribute significantly to axonal regeneration in the PNS. In the first few days, the proliferating Schwann cells fill the interval between opposing ends of the nerve fiber. The sheath of Schwann, or **neurilemma**, in conjunction with the endoneurial connective tissue, forms a tube from the proximal fiber end leading to the distal end. This neurilemmal tube guides the growth of the peripheral axon. As the proximal end of the axon regenerates, many sprouts (regenerated processes of axons) form. One or more axonal sprouts may grow along the tube and pass through the cleft. Some axonal sprouts that cross the scar may grow to connect to the distal portion of the axon at a rate of 4 mm a day. Axonal regeneration is not a simple process, and as such it is not always successful. There is a low probability that the regenerated axon will reach its previously attached fiber; instead, it might attach to a different sensory or motor fiber. This improper connection can be problematic: a pain-mediating fiber connected to a touch receptor, for example, results in the sensation of pain from touch. The nerve fibers that are connected incorrectly usually atrophy. An added factor is that an injury closer to the cell body is more damaging than a distant nerve lesion in which case potential for connecting with a functionally incorrect structure is less existent.

Axonal Regeneration in the CNS

Nerve growth in the CNS would have tremendous implications for the natural and assisted recovery in brain-damaged patients with acquired higher mental dysfunctions. The physiologic concept that most intrigues and frustrates health professionals is the minimal restoration of function after a lesion in the brain. As a result, the prognosis for recovery of axotomized neurons in the brain is always poor. Axons severed in the CNS also undergo regrowth and sprouting similar to those in the PNS; however, unknown factors prevent damaged neurons from reconnecting to the distal axonal segments and reinnervating their target structures. One factor may be the lack of the growth protein in the CNS that is present in the PNS. The proximal ends of axons in the CNS exhibit some growth (sprouting). However, this growth is not significant because the regenerated axons cannot cross the astrocytic scars. Furthermore, there are no Schwann cells and no endoneural tissue tubes (Fig. 5-4) to guide axonal growth. With no guiding structure, the regenerated axons form an axonal ball. In addition, central myelin is a potent inhibitory of axon outgrowth, which is why myelination occurs late in development. Inflammatory responses and scar tissue also inhibit regeneration. Last, there are intrinsic differences between peripheral and central neurons, such as differences in protein expression.

Despite the limited regeneration of the CNS, recovery is highly dynamic and may involve multiple steps, such as restitution of partially injured adjacent neuronal structures and functional reorganization within and across the hemispheres involving the homotopic cortex (Box 5-5).

Key Terms:

Acetylcholine
Acetylcholinesterase
Dopamine
γ-aminobutyric acid (GABA)
Norepinephrine
Serotonin

BOX 5-5

Cellular Connectivity and Axonal Reorganization

The excitatory or inhibitory effect a nerve cell has on the target cell depends on the identity of the neurotransmitter released by the neuron. Nerve cells are highly specialized in responding to excitatory and inhibitory neurotransmitters. The operational power of nerve cells is enhanced by the various ways in which the cell bodies are interconnected and respond to electrochemical signals.

Axonal sprouting in the nervous system is a common observation after a lesion. Once the damaged axons degenerate and their waste is removed by scavenger cells, new growth in the affected area is visible within a short period. This is marked by the growth of button-like swellings on axons. The boutons are the site of synapse formation. The new growth has been attributed to the trophic elements that are released by the affected neurons. While there is no evidence that this sprouting can restore the lost function, it does raise hopes for restitution through rehabilitation.

The general rule is that in the mammalian central nervous system (CNS), any damaged or sectioned axon does not effectively regenerate. Any potential axonal regeneration in the CNS is limited to initially sending sprouts, but that ends within a week or two. This limited growth in the CNS is largely due to inadequate provision of growth proteins. Multiple other factors have also been identified for inhibiting axonal growth in the CNS. With no endoneural membrane, there is no guiding structure for regeneration in the CNS. Further, the growth of axons in the CNS is inhibited by specific myelin-associated proteins secreted by oligodendroglia cells. The CNS myelin is inherently a potent inhibitor of axon outgrowth, which is why myelination occurs late in development after the establishment of neuronal connections. Inflammatory responses and scar tissue also inhibit regeneration. Last, there are intrinsic differences between neurons in the peripheral nervous system (PNS) and the CNS, such as in protein expression. Research focusing on how to simulate the growth environment of the PNS to promote reconnectivity in the CNS has promising implications.

NEUROTRANSMITTERS

Neurotransmitters help regulate brain mechanisms that control cognition, language, speech, moods, attention, memory, personality, motivation, and the tuning of the brain and its pathway (Fig. 5-7). A familiarity with neurotransmitters and their functions is essential.

A neurotransmitter is released at a synapse and it transmits signals across neurons (Table 5-4). There are two types of transmitters in the nervous system: **small molecule** and **large molecule (peptides)**. Small-molecule neurotransmitters include **acetylcholine, dopamine, norepinephrine, serotonin, glutamate**, and **γ-aminobutyric acid** (GABA). The latter five are called **monoamines** because they are derived from **amino acids**. They are known to have short-lasting effects in contrast to long-lasting effects on postsynaptic nerve cells by large-molecule neurotransmitters. Most neurotransmitters have more than one receptor type and may have different effects on different synapses. Also, more than one neurotransmitter may be secreted at a single synapse. It is, therefore, difficult to identify definitively the specific behavioral effect of a given neurotransmitter at all times.

Acetylcholine

Acetylcholine is synthesized from **choline** and **acetyl-coenzyme A (acetyl Co-A)** by the enzyme **choline acetyltransferase**. When released in synapses, it is broken down by the enzyme **acetylcholinesterase**. This disintegration of acetylcholine is necessary to make repetitive nerve impulses to be effective and to allow for muscle repolarization. It is one of the primary neurotransmitters of the PNS regulating muscular activities. Acetylcholine is also functional in the CNS; cholinergic neurons are concentrated in the reticular formation, basal forebrain, and striatum (Fig. 5-7A).

The action of acetylcholine on muscle contraction is measured easily, whereas its effects in the CNS are more

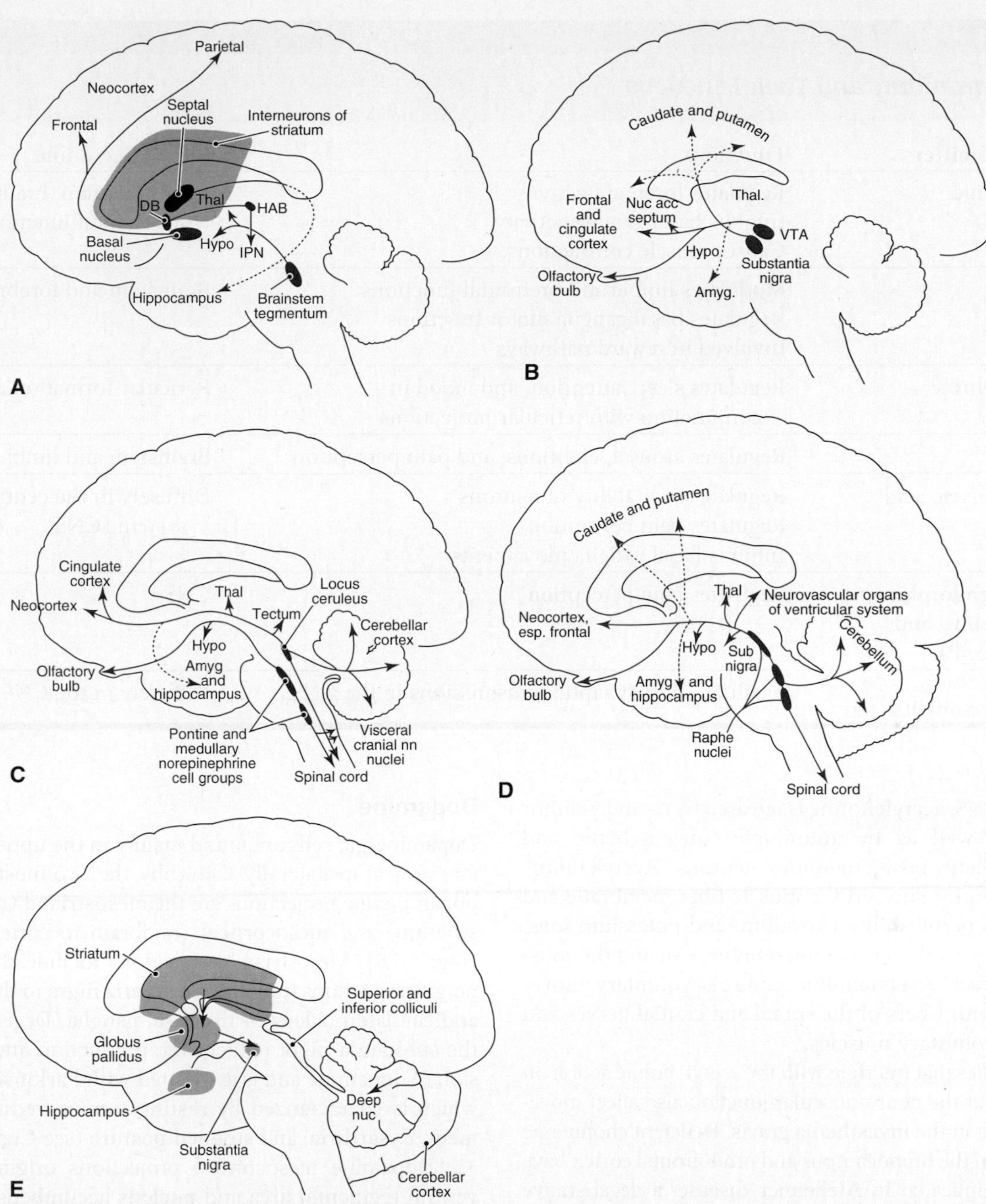

Figure 5-7 Sites of cell bodies and their projections in the brain for acetylcholine (A), dopamine (B), norepinephrine (C), serotonin (D), and γ-aminobutyric acid (E). Amyg., amygdala; DB, diagonal band of Broca; esp., especially; HAB, habenula; Hypo, hypothalamus; IPN, interpeduncular nucleus; nn, nerves; nuc, nucleus; Nuc acc, nucleus accumbens; Sub, substantia; Thal, thalamus; VTA, ventral tegmental area.

difficult to decipher. Thus the direct behavioral effects of acetylcholine are better characterized in the PNS than in the CNS. The cholinergic neurons in the forebrain (**nucleus basalis of Meynert**), together with related nuclei in the nearby septal area, supply the neocortex, hippocampus, and amygdala. These cholinergic projections are thought to participate in regulating levels of forebrain activity. In addition, together with the projections from the reticular formation to the thalamus, they are critical in the cycle of sleep and wakefulness. The reticular cholinergic neurons of the forebrain, with their connections with the basal ganglia, also influence stereotyped movements.

Table 5-4

Neurotransmitters and Their Functions

Neurotransmitters	Functions	Site of Secretion
Acetylcholine	Regulates forebrain activity Inhibits basal ganglia activity Causes muscle contractions	Basal forebrain, brainstem, and myoneural junctions
Dopamine	Modulates limbic and prefrontal functions Regulates basal ganglia motor functions Involved in reward pathways	Brainstem and forebrain
Norepinephrine	Regulates sleep, attention, and mood in conjunction with reticular projections	Reticular formation and ANS
Serotonin	Regulates arousal, emotions, and pain perception	Brainstem and limbic system
γ-Aminobutyric acid	Regulates excitability of neurons Regulates pain perception Inhibits basal ganglia movements	Diffusely in the central nervous system (CNS)
Peptides (endorphins, enkephalins, and substance P)	Regulates pain perception	CNS
Glutamate	Facilitates fast synaptic transmissions in the CNS	Diffusely in the CNS

In the PNS, acetylcholine is released by α- and γ-motor neurons as well as by autonomic (preganglionic and parasympathetic postganglionic) neurons. Acetylcholine binds to receptor sites on the muscle fiber membrane and increases its permeability to sodium and potassium ions. This depolarizes the muscle membrane, causing the muscle to contract. Acetylcholine controls voluntary movements of motor fibers of the spinal and cranial nerves and of many involuntary muscles.

Antibodies that interfere with the acetylcholine action on muscle cells at the neuromuscular junction also affect movement, as seen in the **myasthenia gravis**. Deficient cholinergic projections in the hippocampus and orbitofrontal cortex have also been implicated in **Alzheimer disease**, a degenerative condition characterized by atrophy of the neocortex and hippocampus that causes memory loss, personality change, and dementia. In Alzheimer disease, however, acetylcholine-replacement therapy has not been successful because multiple transmitter systems, such as somatostatin-containing neurons, also are implicated in the degenerative process.

Monoamines

Consisting of norepinephrine, epinephrine, dopamine, and serotonin, the monoamines are a subgroup of small-molecule transmitters derived from amino acids. All monoamine-producing cell clusters lie in the brainstem (Fig. 5-7). Despite the restricted area of origin, these neurons have projections to the wider areas of brain and participate in regulating the activity of large portions of the CNS.

Dopamine

Dopaminergic cells are found mainly in the upper midbrain and project ipsilaterally. Clinically, the two most important dopaminergic projections are the **mesostriatal** (midbrain to striatum) and **mesocortical** (midbrain to cortex) systems (Fig. 5-7*B*). Mesostriatal projections include the dopaminergic projections from the **substantia nigra** to the **putamen** and caudate nucleus of the basal ganglia. Degeneration of the substantia nigra reduces the production and transmission of dopamine and is associated with **Parkinson disease**, which is characterized by **resting tremor, reduced movement, dysarthria**, and **stooped posture** (see Chapter 13).

Dopamine mesocortical projections originate in the **ventral tegmental area** and **nucleus accumbens**, and their terminals are in the cortex, and amygdala. The cortical projections innervate the medial, frontal, anterior cingulate, and olfactory cortices. Dopamine projections to the cortex and limbic structures support their involvement in cognition, emotion, and motivation. Impairments of the mesocortical projections are involved in some mental illnesses (see Chapter 15). Drugs of abuse directly or indirectly cause dopamine release in the nucleus accumbens, suggesting that mesolimbic (midbrain to limbic lobe) projections are involved in pleasurable feelings. Excessive dopamine activity in the forebrain contributes to schizophrenia. **Thorazine** and related drugs that block dopamine receptors are used in the treatment of schizophrenia, which suggests that the midbrain–limbic and midbrain–cortical dopaminergic projections contribute to this psychiatric disorder.

Norepinephrine

Norepinephrine is one of the primary neurotransmitters in the PNS. It is released by the **postganglionic sympathetic neurons** and is responsible for the flight-or-fight reaction. In the CNS, norepinephrine-containing neurons are in the pons and medulla (Fig. 5-7*C*).

Noradrenergic (norepinephrine-containing) cells are located in the reticular formation of the brainstem, **locus ceruleus**, and **lateral medullary reticular formation**. Noradrenergic neurons project to the thalamus, hypothalamus, limbic forebrain structures, and cerebral cortex. Descending noradrenergic fibers project to other parts of the brainstem, cerebellar cortex, and spinal cord.

Clinically, noradrenergic neurons are thought to be involved in generating paradoxical sleep (with brain wave patterns similar to wakeful state, random eye movement (REM)) and maintaining attention and vigilance. Drugs used for the treatment of depression act by enhancing norepinephrine transmission. When examined in postmortem brains, norepinephrine has been found to be distributed richly in the left pulvinar and right ventrobasal nuclear complex of the thalamus. This norepinephrine asymmetry at the thalamic level is intriguing because it may be related to handedness and the prevalence of one-sided vascular lesions.

Serotonin

Although serotonin is an important neurotransmitter of the CNS, 95% of it is found peripherally in blood platelets and the gastrointestinal tract. The highest concentrations of serotonin neurons are found in the **raphe nuclei** (Fig. 5-7*D*). The serotonergic terminals are in the reticular formation, hypothalamus, thalamus, **septum**, hippocampus, **olfactory tubercle**, cerebral cortex, basal ganglia, and amygdala. The rostral reticular serotonergic projections are active in sleep; the caudal reticular serotonin terminals, with afferents from the periaqueductal gray matter, interact with spinal enkephalin interneurons and exert some control over pain input.

Clinically, the firing rate of serotonin and noradrenergic neurons fluctuates with sleep and wakefulness and thus may be involved in the general activity level of the CNS. Serotonin is thought to be involved with the overall level of arousal and slow-wave sleep. It also contributes to the descending pain-control system. Severe depression and mental illnesses are thought to be associated with low levels of serotonin. Serotonin levels were lower in individuals who died from suicide. Since serotonin is an important neurotransmitter regulating mental conditions, antidepressant drugs (e.g., Prozac) work by enhancing the serotonin concentration at the synapse through reducing its uptake.

γ-Aminobutyric Acid

GABA, a derivative of glutamate, is the major inhibitory neurotransmitter for the CNS. Neurons containing GABA are widespread in the nervous system. Examples of GABA local-circuit neurons are cells found in the hippocampus, cerebral cortex, basal ganglia, and cerebellar cortex (Fig. 5-7*E*). GABA serves as the inhibitory neurotransmitter from the striatum to the globus pallidus and substantia nigra, from the globus pallidus and substantia nigra to the thalamus, and from the cerebellar Purkinje cells to the deep cerebellar nuclei. GABA projections suppress the firing of projection neurons and sharpen contrast by inhibiting nearby elements.

Pharmaceutical agents that interact with GABA receptors are widely prescribed for clinical conditions such as epilepsy, anxiety, and insomnia as well as for anesthesia. GABA is implicated in **Huntington chorea**, a degenerative disease characterized by involuntary movements secondary to the loss of GABA-producing neurons in the caudate and putamen (Fig. 15-6*B*). Decreased GABA-containing **striatonigral** (striatum to substantia nigra) projections result in lower GABA levels to the substantia nigra. A reduction in GABA causes an elevation of the ratio of dopamine to acetylcholine, which produces abnormal movements (see Chapter 15). In contrast, a lower ratio of dopamine to acetylcholine ratio, resulting from loss of nigral dopaminergic cells, is associated with the reduced movement (**bradykinesia**) or lack of movements of **Parkinsonism**.

Glutamate

Glutamate is the main excitatory neurotransmitter in the mammalian CNS. Most of the other neurotransmitters discussed in this chapter mediate slower, modulatory effects in the CNS. Glutamate mediates fast synaptic transmissions in the CNS, much in the same way that acetylcholine mediates muscle contractions in the periphery. It is produced by all excitatory neurons in the CNS, and the majority of neurons have receptors for this compound. Its concentration in the extracellular space is regulated tightly by re-uptake pumps in the surrounding glia cells because too much glutamate causes excitotoxicity and excessive calcium influx. Brain damage secondary to stroke or degenerative disorder may be the result, in part, of excessive release or insufficient reuptake of glutamate by astrocytes. In addition to mediating fast transmission, glutamate can also mediate its aforementioned slower, modulatory effects through a different class of receptors.

Peptides

Peptides are large-molecule chemicals that can function as neurotransmitters or neuromodulators. Most neurons that contain a neuropeptide also contain one of the classic small-molecule transmitters. For example, GABA-ergic striatal neurons that project to the globus pallidus also contain peptides, such as **enkephalin**, **endorphins**, and **substance P**. This suggests that a single synapse can mediate multiple effects. Many of these peptides consist of opioid-like compounds, and their projections are important in pain management.

CLINICAL CORRELATES

Brain Tumors

A **neoplasm** (or tumor) refers to an uncontrolled and unregulated growth of body tissue including glia. Tissue involved with a tumor may retain some of its original functions or may revert to a primitive functional state, depending on the severity of tissue infiltration. The underlying cause may have to do with an improper expression of **oncogenes** (coding proteins involved with cellular growth) and a loss of tumor-suppressor genes. What further adds to the growth of a tumor is **angiogenesis**, the formation of new blood vessels promoting growth in tumorous tissue.

Among the notable characteristics of brain tumors are their locations and rates of growth. A tumor can be **primary** or **metastatic**. Primary tumors arise from glia or meninges within the central nervous system. Metastatic tumors arise elsewhere in the body and spread to the brain from the area outside the brain. Most of the spreading tumors in the brain come from cancer of the breast, lung, colon, or from melanoma (melanin containing dark skin cells). This spread from the remote sources occurs through the lymphatics or blood vessels.

Moreover, tumors in the brain are either **malignant** or **benign**. Most malignant tumors grow fast, invade the surrounding tissue, and are fatal. These tumorous tissues are often multifocal and microscopically undifferentiated from the surrounding healthy tissue, which makes their complete removal difficult (Fig. 5-8). Malignancy is determined by grading a tumor on a scale (I–IV). Tumors with a low grade are benign, and their cells are segregated and are differentiable from the surrounding cells; higher grade tumors are more malignant, and their tissue is undifferentiated from the surrounding areas.

Astrocytomas, ependymoma, and **oligodendrogliomas** are the common malignant tumors of the brain (Table 5-5). Astrocytomas arise from astrocytes. Glioblastoma multiforme, a type of astrocytoma, is the most malignant brain tumor; half of patients die within 18 months. Ependymoma arises from the ependymal cells lining the ventricles and obstructs the ventricular functions. Oligodendrogliomas arise from the oligodendroglia and are often seen in the frontal region of the adult brain.

Benign tumors grow slowly and do not infiltrate. The **meningiomas, acoustic neuromas, vestibular schwannomas**, and **pituitary adenomas** are common benign tumors of the brain. Slow-growing meningiomas arise from the meninges, which are the protective membranes of the brain and spinal cord. Meningiomas may lead to increased intracranial pressure. Adenomas of the pituitary glands can cause hormonal dysfunctions and produce visual symptoms by compression of the **optic chiasm**. Acoustic neuromas and vestibular schwannomas arise from the nerve sheath and are located at the cerebellopontine angle. They contribute to impairments of audition and equilibrium. Due to proximity to the lesion site, facial nerve involvement is commonly seen.

Symptoms of these tumors are related focally to the affected brain area but develop slowly. It is the gradual appearance of the symptoms that differentiates it from stroke, which results in a sudden emergence of symptoms. Tumors that initially involve the silent brain regions become symptomatic in later stages. Besides focal symptoms, common clinical symptoms of a brain tumor include progressive weakness, speech or visual loss, anomia,

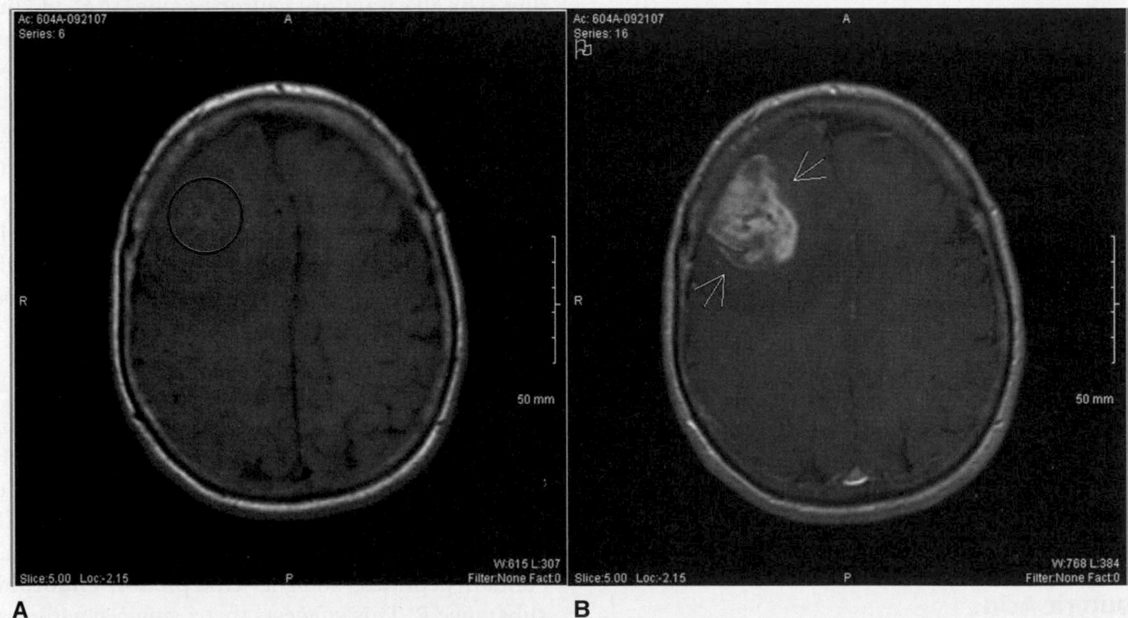

Figure 5-8 Astrocytoma, a high-grade tumor. A grade IV astrocytoma, biopsy-proven glioblastoma multiforme visible on two images; both are T1 MR images, without contrast (A) and with contrast (B).

Table 5-5

Brain Tumor Types

Tumors inside the brain
Astrocytoma Arise from undifferentiated astrocytes. Glioblastoma multiform is the most malignant form of the tumor that grows rapidly and invades extensively and is most frequent in the brains of adults
Oligodendroglioma Arise from the oligodendroglia cells most often in the frontal cortex
Ependymoma Arise from the ventricular lining ependymal cells; the most common form, medulloblastoma, arises in the posterior fossa from the roof of the fourth ventricle
Tumors outside the brain, mostly benign
Meningioma Arise from the meningeal membranes
Acoustic neuroma and vestibular Schwannoma Often located at the cerebellopontine angle, arise from the sheath of the nerve
Pituitary adenoma Most common cause of hormonal and visual deficit, it arises from the pituitary gland

headache, impaired concentration, forgetfulness, and altered personality. The most notable complications of a tumor are seizures and increased intracranial pressure. Increased intracranial pressure, if not treated, can be fatal as it causes midline shift and cortical herniation. Medical treatment of tumors involves surgical excision, radiation therapy (gamma γ-knife), and/or chemotherapy.

DISEASES

Multiple Sclerosis

As an autoimmune central demyelinating disease, multiple sclerosis (M.S.) has been linked to viral infections and abnormalities in the immune system, which reacts improperly to antigens, causing antibodies to attack the body's own myelin at random locations in the central nervous system (Fig. 5-9). Initially, the myelin sheath degenerates, and later on the axon also becomes involved. The initial sparing of axons accounts for the periods of remission (recovery) followed by symptom relapse, which, in the early stages, is seen among 80% of the subjects. Demyelination also promotes glial proliferation, and the broken-up myelin is transported by microglial cells to the regional perivascular spaces. Intense proliferation of glia exceeds the ordinary reparative process; as a result, the glia form dense plaques, or patches, in the white matter of the brain and/or spinal cord. Plaques are a few millimeters to several centimeters in diameter. The demyelination affects the speed of nerve conduction. In advanced cases, the plaques cause secondary degeneration of the axons, which results in weakness, spasticity, and progressive neurological symptoms. Common sites of plaque formation in the brain are the periventricular areas, brainstem, and cerebellar peduncles. Plaque often forms in the optic nerves and optic chasm, as well.

The clinical symptoms vary, depending on the part of the brain being affected. Early symptoms are vision loss, double vision, vertigo, loss of balance, weakness, and numbness in the limbs. The diagnostic triad described by Charcot in 1862 (nystagmus, scanning speech, and intention tremor) is seen in the later stages of illness. Patients with multiple sclerosis are known to exhibit delayed or nonexistent evoked responses to visual, auditory, and somatic stimuli.

The exact antigen responsible for the immune attack seen in M.S. remains unknown. Nonetheless, pathogenesis has implicated **cytokines**, which are proteins that regulate the intensity and duration of an immune response within the plaque. **Tumor necrosis factor α (TNF-α)** has also been associated with inflammation and demyelination; this raises the hope that its inhibition might prevent and/or slow acute demyelination.

Most of the treatment for multiple sclerosis is symptomatic, addressing the inflammatory symptoms. Treatment involves drug use for reducing pain, fatigue, and spasticity. Corticosteroid drugs have been used to alleviate inflammatory symptoms, shorten attacks, and promote remission. Also, **β-interferon and copaxone injections** recently have been used to reduce the frequency and severity of new attacks and slow the progression of the disability by inhibiting the immune processes (Box 5-6).

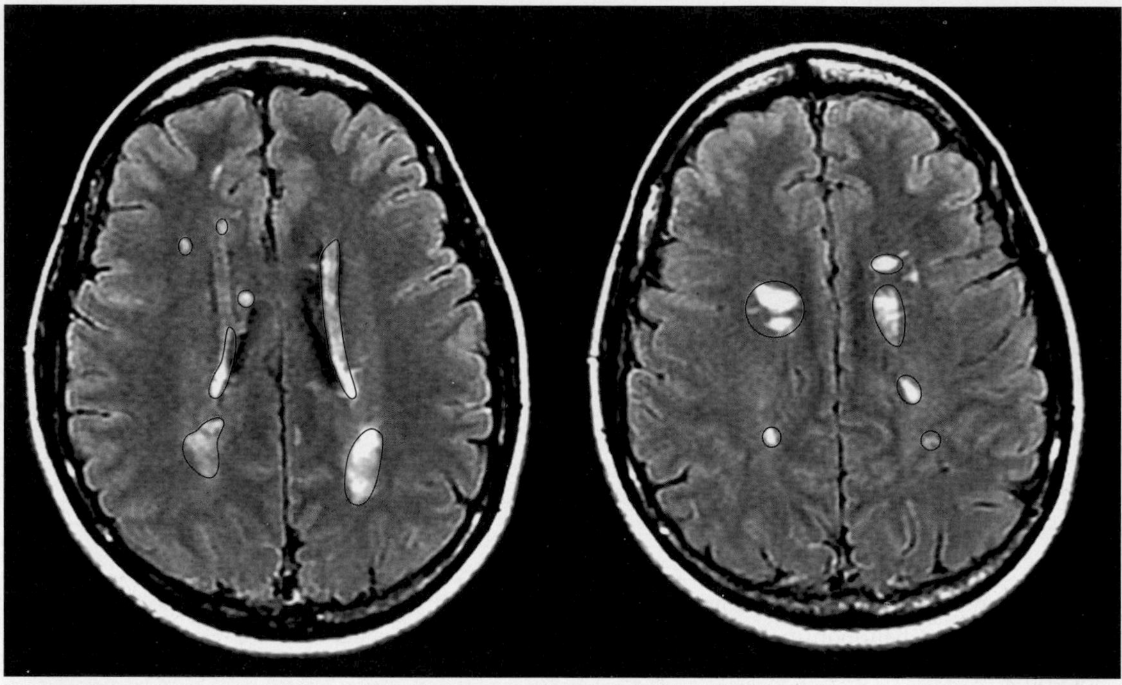

Figure 5-9 Multiple sclerosis. Multiple periventricular and deep white matter foci of abnormal increased signal. Axial FLAIR images show hyperintense lesions perpendicular to the ventricles and within the white matter.

BOX 5-6

Neuronal Transplant

Stem cell research has triggered an immense interest and hope for treating many degenerative and eventually fatal conditions. The basis of this hope is that the embryonic cell can be implanted in the brain to replace the lost neurons and augment the diminished physiologic or chemical activity. Stem cells are best for this replacement because they have not yet been affected by myelin-associated factors and have not grown the axonal process. The success of transplanted embryonic cells is variable, and their promise of clinical application is still being explored. The microenvironment into which the cells are transplanted helps determine the cell's success in surviving and contributes to clinical improvement. In addition, stem cells have the potential to become neuroblasts and thus to evolve into different types of nerve cells.

Stem cells have shown potential for the treatment of Parkinson disease and in the management of spinal cord injuries. In addition, they may offer some hope for Huntington disease and Alzheimer disease. However, their utility in restoring language and higher mental functions in stroke patients remains remote because the higher cortical functions relate to the intracortical connections that are precise, multiple, and have been established with repeated activation. While stem cell replacement holds the key to the future, it has triggered an ethical controversy because many such cells are obtained from human embryos. Research is focusing on alternate sources of stem cells, such as neurons grown in controlled cultures and finding potential cells already in the system. Other cells with potential for growth and multiplication, undifferentiated from stem cells, have been identified in the human olfactory bulb, around the ventricles, in the regions of the hippocampus, bone marrow, as well as adult tissue of any kind. The difference between embryonic and alternate cells is that the numbers of alternate stem cells per unit weight of tissue are smaller and that they have to be grown under different conditions to assume stem cell potential in contrast to embryonic stem cells.

Generally, multiple sclerosis was not considered to be associated with cognitive dysfunction. Recent studies however that have included neuropsychological test batteries have suggested that most patients with chronic multiple sclerosis have significant cognitive impairments.

Guillain–Barré syndrome is also an autoimmune demyelinating syndrome that affects peripheral myelin. It is triggered by an infection which can be with *Campylobacter jejuni*, a food-borne pathogen. This neuropathy affects the nerve conduction by slowing its speed. As a recoverable condition, it is typified with an ascending pattern of sensorimotor deficit that begins with weakness and tingling in toes, fingers, and leg, which spreads to the upper limbs and face along with a loss of deep tendon reflexes. Sensations remain intact. It can be life threatening in case of respiratory or bulbar palsy. For most patients, symptoms can progress up to 4 weeks.

Myasthenia Gravis

Myasthenia gravis is a neuromuscular junction disorder and it is characterized by progressive fatigue and muscle weakness that worsens with exercise and improves with rest. Impaired impulse transmission is caused by an underactivity of acetylcholine secondary to the loss of acetylcholine receptors at the neuromuscular junction. In this autoimmune condition, the antibodies bind with the acetylcholine receptors at motor end plates and prevent the normal effects of acetylcholine. Antibody binding also causes degeneration of the acetylcholine receptors so that lesser receptors remain on the muscle cells. The antibody-producing cells seem to recognize antigens derived from the **thymus**. About 50% of patients with myasthenia gravis have enlarged thymus glands.

Symptoms appear at any age. They are more prevalent in females during the first 30 years of life but, thereafter, are more prevalent in men. Onset is gradual, and muscles may be focally or generally involved. The first signs of the disease often appear in constantly used muscles, such as the muscles of the eye and of respiration. Ptosis and diplopia are the most common early manifestations of the illness. Involvement of the cranial nerves also causes altered facial expression, regurgitation, choking, and hypernasality. Bulbar symptoms in which speech and breathing are involved along with generalized weakness require hospitalization.

Diagnosis is made predominantly based on clinical symptoms, the presence of serum antibodies to the acetylcholine receptor, and electrophysiologic testing. Improvement after testing with an anticholinesterase drug confirms the diagnosis. Drug treatment consists of drugs that inhibit acetylcholinesterase, allowing a higher concentration of the acetylcholine in the synaptic cleft. Overdoses of medication, however, result in cholinergic crises consisting of muscular fasciculation, salivation, and miosis (contraction of the pupil). Myasthenic crisis is treated best by plasmapheresis, steroids, or infusion of immunoglobulins. Prognosis is good for those in whom the disease is not progressive. Long periods of remission do occur, but some patients undergo a progressive course that may result in bulbar and respiratory paralysis.

CASE STUDIES FOR PROBLEM SOLVING

CASE ONE (5-1)

A 60-year-old man presented with the complaint that he was easily tired and needed rest even after a mild exertion. The neurologist who interviewed and examined the patient noted the following:

- A 6-month history of double vision
- Respiratory weakness with shallow breathing and limited vital capacity
- Progressive weakness including slurred speech after a brief period of physical activity
- Near-normal muscular strength after rest
- No cognitive or linguistic deficit except speech intelligibility after exertion
- The neurologist noted that the administration of edrophonium (Tensilon), an acetylcholinesterase inhibitory drug, resulted in improved physical strength of the patient. This led him to suspect a myoneural problem.

Question: How can you relate this motor weakness and speech unintelligibility after sustained physical activity to the suspected diagnosis?

Case (5-1) Discussion: See discussion of case studies

(Continued)

CASE TWO (5-2) *(CONTINUED)*

A 47-year-old woman with a 3-week history of neurological symptoms including double vision, numbness in the left leg, dizziness, and gait imbalance was taken to a hospital where the examining neurologist noted the following:

- A reported history of a 10-day episode of blindness and pain involving the right eye about 2 years ago
- Right optic disc paleness
- Internuclear ophthalmoplegia (failure of adducting eyes in horizontal gaze)
- Decreased pinprick on the left lower abdomen down to the left knee
- Signs of mild cerebellar dysfunction involving the right extremities with gait ataxia
- Mild weakness of the left lower extremity
- A mild form of scanned speech which the patient reported to increase in the afternoon; the articulators looked near normal.
- No sign of impaired cognitive or linguistic functions

Brain MRI revealed multiple white matter hyperintensities (plaques), some perpendicular to the ventricles and one in the brainstem involving inferior cerebellar peduncle.

Question: Can you identify the associated slowly progressive neurological disease?

Case (5-2) Discussion: See discussion of case studies

CASE THREE (5-3)

A 45-year-old woman complained of feeling tired and weak in her legs after short walks or small amount of motor activity. Her speech became unintelligible within a few minutes of talking, and she reported that she regularly cleaned her throat after eating, particularly after a liquid intake. She was seen by a neurologist, who noted the following:

- Minor bilateral ptosis
- Incomplete lateral movement of the right eye (medial strabismus)
- Expressionless and droopy face
- Progressive and fatigable motor weakness
- Progressive speech unintelligibility after continuous speaking
- Signs of swallowing problems

Based on the patient's history, age, and progressive fatigue as well as improvement after an acetylcholinesterase drug, the neurologist suspected that this was a case of an autoimmune disorder, in which the patient's own immune system was attacking the postsynaptic receptor sites at the neuromuscular junction.

Question: This patient is suspected to suffer from which of the following diseases?

a. Graduate school ambition syndrome
b. Myasthenia gravis
c. Multiple sclerosis
d. Huntington chorea
e. Stroke

Case (5-3) Discussion: See discussion of case studies

CASE FOUR (5-4)

A 28-year-old painter began experiencing weakness along with a tingling sensation in both of his lower extremities while climbing a ladder at work in the morning and was sent home to rest. He was immobile by the afternoon as he could not get up and also found it difficult even to sit. By the next morning, he could not raise his arms and was taken to the ER where he reported an episode of respiratory infection about 7 days ago. The examining physical noted the following:

- Weakness involving all four limbs with a greater involvement of the proximal than distal limbs
- Absent deep tendon reflexes
- Near-normal responses to the sensations of pain, touch, and temperature
- Drooling from the both corners of the mouth
- Inability to blow out the cheeks and protrude both lips

An SLP consultation revealed a dysarthric component largely because of imprecise articulation and reduced loudness.

A laboratory work revealed an elevated level of proteins in the CSF.

Looking at the history involving the earlier episode of the infection and the pattern of progressive weakness, the physician suspected this to be a case of postinfectious neopathy by demyelination which predominantly affected the motor functions of the proximal limbs.

Question: Based on your understanding of the neuropathy in this and in Chapter 2, can you relate this to the underlying disease process and explain the criteria for your diagnosis?

Case (5-4) Discussion: See discussion of case studies

SUMMARY

The neuron is the fundamental unit of the nervous system. Its major characteristic is the ability to communicate within the nervous system, with other parts of the body, and with the environment. Neurons in embryogenesis follow a patterned migration and undergo growth of synapse development. A substantial number of neurons, most with incomplete synapses with target neurons, undergo elimination. With billions of multisynaptic connections, the nerve cells serve higher mental functions that include memory, thinking, reasoning, calculation, speech, and language. Neuroglial cells, which support and protect nerve cells, are important in tissue repair and participate in phagocytizing cellular debris. This contributes to natural restitution seen after brain injuries. Nerve cells communicate with one another through nerve impulses that represent all neuronal activity. The nerve impulses have a chemical component that underlies the electric potential of the cells. A neurotransmitter is a chemical substance released at a synapse that transmits signals across neurons. Potential for functional reorganization and potential for progressively connecting axons add to the brain plasticity, which adds to a better natural restitution.

There are two types of transmitters in the nervous system: **small molecules** and **large molecules** (peptides). Small-molecule neurotransmitters include **acetylcholine**, **dopamine**, **norepinephrine**, **serotonin**, **glutamate**, and **GABA**. They are known to have short-lasting effects. Large-molecule peptides produce long-lasting effects on **postsynaptic nerve cells**.

REVIEW QUESTIONS

1. Complete the following statements using the appropriate technical terms:
   A. A cellular depolarization from a resting membrane potential to a less negative state by 10 to 15 mV results in the generation of an ________ ________.
   B. Besides reacting to brain injuries by proliferating in size (________) and numbers (________), the astrocytes also contribute to the________ ________ ________, the first line of defense for the brain from harmful substances.
   C. The ________ cells contribute to the natural recovery process by ingesting and removing the cellular debris.
   D. Two types of degenerative changes follow an axonal sectioning: in________ ________, the retrograde degenerative changes extend to the cell body, while in the ________ ________ degeneration involves the axonal region detached from the cell body.
   E. Acetylcholine, dopamine, norepinephrine, serotonin, glutamate, and γ-aminobutyric acid (GABA) are the ________ ________ neurotransmitters; they are known to have short-lasting effects, in contrast to long-lasting effects on postsynaptic nerve cells by ________ ________ neurotransmitters.
   F. The ________ ________, a multilayered lipid material not only protects the nerve fibers by insulating them but it also regulates the speed of ________ ________
   G. Abnormalities of the cellular cytoskeletal (microtubules, neurofilaments, and microfilaments) structures in the form of tangles and, subsequently, the reduced intracellular protein transfer has been associated with the________ ________.
   H. The ________ are the short cytoplasmic extensions that transmit information to the cell body from other cells via synaptic sites; the ________ are efferent structures that transmit information away from the cell body to other neurons or target organs.
   I. The condition in which antibodies attack the body's own normal tissues is called an ________ ________.
   J. ________ refers to cellular changes marked by swelling, dissolution of cellular organelles (specifically Nissl bodies), and shifting of the nucleus peripherally in soma in response to an injury.
   K. Microphagic cells that ingest cellular debris are called ________.
   L. ________ ________ ________ form myelin around the axons in the peripheral nervous system (PNS).
   M. The point of contact between two neurons is called a________.
2. How does myelin loss in the CNS lead to neurological symptoms?
3. How does the blocking of postsynaptic receptor sites lead to neurological symptoms as seen in myasthenia gravis?
4. Match each of the following functions with its associated glia type.

A. support for primary brain cells	a. astrocytes
B. seal cavity and form scar	b. oligodendrocytes
C. remove the debris by digesting them	c. microglia
D. myelin formation in the CNS	d. Schwann cells
E. contribute to blood–brain barrier	e. glia cells
F. myelin formation in the PNS	

5. Match each of the following neurotransmitters with its associated function.

A. acetylcholine	a. voluntary movements
B. dopamine	b. Parkinson disease
C. norepinephrine	c. sleep, attention, and moods
D. GABA	d. Huntington chorea

6. Name the roles of growth cone and chemical affinity in the synapse development.
7. What is the difference between cellular apoptosis and necrosis?
8. What is the saltatory nerve conduction?
9. List three common malignant types of brain tumors.
10. List four slow-growing tumors of the brain.

6

Diencephalon: Thalamus and Associated Structures

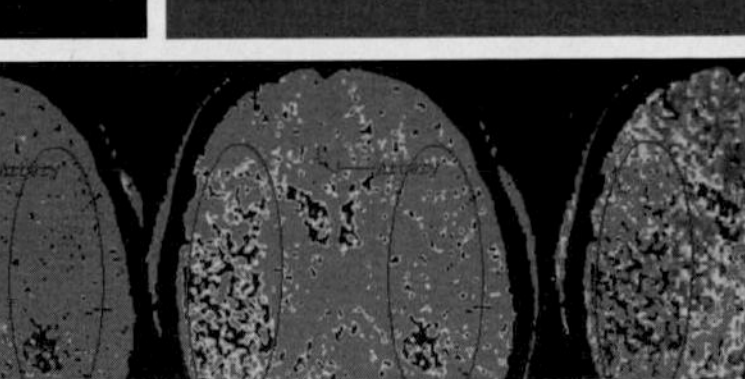

LEARNING OBJECTIVES

After studying this chapter, students should be able to:

- Identify structures of the diencephalon and describe their functions
- Discuss the functional importance of the thalamus
- Identify the locations of major thalamic nuclei and describe their functions
- Describe the sensorimotor and higher mental functions of the thalamic nuclei
- Relate thalamic nuclei to their functional circuits by taking into consideration their afferent and efferent projections
- Discuss sensorimotor and higher mental functions of the thalamus
- Outline thalamic and hypothalamic syndromes

GROSS ANATOMY OF THE DIENCEPHALON

The diencephalon, located beneath the cortex, has well-marked boundaries. Anteroposteriorly, it extends from the interventricular foramen to the posterior commissure. The lateral ventricle and fibers of the corpus callosum form the superior boundary, whereas the third ventricle serves as the medial boundary of the diencephalon. The posterior limb of the internal capsule marks the lateral limit of the diencephalon, while an arbitrary line drawn from the hypothalamic mammillary bodies to the pineal gland forms the ventral limit (Fig. 6-1; see Figs. 2-11 and 2-18). The diencephalon is composed of four parts: thalamus, **epithalamus**, **subthalamus**, and hypothalamus.

Key Terms :

Epithalamus	**Intralaminar nuclei**
Internal medullary lamina	**Subthalamus**

The thalamus serves as a sensorimotor integrator and gateway for information projected to the forebrain. The epithalamus, the oldest part of the diencephalon, includes the habenula and pineal gland; it is concerned with **diurnal** and autonomic bodily functions. The subthalamus, a small region ventral to the thalamus, is important in motor functions through its connections with the brainstem, basal ganglia, and diencephalic structures (see Fig. 3-23). The hypothalamus, located below the thalamus, is part of the **autonomic nervous system** (ANS), which mediates endocrine and other metabolic states, such as body temperature, water balance, and sugar and fat metabolism (see Chapter18). This chapter provides a simplified functional description of the thalamus, focusing on its anatomical circuitry of sensorimotor and cognitive functions.

THALAMUS

The thalamus, an ovoid nuclear mass measuring 3 cm anteroposteriorly and 1.5 cm mediolaterally, lies beneath the cortex in each hemisphere along the midsagittal line. The general location of the thalamus with respect to other surrounding structures can best be seen on horizontal (see Figs. 2-15 and 2-18), coronal (see Fig. 2-19), and midsagittal (Fig. 6-1) sections of the brain. Removal of the overlying lateral ventricles, including the corpus callosum and the cortical mantle, exposes the lateral extent of the dorsal thalamus. The boundaries of the thalamus are identical to those of the diencephalon, except that the ventral limit is marked by the hypothalamic sulcus (Fig. 6-1).

Functionally, the thalamus is an important part of the forebrain neural circuitry, which involves cerebral cortex–basal ganglia and thalamic projections. The reverberating circuits provide means of both retaining information through time and connecting it with the forebrain regions.

Consisting of a collection of subcortical nuclei (Fig. 6-2), the thalamus and its circuit serve three important functions. First, they channel the projections of sensory (pain, taste, temperature, audition, and vision) information entering the lower levels of the nervous system to specific cortical areas. Second, they integrate

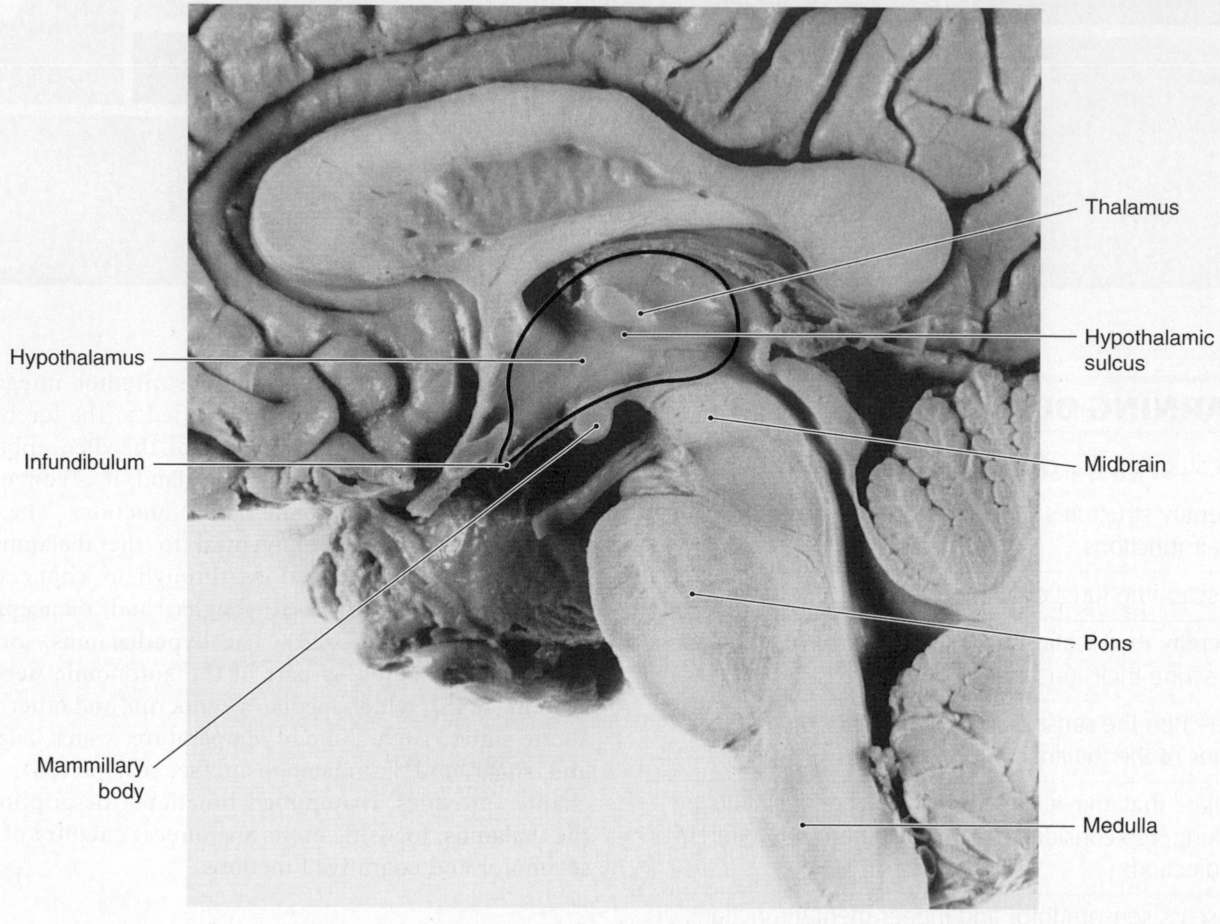

Figure 6-1 An illustration of the boundaries of the diencephalon on a midsagittal section of the brain.

sensorimotor information and project afferents from the basal ganglia, limbic system, and cerebellum to the primary and premotor cortices (see Chapter 15). Third, with the brainstem reticular afferents to multiple targets within the thalamic nuclei, the thalamus and its circuit regulate functions of the associational cortex as well as cortically mediated cognitive functions.

The thalamus is divided into many nuclei; each nucleus has bidirectional fiber connections to specific cortical areas (Fig. 6-2). Some thalamic nuclei are known for their active participation in higher mental functions such as language, speech, and memory, whereas others participate in somatosensory functions alone. Neuropathologic observations and histochemical techniques illustrating retrograde degeneration of the thalamic nuclei have helped researchers develop detailed maps of the nuclei and their projections to the cortex (Figs. 6-3 and 6-4).

Thalamic Structure

The thalamus consists of three tiers of nuclei: medial (mediodorsal), lateral, and ventral (Fig. 6-2). Each tier contains multiple nuclei:

- Medial nuclear complex
  - Dorsomedial (DM) nucleus
  - Midline nuclear complex
- Lateral nuclear complex
  - Lateral dorsal (LD) nucleus
  - Lateral posterior (LP) nucleus
  - Pulvinar
- Ventral nuclear complex
  - Ventral anterior (VA) nucleus
  - Ventrolateral (VL) nucleus
  - Ventral posterior nucleus (lateral and medial)
  - Lateral geniculate body (LGB)
  - Medial geniculate body (MGB)

Additional thalamic nuclei:

- Anterior nucleus (AN)
- Reticular nucleus (RN)
- Intralaminar (centromedian and parafascicular) nuclei

Running anteroposteriorly, the **internal medullary lamina** (a Y-shaped sheath of myelinated fibers) divides the thalamus into mediodorsal and lateral tiers (Figs. 6-1 and 6-2*B*). Rostrally, the two prongs of the internal medullary lamina

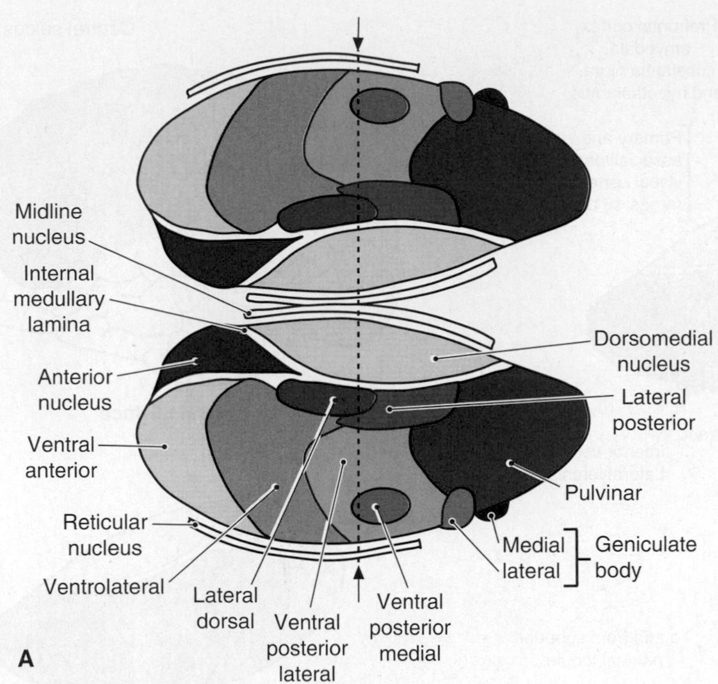

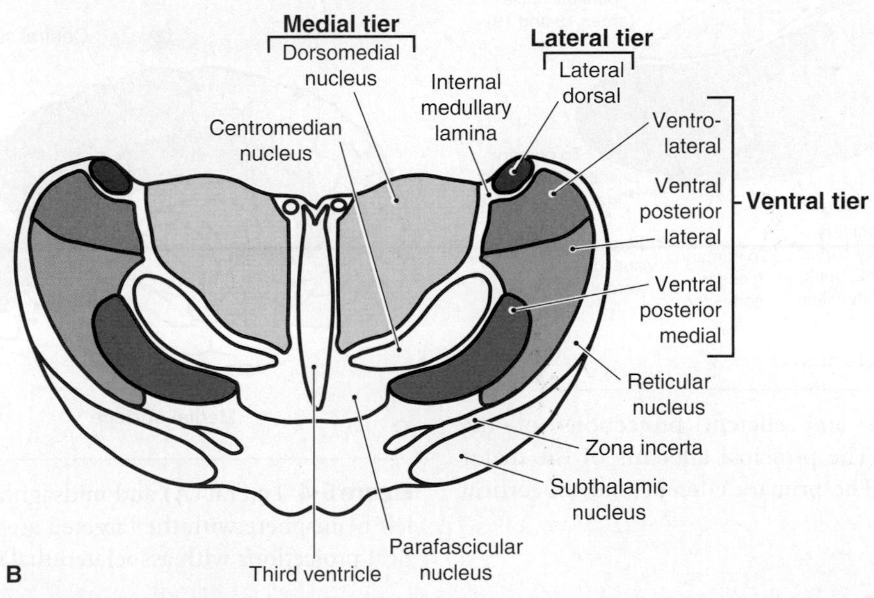

Figure 6-2 Thalamic anatomy. A. Dorsolateral view of the thalamus and its nuclei. B. Cross section of the thalamus with three tiers of nuclei (medial, lateral, and ventral).

surround the **anterior nucleus**; the stem of the internal medullary lamina splits posteriorly and contains the small **intralaminar nuclei**. The ventral tier of the thalamic nuclei is lateral inferior to the lateral tier of the nuclei.

Anatomical Connections and Functions of Thalamic Nuclei

Each thalamic nucleus receives definitive information from thalamic or extrathalamic structures (Fig. 6-3*A*) and screens the information before transmitting it to functionally related areas of the cortex (Figs. 6-3*B* and 6-4; Table 6-1). Familiarity with the afferent and efferent projections is essential for understanding the functional importance of thalamic nuclei in sensorimotor, speech, language, and cognitive functions. These connections also explain the rationale for selecting certain subcortical nuclei in stereotaxic management of intractable pain and movement disorders (see Chapter 15).

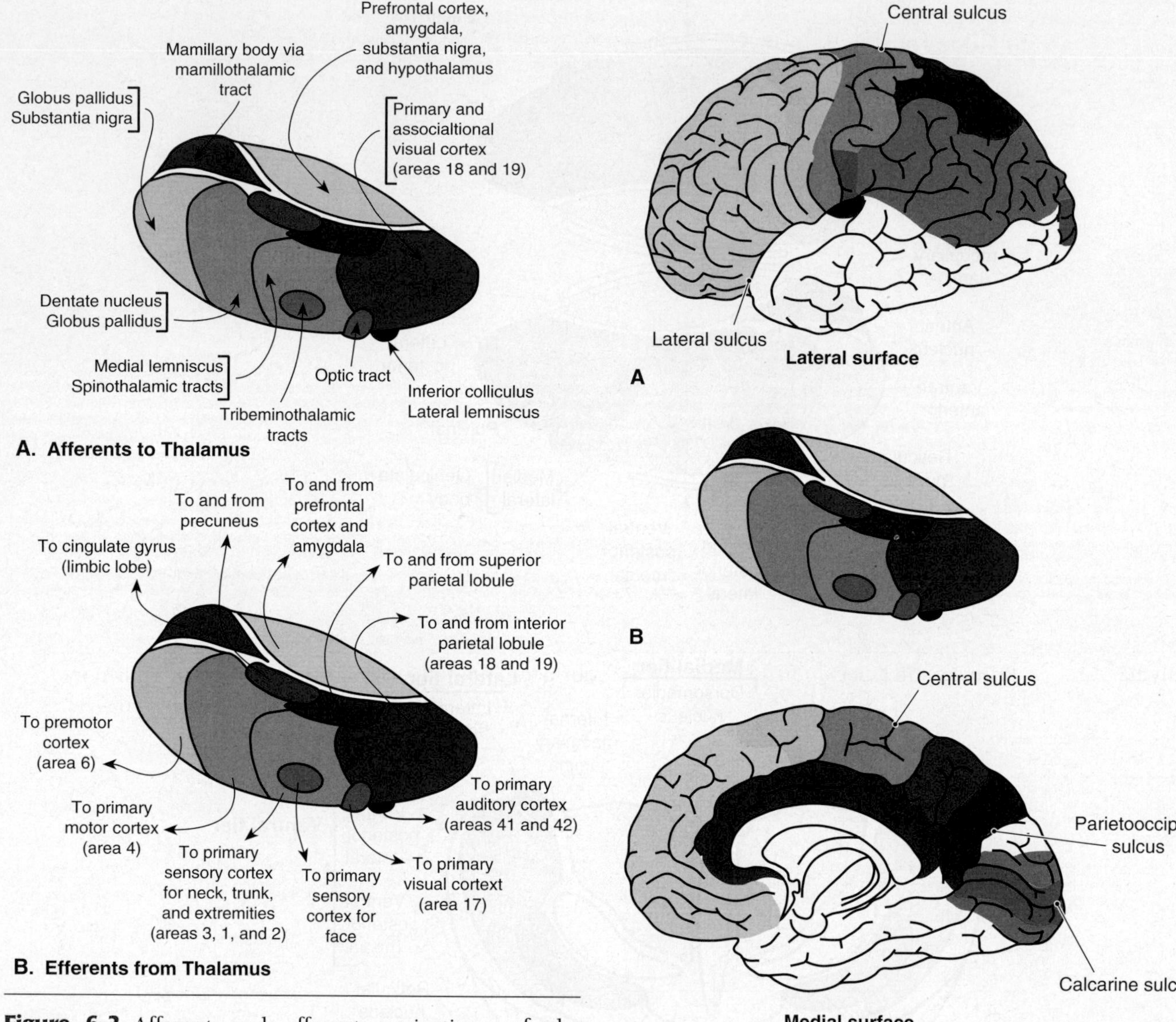

Figure 6-3 Afferent and efferent projections of the thalamic nuclei. A. The principal afferents of the major thalamic nuclei. B. The primary efferent thalamocortical projections.

Figure 6-4 Lateral (A) and midsagittal (C) surfaces of the left hemisphere with the targeted areas of the thalamocortical projections with associated thalamic nuclei (B).

Medial Nuclear Complex

Dorsomedial Nucleus

The DM nucleus occupies the area between the periventricular gray matter of the third ventricle and the internal medullary lamina. The **mammillothalamic tract**, with connections to the structures associated with memory and learning (mammillary bodies and hippocampus), passes beneath this nucleus. The reverberating network of this nucleus is involved with the development of emotion, judgment and reasoning, memory, language, and cognitive functions. The dorsal-level thalamic–cortical networks are also involved in sensory and motor learnings. The afferent and efferent connections are outlined in Table 6-1.

With projections to the prefrontal cortex and limbic structures, the DM nucleus integrates visceral information with affect, emotions, thought processes, personality, and judgment. The DM nucleus may also regulate mood, which can be pleasant, unpleasant, euphoric, or depressive, depending on the nature of the sensory input and stored experiences.

Clinically, the pathology of the DM has resulted in lowering the threshold for rage. Surgical lesions in the DM have been used to ameliorate anxiety-related disorders in humans. Its lesions have also been associated with memory loss in patients with **Wernicke-Korsakoff syndrome**, a personality disorder caused by chronic alcoholism

Table 6-1

Thalamic Nuclei: Afferent and Efferent Projections and Major Functions

Thalamic Nucleus	Afferents From	Efferents To	Major Functions
		Medial nuclear complex	
Dorsomedial nucleus	Prefrontal cortex, substantia nigra, amygdala, and hypothalamus	Prefrontal cortex and amygdala	Integrates visceral information with affect, emotions, thought processes, decision making, and judgment
Midline nuclear complex	Brainstem reticular formation	Cingulate gyrus and hypothalamus	Regulates visceral functions
		Lateral nuclear complex	
Lateral dorsal nucleus	Posterior cingulate gyrus (precuneus)	Precuneus region	May serve visceral–sensory integration
Lateral posterior nucleus	Adjacent thalamic nuclei and superior parietal lobule	Superior parietal lobule	Participates in integrating and transcoding multiple sensory modalities underlying higher mental functions
Pulvinar	Primary and associational visual cortex; inferior parietal lobule	Inferior parietal lobule	Contributes to language functions: formulation, language processing, lexical properties, reading, and writing
		Ventral nuclear complex	
Ventral anterior nucleus	Globus pallidus and substantia nigra	Premotor cortex and primary motor cortex	Facilitates skilled movements; initiates voluntary movements
Ventrolateral nucleus	Dentate nucleus and globus pallidus (basal ganglia)	Primary motor cortex	Coordinates and integrates voluntary motor functions
Ventral posterior nucleus			
Lateral	Medial lemniscus and spinothalamic tracts	Primary sensory cortex: upper two-thirds	Relays somatosensory (protopathic, epicritic) sensation from neck, trunk, and extremities
Medial	Trigeminothalamic tracts	Lower third of the primary sensory cortex	Relays somatosensory (protopathic, epicritic) sensation from face
Lateral geniculate body	Ipsilateral halves of the both retinas via optic tract	Primary visual cortex	Relays visual information from contralateral halves of the visual field
Medial geniculate body	Inferior colliculus and lateral lemniscus	Brodmann areas 41–42; primary and association auditory cortex	Relays auditory information
Anterior nucleus	Mammillary body of hypothalamus via mammillothalamic tract	Cingulate gyrus (limbic lobe)	Mediates visceral and emotional information
Reticular nucleus	Cortex and thalamus	Cortex and other thalamic nuclei	Integrates (presumably) and regulates thalamic neuronal activity
Intralaminar nuclei, centromedian nucleus	Globus pallidus; vestibular nucleus; superior colliculus; brainstem reticular formation; spinal cord (pain and sensory); and motor, premotor, and prefrontal cortices	Basal ganglia and thalamus	Modulates excitability of cortex (related to cognitive functions) and overall function of basal ganglia (related to sensorimotor functions)

characterized by amnesia, disorientation, delirium, confabulations, and hallucinations. Injury to this area may also affect memory with the likely involvement of the underlying fibers of the mammillothalamic tract.

Key Terms :

Dorsomedial nucleus	**Ventral lateral nucleus**
Lateral dorsal nucleus	**Ventral posterior lateral nucleus**
Lateral posterior nucleus	**Ventral posterior medial nucleus**
Mammillothalamic tract	**Wernicke-Korsakoff syndrome**
Pulvinar nucleus	
Reticular nucleus	
Ventral anterior nucleus	

Midline Nuclear Complex

The midline nuclear complex, an important visceral nucleus, is a diffuse and less distinct cluster of nuclei that is located in the periventricular walls of the third ventricle above the hypothalamus. The nuclei are in the region of the massa intermedia fibers and bridge the gray matter across the third ventricle. With afferents from the amygdaloid complex and reticular formation and projections to amygdaloid nucleus and hypothalamus, clinically this nuclear complex is known to serve important visceral and emotional functions.

Lateral Nuclear Complex

The lateral nuclear complex is a narrow cellular strip on the dorsal surface of the thalamus. It consists of three nuclei: the **lateral dorsal nucleus, lateral posterior nucleus**, and **pulvinar nucleus**, arranged in rostrocaudal fashion.

Lateral Dorsal Nucleus

The functions and connections of the LD nucleus are poorly understood. Located immediately caudal to the anterior nucleus, it has reciprocal connections with the precuneus gyrus in the medial parietal lobe (see Fig. 2-10). It also receives afferents from the pretectal region in the midbrain. Clinically the LD nucleus contributes to visceral–sensory integration that is needed for any behavioral responses.

Lateral Posterior Nucleus

Located caudal to the LD nucleus, the LP is another nucleus not well understood for its functions. With its reciprocal connections to the superior parietal lobule, a sensory integrative area, this nucleus is likely involved with the information integration involving multiple modalities including vision, tactile, and audition, prior to formulating any behavioral response.

Pulvinar Nucleus

The pulvinar, the largest and most posterior portion of the thalamic nucleus, lies caudally in the lateral division. It is considered to have a role in higher mental functions, with major afferents from the primary and associational visual cortices, and from the visual–motor integrating area of the superior colliculus, and with projections to the inferior association cortex of the parietal lobule with angular and supramarginal gyri.

Clinically, the pulvinar has been associated with the regulation of mental functions, including language formulation, lexical storage and processing, reading, and writing. The association of some of these linguistic functions with the pulvinar has been identified by stereotaxic exploration of the subcortex (Ojemann et al., 1968).

Ventral Nuclear Complex

The ventral nuclear complex relays information from sensory surfaces to the sensory cortex and provides feedback from the motor system effectors (muscles and joints) to the primary and secondary motor cortices. This neuronal circuitry is continuously involved in sustained cortical activity related to sensation and precise motor control.

Ventral Anterior Nucleus

The VA nucleus lies in the most rostral area of the ventral nuclear complex. With afferents from the globus pallidus of the basal ganglia (see Chapter 15) and substantia nigra and projections to the premotor cortex, this nucleus has a definitive role in the execution and planning of skilled and sequential movements.

Ventrolateral Nucleus

The VL is another important nucleus in the regulation of volitional movements. Both the afferents from the contralateral cerebellar hemisphere (via the superior cerebellar peduncle and inner segment of the globus pallidus) and the efferents to the primary motor cortex underlie the VL's role in regulating cortically generated movements.

This nucleus is important in coordinating different aspects of motor functions because it integrates input from the basal ganglia (caudate nucleus, putamen, and globus pallidus) with feedback from the cerebellum before projecting the integrated information to the primary motor cortex. Clinically, a disruption of its neuronal circuitry results in abnormal (involuntary) movements. This nucleus, because of its role in relating the basal ganglia to the motor cortex, has consistently been targeted for stereotaxic management of movement disorders.

Ventral Posterior Nucleus

Consisting of two subnuclei (lateral and medial), the **ventral posterior nucleus** serves as a thalamic relay center for somatosensation (pain, temperature, and discriminative touch) from the body and face (see Chapter 11).

Ventral Posterior Lateral Nucleus

The **VPL nucleus** relays information related to somatic (pain, touch, and temperature) sensation from the body.

With afferents from the body via the ventral and lateral spinothalamic tracts and the medial lemniscus, and efferents to the dorsal two-thirds of the primary somesthetic cortex in the postcentral gyrus (Brodmann areas 3, 1, 2), this nucleus is uniquely situated to modulate somatic sensation.

Ventral Posterior Medial Nucleus

The **VPM nucleus** serves as the thalamic sensory relay center for the sensations of taste, pain, temperature, and discriminative touch for the head and face. With afferents from the secondary fibers of the trigeminal (CN V) nerve and efferents to the lower third of the primary somesthetic cortex, the VPM is important in facial sensation, where sensory information reaches consciousness and is analyzed.

The projection fibers from the ventral nuclear complex travel through the internal capsule and extend to the primary somesthetic cortex in the parietal lobe (Brodmann areas 3,1,2). Even though cortical participation is necessary for the refinement of these sensations and for their interpretation in the context of previous experiences, some awareness of pain, temperature, and discriminative touch sensations has been demonstrated at the thalamic level.

Lateral Geniculate Body

Located beneath the pulvinar, the **LGB** serves as the thalamic relay center for the sensation of vision. With afferents from the ipsilateral halves of both retinas/eyes (representing contralateral halves of the visual fields) and efferents to the primary visual cortex (Brodmann area 17; see Chapter 8), the LGB mediates in transmission and integration of the visual information. Clinically, pathology of the LGB and/or its projections results in the loss of vision in contralateral halves of the visual fields, also called homonymous hemianopsia (see Chapter 12).

Medial Geniculate Body

The **MGB** is the circular area adjacent to the LGB beneath the pulvinar; it is the primary relay center for auditory information. With afferent fibers from the organ of Corti in both ears via the fibers of the lateral lemniscus and brachium of the inferior colliculus, it projects to the primary auditory cortex (Brodman areas 41–42). The fibers leaving the MGB constitute auditory radiations (**geniculo-Heschl fibers**) traveling through the internal capsule before terminating in the primary auditory cortex on the superior surface of the lateral fissure, the transverse gyri of Heschl. Clinically, a pathology of the MGB and/or its efferents affect verbal processing and the ability to discriminate speech sounds in addition to a minimum attenuation of hearing sensitivity in both ears.

Additional Nuclei in the Thalamus

Anterior Nucleus

The anterior nucleus (AN) protrudes as an anterior tubercle in the floor of the lateral ventricle and is surrounded by the forks of the internal medullary lamina. The AN is functionally related to the limbic brain (hippocampus, cingulate gyrus, and hypothalamus) and, in part, contributes to digestive, respiratory, urogenital, emotional, and endocrine functions. With afferents from the ipsilateral and contralateral mammillary bodies of the hypothalamus through the mammillothalamic tract (with input from reticular formation, hippocampus, and septum pellucidum), the AN projects to the cingulate gyrus, an important structure in the limbic circuitry.

Besides mediating visceral and emotional information, clinically the AN also regulates the hypothalamic and limbic influence on the neocortex. Mammillary (hypothalamic) afferents to the AN also imply its role in memory function, because the degeneration of the mammillary bodies is usually noted in alcoholics as part of Wernicke-Korsakoff syndrome. Electrical stimulation and ablation of the nucleus induce changes in blood pressure, anxiety levels, and emotional drive.

Reticular Nucleus

The **reticular nucleus (RN)** consists of a thin layer of nerve cells that covers the entire lateral thalamus. These scattered nuclei of the RN receive input from virtually all ascending systems as well as from other thalamic nuclei. With collateral afferents from thalamocortical and corticothalamic projections, it sends projections diffusely to the brain. Functionally, this nucleus is thought to regulate thalamic neuronal activity participation, which influences cortical functions by inhibiting or facilitating the thalamocortical relay.

Key Terms:

Habenular nucleus	**Prerubal area**
Intralaminar nuclear complex	**Tuber cinereum**
Parafascicular nucleus	**Zona incerta**

Intralaminar Nuclei

The **intralaminar nuclear complex** consists of several nuclei interspersed in the core of the internal medullary lamina (Fig. 6-2). The centromedian nucleus and **parafascicular nucleus**, two important intralaminar nuclei, indirectly contribute to the diffuse reticular–brain activation system.

- **Afferent connection:** The intralaminar complex receives afferents from the globus pallidus, vestibular nucleus, superior colliculus, and most importantly the brainstem reticular formation. The centromedian and parafascicular nuclei also receive cortical afferents from the motor, premotor, and prefrontal cortical areas. The rostral intralaminar complex receives input from the brainstem reticular formation and pain and other sensory inputs from the spinal cord.
- **Efferent projection:** The intralaminar nuclei predominantly project to the basal ganglia (putamen and caudate) and sparsely to the entire cerebral cortex.

The intralaminar system as a whole influences the excitability of the association cortex with both its intrathalamic projections and striatal collaterals to the cortex. With its afferent and efferent connectivity, the intralaminar system is in a prime position to modulate the excitability and overall function of both the cortex and basal ganglia related to cognitive and sensorimotor functions. Intralaminar nuclei, in particular the centromedian, are also known to evoke a cortical recruiting response when directly stimulated with electrical impulses (Bhatnagar and Buckingham, 2010; Bhatnagar and Mandybur, 2005; Bhatnagar et al., 1989, 1990a). The stimulation of the centromedian nucleus has been noted to have positively affected human performance in many cortically mediated higher mental functions involving the frontal, parietal, cingulate, and orbital areas of the association cortex (Bhatnagar et al., 1989, 1990a,b).

EPITHALAMUS

The epithalamus consists of two small structures: **habenular nucleus** and pineal gland (see Figs. 2-12 and 2-18). The cone-shaped pineal gland, an endocrine structure, renders an inhibitory influence over gonadal (sex gland) functions. It also secretes melatonin in response to the day–night cycle (as sensed by the visual system), regulates diurnal rhythms of the brain, and controls endocrinic activity related to the sleep cycle. Located lateral to the pineal gland, the habenular nuclei—with afferent and efferent projections to the anterior hypothalamus, limbic lobe, orbital cortex, and brainstem reticular formation—serve autonomic functions, such as emotional experiences and drives, and possibly the sense of smell.

SUBTHALAMUS

Subthalamic structures, although anatomically included in the diencephalon, are functionally related to the basal ganglia and are discussed in Chapter 15 (see Figs. 15-3, 15-6, and 3-23). The subthalamus refers collectively to several nuclei between the thalamus and the midbrain. The subthalamus includes primarily the subthalamic nucleus and secondarily the **prerubral** (fields of Forel, or H fields) **area** and **zona incerta**.

The subthalamic nucleus is connected to the globus pallidus via bidirectional fibers and it makes substantial contributions to motor functions. A lesion in this nucleus results in contralateral hemiballism, a motor disorder characterized by sudden involuntary movements that emerge with force and rapidity; these movements persist during wakefulness but disappear during sleep (see Chapter 15).

The fields of Forel are the regions through which various motor fibers pass before terminating in the thalamus (see Fig. 15-5). The zona incerta, a thin area of gray mater, lies in the subthalamus between the thalamic and the lenticular fasciculi. With afferents from the motor cortex and cerebellum, it serves as a visuomotor coordinator by projecting to the superior colliculus and pretectal area.

HYPOTHALAMUS

The hypothalamus contains important nuclei and a tract that forms the crossroads among the limbic system, brainstem, and thalamus. Located below the thalamus (Fig. 6-1; also see Figs. 2-11, 2-12), it forms the VL walls of the third ventricle. It also includes many specific nuclei and several structures, such as the optic chiasm, mammillary bodies, hypophysis (pituitary gland), infundibular stem (pituitary stalk), and **tuber cinereum** (see Chapter 18). The hypothalamus is a functionally unique organ because its afferents and efferents involve two modes of communication: neural and hormonal. Using the neural impulses, the hypothalamus connects with the brain and spinal structures; the hormonal efferents, mostly regulated by the pituitary gland, allow the hypothalamus to communicate with the body by releasing selected proteins into the blood circulation. The released proteins influence various body activities (see Chapter 18).

Closely connected with the forebrain and the limbic system, the hypothalamus serves three partly overlapping functions. First, it is the controlling center for the ANS. Second, it is the regulating center of the endocrinic activities, by means of neurosecretions (through neurophysis) that control important metabolic activities of the body and provide homeostasis (constant internal environment necessary for reproduction). Third, it controls body temperature, water and food intake, sugar metabolism, sexual behavior, and emotional states (e.g., feelings of well-being, anger, and aggression). Lesions involving the hypothalamus and /or its projections result in a variety of autonomic and hormonal disturbances. It additionally results in diabetes insipidus, which is characterized by increased urinary output and excessive thirst, disturbances of temperature control and food and water intake, and hormonal abnormalities.

COGNITIVE FUNCTIONS OF THE THALAMUS

The belief that the thalamus plays only a precognitive sensorimotor role is no longer accepted. In the past 40 years, evidence from neurolinguistic and neurosurgical research has shown that some language and speech functions, along with cognitive processes, are asymmetrically lateralized at the thalamic level. In addition, a less discussed fact is that the thalamus with afferents from the brainstem reticular formation mediates overall cortical alertness, information flow, and tuning of cortical structures. The thalamus, in conjunction with adjacent basal ganglia structures, participates in sensorimotor processes that underlie speech and language processing.

Penfield and Roberts (1959) first proposed that the thalamus, with its extensive projections, has an integrative role in speech and language functions. More recently, radiographic images have helped identify many cases of spontaneous thalamic lesions with subsequent speech–language disturbances. Using evidence from patients with hemorrhage in the dominant thalamus, researchers have found persisting aphasic symptoms, such as verbal paraphasia, anomia, and jargon, with otherwise intact comprehension and repetition. Evidence supporting thalamic participation in language function has also come from intraoperative language and speech testing by the focal stimulation of the thalamic nuclei, which was used for functional mapping during stereotactic operations. Stereotactic destructive lesions in the VL nucleus and pulvinar of the thalamus for the treatment of dyskinetic behavior further support the belief that there are language-specific functions in the left dominant thalamus (Ojemann, 1983). Evaluation of language function in patients with lesions in the left VL thalamic nucleus and the pulvinar revealed transient and lasting aphasia, including naming disturbances, speech-related disorders, and reduced word fluency.

Thalamic stimulation has been found to facilitate verbal recall (Bhatnagar and Andy, 1989; Bhatnagar and Mandybur, 2005; Bhatnagar et al., 1989, 1990a,b; Ojemann, 1978). Facilitatory effects have been noted on verbal memory, lexical retrieval, and nonverbal functions from stimulation of the left centromedianus, a neurolinguistically unexplored and previously unimplicated intralaminar thalamic nucleus. Some facilitatory effects on verbal memory were also found after stimulation of the right centromedian nucleus, but they were not as dramatic as the ones observed from the stimulation of the left centromedianus (Bhatnagar et al., 1990a).

In at least one case, the mechanical intraoperative perturbation of the left thalamus, preparatory to a therapeutic lesion placed for chronic pain, resulted in the elicitation of stutter-like syllabic reiterations (Andy and Bhatnagar, 1991). It is interesting that stimulation in the same area of the intralaminar thalamic nuclei in neurosurgical patients also led to amelioration of the acquired stuttering (Andy and Bhatnagar, 1992; Bhatnagar and Buckingham, 2010). This thalamic influence on cortically mediated higher mental functions has been judged to be a facilitatory one.

CLINICAL CORRELATES

Thalamic Syndrome

Although the most discriminating analysis of somatosensory information and its integration with tactile, visual, and auditory information occurs in the sensory cortex at the parietal lobe, crude sensations of pain, touch, temperature, vibration, and taste can be appreciated at the thalamic level.

Thalamic syndrome (depending on the location and extent of the lesion) represents a disorder of somatosensory functions. It is characterized by increased or decreased thresholds for the sensations of touch, pain, and temperature on the contralateral half of the body. Thalamic pathologies may alter the perception of somatic sensation for some patients, so that a contact with a wisp of cotton can be quite painful. In other cases, the threshold to pain is high; but once that threshold is reached, the sensation is exaggerated and more painful than normal. For example, a pinprick may provoke a burning sensation of pain, and pleasant musical tones may sound like uncomfortable discord. Spontaneous pain sensation can also emerge from a thalamic lesion. This pain is usually poorly localized and intractable to analgesic agents. There are also cases of reported sensation of paresthesia (ants crawling on the skin). A large and diffuse thalamic lesion can cause emotional instability, which is marked by spontaneous and uncontrollable laughing and crying responses; this most commonly results from the occlusion of the thalamogeniculate branch of the **posterior cerebral artery**.

Linguistically impaired motor speech (dysarthria), anomia, and a variable degree of reading and writing disorders have been observed to occur after thalamic lesions (Alexander, 1989).

CASE STUDIES FOR PROBLEM SOLVING

CASE ONE (6-1)

A 45-year-old man fell while taking a shower and was found by his wife lying on the floor, fully conscious. Realizing that something was not right, she advised him to take a rest. Within a few hours, his speech became unintelligible and he told his wife about the pain and weakness he experienced in his right arm. At this point, the wife drove him to the hospital emergency room, where the attending physician noted the following signs:

- Paresis in the right arm
- Severe pain in the right shoulder and arm
- Sensation of paresthesia (burning and pricking) in the right arm
- Lowered pain threshold (a slight touch caused sharp pain sensation)
- Speech unintelligibility because of dysphonia and imprecise articulation
- Some emotional instability marked by frequent bursts of crying and panic
- Some word-finding deficit
- Excellent comprehension for written and spoken language

The presence of sensorimotor impairments without any sign of aphasia (except a mild anomia) led the physician to suspect a subcortical lesion. The brain MRI study revealed a left diencephalic cerebrovascular accident involving a part of the adjacent internal capsule.

Question: How can you relate these symptoms with the observed pathology?

Case (6-1) Discussion: See discussion of case studies.

CASE TWO (6-2)

A 55-year-old female truck driver began experiencing difficulty seeing while driving particularly on the left side. She made an appointment with a neurologist, who noted the following:

- Left homonymous hemianopia, manifested as loss of vision in contralateral left fields for both eyes
- Definitive difficulty in understanding spoken language
- Noticeable confusion in identifying the directions of sound sources
- Increased confusion in focusing on the physician when there were noises outside the room and when an announcement came on the intercom system
- Normal pure tone threshold on audiometric testing
- Normal visual acuity
- No sign of speech, language, or cognitive disorder on a speech-language pathology (SLP) assessment

The brain MRI study revealed a small infarct involving the lateral posterior inferior area of the right thalamus.

Question: What thalamic nuclei are in the posterior ventral region of the thalamus? How can you relate these selective visual and auditory symptoms with this involved thalamic region?

Case (6-2) Discussion: See discussion of case studies.

CASE THREE (6-3)

A 55-year-old man presented with slurred and slowly articulated speech with the sensation of numbness but no pain in his mouth. There was no other symptom present. There was no limb weakness, aphasia, or any sign of reduced cognitive functioning. The brain MRI study revealed a small infarct in the caudal region of the ventral posterior nucleus in the left thalamus.

Question: Of the following thalamic nuclei that mediate somatosensation from the face, which is likely to be involved?

- Ventral lateral
- Ventral anterior
- Ventral posterior lateral
- Ventral posterior medial
- Dorsal lateral

Case (6-3) Discussion: See discussion of case studies.

CASE FOUR (6-4)

A 70-year-old patient with Parkinson disease, with a deep brain stimulator implanted in the left subthalamic nucleus, was seen by an SLP for the assessment of his speech unintelligibility. The goal of the implant was to modulate the thalamic (ventral lateral) projections to the motor cortex so that tremor and rigidity would no longer be disabling to the patient.

Question: Which of the cortical areas, exclusively receiving afferents from the VL, was likely to be affected?

- Brodmann area 4
- Brodmann area 17
- Brodmann areas 9–10
- Brodmann areas 41–42
- Brodmann areas 3, 1, 2

Case (6-4) Discussion: See discussion of case studies.

SUMMARY

The diencephalon consists of four major structures: thalamus, subthalamus, epithalamus, and hypothalamus. The thalamus, the largest and the most prominent diencephalic nucleus, serves as the sensorimotor relay center to screen all sensory and motor information before channeling it to the cerebral cortex. The thalamus is divided into many functionally specific nuclei, and each of these nuclei makes direct anatomic projections to corresponding functional areas of the neocortex. The subthalamus is important in the organization of motor functions and is functionally related to the basal ganglia. The epithalamus, the oldest part of the diencephalon, consists of the habenular nucleus and pineal gland. The pineal gland, an endocrine organ, mediates its influence on sex glands and diurnal rhythm. The hypothalamus is a major diencephalic structure for controlling activities of the autonomic and endocrine systems.

REVIEW QUESTIONS

1. Complete the following statements using the appropriate technical terms:
   A. The ________ is composed of four parts: thalamus, epithalamus, subthalamus, and hypothalamus.
   B. As a sensorimotor integrator, the ________ is the gateway for projecting sensorimotor information to the ________.
   C. As the regulator of the autonomic nervous system, the ________ also mediates endocrine functions, fat metabolism, and the metabolic states including the functions like body temperature, water balance, and sugar presence in the blood.
   D. With projections to the prefrontal cortex and limbic structures, the ________ nucleus of the thalamus is known to integrate visceral information with affect, emotions, thought processes, personality, and judgment.
   E. Caused by chronic alcoholism, ________ syndrome is characterized by amnesia, disorientation, delirium, confabulations, and hallucinations.
   F. In ________, a commonly seen symptom after thalamic lesion, patients become hypersensitive to the sensations of touch, pain, and temperature on the contralateral half of the body.
2. Name the thalamic nuclei that are marked with letters in the figure (Exercise Fig. 6-1 given below):

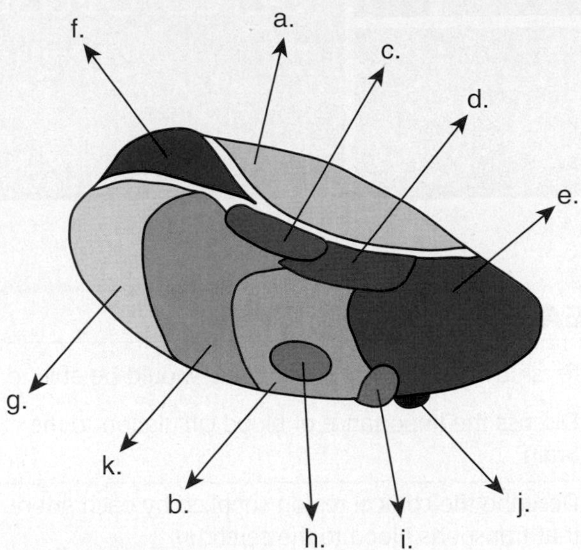

3. Match each of the following thalamic nuclei with its associated area of projection in the brain.

A. ventral lateral	a. transverse gyri of Heschl
B. ventral anterior	b. premotor cortex
C. pulvinar	c. cingulate gyrus
D. dorsal medial	d. prefrontal cortex
E. anterior nucleus	e. inferior parietal lobule
F. lateral geniculate	f. calcarine cortex
G. medial geniculate	g. precentral gyrus

4. List three characteristics of the thalamic syndrome:
5. List three symptoms of the hypothalamic syndrome:
6. What thalamic structures and pathway are affected in Wernicke-Korsakoff syndrome?
7. Which thalamic nucleus mediates afferents from the medial lemniscus to the cerebral cortex?
8. Which thalamic nucleus is dedicated to mediating trigeminal projections to the cerebral cortex?
9. A patient presenting with altered (increased or decreased) thresholds for the sensations of touch, pain, and temperature on the contralateral half of the body is likely to have what syndrome?
10. What thalamic nucleus is reciprocally connected with the language cortex in the inferior parietal lobule?

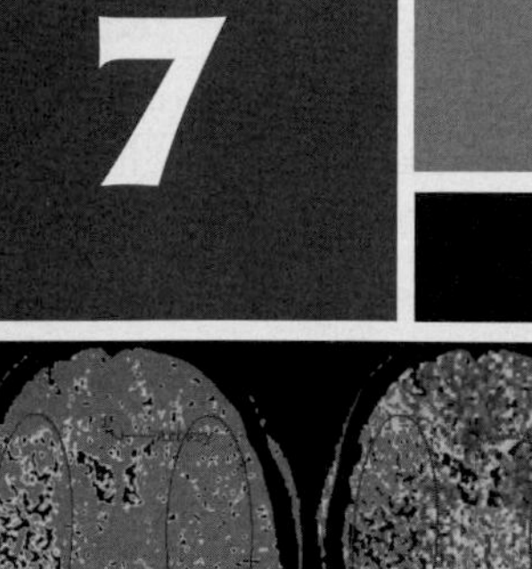

7 Cerebrovascular System

LEARNING OBJECTIVES

After studying this chapter, students should be able to:

- Discuss the importance of blood circulation to the brain
- Describe the cortical region supplied by each artery that transports blood to the cerebrum
- Be familiar with the blood supply to the subcortical structures and brainstem
- Outline clinical symptoms associated with involvement of major arteries
- Explain the significance of potential collateral circulation
- Describe the venous–sinus system
- Explain common types of cerebrovascular accidents (CVAs) and associated risk factors
- Describe the physiology of CVAs
- Appreciate the concept and clinical significance of the blood–brain barrier

Blood supplies brain cells with needed nutrition, such as glucose and oxygen, and it also removes the metabolic waste, carbon dioxide, from nerve cells. Nerve cells depend on an uninterrupted supply of oxygenated blood. They cannot use any other source of energy, and they do not have the mechanism for storing this glucose and oxygen energy source; therefore, the effects of **ischemia** on brain cells are rapid and functionally disabling.

Although its mass comprises only 2% of body weight, the brain consumes approximately 20% of the total cardiac output and uses more than 20% of oxygen and metabolized glucose. An average of 750 mL of blood is pumped to the brain per minute, which ensures an optimal level of blood flow to approximately 50 to 60 mL per 100 g tissue per minute to the brain. This blood flow volume is needed for the optimal functioning of the cells in the brain. A reduction in the blood flow volume, particularly below 20 mL/100 g/min, has clinical implications that range from impaired cellular functioning to electrical silence and, finally, to irreversible damage to cells in the brain. After perfusion in the brain, the circulated blood is drained through the veins and sinuses back to the heart and pumped through the lungs for the reoxygenation of hemoglobins.

Without adequate blood supply, the brain can function for only a short time before the cell bodies are damaged irreversibly. Vascular interruption for 4 to 6 minutes results in irreversible brain damage affecting the cells in the center of the infarct, called the "core." The area surrounding the "core" infarct is called the "**ischemic penumbra**," which contains "idle" neurons; the idle cells may survive about 20 minutes in the absence of collateral circulation, and up to 6 to 8 hours if there is some degree of collateral supply, which is the most common vascular arrangement (Box 7-1).

Key Terms:

Arteriole	**Core nuclei**
Artery	**Ischemic penumbra**
Basilar artery	**Vein**
Capillary	**Venules**
Circle of Willis	**Vertebrobasilar system**
Carotid system	

VASCULAR NETWORK

Blood circulation to the brain depends on an elaborate network of **arteries**. Arteries carry oxygenated blood to the brain and **veins** return the deoxygenated and circulated blood back to the heart. Large arteries divide into **arterioles** that deliver blood to the **capillaries**, the terminal extensions of the arterial network. Unlike large arteries, capillaries do not permit rapid flow of blood. This slow blood circulation at the capillary level allows blood and brain cells to exchange nutritive substances. Capillaries also connect the arterioles with **venules**, the smaller extensions of the **venous system** deep in the cortical substance. The

BOX 7-1

Cellular Sensitivity to Anoxia

Without adequate blood supply, the brain can function for only a short time before causing irreversible damage to its cell bodies. The conventional understanding is that approximately 5 to 8 seconds of circulatory interruption to the brain may results in loss of consciousness, and vascular deprivation sustained for 20 to 25 seconds eliminates the electrical activities in the affected brain cells. Vascular interruption for 4 to 6 minutes results in irreversible brain damage. This rule of anoxia applies only to the cells in the center of the infarct, called the "core." Not all affected brain cells die immediately after stroke. The area surrounding the "core" infarct is called the "ischemic penumbra," and contains "idle" neurons; these cells may be electrically silent but metabolically active to sustain membrane potentials. The "idle" neurons may survive about 20 minutes in the absence of any collateral circulation and up to 6 to 8 hours (with 2–4 being the most critical window) if some degree of collateral vascularization becomes operational. The revascularization is the most common poststroke vascular arrangement. The time period immediately after the stroke is of immense therapeutic value. Revascularization in this restricted period minimizes the functional loss. Recognition of the value of this time period has led to the development of many reperfusion interventions, such as tPA and clot retrieval through the Mercy device. These techniques have targeted the "idle" cells, which are located within the "ischemic penumbra."

The reperfusion failure in the critical window of the first 4 hours has a variable effect for the cells at different sites in the brain as these have a variable sensitivity to anoxia. Generally the brain cells, which are active at all times, are the most susceptible to anoxia. This accounts for the high vulnerability of cells in the cerebral cortex, cerebellum (Purkinje cells), and hippocampus. The cells in the brainstem and spinal cord can sustain oxygen deprivation for a longer period.

venules receive the deoxygenated blood from the capillaries and transport it to larger veins on the cortical surface that, in turn, empty blood into the sinuses, which transport it back to the heart for reoxygenation. Since they do not have smooth muscles, veins are thinner than arteries. Consequently, average blood pressure (BP) is considerably lower in veins than in arteries; this is one reason why more strokes occur in arteries than in veins.

Cerebrovascular Supply

The brain receives its blood supply from two arterial systems: the **carotid** and the **vertebral basilar**. These two arterial channels join in the **circle of Willis** at the base of the brain (Figs. 7-1 and 7-2). Cortical and subcortical (penetrating) arteries that originate from the circle of Willis supply blood to the external and internal structures of the forebrain.

Carotid System

The carotid system begins with the **common carotid artery**, which ascends on each side of the neck. Posterior to the jaw, the common carotid artery divides into the **external carotid** and **internal carotid** (Fig. 7-1A). The external carotid artery and its branches supply blood to the facial muscles and forehead as well as to the oral, nasal, and orbital cavities. The internal carotid artery, a major source of blood to the brain, enters the cranium through the **carotid foramen** in the **petrous bone** and curves forward and medially to enter the **cavernous sinus**. At this point, two important arteries branch off the internal carotid: the **anterior choroidal** and **ophthalmic**. The ophthalmic artery supplies blood to the eyeball and ocular muscles. Its branches connect with branches of the external cerebral artery and form the basis for a potential **collateral circulation** (see discussion under *Collateral Circulation*).

The internal carotid artery emerges from the cavernous sinus, joins the circle of Willis, and divides to form two cortical arteries, the **anterior cerebral artery** (ACA) and **middle cerebral artery** (MCA).

Vertebral Basilar System

Arising from the **subclavian arteries**, two **vertebral arteries** ascend through the bony foramen of the upper cervical vertebrae. They enter the posterior cranial fossa of the skull through the **foramen magnum** and continue along the ventrolateral surface of the medulla oblongata (see Fig. 2-31). At the level of the caudal pons, both vertebral arteries merge to form a single **basilar artery** that courses upward along the pontine midline, eventually joining the circle of Willis (Figs. 7-1 and 7-2).

Before terminating in the circle of Willis, the vertebral basilar arteries give rise to numerous branches that supply blood to the spinal cord, medulla, pons, midbrain, and cerebellum (Tables 7-1 and 7-2). A familiarity with the vascular distribution of the brainstem is important, as the brainstem houses cranial nerve nuclei, sensorimotor fibers, and the reticular formation. Each vertebral artery gives rise to three major arteries: **posterior spinal**, **anterior spinal** (Figs. 7-1 and 7-6), and **posterior inferior cerebellar** (Figs. 7-1 and 7-2). Some of the branches of the posterior spinal artery also supply the dorsal medulla,

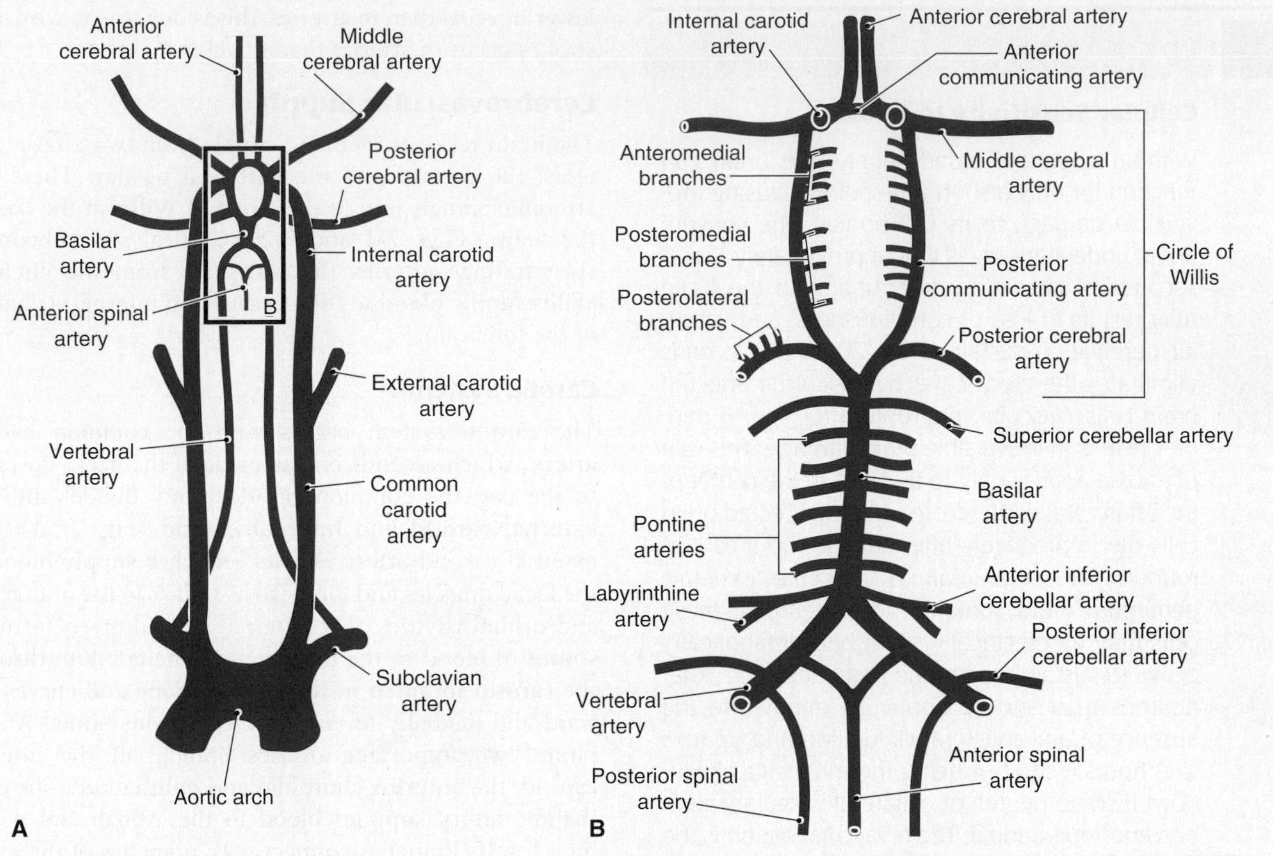

Figure 7-1 Vascular network to the brain. A. Carotid and vertebral basilar systems. B. An enlarged view of the circle of Willis.

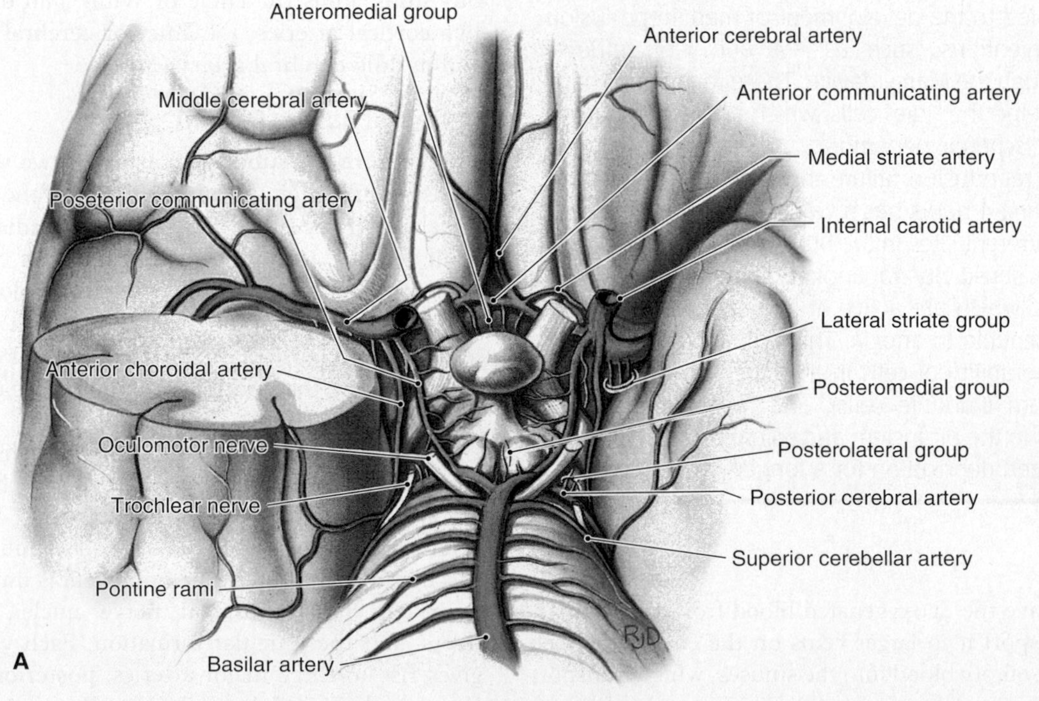

Figure 7-2 Cerebral arterial structure at base of brain (A);

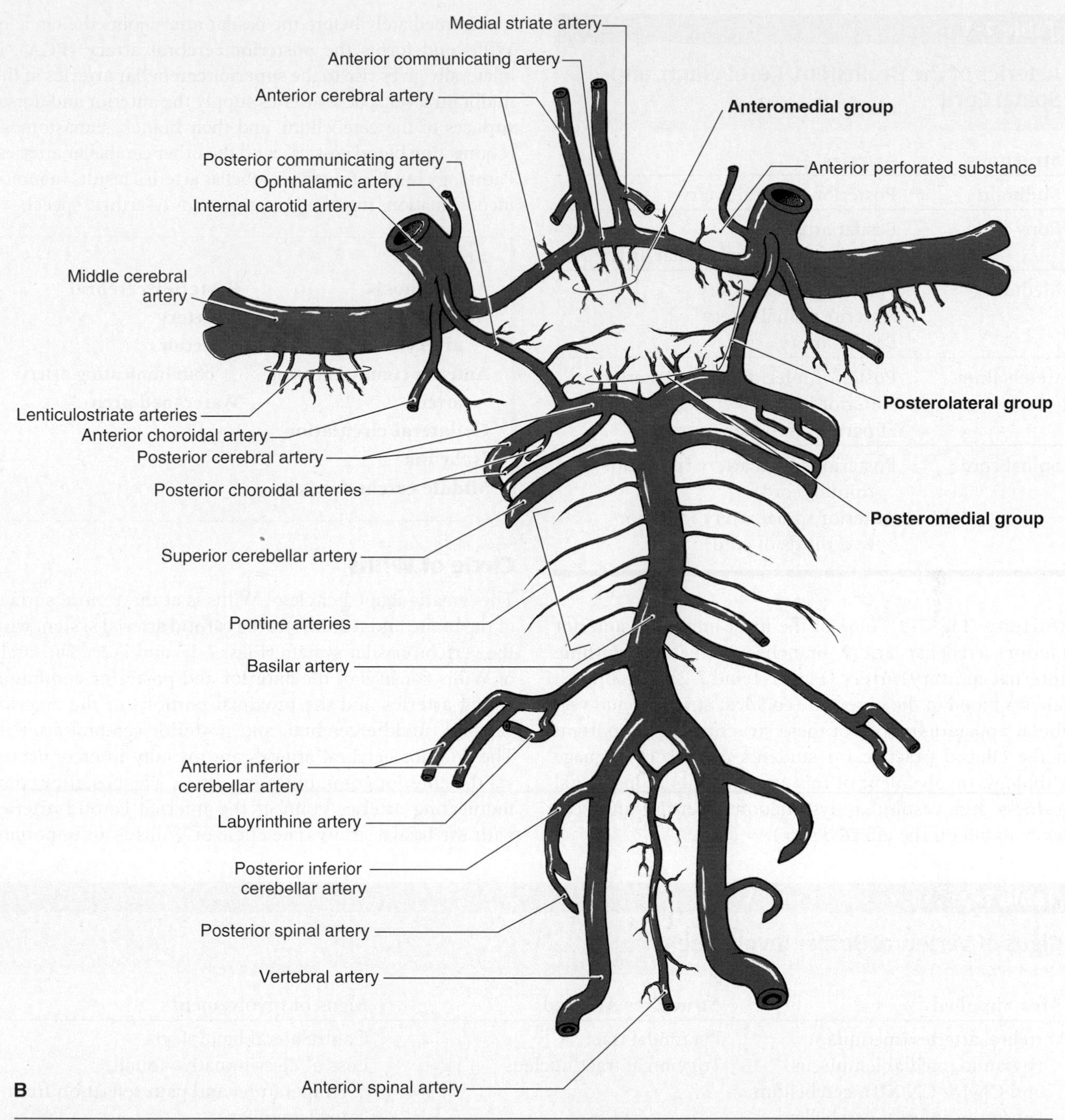

Figure 7-2 *(Continued)* a schematic illustration of the circle of Willis (B).

while the remaining branches travel caudally to supply the dorsal third of the spinal cord.

The anterior spinal artery emerges from each vertebral artery and descends along the midline. Some of its branches also supply the lower median medulla, which contains the pyramidal fibers, pyramidal decussation, and medial lemniscus fibers (see Figs. 3-7 and 3-9). The remaining branches supply the ventral two-thirds of the spinal cord. Occlusion of the anterior spinal artery branches that supply the medulla also results in **alternating hemiplegia**, which is associated with ipsilateral paralysis of the face and tongue as well as contralateral paralysis of the extremities (see Chapter 16). Each posterior inferior cerebellar artery supplies a large part of the cerebellum.

Immediately after its formation, the basilar artery gives rise to **anterior inferior cerebellar arteries**, which proceed laterally to serve the anterior and lateral surfaces of the cerebellum. At the pontine level, the basilar artery gives rise to many rami bilaterally that supply the pontine

Table 7-1

Arteries of the Brainstem, Cerebellum, and Spinal Cord

Structures	Arteries
Midbrain	Posterior cerebral artery
Pons	Basilar artery Anterior inferior cerebellar artery
Medulla	Posterior spinal artery Anterior spinal artery Basilar artery
Cerebellum	Posterior inferior cerebellar artery Anterior inferior cerebellar artery Superior cerebellar artery
Spinal cord	Posterior spinal artery (posterior third of cord) Anterior spinal artery (anterior two-thirds of cord)

structures (Fig. 7-2). One of the most important anterior inferior cerebellar artery branches is the **labyrinthine (internal auditory) artery** (Figs. 7-1 and 7-2). This branch delivers blood to the inner ear (cochlear structure and vestibular apparatus); both of these structures are important in the clinical practice for students of speech–language pathology. Involvement of this artery results in ipsilateral deafness and vestibular dysfunctions (vertigo and tendency to fall on the affected side).

Immediately before the basilar artery joins the circle of Willis and forms the **posterior cerebral artery** (PCA), it bilaterally gives rise to the **superior cerebellar arteries** at the midbrain level. These arteries supply the anterior and dorsal surfaces of the cerebellum, and their branches anastomose (connecting blood vessels) with the other cerebellar arteries. Pathology implicating the cerebellar arteries results in motor incoordination, impaired balance, and dysarthric speech.

Key Terms:

- **Anastomosis**
- **Anterior cerebral artery**
- **Anterior communicating artery**
- **Collateral circulation**
- **Ischemia**
- **Middle cerebral artery**
- **Posterior cerebral artery**
- **Posterior communicating artery**
- **Watershed area**

Circle of Willis

The wreath-shaped circle of Willis is at the ventral surface of the brain, and it connects the carotid arterial system with the vertebrobasilar system (Figs. 7-1B and 7-2). The circle of Willis consists of the **anterior** and **posterior communicating arteries** and the proximal portions of the anterior cerebral, middle cerebral, and posterior cerebral arteries. The anterior cerebral arteries are rostrally interconnected via the anterior communicating artery. The posterior communicating arteries connect the internal carotid arteries with the basilar artery. The circle of Willis is an important

Table 7-2

Signs of Vertebral Basilar Involvement

Area Supplied	Structures Affected	Signs of Involvement
Vertebral arteries: medulla (pyramid, medial lemniscus, and CN IX–CN XII), cerebellum (posterior inferior cerebellar arteries), and choroid plexus of fourth ventricle	Pyramidal tract	Contralateral hemiplegia
	Trigeminal tract/nucleus	Loss of discriminative touch, temperature, and pain sensation from ipsilateral face
	Lateral spinothalamic tract	Loss of pain and temperature sensation from contralateral trunk and limb
	Cerebellum	Ipsilateral ataxia
	CN VIII: vestibular portion	Vertigo, nystagmus, and vomiting
	CN IX, CN X, and CN XII (pharynx, palate, glottis, and tongue)	Dysphagia and dysarthria
Basilar artery: lateral pons, cerebellum (anterior inferior cerebellar and superior cerebellar arteries), and CNs (V, VII, VIII, and X)	Pyramidal tract	Hemiplegia
	Cerebellum	Ataxia
	CN V and nucleus	Loss of facial sensation
	CN VII and nucleus	Facial paralysis
	CN VIII and nucleus	Deafness, nystagmus, and vertigo
	CN X and nucleus	Vomiting

CN, cranial nerve.

BOX 7-2

Anastomosis

Anastomosis is the site of a natural interconnection between two blood vessels. Besides the interconnection, it also provides the mechanism for revascularization in the brain through collateral circulation in the case of vascular insufficiency. A functional collateral circulation is associated with better recovery and good clinical outcome for patients with stroke. Many factors affect the development of the collateral circulation. In general, a slowly developing arterial insufficiency facilitates the maximum development of compensatory vascular circulation. A sudden arterial occlusion usually does not lead to an effective alternate circulation. Serving to equalize the vascular blood supply to both sides of the brain, the circle of Willis is the most important anastomotic point for revascularization; nonetheless, the arterial system from one hemisphere can never adequately perfuse the other hemisphere through the communicating arteries of the circle. Further, a systematic hypotension not only prevents the development of a collateral circulation, but it also adds to a global cerebral ischemia involving the connected arteries, which is marked with a "watershed" infarct.

anastomotic point that serves to equalize the vascular blood supply to both sides of the brain. However, because of usual pressure equalization in both arterial systems, very little blood normally flows through the communicating arteries to the left and right sides of the circle (Box 7-2).

Two types of arteries, **cortical** and **central**, arise from the circle of Willis. The cortical branches are major arteries that largely supply the external brain structures (Table 7-3) and give rise to branches that anastomose with other cortical arteries. The central branches are small arteries that penetrate the ventral surface of the brain to supply the internal and subcortical brain structures.

Cortical Arteries

Anterior Cerebral Artery

After arising from the bifurcation of the internal carotid artery at the circle of Willis, the ACA travels rostrally in the interhemispheric fissure along the midsagittal surface of the brain. It follows the genu of the corpus callosum and continues posteriorly along its dorsal surface (Fig. 7-3). With **orbital**, **frontopolar**, **callosomarginal**, and **pericallosal** branches, it supplies the orbital and medial cortical surfaces of the prefrontal, frontal, and parietal lobes. It also provides a part of the blood supply to the corpus striatum and the internal capsule. In the posterior medial cortical area, the branches of the ACA anastomose with the branches of the PCA. Many terminal branches of the ACA cross over to the lateral cortical surface and develop anastomosing continuity with the branches of the MCA in the **watershed area**, where the distribution of major cerebral arteries overlaps (see the discussion under *Collateral Circulation*). The watershed area is located at the end of the arterial distribution and is most affected in the case of critically low cerebral blood flow. This region can also serve as the point of **anastomosis**, and it has significant implications for recovery after stroke.

Clinical Correlates: The interruption of blood circulation involving the ACA usually results in a decreased blood supply to the midsagittal extension of the sensory and motor cortices, causing sensory loss and paralysis in the legs, feet, and toes (Table 7-4; see Figs. 2-6 and 16-1). The vascular impairments of this artery may also lead to many prefrontal lobe symptoms, which include disorders of thinking, reasoning, abstracting, self-monitoring, memory, and planning. Additional impairments include decreased spontaneity, motor inaction, impaired judgment, reduced concentration, and impaired executive function. Since the ventral and medial part of the prefrontal cortex is responsible for social interaction, acquired sociopathic behavior is seen following bilateral damage to this region of the prefrontal cortex.

Table 7-3

Vascular Supply to the Brain Surface and Lobes

Brain Area	Artery
Frontal lobe	
Lateral surface	Middle cerebral artery
Medial surface	Anterior cerebral artery
Inferior surface	Middle and anterior cerebral arteries
Parietal lobe	
Lateral surface	Middle cerebral artery
Medial surface	Anterior cerebral artery
Occipital lobe	
Lateral and medial surfaces	Posterior cerebral artery
Temporal lobe	
Lateral surface	Middle cerebral artery
Medial surface	Jointly by middle cerebral, posterior cerebral, posterior communicating, and anterior choroidal arteries
Inferior surface	Posterior cerebral artery

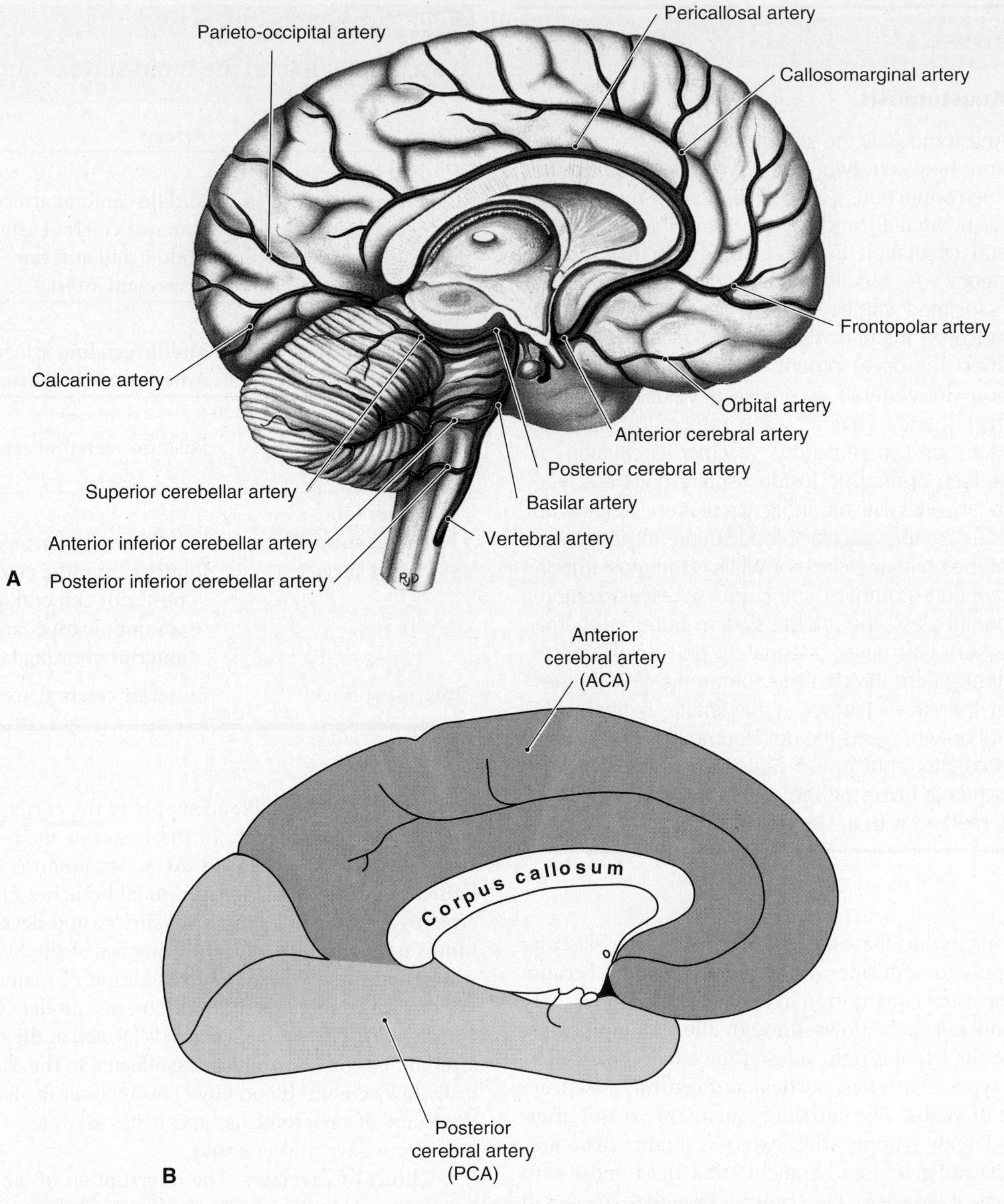

Figure 7-3 A. Anterior and posterior cerebral arteries together with cerebellar and brainstem arteries on midsagittal brain surface. B. Diagram of the midsagittal territory covered by the anterior cerebral and posterior cerebral arteries.

Middle Cerebral Artery

The MCA is the direct continuation of the internal carotid artery. After leaving the circle of Willis, it runs laterally and emerges through the sylvian fissure on the lateral brain surface. On the lateral surface, it divides into the temporal, frontal, and parietal branches (Fig. 7-4AB). The MCA branches supply blood to the entire lateral surface of the brain, which includes the sites for speech, language, and a large part of sensorimotor areas. The important areas are the somatosensory cortex in the postcentral gyrus, the

Table 7-4

Signs of Involvement of the Cortical Arteries

Area Supplied	Structures Affected	Signs of Involvement
Anterior cerebral artery: medial aspect of frontal lobe, anterior 80% of corpus callosum, and partial supply to basal ganglia (caudate head and putamen)	Sensory and motor cortices (medial surface)	Loss of somatic sensory and paralysis of opposite leg and foot
	Prefrontal cortex	Mental impairments: lack of spontaneity, easy distraction, problem-solving deficit, indecisiveness, and altered personality
Middle cerebral artery: entire lateral surface of cerebral hemisphere (including sensorimotor area, premotor area, language cortex, and associational cortex), inferior frontal lobe, basal ganglia (body and head of caudate, lateral globus pallidus, and putamen), and internal capsule	Precentral gyrus	Contralateral hemiplegia with spared leg and foot
	Postcentral gyrus	Contralateral hemianesthesia
	Visual radiation fibers in temporoparietal lobes	Homonymous hemianopsia
	Dominant hemisphere	Aphasia
	Nondominant hemisphere	Visual–spatial deficit and constructional apraxia
	Prefrontal lobe	Cognitive impairments
	Internal capsule: lateral striate arteries	Hemiplegia and hemianesthesia without aphasia
Posterior cerebral artery: medial surface of occipital lobe and inferior surface of occipital and temporal lobes	Calcarine cortex	Contralateral homonymous hemianopsia
	Thalamus	Thalamic syndrome: low pain threshold
	Upper midbrain	Coma and cranial nerve symptoms
	Subthalamic nucleus	Hemiballism
	Hippocampus	Memory impairment

motor cortex in the precentral gyrus, the Broca area in the premotor region, the prefrontal cortex, the primary auditory cortex in the transverse Heschl gyrus on the superior surface of the first temporal gyrus, the Wernicke area in the superior posterior temporal lobe, and the angular and supramarginal gyri in the inferior parietal lobe.

While passing through the lateral sulcus, the MCA gives off **lateral** and **medial lenticulostriate** branches that supply the basal ganglia and diencephalon (Fig. 7-5). The medial lenticulostriate artery supplies blood to the globus pallidus, the posterior internal capsule, and the medial ventral area of the thalamus. The lateral lenticulostriate artery supplies the entire pulvinar and caudate nucleus. Clinically, the branches of the lenticulostriate artery are the common sites of bleeding in the brain. Hypertension is one of the common causes of this bleeding.

Clinical Correlates: Impaired vascular circulation involving the MCA results in contralateral hemiplegia and impaired sensory functions that include discriminative touch, tactile agnosia, and reduced pain and temperature (Table 7-4). Other symptoms, depending on the hemisphere involved, are aphasia, constructional apraxia, temporospatial deficits, homonymous hemianopia, as well as reading and writing deficits. Lenticulostriate artery damage results in involuntary motor movements and sensorimotor symptoms.

Posterior Cerebral Artery

The basilar artery bifurcates to form two posterior cerebral arteries. With a potential anastomotic flow from the posterior communicating artery, each PCA curves along the inferior brain surface to supply blood to the anterior and inferior temporal lobe; it covers important structures, such as the uncus, inferior temporal gyri, hippocampus, and inferior and medial occipital lobe, including the primary visual cortex in the calcarine region. The end branches of the artery also cross over to the lateral surface and anastomose in the watershed region with the terminal branches of the MCA.

Clinical Correlates: Occlusion of the PCA results in homonymous hemianopsia. Occlusion of the basilar artery, which provides blood to both posterior cerebral arteries, results in total blindness as well as numerous pontine and cerebellar symptoms (Table 7-4). Bilateral involvement of the occipital lobe is associated with cortical blindness where the patient cannot see but can detect light. Bilateral involvement of the visual association cortex, which deals with recognition and object appreciation, results in visual agnosia. Medial temporal involvement may also cause memory impairments.

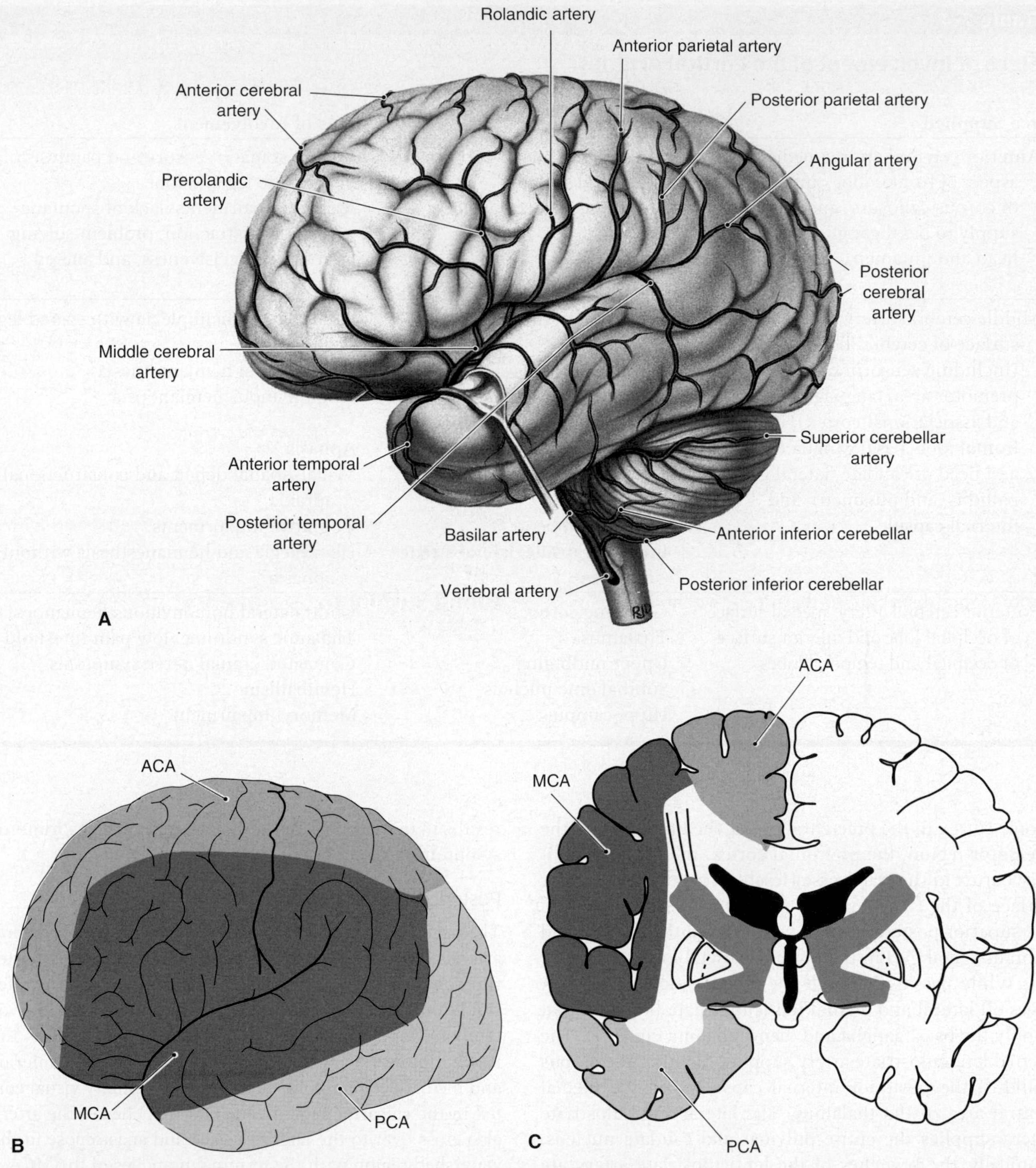

Figure 7-4 A. Blood circulation to the lateral surface of the cerebral hemisphere and cerebellum. B. Diagram of the lateral cortical surface marking the territories of three cortical arteries. C. Coronal illustration of the territories of three cortical arteries. ACA, anterior cerebral artery; MCA, middle cerebral artery; PCA, posterior cerebral artery.

Central Arteries

The central arteries are the branches that arise either from the proximal portions of the cortical arteries or from the circle of Willis, and they penetrate the inferior surface of the brain (Fig. 7-2). These penetrating branches supply blood to the subcortical structures that include the thalamus, hypothalamus, caudate nucleus, putamen, globus pallidus, internal capsule, choroid plexus, and others (Table 7-5). One important aspect of the central arteries' circulation is the marked overlapping of blood supply as

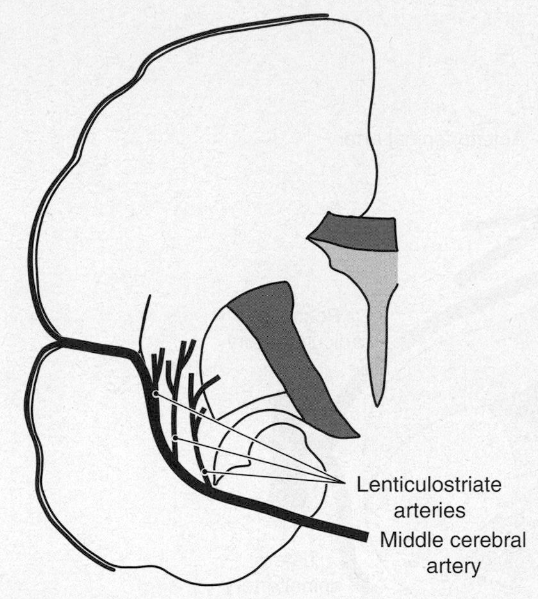

Figure 7-5 Diagrammatic illustration of the lenticulostriate arteries.

Table 7-5

Vascular Supply to the Subcortical Structures

Structure	Artery
Thalamus	Posteromedial, posterolateral, and choroidal
Hypothalamus	Anteromedial and posteromedial
Caudate nucleus	Anterolateral, medial striate, and lenticulostriate
Putamen	Lenticulostriate, medial striate, and anterior choroidal
Globus pallidus	Anterior choroidal
Subthalamus	Posteromedial
Red nucleus and substantia nigra	Posteromedial

the branches distribute to the subcortical areas. The overlapping blood supply facilitates the development of anastomotic channels in response to occlusive or ischemic vascular problems. Important central arteries are the **anteromedial**, **medial striate**, **anterior choroidal**, **posterior choroidal**, **posteromedial**, and **posterolateral** (Fig. 7-2).

The anteromedial arteries arise from the anterior communicating and anterior cerebral arteries and supply the hypothalamus and suprachiasmatic regions of the brain; their involvement results in disorders of the autonomic nervous system. The medial striate arteries arise from the ACA and supply blood to parts of the caudate nucleus, putamen, and anterior limb of the internal capsule. Its impaired circulation results in involuntary movements.

The anterior choroidal artery supplies blood to the choroid plexus, hippocampus, and portions of the globus pallidus, posterior internal capsule, putamen, and geniculate bodies. Signs of its occlusion consist of contralateral hemiplegia, contralateral hemianesthesia, involuntary movements, and cerebrospinal fluid (CSF) secretion disorder. The involvement of the hippocampus results in impaired memory consolidation.

The posterior choroidal artery (not shown) supplies blood to the choroid plexus of the third ventricle, tectum in the midbrain, and pineal gland. The posteromedial arteries supply blood to the red nucleus, substantia nigra, medial portion of the cerebral peduncle, subthalamic nucleus, midbrain reticular formation, and superior cerebellar peduncle. Occlusion of the posteromedial arteries results in multiple sensorimotor symptoms including contralateral ataxia (red nucleus involvement), involuntary movements (substantia nigra involvement), hemiballism (subthalamic nucleus dysfunctioning), and altered consciousness as well as coma (midbrain reticular involvement).

Blood Supply to Spinal Cord

Blood is supplied to the spinal cord by two major longitudinal arteries, the anterior and posterior spinal arteries, both of which originate from the vertebral arteries (Figs. 7-1 and 7-6). The anterior spinal arteries from each vertebral artery join to form a single descending artery along the midline, giving rise to branches on the left and right to perfuse the anterior two-thirds of the spinal cord. This spinal region contains sensorimotor fibers from extremities and spinal motor neurons. Vascular flow interruption of the anterior spinal artery affects the ascending sensory and descending motor fibers and causes hemiplegia and protopathic (pain and temperature) hemisensory loss.

The posterior spinal arteries descend on the dorsal surface of the cord and supply the dorsal spinal area (Fig. 7-6), which contains the dorsal lemniscal fibers and dorsal gray column (see Chapter 11). The circulatory disorders of this artery result in a loss of epicritic sensation, which is marked by impaired two-point touch and the loss of proprioceptive and kinesthetic awareness from the limbs.

The vascular supply to the spinal cord is augmented further by the segmental radicular arteries; these arteries descend from the aorta and enter the spinal column through the intervertebral foramina along with the spinal nerves. Each radicular spinal artery supplies blood to about six spinal segments, except the great radicular **artery of Adamkiewicz**, which supplies most of the caudal third of the cord. The artery of Adamkiewicz is formed at the lower thoracic and upper lumbar level by one enlarged radicular artery. Since the spinal cord controls the movement of the muscles of respiration, it is important to understand its vascular supply.

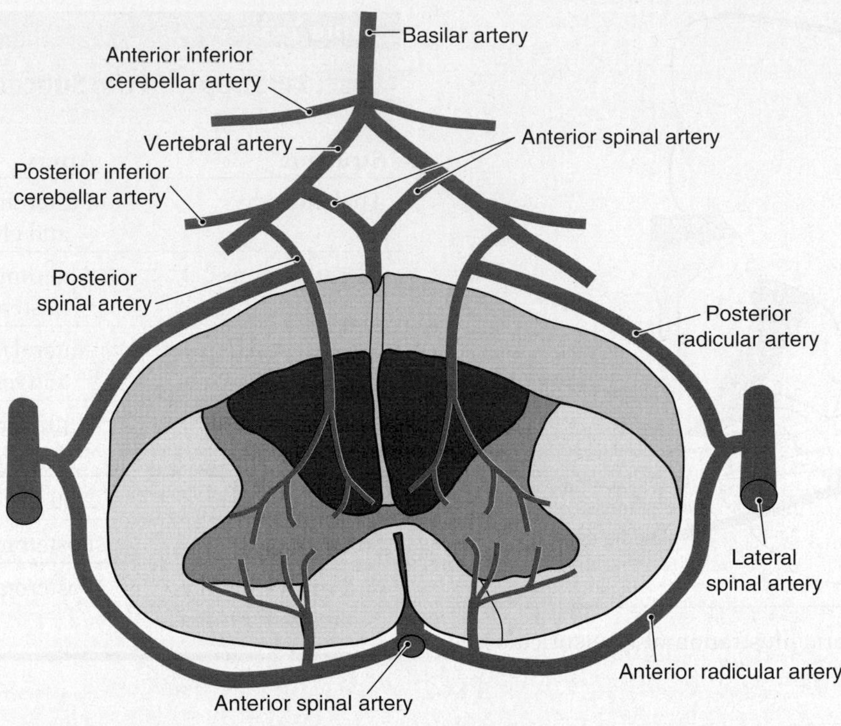

Figure 7-6 Spinal blood distribution through posterior and anterior spinal arteries and its augmentation by the radiculospinal arteries.

Collateral Circulation

Collateral circulation refers to the provision for the alternative vascular supply to a given structure after it has lost its primary arterial blood supply (Box 7-2). It is an important clinical concept with significant implications for the natural recovery process following brain injuries, since a provision for good collateral circulation results in a good clinical outcome. There are many potential channels for alternative blood circulation; however, not all are always effective. The variability in arterial anatomy and the degree of vascular pathology both contribute to the development of collateral circulation. In general, better collateral circulation develops if the arterial occlusion is gradual and if the blocked artery is closer to the main arterial trunk. Obstruction of the terminal arteries or capillaries, after they have penetrated deep into the brain, reduces the arterial potential for developing collateral circulation.

There are four potential points of collateral circulation within one hemisphere or across both. First, the anterior communicating artery connects the vascular supply for both hemispheres by linking two anterior cerebral arteries. Second, the vertebral basilar system can potentially feed through the posterior communicating artery, if there is a significant vascular insufficiency involving the internal carotid artery. The posterior communicating arteries may also draw from the internal carotid artery and feed into the posterior cerebral arteries if the vertebral basilar arterial system is occluded. Third, thromboembolic involvement of the internal carotid artery can trigger a retrograde blood flow from the external carotid artery through the ophthalmic artery branches in the eye. Fourth, the terminal branches of all three cortical (anterior, middle, and posterior cerebral) arteries may anastomose in the watershed (end) area on the lateral brain surface, which is highly probable in the case of reduced blood volume through any one of the three cortical arteries. The watershed area is clinically an important area. Depending for its perfusion on all three cortical arteries, the end distributional area of the three cortical (anterior, middle, and posterior) cerebral arteries is highly susceptible to global ischemia. A **watershed infarction** syndrome consists of paralysis and sensory loss predominantly involving the arm; the face and speech are spared.

Key Terms :

Aneurysm	**Embolism**
Anoxia	**Hemorrhage**
Arteriosclerosis/ Atherosclerosis	**Hypertension**
	Ischemia
Arteriovenous malformations	**Thrombosis**
	Transient ischemic attack
Cerebrovascular accident	**Watershed infarction**

Vascular Pathology

Vascular diseases of the brain are the most frequent causes of neurological deficits and adult disabilities. In the

BOX 7-3

Effects of Ischemia on Brain Cells

Once the cerebral blood flow falls below 15 mL/100 g tissue/min, it has a drastic impact on the functioning of brain cells, with cells dying. Initially, the brain responds to a clinically significant ischemia by activating its two autoregulatory mechanisms: vasodilation and opening of alternate channels for potential collateral circulation. In the absence of the reperfusion availability within a critical time period of 2 to 4 hours and possibly extending to 7 to 8 hours, the cells undergo a series of micromolecular changes before necrotizing. Cells subjected to ischemia quickly lose their energy that is needed to maintain the ionic balance and move ions across the cellular membrane. The brain responds to the loss of cellular energy by releasing glutamate and aspartate, two facilitatory neurotransmitters which is called "excitotoxicity." This extracellular presence of glutamate (as well as aspartate) causes the opening of the calcium channels in the cellular membrane triggering the influx of calcium (as well as the ions of sodium and chloride) and expulsion of potassiums. The excessive calcium presence within the cells causes the release of many destructive enzymes which further adds to the injury and the cells undergo inflammatory changes followed by chromatolysis and necrosis.

The availability of the collateral circulation for reperfusion is extremely important in the functional restitution. Every minute and hour of ischemia after the stroke onset is critical. By one estimate (Saver, 2006), a large vessel stroke risks causing the loss of about 120 million neurons, 830 billion synapses, and 447 mi. of myelinated fibers for each hour of stroke. This roughly translates into a loss of about 1.9 million neurons, 14 billion synapses, and 7.4 mi. of myelinated fibers for each minute poststroke. This is a considerable loss when the brain is considered to have 20 to 100 billion of cells.

United States, vascular accidents are ranked as the third-most common cause of death after cancer and heart disease; this may also universally be true. Vascular interruption not only deprives the brain cells of life-sustaining oxygen but it also disconnects the axonal pathways in the brain. Without oxygen, some brain cells die (infarction) immediately while others become idle and remain somewhat functional. However, if not reperfused within a short window of time, they also infarct (Box 7-3).

Cerebrovascular accidents (CVA/stroke) are characterized by a sudden development of focal—as opposed to gradual—neurological deficits, which fall into two common types: **occlusive vascular**(**thrombosis** or **embolism**) and **hemorrhagic** (bleeding from ruptured vessels including aneurysm and **arteriovenous malformations**) strokes (Table 7-6; Box 7-4).

Occlusive Vascular Pathology

Atherosclerosis, hardened arterial walls, is the primary cause of local arterial occlusion, and it accounts for over 80% of cerebral vascular accidents (CVAs). It is a slow process that takes years to develop in which various lipids, blood platelets, calcium deposits, fatty particles, and other undissolved substances in the blood gradually accumulate along the inner walls of blood vessels and cause narrowing of the arterial lumen. The adherence of lipids and blood

Table 7-6

Principal Types of CVAs

Type	Location	Time of Occurrence	Warning Signs
Thrombosis	Occlusion at atherosclerotic lesion	During sleep and periods of low physical activity	Transient ischemic attacks, headaches, and seizures
Embolism	Occlusion of smaller artery by displaced clot moving peripherally	When awake and active	None; possible headaches and seizures
Hemorrhage	Rupture of arterial wall or aneurysm and arteriovenous malformations	Bleed anytime, usually during awake hours	None

BOX 7-4

Cerebral Vascular Accidents

There are two types of strokes: ischemic and hemorrhagic. In ischemic strokes, which happen suddenly, a blood vessel in the brain gradually blocks and the oxygen-deprived regions of the brain develop an infarct. Thrombotic and embolic are two examples of this occlusive type of stroke.

In hemorrhagic strokes, the weakened arteries in the brain are ruptured and the escaped blood impairs the cells and pathways with increased intracranial pressure. Intracerebral hemorrhage involves the deep penetrating arteries. These arteries have thin walls, supply to the basal ganglia and internal capsules, and are highly susceptible to damage. Trauma and hypertension are two most frequent causes of hemorrhage in the brain. The escaped blood within the brain not only reduces the oxygen source for the brain cells but it also cuts or disrupts axonal pathways and damages the surrounding tissues. Massive intracerebral hemorrhages result in focal contralateral sensorimotor (hemiplegia and hemianesthesia) symptoms. Large veins as they pass outward through arachnoid and dura membranes are prone to damage. Usually seen in cases of traumatic brain injuries, their rupture is the common cause of subdural hematoma which usually appears long and crescent shaped. Large hematomas require surgical evacuation. Rupture of dural vessel like the middle meningeal artery is commonly involved with epidural hematoma. In this case, the escaped blood accumulates between the skull and the dura (extradural hemorrhage) mater. Untreated hematoma can lead to the herniation of the brain into the vertebral column possibly causing death.

BOX 7-5

Transient Ischemia and Watershed Infarct

These two important concepts are associated with vascular dysfunction. The transient ischemic attack, often an indicator of a major impending stroke, is a temporary vascular dysfunction secondary to a focal occlusion or narrowing of the blood vessels. Clinically, this vascular dysfunction is marked by short-term symptoms of weakness, numbness, double vision, speech difficulty, and word-finding problem that last for 3 to 5 minutes and do not involve a permanent brain damage. Clinical signs lasting more than 30 minutes or so are considered to have resulted from a stroke with a permanent structural infarct.

The territory located at the end of the vascular distribution for three major (anterior, middle, and posterior) cerebral arteries, called the watershed area, receives blood circulation through the cortical arteries and is the site where all three arteries are connected. This borderzone territory becomes highly susceptible to anoxia secondary to a generalized hypoperfusion involving all three major arteries.

platelets usually occurs at an ulcerated or injured site, commonly a point of bifurcation. Increased blood coagulability also contributes to an occlusive disease.

Since a narrowed or blocked arterial lumen (channel) reduces or stops blood flow, the brain suffers from ischemia (insufficient blood supply). A **transient ischemic attack** (TIA) is a temporary interruption of blood circulation to the brain. This is caused by mechanisms that interfere with blood supply to the brain, such as occlusive carotid disease, emboli from the heart or proximal part of an artery, and infrequently spasms of arterial muscles. The exact symptoms are focal and depend on the brain area affected. A patient with TIA may have several of the following suddenly emerging symptoms: focal weakness, double vision, headache, paresthesia, hemianesthesia, dysarthria, and dizziness. These may last from a few minutes to an hour. If these symptoms last longer than 30 minutes or so, it is a full stroke (Box 7-5).

The symptoms of a TIA are clinically significant, since their short-lived presence indicates that a larger stroke may be in progress (Table 7-7). Not all strokes are preceded by a TIA; only about one-third of individuals with TIA later

Table 7-7

Warning Signs of Stroke

Warning Signs of Stroke
Sudden onset of numbness or weakness on one side of body
Sudden inability to speak and understand others
Sudden difficulty in seeing with one or both eyes; double vision
Sudden loss of balance and dizziness
Headache with no cause

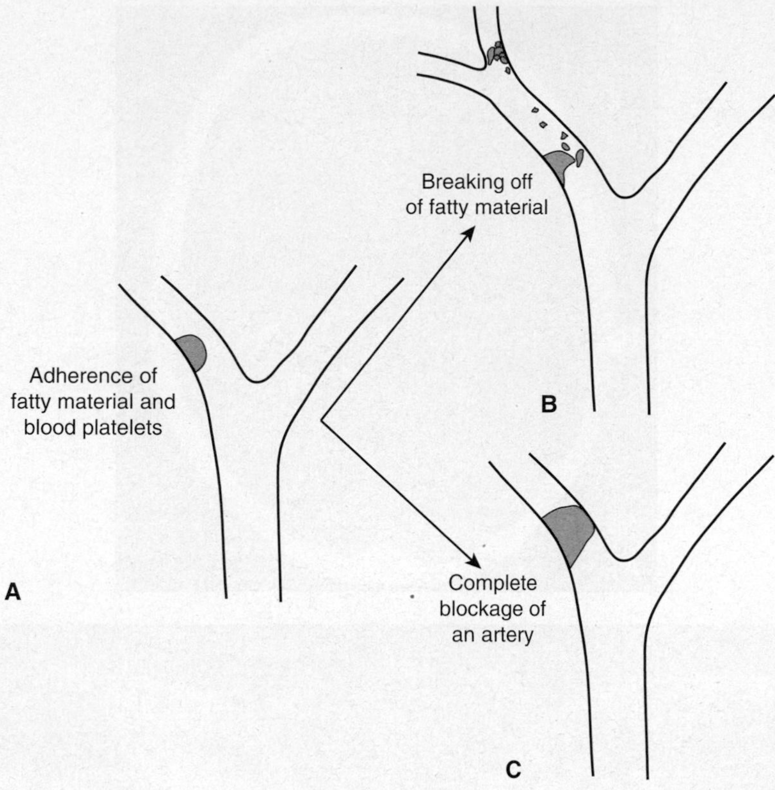

Figure 7-7 A Graphic illustration of thromboembolism. **A.** Thromboembolism forms in vascular system. **B.** Embolus is a detached part of thrombosis, which occludes a smaller vessel. **C.** Thrombotic occlusion of a large blood vessel.

have a major stroke. Administration of blood-thinning medication at this stage may prevent a major CVA. In arteriosclerosis, the heart initially compensates for the reduced blood flow by pumping blood with greater force. However, this compensatory pumping leads to **high blood pressure** (**hypertension**), another critical neurological condition. Once the atherosclerotic process has begun (Fig. 7-7A), it reduces the arterial blood supply by forming either an embolus (Fig. 7-7B) or a thrombus (Fig. 7-7C).

Comprising 25% of the CVAs, embolism is blockage in a distal artery with a narrow lumen. An embolus is a clot that breaks free from a thrombus and enters the bloodstream, eventually blocking a small end artery. Cerebral emboli produce rapid development of neurological signs that mostly do not progress. Embolic strokes usually occur during a period of activity and often affect young people.

Accounting for 65% of the CVAs, thrombosis is a local build-up of fatty substances and blood platelets in a cerebral vessel that is caused by an atherosclerotic plaque; the build-up mostly occurs at sites of arterial bifurcation or at sites subjected to injury and inflammation. The presence of plaque causes the degeneration of the vessel wall, and damage to the endothelial layer attracts fibrin and blood platelets to the site. The thrombosis grows slowly; it can take several years for the arterial lumen to close. A thrombosis becomes symptomatic only in the mid and late years. By then, the arterial lumen is mostly blocked, which results in an infarct (Fig. 7-8A). Most thrombotic strokes occur during sleep or a period of inactivity, because the lower BP during inactivity allows vessels to narrow or close. One warning sign of a thrombotic stroke is TIA (occurring in 30% of patients who later develop stroke).

Hemorrhage

Accounting for about 10% to 15% of CVAs, hemorrhagic strokes are associated with sudden onset of neurological symptoms and may cause coma and stupor that may progress with time. Hemorrhagic strokes result from the bleeding of rupturing of weakened blood vessel walls under the pressure of constant blood flow. Hemorrhages can occur anywhere in the arterial system; however, the lenticulostriate arteries that supply the thalamus and basal ganglia are the most common sites (Fig. 7-5). The major locations of hemorrhagic strokes are the **intracerebral**, **extradural**, **subdural**, and **subarachnoid** areas (Fig. 7-9). Lacunar infarcts and intracerebral hemorrhage are traditionally considered strokes, while extradural and subdural hematoma is subsequent to trauma and arachnoid hemorrhage results from a rupture of an aneurysm as well as arteriovenous malformation.

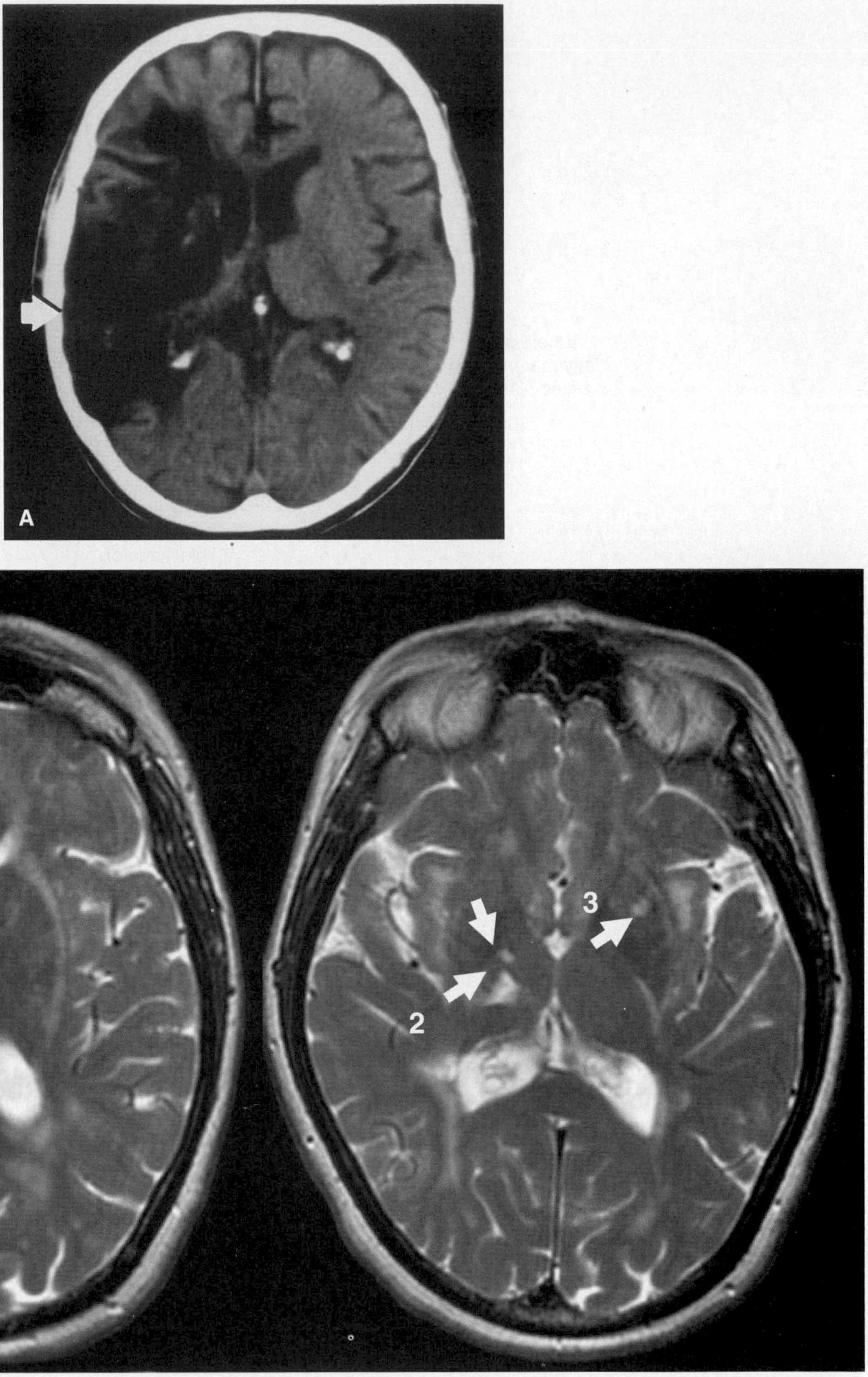

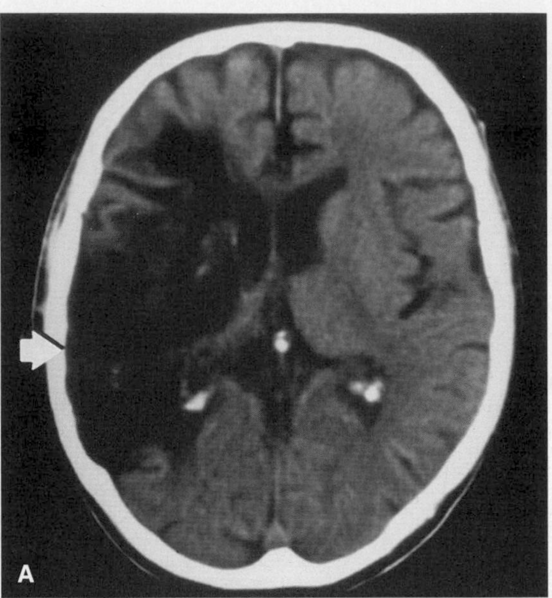

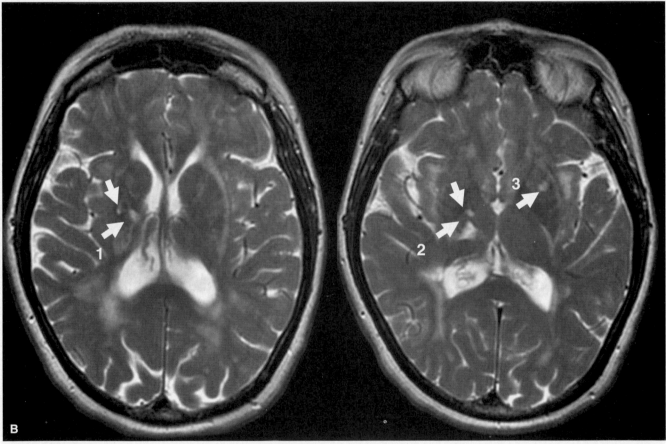

Figure 7-8 A large right middle cerebral artery infarct *(arrow)*, an axial CT image (**A**). Multiple lacunar infarcts in the right thalamus (1), the right (2) internal capsule, and the left (3) putamen on axial MR images (**B**).

Lacunar strokes involve small arteries of the basal ganglia and thalamus (Fig. 7-8B,C). They develop abruptly or in spurts over days and are commonly found in individuals with idiopathic hypertension. Intracerebral hemorrhages are space-occupying lesions involving the rupturing of an intracranial artery. Blood released from the ruptured artery, if not surgically drained, accumulates to form a hematoma, which encroaches on vital cortical centers. Intracerebral hemorrhages usually occur during an active or awake state. The full extent of deficit

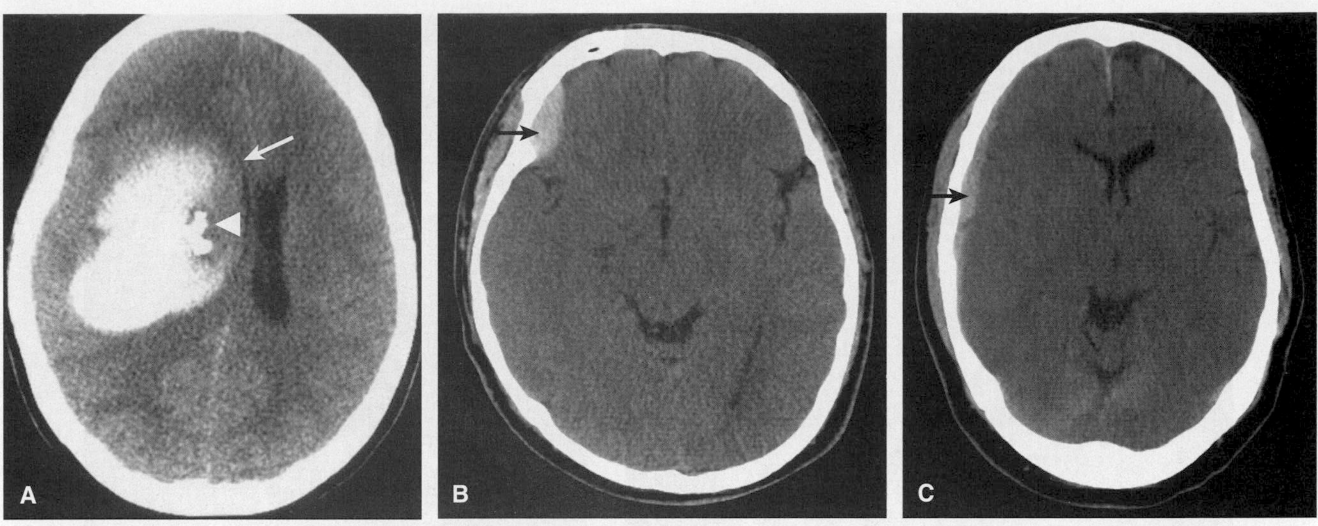

Figure 7-9 Cerebral hemorrhagic stroke (A). CT scan of a large intracerebral hemorrhage with notable embolic material is present in the deep component of the ruptured AVM (*arrowhead*); also evident is the mass effect causing midline shift (*long arrow*); CT images of an epidural (B) and a subdural (C) hematoma.

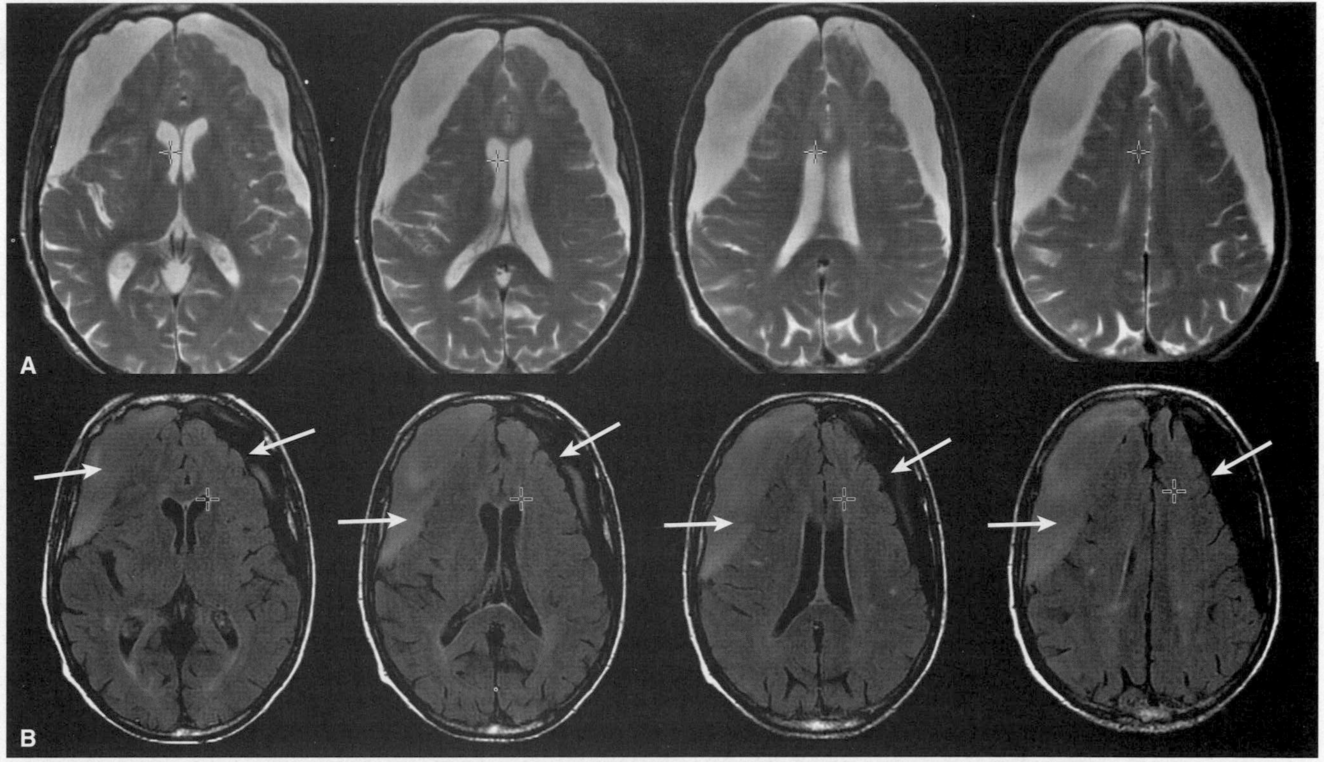

Figure 7-10. MR Image of bilaterally located subdural hematomas (A). The hypodensity in the left side of the FLAIR image (B) indicating a more acute hematoma than on the right sided.

is seldom present at the outset but develops over several hours.

Extradural and subdural hematomas result from a traumatic injury. In extradural (epidural) hematoma, a blood vessel (the meningeal artery) ruptures between the dura mater and skull. The extravasated blood separates the dura from the inner skull and forms a large lens-shaped accumulation of blood. In subdural hematoma, mostly affected are the bridging veins that go outward from the dura and arachnoid, and the blood accumulates outside the arachnoid tissue beneath the dura mater (Fig. 7-10). The accumulated blood, if not surgically drained, gradually

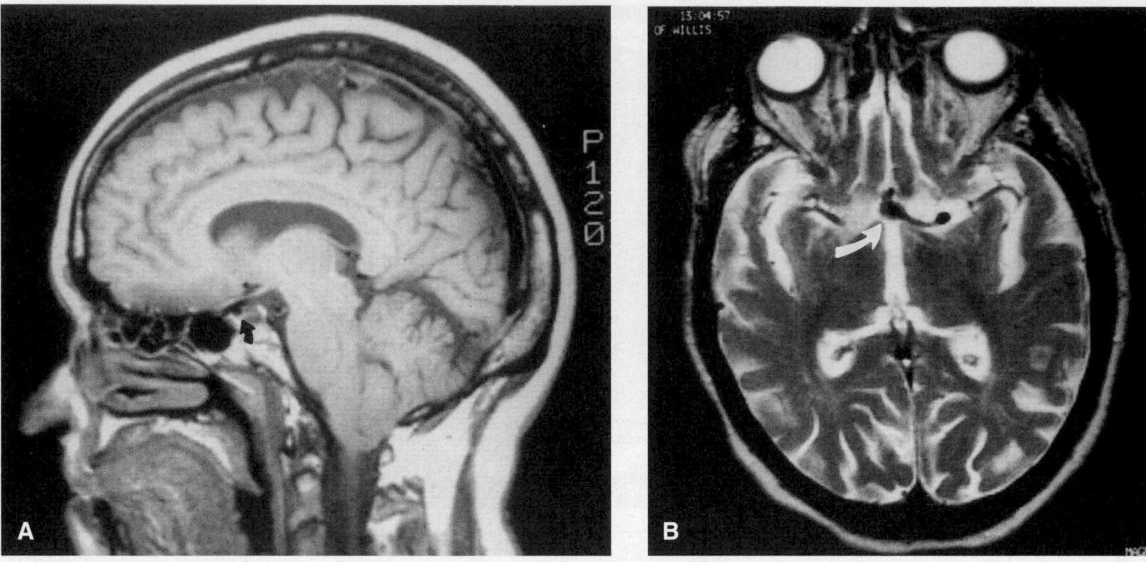

Figure 7-11. Sagittal T1-weighted MRI of an aneurysm (**A**, *arrow*) involving the internal carotid artery. A T2-weighted axial MRI of the anterior communicating artery aneurysm (**B**, *curved arrow*).

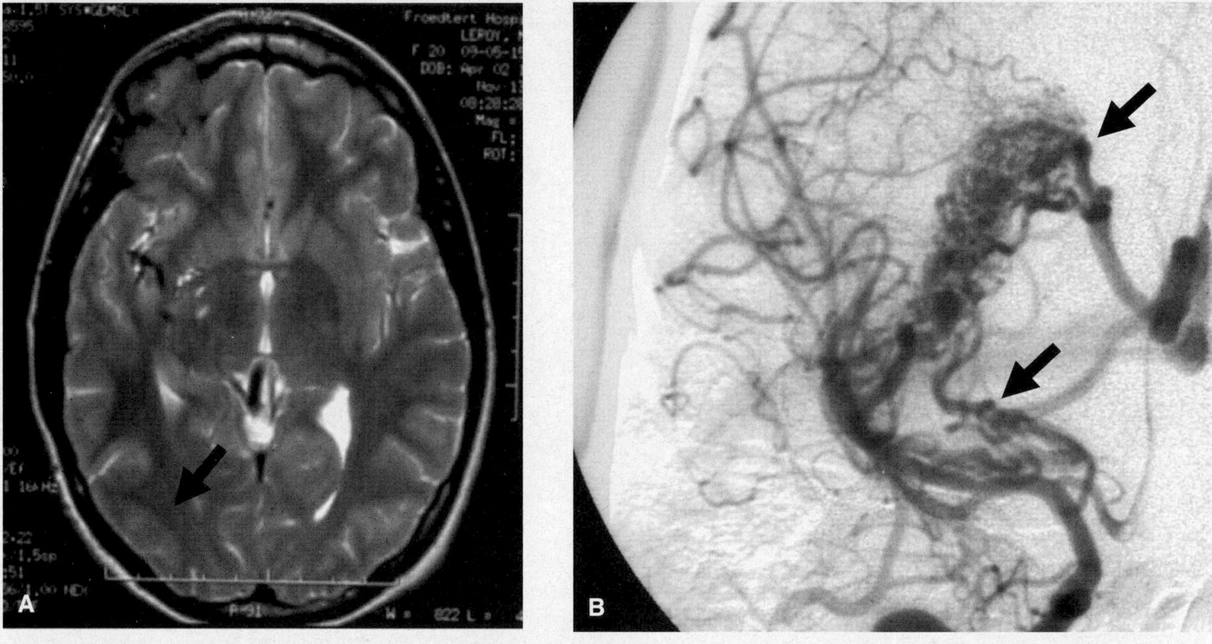

Figure 7-12 MRI scan, axial T2 weighted, shows enlarged arteries, veins, and AVM nidus (*arrowheads*) in the right sylvian choroidal region (**A**); **B.** AVM in the anterior choroidal artery (*small arrow*) and deep portion of the AVM (*large arrow*).

expands and begins to compress the soft underlying brain tissues, causing irreversible brain damage. Another potential site for hemorrhage is the subarachnoid space, which is commonly seen with the bleeding of an arteriovenus malformation (AVM) or aneurysm.

An **aneurysm** is a local balloon-like dilation of an artery that is considered to be a congenital pathology (Fig. 7-11). It usually occurs at points of bifurcation of major cerebral arteries. The outpouchings of an aneurysm are due to either weakness in the vessel wall or congenital arterial defect. An aneurysm can be neurologically symptomatic in two ways: first, the mass effect of arterial dilation compresses the surrounding structures; second, the aneurysm, no longer able to withstand the blood flow pressure, ruptures and releases blood into the brain or onto its surface.

An AVM is a congenital condition in which a tangled dilated artery or vein becomes connected in a local area (Fig. 7-12); thus the arterial blood bypasses the cortical tissue and directly drains into the veins, depriving the underlying tissue of oxygen. With age, the AVMs may become large and are susceptible to hemorrhage because of their thin walls. These malformations often cause seizures and recurrent headaches (mimicking migraines). Depending on the location of the malformations, they can also cause language impairments, motor speech problems, visual disorders, sensory loss, and hemiplegia.

ISCHEMIA RISK FACTORS

There are two types of risk factors for stroke: modifiable and nonmodifiable (Table 7-8). Medical conditions and lifestyle-related issues can be controlled either medically or by changing living habits; these include hypertension, heart disease, diabetes mellitus (also called type II diabetes), and high cholesterol. Lifestyle-related modifiable risk factors are smoking, obesity, eating habits, and physical inactivity. Advancing age, gender, hereditary predisposition, and ethnic composition are the risks that cannot be treated. Untreated hypertension can damage the arterial walls so that they become sites of atherosclerotic plaques. High BP is the single-most common risk factor for strokes, and controlling hypertension contributes to a significant decline in the incidence of stroke (Box 7-6).

Heart disease is another frequent cause of the embolic stroke, as clots leaving the heart can block brain arteries. Persons with **coronary artery disease (CAD)** are at twice as much risk of having a stroke as the general population. **Diabetic mellitus** is known to accelerate the development of atherosclerosis. Also, high cholesterol levels cause build-ups on arterial walls, narrowing their passageways and leading to heart attack and stroke (Box 7-7). Lifestyle-related habits, such as smoking and unhealthy eating, substantially increases the risk for CAD; quitting smoking alone can lower the risk for CVA by 50% to 70% within 5 years.

BOX 7-6

Blood Pressure

Blood pressure (BP) is the most clinically important indicator of the healthy functioning heart and adequate blood circulation to the brain. It is recorded with two numbers; for example 120/80 mm Hg which is the normal BP. The upper number indicates the **systolic pressure** which is present when the heart pushes the blood out and away. The lower number marks the **diastolic pressure** when the heart rests between two beats. Elevated BP to a certain extent may not have any clinical symptoms, but if not treated, it adds to the risks of coronary artery disease, cardiac failures, and atherosclerosis (hardening of arteries). It is the atherosclerosis that can eventually lead to cerebral vascular accidents. Family history, physical inactivity, obesity, diabetes, constant tension, and kidney diseases are common causes of high BP, which can also be idiopathic.

Table 7-8

Modifiable and Nonmodifiable Risk Factors for Stroke

Modifiable	Nonmodifiable
Medical	Age
Hypertension	Gender
Hypercholesterolemia	Ethnicity
Hyperlipidemia	Heredity
Carotid artery disease	
Diabetes	
Lifestyle	
Physical inactivity	
Oral contraceptive use	
Cigarette smoking	
Obesity	

VENOUS SINUS SYSTEM

Veins and sinuses collect deoxygenated blood and transport it back to the heart and lungs for reoxygenation. Drainage of the blood first begins at the capillary level, where the intracerebral capillaries unite to form small veins that are called venules. Venules collect the blood and transfer it to the network of large veins. Veins that drain the surface and the deep brain structures empty the blood into large dural sinuses. The sinuses, which consist of spaces between the periosteal and meningeal layers of dura mater, are in the cranium (Fig. 7-13; see Fig. 2-43).

Dural Sinuses

The dural sinuses form a network of cavities in and around the brain (Figs. 2-43 and 7-13). The **superior sagittal sinus** runs along the dorsomedial line on the vertex in the falx cerebri, receiving blood from the superior cerebral veins and CSF drained through the **arachnoid villi**. The **inferior sagittal sinus** runs in the inferior margin of the **falx cerebri** over the dorsal edge of the corpus callosum. Posteriorly, it joins the straight (rectus) sinus, which empties into the **sinus confluence**. The paired **transverse**

BOX 7-7

Cholesterol and Stroke Risks

A moderate amount of cholesterol is essential for the healthy body because it contributes to the production of hormones and formation of cell membranes. However, an excessive level of blood cholesterol (hypercholesterolemia) poses a major risk factor for CAD and CVA. Cholesterol is combined with proteins (lipoproteins) before it can be transported to and from the cells. Among others, two important lipoproteins are high-density lipoprotein (HDL) and low-density lipoprotein (LDL).

HDL removes excessive cholesterol from the cells and transports it to the liver for the final disposal. Thus, HDL, also called good cholesterol, not only reduces the risk of arteriosclerosis by controlling blood lipids, but it also prevents plaque formation in arterial walls. LDL is considered bad cholesterol, since it has a tendency to stick to the arterial walls in the brain and heart; this build-up leads to sticky deposits called atherosclerotic plaques. The plaque formation interrupts the flow of blood by narrowing or completely blocking the arteries, which leads to stroke.

There are two main sources of cholesterol in the blood: liver and food. The liver synthesizes about 75% of cholesterol to meet the energy needs of the body cells. The remaining 25% of cholesterol comes from secondary sources of food high in saturated fat, and it includes dairy products, red meats, and eggs. Most plant foods, such as grains and vegetables, are free of cholesterol. The body produces whatever amount of cholesterol it needs, and, once the cell need is filled, all the excessive cholesterol flows to the blood.

Measured in milligrams per deciliter (mg/dL), the normal range for total blood cholesterol is between 140 and 200 mg per dL of blood. Any blood cholesterol above 200 increases the risk for coronary artery disease. Within the total cholesterol value, it is desired to have a higher HDL (good) cholesterol, since it protects against CAD by keeping bad cholesterol (LDL) from building up in the arteries.

Cholesterol values have different interpretations depending on many factors, such as risk, genetics, and ethnic groups, but professionals have made the following recommendations:

1. Total cholesterol
   - Optimal if <200 mg/dL
   - High risk if >200 mg/dL
2. LDL cholesterol
   - Optimal if 100 mg/dL or lower
3. HDL cholesterol
   - Optimal and low risk for CAD if >60 mg/dL
   - High risk for coronary diseases if <40 mg/dL

There is a close relationship between higher blood cholesterol and heart diseases. Excessive blood cholesterol usually builds up in the arteries, leading to atherosclerosis that begins with damage to the internal lining of the arteries, usually due to high BP. This is followed by the accumulation of lipids, such as cholesterol, triglycerides, red blood cells, and blood platelets, at the damaged site. The plaque leads to the narrowing of the arterial passage and can cause stroke. High blood cholesterol can be treated using a series of drugs that include statins (Atrovastatin (Lipitor), Simvastatin (Zocor), Fluvastatin (Lescohl), Provastatin (Pravacohl), and Lovastatin (Mevacor)), nicotine acids, fibric acids, and bile acid sequestrates. Some of these medicines manage the cholesterol by not only lowering the LDL but also by increasing the count of HDL.

sinuses, which arise from the **confluence of sinuses**, course downward to form the **internal jugular vein**, which returns blood to the heart.

Cerebral Veins

The superficial and deep veins collect the circulating blood from the cortical and subcortical areas and empty it into the sinus network. The superficial cerebral (**superior**, **inferior**, and **superficial middle cerebral**) veins collect circulated blood from the neocortex and subcortical white matter and drain it into the superior sagittal sinus (Fig. 7-14).

The deep cerebral veins that include numerous smaller veins (the internal cerebral, basal, choroidal, and thalamostriate) drain blood from the subcortical structures (including the striatum, thalamus, choroid plexus, and hippocampus) and empty into the **great cerebral vein of Galen** that opens into the **straight sinus**.

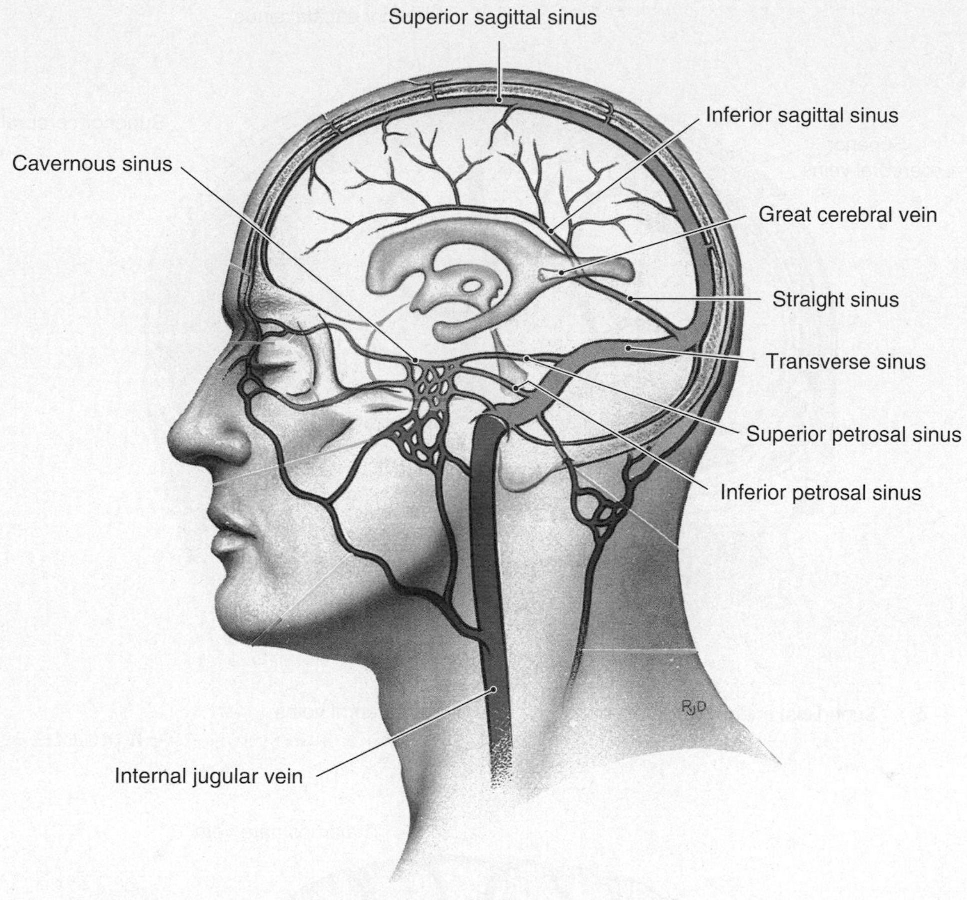

Figure 7-13. Dural venous sinuses system with connections.

The venous drainage of the spinal cord is similar to the arterial network. The anterior and posterior spinal veins are joined by the anterior radicular veins.

CEREBRAL BLOOD FLOW REGULATION

The brain–blood circulation requires the maintenance of a constant BP. The arterial response that regulates blood flow is autoregulated depending on the brain's metabolic needs. The muscle cells in the arterial walls respond by contracting to increased BP while they relax in response to a lower BP. The autoregulation maintains a constant blood flow with a mean arterial pressure in the range of 60 to 140 mm Hg. On average, for normal functioning, the brain needs the blood supply of 50 to 60 mL per 100 g brain tissue per minute. If this flow amount is reduced, the brain cannot optimally function (Table 7-9).

With increasing age, the arteriosclerosis causes the arteries to lose their elasticity, in which case, not only the flow of blood in arteries is reduced but it also flows in spurts, causing an increase in internal BP. The arteries also respond to brain tissue metabolic states. Increased carbon dioxide content in the brain causes the dilation of the arterial walls, allowing greater blood flow to the active gray matter in the brain.

Cushing and **Monroe-Kelly** reflexes become operational in the case of pathologies, such as stroke and traumatic brain injuries, and contribute to the **autoregulation** of blood flow and controls its volume in the brain. The Cushing reflex is a systematic rise in the pressure of blood in case of increased intracranial pressure. This elevated BP overcomes the effect of increased intracranial pressure and ensures adequate vascular perfusion in the brain. The Monroe–Kelly reflex adjusts intracranial volumes of blood, CSF, and tissue content. It decreases blood flow in the case of hydrocephalus and reduces CSF in the case of vessel constriction due to lower blood CO_2.

Key Terms :

Anticoagulant
Blood–brain barrier
Blood platelet inhibitor
Thrombolytic agent
Tissue plasminogen-activating agents (t-PAs)
Vasodilator
Vessel permeability

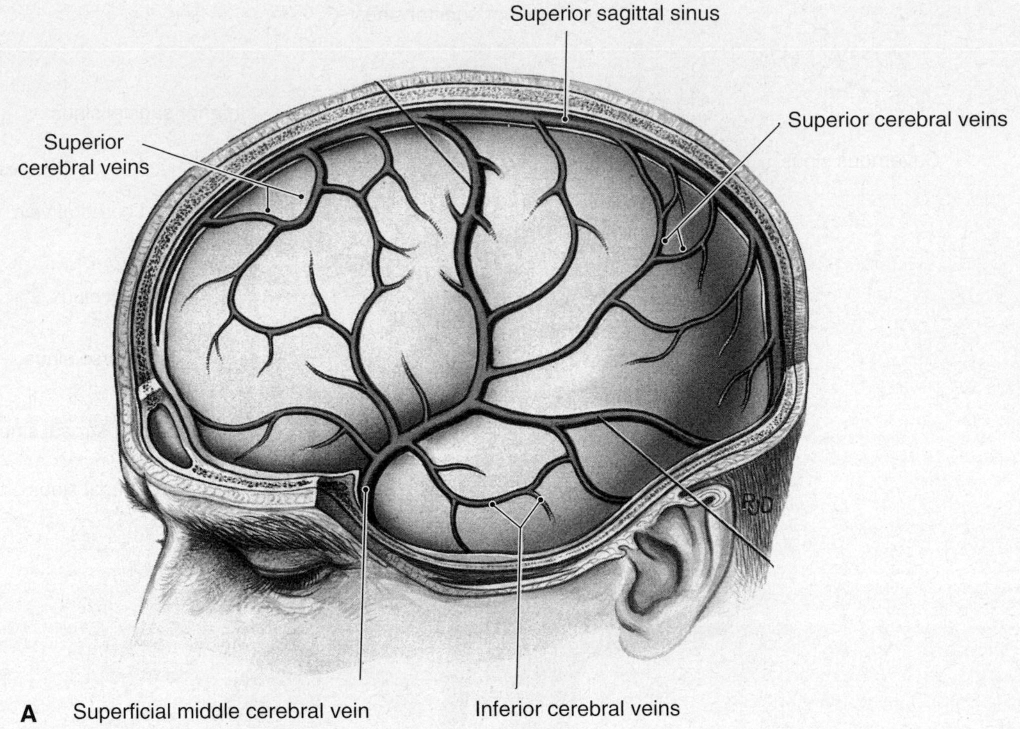

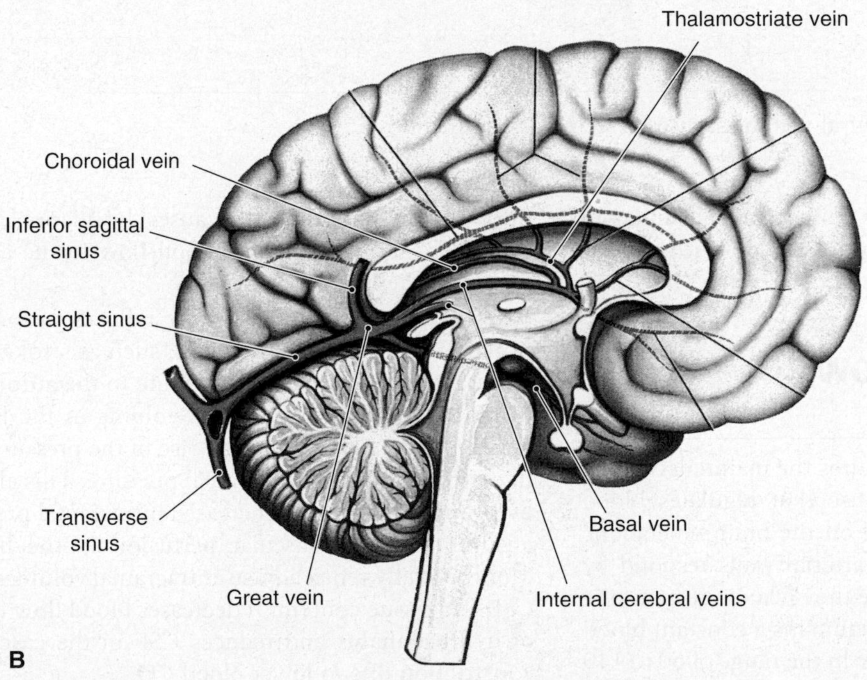

Figure 7-14. Superficial and deep veins. A. Large veins on the lateral surface include branches of superior cerebral, inferior cerebral, and superficial middle cerebral veins. B. Midsagittal view of the internal cerebral veins.

Table 7-9

Blood Flow Volume and Brain Functioning

Flow (mL/100 g brain tissue/min)	Levels of Brain Functioning
50–60	Normal level of brain function
20–45	Lower efficiency of brain function
15–20	Significantly impaired brain function with electrical silence
Consistently < 15	Loss of function with permanent tissue damage

CLINICAL CORRELATES

Treatment of Vascular Diseases

The important goals of medical management of a stroke, including medication and/or surgical intervention, are: (1) decrease morbidity, (2) restore normal blood circulation, (3) contain the infarct size, and (4) reduce poststroke complications. The exact treatment, which is managed by trained professionals, depends on the location of the lesion in the brain and whether the disease is occlusive or hemorrhagic. In the treatment extended in case of cardiac thromboembolic etiology, blood-thinning **anticoagulant** drugs, such as **heparin** or **warfarin** (Coumadin), are used to reduce stroke by preventing further embolization.

Platelet-inhibiting drugs, such as **acetylsalicylic acid** (aspirin), **dipyridamole** (Aggrenox, Persantine), **clopidogrel bisulfate** (Plavix), and **ticlopidine** (Ticlid), are used to control the risks of recurrent TIAs; these drugs achieve their goals by inhibiting thrombus formation by decreasing the aggregation of blood platelets. Cerebral vasodilating drugs, such as **papaverine**, when used on patients with thromboembolic strokes, have had some success. The discovery of **thrombolytic agents**, such as recombinant **tissue plasminogen-activating agents (t-PAs)**, has been very effective in restoring blood flow to the affected area. The tPA opens the clogged vessels within hours by dissolving the thrombotic clot. However, this clot-busting tPA-based treatment is effective only if it is administered intravenously within 3 hours or interarterially within 6 hours of the onset of a stroke; less than 5% of stroke patients are suitable for receiving t-PA treatment. Tissue plasminogen activator is very potent and can cause hemorrhage into the brain, lungs, and abdomen. Thus its administration requires ruling out any predisposition for a hemorrhage.

Treatment for patients with carotid atherosclerosis requires surgical removal of the plaque (endarterectomy). This procedure is highly favorable for symptomatic patients with 70% to 99% stenosis of the culprit carotid artery. Large-scale, randomized, controlled trials also support carotid endarterectomy for primary stroke prevention in asymptomatic patients with 80+% internal carotid artery stenosis (Box 7-8).

Recently, two newer invasive endovascular treatments have become available: carotid **angioplasty/stenting** and the **Merci retrieval system**. Carotid artery angioplasty combined with stent placement using a filter for intracerebral embolic protection can be an alternative to endarterectomy in high-risk surgical patients. The Merci retrieval system can be used in patients with acute stroke to remove fresh clot from the intracerebral branches of the internal carotid artery. This involves the threading of a corkscrew-like device into the blood vessel to restore blood flow by snaring and removing the clot.

Aneurysms that can rupture and cause hemorrhage or neurologic deficit and/or seizures require immediate attention. In the case of a hemorrhagic condition, medically optimal treatment is the reduction of elevated BP. The medical management of an aneurysm involves lowering BP to prevent bleeding. Clipping is used to obliterate the neck or attachment of the aneurysm to the blood vessels, thus disabling it; clipping is undertaken mostly to treat aneurysms that are outside the brain. Hard-to-access aneurysms are treated without opening the skull through coiling, which involves placing a platinum coil in the aneurysm. This coil causes a blood clot to form, sealing off the aneurysm.

Blood–Brain Barrier

The **blood–brain barrier (BBB)** is an important clinical concept and serves as a line of defense for the brain. It restricts the movement of harmful substances, such as infectious microorganisms, from the bloodstream to the brain tissue and extracellular fluid, which is similar to CSF. The BBB regulates the arterial permeability in only the CNS. Brain capillaries, unlike the muscle capillaries, are lined by endothelial cells, which join tightly and leave no intracellular pores or fenestrations. The endothelial cell membrane is surrounded further by the end feet of astrocytes outside the capillary wall (Fig. 7-15). Both of these add to the selective membrane permeability, restricting the flow of harmful substances in the blood to the extracellular space.

Information regarding which substances cross the BBB is important in the medical management of brain diseases. While the BBB keeps harmful microorganisms out of the brain, the BBB can also keep many helpful drugs and antibiotics out, making the treatment of many cerebral infections difficult. Only lipid-soluble substances cross the BBB. The BBB is not fully developed in infants; it makes them vulnerable to more drugs and microorganisms.

Some diseases in the brain enable some normally excluded substances to enter into the CSF and cellular interstitial fluid by disrupting the BBB. Meningitis, stroke,

BOX 7-8

Carotid Endarterectomy

Endarterectomy is a surgical procedure used to remove atherosclerotic plaque from the walls of the internal carotid artery. The plaque, formed by the gradual accumulation of cholesterol, undissolved fatty, lipid-rich substances, cellular deposits and calcium elements, causes stroke by either impeding flow to the brain or by rupturing and releasing debris into the cerebral bloodstream. When this occurs, small particles of the plaque migrate upstream and occlude the smaller arteries within the brain. Localized lack of blood flow to the affected portions of the brain results in stroke. Endarterectomy is performed to physically remove the plaque to reduce the risk of subsequent stroke. The risk of stroke has been found to increase with increasing amount of plaque present within the artery measured as a percent narrowing (stenosis). Large-scale, multi-institutional randomized controlled trials have shown that endarterectomy is indicated in symptomatic patients with 70% to 99% stenosis and in asymptomatic patients with more than 80% stenosis (North American Symptomatic Carotid Endarterectomy Trial Collaborators, 1991; Executive Committee for the Asymptomatic Carotid Atherosclerosis Study, 1995). An alternative method for the treatment of carotid artery disease is percutaneous stent insertion (Executive Committee for the Asymptomatic Carotid Atherosclerosis Study, 1995). This is a less invasive procedure which treats the plaque by "trapping" it under a metal scaffold stent. However, several recent clinical trials comparing stenting against endarterectomy have not demonstrated any major benefit to stenting with higher peri-procedure stroke rates (The SPACE Collaborative Group, 2006; Mas et al., 2010). Therefore, presently, for most patients, endarterectomy remains the standard of care in treatment of carotid artery disease.

Carotid endarterectomy can be performed with the patient under general anesthesia or partially awake. An incision is made in one of the skin folds of the neck to access the affected carotid artery. The common, internal, and external carotid arteries are controlled with vascular clamps. Blood flow to the brain is temporarily occluded and a longitudinal incision is made through the area of the plaque. Patients under general anesthesia are checked to ensure cerebral perfusion is adequate. Several methods can be employed, but if perfusion is low, a temporary silastic tube is placed to "shunt" blood from the common carotid artery to the internal carotid artery upstream from the area of the plaque. The plaque is then completely removed from the artery. The artery is then closed using an intervening patch to repair the incision. This patch technique helps to prevent re-narrowing as the artery heals. The operation lasts approximately one and a half to two hours, does not involve much blood loss, and is typically well tolerated by even high-risk patients. Two main complications can occur with endarterectomy, which have implications for students of communicative behaviors: stroke and nerve injury. The peri-procedural stroke risk is about 1% to 2% in asymptomatic patients and 3% to 5% in symptomatic patients. Permanent or temporary nerve injury can occur to the hypoglossal, marginal mandibular, and recurrent laryngeal nerves, which leads to dysarthria and affects speech intelligibility. Rarely, nerve injury can also occur to the glossopharyngeal, spinal accessory, and superior laryngeal nerves if dissection of the artery is more extensive due to anatomical concerns. Most nerve injury is temporary and resolves by 6 months postoperatively.

and brain tumors are a few conditions that disrupt the BBB and allow toxic substances to enter the brain. In brain tumors, new proliferating capillaries are known to have intracellular pores, which affect the capillary permeability. This has some diagnostic significance, because radioactive amino acids can exit through pores into the brain, allowing the identification of tumor localization.

Lesion Localization

RULE 3: Symptoms Suggesting a Vascular System Disorder

Presenting Symptoms. Sudden development of contralateral hemiplegia of the face (mostly), arm, and upper extremity, more than the leg, with accompanying sensory loss results from occlusion (thrombosis or embolism) of the MCA. Additional symptoms may include the ones discussed under rule 1 in Chapter 2. (An abrupt onset of symptoms indicates vascular pathology, while gradual progression of symptoms indicates a mass lesion, like a tumor.)

Rationale. The regions of the motor cortex involved with the representation of different body parts are perfused by two arteries: the MCA and the ACA. The MCA supplies the area of motor control for the face, hand, and upper extremity, while the ACA serves the motor cortical area with the representation of legs and toes (Fig. 7-4; also see Fig. 16-1). Involvement of the corticospinal fibers accounts for the contralateral paralysis of the face, trunk, and upper extremity. Involvement of the somatosensory cortex and thalamocortical fibers results in hemianesthesia for the trunk, face, and upper extremity.

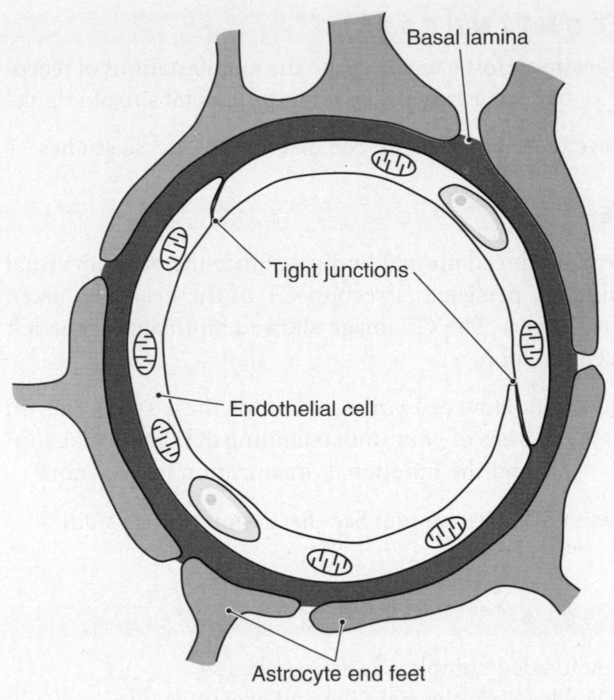

Figure 7-15. The arterial structure contributing to the blood-brain barrier in the brain.

Presenting Symptoms. Toe, foot, and leg paralysis as well as sensory loss and mental impairments (distractibility, indecisiveness, personality changes, and lack of spontaneity) are associated with ischemia due to embolism or thrombosis in the ACA distribution.

Rationale. This artery supplies the medial frontal cortex, which serves personality, higher mental functions, and motor control for the leg (Figs. 16-1, 7-3, and 7-4).

Presenting Symptoms: Homonymous hemianopsia (blindness in contralateral eye and memory impairments are associated with the PCA involvement). Visual agnosia, if present, requires a bilateral involvement of this artery.

Rationale. The PCA supplies the visual cortex in the occipital lobe, inferior-medial temporal lobe, and the thalamus (Fig. 7-3). Low pain threshold also is seen because of the thalamic involvement.

CASE STUDIES FOR PROBLEM SOLVING

CASE ONE (7-1)

A 55-year-old woman was admitted to a hospital for high blood pressure. She had a stroke while sleeping. When she awoke, her right hand and leg would not move, and her head felt heavy. She could not find appropriate words to explain the loss of motor control. She was examined by a neurologist and, at his recommendation, a speech language pathologist. They observed the following:

- Right hemiplegia with intact sensation for touch, pain, and temperature
- Moderate difficulty finding words
- Limited verbal output
- Impaired verbal repetition
- Impaired reading and writing
- Near-normal auditory comprehension

Within a few days, her speech improved, but it still was sparse and consisted of only a few words. She used many gestures and pointed with her left arm. Failure to communicate frustrated her, and she appeared depressed. The brain MRI revealed a large infarct in the left frontal lobe anterior to the central sulcus that involved the anterior language cortex and a large part of the motor cortex.

Question: How can you relate paralysis and the manifestations of aphasia with the identified infarct?

Case (7-1) Discussion: See discussion of case studies

CASE TWO (7-2)

A 65-year-old right-handed man was admitted to a hospital after sudden development of confusion. Initially, the man did not speak much except some jargon and stereotyped expressions. After 3 weeks of care and recovery, he exhibited the following:

- Severe receptive aphasia
- Fluent and copious verbal output
- Severe anomia marked with many (related and unrelated) paraphasic errors and perseverations and excessive usage of general pronouns
- Semantically empty speech
- Impaired ability to repeat stimuli longer than five words
- Severe difficulty in understanding others
- Moderate alexia
- Poor writing, mostly jargon
- Intact somatosensory and motor functions
- Right visual field defect

(Continued)

CASE TWO (7-2) (CONTINUED)

The brain MRI revealed an infarct in the left posterior superior temporal gyrus and parts of the left inferior parietal lobe.

Question: How can you relate the manifestations of receptive aphasia with the temporoparietal site of infarct?

Case (7-2) **Discussion:** See discussion of case studies

CASE THREE (7-3)

A 59-year-old woman woke up blind in the right eye. She was taken to a hospital, where the attending physician noted the following:

- A history of elevated blood pressure
- No history of trauma
- No previous episode of transient ischemic attack
- Right homonymous hemianopia

With selective visual symptoms, a vascular cause was suspected. However, computed tomography (CT) of the head produced normal findings. Since the patient's visual difficulty persisted, a second CT of the head was taken after 3 days. The CT image showed an infarct in the left occipital lobe.

Question: How can you account for these symptoms on the basis of your understanding of the vascular supply and the functional organization in the brain?

Case (7-3) **Discussion:** See discussion of case studies

CASE FOUR (7-4)

A 60 year-old priest was taken to an emergency room for sensorimotor problems that developed abruptly while he was getting ready to go to church to speak for a Sunday service. The attending physician noted the following:

- Unintelligible dysarthric speech
- Hypernasality (with lowered left palate)
- Dysphagia with liquid diet
- Sensation loss on the left side of the face
- Difficulty balancing with falling to the left
- Difficulty hearing in the left ear
- Left-sided complete facial paralysis
- Weakness in the right leg and arm

The brain MRI revealed an infarct in the left caudal lateral–ventral pons extending to the medulla.

Question: How can you account for these symptoms of the left face and paralysis of the right half of the body? Can these symptoms be related to the involvement of the blood supply to the pontomedullary area? If so, how?

Case (7-4) **Discussion:** See discussion of case studies

CASE FIVE (7-5)

A 55-year-old man suffered a stroke while sleeping. He woke up with a headache and was perspiring. In the morning, he appeared confused, could not walk, and had difficulty talking. He was taken to the ER where he presented with the following:

- Paralysis of the right side of the body
- Loss of pain and temperature on the right side of the body
- Lower facial palsy
- Paralysis of the right tongue
- Unintelligible speech marked with distorted consonants, slow rate of speech, hypernasality, aphonic, and breathy voice
- Impaired swallow marked with premature swallow and poor bolus control
- Nearly intact ability to wrinkle forehead
- No aphasic or cognitive impairments

The brain MRI revealed an infarct of the left internal capsule (genu and posterior limb) extending to the medially located thalamus.

Question: How can you explain these symptoms subsequent to a subcortical stroke and explain why the patient did not have aphasia?

CASE (7-5) **Discussion:** See discussion of case studies

CASE SIX (7-6)

A 75-year-old right-handed man, who was diagnosed with stroke and aphasia, was seen by an SLP, who noted the following:

- Fluently spoken and well-articulated speech
- Speech consisting of meaningless strings of words
- Poor repetitions particularly involving longer stimuli
- Impaired comprehension for both spoken and written language
- Moderate-to-severe anomia
- Highly optimistic attitudes

An MRI revealed a large infarct lesion in the left temporal parietal cortex involving Brodmann areas 39, 49, and 22.

Question: How can you identify the aphasia type and account for its association with the lesion site?

Case (7-6) **Discussion:** See discussion of case studies

SUMMARY

The nerve cells in the CNS depend on an adequate and uninterrupted supply of blood and oxygen. The heart pumps oxygenated blood to the CNS through two arterial systems, vertebrobasilar and the carotid. Both of these arterial networks join the arterial circle of Willis at the base of the brain, the major anatomic point for developing a potential collateral circulation. Three cortical branches and numerous penetrating subcortical branches arise from the circle of Willis and supply blood to cortical and subcortical (basal ganglia, thalamus, hypothalamus, and ventricles) structures in the brain. After perfusion, the deoxygenated blood is collected by veins and drained into the sinus system responsible for transmitting the collected blood and CSF back to the heart for reprocessing. Vascular interruptions in CVAs cause injury to neurons and result in focal neurological symptoms. While there is no cure for strokes, the medical treatment is geared to preserve life, minimize damage, restore vascular supply, and prevent future strokes.

REVIEW QUESTIONS

1. Complete the following statements using the appropriate technical terms:

   A. _____ marks a natural link between two blood vessels.

   B. The development of _____ _____ to an ischemic tissue plays an important role in the natural recovery.

   C. Subsequent to a congenital weakness in the arterial wall, _____ results in a localized dilation of an artery.

   D. A _____ _____ _____ results in temporary focal neurological symptoms that can last up to 30 minutes.

   E. The vascular volume that is needed for the optimal brain functioning is approximately _____–_____ ML per minute _____ _____ grams of brain tissue.

   F. The _____ drugs are used to reduce or prevent intravascular clotting in the brain.

   G. Representing the selective permeability of the blood vessels in the brain, the _____ _____ _____ restricts the movement of harmful substances from the _____ to the brain tissue.

   H. In _____ _____, the blood leaks from a ruptured artery and increases pressure in the brain by occupying an intracranial space.

   I. In _____, the sustained presence of elevated arterial blood pressure can cause damage to the heart and the brain.

   J. Thrombolytic drug like tPA (*tissue plasminogen activator*) restores blood circulation by _____ _____ _____.

   K. Three cortical (middle, anterior, posterior) arteries originate from the_____ _____ _____.

   L. _____ _____ is a congenital condition in which the arterial blood shunts to the veins, bypassing the underlying cortical tissue.

   M. In _____, a clump detached from the atherosclerotic plaque flows in the bloodstream and blocks a smaller and distal artery.

   N. A _____ refers to a localized clot that blocks the lumen of a blood vessel.

   O. _____ is the process of narrowing of the arterial lumen owing to accumulation of fatty substances (cholesterol and triglycerides) and lipids along the intimal walls of the blood vessels.

   P. By joining the _____ _____ _____ at the base of the brain, the carotid and vertebrobasilar systems form a major _____ point.

   Q. As an indicator of generalized hypoperfusion cellular death in the area peripheral to the primary distribution zones for the three cerebral arteries is the_____ _____.

   R. _____ pathologies are located beneath the dura mater.

   S. _____ vascular pathologies are located external to the dura mater.

   T. In stroke, an_____ _____ _____ _____ kills brain cells by affecting the oxygen supply.

2. Match each of the following cortical arteries with the brain region it supplies:

a. Anterior cerebral artery (ACA)	a. occipital lobe
b. Posterior cerebral artery (PCA)	b. lateral cortical surface
c. Middle cerebral artery (MCA)	c. midsagittal and ventral frontal surface

3. List three clinical symptoms that are likely to result from a cerebrovascular accident involving the ACA.
4. List three clinical symptoms that are likely to result from a cerebral vascular accident involving the MCA.
5. List two clinical symptoms that are likely to result from a cerebral vascular accident involving the PCA.
6. What is ischemic penumbra? How does it relate to recovery?
7. Define stroke.
8. Why is the blood brain barrier important for the brain?
9. Name the mechanism that maintains a stable blood flow to the brain?
10. List two goals of the medical management of a cerebral vascular accident.

8 Ventricles and Cerebrospinal Fluid

LEARNING OBJECTIVES

After studying this chapter, students should be able to:

- Describe the functions of cerebrospinal fluid (CSF)
- Outline the circulation path of CSF
- Discuss the circulatory disorders of CSF
- Explain the diagnostic significance of CSF

Cerebrospinal fluid (CSF) is a clear, colorless fluid. It is produced by the choroid plexus in the ventricular system and circulates from the ventricles to the subarachnoid space around the CNS. By forming a mechanical cushion around the CNS, the CSF protects the brain and spinal cord from sudden and violent body movements. The buoyancy of the floating CSF, an important protective mechanism, reduces the brain's weight by more than 95%. Thus, a brain weighing 1,400 to 1,500 g in the air would weigh only about 70 to 75 g when floating in CSF. As an active transport mechanism, CSF may also participate in the removal of harmful substances and waste resulting from cellular metabolic activities.

Key Terms:

Cisterns	**Subarachnoid space**
Choroid plexus	**Ventricles**
Collateral trigone	

CHOROID PLEXUS

Extending from the ventricular surface into the ventricular cavity, the **choroid plexus** is formed by an extensive network of infolded vascular capillaries, which are covered by the **vascular pia mater (tela choroidea)** and connective tissue. This also receives an **epithelium layer** from the **ependymal lining** of the inner ventricular surface. The choroid plexus, with a minutely folded surface, is a fenestrated structure with tight junctions around its apical regions. The pores are formed by epithelial cells. The tight junctions between adjacent cells contribute to the barrier for the exchange of dissolved substances between the blood and CSF. The choroid plexus is located primarily in the center of the lateral and fourth ventricles; its largest formation is around the collateral trigone region of the lateral ventricles (Fig. 8-1). No choroid plexus is present in the small opening of the cerebral aqueduct of Sylvius or in the anterior or posterior horns.

Cerebrospinal Fluid Volume

The average total volume of CSF present in the human brain is 120 to 140 mL. The choroid plexus in the human brain secretes about 500 mL/CSF/d (~ 0.35 mL every minute) through passive diffusion from blood. CSF is normally replaced three times every 24 hour and is secreted through the modified capillary–pia membranous network of the choroid plexus. The CSF contains blood plasma but differs from blood in its molecular composition—for example, CSF contains less protein (15–45 mg/dL) and less than half the blood glucose (50–70 mg/dL) and has almost no white or red blood cells. Diseases of the CNS can change the constituent composition of CSF, which has diagnostic importance for identifying pathologic changes in the CNS.

CEREBROSPINAL FLUID CIRCULATION

CSF circulates in the ventricles and the subarachnoid space. There are four ventricles in the brain (Fig. 8-1; also see Fig. 2-36): two lateral ventricles (one in each hemisphere), the third ventricle (between two thalami), and the fourth ventricle (in the brainstem). CSF flows from both lateral ventricles in the cerebral hemispheres to the third ventricle via the interventricular foramen (of Monro). The third ventricle, which is located vertically between the two thalami, drains its fluid to the fourth ventricle through the cerebral aqueduct (of Sylvius). From the fourth ventricle, CSF enters the subarachnoid space through three openings: two lateral openings of foramina of Luschka and one mediodorsal opening of foramen of Magendie (Fig. 8-1).

The subarachnoid space wraps around the entire CNS between the arachnoid membrane and pia mater. The subarachnoid space varies from region to region: it is

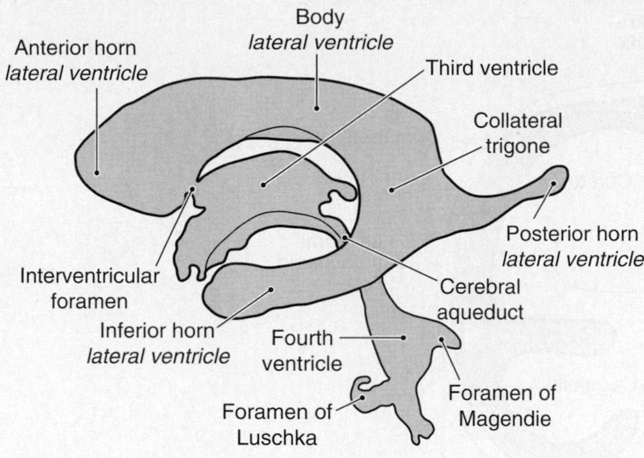

Figure 8-1 Lateral view of the ventricles.

narrow over the gyri and wide over the fissures. The arachnoid, which rests under the dura mater, is separated from the dura by a potential **subdural space**, whereas the pia mater closely adheres to the cortical surface. Arachnoid trabeculae extend from the arachnoid to the pia mater and contribute to the maintenance of the subarachnoid space (Fig. 8-2; see Fig. 2-46A).

The subarachnoid space houses many **cisterns** that serve as large pockets of CSF. The important cisterns are the **cerebellomedullary**, **superior**, **interpeduncular**, **chiasmatic**, **pontine**, and **lumbar**. These cisterns receive fluid from the fourth ventricle. The lumbar cistern, the largest of these, extends from L2 to S2 and contains fibers of the cauda equina and filum terminale (Fig. 8-2).

Once in the subarachnoid space, CSF flows up toward the convexity of the brain or down toward the spinal cord. Some CSF infiltrates the depths of the cerebral cortex along the blood vessels that penetrate the brain. This area around the penetrating blood vessels is the perivascular space, the site for possible diffusion of metabolic solutes from the CSF into the extracellular fluid (see Fig. 2-46). The diffusion of metabolites has important implications for medical treatment.

ABSORPTION OF THE CEREBROSPINAL FLUID

CSF is absorbed through the **arachnoid granulations**, which are one-way openings. These tufted structures are dorsal along both sides of the superior sagittal sinus

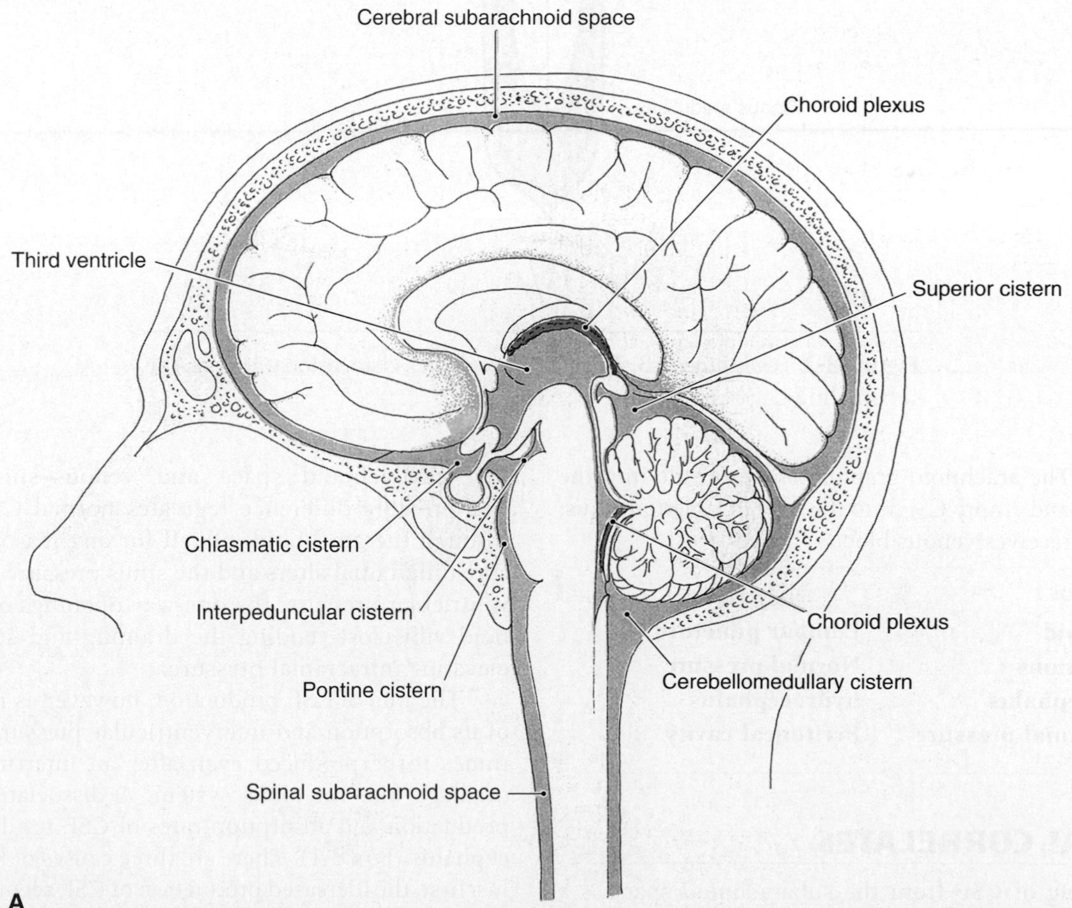

Figure 8-2 A. Sagittal view of the subarachnoid space and major subarachnoid cisterns.

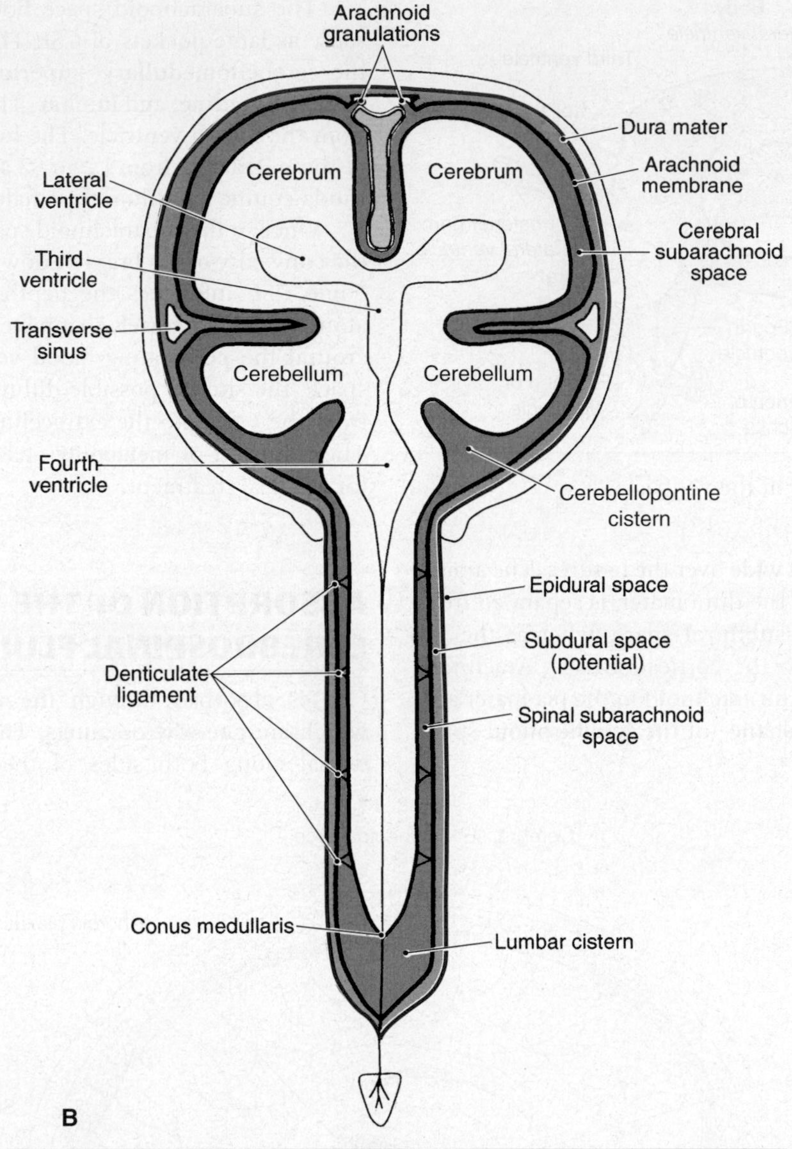

Figure 8-2 (*Continued*) B. Frontal view of the cistern locations of the subarachnoid spaces.

(Fig. 8-3). The arachnoid granulations protrude into the dural sinus and empty CSF into the superior sagittal sinus, which also receives venous blood.

> ***Key Terms :***
>
> **Arachnoid granulations**
> **Hydrocephalus**
> **Intracranial pressure**
> **Lumbar puncture**
> **Normal pressure hydrocephalus**
> **Peritoneal cavity**

CLINICAL CORRELATES

The draining of CSF from the subarachnoid space is a pressure-sensitive process. Emptying CSF into the superior sagittal sinus requires a pressure differential between the subarachnoid space and **venous–sinus system**. The pressure difference regulates normal CSF drainage through the arachnoid villi. If for any reason this pressure differential alters and the sinus pressure exceeds the ventricular pressure, the one-way openings of the arachnoid villi close, ending the draining and subsequently elevating intracranial pressure.

The rate of CSF production, however, is independent of its absorption and interventricular pressure. CSF continues to be produced even after an interruption in its drainage into the sinus system. A dissociation between production and absorption rates of CSF results in **hydrocephalus** (Box 8-1). There are three causes of hydrocephalus: first, the increased production of CSF, second, blocking of the draining path from the ventricles to the subarachnoid space, and third, impaired CSF absorption in the

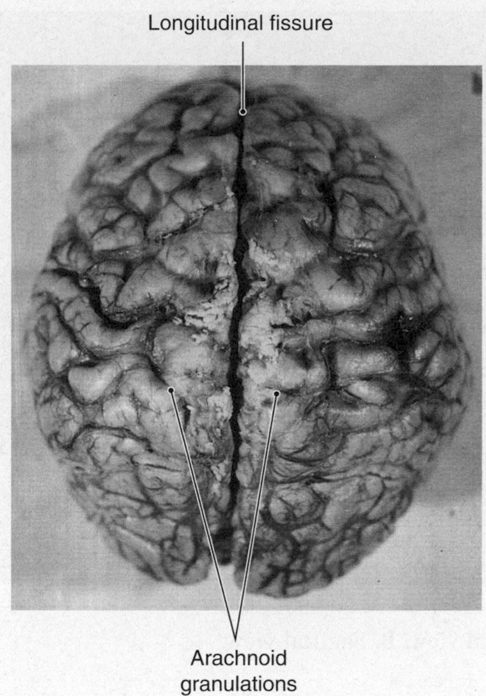

Figure 8-3 An image of the tufted prolongations of pia-arachnoid villi (granulation), which drain CSF into the superior sagittal sinus.

subarachnoid space. Regardless of the underlying cause, in hydrocephalus, an excessive amount of CSF leads to an increased pressure in the brain. Sustained pressure increase causes enlargement of the ventricles and damage to the surrounding cortical tissue (Fig. 8-4). If hydrocephalus begins in infancy, the increased CSF pressure also enlarges the cranial vault.

Circulatory Disorders

Obstruction in the path of CSF flow or its impaired absorption in the subarachnoid space leads to hydrocephalus; the subsequent CSF accumulation causes the ventricles to enlarge. There are two primary (communicating and obstructive) and two secondary (**normal pressure** and **ex vacuo**) types of hydrocephalus.

Primary Types

In communicating hydrocephalus, the problem relates to an inadequate drainage of the CSF into the sinus; its access to the subarachnoid space through the foramina of Magendie and Luschka is open and functional. Choroid tumor and inflammation (meningitis) of the brain are two common causes of communicating hydrocephalus.

In obstructive (noncommunicating) hydrocephalus, the CSF flow from the ventricles to the subarachnoid space is blocked. The obstruction can occur either in the ventricular system itself or in apertures (Luschka and Magendie foramina) from the fourth ventricle. The most common site of blockage is the narrow aperture of the cerebral aqueduct in the midbrain. A mesencephalic tumor also can cause hydrocephalus by contributing to the narrowing (stenosis) of the cerebral aqueduct.

Regardless of the hydrocephalic type, the final result affects brain functions. An increased CSF pressure enlarges the ventricles and elevates the intracranial pressure. This compresses the surrounding white and gray matters (Fig. 8-4), affecting vital cortical functions, including sensorimotor and higher mental functions. In children with hydrocephalus, the head becomes pyramidal, and the face is disproportionately small with the eyes turned outward. In the most advanced cases of hydrocephalus, a coronal section of the brain would reveal two large compartments of the lateral ventricles, and the cortical mantle is substantially reduced to a thin layer between the ventricles and skull. In children, developmental abnormalities can cause

BOX 8-1

Hydrocephalus

Hydrocephalus is a neurological condition of abnormal circulation and/or absorption of the CSF. An obstruction in the flow of the CSF from the choroid plexus ventricles to the site of its absorption into the venous system through the arachnoid granulations (villi) in the superior sagittal sinus causes excessive accumulation of CSF within the ventricular cavity of the brain. This makes the ventricles dilate and enlarges the cranium in children. Untreated hydrocephalus also contributes to brain atrophy and results in mental deficiency. The adult skull does not increase in size; rather the ventricles enlarge at the expense of the surrounding cortical tissues, and there is a substantially higher intracranial pressure.

A major cause of congenital hydrocephalus in infants, particularly in the fetal period, is the Arnold Chiari malformation, in which the posterior cranial fossa does not normally develop, and the cerebellum herniates into the vertebral canal (see Chapter 4). Meningitis is another cause of hydrocephalus, as it impairs the draining outlets of the arachnoid granulations.

Clinically the circulatory failures of the CSF are marked by abnormal behavioral symptoms, such as slow thinking and decreased responsiveness, lethargy, stupor, and coma in some severe cases. Hydrocephalus can be treated surgically by diverting CSF into the blood stream.

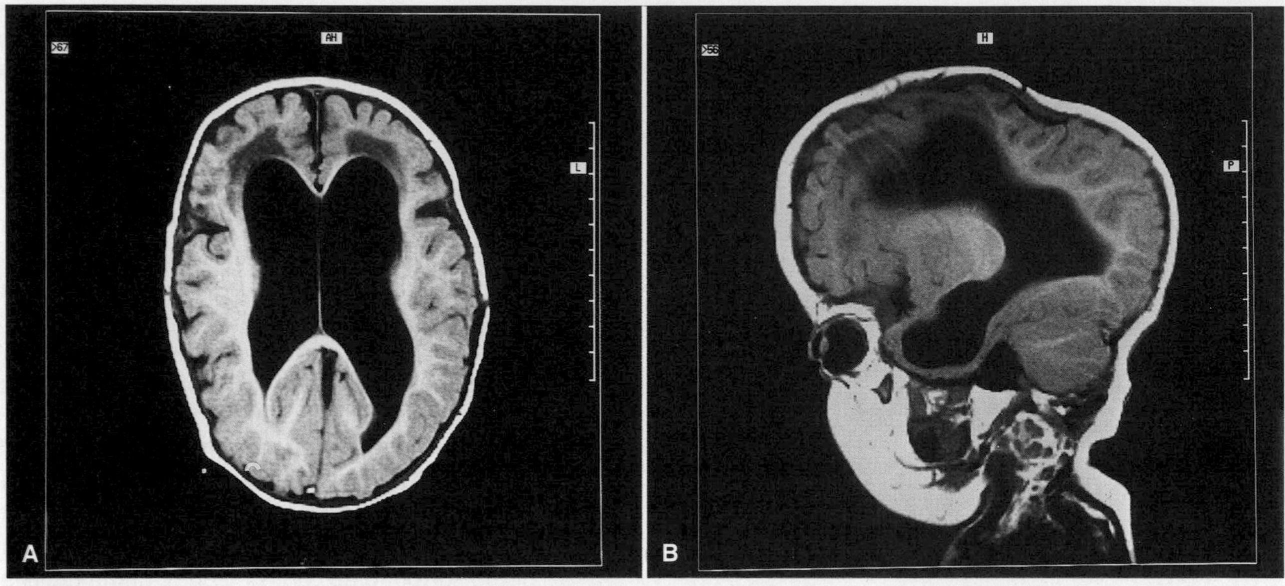

Figure 8-4 MRI of the enlarged lateral ventricles in a child: A. Axial view. B. Sagittal view.

congenital hydrocephalus that is present even during the fetal period.

Secondary Types

Ventricular dilation can also occur subsequent to other brain pathologies, such as brain atrophy (hydrocephalus ex vacua), traumatic injuries, and brain inflammation (normal pressure hydrocephalus). The secondary hydrocephalic conditions are commonly present in the elderly population.

Although not a true hydrocephalic condition, hydrocephalus ex vacuo causes a generalized cortical atrophy. With the atrophy of the gray and white matter, the ventricular space is larger but without any significant increase in CSF pressure. It may take years to develop this condition; symptoms may relate to generalized atrophy of the brain.

Commonly seen among elderly individuals, normal pressure hydrocephalus can result from meningitis, subarachnoid hemorrhage, and/or trauma. The ventricular space is enlarged, though CSF pressure fluctuates from time to time. Common problems seen in patients with normal pressure hydrocephalus are frequent urination, impaired gait, and dementia.

Treatment

Hydrocephalus is no longer a fatal and hopeless condition. If diagnosed early, it can be corrected by surgical procedures. Treatment involves diverting the blocked ventricular CSF into the blood stream or to another body cavity for absorption. A thin rubber tube is inserted surgically into the enlarged ventricular cavity and is used to divert CSF flow to the abdominal peritoneal cavity, pleural space, or right atrium of the heart. Usually, the tube has a valve system to help regulate the pressure inside the skull, preventing complete collapse of the brain. This is called a shunt. Draining into the peritoneal (potential fluid-filled gap between the abdonial muscle and abdominal organs) cavity is the most common procedure.

Diagnostic Significance of Cerebrospinal Fluid

Changes in the pressure and composition of CSF have diagnostic significance. CSF pressure is measured by **lumbar puncture**. A needle is inserted into the lumbar subarachnoid space between the L3 and S1 (Fig. 8-5; Box 8-2) vertebrae, because spinal penetration at this point does not injure any nerve fibers. Once CSF starts flowing, the needle hub is attached to a manometer or other pressure-sensitive device. The normal CSF pressure range in an adult is 80 to 180 mm H_2O. A pressure level higher than normal is an indicator of a pathologic process and can occur in response to increased amounts of CSF, brain swelling, and brain tumors. Further, on a chemical analysis, any deviation from the normal compositional values (protein = 15–45 mg/dL, glucose = 50–70 mg/dL, and white blood cells = 1–5/mL) are considered diagnostically important and help in the differential diagnosis of infections of the brain and meninges—**multiple sclerosis, neurosyphilis, Guillain–Barré syndrome, carcinomatous meningitis**, and **neuropathies**. Lumbar puncture is contraindicated in cases of increased intracranial pressure because of the possibility of a brainstem herniation.

Spinal puncture also is used to administer anesthesia in the lower spinal region.

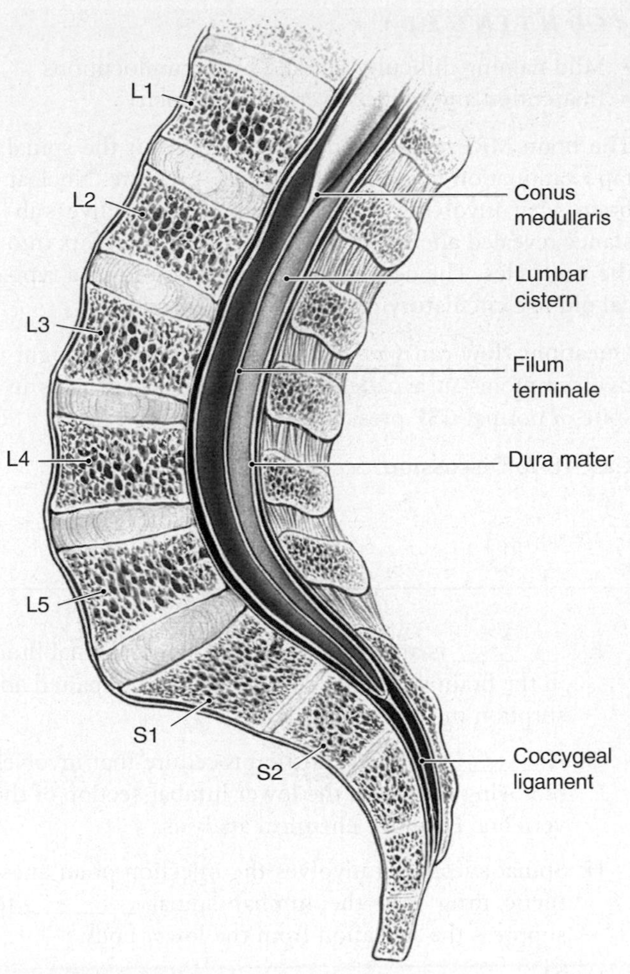

Figure 8-5 The lumbar cistern, the site used for removing CSF during the lumbar puncture.

BOX 8-2

Lumbar Puncture

Lumbar puncture is an invasive procedure that involves removing a small amount of CSF for diagnostic purposes. The fluid is removed through a puncture into the subarachnoid space of the lumbar region by inserting a needle between L3 and S1. A CSF pressure level higher than normal can be an indicator of brain swelling or brain tumors. A chemical analysis of the removed fluid provides important diagnostic information. For example, bacterial meningitis, infection, or cerebral infarct causes the white blood cell count to increase. Elevated CSF protein content suggests a block in the subarachnoid space. Presence of blood pigments may indicate an intracranial hemorrhage. Deviations from the normal compositional values (protein = 15–45 mg/dL, glucose = 50–70 mg/dL, and white blood cells = 1–5/ mL) are considered diagnostically important. The other function of this procedure is the administration of anesthetic drugs into the spinal subarachnoid space that leads to suppression of pain in the lower body.

CASE STUDIES FOR PROBLEM SOLVING

CASE ONE (8-1)

A 25-year-old graduate student had not felt well for 3 months as she reportedly suffered from severe headache, lethargy, slow thinking, forgetfulness, and frequent attacks of nausea. She was seen by a neurologist who noted near-normal sensorimotor and cranial nerve functions. Further testing revealed that the woman was somewhat lethargic and exhibited some confusion and a slow ability to process language. The brain MRI revealed a large lateral–ventricular and third ventricular cavity. She also reported experiencing some autonomic dysfunctioning, such as insomnia and irregular menses.

Question: How can you relate these symptoms with the blocked cerebrospinal fluid (CSF) system and underlying diseased condition?

Case (8-1) Discussion: See discussion of case studies

(Continued)

CASE TWO (8-2) *(CONTINUED)*

A 75-year-old retired professor who had been experiencing memory problems and difficulty in walking straight due to imbalance was examined by a neurologist who noted the following:

- Unsteady gait marked by wavering and tendency to fall
- Frequent need for urination
- Indifferent personality

SLP consultation revealed:

- Normal comprehension
- Well-articulated speech
- Short-term memory problem
- Difficulty in learning new information
- Incoherence in spontaneous discourse
- Reduced pragmatics marked by impaired topic maintenance and turn-taking ability
- Mild naming difficulty marked by circumlocutions
- Inattention and reduced verbal spontaneity

The brain MRI revealed large ventricles, but the spinal tap examination revealed normal CSF pressure. Nuclear brain scan involving the injection of radioactive substance revealed altered absorption with a CSF reflux into the ventricles. The neurologist diagnosed it to be a typical old-age circulatory problem.

Question: How can you explain these prefrontal cognitive symptoms in a patient with enlarged ventricles in spite of normal CSF pressure?

Case (8-2) Discussion: See discussion of case studies

SUMMARY

CSF, produced by the choroid plexus, circulates from the ventricles to the subarachnoid space before its absorption into the sinus system. Along with the meningeal membranes, CSF, with its buoyancy, protects the brain and spinal cord. Its other function is to regulate extracellular environments by removing harmful substances and waste products that result from cellular metabolic activities. Inadequate drainage of the CSF results in excessive accumulation of CSF followed by increased intracranial pressure and hydrocephalus. Hydrocephalus can be treated by surgically implanting a shunt. However, if not adequately treated, the increased intracranial pressure that accompanies hydrocephalus enlarges the ventricular cavity and causes irreparable brain damage.

REVIEW QUESTIONS

1. Complete the following statements using the appropriate technical terms:

   A. At the ________, the ventricular body enlarges before diverging into the posterior and inferior horns.

   B. A blockage of the draining passage through which CSF reaches the subarachnoid space causes ________ type of hydrocephalus.

   C. A pressure difference between the sinus system and ventricular cavity regulates normal CSF drainage through the ________ into the superior sagittal sinus.

   D. If the sinus pressure exceeds ventricular pressure, the arachnoid villi close, causing an ________ in the brain.

   E. The ________ covered with ependymal cells secretes CSF through a ________ from the blood.

   F. ________ is an accumulation of cerebrospinal fluid in the brain ventricles secondary to its impaired absorption in the sinus system.

   G. A ________ is a diagnostic procedure that involves removing CSF from the lower lumbar section of the vertebral canal for chemical analysis.

   H. Spinal anesthesia involves the injection of an anesthetic drug into the lumbar spinal ________ to suppress the sensation from the lower body.

   I. The ________ are the sites for the secretion and storage of CSF.

   J. The common midbrain site associated with obstructive hydrocephalus and the enlargement of the lateral ventricles is the ________.

2. Match the type of hydrocephalus with its associated description:

A. Communicating sagittal sinus	a. impaired CSF drainage into the superior
B. Obstructive (noncommunicating)	b. large ventricular cavities subsequent to brain atrophy
C. Normal pressure hydrocephalus	c. blocked access of the CSF to the subarachnoid space
D. Hydrocephalus ex vacuo	d. hydrocephalus with impaired gait, frequent urination, and dementia

3. What is the major complication of increased intracranial pressure in the brain?

4. Name the spinal site used for lumbar puncture.

5. Name two clinical functions of the lumbar puncture.
6. Name the foramina that are associated with the following functions:
   A. Connecting lateral ventricles to the third ventricle
   B. Connecting the third ventricle to the fourth ventricle
   C. Discharging CSF from the fourth ventricle to the subarachnoid space
7. Which of the ventricles in the brain has cavities in both hemispheres?
8. How does a cerebral aqueduct stenosis contribute to hydrocephalus?
9. Name the structure that drains CSF into the superior sagittal sinus.

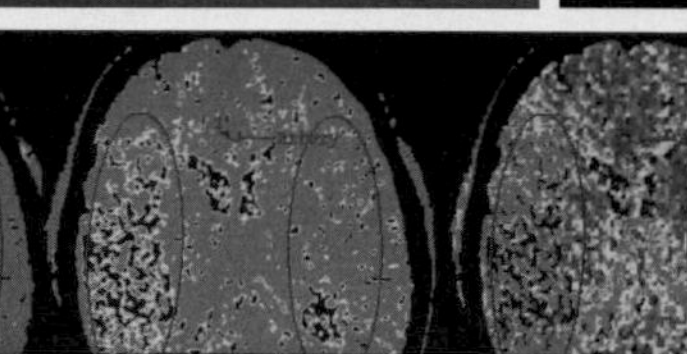

9 Auditory System

LEARNING OBJECTIVES

After studying this chapter, students should be able to:

- Discuss the inner ear response to transmitted sounds
- Discuss the brain's mechanism used for localizing sound sources
- Describe the central auditory mechanism outlining the central auditory pathway
- Explain distinctive characteristics of the auditory mechanism
- Discuss the potential reticular role in auditory processing
- Outline the effects of cortical and subcortical lesions on hearing
- Differentiate between conductive and sensorineural hearing losses
- Describe the clinical importance of common audiometric/special hearing tests
- Discuss the role of the descending auditory pathway

Essential to spoken language, the sense of hearing serves as a foundation for verbal communication and, along with other senses contributes to the social quality of life. Hearing impairments, congenital or acquired, restrict human communication by affecting the transmission and/or perception of sound signals.

The process of audition (hearing) begins as the sound waves strike the **tympanic membrane**. The vibration of the tympanic membrane converts the pressure waves into mechanical energy, setting the middle-ear **ossicles** into motion. This mechanical energy is further transformed into a hydraulic energy in the cochlear fluid of the **inner ear**. The inner ear patterned hydraulic waves stimulate the **cochlear hair cells**, which send the coded impulses through the fibers of the vestibulocochlear (CN VIII) nerve to the **cochlear nuclear complex** in the brainstem. The **cochlear complex** nuclei transmit nerve impulses to multiple synaptic points in the brainstem and the thalamus before projecting to the primary auditory cortex. The combined signals from both ears, their intensity, and interaural time difference are integrated for sound localization. Auditory impulses travel to the primary auditory cortex on the superior surface of the temporal lobe in the Heschl gyri. The primary cortical area is involved with the sound pattern analysis that is needed for auditory discrimination and sound perception. The perceived auditory impulses finally travel to the Wernicke (language cortex) area in the left hemisphere, where auditory signals are interpreted into language-specific meaningful messages for the comprehension of spoken language. This chapter provides a functional description of the anatomy and physiology of hearing from the ear to the primary auditory cortex.

Key Terms :

Cochlear hair cells	**Intensity**
Decibel	**Ossicles**
Frequency	**Pitch**
Hearing level	**Sound pressure level**

SOUND AND PROPERTIES

Sound is created when a force sets a molecular vibration in the medium that propagates a pressure wave. It is the movement of the molecules in the medium that transmits sound and it is characterized by two major attributes: frequency and intensity.

Frequency, the speed of particles vibration is measured in cycles per second, or Hertz (Hz). The cochlea is uniquely equipped to identify the individual frequency components of a complex sound. Frequency analysis determines if the sound is a pitch (harmonically related tones) or a noise (random tones). The human ear can detect sounds within a range of 20 to 20,000 Hz. The frequencies that are important for human speech fall in the range of 250 to 8,000 Hz, with most sensitive frequencies range being 1,000– to 3,000 Hz. Low- and high-frequency sound are perceived respectively as having a low and high pitch. However, the relationship between frequency and pitch is not always linear.

Similarly, the human hearing apparatus is also sensitive to a selected intensity range over a large dynamic range. Represented by the amplitude of the sound waves, the intensity is the strength of molecular movement, and it correlates with perceived loudness. The sound intensity is measured in decibels (dB), which are defined as the log of the ratio between the **measured sound pressure** (P_x) at the tympanic membrane and a well-defined **reference sound pressure** (P_r). The formula for calculating the **sound pressure level** (SPL) in decibels is: SPL (dB) = 20 log P_x/P_r.

The reference sound pressure is always 0.0002 dyne/cm², or 20 μPa, which represents the SPL that is required to make a 1,000 Hz sound just audible to the human ear. If P_x equals P_r, the SPL is 0 dB. A measure of 0 dB does not mean that there is no sound; rather, it means that the measured sound pressure is equal to the reference sound pressure.

A sound that is 10 times the power of 20 μPa (level of a just audible sound) has a 20 dB SPL. If the measured sound pressure is 100 times the reference sound pressure (just audible level), the intensity of the measured sound would be 40 dB, because log 100 = 2.

The human ear is sensitive to an SPL intensity range of 0 to 140 dB, with most spoken communication taking place at 60 dB. Prolonged and repeated exposure to sounds >90 to 100 dB may cause permanent structural damage to the cochlear hair cells; this is commonly seen in industrial workers. Sounds >140 dB cause pain.

Changes in intensity are perceived as changes in loudness. However, there is not always a 1:1 relationship between loudness and intensity. This is because the human ear is not equally sensitive to all sound frequencies. More intensity is required at some frequencies for a listener to detect the presence of that sound than at others. For example, the average normal-hearing listener needs 45.5 dB to hear a 125 Hz sound but requires only 8.5 dB to hear a 2,000 Hz sound. Thus, the best known reference for decibels is hearing level (HL), which indicates sound intensity in relation to average normal hearing. An HL of 0 dB denotes an intensity level that is barely heard by the human ear.

Key Terms:

External auditory meatus	**Malleus**
Eustachian tube	**Stapes**
Incus	**Tympanic membrane**

ANATOMY AND PHYSIOLOGY

Transmission of Sound

The **external ear** (the cartilaginous **pinna, external auditory meatus**, and tympanic membrane) (Fig. 9-1) contributes to sound detection by collecting and then channeling the collected sound waves in the external auditory meatus to the tympanic membrane. The pinna and canal enhance the peak resonance of the sound particularly those coming from the back of the head and they also play a role in sound localization.

The air-filled cavity of the middle ear contains three interconnected ossicles (the **malleus, incus**, and **stapes** that are suspended by ligaments), which connect the tympanic membrane to the **oval window** of the inner ear. The **eustachian tube**, which runs from the middle ear to the nasopharynx, ventilates the middle ear by equalizing middle-ear pressure with the atmospheric pressure.

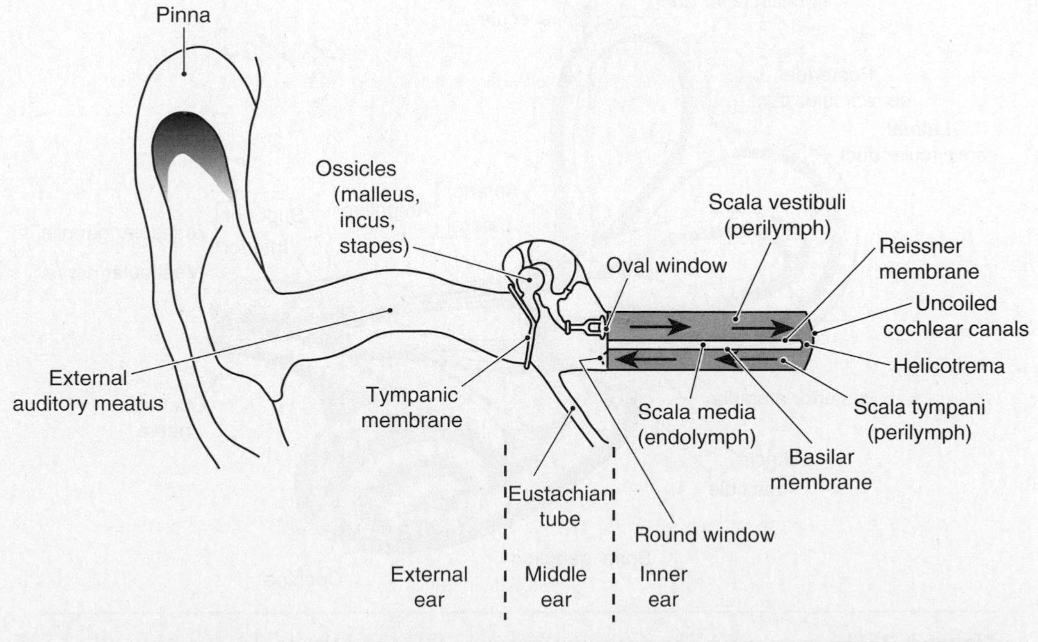

Figure 9-1 Anatomy of the external, middle, and inner compartments of the human ear.

The middle ear regulates its energy transmission to the inner ear using the stiffness of the ossicles to compensate not only for the difference in impedance between air and fluid, but also for the size discrepancy between the tympanic membrane (50 mm^2) and the oval window (3.5 mm^2). It does so by reducing the movement of the tympanic membrane and by increasing its force on the cochlear oval window to ensure an optimal transmission of sound. The mass and stiffness of the ossicular action restrict the motion speed, which limits the range of sound frequencies that can be efficiently transmitted through the middle ear. Thus, we hear only the sound frequencies that are not dampened by these motion limitations imposed by the mass and stiffness.

The motion of the middle-ear ossicles is reflexively controlled by two muscles: **tensor tympani** and **stapedius**. These muscles reflexively protect the auditory mechanism from damage by controlling the ossicular motion when exposed to high-intensity sounds. The stapedius muscle, controlled by the facial (CN VII) nerve, inserts into the stapes and contracts to restrict the stapes' movement in response to sounds louder than 70 to 80 dB. The tensor tympani muscle, controlled by the trigeminal (CN V) nerve, inserts into the malleus and participates in restricting ossicular movements in response to louder sounds, specifically noises (Moor and Linthicum, 2004). Together, both muscles stiffen the ossicular system and attenuate the transmission of energy for high-intensity sounds to the inner ear (attenuation reflex) with a reflex latency time of 50 to 150 ms. This latency is too long to fully protect the inner ear from any loud noise. Further, the sound intensity is attenuated by only approximately 10 to 15 dB, which is largely caused by the action of the stapedius muscle and affects only low-frequency sounds. The extent of noise attenuation by the tensor tympani is small, as this muscle is more involved with the flexibility of the tympanic membrane.

> ***Key Terms:***
> **Endolymph**
> **Depolarization**
> **Graded potentials**
> **Inner hair cells**
> **Nerve impulse**
> **Outer hair cells**
> **Perilymph**

Inner Ear

The inner ear consists of a dual-functional mechanism for serving the special sensory modalities of audition and equilibrium which are served by the interconnected fluid-filled **membranous labyrinth ducts** (Fig. 9-2). The dual-function membranous labyrinth is encased in a series of cavities in the petrous portion of the temporal bone (**bony labyrinth**). The membranous labyrinth contains the fluid-filled saccule, utricle, **semicircular ducts**, and the cochlear duct. The vestibular apparatus (saccule, utricle, and semicircular ducts) mediate equilibrium (see Chapter 10), whereas the cochlear duct (**scala media**) of the membranous labyrinth serves hearing and other special sensory functions.

Cochlear Structure

The cochlea is a snail-shaped structure coiled 2.5 times around the **modiolus**, the central bony core of the cochlea

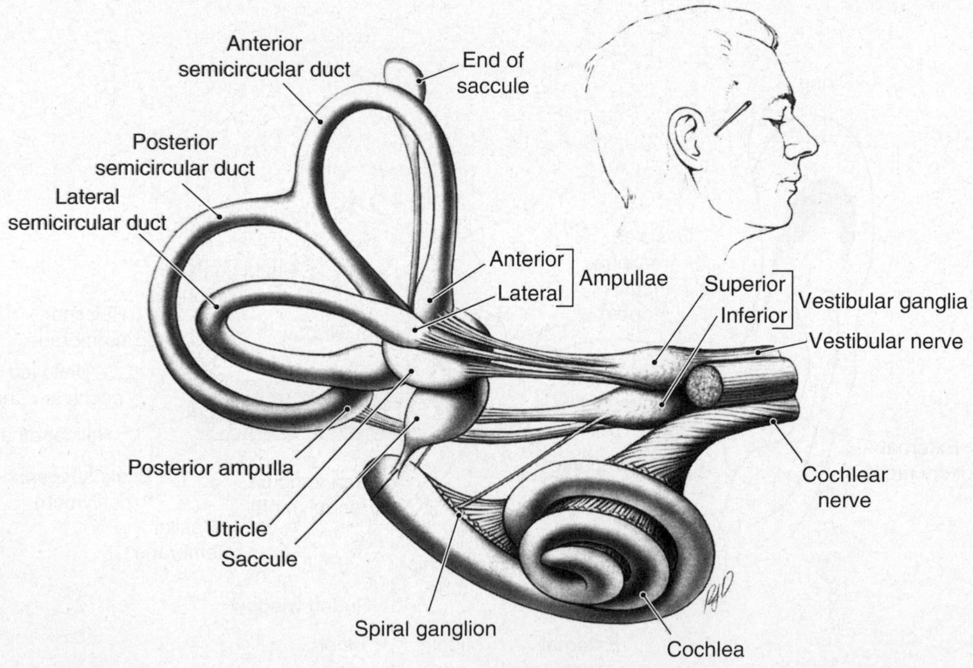

Figure 9-2 The vestibular labyrinth, circuitous cochlea and the cochlear and vestibular nerves.

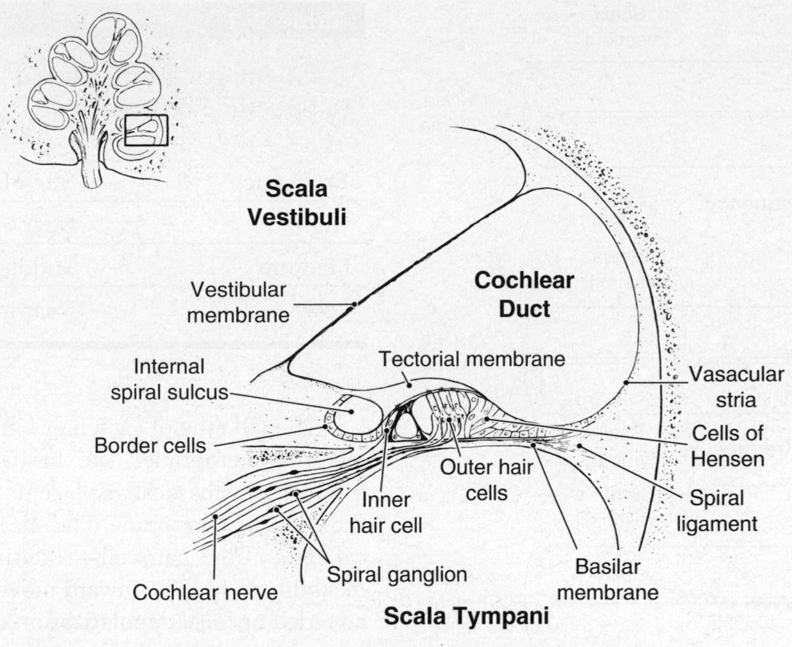

Figure 9-3 The cochlear duct on a radial section of the cochlea showing the cavities of the scalae vestibuli, media, and tympani and the structures of the cochlear duct. The location of the section is given in the inset.

(Fig. 9-2). It is shown in cross-sectioned Figure 9-3 and uncoiled in Figures 9-1 and 9-4. The cochlea consists of three fluid-filled scalae: the **scala vestibuli** (upper compartment), scala media, and **scala tympani** (lower compartment). The scala vestibuli follows the inner contour of the cochlear duct and joins the scala tympani at the apex of the cochlea though the **helicotrema**. The scala media, which ends near the cochlear apex, is between the scala tympani and scala vestibuli.

The scala vestibuli and tympani are filled with **perilymph**, a fluid similar to the CSF in composition with high sodium (Na^+) concentration. As part of the membranous labyrinth, the scala media is filled with **endolymph**. With a high concentration of potassium (K^+), this is similar in composition to intracellular fluid, and it is largely maintained by **stria vascularis** located on the outer wall of the cochlea (Box 9-1). The scala media (cochlear duct) contains the sensory organ of Corti with sensory hair cells, the primary receptor cells. Hair cells in humans are arranged in three rows of **outer hair cells (OHCs)** and one row of **inner hair cells (IHCs)**, which run along the length of the basilar membrane. There are approximately 12,000 OHCs and 3,500 IHCs. Projecting from each OHC are 40 to 150 **stereocilia**, and projecting from each IHC are 50 to 70 bands of stereocilia. The taller **cilia** (apical ends) of the hair cells project to the overlying **tectorial membrane**, which extends over the entire organ of Corti. The IHCs and OHCs differ in terms of their innervation. The bases of the IHCs are innervated by the cochlear nerve endings, whereas the OHC are connected to the projections from the descending auditory pathways, particularly the **olivocochlear bundle** (OCB).

Cochlear Function

The cochlea absorbs the mechanical energy and is concerned with transferring sound vibrations into neural impulses. Since the basilar membrane is structurally flexible, it responds to the transmitted pressure in the cochlear perilymph by its displacement. The basilar membrane is known for its tonotopic representation, which ranges from 20 to 20,000 Hz, with higher frequency representation in the base, which is narrower in comparison to its apex, the site of low frequencies. As the basilar membrane is displaced at its base, the deformation moves toward the apex of the cochlea as a traveling wave. As the pressure wave moves, its velocity slows, but the amplitude increases toward the apex, eventually reaching its maximum. Different sound frequencies produce different traveling wave patterns, with peak amplitude at different regions of the cochlea (Table 9-1). The peak amplitude of the traveling wave for high-frequency sound occurs near the base of the basilar membrane.

As the frequency of the stimulus decreases, the peak amplitude of the traveling wave moves toward the helicotrema. A signal consisting of many frequencies causes a sound wave to have multiple peaks along the basilar membrane. Hair cells are most stimulated at the point of the maximum peaks (Fig. 9-4); the differential displacement of the basilar membrane suggests cochlear frequency selectivity/tuning to its mechanical properties.

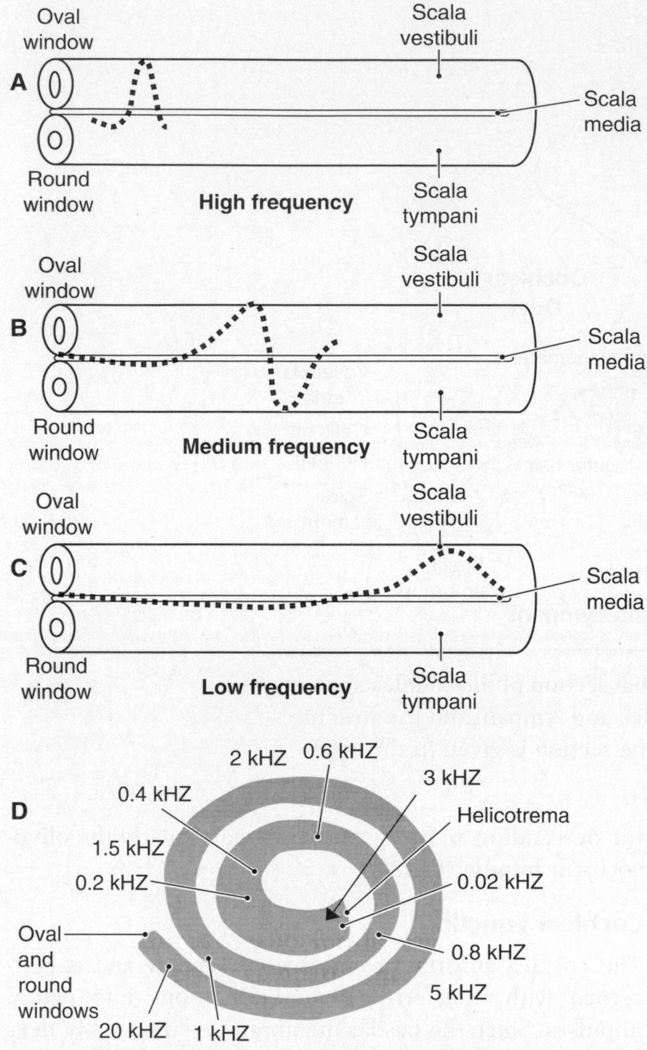

Figure 9-4 Traveling wave patterns of high (A)-, medium (B)-, and low-frequency (C) sounds and the corresponding basilar membrane points (D) of displacements.

Table 9-1

Cochlear Locations Tuned to Specific Frequencies

Frequency	Site of Maximum Amplitude
High	Near oval window
Medium	Middle
Low	Near helicotrema

The tall cilia of each hair bundle are embedded in the tectorial membrane. The basilar membrane movement produces mechanical displacement of these cilia relative to the tectorial membrane. The shearing effect bends the apical ends of the hair cells, resulting in increased cilia permeability to K^+. The inward movement of the ions leads to a graded or local depolarization of the hair cell; the depolarized cell causes the synaptic vesicles to release a neurotransmitter in the synaptic cleft between the hair cells and the cochlear nerve fibers. This depolarizes the afferent cochlear nerve terminals, and the generated action potentials travel to the brainstem through the fibers of the vestibulocochlear nerve (CN VIII).

Electrical Transduction

The chemical properties of action potentials include the ionic properties of the hair cells and transmission of the charged particles through the cell membranes (see Chapter 5). There is an ionic gradient between the endolymph and intracellular potential of the hair cells. With a potential difference of +80 mV between endolymph and perilymph and intracellular potential of −70 mV (resting state), there is a 150 mV gradient difference across the cilia of a hair cell. This difference is considered essential for normal functioning of the hair cell. As the basilar membrane moves against the tectorial membrane, deformation of the stereocilia of the hair cell bundle increases potassium ion permeability and opens K^+ sensitive pores in the tips of cilia.

The mechanical deformation of the receptive ends in the cochlea cells opens ion-specific channels, allowing the movement of potassium into the cell bodies through the cilia in the scala media. With K^+ influx, the depolarized hair cell opens the calcium (Ca^{2+}) channels, causing calcium ions to move into the cell. The calcium movement causes synaptic vesicles at the base of the cell to release glutamate (a fast excitatory neurotransmitter) in the synaptic space, which is picked up by the appropriate receptors in the cochlear nerve terminals (Fig. 9-5). The action potential discharges that are generated in the nerve terminals travel through the (peripheral and central) fibers of CN VIII to the cochlear nuclear complex located at the pontomedullary junction.

BOX 9-1

Role of Stria Vascularis

Located laterally in the scala media, stria vascularis not only produces endolymph, a fluid with low sodium/high potassium, but it also contributes to the maintenance of the ionic difference between endolymph and perilymph, which is essential for the optimal functioning of the inner ear. Structural and function abnormalities related to stria vascularis have an effect on the optimal functioning of the cochlear hair cells. Its degeneration causes a proportionate hearing loss involving all frequencies.

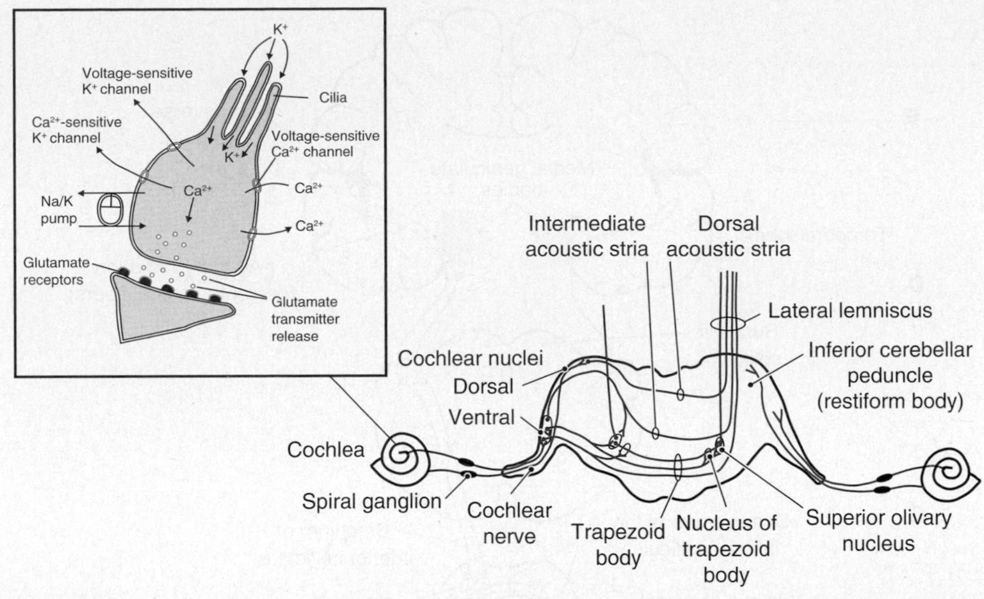

Figure 9-5 Retrocochlear neural mechanism. Peripheral processes of the spiral ganglions project to hair cells in the cochlea. Inset, the impulse transduction by which the glutamate release depolarizes the cochlear nerve terminals.

Neural Coding of Auditory Information

In the transmission of audition, all the properties of sound (e.g., timing, intensity, frequency) are fully retained throughout the path to the brain. The mechanism used to code these attributes is not well understood; however, it is likely that information is coded in a variety of ways with some or substantial redundancy. For instance, the cochlear frequency represented by the stimulation of hair cells at specific regions along the basilar membrane may only be one way of tonal coding. Other ways to code this information could also be the number of cochlear units responding adequately to a specific frequency and/or the synchronous firing patterns of auditory nuclei. Sound intensity could possibly be coded by the number of related neural units stimulated along the basilar membrane, by the intensity of discharging rates of fibers, or by the number of axons involved in the information transmission. Furthermore, the central pathway may regulate which fibers are active in transmitting auditory signals, the properties of the sound (intensity, frequency), and information related to binaural or monaural interactions (Kingsley, 1999).

Key Terms :

Inferior colliculus	**Medial geniculate body**
Internal auditory meatus	**Spiral ganglia**
	Superior olivarynucleus
Lateral lemniscus	**Temporal planum**

Retrocochlear Auditory Mechanism

The **retrocochlear** (post cochlea) auditory system transmits signals from the hair cells in the organ of Corti to the brainstem cochlear nuclear complex (Fig. 9-5). The hair cells transmit nerve impulses to the peripheral (many unmyelinated) axons of the unipolar **spiral ganglia** (first-order neuron in bony modiolus). The central (myelinated) processes of the spiral ganglion cells form the acoustic branch of the vestibulocochlear (CN VIII) nerve and pass through the internal auditory meatus, a canal in the petrous portion of the temporal bone that opens into the cranial cavity at the side of the junction of the pons and medulla (see Fig. 17-4). The afferent axons synapse in the cochlear nuclear complex (Figs. 9-3 and 9-5). There are approximately 30,000 spiral ganglia cells in the modiolus, which can be divided into types I and II. Type I cells, which amount to about 90% of the total spiral ganglion cells, respond to a narrow range of frequency by being connected to only a few select hair cells in the cochlea, indicating a selectivity of processing. On the other hand, the axonal processes, originating from type II cells in the spiral ganglion, synapse with 10 or more hair cells, suggesting their sensitivity to a wider range of frequencies and with less precision (Kingsley, 1999).

CENTRAL AUDITORY PATHWAYS

The central auditory pathway extends from the cochlear nuclear complex and all its relay nuclei up to and including the primary auditory cortex (Fig. 9-6; Table 9-2). In contrast to a three-neuron organization (see Chapter 11), the auditory pathway contains multiple synapses between the cochlear nuclei (second-order neurons) and the thalamus (third-order neurons). The myelinated fibers of the

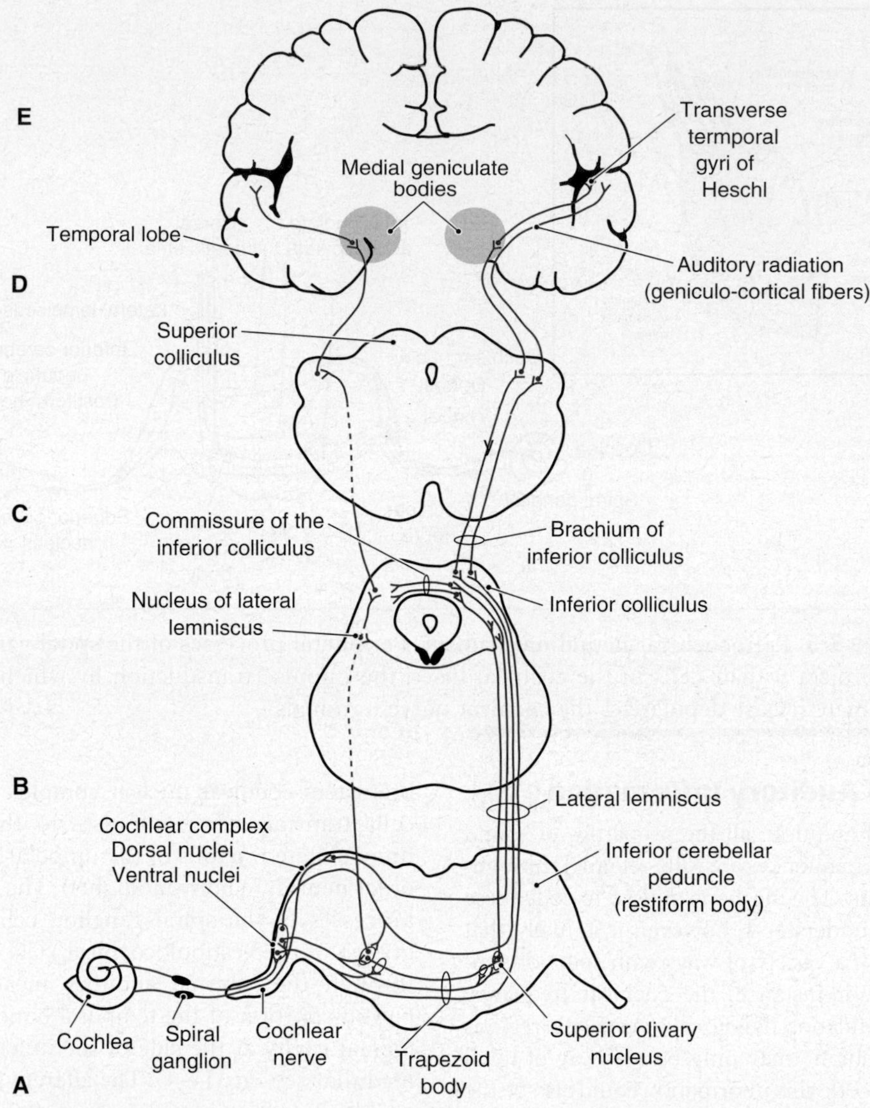

Figure 9-6 A schematic illustration of the auditory pathway. The central auditory pathway begins as secondary fibers arising from the cochlear nuclear complex and forming crossed and uncrossed stria. These fibers synapse on the superior olivary nucleus and ascend through the brainstem to the auditory cortex. A. Medulla. B. Pons. C. Inferior colliculus level. D. Medial geniculate body of thalamus. E. Transverse gyri of Heschl.

vestibulocochlear (CN VIII) nerve enter the brainstem laterally at the pontomedullary junction and synapse on the cochlear nuclear complex (see Fig. 17-5). Structures included in the central auditory pathway are the cochlear nuclei, superior olivary nuclei, lateral lemniscus, inferior colliculus (IC), **brachium of inferior colliculus**, medial geniculate body (MGB), auditory radiations (geniculocortical fibers), and primary auditory cortex in the transverse gyri of Heschl (Tables 9-2 and 9-3).

There are two basic parts of information transmission in the central auditory pathway: one is preserving information and the other is processing information. Preserving information involves the retention of the tonotopic representation from the cochlear hair cells to the primary auditory cortex. The processing, a hierarchically interactive system, refers to the contralaterality of auditory projections, incorporation of monaural and binaural afferents, and integration of audition with other information including attention in signal processing. The contralaterality of audition relates to the preponderance of projections that originate in one ear and after multiple crossings travel to the auditory cortex on the opposite side; the projections to the ipsilateral auditory cortex, though real, are fewer and clinically less significant. The processing rule also concerns gradually increased processing complexity marked by elaboration, abstraction,

Table 9-2

Summary of the Auditory System

Auditory Functions	Structures
Signal amplification and impedance matching	External and middle ear
Fluid motion conversion in neural impulses	Cochlea (hair cells)
First-order nerve cells	Spiral ganglia
Signal transmission to CNS	Auditory nerve
CNS structures involved with transmitting, integrating, and processing (perception and recognition) of auditory signals	Cochlear nuclear complex Trapezoid body Superior olivary nucleus Inferior colliculus Brachium of inferior colliculus Medial geniculate body Primary and association auditory cortices

CNS, central nervous system.

and synthesis at the higher neuraxial levels. The primary auditory cortex has over 100,000,000 neurons in contrast to merely 900,000 functional units in the cochlear nucleus (Worden, 1971).

Cochlear Nuclear Complex

Fibers of the vestibulocochlear (CN VIII) nerve enter the brainstem at the pontomedullary junction dorsolateral to the inferior cerebellar peduncle (restiform body). They terminate in the cochlear nuclear complex (second-order neuron), which is divided into dorsal and ventral nuclei (Figs. 9-5–9-7A; see Fig. 3-11). The dorsal cochlear nucleus lies dorsolateral to the restiform body, whereas the ventral cochlear nucleus is ventral and lateral to the restiform body. The entering fibers of the vestibulocochlear nerve divide into dorsal and ventral branches and synapse onto the respective cochlear nuclei. Specialized cochlear cells, such as bushy and multiform, have been identified in the cochlear complex (Kingsley, 1999). Some of these cells may provide a sustained response to tones mediating important sound attributes such as phase and timing, whereas others may exclusively be responsive to changes in SPL.

Table 9-3

Auditory Structures and Associated Processing Disorders

Structures	Clinical Characteristics
Outer and middle ear	Interruption of sound transmission by air (conductive hearing loss), marked by air–bone gap, fluctuating hearing loss, softly spoken speech, and hearing well in noise
Cochlear hair cells	Interruption of sound transmission to the same degree by air and bone (sensorineural hearing loss), marked by difficulty in hearing and understanding particularly in noise, speaking loudly, and loudness recruitment
Auditory nerve and related structures	Largely preserved hearing sensitivity but reduced understanding of speech and difficulty hearing in noisy environments
Cochlear nuclear complex	Altered hearing sensitivity leading to impaired hearing (deafness) in ipsilateral ear
Superior olivary nucleus	Profoundly impaired ability to identify sound sources; some attenuation in bilateral hearing sensitivity
Lateral lemniscus	Impaired ability to process speech in noise, identify sound source, and grasp crucial linguistic information in discourse; bilateral attenuation in hearing sensitivity
Inferior colliculus	Reduced ability to process and screen patterns of speech; impaired integration of audition with visual-motor functions for reflexive responses and reduced auditory attention
Medial geniculate body	Reduced ability to incorporate attention in screening auditory information, regulate information processing speed, and activate audition-triggered visceral functions; minimal effect on hearing sensitivity
Gyri of Heschl	
Unilateral lesion	Impaired ability to discriminate and process complex time-based sound patterns typifying phonemic units of human speech; minimal to no effect on hearing sensitivity
Bilateral temporal lesions isolating Wernicke area	Profoundly impaired speech comprehension (pure word deafness) owing to speech stimuli imperception; preserved spoken language, naming, reading, and writing functions

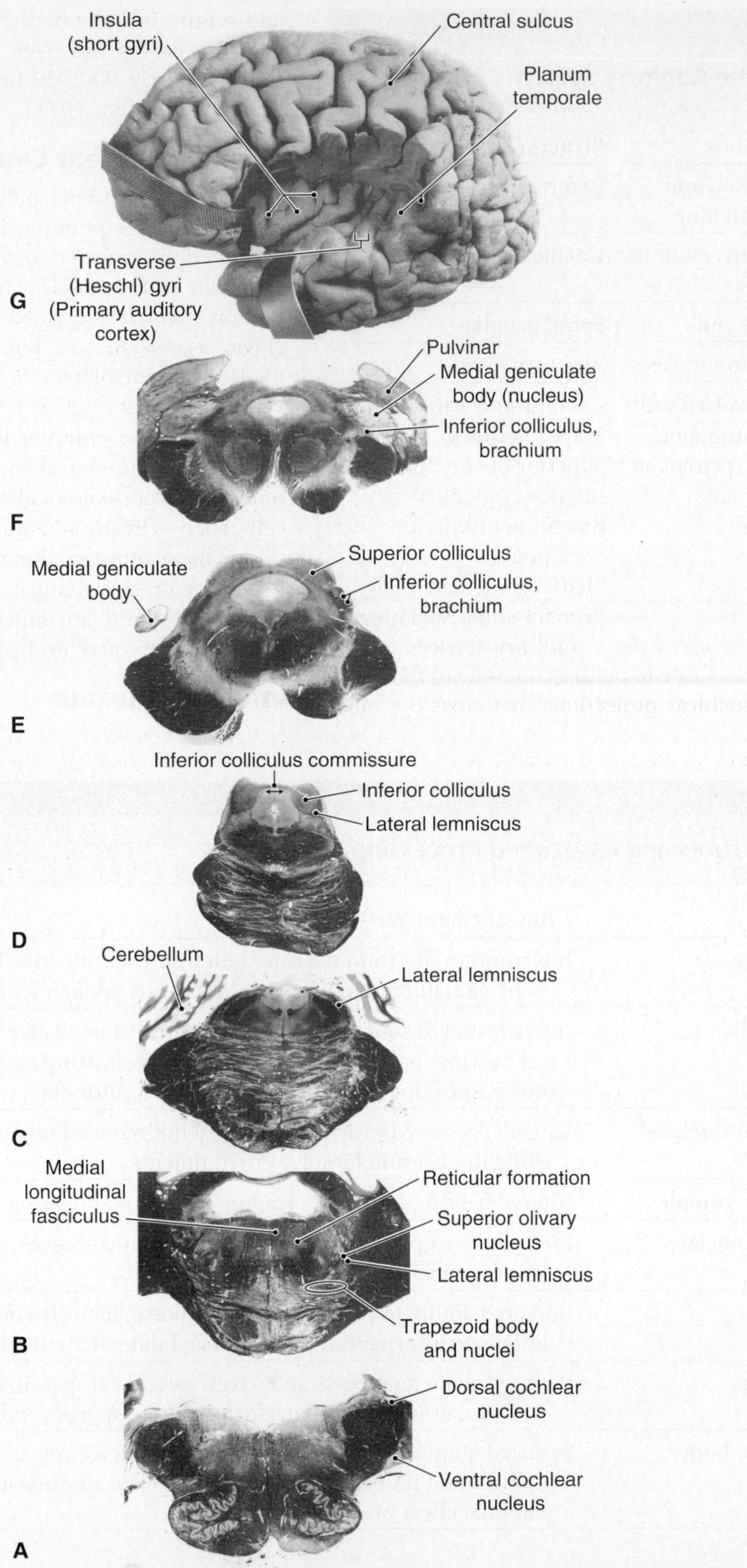

Figure 9-7 Illustration of the central auditory pathways from the cochlear nuclei in the brainstem to the primary auditory cortex on axial sections using the tissue slices from the brainstem, and diencephalon; A. Medulla; B. Lower pons; C. Rostral pons; D. Pontine–midbrain junction; E. Midbrain; F. Midbrain–diencephalon junction; G. Forebrain, exposed primary auditory cortex and planum temporale after the removal of tissue from the overlying operculi of the frontal and parietal lobes.

The discrete tonotopic organization is an important principle governing the functional representation at the cochlear nuclear complex and through the auditory pathway. There is a 1:1 relationship between the tonal representation of the hair cells in the organ of Corti and the cells in the cochlear nuclear complex. The fibers from the apex of the cochlea, which carry low-frequency information, terminate at the superficial layers of the cochlear nucleus, whereas fibers from the base of the cochlea, which carry high-frequency information, penetrate deeper in the cochlear nuclear complex and thus preserve the tonal correspondence. This discrete tonotopic representation is retained throughout the ascending fibers of the central auditory pathway and all its nuclei up to the auditory cortex.

Cochlear Nuclear Projections

The cochlear nuclear complex sends multiple projections to both the ipsilateral and contralateral ascending auditory pathways. The exact nature of these projections is not as clear as it seems to be in published diagrams. In general, although most auditory fibers cross the midline to project to the opposite cortical areas, a small number of fibers remain ipsilateral and ascend on the same side to the auditory cortex. The cochlear projections that cross the midline travel in three bundles: **dorsal acoustic stria, intermediate stria**, and **trapezoid body**. Again, there may be a function for each of these channels in mediating specific auditory attributes; however, our knowledge of those attributes is incomplete. The cells along the crossing fibers of the trapezoid body form the nucleus of the trapezoid body. The fibers of the dorsal acoustic stria cross the midline and terminate in the contralateral lateral lemniscus without sending projections to any of the olivary nuclei. The collaterals from the fibers of the intermediate acoustic stria may project to the ipsilateral and/or contralateral superior olivary complex, while the main body of fibers joins the contralateral lateral lemniscus. The fibers of the trapezoid body, by far the most important and largest stria, cross the midline to terminate in the superior olivary nucleus, which is located laterally in the dorsal pons. The auditory fibers that are ipsilateral either send projections to the ipsilateral superior olivary nucleus or bypass it on their way to the ipsilateral lateral lemniscus.

Superior Olivary Nucleus

The superior olivary nucleus, a collection of nuclei in the pons, is the first structure to receive auditory inputs from both the ipsilateral and the contralateral cochlear nuclei. It contains binaural cells (lateral superior olive and medial superior olive) that are uniquely equipped to calculate differences in the time and intensity of auditory stimuli from both ears. The superior olivary nucleus contains two large dendrites extending from the opposite sites of the soma. The medial dendrite receives projections from the contralateral cochlear nuclei, whereas the lateral dendrite receives input from the ipsilateral cochlear nuclei. This structural arrangement allows the superior olivary nucleus to compare, millisecond by millisecond, the auditory signals arriving from both ears. By integrating time differences of as little as 400 μs and the slightest intensity differences received from both ears, the superior olivary nucleus contributes to the spatial localization of the sound. This ability to localize sound is remarkable, as the path difference between the ears is approximately 5 in.

Lateral Lemniscus

The lateral lemniscus, the primary ascending auditory pathway, extends from the superior olivary nucleus to the IC of the midbrain (see Fig. 3-14). Its fibers climb laterally in the pontine tegmentum. The cell bodies along the fibers form the nucleus of the lateral lemniscus. The lateral lemniscus receives crossed and uncrossed projections from the dorsal, ventral, and intermediate striae. Thus, it retains a bilateral representation with a stronger representation from the opposite ear. This bilaterality of projections explains why the pathology of the central auditory pathway at any level does not lead to a profound hearing impairment in one ear.

Inferior Colliculus

On their way to the midbrain, the fibers of the lateral lemniscus pass dorsolaterally through the pontine tegmentum, potentially making numerous connections, before synapsing on nuclei in the IC in the midbrain (Figs. 9-6 and 9-7). Virtually all of the lateral lemniscus fibers synapse on the nuclei in the IC; the remaining few fibers pass without synaptic relays to it. Both inferior colliculi are connected through the commissural fibers, permitting further crossing and integration of monaural and binaural properties of the auditory input. This integration has additional implications for the localization of a sound source. While the cellular organization in the IC is known to retain frequency-specific regions with increased neuroanatomic complexity and projectional diversity, the central and pericentral cells of the IC respond to complex patterns of auditory stimuli, indicating a higher level of signal analysis and information processing beyond the level of tonal processing. The primary output of the IC is to the thalamus, as its projections travel through the brachium to the MGB (Figs. 9-6 and 9-7; see Fig. 2-21).

A largely ignored part of the IC is that along with the superior colliculus and sensorimotor afferents, it is a part of the tectal neuronal circuitry in the brainstem, which provides the organism with a three-dimensional neurologic map of the external environment. According to this neurologic map, eye movements and/or head turns and body turns occur in response to visual stimuli (superior colliculus), loud or unexpected directional sounds (IC), or sudden or unexpected tactile stimuli. These startle reflexes are quite rapid and can occur even if the thalamus or cerebral cortex is nonfunctional. The outer layers of the superior colliculus receive ganglion cell axons from the retina in an organized map of the environment, by which a stimulus activates specific areas of the retina. Ascending auditory signals send collateral information into the IC, providing a similar spatial orientation. The IC projects fibers to the deep layers of the superior colliculus, where the common output for the visual and auditory startle reflexes uses tectobulbar and tectospinal pathways to reach the spinal and brainstem motor apparatus.

The IC also sends fibers to the midbrain reticular formation. With a reticular integration, the circuitry of the tectum also has a cognitive role to play by incorporating attentional processes for selecting, screening, analyzing, inhibiting, and/or enhancing the processing of auditory information, and for multisensory integration, and audition-based learning. This also explains how audition contributes to the automatic survival mechanism that includes auditory-motor reflexes.

Medial Geniculate Body

The MGB is the thalamic relay nucleus for the transmission of auditory information. Located in the lateral–caudal portion of the lower layer of thalamic nuclei, it receives its tonotopic input from the ipsilateral IC (Figs. 9-6 and 9-7). There is no known crossing of impulses directly at the level of the MGB. Nonetheless, the possibility remains for some information to cross to the other side through thalamic commissural (massa intermedia) fibers. The projection fibers from the MGB (auditory radiations or geniculocortical) pass ventrally (sublenticular) and caudally (retrolenticular) to the lenticular portion of the internal capsule. They terminate in the ipsilateral primary auditory cortex, the gyri of Heschl in the superior temporal lobe (Figs. 9-7 and 9-8).

With its strategic location between the basal ganglia and the thalamic nuclei, and with its multiple and diverse projections, the MGB is involved with issues beyond the transmission of information to the cortex. With its projections to the adjacent putamen (basal ganglia), amygdaloid nucleus (limbic lobe), and tertiary regions of the temporal and parietal cortex and its afferents from the brainstem reticular-activating system, the MGB is likely to help integrate attentional processes with auditory information as well as use auditory afferents to regulate visceral functions, emotional expression, and the pain mechanism.

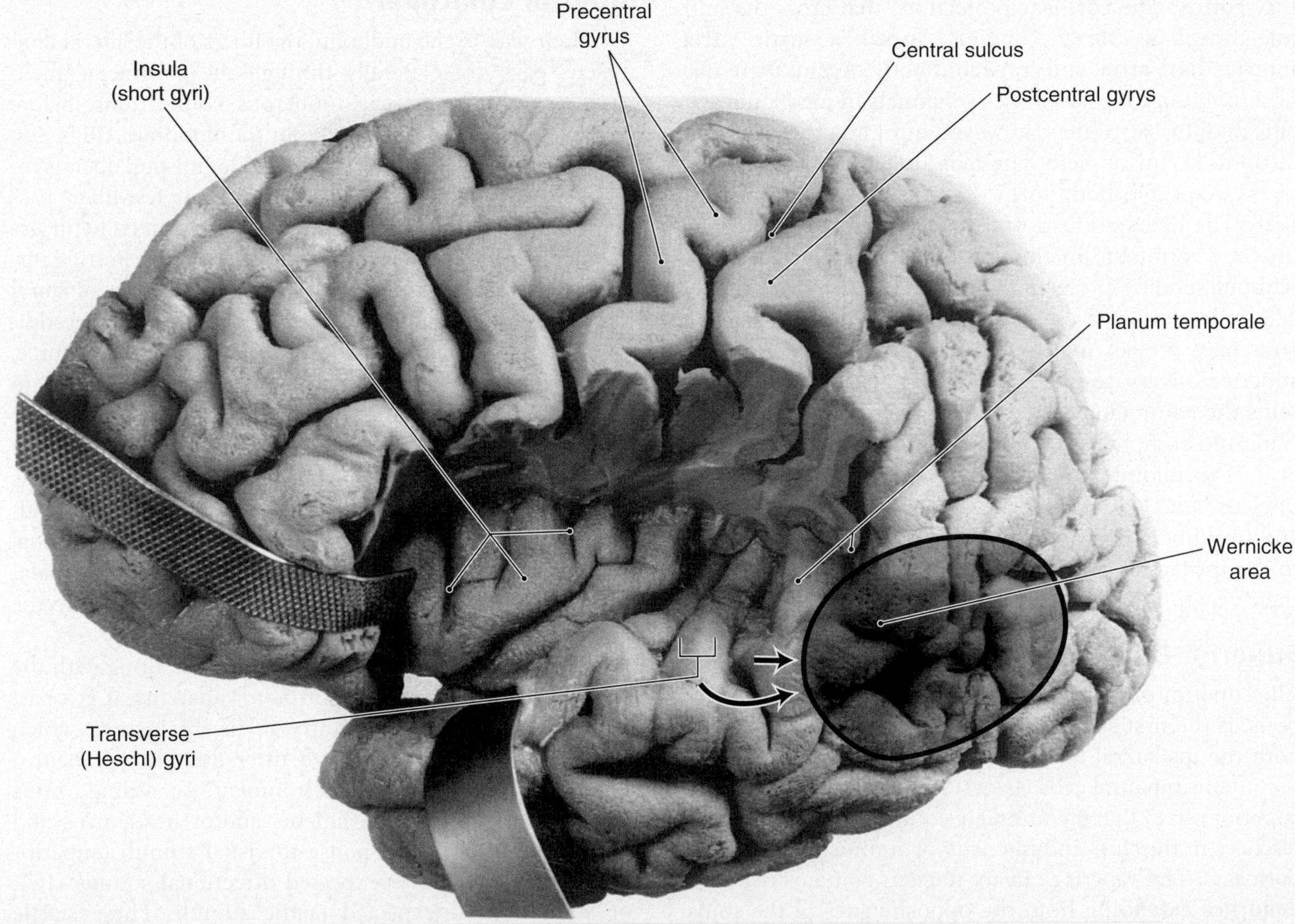

Figure 9-8 Exposed primary auditory cortex in the gyri of Heschl with projections to the language association cortex of Wernicke, which is located in the posterior superior temporal region.

Primary and Auditory Association Cortex

The primary auditory cortex (Brodmann area 41), with its well-developed inner granular layer, is located in the transversely oriented gyri of Heschl, which are buried in the lateral sylvian sulcus on the dorsal surface of the superior (first) temporal gyrus. This area is surrounded by the secondary auditory area (Brodmann area 42), which extends onto the lateral surface of the superior temporal gyrus.

Receiving impulses through crossed and uncrossed fibers from both ears, the primary auditory cortex is known to retain the cochlear tonotopic representation with a representation for higher frequencies in the posteromedial region and lower frequencies in the anterolateral region of the gyri of Heschl. The area in between receives fibers carrying the middle range of frequencies. Experimental studies in animal brains suggest that the tonal representation is not fully mapped in the human brain (Bhatnagar and Andy, 1988). The primary auditory cortex is not absolutely essential for frequency discrimination; rather, it screens for those patterned acoustic properties that are important in auditory discriminations based on the timing patterns of auditory events, such as human speech perception. Some of its neurons also respond to loudness and spatial locations.

The secondary auditory cortex receives some input from the thalamic MGB. Along with the primary auditory cortex, it processes other essential properties of audition, such as timing patterns and spatial attributes typical of human speech. A pathologic involvement of the auditory cortex leads to acoustic form of aphasia and is characterized by an impaired ability to perceive and discriminate speech sounds. The primary auditory cortex has also been known to retain functional plasticity beyond early years (Box 9-2).

The area posterior to the auditory cortical region is the area of planum temporale (temporal planum) which is hidden by the overlying operculum of the temporal, parietal, and frontal lobes. In most individuals, the left planum temporale area is larger than in the right brain, a fact that has been associated with the cerebral dominance (Geschwind and Levitsky, 1968).

An extensive axonal bundle connects the auditory (primary and secondary) cortex to the language association cortex, also called Wernicke area (Brodmann area 22). This association cortex includes part of the planum temporale, posterosuperior first temporal gyrus, and the inferior parietal lobe; it is concerned with the comprehension of spoken language, which involves recognizing language stimuli, interpreting their meanings, and recognizing social/paralinguistic properties of language with respect to previous memories and linguistic experiences and knowledge. The Wernicke area, as part of the larger language interpretative cortex involving the temporal and parietal lobes, also contributes to language formulation.

BOX 9-2

Plasticity in the Auditory Cortex

The brain's ability to reorganize in response to an injury is mostly prevalent in younger brains. However, some neuronal plasticity continues even in adult life. In an example to demonstrate this, Kilgard and Merzenich (1998) installed an electrode in the nucleus basalis of Meynert below the globus pallidus in a rat brain and reinforced the cholinergic projections to activate cortical auditory neurons. The rats were exposed to a 9-kHz tone in 8- to 40-second intervals. This exposure was paired with a brief electric stimulation of the nucleus. The rats' auditory cortexes were later examined for tonotopic representation using a single neuron recording. Most auditory neurons in experimental rats were found to respond to tones near 9 kHz. The neurons responsible for the other tones were confined to a small area in the remaining auditory cortex. Externally applied current for mapping the cortical tissues has further revealed a progressive reorganization in the human adult brain. A deficit elicited in the beginning of the stimulation trials was noted to have faded away from the same cortical tissue on repeated stimulations (Lesser et al., 1987). In another experiment of functional reorganization, the stimulation of the cortical area that originally controlled a set of muscles innervated by a specific nerve was later noted to have switched its control to adjacent muscles after the motor-nerve transection (Donoghue and Sanes, 1988).

AUDITORY REFLEXES

Auditory reflexes coordinate head and eye movements toward sound and influence vestibular functions. This reflex mechanism primarily involves three anatomic pathways.

The first pathway includes the projections from the IC to the superior colliculus and tectum; this integrates the auditory and visual systems and controls extraocular movements and is also involved with the startle and attention reflexes.

The second pathway from the superior olivary nucleus to the medial longitudinal fasciculus projects to the nuclei of the following cranial nerves: occulomotor (CN III), trochlear (CN IV), and abducens (CN VI). Impulses traveling on these two pathways regulate directional ocular movements in response to auditory stimuli.

The third pathway includes the auditory projections to the vestibular nuclear complex and participates in equilibrium.

VASCULAR SUPPLY TO THE AUDITORY MECHANISM

The auditory mechanism is also susceptible to damage from a variety of pathologies including the cerebrovascular accidents. The oxygen supply to the neuronal circuitry of audition comes from an intricate arterial network of the brainstem. The inner ear cochlear mechanism, semicircular canals of the vestibular mechanism, and spiral ganglia and their central and peripheral processes receive their vascular supply from the basilar artery, in particular the internal auditory (labyrinthine) artery, a branch of the anterior inferior cerebellar artery (AICA) (see Fig. 7-1b). Any vascular interruption involving the AICA is likely to result in a monaural hearing loss. With proximity of the facial nerve (CN VII), this also results in facial paralysis. Ocular movements may also be impaired depending on the involvement of the abducens nerve (CN VI).

The ascending auditory path, involving the superior olivary nucleus and the lateral lemniscus fibers, receives its blood through the smaller bilateral circumferential branches of the basilar artery (Fig. 7-1b). Branches of the superior cerebellar artery and quadrigeminal artery provide blood to the IC. An occlusion of the lateral basilar artery branches or superior cerebellar artery is likely to affect the auditory projections ascending from both ears, resulting in a binaural attenuation of hearing sensitivity. The thalamic medial genicular body relies on the thalamogeniculate artery (branched off the posterior cerebral artery) for its blood supply. The blood supply to the primary and secondary auditory cortex flows through the branches of the middle cerebral artery (see Chapter 7). These multiple sources of vascular circulation associate the auditory processing deficits with the CVA involving different blood vessels.

DISTINCTIVE PROPERTIES OF AUDITORY SYSTEM

Four distinctive properties of the auditory system are: (1) bilateral auditory representation, (2) tonotopic representation, (3) sound source localization, and (4) descending auditory projections for the tuning of the receptors.

Bilateral Auditory Representation

The multiple crossings of auditory information through ascending interconnections at the levels of the cochlear nuclei, lateral lemniscus, and IC contribute to the bilaterality of cortical auditory representation. The primary auditory cortex in each hemisphere receives input from both ears with greater afferents from the opposite ear and fewer projections from the ipsilateral ear. A lesion at any point along the central auditory pathway extending from the pons to the auditory cortex would not result in complete hearing loss involving either of the ears; it causes only a mild loss of hearing.

Tonotopic Representation

Discrete tonal representation at the cochlear level is maintained throughout the central auditory pathway. Despite the multiple interconnections and crossings in the ascending pathways, the tonal representation from the hair cells in the cochlea is retained throughout the auditory system. Tones are represented even in the primary auditory cortex, where a single neuron responds best to certain sound frequencies.

Sound Source Localization

The interaural difference between the times of arrival and intensities of acoustic impulses is important in localizing the sound source. When each ear receives a particular sound but at different times, the difference is known as the interaural time delay. The ear nearest the source receives the information first. The intensity difference is the differentially perceived loudness of a sound. Since the sound is less intense in the ear farther from the source, individuals use the loudness difference to determine a sound's location, which begins at the level of the superior olivary nucleus.

Descending Auditory Projections

Parallel to the ascending projections, descending auditory fibers are known to exist from the primary auditory cortex to the cochlear hair cells. These fibers provide feedback circuits to refine the perception of pitch and loudness and to sharpen the reception of specific frequencies through the process of lateral inhibition, which also improves the signal-to-noise ratio. The descending connections (corticogeniculate, corticocollicular, colliculo-olivary, olivocochlear, and colliculo-cochlear fibers) contribute to better hearing in noisy situations through the suppression of competing background sounds. These fibers attenuate the transduction of certain sound frequencies through the regulation of the contractile properties of the OHCs by changing their length and influencing their responsiveness. By reducing their bend during a basilar membrane movement, the olivocochlear projections can contribute to a reduction in hearing sensitivity by 20 to 25 dB (Kingsley, 1999) and also participate in focused auditory attention.

Key Terms:

Central auditory impairments
Conductive hearing loss
Ménière disease
Otitis media
Otosclerosis
Presbycusis
Sensorineural hearing loss

CLINICAL CORRELATES

Hearing Impairments

Clinically, hearing impairment is categorized into four types: conductive, sensorineural, mixed, and central (Table 9-3).

Conductive Hearing Loss

Middle-ear pathologies affect sound transmission to the cochlea and cause a conductive hearing loss (CHL), which is characterized by fluctuating hearing loss; good word–speech recognition ability, specifically at high intensities; softly spoken speech; impaired auditory reflex; and, most important, an air–bone gap. CHL has a less severe communicative effect. **Otosclerosis** and **otitis media** are two common causes of CHL. In otosclerosis, a dominant autosomal condition, a pathologic growth of bone near the oval window impedes the movement of the stapes. In otitis media, an accumulation of the fluid in the middle ear causes the eustachian tube to malfunction; this leads to a fluctuating hearing impairment.

Sensorineural Hearing Loss

Sensorineural hearing loss (SNHL) is associated with damage to the cochlear hair cells and/or the auditory nerve. Sensorineural loss is usually permanent and can range from mild to complete in the affected ear. Clinically, it is characterized by difficulty in understanding speech, particularly in noise, and frequently by tinnitus; cochlear involvement is also marked by recruitment (abnormally rapid growth of loudness after the hearing threshold is reached). Patients usually speak loudly as a result of their reduced self-monitoring ability.

Prolonged exposure to noise (industrial environment, loud music, and engine noise) can damage hair cells and is a common cause of SNHL. The noise-induced effect is noticeable generally for high frequencies. Toxicity owing to the accumulation of certain antibiotics in endolymph can also be damaging to hair cells. Other causes include **Ménière disease** and **presbycusis**. Ménière disease, a chronic condition associated with edema and excessive endolymphic pressure in the membranous labyrinth, is marked by progressive and fluctuating hearing loss, sensation of ringing in the ears, and vertigo (spinning sensation). Presbycusis, an age-induced and progressive hearing impairment, affects perception and discrimination of sound. It primarily affects the high frequencies and results from the degeneration of hair cells in the first turn of the cochlear duct (Boxes 9-3 and 9-4).

Disease, irritation, or pressure on the nerve trunk can structurally affect the vestibulocochlear (CN VIII) nerve fibers and cause hearing impairment. It usually results in tinnitus and can cause mild-to-profound hearing impairment. The clinical picture is similar to that of general SNHL, except that in this case a patient's ability to understand speech is more reduced than expected based on the degree of hearing loss. Extensive damage to the nerve usually results in unilateral or asymmetrical hearing loss.

Tumors of the sheath (Schwann cells) of the vestibulocochlear nerve (CN VIII) are also associated with hearing impairment. Such tumors (**vestibular schwannoma** or **acoustic neuroma**) are located at the

BOX 9-3

Noise and Age-Induced Hearing Loss

Sustained exposures to loud noise as well as trauma to the head are known to cause degeneration in the base region of the cochlea, which is responsible for processing high-frequency tones. Noise-induced hearing loss represents high-frequency tone deafness, which is noted mostly among those who are employed in factories or work around jet noises.

Presbycusis is an age-associated hearing loss. It begins in the middle age with the degeneration of outer hair cells in the basal end of cochlea. It becomes symptomatic when the degeneration involves the hair cells for the upper speech range frequencies.

It is marked with a diminished ability to discriminate sounds, particularly high-pitched fricative (s, sh, th, and ch) sounds, difficulty communicating in noisy environment, easier comprehension of male than female voice, and the sensation of tinnitus (a ringing or hissing sound).

BOX 9-4

Cochlear Implants

A cochlear implant procedure is frequently used to treat profound sensorineural hearing loss (SNHL). It involves the implantation of 12 to 22 pairs of electrodes in the cochlea. An integrated speech-processing algorithm converts incoming sound into electrical impulses, which are sent to these electrodes, resulting in stimulation of different regions of the cochlea. If applied early, cochlear implants provide significant improvement in speech and language development for congenital profound SNHL.

cerebellopontine angle and are clinically associated with hearing impairment and disequilibrium. In later stages, tumorous growth can involve the intracranial roots of the trigeminal nerve (CN V) and facial nerve (CN VII), which results in the loss of pain and temperature sensation from the ipsilateral face (spinal tract of trigeminal nerve), facial weakness (facial nerve), loss of taste from the anterior part of tongue (chorda tympany of the facial nerve [CN VII]), and cerebellar symptoms (unstable gait and ataxia).

Mixed

The presence of both—conductive and sensorineural—hearing losses is referred to as mixed hearing loss. Clinically, it is characterized by a lower sensitivity to both bone- and air-conducted stimuli. The audiogram reveals an air–bone gap, with bone conduction invariably being better.

Central Auditory Impairment

The central auditory system includes the lower brainstem (cochlear nuclei, superior olivary nucleus, and lateral lemniscus), upper brainstem (IC and MGB), and the primary auditory cortex (Figs. 9-7 and 9-8; Box 9-5). Clinically, the most identifying feature of central auditory dysfunction is the near-normal sensitivity/thresholds to auditory stimuli but impaired processing of linguistic and metalinguistic signals.

Lower Brainstem Symptoms

A lesion involving the superior olivary nucleus has a minimal effect on hearing sensitivity, but it has a profound effect on the ability to identify and localize the source of sound, an ability of summating temporal information received from both ears. Similarly, a unilateral involvement of the lateral lemniscus is not likely to cause a severe hearing impairment in either of the ears. However, it causes subtle symptoms, such as impaired processing of speech in noise and retaining of crucial and critical linguistic information in a conversational setting.

Upper Brainstem Symptoms

Reflecting an increased neuroanatomic processing complexity, reticular integration, and projectional diversity, the central and pericentral cells of the inferior colliculi play an important role in screening, channeling, and responding to complex auditory patterns and processing. Their pathological involvement affects the transmission of auditory signals and the integration of audition with visual-motor functions for reflexive responses. It also has implications for the metacognition of self-awareness in three-dimensional space. With multiple crossed and uncrossed input and diverse projections, the MGB, besides relaying information, has an important role in integrating complex auditory patterns with the reticular arousal system (Bhatnagar et al., 1989 and 1990). Pathology of the diencephalic MGB might restrict a patient's ability to select and attend to auditory information, regulate the processing speed, and activate emotional and visceral functions associated with audition. The attenuated integration of attention might also result in delayed, degraded, and subnormal linguistic processing of speech.

Cortical Involvement

Patients with unilateral cortical lesions usually exhibit near-normal-hearing thresholds. However, they display an impaired ability to perceive and discriminate speech. Both hearing sensitivity and speech perception are known to be profoundly impaired after bilateral cortical lesions. The secondary auditory cortex, along with the primary auditory cortex, processes other essential properties of audition typical of human speech, such as timing patterns and spatial attributes. A pathologic involvement of the primary and secondary auditory cortices leads to acoustic aphasia, which is marked by an impaired discrimination of speech sounds, a skill essential for learning phonemes and understanding language (Fig. 9-8).

Involvement of the language association cortex (Brodmann area 22) results in aphasic deficits. This produces a syndrome of paragrammatism (Wernicke aphasia), which is characterized by impaired comprehension of spoken and written language, reduced ability to write, substantial word-finding difficulty, euphoria, asemantic though fluent verbal output, and poor self-monitoring

BOX 9-5

Central Auditory Disorder

Multiple relay nuclei and many potential points of fiber crossing in auditory transmission have significant clinical implications. A unilateral pathology of the cochlear nuclear complex and/or the acoustic nerve results in a complete monaural deafness. However, any unilateral damage to the central auditory pathway at or above the superior olivary nucleus leaves some projections from each ear intact. Thus, involvement of the central auditory pathway does not result in a unilateral hearing loss, but rather partially affects hearing bilaterally because of the affection of the binaural projections. Further, depending on the level involved in the central pathway, inattention and impaired information screening may contribute to additional processing deficits.

skills. Lexical retrieval disorder is profound and it is marked by verbal confusion, verbal paraphasia, and frequent neologisms (unrecognized word formations) that make all verbal output disjoined speech, which is referred to as jargon aphasia. Words can be spoken fluently, although speech remains largely meaningless (see Chapter 19).

Right hemispheric temporal lesions affect the processing of environmental sounds, nonverbal memory, and musical and prosodic interpretation. Supporting evidence has come from research on patients undergoing temporal lobotomy for medically intractable epilepsy; tonal processing was not disrupted after a left temporal lobectomy.

Word Deafness

Word deafness is another language-based syndrome. This uncommon disorder is manifested by a severe loss of language comprehension, though speech production, naming, reading, and writing are spared. The associated pathology involves a bilateral temporal lesion, which causes an isolation of the primary auditory cortices from the Wernicke area by interrupting the fibers bilaterally radiating from the gyrus of Heschl (see Chapter 19).

Evaluation of Hearing Disorders

There are many diagnostic tests of hearing. **Tuning fork tests** are the simple bedside tests of hearing and are frequently used as the first level of testing. **Pure tone audiometry** is the most reliable test for evaluating hearing sensitivity. **Tympanometry**, **evoked otoacoustic emissions**, and **auditory brainstem response (ABR) audiometry** are a few specialized tests of hearing with specific diagnostic applications.

Tuning Fork Tests

Tuning fork (**Rinne** and **Weber**) tests are used for an initial impression of the hearing impairment and differentiate CHL from SNHL (Table 9-4; Fig. 9-9).

Rinne Test

In the Rinne test, the stem of a vibrating tuning fork (512 Hz) is placed on the mastoid process and the patient is asked to listen to the tone (by bone conduction). When the tone from the fork is no longer heard by the patient, the fork is placed in front of the ear to determine if the patient can still hear the sound, this time by air conduction.

Clinical Information: A patient with normal hearing or SNHL should hear the tone longer by air conduction than by bone conduction (positive Rinne). A patient with a CHL hears the sound longer by bone conduction (negative Rinne).

Weber Test

In this test, a vibrating tuning fork is placed on the scalp at vertex, and the patient is asked to lateralize the sound by indicating whether the tone is louder in one ear.

Clinical Information: In patients with normal hearing or bilaterally symmetrical hearing loss, the sound is sensed at the midline. Those with a unilateral CHL hear the sound in the affected ear. Patients with a unilateral SNHL hear the sound mainly in the unaffected ear.

Pure Tone Audiometry

Pure tone audiometry is used to establish the threshold of hearing across the frequency range that is most important for human communication. A pure tone audiometer generates pure tones at various frequencies and intensities. The calibration of the audiometer takes into consideration the differential sensitivity of the human ear to various frequencies by making 0 dB HL at each frequency equal to the lowest intensity level in SPL decibels required by the average normal listener to hear that frequency. In audiometry, hearing is tested by determining air- and bone-conduction thresholds to each frequency.

Table 9-4

Clinical Finding of Tuning Fork Test

Tests	Normal Hearing	Conductive Loss	Sensorineural Loss
Rinne: Tuning fork placement on the mastoid process	Air better than bone conduction	Better hearing through bone conduction than air conduction	Reduced sensitivity to both air and bone conductions
Weber: Tuning fork placement on the scalp vertex	Lateralized to both ears	Sound lateralized to the affected ear	Sound lateralization to the better ear

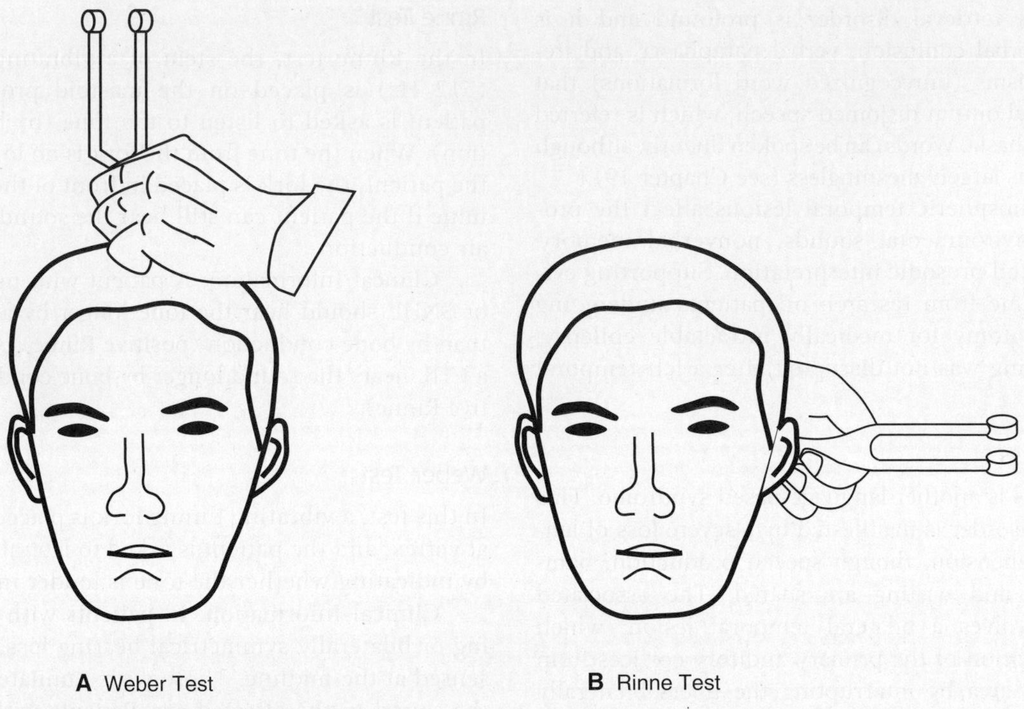

Figure 9-9 Tuning fork testing. A. In the Weber test, louder sound in the poorer hearing ear indicates a CHL. B. In the Rinne test, the patient's ability to hear longer through air conduction indicates the absence of a CHL.

Hearing loss refers to an increase in intensity above the normal sensitivity required to reach the threshold. For example, a 50-dB loss at 1,000 Hz means that the patient requires 50 dB of sound pressure above normal sensitivity to obtain the threshold. In a CHL, the threshold for bone conduction is normal and better than that for air, also called the air–bone gap. Hearing sensitivity by bone and air is, however, decreased to the same degree in SNHL.

Tympanometry

Tympanometry measures the compliance of the tympanic membrane and middle-ear pressure under the conditions of changing air pressure (relative to atmospheric pressure) in the external auditory meatus. Impaired tympanic membrane compliance is an indicator of middle-ear pathology (e.g., middle-ear fluid, ossicular abnormalities, or eustachian tube dysfunction).

Otoacoustic Emission

The cochlear OHCs in normally hearing individuals expand and contract in response to sound stimulation. This movement produces minute pressure waves that are transmitted through the cochlear fluids and can be recorded in the external ear canal. These are known as otoacoustic emissions. Absence of these minute subclinical signals indicates dysfunction of the OHCs, thus suggesting a hearing loss, either conductive or sensorineural.

Auditory Brainstem Response Audiometry

ABR audiometry measures neuronal activity (synchronous neural firings) from the brainstem auditory pathway within 10 ms after the onset of controlled stimuli, such as clicks. Within this period, five vertex positive wave peaks are identified from the event-based electrical activity recorded from scalp electrodes (see Fig. 20-18). Each of these waveforms is thought to be generated at a different anatomic point in the auditory pathway (see Table 20-6). By taking into consideration the altered interpeak latency or changes in the peaks of amplitude, one can identify potential lesion sites in the vestibulocochlear (CN VIII) nerve or brainstem. ABR audiometry is a reliable and clinically powerful test; it does not require the patient's participation and because the response is intensity dependent, it can be used to assess hearing-processing in infants, subclinical patient population, and uncooperative patients (see Chapter 20).

CASE STUDIES FOR PROBLEM SOLVING

CASE ONE (9-1)

A 65-year-old university professor complained of a sudden difficulty in hearing with her left ear accompanied by ringing, nausea, and dizziness. She was taken to a hospital. On testing, she exhibited the following signs:

- Hearing loss in the left ear
- Tendency to fall to her left side
- Loss of pain and temperature sensation on the left side of the face and right side of the body
- Difficulty in swallowing

A brain MRI study revealed a small infarct in the dorsolateral region of pons and medulla on the left side.

Question: How could a dorsal pontomedullary lesion cause problems with hearing and equilibrium and account for the sensory loss and difficulty in swallowing?

Case (9-1) Discussion: See discussion of case studies

CASE TWO (9-2)

A 50-year-old man lost hearing in his right ear and had right-sided imbalance. At first, he compensated by using his left ear when using the telephone. As his equilibrium-related difficulty worsened, he began hearing a high-pitched ringing in the right ear and noticed right facial weakness. He decided to see his physician, who observed the following symptoms:

- Right-sided facial weakness
- Mild unsteadiness while walking
- Right ear SNHL of 45 dB, which increased to 65 dB for higher frequencies (pure tone audiometry)
- Marked reduction in right ear speech discrimination

Positive Rinne findings, absence of air/bone gap on audiometry, and poor speech discrimination in the right ear ruled out a CHL. A brainstem MRI study confirmed a right acoustic schwannoma at the cerebellopontine angle. Surgical removal of the tumor relieved the pressure and largely restored the impaired functions.

Question: How can you account for this clinical picture by relating the symptoms to the involved pathways?

Case (9-2) Discussion: See discussion of case studies

CASE THREE (9-3)

A 25-year-old teacher fell in front of her students while teaching and was taken to the ER, where the attending neurologist noted the following:

- Headache and vomiting
- Profound hearing loss in the right ear, determined by pure tone audiometry
- Disequilibrium with a tendency to fall to the right
- No other sensorimotor or cognitive impairment

A magnetic resonance arteriography study indicated a thromboembolic occlusion of an artery originating from the anterior inferior cerebellar artery on the right.

Question: How can you explain these symptoms?

Case (9-3) Discussion: See discussion of case studies

CASE FOUR (9-4)

A 27-year-old woman with a 3-week history of an auditory problem and double vision was taken to the hospital, where the examining neurologist noted the following:

- A reported history of a 10-day episode of impaired vision and understanding of spoken language
- Right optic nerve paleness
- Tendency to run into things because of her inability to see objects on the floor
- Mild signs of cerebellar dysfunction involving the right extremities with gait ataxia

A speech–language pathology consultation revealed the following:

- Some auditory incomprehension marked by inattentiveness to details, missing information, inconsistencies in response, and difficulty in making sense out of speech in noise
- No signs of impaired language (aphasia), cognitive dysfunction (dementia), or unintelligible speech (dysarthria)

(Continued)

CASE FOUR (9-4) *(CONTINUED)*

An audiologic consultation revealed the following:

- Difficulty with sound localization
- Mild bilateral SNHL on pure tone audiometry
- Poor comprehension of speech in noise
- Presence of acoustic reflexes at appropriate hearing levels
- Normal evoked otoacoustic emission responses, suggesting a structurally intact cochlea
- Normal brainstem auditory-evoked responses, testifying to a normal functioning of the auditory brainstem

The attending neurologist suspected that the patient had a progressive degenerative disease of the nerve coverings, which was confirmed by the presence of multiple white matter hyperintensities (demyelinated plaques) on brain MRI studies, which revealed one in the cerebellum and two in the posterior lateral thalami involving the geniculate bodies.

Question: Based on your anatomic knowledge, can you relate the auditory symptoms with the identified pathology sites?

Case (9-4) Discussion: See discussion of case studies

SUMMARY

Audition begins in the external ear, when collected sound waves strike the tympanic membrane. The resulting vibration of the tympanic membrane converts sound waves into mechanical energy, causing the ossicles in the middle ear to move back and forth. This mechanical energy is further transformed to a hydraulic form of energy in the cochlear fluid of the inner ear, which activates the sensory hair cells in the cochlea and transforms the hydraulic energy to electrical nerve impulses. The nerve impulses are transmitted by the vestibulocochlear nerve (CN VIII) fibers to the cochlear nuclei in the brainstem. The cochlear cells project these nerve impulses to multiple synaptic points in the brainstem and thalamus before transmitting the impulses to the primary auditory cortex in the temporal lobe. The auditory impulses travel from the primary and secondary auditory cortex to the Wernicke (associational language) area, where the auditory signals are analyzed and interpreted into meaningful language-specific messages.

REVIEW QUESTIONS

1. Complete the following statements using the appropriate technical terms:

   A. The endolymph-filled cavities of saccule, utricle, semicircular ducts, and the scala media form the ________ ________.

   B. Located in the ________ ear, the ________ ________, and ________ muscles reflexively protect the auditory mechanism from damage by controlling ossicular motion.

   C. The stapedius muscle, controlled by the ________ ________, restricts stapes movement. The *tensor tympani* muscle, controlled by the ________, participates in restricting ossicular movements.

   D. The ________ auditory system includes the signals from hair cells in the organ of Corti to the brainstem cochlear nuclear complex.

   E. The ________ ________ ________ is the first structure to receive auditory inputs from both (ipsilateral and the contralateral) ________ nuclei.

   F. The ________ ________ contains the brainstem auditory fibers that originate from the superior olivary nucleus and project to the ________ ________.

   G. A lesion above the ________ ________ ________ is not likely to cause a profound hearing loss in either of the ears because of multiple ________ of the fibers.

   H. The transverse Heschl gyri are the site of the ________ ________ ________.

   I. ________ ________ ________ mediates auditory information from the thalamus to the ________ ________ ________.

   J. The labyrinthine artery that supplies blood to the inner ear and cochlear complex is a branch of the ________ ________ ________, which originates from the ________ ________.

   K. The ________ ________ ________ is not absolutely essential for frequency discrimination; rather, it screens properties that are important in auditory discriminations.

   L. In most right-handed individuals, the ________ ________ is larger in the left brain and this in humans has been related to the ________ ________.

2. List two functions of the superior olivary nucleus.
3. Match each of the following clinical concepts with its associated statement.

A. CHL	a. with a tuning fork placed on the vertex, the subject reports in which ear the tone was perceived better
B. SNHL	b. with a tuning fork pressed against the mastoid process, the subject hears by bone conduction
C. Rinne test	c. pathologies of hair cells in the cochlea
D. Weber test	d. impaired sound transmission in the middle ear

4. Match each of the following structures with its associated vascular sources:

A. hair cells in the cochlea and three semicircular canals (c)	a. middle cerebral artery
B. lateral lemniscus	b. pontine branches
C. inferior colliculus	c. labyrinthine artery
D. medial geniculate body	d. thalamogeniculate artery
E. primary auditory cortex	e. superior cerebellar artery

5. Order these auditory relay nuclei (superior olivary nucleus, cochlear nuclear complex, eighth cranial nerve, lateral lemniscus, inferior colliculus, primary auditory cortex, medial geniculate body, auditory radiation fibers) in a hierarchic sequence reflecting the transmission of the ascending auditory information from the ear to the cortex:

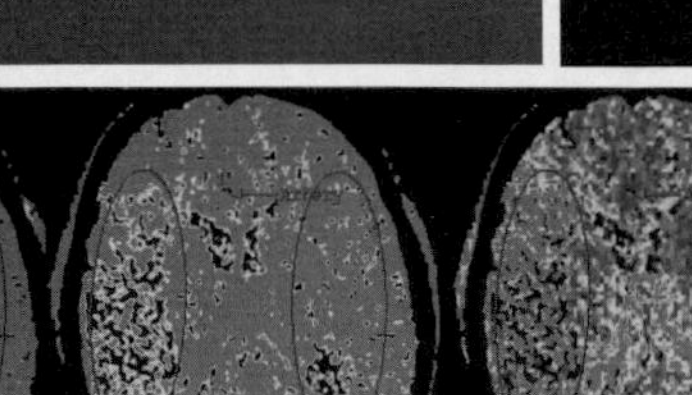

10 Vestibular System

LEARNING OBJECTIVES

After studying this chapter, students should be able to:

- Describe the role of the vestibular system in equilibrium
- Discuss the anatomy of the vestibular system
- Explain the functioning of the vestibular mechanism
- Describe the mechanism of nystagmus
- Discuss the mechanism that controls rotational and ocular movements
- Outline the methods used for assessing the vestibular mechanism integrity
- Discuss vestibular dysfunctions
- Describe the role of voluntary control on eye movement

With adequate proprioceptive and visual inputs, the vestibular system, with sensitivity to angular and linear acceleration, performs two important tasks: equilibrium and eye fixation. Regulation of the body's equilibrium ensures a normal upright posture in space through postural reflexes. The eye movement coordination is needed to maintain eye fixation on objects during body and head movements. Both of these functions are controlled subconsciously and are regulated by integrating information received from receptors in the semicircular membranous ducts of both inner ears.

Key Terms :

Cristae	**Saccadic**
Cupula	**Semicircular ducts**
Macula	**Vestibule**

ANATOMY OF THE VESTIBULAR SYSTEM

The major components of the vestibular system are the **semicircular ducts**, **vestibule** (**saccule** and **utricle**), and **vestibular nuclei** (Figs. 10-1–10-4). Other functionally associated structures are the **medial longitudinal fasciculus** (MLF), cranial (oculomotor, trochlear, abducens) nerves for controlling ocular movement, brainstem reticular formation, and vestibular projections to the spinal cord and cerebellar nuclei. The sensory receptors (hair cells) in the semicircular ducts respond to rotations of the head and changes in body position. They project impulses to the brainstem vestibular nuclei, which in turn transmit the information to the MLF, cerebellum, and spinal motor neurons to coordinate posture and eye, head, and neck movements.

Semicircular Ducts and Vestibular Sacs

The three endolymph filled semicircular ducts in the inner ear are connected to the vestibule (utricle and saccule). The semicircular ducts are at right angles to one another and are named according to their relative positions: anterior, posterior, and lateral (Fig. 10-2). Different space positions enable the receptors in the ducts to detect acceleration of the body in various planes. Each semicircular duct has an enlarged end area called the **ampulla (dilation)**, which contains **cristae**. The cristae (the sensory hair cells or **cilia**) are covered by **cupula**, a gelatinous, mass-filled capsule (Fig. 10-3B). Inside the vestibule are two sacs, the utricle and saccule. Both ends of the semicircular canals are connected to the utricle. The **maculae** of the utricle and saccule also contain sensory receptors (hair cells). A thin layer of gelatinous mass, the **otolithic membrane**, covers these hair cells (Fig. 10-3C). The otolithic membrane also contains calcium crystals and proteins; these, also called otoliths, add mass and gravity to the membrane. The maculae lie in the horizontal plane when the head is held horizontal, so that the otolithic membrane sits directly on the hair cells. In this case, if the head tilts or linearly accelerates, the membrane lags behind, bending the cilia. The subsequent increase or decrease in the firing rate of cells results in the sensation of up and down.

The **vestibular labyrinths** and the receptors of both sides interact in harmony in a normal functioning vestibular system. The vestibular receptors, like cochlear terminals, do not exhibit significant adaptations. Thus, the endings in the utricular and saccular maculae signal steady-state gravitational information and some dynamic

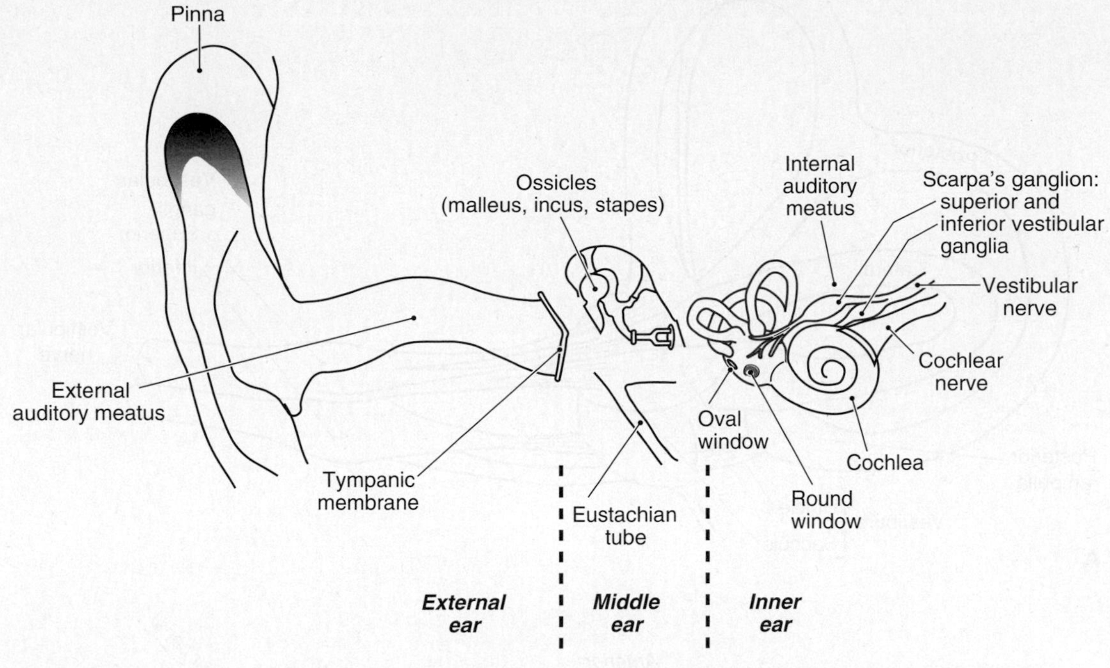

Figure 10-1 Frontal view of the anatomic relationship among the external, middle, and inner parts of the ear.

changes in **inertia** during linear acceleration and deceleration of head movements.

Vestibular Nerve and Nuclei

The vestibular nerve is formed by the fibers of the first-order sensory neurons in the unipolar vestibular (**Scarpa**) ganglia. The peripheral processes of the Scarpa ganglion connect to the hair cells in the utricle, saccule, and semicircular canals, and its central projections form the vestibular nerve (Figs. 10-3 and 10-4). The vestibular ganglion of Scarpa consists of **superior** and **inferior** ganglia. Located in the bony cavity of the petrous bone, the central processes of the Scarpa ganglion enter through the internal auditory meatus to reach the junction of the medulla and pons.

The vestibular nerve fibers, which carry information concerning body equilibrium, join the auditory afferents to form the vestibulocochlear nerve (CN VIII) before they emerge from the internal auditory meatus to enter the **pontocerebellar junction** of the brainstem. Besides the vestibular and cochlear fibers, the fibers of the facial nerve (CN VII) also pass through the internal auditory meatus. Thus a lesion at this point has significant implications for a series of symptoms that include **vertigo, tinnitus**, sensorineural hearing loss, and facial palsy.

In the brainstem, the vestibular and auditory (CN VIII) nerve fibers separate and project to different groups of nuclei. Vestibular fibers terminate in the **vestibular nuclear (superior vestibular, lateral vestibular, medial vestibular**, and **inferior vestibular) complex** in the lateral–dorsal area of the medulla (Fig. 10-4). The auditory nerve fibers project to the cochlear nuclei (see Chapter 9).

Vascular Supply to the Membranous Labyrinthine

The labyrinthine artery, which originates from the anterior inferior cerebellar artery, supplies blood to the membranous labyrinth, which includes the cochlear structure, the semicircular canals, and their first-order neurons (Fig. 7-1b, see Chapter 9). Any vascular accident involving these arteries will affect the functioning of the membranous labyrinth and produce nystagmus, dizziness, and unsteady gait in addition to hearing impairment. The involvement of the anterior inferior cerebellar artery also results in symptoms involving multiple cranial nerves (spinal tract of trigeminal [CN V] plus the facial [VII], vagus [X], and hypoglossal [XII] nerves).

Vestibular Projections

The vestibular nerve fibers enter the brainstem and terminate in the vestibular nuclear complex. The vestibular complex then distributes multiple secondary projections to the cerebellum, spinal cord, and nuclei of the extraocular (oculomotor [CN III], trochlear [CN IV], and abducens [CN VI]) nerves through the MLF (Fig. 10-4). Some fibers bypass the vestibular nuclei; many of these instead enter the cerebellum through the **juxtarestiform body**, which is located medial to the inferior cerebellar peduncle (Restiform body).

Projections to the Cerebellum

The major projections from the vestibular nuclei go to the older cerebellar structures, including the **flocculonodular lobe, vermis**, and **fastigial nucleus**. Most of these bidirectional projections, arising from the superior and inferior

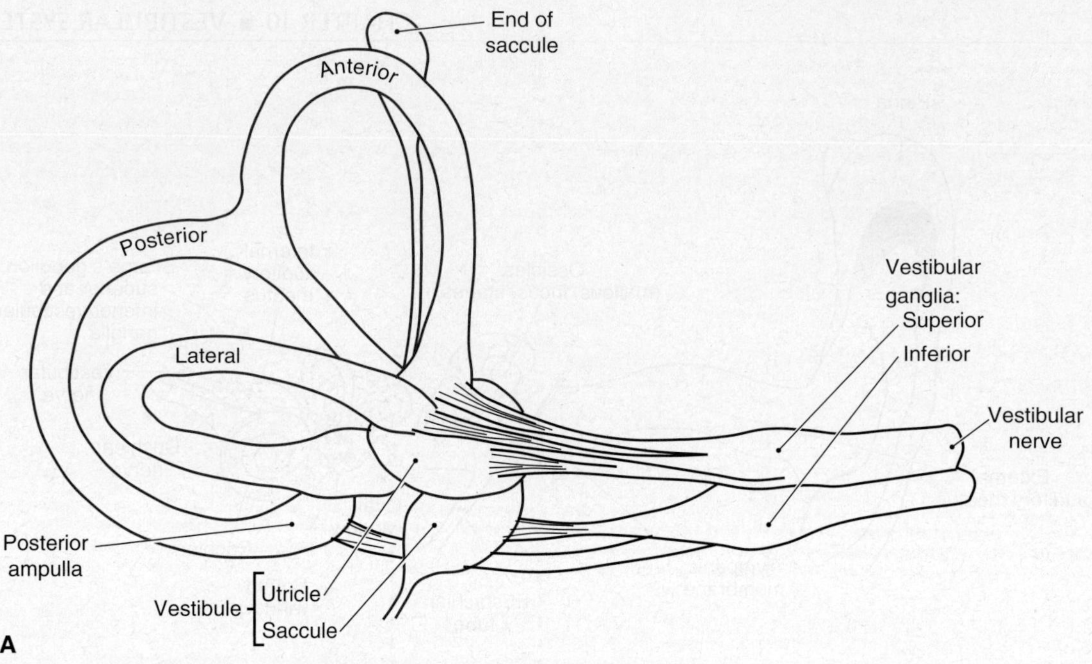

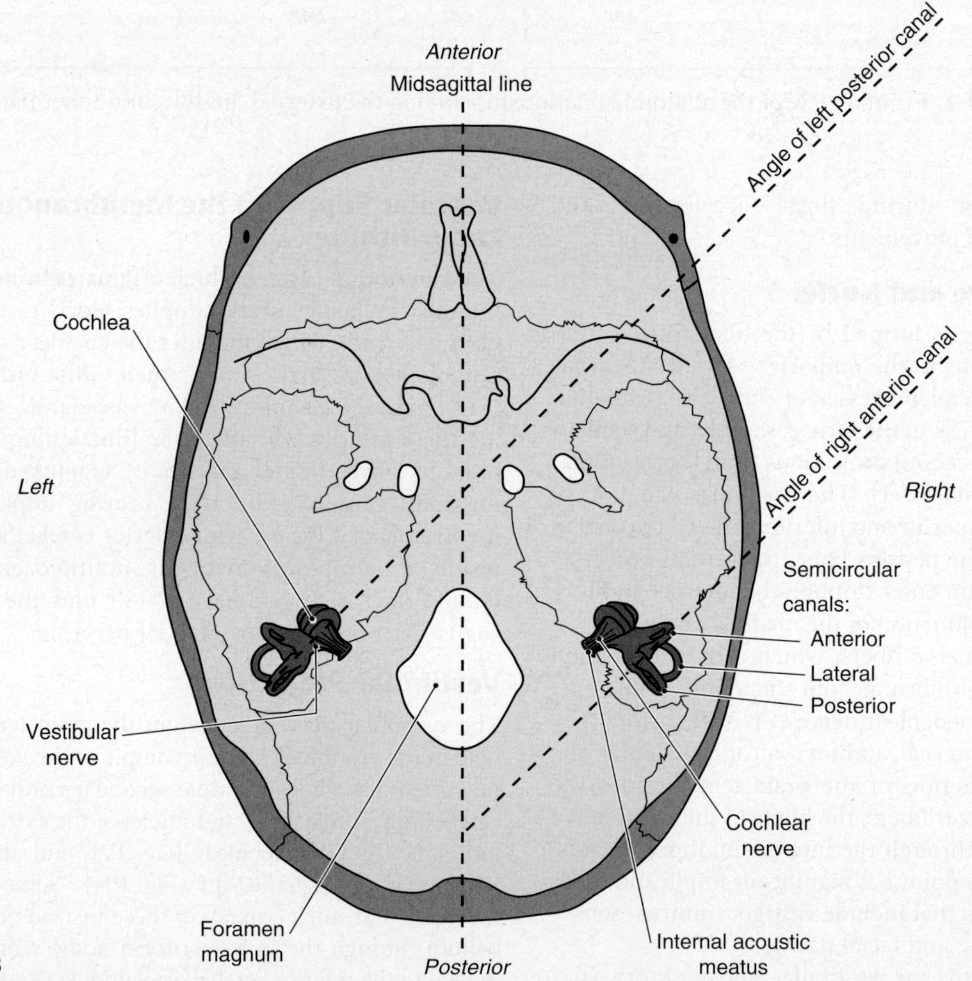

Figure 10-2 A. Structures important for equilibrium: the membranous labyrinth made up of interconnected tubular ducts, the semicircular ducts containing the endolymphatic fluid, the utricle, the saccule with an extension (not shown), and the cochlear duct. The vestibular ganglia and vestibular nerve are also shown. B. Orientation of the anterior, horizontal, and posterior semicircular canals in the base of the skull. The planes of vertical orientation for the anterior and posterior canals form similar angles in relation to the midsagittal line.

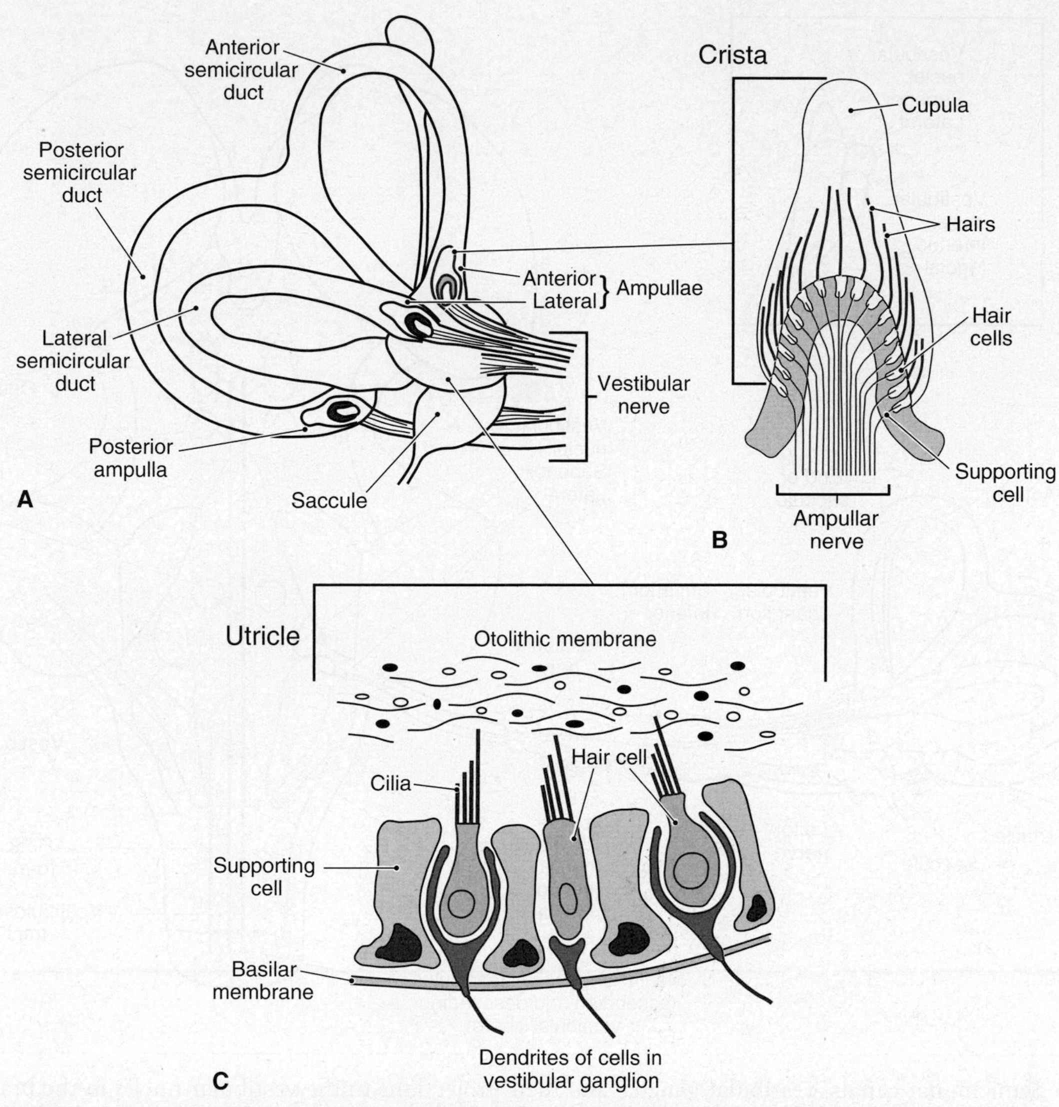

Figure 10-3 A. The semicircular canals and enlarged ampullae house the cristae. B. Hair cells, nerve, and cupula in the ampulla. C. Hair cells and the otolithic membrane arrangement of maculae of the saccule and utricle.

vestibular nuclei, connect the vestibular system and cerebellum and play an important role in the maintenance of body equilibrium. With constant and updated vestibular feedback coupled with cerebellovestibular projections and spinocerebellar proprioceptive input, the cerebellum not only participates in monitoring body and head positions but also regulates the necessary muscular adjustments.

Projections to the Spinal Cord

Fibers originating from the lateral vestibular nucleus descend through the medulla, enter the ventral column of the spinal cord, and terminate at different spinal levels as they supply the motor units of the axial muscles and the limbs. The primary function of the vestibulospinal projections is to maintain the muscle tone that is needed to counteract the pull of gravity.

Projections to the Medial Longitudinal Fasciculus

Located in the midline of the pons, medulla, and midbrain, the MLF fibers from the medial vestibular nuclei project bilaterally to the motor nuclei of the oculomotor nerve (CN III), trochlear nerve (CN IV), abducens nerve (CN VI), and spinal accessory nerve (CN XI). As part of the **pontine gaze center**, these cranial nerves regulate patterned vertical and horizontal movements of the eyes and coordinate them with head movements through the regulation of the ocular and neck muscles. Crossed and uncrossed projections from the MLF synchronize extraocular muscles for controlling conjugate eye movements and regulating visual fixation. The right conjugate movement, for example, would involve the coordination (contraction) of the **lateral rectus** (in the

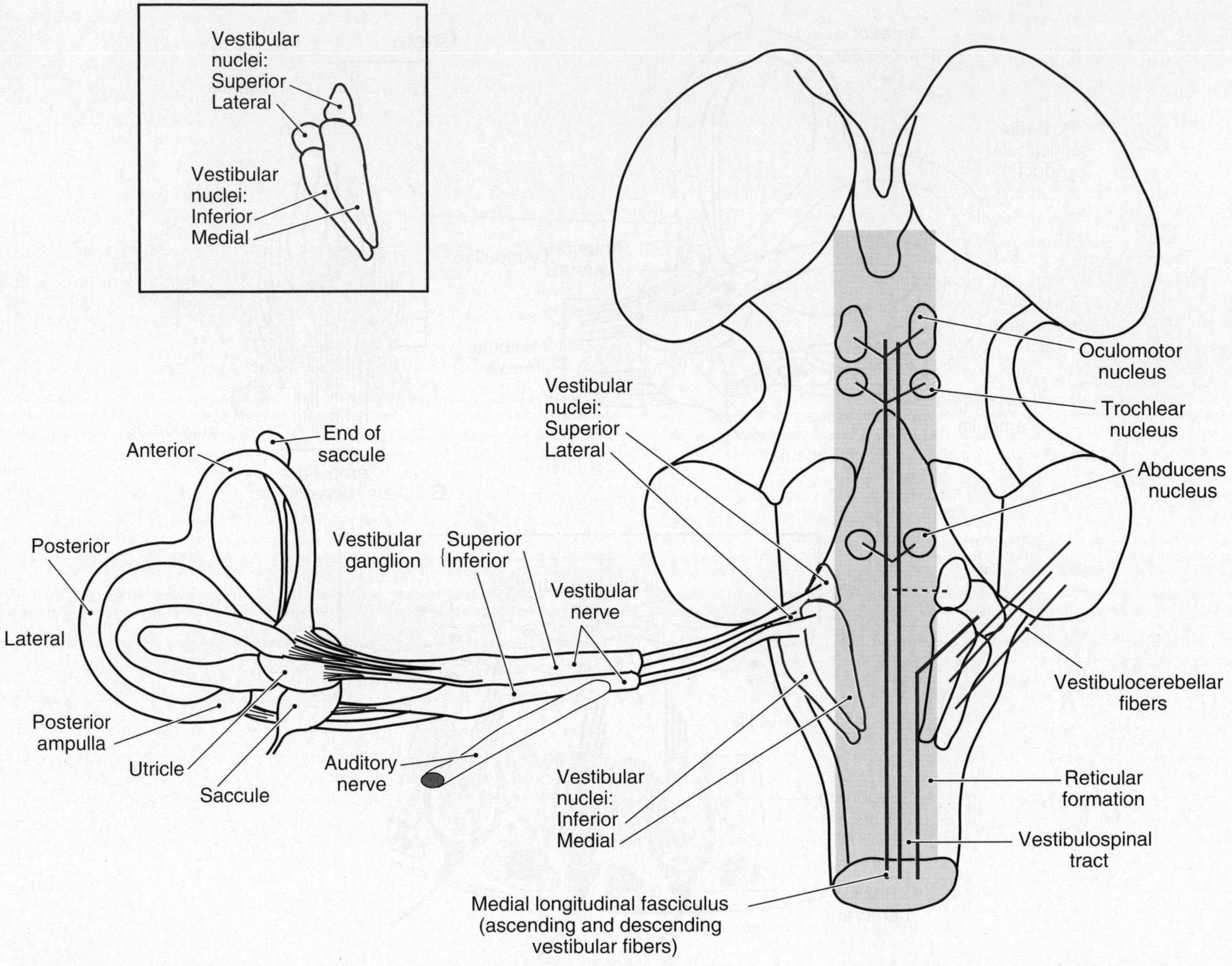

Figure 10-4 Semicircular canals, vestibular ganglia, and their projections to the vestibular nuclei in the brainstem.

right eye) and **medial rectus** (in the left eye) for avoiding double vision.

The left conjugate movement, on the other hand, would involve the coordination (contraction) of the lateral rectus (in the left eye) and medial rectus (in the right eye) for avoiding double vision.

Additional Vestibular Projections

Additional vestibular fibers—with projections to the brainstem reticular formation and ascending reticular activating system—mediate several important functions, including tonal control, maintenance of body equilibrium, and regulation of visceral–automatic activities (e.g., dizziness, nausea, and vomiting with excessive labyrinthine stimulation).

CONTROLLING EYE MOVEMENTS

There are two neural mechanisms for controlling eye movements: **vestibular-ocular** and **cortical-voluntary**. The vestibular-ocular network regulates the reflexive control of conjugate and vertical eye movements through the crossed and uncrossed projections of the MLF (Fig. 10-4). The frontal eye field in the middle frontal gyrus (Brodmann area 8) regulates voluntary control of **saccadic** (quick rotation of the eyes from one fixation point to another that is used in reading) eye movements (Fig. 10-5).

Vestibular Control of Conjugate Eye Movement

We constantly make slow or quick movements with our heads. If our eyes were fixed with no compensatory mechanism for head movements, it would be difficult for us to see clearly. Everything that we see would appear out of focus and distorted by fluctuating movements if not for the important vestibulo-ocular connections that serve as the neurally controlled **gyroscopic** compensatory mechanism for stable eye movements. Lesions of the MLF (usually the result of multiple sclerosis or a stroke) dysconjugate eye movements.

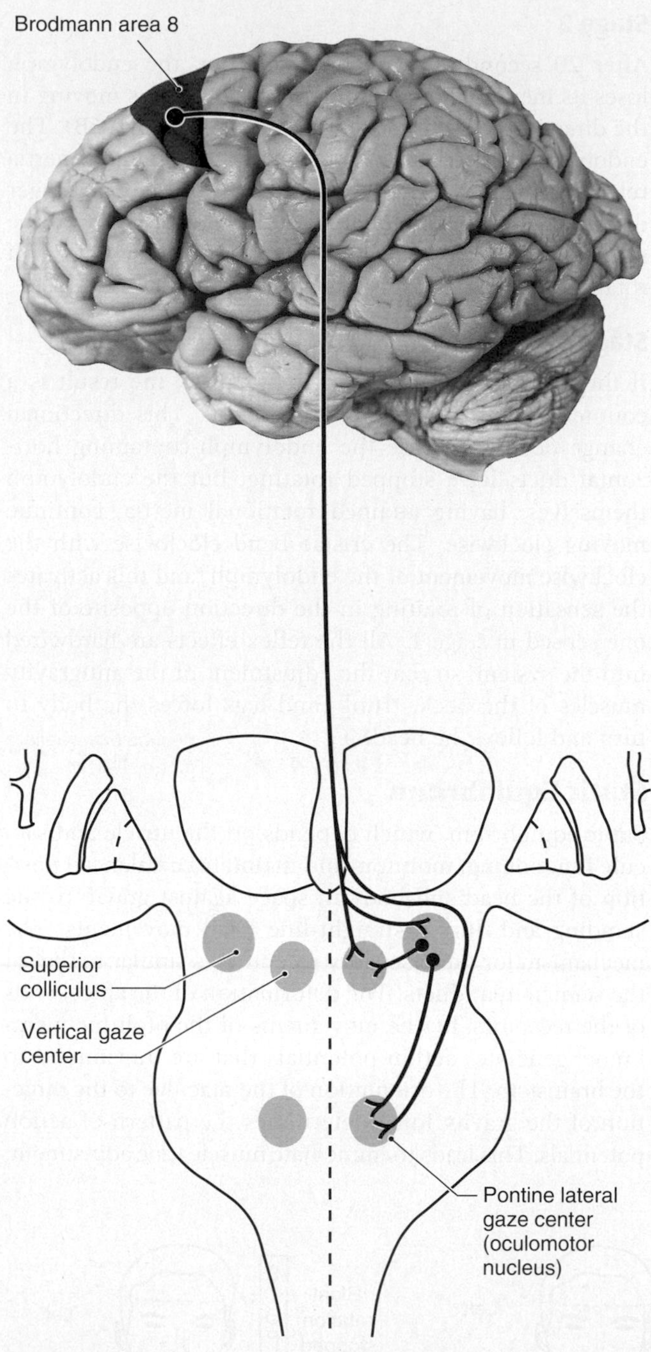

Figure 10-5 The cortical and brainstem mechanism for controlling eye movements.

Triggered by rapid (accelerating and decelerating) head movement, the vestibular (semicircular canals) component of the inner ear sends signals to the medial vestibular nucleus, which provides input to the abducens (CN VI) nucleus within the **pontine horizontal gaze center**. This input, inhibiting ipsilateral conjugate eye movement while facilitating contralateral eye movement, ensures a smooth conjugate ocular movement. With its ascending projections to the trochlear (CN IV) nuclei in the vertical gaze center, the vestibular input also regulates any vertical ocular movement (Fig. 10-4).

If for any reason, normal or pathologic, the vestibular input is reduced, the eyes as a rule deviate to the side of the reduced vestibular input. This is commonly seen in case of a lesion involving the vestibular mechanism and with stimulation of the external auditory canal with cold water. Even in case of a head movement to the opposite side, the activation of the ipsilateral eye compensates and keeps the visual image fixed on the retina, thus avoiding any visual blurring.

Cortical Mechanism for Controlling Voluntary Eye Movement

Gaze control involves coordinated movements of the eyes for maintaining objects on the central retina (**fovea**) for clarity. These movements are saccadic and are either quick or smooth. The quick movements cover up to 400 to 450 degrees per second and track stable objects. Smooth movements cover 50 to 60 degrees per second and keep a moving target focused on the retina. Voluntary control of eye movements comes from the frontal eye field (Brodmann area 8) by way of the superior colliculus in the midbrain. With afferents from the parietal lobe (Brodmann area 7), prefrontal cortex, and the deep layers of the superior colliculi, the frontal eye area activates the brainstem gaze (vertical and horizontal) centers (Fig. 10-5).

The parietal afferents, with links to the visual association cortex, lead us to exploring the novelty of visual stimuli, whereas the frontal afferents regulate the direction of the gaze. The afferents from the superior colliculus, representing the integration of the visual, auditory, and reticular reflexive functions, provide the basis for integrating attention with visual pursuit in saccadic ocular movement.

> ***Key Terms:***
>
> **Dynamic equilibrium** **Static equilibrium**
> **Inertia**

PHYSIOLOGY OF EQUILIBRIUM

Two physiologic mechanisms control equilibrium: **dynamic** and **static**. Dynamic (kinetic) equilibrium regulates the maintenance of body and head positions during rotational and angular acceleration and deceleration. Static equilibrium regulates straight-line (linear) movements of the head in space and both head and body position during rest.

Dynamic Equilibrium

The hair cells of the cristae in the maculae of the semicircular ducts regulate dynamic equilibrium. Each semicircular duct is situated in planes at right angles to each other covering the entire space. The sensory cells in the semicircular ducts respond to angular and rotational head movements. However, each group of receptors responds maximally when the movement is oriented in the plane of the duct. When receptors in the duct of one side are excited, receptors in the corresponding semicircular duct of the opposite side are simultaneously inhibited (Fig. 10-2). On rotation of the head, the moving endolymph in the canal deforms the cristae. Deformation of hair cells generates action potentials, which travel to the brainstem (Fig. 10-3).

The bipolar neurons in the vestibular ganglion that innervate the cristae are constantly active, firing even without a stimulus. This neuronal firing either increases or decreases depending on the direction of their deformation. The frequency of firing increases when the crista bends toward the utricle, and the rate decreases when the crista bends away from the utricle.

Sensation of Rotation

Three events in body rotation represent three stages of the endolymph inertia in the semicircular canals, with each relating to a different rotatory sensation. This is best demonstrated with a rotating (Bárány) chair.

Stage 1

At the beginning of a rotation to the right (clockwise), the endolymph in the horizontal canal tends to lag behind because of inertia. The momentum of endolymph swings the hair cells and cupula in the opposite direction (counterclockwise) of the head movement (Fig. 10-6A). The directional bending and movement of the cristae influence the impulses that are transmitted to the brainstem vestibular nuclei. The brainstem vestibular nuclei interpret the resulting sensation as a clockwise rotation—the opposite direction of the endolymph movement and of the bending of the cristae. The slow phase of bilateral eye movement is always in the direction of the deviation of the cristae.

Stage 2

After 20 seconds of moderate rotation, the endolymph loses its inertia, gathers momentum, and starts moving in the direction of the rotation of the body (Fig. 10-6B). The endolymph and cristae also acquire a new state of inertia related to the turning body, and the hair cells are no longer distorted. With the endolymph at this stage rotating at the same speed and direction as the head, the sensation of rotation is minimal with eyes closed.

Stage 3

If the chair suddenly stops (Fig. 10-6C), the result is a counterclockwise sensation of rotation. This directional change occurs because the endolymph-containing horizontal ducts have stopped rotating, but the endolymph themselves, having attained rotational inertia, continue moving clockwise. The cristae bend clockwise with the clockwise movement of the endolymph, and this activates the sensation of rotating in the direction opposite of the one sensed in stage 1. All the reflex effects are hardwired into the system, so that the adjustment of the antigravity muscles of the neck, trunk, and legs forces the body to turn and follow the head.

Static Equilibrium

Static equilibrium, which depends on the utricle and saccule functioning, monitors and maintains a balanced position of the head and body in space against gravity while standing and during straight-line head movements. The mechanism for these sensory receptors is similar to that of the semicircular ducts. The deformation of the apical ends of the receptors, by the movements of the otolithic membrane, generates action potentials that are transmitted to the brainstem. The orientation of the maculae to the direction of the gravity force determines the pattern of action potentials. This leads to immediate muscle tone adjustment,

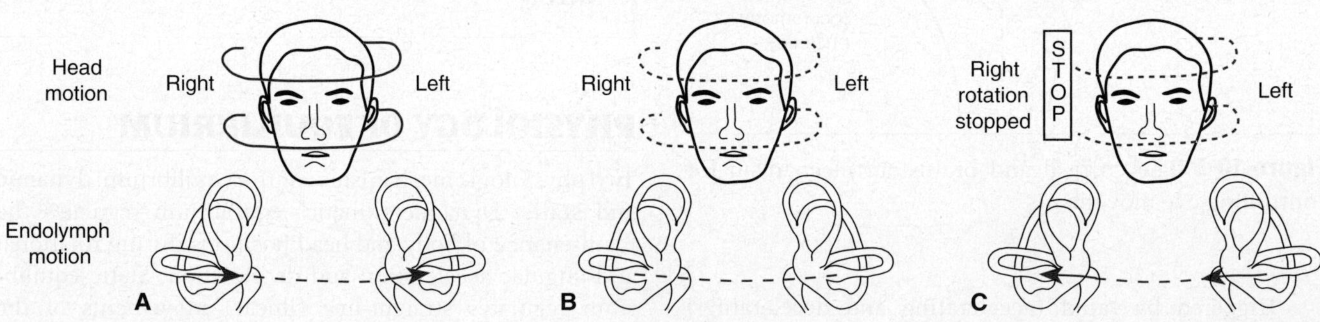

Figure 10-6 The three stages of endolymph movement in relation to the sensation and direction of body rotation with the eyes closed. These head rotations involve endolymph in the horizontal (lateral) semicircular canals. A. At the beginning of rotation, the counterclockwise movement of the endolymph induces a clockwise sensation of rotation. B. With constant rotation after a period of head turning, the endolymph and bony canals rotate at the same rate, and sensory cells in the ampullae are not stimulated; thus there is no longer any sensation of rotation. C. When the clockwise rotation suddenly stops, the endolymph continues to flow clockwise because of inertia; this induces a sensation of counterclockwise rotation. Arrows, direction of motion.

which is needed for the maintenance of equilibrium. Gravity acting on the otolithic membrane causes the maculae to respond quickly to any movement (tilting, acceleration, and deceleration) of the head; fluctuating activation of the maculae for a longer period produces motion sickness.

The vestibular ducts supplement the control of static equilibrium through predictive functions. An example of such a function is the detection of a slight change in head position that prevents a fall while a person is running. The postural reflexes automatically adjust the tone of antigravity muscles. In contrast, the utricle cannot detect loss of balance until it actually occurs. Being off balance must be detected quickly if the person is to initiate appropriate adjustments.

Key Terms :

Nystagmus **Vertigo**

Nystagmus

Nystagmus represents a series of reflexive rhythmic conjugate eye movements. The function of the vestibular reflexes is to maintain a stable, conjugate visual fixation point. If the head slowly rotates in any plane, the vestibular reflexes produce the opposite conjugate eye rotation, retaining the fixation point. These slow rotatory eye movements and the reflex wiring involve the vestibular nuclei and their ocular projections through the MLF.

The rhythmic movement of the eyeballs in nystagmus, the most common vestibular reflex, is a normal compensatory reflex. It consists of two phases: a slow phase in which the eye slowly drifts away from the central field of gaze toward the periphery and a fast phase in which the eye, with a sudden jerk, returns to the central field of gaze. Nystagmus is identified according to the direction of its quick phase (e.g., left nystagmus occurs when the quick component is to the left).

The absence of nystagmus with continued head turn is abnormal, and so is its presence without any head rotation. A new method of assessing nystagmus is electronystagmography, which is based on electro-oculography and involves placing skin electrodes at the outer canthi (outer angle of each eye) to register horizontal or vertical nystagmic movements.

Induced Nystagmus

The influence of the vestibular system on eye movements is best illustrated by spinning a person in a rotating chair about 10 times in 20 seconds. The rotation induces ocular nystagmus, a rhythmic eye movement with slow and fast components. During clockwise rotation of the vestibular ducts (with counterclockwise flow of endolymph in the horizontal semicircular ducts), the eyes move slowly counterclockwise. The fast component of nystagmus is clockwise in the direction of rotation. During a counterclockwise rotation, the fast component of nystagmus is counterclockwise.

Nystagmus can originate in the occipital lobe or in the vestibular apparatus. **Opticokinetic nystagmus** is vision dependent and not vestibular instigated. It can be activated by visual fixation on a moving pattern and can be induced in any dimension—horizontal, vertical, and oblique. Vestibular nystagmus is independent of visual input.

However, visual input can be used to suppress vestibular nystagmus, which is best illustrated by ice skaters and ballet dancers. Professional figure skaters and ballet dancers develop the capacity to control their eye movements independent of vestibular feedback. These do not show any reactive nystagmic movements during or after body rotations. They prevent reactive nystagmus by learning to use visual feedback to suppress vestibular input by quick head rotations laterally over their shoulders. This facilitates continued eye fixation on the same object while the body continues to turn more slowly (Box 10-1).

CLINICAL CORRELATES

Motion Sickness

Motion sickness, the most common disorder of the vestibular system, is characterized by vertigo, the subjective sensation of body rotation. It is also associated with dizziness (fainting and light-headedness), nausea, and vomiting, all of which can be disabling. This is true especially after repeated up and down movements, such as in an airplane in rough weather or on a boat in high waves. Most people adapt to these circumstances, and those who do not can be treated with an antihistamine, such as dimenhydrinate (Dramamine).

Vertigo

Vertigo, the sensation of spinning through space (**subjective vertigo**) or of the environment spinning around oneself (**objective vertigo**), can be very disabling. It is mostly

BOX 10-1

Localizing Value of Vestibular Symptoms

Originating from the anterior inferior cerebellar of the basilar artery, the labyrinthine artery supplies the inner ear containing the vestibular and cochlear mechanisms. Its selective occlusion not only causes deafness in the corresponding ear, but it also affects equilibrium. The patient tends to fall toward the side of the artery occlusion, and there is no response to caloric test in the affected ear. This ipsilaterality of symptoms plays a role in lesion localization.

associated with impaired function of the vestibular apparatus and is commonly found in people who suffer from **Ménière disease**, a condition of obscure origin characterized by abnormally high endolymphatic pressure and later by mixing of endolymph and perilymph secondary to a rupture in the vestibular apparatus. Ménière disease also involves the organ of hearing and includes tinnitus (ringing, humming in the ear), hearing loss, and eventual deafness.

Labyrinth Dysfunction

Labyrinthitis is the irritation of the intercommunicating semicircular ducts and vestibule of the vestibular apparatus secondary to a viral infection or inflammation. It is a common labyrinth dysfunction and often a cause of vertigo. Impairment of the labyrinth on one side (unilateral) causes a short period of vertigo, disequilibrium, nystagmus, and some nausea and vomiting (Box 10-2). The patient tends to fall toward the side of the lesion. This is likely to result from impaired downward pressure on one foot secondary to unopposed vestibulospinal activity on the normal side. The disequilibrium that occurs after bilateral destruction of the labyrinth is generally transient, although it sometimes persists and recurs for many months. Labyrinthine irritation is also a part of Ménière disease (see Chapter 9).

Benign Positional Vertigo

The condition of benign vertigo, which is induced by changes in head position, is commonly seen in the elderly population. The underlying causes include oversensitive vestibular cilia and otolithic degeneration.

Diagnostic Tests

The **acceleration–rotation chair** and **caloric stimulation** are used to evaluate vestibular functions.

BOX 10-2

Vestibular Dysfunctioning

Tumor and stroke involving the labyrinthine artery are two common causes of the vestibular dysfunction. A unilateral vestibular disease is marked with the rotation of both eyes and tendency to fall to the side of lesion. The patient also tilts the head to the same side in order to compensate for the horizontal gaze.

Patients with a bilateral vestibular disease/dysfunction heavily rely on the visual input in place of the lost vestibular input. However, such patients are likely to fall with distractions that compromise the visual input. Such patients also have difficulty in fixating their gaze on an object while the body is in motion.

Acceleration–Rotation Chair

The integrity of vestibular projections to the cranial nerve nuclei can be examined by stimulation of the labyrinth in a rotating subject, also called the **Bárány test**. It is performed on a seated patient with the head tilted forward at 30 degrees so that the lateral semicircular canals are in horizontal plane. After turning clockwise for 20 seconds, the chair is suddenly stopped. With acquired inertia, the endolymph continues to move in the direction (clockwise) of rotation causing the cilia to bend in the same clockwise direction. Subsequent to the cessation of the movement, the vestibular projections to the MLF cause reflexive nystagmus, the oscillatory movements of the eyes (with fast component) in the direction (counterclockwise) opposite to the rotation. Additionally, if asked to walk at this point, the subject deviates to the direction of movement.

Caloric Stimulation

The vestibular end organ functions can also be independently assessed by caloric stimulation of the semicircular ducts. This involves the irrigation of both ear canals with water of different temperatures to induce a convection current in endolymph and measure the system response. This assessment is particularly important in patients with symptoms of dizziness and vertigo. Caloric assessment can be performed using warm (40°C) or cold (30°C) water. In a normal patient, cold water in the external auditory meatus induces nystagmus to the side opposite the canal/ear tested, whereas warm water causes nystagmus to the same side. There is either reduced or absent nystagmus on the side of the lesion in the case of a unilateral vestibular pathway lesion In a normal subject, both ears are likely to respond equally.

A caloric test with ice water is used to differentiate bilateral cortical (frontal) lesions from brainstem damage in comatose patients usually after a head injury. The external canal is filled with cold water for 20 seconds. In the case of a bilateral cortical lesion, there is no nystagmus, and the eyes deviate to the side of the instilled ear. If coma is secondary to a brainstem lesion, the instillation of cold water will not affect the conjugate gaze.

Doll's Eye Reflex

It is used to evaluate the functionality of the brainstem in patients with traumatic brain injury or in a coma. The underlying principle is that the weighted eyeballs in a doll move in response to the doll's head being turned, as opposed to staying on a fixed point. It is tested by turning the patient's head from side to side. If the eyes move laterally in the direction opposite to the head movement, the reflex is positive and the brainstem is functional. However, if the eyes do not turn and remain on a fixed point in the same direction, the reflex is negative and is an indicator of injury in the midbrain involving ocular cranial nerves (CN III, CN IV, and CN VI).

CASE STUDIES FOR PROBLEM SOLVING

CASE ONE (10-1)

A 50-year-old woman had sudden episodes of ringing in the ears, dizziness, vomiting, and vertigo. Every time she got up, she felt unsteady. She was taken to the hospital and, on testing, exhibited the following:

- No vestibular response in the left ear on caloric testing
- Head posture tilted to the left
- Severe vertigo
- Deafness in the left ear
- Loss of pain and temperature sensation on the left side of the face

A brain MRI study revealed an infarct in the dorsal lateral region of the left medulla and caudal region of the left pons.

Question: How can you relate the vestibular symptoms with the left medullary-pontine lesion?

Case (10-1) Discussion: See discussion of case studies

CASE TWO (10-2)

A 45-year-old schoolteacher woke up feeling dizzy. She experienced unsteadiness while standing, the sensation of the room spinning, and did not hear in her right ear. She consulted a neurologist who noted the following:

- Profound hearing impairment in the right ear
- Unsteady posture
- Gait ataxia with a tendency to fall to the right side
- Left nystagmus
- No sign of limb or pharyngeal paralysis

An SLP evaluation revealed no cognitive, linguistic, or speech-related deficit. The only clinically significant point was that she used only her left ear for listening.

A magnetic resonance angiogram revealed the absence of a branch of the anterior inferior cerebellar artery, which is a sub-branch of the basilar artery on the right side.

Question: Based on your understanding of the vestibular vascular supply, can you provide an explanation for these selective symptoms?

Case (10-2) Discussion: See discussion of case studies

CASE THREE (10-3)

A 35-year-old student had a ringing sensation in the right ear and had suffered two disabling attacks of vertigo associated with nausea within 3 months. She was seen by a neurologist, who noted the following:

- Signs of fluctuating hearing loss
- Reported sensation of tinnitus
- Repeated attacks of vomiting and nausea
- Normal somatosensory functions outside of these attacks

The brain MRI study was normal. With no evidence of structural changes, the neurologist suspected this to be a case of excessive or fluctuating endolymphic pressure in the inner ear.

Question: Can you comment on the pathophysiology of these symptoms?

Case (10-3) Discussion: See discussion of case studies

CASE FOUR (10-4)

A 28-year-old woman, who suddenly fell sick, was taken to the ER where she presented with the following:

- Dizziness, nausea, and vomiting
- A tendency to fall to the right
- Left nystagmus
- Decreased hearing sensitivity in the right ear
- Breathy and hoarse voice
- Nasal emission and difficulty swallowing
- No cognitive or language disorder
- No asymmetry involving the lingual and facial muscles

Which of the following lesion sites could account for these clinical symptoms?

a. right pons and left frontal cortex
b. caudal pons and rostral medulla on the right
c. rostral medulla and caudal pons on the left
d. bilateral spinal lesions
e. bilateral midbrain lesions

Case (10-4) Discussion: See discussion of case studies

SUMMARY

The vestibular system is a reflexive sensorimotor system. It controls two important functions: equilibrium and conjugate eye movements. With sensory receptors in the semicircular canals of the inner ear, nuclei in the brainstem, and direct connections to other brainstem systems including the cranial nerves for ocular movements, the vestibular apparatus helps humans maintain a balanced upright posture, coordinate head and body movements, and control eye fixation on a point in space, even during body and head movements. The vestibular system is closely linked with the visual and proprioceptive systems; it constantly integrates incoming visual and proprioceptive cues, which contribute to the execution of skilled and coordinated activities like dancing, skating, and acrobatics. The functional importance of the vestibular system becomes evident in patients whose body balance is impaired by Ménière's disease, labyrinthis, or tumors (acoustic neuroma or vestibular schwannoma) of the vestibulocochlear (CN VIII) nerve. Clinically, its assessment provides important diagnostic information about the brainstem and brain functioning.

REVIEW QUESTIONS

1. Complete the following statements using the appropriate technical terms:
   A. __________ __________ regulates the maintenance of body and head positions during rotational and angular acceleration and deceleration.
   B. __________ represents a tendency of fluid to oppose any movement from a rest position.
   C. __________ is the oscillating movements of the eye, which is caused by dysfunctioning of the vestibular mechanism.
   D. The dysfunction of the __________ __________ __________, which integrates the vestibular input with the coordinated eye movement, leads to double vision.
   E. Characterized by vertigo, nausea, vomiting, tinnitus, and progressive but fluctuating sensory hearing loss, __________ __________ is associated with increased endolymphatic pressure in the __________ __________.
   F. __________ regulates straight-line (linear) movements of the head in space and both head and body position during rest.
   G. As a disorder of the vestibular system, __________ refers to a sensation of self-rotation or the spinning of the space around.
   H. The __________ regulates the position of the head and neck in space besides monitoring upright posture reflexes.
2. A 28-year-old woman was seen for a complaint of dizziness, nausea, and vomiting. On examination, she exhibited a tendency of falling to the right, left nystagmus, and deafness in the right ear, analgesia on the left body, hoarseness, and swallowing difficulty. Name the side and location of the lesion.
3. Professionals participating in which two activities do not exhibit reflexive rotational nystagmus?
4. Provide three cardinal clinical symptoms that are associated with the Ménière disease.
5. Name the purpose of irrigating the external auditory canal with warm and cold water.

11 Somatosensory System

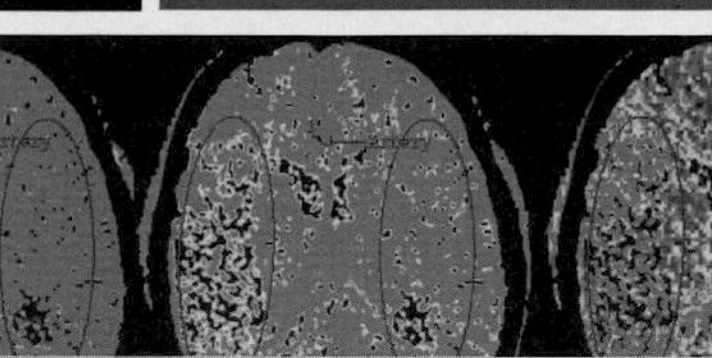

LEARNING OBJECTIVES

After studying this chapter, students should be able to:

- List the major modalities of sensation
- Explain the three-neuron organization for somatic sensation
- Describe the neural pathways for the epicritic systems of the face and body
- Describe the neural pathways for the protopathic systems of the face and body
- Describe the neural pathways of conscious and unconscious proprioception
- Outline common disorders of somatosensation
- Explain the concepts and mechanisms of referred and phantom pain
- Solve clinical problems by relating somatosensory disorders to plausible lesion sites
- Outline the methods and stimuli for assessing somatic sensation

SOMATOSENSATION

Somatosensation refers to the bodily experienced external and internal sensations and include pain, temperature, touch, and **proprioception**. It begins with specialized receptors in the skin, muscles, joints, and blood vessels that convert sensation to neural signals and transmit them through the spinal cord to the sensory cortex in the parietal lobe. Localized receptors in the skin and muscles feed into a single sensory nerve fiber, which combines with other sensory nerve fibers to form a fiber bundle.

Closer to the spinal cord, the afferent and efferent fiber bundles of the spinal nerve separate forming dorsal and ventral spinal nerve fibers (Fig. 11-1). There are two types of afferent nerve fibers that have their cell bodies in the dorsal root ganglion (DRG). Only stretch afferent neuronal terminals (A1) synapse with a lower motor neuron (LMN) dendrite or cell body and mediate the stretch reflex; all other afferents terminate in the dorsal horn association nucleus. The LMN circuitry not only distributes to local (segmental and intersegmental) reflex output but also integrates other ongoing output activity descending from the higher CNS levels.

The dorsal horn circuitry modifies and integrates the input information before distributing collaterals to the brainstem reticular formation, the higher sensory centers on the opposite side, and the rostral intersegmental reflex circuits. The ascending fibers carry information regarding pain, touch, temperature, and sense of position and travel through the spinal cord, brainstem, and thalamus before projecting to the primary sensory (postcentral gyrus) and the associational sensory (superior parietal lobule) cortices in the parietal lobe. The primary cortex analyzes information for a conscious perception of the sensation. In the sensory associational region, on the other hand, the lower-order tactile sensations are analyzed, elaborated on, integrated with previous experiences, and raised to the highest conscious level for cognitive elaboration. The somatosensory system is discretely organized; each tract separately mediates its respective modalities of sensation maintaining the point-to-point representation of its corresponding body surface (see Fig. 2-6*A*). Also see chapters 2 and 19 for the cognitive functions of the parietal association region.

Basis for Clinical Information

Knowledge of the sensory receptors, ascending paths taken by sensory fibers, points of fiber crossing, and cortical areas related to underlying conscious perceptual experiences provides the groundwork needed for understanding the organization of the somatosensory system. This knowledge of the modalities of pain, touch, and temperature also helps relate patterns of sensory deficits to lesion sites in the central pathways.

Types of Sensation

There are three primary types of somatic sensation: **mechanoreception**, **thermoreception**, and **nociception** (Table 11-1). Mechanoreception implies the displacement of the nerve endings and includes touch, pressure, vibration (tactile), and

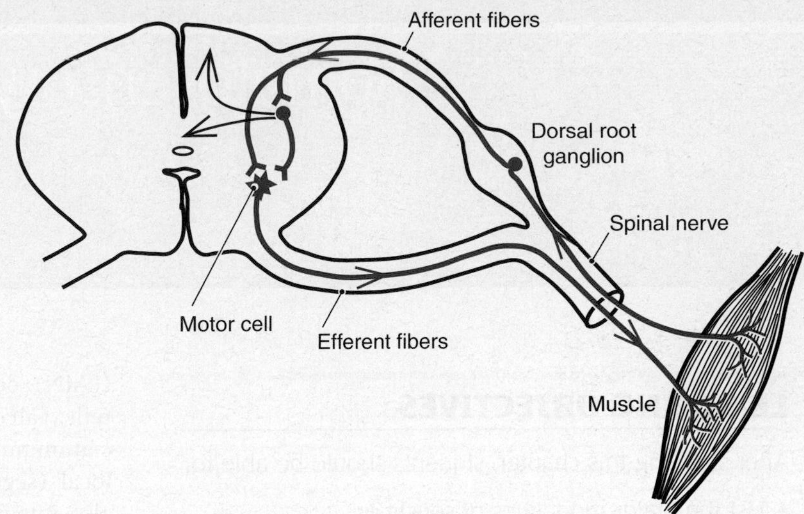

Figure 11-1 Cross section of a spinal cord showing the afferent and efferent spinal fibers that join to form the spinal nerve.

kinesthesia (limb position and movement). Touch is further divided into fine discriminative (localizable) and diffuse (unlocalizable) types. Thermoreception includes the sensation of cold and heat. Nociception refers to pain related to tissue destruction.

Specialized Receptors

Various structurally different receptors, including the somatosensory end organs, are located in the skin, limb joints, blood vessels, and muscles. Primarily, the modality of receptor type is identified by its maximal sensitivity (responsiveness) to the smallest amplitude of sensory stimuli of heat, pain, and touch. Receptors can also be identified by their adaptiveness to stimuli. Quickly adapting receptors respond strongly at the onset of the stimulus; however, as they adapt to the stimulus strength, their responses become weaker, eventually dying out. The nonadapting receptors may not respond so vigorously to the stimulus onset. Once activated, however, they continuously provide signals to the brain as long as the stimulus remains present. The basic types of sensory receptors in the body are **encapsulated endings**, **free nerve endings**, and **expanded tip endings** (Fig. 11-2; Table 11-2). An additional class of receptors that mediate olfaction and taste are not discussed here.

Table 11-1

Types of Sensation

Somatic Senses	Mediated Modalities
Mechanoreception	Touch, pressure, vibration, and proprioception
Thermoreception	Cold and heat
Nociception	Pain

Encapsulated Endings

Commonly distributed in subcutaneous tissues, skin, fingertips, palms, lips, and external genitals, these most sensitive and rapidly adapting mechanoreceptors mediate sensations of vibration and fine discriminative touch. These consist of concentric layers of tissue around a nerve ending. Any deformation of the external layer compresses all of the fluid-filled inner layers, altering the contour of the capsule. The receptors in this category are **Meissner corpuscles** and **Pacinian corpuscles** (Fig. 11-2).

Free Nerve Endings

Distributed throughout the body, skin, cutaneous tissue, and visceral organs, these nonadapting free nerve ending receptors consist of fine branchings of fiber and mediate the sensations of pain and temperature. They respond by sending signals at a slow rate for long periods (Fig. 11-2).

Expanded Tip Endings

Merkel receptors and **Ruffini endings** consist of nerve endings with knobs that mediate touch, temperature, and pressure. Located in the dermis and joints, these mechanoreceptors transmit slowly and are moderately adaptive (Fig. 11-2).

Three-Neuron Organization

All somatosensory pathways are anatomically organized in such a manner that a given sensory impulse enters the CNS, crosses the midline, and then ascends to the contralateral sensory cortex. This impulse transmission involves three-neurons and their fibers (Fig. 11-3). The first-order neurons, with their cell bodies in the spinal DRG, collect sensory information from the periphery and transmit it to the second-order neurons in the CNS. The second-order neurons, depending on the modality of sensation, are either in the spinal cord or in the brainstem. The second-order fibers consistently cross

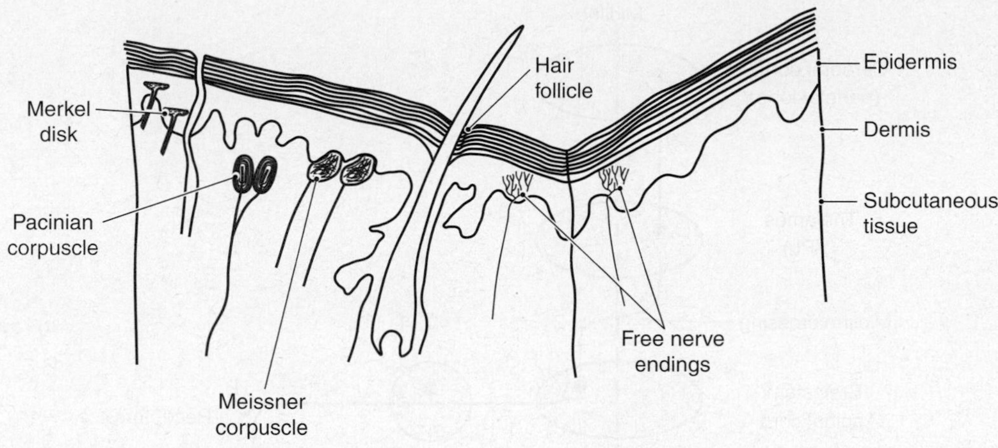

Figure 11-2 Common sensory receptors. Meissner and Pacinian corpuscles (fine discriminative touch); Merkel end organs, with expanded tips (diffuse touch); Receptors with free nerve endings (pain and temperature).

the midline and ascend to the opposite thalamus, which contains the third-order neurons. The third-order fibers project from the thalamus to the primary sensory cortex.

Innervation Pattern

The spinal organization of the sensory pathway is mixed. Pathways mediating discriminative touch, which represents relatively late development, have the input axon proceeding up the ipsilateral side, and decussation is delayed to the medullary level. However, the earlier developed pathways, which mediate pain, temperature, and diffuse (nonlocalized) touch, decussate in the spinal cord at multiple sites and proceed rostrally on the contralateral side.

Table 11-2

Receptors for Somatic Sensation

Receptor Types	Suggested Mediated Modalities
Encapsulated endings Pacinian corpuscles Meissner corpuscles	Tactile (discriminative touch, vibration)
Free nerve endings	Pain and temperature (heat, cold); some tactile
Expanded tip endings Merkel receptors Ruffini endings	Tactile (touch, pressure); temperature

Consequently, a spinal lesion has different clinical implications for both of these sensation types. A spinal lesion would result in the loss of discriminative touch on the body ipsilateral to the lesion and loss of pain and temperature on the side contralateral to the lesion.

Key Terms:

Agnosia	**Proprioception**
Epicritic sensation	**Protopathic sensation**
Kinesthesia	

Spinal Anatomic Division

The somatosensory system is divided into the **dorsal column–medial lemniscal system** and the **anterolateral system** (Fig. 11-4). The dorsal column–medial lemniscal system, also called the **epicritic system**, is phylogenetically newer. The large myelinated fibers of the dorsal column system not only conduct impulses rapidly but also represent a precise map of the body surface. Located in the dorsal spinal region and maintaining a high degree of precision and intensity resolution, the epicritic sensation includes the sensations of fine discriminative touch, vibration, limb position, kinesthesia, and proprioception.

The anterolateral system, a phylogenetically older system, is also called the **protopathic system** (Table 11-3). This system is further divided into the **lateral spinothalamic** (pain and temperature) and the **anterior spinothalamic** (high threshold and poorly nonlocalizable touch) **tracts**.

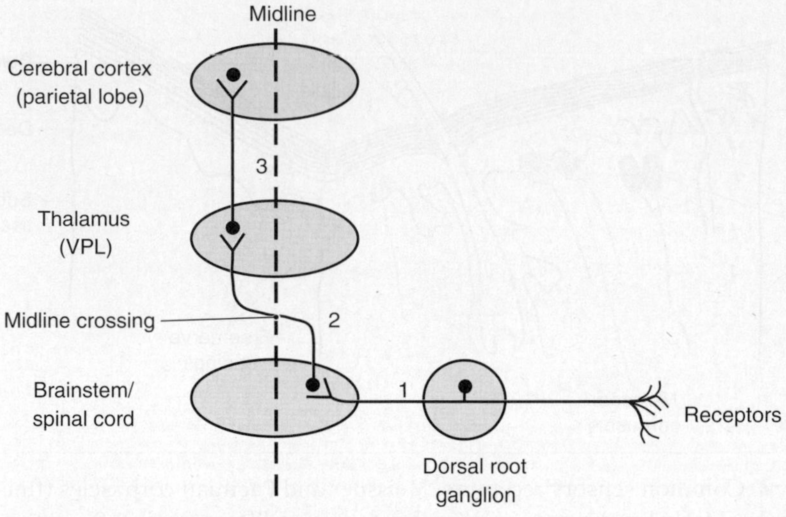

Figure 11-3 The three-neuron organization of somatosensory system. First-order neurons (*1*), with their cell bodies in the dorsal root ganglion, collect sensory information from the body surface. First-order fibers transmit sensory information to second-order neurons (2) in the CNS. Depending on the mediated modality, second-order neurons are in either the spinal cord or the brainstem. Second-order fibers cross the midline and terminate in the third-order neurons (3) of the contralateral thalamus. Third-order fibers project to the primary sensory cortex in the parietal lobe. *VPL*, ventral posterior lateral.

Dorsal Column–Medial Lemniscal System

The dorsal column–medial lemniscal system mediates postural position sense, fine discriminative touch, and vibration. Position sense, which is mediated consciously and unconsciously, is divided into two types: proprioception and kinesthesia. Proprioception, the internal awareness of limb position in space, is essential in the acquisition of skilled movements, such as speech and writing, and it provides the cortex with a conscious awareness of the spatial position of body parts and the body during motion. Kinesthesia, the internal awareness of limb movement, is essential to the acquisition of skilled movements and provides information related to the direction and range of limb movements. Fine discriminative touch is involved with the analysis and identification of objects through tactual manipulation (**stereognosis**), the recognition of figures and numbers written on the body (**graphesthesia**), the discrimination between two or multiple points of touch, and the awareness of touch.

Receptors

Meissner and Pacinian corpuscles, both of which are exceedingly sensitive and highly adaptive encapsulated end receptors, primarily serve epicritic sensation. They mediate discriminative touch and vibration. Additional receptors such as **muscle spindle organs** are the most sensitive (lower threshold) receptors to vibration, kinesthesia, and proprioception.

Neural Pathways

The dorsal column–medial lemniscal system consists of two fasciculi: fasciculus gracilis and fasciculus cuneatus (Fig. 11-4; Table 11-4). Each fasciculus mediates discriminative touch from different body regions; however, both follow a similar three-neuron sensory organization and innervation pattern (Fig. 11-5*A*). The first-order fibers, with their cell bodies in the DRG, collect sensory information from the body and enter the spinal cord. After entering the cord, the afferent axons divide into short and long branches. The short axons extend to the spinal dorsal gray horn and mediate reflexive activity. The long axonal fibers ascend ipsilaterally in the gracilis and cuneatus fasciculi and synapse on the gracile and cuneate nuclei in the medulla, then cross the midline and project to the primary sensory cortex in the parietal lobe.

Fibers in the dorsal column–medial lemniscal system are arranged in a laminar fashion; the sacral fibers are the most medial in the dorsal column. Lumbar fibers travel parallel to sacral fibers in the dorsal column and are laterally joined by fibers from the thoracic and cervical levels. Therefore, the fibers mediating sensation from the leg are medial, whereas the fibers from the arm are most lateral.

Fasciculus Gracilis

The fasciculus gracilis transmits epicritic sensations from the lower half of the body and includes the afferent fibers entering the dorsal column approximately from the sacral to midthoracic sections of the spinal cord (Fig. 11-5*B*). After projecting short axons to the dorsal horn for reflexive activity, the first-order fibers, with neurons in the DRG, ascend medially in the dorsal column of the spinal cord. Fibers of the fasciculus gracilis terminate in the nucleus gracilis, the

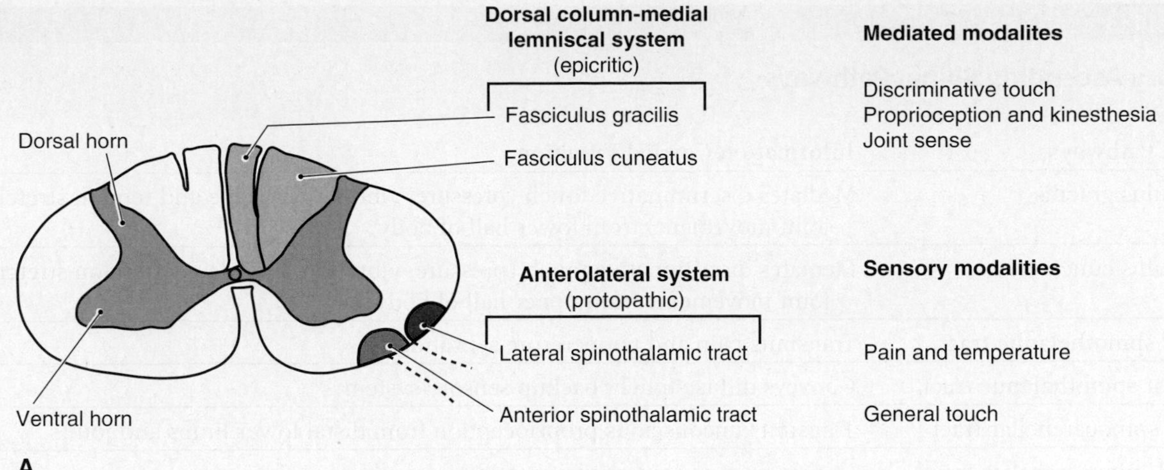

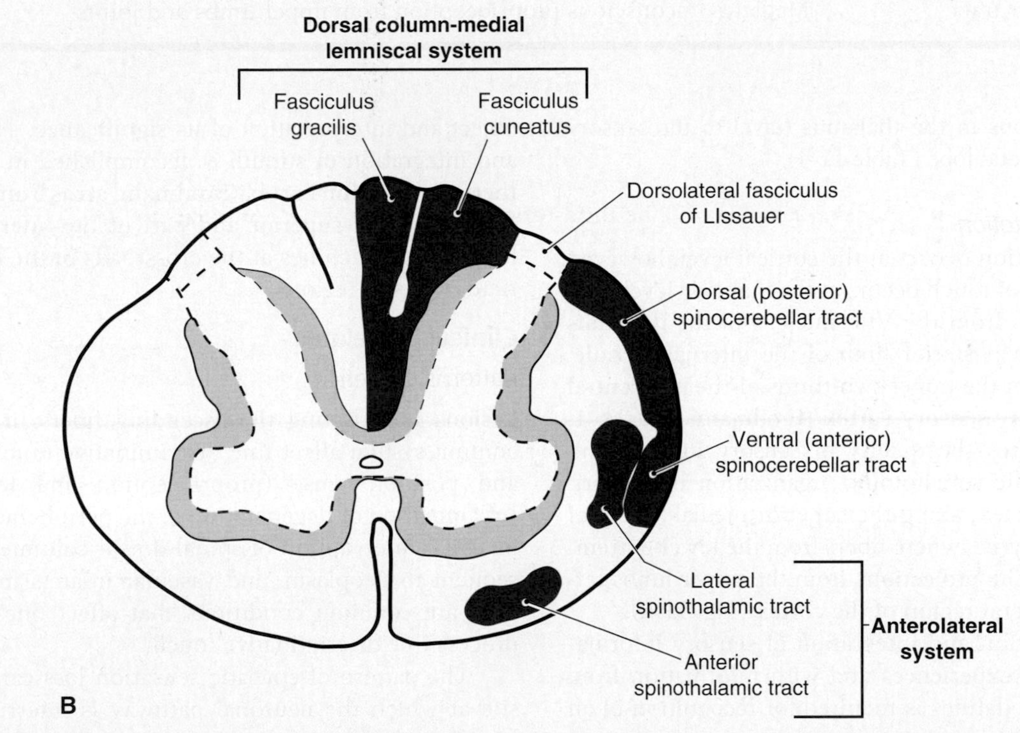

Figure 11-4 A. Anatomic division of the somatosensory system. B. Spinal locations of the sensory pathways.

second-order sensory neuron in the dorsal caudal medulla. From this point, the internal arcuate (the second order) fibers cross the midline to merge with the fasciculus cuneatus in the medial lemniscus. The medial lemniscus, formed by the crossed dorsal column fibers, ascends and terminates on the ventral posterior lateral nucleus (VPL), the third-order neurons in the thalamus. The projections from the third-order neurons in the thalamus travel to the sensory cortex in the parietal lobe (Table 11-4).

Fasciculus Cuneatus

Fibers of the fasciculus cuneatus, which are lateral to the fasciculus gracilis in the dorsal column, carry epicritic sensations from the upper body and enter the spinal cord above the midthoracic level (Fig. 11-5*B*). These fibers ipsilaterally ascend the spinal cord dorsal column toward the brainstem and terminate at the nucleus cuneatus, the second-order neuron which is lateral to the nucleus gracilis in the dorsal caudal medulla.

The internal arcuate fibers, the second-order fibers from the nucleus cuneatus, travel medially and cross the midline just above the pyramid in the medulla (Fig. 3-8). After the crossing (decussation), the internal arcuate fibers form the medial lemniscus, a fillet-shaped bundle of fibers. The medial lemniscus fibers ascend along the midline through the medulla and the pontine tegmentum (see Figs. 3-9–3-11 and 3-14). Later they migrate dorsolaterally in the midbrain to enter the VPL of the thalamus, the third-order sensory relay nucleus (see Fig. 3-18). The projections from the

Table 11-3

Primary Ascending Spinal Pathways

Spinal Pathways	Information Carried/Function
Fasciculus gracilis	Mediates discriminative touch (pressure, vibration, muscle and tendon stretch, and joint movement) from lower half of body
Fasciculus cuneatus	Mediates discriminative touch (pressure, vibration, muscle and tendon stretch, and joint movement) from upper half of body
Lateral spinothalamic tract	Transmits pain and temperature sensation
Anterior spinothalamic tract	Conveys diffuse touch; backup sensory system
Dorsal spinocerebellar tract	Transmits unconscious proprioception from distal lower limbs and joints
Ventral spinocerebellar tract	Carries unconscious proprioception from muscles of lower extremities, proximal limbs, and axial muscles
Cuneocerebellar tract	Mediates unconscious proprioception from upper limbs and joints

third-order neurons in the thalamus travel to the sensory cortex in the parietal lobe (Table 11-4).

Cortical Representation

Conscious sensation occurs at the cortical level; however, crude awareness of touch occurs at the thalamic level. The third-order fibers from the VPL nucleus of the thalamus pass through the posterior limb of the internal capsule. They terminate in the upper two-thirds of the postcentral gyrus, the primary sensory cortex (Brodmann areas 3, 1, 2), which analyzes the quality of sensory information. There is a specific somatotopic organization in the primary sensory cortex, along the superior medial aspect of the postcentral gyrus, where fibers from the lower extremities terminate. The projections from the upper limbs terminate in the lateral region of the cortex (Fig. 11-6).

The elaboration and integration of sensory information with stored experiences and with information from other sensory modalities is required for recognition of an object and interpretation of its significance. This analysis and integration of stimuli is accomplished in the **somesthetic association cortex** (Brodmann areas 5 and 7), which consists of the superior and part of the inferior parietal lobule and which lies at the crossroads of the temporoparieto-occipital regions.

Clinical Correlates

Patterns of Deficit

Lesions interrupting the ascending fibers in the dorsal column system affect fine discriminative touch sensation and position sense (proprioception and kinesthesia). Inflammation or degeneration of the peripheral nerve and/or DRG, interruption of spinal dorsal column fibers consequent to neoplasm, and vascular infarcts in the spinal cord are common conditions that affect one's ability to process fine discriminative touch.

The pattern of epicritic sensation loss can reveal the site at which the neuronal pathway is interrupted. This

Table 11-4

Components of the Epicritic System: Fine Discriminative Touch

Nerve Cell Order	Associated Fibers	Target Nucleus
First-order neuron (DRG)	With cell bodies in DRG, first-order central fibers enter spinal cord to form dorsal funiculus and ascend ipsilaterally to medulla	NG and NC in caudal medulla
Second-order neuron (NG, NC)	With cell bodies in NG and NC, internal arcuate fibers cross midline in medulla and ascend as medial lemniscus to thalamus	VPL of thalamus
Third-order neuron (VPL of thalamus)	With cell bodies in the VPL, thalamocortical projections ascend from thalamus to cortex	Primary sensory cortex (body area)

DRG, dorsal root ganglion; *NC*, nucleus cuneatus; *NG*, nucleus gracilis; *VPL*, ventral posterior lateral nucleus.

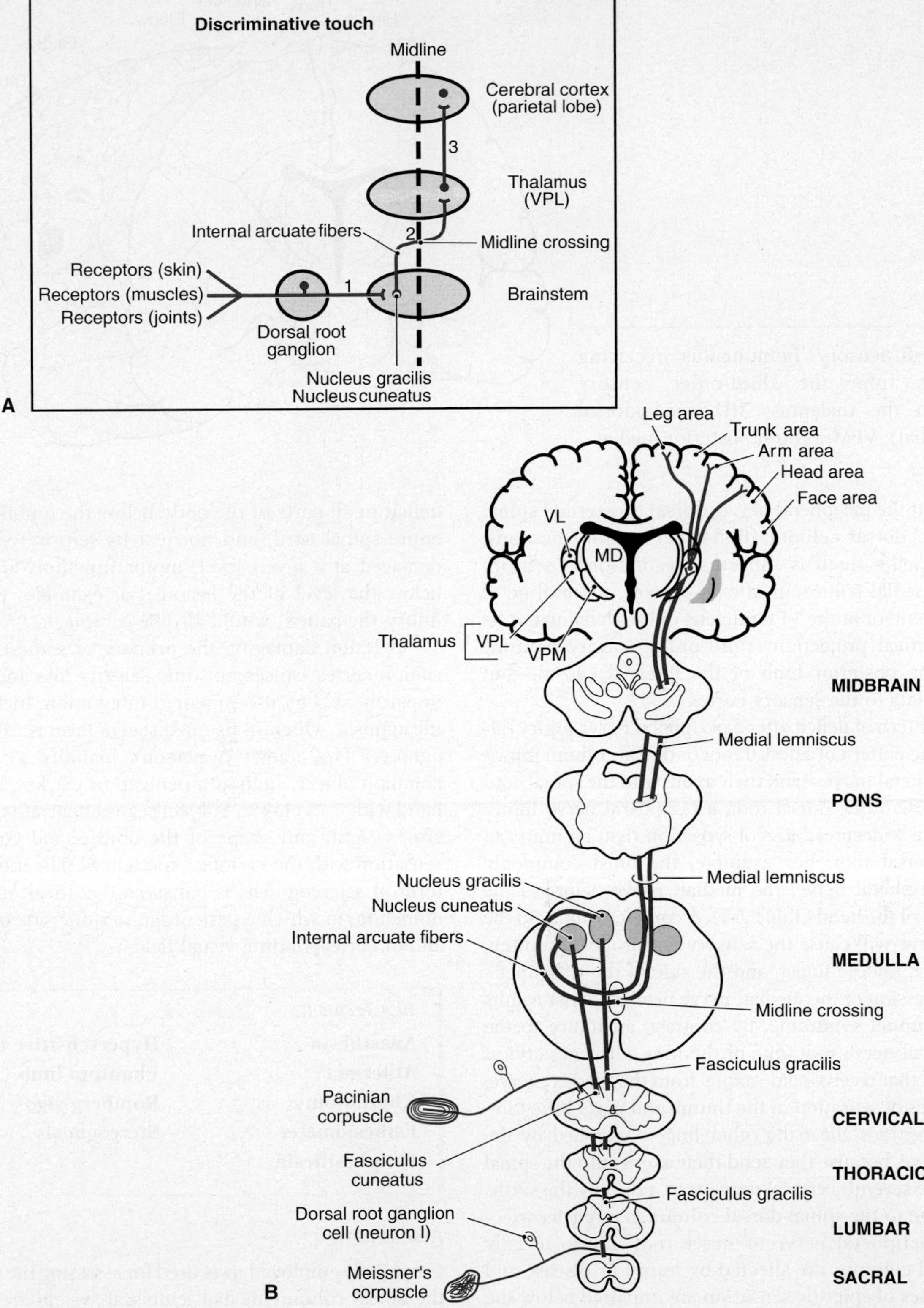

Figure 11-5 A. The three-neuron organization of the dorsal column–medial lemniscal system. B. The dorsal white column. MD, mediodorsal (dorsomedial); *VL*, ventrolateral; *VPL*, ventral posterior lateral; *VPM*, ventral posterior medial.

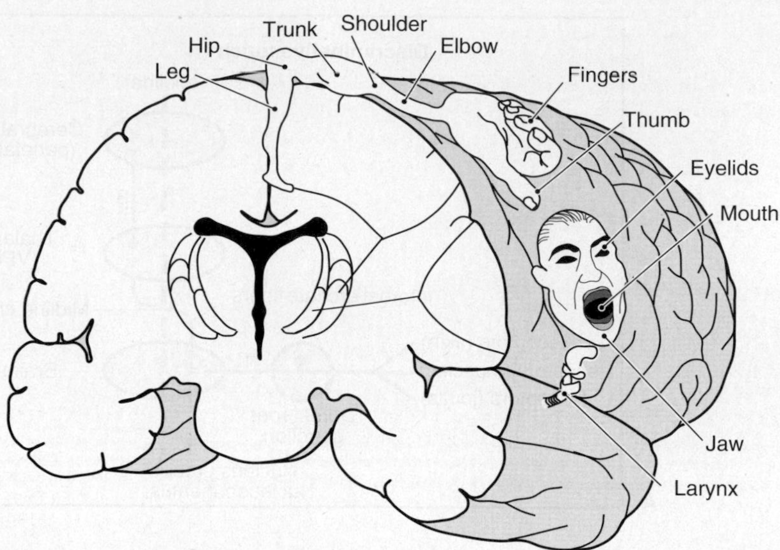

Figure 11-6 Sensory homunculus receiving projections from the third-order sensory nucleus in the thalamus. *MD*, mediodorsal (dorsomedial); *VPM*, ventral posterior medial.

can occur at the peripheral nerve, dorsal (posterior) spinal nerve root, dorsal column (first-order sensory neuron), nucleus gracilis, nucleus cuneatus (second-order sensory neuron), medial lemniscus after it crosses the midline of the brainstem, or at the VPL nucleus of the thalamus or its thalamocortical projection (third-order sensory neuron) through the posterior limb of the internal capsule and corona radiata to the sensory cortex.

The pattern of deficit after a peripheral nerve injury differs from the pattern of a dorsal root or dorsal column injury. Since peripheral nerves send their axons into the spinal cord over more than one dorsal root, a peripheral nerve injury causes more widespread loss of sensation than an injury to a single dorsal root. For example, the most commonly injured peripheral nerve, the **median nerve**, supplies the thumb side of the hand (Table 2-5). A complete injury to the median nerve will cause the sensory loss from the thumb, index finger, middle finger, and the side of the ring finger. The compression of the median nerve near the wrist results in **carpal tunnel syndrome**. By contrast, an injury to the sixth cervical nerve root, one of the four adjacent cervical nerve roots that receive some axons from the median nerve, creates a loss of sensation in the thumb and part of the forearm but does not affect the other fingers supplied by the median nerve, because they send their axons into the spinal cord via the seventh cervical nerve root, not only the sixth.

Damage to the spinal dorsal column is rarely as selective as a peripheral nerve or nerve root injury; usually both dorsal columns are affected by injury or disease and all modalities of epicritic sensation are impaired below the level of the lesion on the same (ipsilateral) side. Any lesion affecting the internal arcuate fibers or anything past them will result in a contralateral pattern of loss.

The key to clinically identifying the spinal cord as the site of injury is to find a level on the body below which sensation is abnormal (impaired, altered, or lost). For example, a lesion that completely interrupts the sensory pathways at the level of the T10 would cause a sensory deficit in all parts of the body below the umbilicus. If the entire spinal cord, and not just its sensory pathways, is damaged at a given level, motor functions are also lost below the level of the lesion. For example, with a T10 injury, the patient would also be paraplegic.

A lesion damaging the primary or somesthetic association cortex causes not only sensory loss and cognitive impairments but also impaired integration, including tactile agnosia, which in its most severe form is called astereognosis. This shows a person's inability to identify a common object, such as a pen cap or car key, held in the hand with eyes closed. Subjects cannot narrate the texture, size, weight, and shape of the objects and compare the sensation with the various experiences. The most extreme form of astereognosis is considered cortical neglect phenomenon, in which a patient ignores one side of the body, and/or corresponding visual fields.

Key Terms:

Anesthesia	**Hypersensitive tangle**
Athermia	**Phantom limb**
Chordotomy	**Romberg sign**
Esthesiometer	**Stereognosis**
Graphesthesia	

Assessment

Commonly employed tests used for assessing the integrity of the dorsal column–medial lemniscal system are two-point tactile discrimination, vibratory sense, position sense, stereognosis, and graphesthesia. The two-point discrimination test assesses the individual's ability to identify two close points of stimulation. Pencil tips or a special instrument, an **esthesiometer**, are used for stimulating two closely spaced points. The patient, with eyes closed, is asked to differentiate between the two points of touch. The distance between the two points is gradually decreased until the subject can no longer tell which two points were touched. For stereognosis, the patient, with eyes closed, is required to identify an object by feeling its contour, weight, shape, and texture. Graphesthesia tests a patient's ability to identify, with eyes closed, a number or letter written on the skin. Vibratory sense is assessed via a tuning fork held against a bony surface. The patient describes when and where the vibration was felt. Impaired vibration sense is an important indicator of a disease affecting the large myelinated fibers.

The **Romberg test** is used to evaluate proprioceptive function. With eyes closed, the patient stands with feet together. Unsteadiness in this position indicates a lack of proprioception in the lower extremities. Kinesthetic awareness is tested by moving the individual's fingers and toes while he or she reports on the direction of joint movements. Kinesthetic proprioception concerning position sense is also tested by moving the patient's arm to an angle 45 degrees or more and then asking him or her to duplicate the shoulder angle with the other arm. Separate assessments of the upper and lower limbs can be used to evaluate the integrity of the fasciculi gracilis and cuneatus.

Anterolateral System

Involved with protopathic sensation and named for the location of its fibers within the spinal white column, the anterolateral system is divided into the lateral and anterior spinothalamic tracts. The lateral spinothalamic tract mediates the sensations of pain and temperature. The anterior spinothalamic tract mediates diffuse or unlocalized touch.

Lateral Spinothalamic Tract

Receptors

End organs with free nerve endings are the mediators of pain and temperature sensations. Some encapsulated receptors may also secondarily contribute to the modalities of pain and temperature (Table 11-5).

Neural Pathway

The pathway carrying the sensations of pain and temperature (hot and cold) begins at the nociceptive receptors in the skin (Fig. 11-7*A*). The first-order fibers, with their nuclei in the DRG, carry sensations from the free nerve ending receptors in the skin and enter the dorsolateral spinal cord. After entering the cord, these fibers travel up or down a few spinal segments in the **dorsolateral fasciculus (Lissauer tract)** before penetrating the dorsal spinal gray matter. After penetration, the fibers terminate in the **substantia gelatinosa** and **nucleus proprius**. Collaterals from the substantia gelatinosa and nucleus proprius project via interneurons to motor neurons in the ventral gray horns and mediate withdrawal reflexes.

The second-order fibers cross the midline in the ventral white commissure to ascend in the lateral spinothalamic tract (Fig. 11-7*B*). Fibers carrying pain and temperature sensation from the entire body travel in the lateral spinothalamic tract and ascend toward the brainstem on the way to the thalamus. After traveling through the medulla (see Fig. 3-11), ventrolateral pons (see Fig. 3-14), and midbrain tegmentum (see Fig. 3-16), the spinothalamic fibers terminate on the third-order neurons in the VPL nucleus of the thalamus. Thalamocortical fibers travel through the internal capsule and corona radiata, then project to the upper two-thirds of the postcentral gyrus in the parietal lobe (Fig. 11-6). The primary sensory cortex is responsible for a fine analysis of sensation and determines its quality and source.

Cortical Representation

Note that the stimulation of the primary sensory cortex does not result in the experience of pain. This primary cortex determines where the pain is (localization) but is not involved in the intensity of the pain. Pain may be characterized as sharp or dull (diffuse). The neuronal mechanism of sharp pain is well understood, as it is projected to the cortex by way of specific thalamic (VPL and **ventral posterior medial [VPM]**) nuclei (see Chapter 6). It involves faster conduction and is precisely localizable. However, dull pain involves multisynaptic pathways. The lateral spinothalamic tract mediating nociceptive afferents from the body, viscera, or face gives off many collaterals that terminate on the reticular nuclei in the brainstem; these reticular nuclei project to the thalamus, hypothalamus, and hippocampus.

Table 11-5

Components of the Protopathic System: Pain, Temperature, and Touch

Nerve Cell Order	Associated Fibers	Target Nucleus
First-order neuron (DRG)	With cell bodies in DRG, first-order fibers enter spinal cord	NP and SG in spinal dorsal horn
Second-order neuron (NP, SG)	With cell bodies in NP and SG, second-order fibers cross midline in spinal cord, form lateral and ventral spinothalamic tracts, and ascend to thalamus	VPL of thalamus
Third-order neuron (VPL of thalamus)	With cell bodies in VPL, thalamocortical projections ascend from thalamus to cortex	Primary sensory cortex (body area)

DRG, dorsal root ganglion; *NP*, nucleus proprius; *SG*, substantia gelatinosa; *VLP*, ventral posterior lateral nucleus.

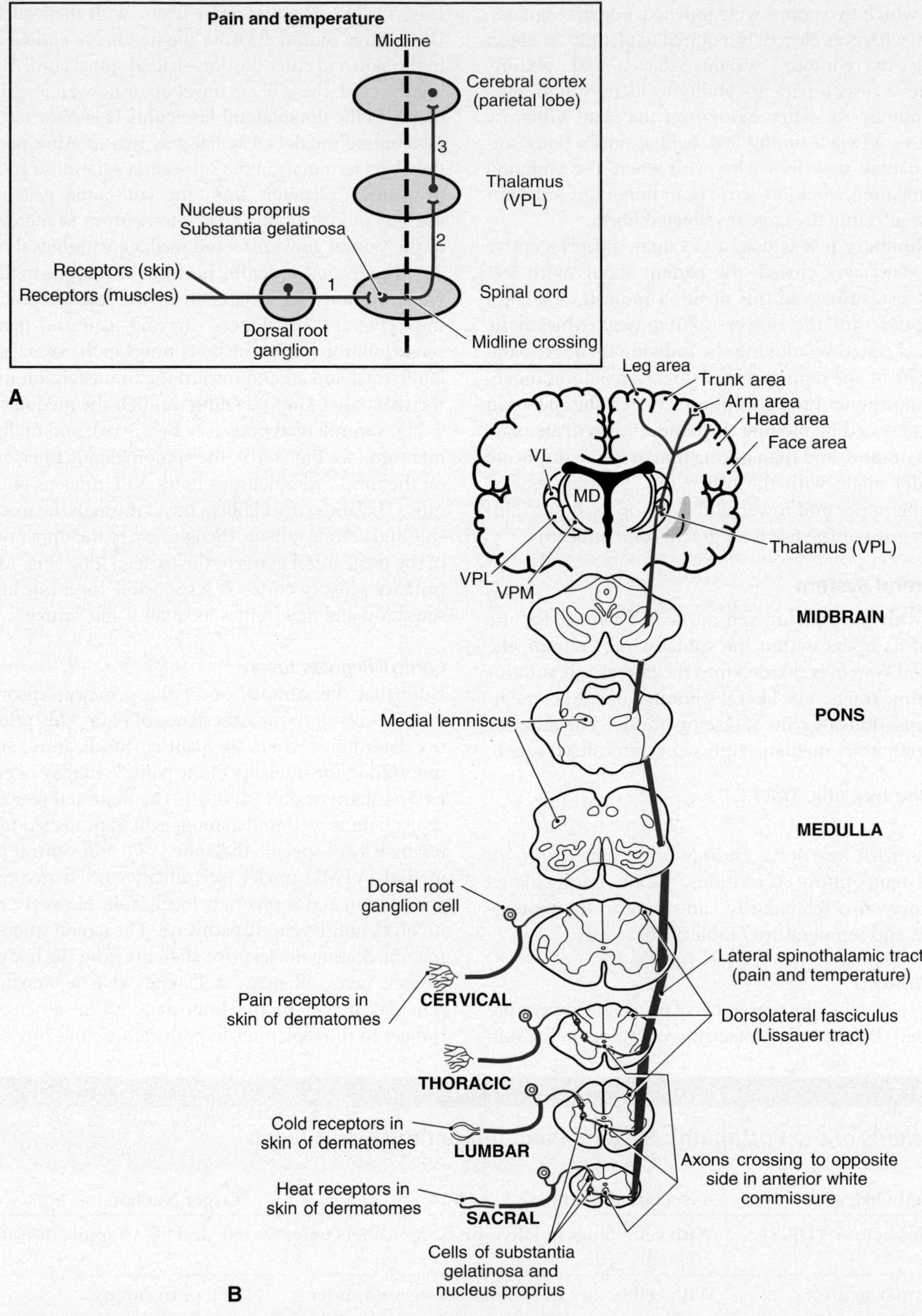

Figure 11-7 A. The three-neuron organization of the anterolateral system. B. The lateral spinothalamic tract. MD, mediodorsal (dorsomedial); *VL*, ventrolateral; *VPL*, ventral posterior lateral; *VPM*, ventral posterior medial.

Clinical Correlates and Assessment

The emotional response to the hurting experience of pain includes the limbic system. The nociceptive afferents from the body, viscera, or face reaching the thalamus also innervate the intralaminar nuclei of the thalamus (see Chapter 6). The intralaminar nuclei project into the limbic system, including the hippocampus, amygdaloid complex, and associated old brain regions. The experience of the affective (hurt) aspect of pain is undoubtedly associated with these projections

The descending reticular (periaqueductal gray matter) projections are known to modulate pain perception. The reticular projections, along with other brainstem nuclei, project to the dorsal horns of the spinal cord to inhibit the pain-mediating pathways. By regulating the transmission of pain, the reticular projections participate in mediating many somatic and visceral responses to pain, such as nausea, fainting, changes in heart rate, and alterations in the frequency and depth of respiration.

Key Terms :

Analgesia	**Phantom pain**
Analgesics	**Referred pain**
anesthesia	**rhizotomy**
anesthetics	**tractotomy**
Narcotics	

Patterns of Deficit

An interruption of the ascending fibers at any point in the neuraxis alters the perception of pain and temperature. Damage to peripheral (spinal) nerves or the DRG subsequent to compression or reduced local circulation results in reduced pain sensitivity. A pinched nerve root from a herniated intervertebral disk usually results in pain perceived in whichever body area is connected to the compromised neural structure. Damage to spinothalamic fibers also affects the transmission of pain and temperature to the sensorimotor cortex. Because pain and temperature fibers cross the midline in the spinal gray matter, a degenerative lesion in the area around the central canal of the spinal cord would interrupt the fibers carrying pain and temperature as they cross the midline in the ventral white commissure. This is commonly seen in syringomyelia in which the pain and temperature sensations from the opposite sides of the body are lost below the lesion. Similarly, a lesion at the brainstem level affects the contralateral half of the body. However, if the DRG, nucleus proprius, or substantia gelatinosa is damaged, sensation is affected on the ipsilateral half of the body.

Knowing the point of fiber crossing is important in determining which cutaneous area will be affected as a result of a given lesion. This information is the guiding post for choosing the anatomic site for the surgical management (**chordotomy**) of intractable pain. Patients' inability to perceive sensations in delineated body areas allows clinicians to identify the dermatomes involved with the level of the spinal cord damage. Once the affected dermatomes are determined, one can identify which afferent nerves or spinal dorsal roots are damaged (see Fig. 2-34).

Referred pain cannot always be solely attributed to a particular anatomic pathway. The pain known as referred pain occurs at one site but is sensed in another site. Pain sensation in the viscera is poorly localized and serves as a good example of referred pain. The CNS does not contain special pathways devoted to visceral sensation; thus, visceral pain impulses follow the same pathways that are used by somatic pain afferents. Therefore, the brain is likely to interpret visceral pain impulses as somatic pain signals. For example, cardiac pain is referred to the chest and/or inner side of the arm. This is because the area of reference for pain coincides with the body parts served by somatic sensory nuclei from the same spinal segments, which are T1–T8. Thus, sensory nuclei from the same spinal segment mediate sensation from different visceral and somatic areas (Table 11-6).

Phantom limb is another phenomenon related to pain. If a limb or substantial part of a limb is amputated, the patient may, for many months after the surgery, continue to have shooting pain and tingling and may sometimes feel as if the fingers or toes were crossed or that the limb were bent behind the back. The pain or discomfort is interpreted as originating from the missing part of the limb. There are two explanations for **phantom pain**. First, after sectioning, the peripheral process of afferent neurons usually regrows. Often the growth tip encounters scar tissue, where it grows into a **hypersensitive tangle** or knot (neuroma). Irritation from pressure, tightening scar tissue, or prosthesis often results in the generation of action potentials that, on projection to the forebrain, are interpreted as pain in a distal innervation zone that no longer exists. Second, it is difficult to forget a lifetime of learning the association between the distal, now missing, part of the limb and the touch, pain, and position experiences associated with that part.

Table 11-6

Principal Dermatomes Commonly Cited for Referred Pain

Somatic Projection	Visceral Organ(s)
C3–C4	Diaphragm
T1–T8	Heart
T10	Appendix
T10–T12	Testes and prostate
T10–T12	Ovaries and uterus

With its somewhat unlocalizable cortical representation, pain has proven to be a mysterious perception. Its medical treatment continues to pose challenges. For example, the alleviation of pain by cutting the dorsal root (rhizotomy) or a tract (tractotomy) has usually been transient; the pain has most often returned, and with greater intensity. The ablation of the ventrobasal thalamus (a site associated with thalamic pain syndrome) generally decreases sensation from the contralateral side of the body, but it does not entirely suppress the pain. Intralaminar stimulation has, however, proven to be more beneficial and effective (Bhatnagar et al., 1990; Bhatnagar and Mandybur, 2005); direct stimulation of the exposed brain has resulted in an evoked sensation of tingling, pressure, and numbness, but it has never resulted in the evoked sensation of pain. This finding has allowed neurosurgeons to operate on the brain of awake patients (Bhatnagar et al., 2000; Penfield and Roberts, 1959).

Narcotics (analgesic drugs like meperidine and fentanyl that have effects similar to those of opium), **nonaddictive analgesics**, and local anesthetics are commonly used for pain relief. The best analgesic is morphine, an extract from the opium poppy. These agents suppress pain sensitivity by inhibiting receptor functioning, blocking the transmission of pain impulses, or blocking or slowing the central pain-processing mechanism. Local anesthetic agents are used to control pain by blocking its transmission peripherally or centrally. The human brain is known to contain enkephalin, a morphine-like substance. Released from the nerve endings in the CNS, enkephalin not only serves as an analgesic in the body but also regulates mood and motivation.

Assessment

The modality of pain is assessed by pricking the body surface with a pin or by pinching the skin. The patient is asked to describe the sensation. This is repeated until the area of deficit is mapped. There are three common types of altered responses to pain: **analgesia** (no sensation of pain), **hypalgesia** (decreased sensation to pain or higher pain threshold), and **hyperalgesia** or exaggerated response (increased pain sensation or lower pain threshold).

Thermal sensation is assessed by using hot and cold stimuli. Hot and cold stimuli are applied to various parts of the body, and the patient is asked to differentiate them. Common pathologic responses related to thermal sensation are **athermia** or **thermal anesthesia** (total absence of sensation), **hypothermia**, **thermal hypesthesia** or **hypoesthesia** (raised or elevated threshold of response to thermal stimuli), and **hyperthermia** or **thermal hyperesthesia** (lower threshold to temperature, resulting in an exaggerated response).

Anterior Spinothalamic Tract

Information pertaining to two types of touch, discriminative and diffuse, travels in different neural pathways. Diffuse touch refers to a global sensation that lacks a qualitative description and does not relate to a specific location. As a rudimentary backup system, it is mediated through the anterior spinothalamic tract. Diffuse touch includes collaterals from the dorsal column. Neuronal conduction for diffuse touch sensation follows a three-neuron organizational system, similar to the system that mediates pain and temperature.

Receptors

The identity of nerve endings transducing diffuse touch is not fully resolved. All three types of receptive end organs (encapsulated endings, free nerve endings, and expanded tip endings) and the collaterals from the dorsal column contribute to this nonlocalized touch sensation.

Neural Pathway

The first-order sensory fibers transmit general touch sensations from the skin to the CNS. On entering the dorsolateral spinal cord, the fibers disperse longitudinally in the **dorsolateral fasciculus of Lissauer**. They then travel up and down a few spinal segments before terminating in the nucleus proprius and substantia gelatinosa, the second-order nuclei in the dorsal horn. Some second-order fibers terminate in the adjacent gray matter, which serves spinal reflexes; however, most cross the midline in the ventral spinal gray matter and turn upward to form the anterior spinothalamic tract (Fig. 11-8). The anterior spinothalamic tract fibers ascend in this general location to the brainstem, where they move laterally, getting closer to the lateral spinothalamic tract (see Figs. 3-11, 3-14, and 3-16). Before terminating in the VPL nucleus of the thalamus, the anterior spinothalamic tract fibers give off many types of collaterals to the brainstem reticular formation. The third-order fibers from the thalamus travel through the internal capsule, then project into the upper two-thirds of the postcentral gyrus located in the parietal lobe (Fig. 11-8). The anterolateral spinothalamic tract is known to project bilaterally to the sensory cortex.

Clinical Correlates and Assessment

Since diffuse touch serves as the backup sensory system for the dorsal–lemniscal column, and since it projects to the cortex bilaterally, the interruption of the anterior spinothalamic tract causes no obvious clinical deficit. Diffuse touch is abolished only when the spinal cord is completely severed.

Diffuse touch is tested using a piece of cotton or a wisp of wool. A patient relying on this backup system notices a touch but cannot determine its location or describe its quality. It can be assessed effectively only when the pathway for fine discriminative touch is not functioning.

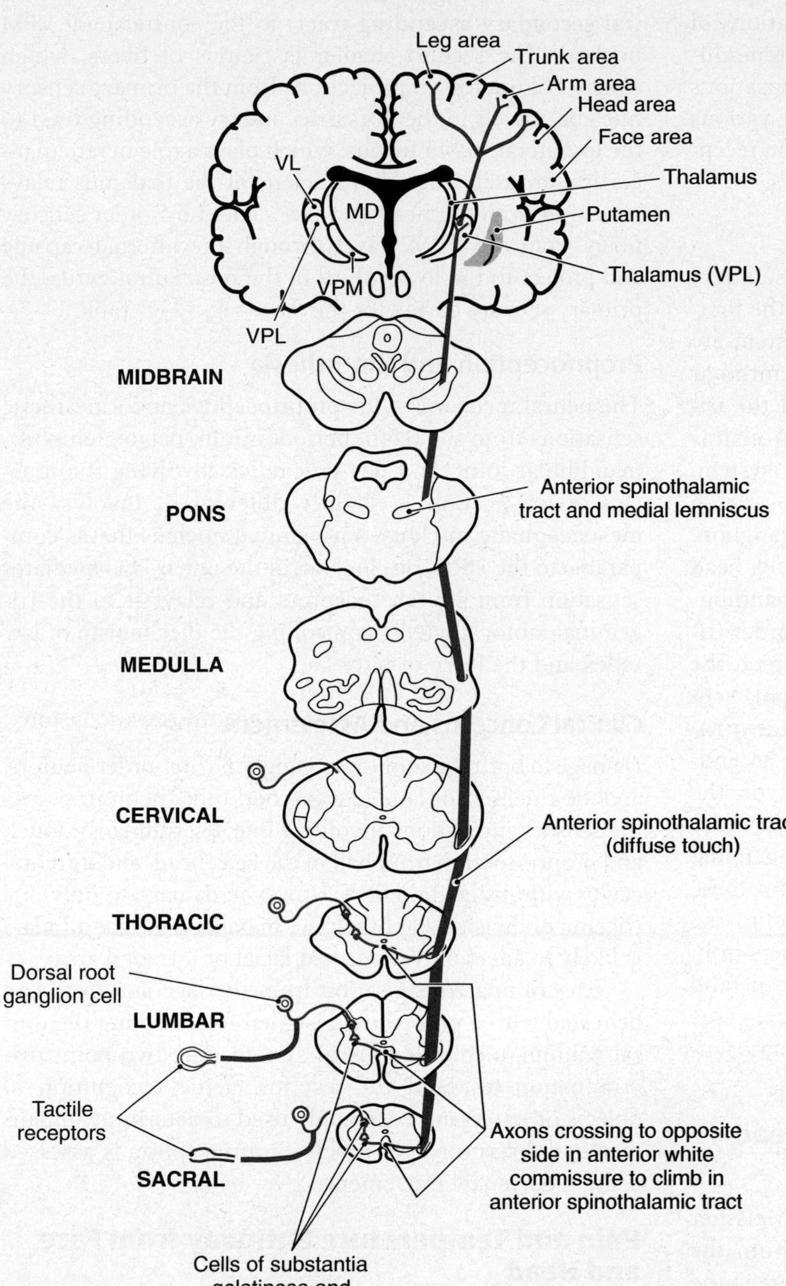

Figure 11-8 The anterior spinothalamic tract, which transmits bodily diffuse touch. MD, mediodorsal (dorsomedial); *VL*, ventrolateral; *VPL*, ventral posterior lateral; *VPM*, posterior medial.

SENSORY PATHWAYS FOR THE HEAD AND FACE

The trigeminal nerve (CN V) is the principal sensory nerve for the face and head. The **maxillary**, **ophthalmic**, and **mandibular branches** of the trigeminal nerve innervate different regions of the head, face, and intraoral structures. These trigeminal branches mediate sensations from the skin of the face, forehead, anterior half of the scalp, and most of the dura mater, orbital cavities, and mucosal membrane in the nasal and oral cavities. Fibers of the trigeminal nerve (CN V) are also joined by the fibers carrying sensation from the following nerves: facial (CN VII), glossopharyngeal (CN IX), and vagus (CN X). Together, these nerves cover the remaining scalp, external ear, ear canal, tympanic membrane region, and pharyngeal and laryngeal areas.

The trigeminal system is comparable to the previously discussed body-somatosensory system. It contains different neural mechanisms for the epicritic system, which is responsible for fine discriminative touch, proprioception, and kinesthesia, as well as the protopathic sensations of pain, temperature, and diffuse touch. In each system, different fibers serve epicritic and protopathic sensations from the head and face. The receptors serving the various sensations for the head and face are identical to the receptors previously discussed for the body.

Three-Neuron Organization

The trigeminal sensory system also follows the standard three-neuron organization; however, locations of the first- and second-order neurons for the trigeminal system are different (Fig. 11-9*A*). The peripherally located **semilunar ganglion** (also called the trigeminal ganglion) of the trigeminal (CN V) nerve serves as the first-order neuron; this is identical to the DRG of the general sensory system. Afferent fibers, except for those associated with stretch receptors, have their cell bodies in the semilunar ganglion. The peripheral fibers have a large distribution to the head and face through the ophthalmic, maxillary, and mandibular branches of the nerve. There are two second-order trigeminal sensory nuclei in the brainstem with which the entering central fibers synapse: the **chief (principal) sensory nucleus** (discriminative touch) and the **trigeminal spinal tract nucleus** (pain and temperature). The ascending first-order trigeminal sensory fibers synapse on the chief sensory nucleus, whereas the descending first-order sensory fibers terminate in the nucleus of the trigeminal spinal tract. The second-order sensory fibers from these two central nuclei cross the midline and ascend to the VPM nucleus of the thalamus. The third-order fibers from the VPM nucleus travel through the internal capsule and terminate in the lower third of the postcentral gyrus (Brodmann area 3,1,2), which serves as the primary sensory cortex for the face.

Discriminative Touch from Face and Head

Receptors

The encapsulated end organs (of Pacinian and Meissner corpuscles) mediate fine discriminative touch from the face and head; these receptors were discussed before in the section "Dorsal Column–Medial Lemniscal System."

Neural Pathway

The encapsulated receptors in the skin of the face and head are the first to receive discriminative touch sensations. The central processes of the first-order trigeminal (ophthalmic, maxillary, and mandibular) fibers, with their cell bodies in the semilunar (trigeminal) ganglion, mediate fine discriminative sensation from the head, intraoral structures, and face. The central processes of the semilunar ganglion terminate in the cells of the chief (principal) sensory nucleus of the trigeminal (CN V) nerve. The second-order trigeminothalamic fibers from the chief (principal) sensory trigeminal nucleus project to the thalamus. The larger fasciculus of fibers crosses the midline and ascends in the medial lemniscus (although it is considered to be part of the **ventral secondary ascending tract**) to the contralateral VPM nucleus. The second smaller fasciculus of fibers, which consists of uncrossed projections from the primary sensory nucleus, travels in the **dorsal secondary ascending tract** to the ipsilateral VPM nucleus, which plays a role in reticular–cortical arousal. The VPM nucleus of the thalamus relays sensation from the head and face. The third-order sensory fibers from the VPM travel through the internal capsule and project to the lower third of the postcentral gyrus, the primary sensory cortex for the face (Fig. 11-9; Table 11-7).

Proprioception and Kinesthesia

The neural mechanism for proprioceptive and kinesthetic sensations from the teeth, periodontium, palate, temporomandibular joint, and jaw-jerk reflex involving the muscles of mastication is slightly different. It involves the **mesencephalic nucleus**, a trigeminal nucleus that is comparable to the DRG, but located in the pons. This mediates sensation from stretch receptors and relays it to the trigeminal motor nucleus, controlling the mechanism of jaw reflex and the force of bite.

Clinical Concerns and Assessment

Damage to both the semilunar ganglion (first-order neuron) and the chief sensory nucleus (second-order neuron) blocks the sensory projections involving fine discriminative touch and proprioception from half of the face, head, and intraoral cavity with ipsilateral effect. However, damage to only one trigeminal division (ophthalmic, maxillary, or mandibular) is likely to affect only a selected facial or intraoral area.

Discriminative sensation from the face and head can be tested with a procedure designed for assessing the dorsal column–medial lemniscal system. The two-point discrimination test and the test for tactile recognition of objects or letters are commonly used to determine impairments of discriminative touch. Proprioception is assessed using passive jaw movement.

Pain and Temperature Pathway from Face and Head

Receptors

Receptors with free nerve endings are discussed in the section "Anterolateral System."

Neural Pathway

The central processes of the ophthalmic, maxillary, and mandibular trigeminal divisions mediate pain and temperature from the nociceptive receptors in the facial and intraoral skin. The first-order trigeminal sensory fibers, with cell bodies in the semilunar (trigeminal) ganglion, enter the mid-pons. They turn downward (caudally), terminating in the **spinal trigeminal nucleus**. The **spinal trigeminal tract** (CN V) also receives general somatic sensation from the facial (CN VII), glossopharyngeal (CN IX), and vagus (CN X) nerves, and it extends up to

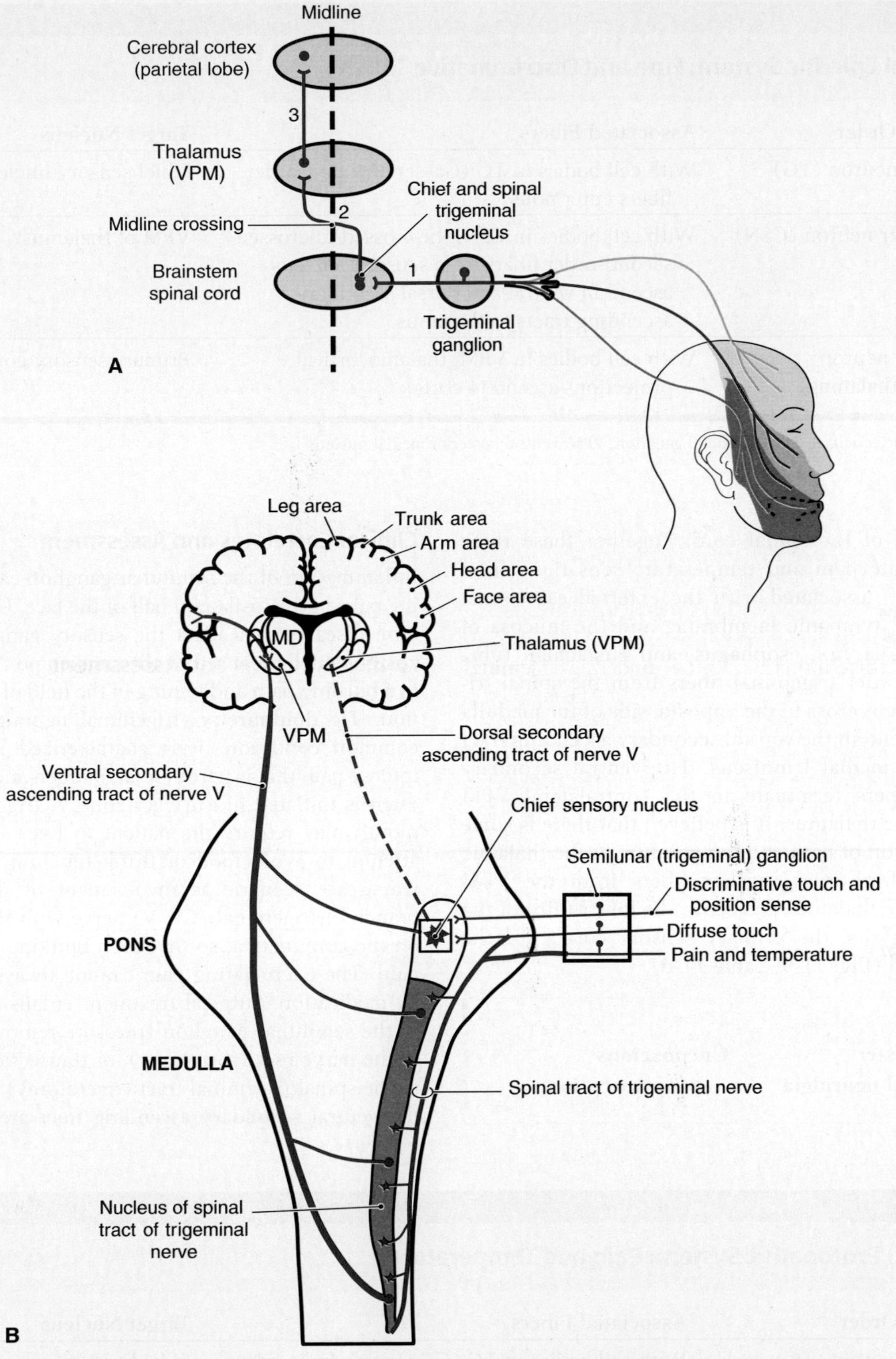

Figure 11-9 A. The three-neuron organization of the epicritic and protopathic systems for the trigeminal cranial nerve. B. Trigeminal fibers. First-order fibers with cell bodies in the semilunar ganglion, the trigeminal nuclear complex (chief sensory or spinal nuclei), a second-order neuron. The contralateral posterior medial nucleus, a third order neuron. Projections of the third-order sensory fibers to the lower third of postcentral gyrus, the primary sensory area for the face. *MD*, mediodorsal (dorsomedial).

Table 11-7

Trigeminal Epicritic System: Fine and Discriminative Touch

Nerve Cell Order	Associated Fibers	Target Nucleus
First-order neuron (TG)	With cell bodies in TG (Gasserian), first-order fibers enter pons	Chief sensory nucleus
Second-order neuron (CSN)	With cell bodies in CSN, the crossed/uncrossed second-order fibers from sensory nucleus ascend in ventral and dorsal secondary ascending tracts to thalamus	VPM of thalamus
Third-order neuron (VPM of thalamus)	With cell bodies in VPM, thalamocortical projections ascend to cortex	Primary sensory cortex (face area)

CSN, chief sensory nucleus; *TG*, trigeminal ganglion; *VPM*, ventral posterior medial nucleus

the C4 level of the spinal cord. Together these three nerves mediate pain and temperature sensations from the structures associated with the external ear (pinna and meatus), tympanic membrane, and the mucosa of the pharynx, larynx, esophagus, and eustachian tube. The second-order trigeminal fibers from the spinal trigeminal nucleus cross to the opposite side of the medulla and then ascend in the ventral secondary ascending tract close to the medial lemniscus. The ventral secondary ascending fibers terminate in the contralateral VPM nucleus of the thalamus. It is believed that there is some crude sensation of pain and temperature at the thalamic level. The third-order sensory fibers from the VPM nucleus in the thalamus project to the lower third of the postcentral gyrus, the primary sensory cortex for the face and head (Fig. 11-9; Table 11-8).

Key Terms :

Herpes zoster
Trigeminal neuralgia
Unconscious proprioception

Clinical Correlates and Assessment

Inflammation of the semilunar ganglion causes excruciating pain in the ipsilateral half of the face. One of the common diseases that affect the sensory ganglion is **herpes zoster**, which is caused by the chicken pox virus. It results in a burning pain and itching in the field of nerve distribution. **Tic douloureux** (trigeminal neuralgia) is another common condition. It is characterized by episodes of intense pain that is paroxysmal (sudden and stabbing) and often is initiated in a trigger zone. A trigger zone in the mouth may require the patient to twist the head in an attempt to avoid food or drink touching the zone. The worst-case scenario is involvement of the ophthalmic branch of trigeminal (CN V) nerve with the trigger zone on the conjunctiva, so that even blinking can trigger the pain. The excruciating pain cannot always be controlled by medication. Surgical treatment entails decompression of the semilunar ganglion (pressure removal), sectioning of the nerve root (rhizotomy), or transection of the fibers in the spinal trigeminal tract (tractotomy). If the fibers in the ventral secondary ascending tract are damaged, the

Table 11-8

Trigeminal Protopathic System: Pain and Temperature

Nerve Cell Order	Associated Fibers	Target Nucleus
First-order neuron (TG)	With cell bodies in TG (Gasserian), first-order (central) fibers enter pons	Spinal trigeminal nucleus
Second-order neuron (TSN)	With cell bodies in TSN, second-order fibers cross midline and ascend in ventral secondary ascending tract to thalamus	VPM of thalamus
Third-order neuron (VPM of thalamus)	With cell bodies in VPM, thalamocortical projections ascend from thalamus to cortex	Primary sensory cortex (face area)

TG, trigeminal ganglion; *TSN*, trigeminal spinal tract and nucleus; *VPM*, ventral posterior medial nucleus

ability to sense pain in the contralateral half of the face is affected.

Pain and temperature are assessed by pricking with a pin or pinching the skin and using warm and cool objects as stimuli. The patient is asked to report the quality and location of the sensation to map its distribution. As noted earlier, analgesia, hypalgesia, and hyperalgesia are the common types of altered pain responses; thermal anesthesia or athermia, thermal hypesthesia or hypothermia, and thermal hyperesthesia or hyperthermia are the common pathological responses to thermal sensation.

Diffuse Touch from Face

Receptors

All types of receptive end organs mediate diffuse touch.

Neural Pathway

Both dorsal and ventral secondary trigeminal tract fibers are involved in bilateral projections of diffuse touch from the face and head. The central processes of the ophthalmic, maxillary, and mandibular trigeminal branches mediate diffuse touch sensation. Fibers of these branches are divided into two groups. One turns caudally in the spinal trigeminal tract and synapses in the spinal trigeminal nucleus. The second terminates in the chief sensory nucleus of the trigeminal (CN V) nerve. As they emerge from the spinal trigeminal nucleus, these second-order fibers are also joined by fibers of the glossopharyngeal (CN IX) and vagus (CN X) nerves. These second-order fibers cross the midline and course along the ventral secondary ascending tract to the VPM nucleus of the thalamus. The crossed and uncrossed second-order fibers from the chief sensory nucleus of the trigeminal (V) nerve travel in the dorsal secondary ascending tract. These fibers terminate in the VPM nucleus of the thalamus. The third-order sensory fibers from the thalamus pass through the internal capsule and terminate in the lower third of the postcentral gyrus, the primary sensory cortex for the face and head (Figs. 11-6 and 11-9).

Clinical Correlates and Assessment

Diffuse touch serves as the backup sensory system; it can be assessed effectively only when the pathway for fine discriminative touch is not functioning. However, damage to either trigeminal ascending tract (dorsal or ventral) causes partial to complete anesthesia in the face and head. Damage to the involved pathway or pathways can be determined by testing the modality of touch and its altered responses over the face.

UNCONSCIOUS PROPRIOCEPTION

Unconscious proprioception mediates stretch afferent information from the lower limb muscles and joints about the position, range, and direction of limb movements to the cerebellum. Serving as the backup for conscious proprioception (dorsal column–medial lemniscal system), unconscious proprioception involves multiple afferent inputs to the cerebellum, which is vital to the acquisition and maintenance of skilled motor activities, such as walking, speaking, writing, and eye movement. The **spinocerebellar tracts** transmit unconscious proprioception and exteroceptive impulses from muscle spindles and limb joints to the cerebellum and help monitor and modify ongoing movement. The spinocerebellar pathways, unlike the other somatosensory pathways, follow a **two-order neuronal system** because they do not directly project to the cortex. The system consists of three second-order fiber tracts: **ventral spinocerebellar**, **dorsal spinocerebellar**, and **cuneocerebellar** (Fig. 11-10).

Innervation Pattern

Unconscious proprioceptive projections to the cerebellum are organized ipsilaterally to the input (and to the output). The developmentally newer and rapidly conducting (dorsal spinocerebellar and cuneocerebellar) pathways proceed on the ipsilateral side to reach the same side of the cerebellum. The older ventral spinocerebellar projections cross twice and remain ipsilateral.

Receptors

Muscle spindles and Golgi tendon organs, which are located in muscles and originate from nerve endings in limb joints, mediate unconscious proprioception.

Neural Pathways

Ventral Spinocerebellar Tract

Projecting bilaterally to the cerebellum, the ventral spinocerebellar tract mediates unconscious proprioception from the lower limbs (e.g., girdles, pelvis, and legs) and body axis. Fibers of this tract enter the cerebellum through the superior cerebellar peduncle and terminate in the cerebellar vermis (midline cerebellar structure) (Table 11-9).

Dorsal Spinocerebellar Tract

The dorsal spinocerebellar tract mediates unconscious proprioception from the lower and middle regions of the body, including the legs, thighs, pelvis, abdomen, and thorax. There is substantial overlapping of innervation for the lower limbs because unconscious proprioception is also mediated by the ventral spinocerebellar fibers. The fibers of the dorsal spinocerebellar tract enter the ipsilateral cerebellar cortex via the **inferior cerebellar peduncle** (Table 11-9).

Cuneocerebellar Tract

A developmentally newer system, the cuneocerebellar fibers mediate unconscious proprioception from the upper limbs and neck. The cuneocerebellar tract enters the

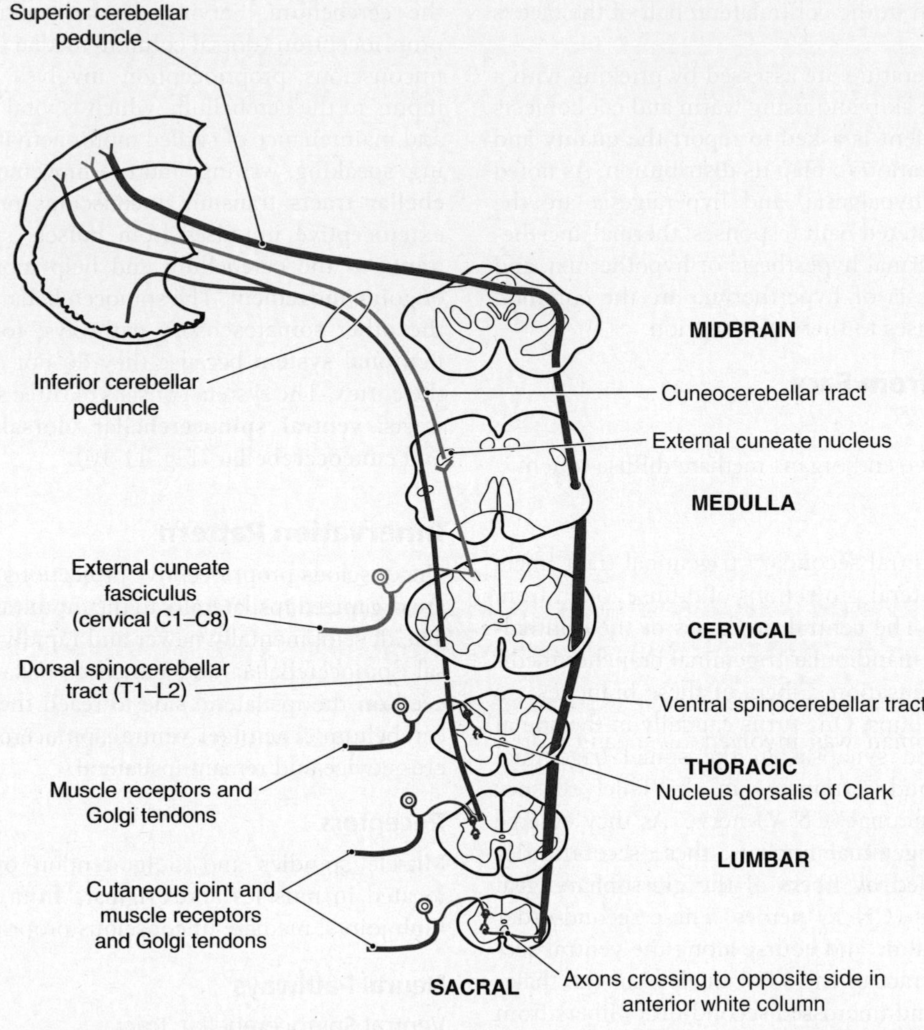

Figure 11-10 Spinocerebellar tracts: ventral spinocerebellar, dorsal spinocerebellar, and cuneocerebellar.

Table 11-9

Spinocerebellar Projections

Pathway	Projection Fibers	Target Structure
Ventral spinocerebellar tract	With cell bodies in DRG, first-order fibers enter spinal cord, terminate on undefined sensory cells Second-order fibers cross midline and ascend to enter cerebellum via crossed fibers of superior cerebellar peduncle	After two crossings, fibers carry unconscious proprioception from lower limbs to ipsilateral cerebellum
Dorsal spinocerebellar tract	With cell bodies in DRG, first-order fibers enter spinal cord and terminate on nucleus dorsalis of Clark Second-order fibers ascend ipsilaterally to enter cerebellum via inferior cerebellar peduncle	Uncrossed fibers mediate unconscious proprioception from distal lower limbs, joints, and middle regions of body to ipsilateral cerebellum
Cuneocerebellar tract	With cell bodies in DRG, first-order fibers enter spinal cord and terminate on external cuneate nucleus Second-order fibers ascend ipsilaterally to enter cerebellum via inferior cerebellar peduncle	Uncrossed fibers mediate unconscious proprioception from distal upper limbs and joints to ipsilateral cerebellum

ipsilateral cerebellum via the inferior cerebellar peduncle (Table 11-9).

Clinical Correlates and Assessment

The rapid conduction of the cerebellar projection of position and movement information is essential for rapid and skilled manipulation of the distal parts of the extremities. Furthermore, because the spinocerebellar pathway serves as merely the backup for the dorsal column–medial lemniscal system, it is not always possible to determine clinically the extent to which kinesthetic and proprioceptive losses result from the interruption of this tract.

The Romberg test is used to assess proprioception-based cerebellar functions; however, it also reflects the functioning of conscious proprioception (dorsal column–medial lemniscal system).

CLINICAL CORRELATES

Lesion Localization

Rule 4: Symptoms Suggesting Spinal Central Gray Lesion

Presenting Symptoms. Bilateral loss of pain and temperature sensation with preserved sense of touch in the same limbs (usually the two upper limbs) implies a lesion (cavitation or syringomyelia) in the spinal central gray. **Rationale.** A segmental cavitation or degeneration in the spinal gray around the central canal region results in a bilateral deficit. This cavitation is most marked in the cervical spinal region and affects the hands and shoulder regions. This lesion interrupts the axons carrying pain and temperature as they cross through the anterior white commissure. Clinically, a burn in this case is no longer a painful stimulus.

CASE STUDIES FOR PROBLEM SOLVING

CASE ONE (11-1)

A 35-year-old woman was involved in an automobile accident and taken to the emergency room. She was examined by a neurologist who noted the following:

- A complete loss of epicritic (two-point touch and proprioceptive) sensation in right lower limb
- Impaired joint position and vibration sensation on right side (once it was determined that the primary sensations are impaired, no cortical sensory assessment involving the two-point discrimination was undertaken).
- Paralysis of the right lower limb
- Loss of pain and temperature from the left lower limb

A spinal MRI study revealed a fractured thoracic vertebra with a bone fragment in the spinal canal, indicating injury to the right half of the spinal cord at the T12 level; this is also called spinal cord hemisection (Brown–Séquard syndrome, Fig. 11-11). A reevaluation of the sensorimotor functions 3 weeks later revealed spasticity in the limb and a positive Babinski sign.

Question: How can you relate these clinical symptoms to the identified pathology?

Case (11-1) Discussion: See discussion of case studies

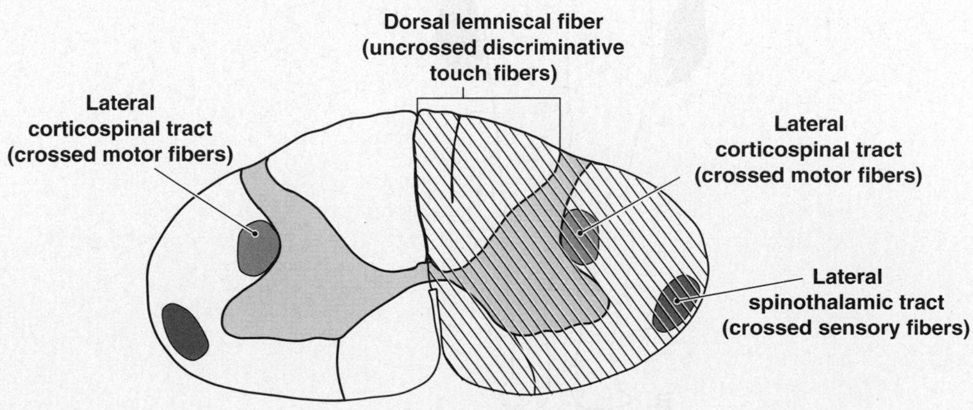

Figure 11-11 Illustration of spinal involvement causing Brown–Séquard syndrome.

(Continued)

CASE TWO (11-2) *(CONTINUED)*

A 55-year-old cook consulted with his doctor regarding the lack of pain and thermal sensation in his hands and forearms. On examination, the physician noted the following:

- A few burn marks on the palms and fingertips bilaterally
- No response to pinpricks and thermal stimuli in the hands and forearms on both sides
- Some weakness and atrophy of muscles of the both hands

A spinal MRI study revealed a small cavity in the C6–C8 and T1 regions of the cord (Fig. 11-12).

Question: How can you explain these pain and temperature symptoms in relation to the identified syringomyelia?

Case (11-2) Discussion: See discussion of case studies

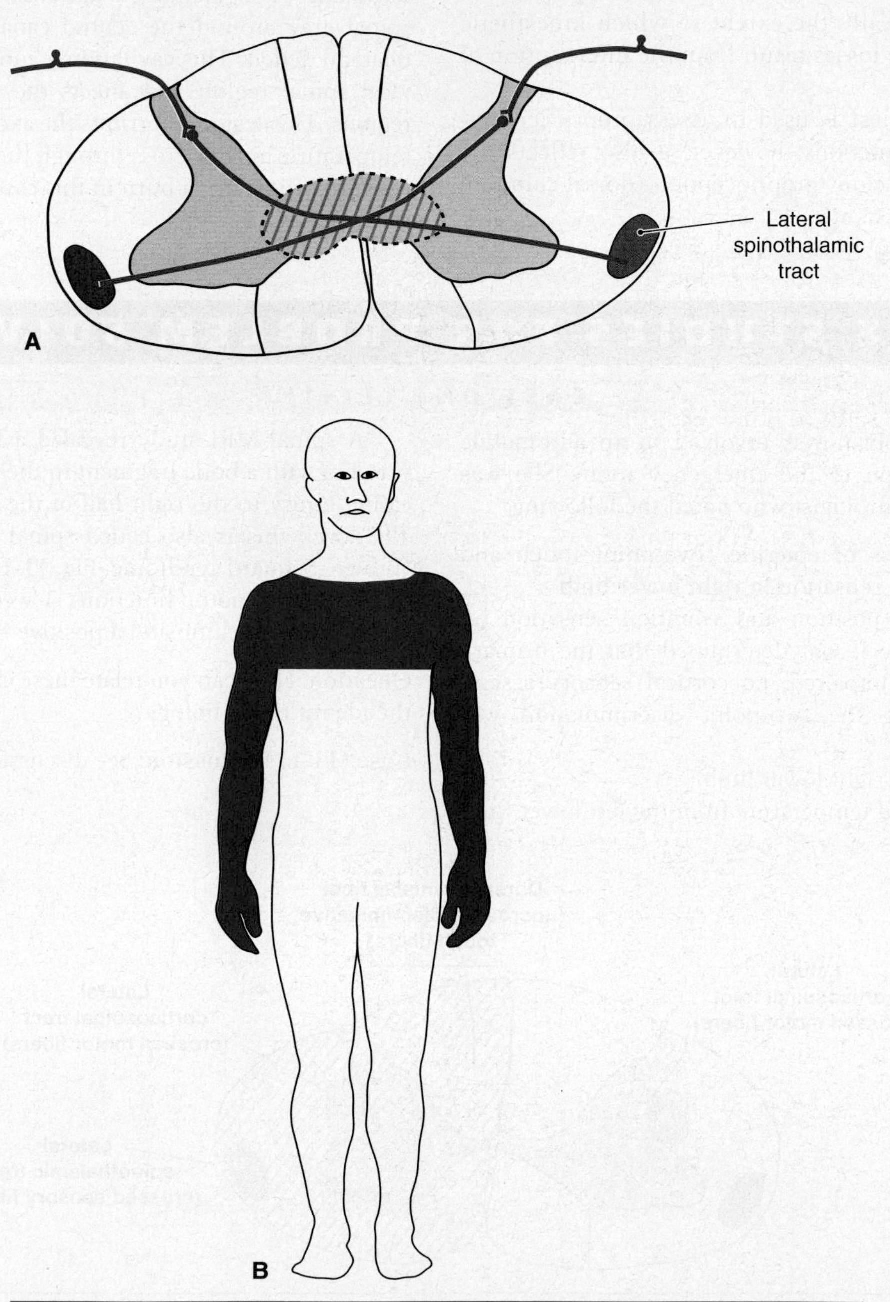

Figure 11-12 A. Diagrammatic illustration of a syringomyelic cavity in the cervical gray matter; B. Diagrammatic illustration of a bilateral loss of pain and temperature reception and possibly flaccid paralysis of the upper limbs muscles subsequent to the interrupted pain and temperature fibers.

(Continued)

CASE THREE (11-3) *(CONTINUED)*

A 62-year-old man who suffered a stroke while asleep was taken to the emergency room. The attending neurologist noted the following:

- Unintelligible dysarthric speech
- Right facial paralysis
- Impaired swallowing with paresis of the right pharyngeal muscles
- Loss of pain and temperature sensation on the right face
- Loss of pain and temperature on the left half of the body
- Intact cognitive and linguistic functions

Question: Can you localize a lesion (somatosensory cortex, motor cortex, internal capsule, basal ganglia, medulla, or spinal cord) that was likely to have produced these dissociated findings?

Case (11-3) Discussion: See discussion of case studies

CASE FOUR (11-4)

A 70-year-old woman complaining of episodic excruciating pain in her face was reported to have gradually become disinclined to speak and began using gestures for communicating. Considering a possible case of a neurological disease in addition to depression, she was taken to a neurologist, who noted the following:

- Malnourished body habitus
- No limb or facial paralysis
- No sensory loss on either side of her face
- Excruciating episodic pain involving the face any time the patient touched the ipsilateral alveolar region with the tip of her tongue

A brain MRI study revealed no abnormality. The attending neurologist suspected this to be a case of cranial nerve dysfunction associated with a trigger zone in the mouth around the alveolar region.

Question: Can you provide an explanation for the patient's disinclination for speaking?

Case (11-4) Discussion: See discussion of case studies

CASE FIVE (11-5)

A 55-year-old man suffered a stroke while sleeping; he presented with altered somatosensory problems and saw a neurologist who noted the following:

- Loss of fine discriminative touch from the right half (upper and lower extremities) of the body
- Loss of sensation from the left side of his face
- No other sensorimotor symptoms were noted, except absence of the left corneal reflex

Question: Which of these clinical signs is most indicative of the lesion site?

Case (11-5) Discussion: See discussion of case studies

CASE SIX (11-6)

A 55-year-old woman woke up perspiring; she was alarmed by experiencing numbness and clumsiness of her left hand. She was taken to a neurologist, who noted the following:

- Intact left arm strength
- No loss of sensation for pain, touch, and temperature
- Impaired tactile recognition of object in the left hand (astereognosis)
- No recognition of anything written on the left palm (agraphesthesia)
- Difficulty with orientation on a map
- Some constructional (drawing and copying) problems
- No sign of motor speech problem and/or aphasia

A brain MRI study revealed a small infarct involving Brodmann area 5 extending to area 7 in the right parietal lobe.

Question: Can you relate these selected symptoms with the cortical area responsible for the cortical sensory integration?

Case (11-6) Discussion: See discussion of case studies

SUMMARY

Somatic sensation includes the physical experiences of pain, temperature, touch, and proprioception. It begins with specialized receptors in the body and terminates in the parietal lobe. Receptors in the skin convert sensory stimuli to neural signals and transmit the stimuli on afferent nerve fibers to the primary sensory cortex in the parietal lobe via the spinal cord, brainstem, and thalamus. This awareness is later transmitted to the sensory association cortex, where the information is analyzed, elaborated on, integrated with previous experiences, and raised to the highest level of consciousness. The somatosensory system is discretely organized; the information collected by specialized receptors is transmitted on separate axonal tracts. Each tract mediates specific modalities of sensation. Within each tract, a point-to-point somatotopic representation of the body surface (somatotopic organization) is maintained. This spatial organization of neurons, tracts, terminals, and nuclei is maintained up to the somesthetic cortex (body homunculus). Knowledge of sensory pathways, sensory receptors, points of fiber crossings, and cortical areas underlying conscious perception for different sensations provides a solid groundwork for understanding sensory organization.

REVIEW QUESTIONS

1. Complete the following statements using the appropriate technical terms:

   A. ________ refers to sensation loss that results either from a neurological disconnection/dysfunction or through a drug induced suppression of nerve activity.

   B. In ________, the patient's ________ recognition is tested by writing letters and drawing shapes on the skin surface.

   C. ________ represents an internal awareness of the range and direction of the movement, whereas ________ is the inner awareness of the limb position.

   D. In ________, one uses the discriminative ability to identify the shape, size, and texture of the object through tactile sensation.

   E. ________ is the state in which painful stimuli are no longer perceived as being hurtful.

   F. ________ sensation includes discriminative touch and proprioceptive awareness.

   G. A sensation of pain in the area of a nerve distribution is an example of ________.

   H. ________ includes the sensation of pain, temperature, and/or nonlocalized sense of touch.

   I. ________ is a surgical procedure that involves sectioning of the lateral spinothalamic tract to relieve medically intractable pain.

   J. Patients' inability to perceive sensation from delineated body areas allows neurologists to identify the involved ________ with the spinal cord damage.

2. Match the following clinical concepts with associated statements.

A. referred pain	a. pain sensation from an amputated limb
B. phantom pain	b. source of pain being different than sensed
C. trigeminal pain	c. evaluation of proprioception
D. carpal tunnel syndrome	d. nerve entrapment syndrome
E. Romberg test	e. neuralgia with trigger point

3. Name the etiology that is often associated with bilateral loss of pain and temperature, usually in the upper extremities.
4. Name the spinal syndrome that is characterized by ipsilateral sensory (proprioception) loss and paralysis as well as contralateral loss of pain and temperature.
5. Match each of the following sensation types with its associated spinal tract:

A. thermal sensitivity	a. lateral spinothalamic tract
B. crude/diffuse touch	b. anterior spinothalamic tract
C. pain sensation	c. spinocerebellar tracts
D. unconscious proprioception	d. dorsal column–medial
E. vibratory sense	
F. position sense	
G. two-point discrimination	

6. A person who tends to fall with eyes closed is lacking what kind of information?

12

Visual System

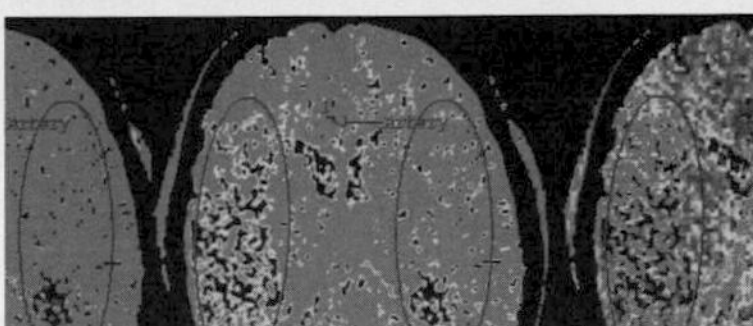

LEARNING OBJECTIVES

After studying this chapter, students should be able to:

- Describe the function of the eyeball structures
- Describe the structures and functions of the retina
- Explain the functional differences between cones and rods
- Outline errors of refraction and the ways to remediate them
- Discuss the central visual pathway
- Relate visual field defects with lesion sites
- Describe the neural mechanism of visual reflexes

Like audition, the visual system is an important sensory modality that is essential for a functional independence, but its disturbances also provide important clues to many neurologic conditions and lesion sites. Visual perception involves a combination of four events: (1) the **refraction** of light rays by the **lens** and **cornea**, (2) the conversion of the electromagnetic energy in light by the **retinal photoreceptor cells** into nerve impulses, (3) the transmission of impulses from the retinal photoreceptors to the visual cortex in the occipital lobe, and (4) the perception of visual images in the primary visual cortex. The primary visual cortex projects to the adjacent visual association region, where visual information is elaborated and synthesized with experiences in memory for its recognition. The organization of this chapter follows the order of neural events as they occur, beginning with the eyeball and ending with the primary visual cortex.

Key Terms :	
Binocular visual field	**Optin nerve**
Monocular visual field	**Retinal field**
Optic tract	**Visual field**

Distinguishing among three sets of terms is essential for understanding the visual system: **optic nerve** and **optic tract**, **visual** and **retinal fields**, and **monocular** and **binocular vision**. The optic (CN II) nerve includes the nerve fibers from the retina to the optic chiasm. The optic tract includes nerve fibers traveling between the chiasm and the lateral geniculate body (LGB) of the thalamus. Thalamic projections to the visual cortex travel via the **geniculocalcarine** (optic radiation) **fibers**.

The visual field is the external area visible to one or both eyes without movement. The retinal field is the focused representation of the visual field. The retinal image is the reverse of the visual field image—that is, up becomes down, and left becomes right.

The retinal field for each eye contains the portions of the visual field that are seen in common with the other eye (binocular) and a portion that is seen only by one eye (monocular). The **monocular visual field** is the lateral portion of the visual field that is perceived in only one eye (Fig. 12-1). By alternately closing the left and right eyes, one can produce a shift between right and left monocular vision. The **binocular visual field** is seen in both eyes as they simultaneously focus on a single object. Light rays from an object strike the corresponding (homonymous) retinal points in both eyes, and the images from the two eyes merge into one image in the cortex. Any slight deviation in the coordination of the eyes would prevent light rays from striking corresponding (homonymous) retinal points, resulting in double (diplopia) vision.

Key Terms :	
Anterior cavity	**Melanocytes**
Aqueous humor	**Posterior cavity**
Canal of Schlemm	**Sclera**
Ciliary body	**Vitreous humor**

ANATOMY OF THE EYE

Eyeball

The eyeball weighs approximately 7.5 g and is 2.4 cm (~1 inch) long. Five-sixths of its surface is concealed within the orbital cavity. The eyeball is divided into a small **anterior** and a large **posterior cavity** (Fig. 12-2A). The anterior cavity contains the **ciliary body**, **suspensory ligaments**,

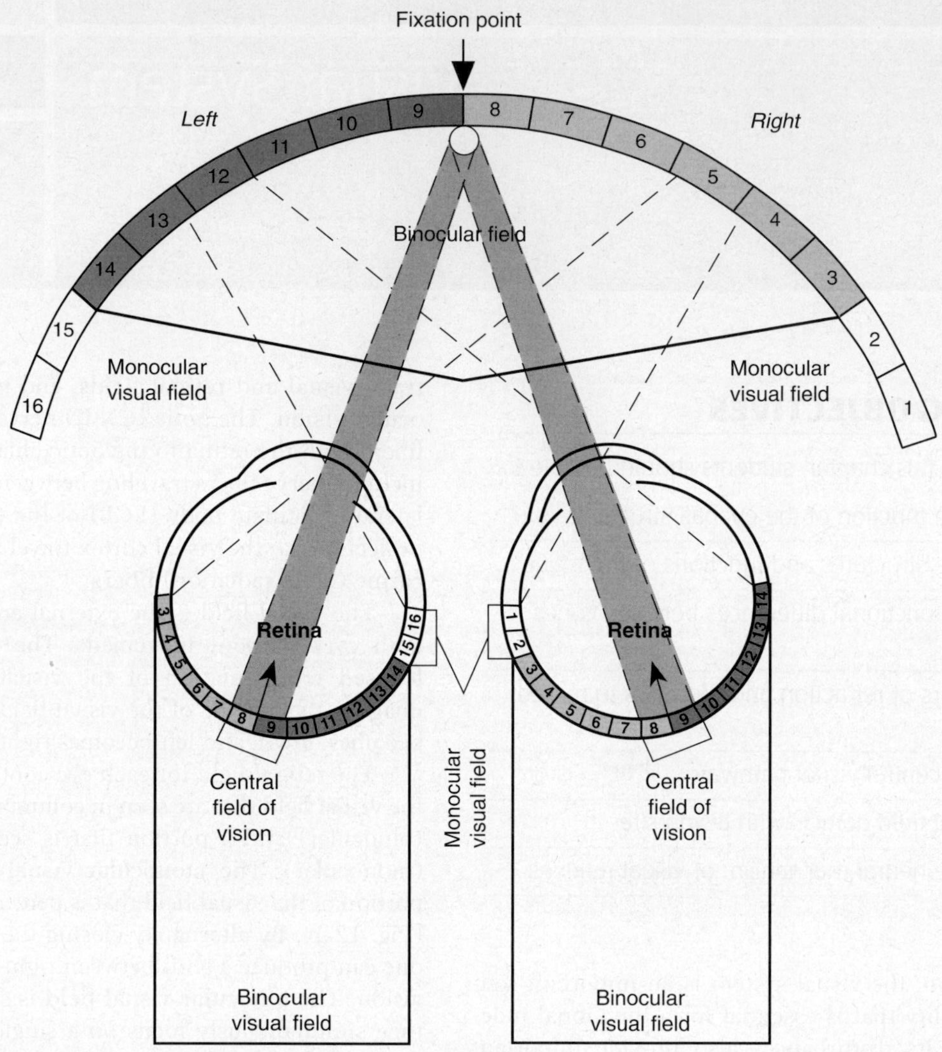

Figure 12-1 Diagrammatic illustration of visual fields. Shaded area, binocular field; open area, monocular field.

iris, and lens (Fig. 12-2*A*). The principal function of these structures is to adequately refract light rays for producing a sharply focused image on the retina. The anterior cavity is divided into **anterior** and **posterior chambers**. The anterior chamber includes the area between the cornea and iris, and the posterior chamber includes the area between the iris and the suspensory ligament. The anterior chamber is filled with **aqueous humor**, a fluid similar to the CSF that is produced behind the iris in the posterior chamber by the **choroid plexus** of the **ciliary processes and it** undergoes constant replacement. The aqueous humor flows through the pupil to the anterior chamber, where its production is balanced by its drainage into the venous system through the **canal of Schlemm**. The fluid passes through the veins of the choroids through a valve-like mechanism, which prevents its back flow. There are two major functions of the aqueous humor: the first is to maintain normal intraocular pressure, the second is to link the lens and cornea with the circulatory system. Any chronic increase in intraocular pressure, wherein the production of aqueous humor exceeds its reabsorption, leads to **glaucoma** (Box 12-1).

The posterior cavity, the area between the lens and the retina, is filled with **vitreous humor**, a jelly-like substance that in part maintains normal intraocular pressure and prevents the eyeball from collapsing. The vitreous humor is formed once in early life and it is never replaced. It has a very a slow rate of turnover; thus, it takes a long time for macrophages to remove blood in case of a hemorrhage involving the vitreous humor. Commonly seen floaters in the visual field are protein molecules that are located in the vitreous humor near the retina.

The eyeball consists of three ocular layers (Fig. 12-2): outer fibrous tunic (**sclera**), middle vascular tunic (**choroid**), and inner nervous tunic (**retina**). The fibrous tunic, an extension of the meningeal dura mater, has two divisions: sclera and **cornea**. The sclera, the white dense layer of opaque connective tissue, covers the round section of the eyeball. A larger part of the sclera is concealed within

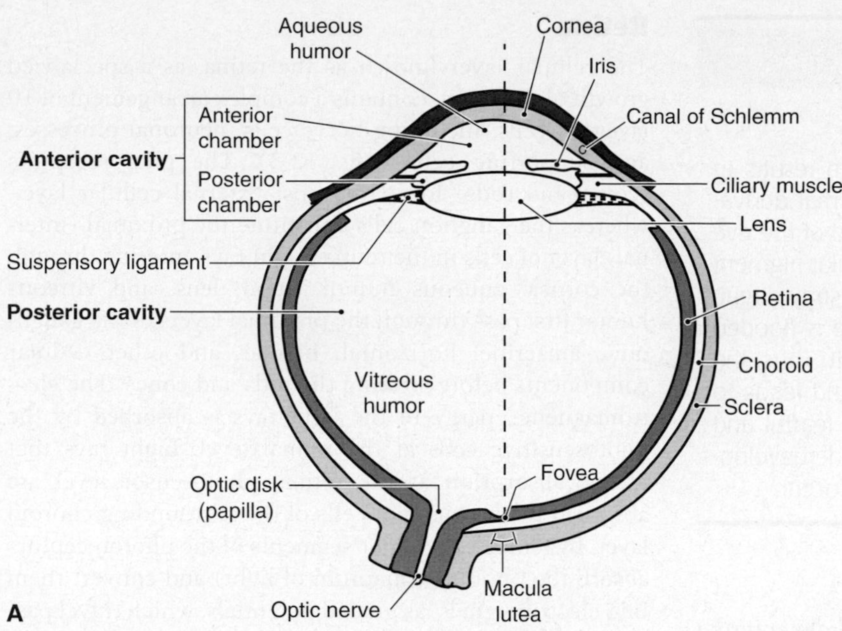

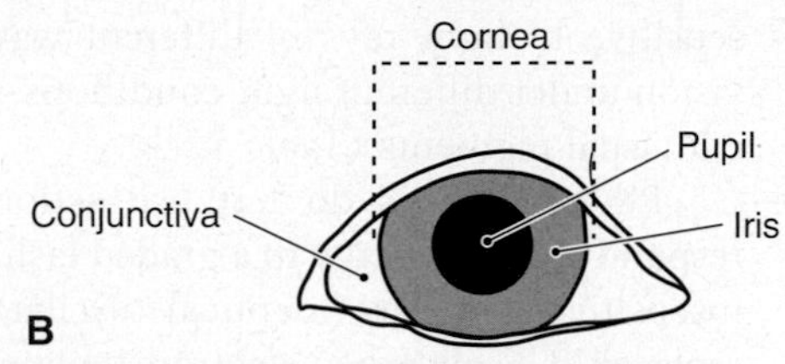

Figure 12-2 Structures of the eyeball. **A.** Cavities and chambers, ciliary muscles, suspensory ligaments, and their attachments to the lens. **B.** Anterior view of the iris around the pupil and cornea.

BOX 12-1

Glaucoma

Glaucoma is an ocular disease involving increased pressure (>22 to 25 mm Hg) in the aqueous humor inside the optic globe. It results in visual defects and eventually in blindness. A commonly held theory is that the increased pressure can collapse the veins that drain the optic globe. Consequently, the venus stasis and the loss of oxygen supply to the optic nerve axons and cause the atrophy of the optic nerve. Reduced blood flow to the optic nerve causes the atrophy of the nerve at the optic disk and subsequently leads to blindness. An alternate theory suggests that high pressure on the nerve axons contributes to the loss of impulse conduction and complete blindness. The perceptual changes in glaucoma are progressive and cause no discomfort. The field defect begins from the periphery and gradually progresses to the central vision. One of the treatments for glaucoma involves controlling the secretion of vitreous humor using vasoconstricting drugs that attenuate the ciliary blood supply.

the orbital cavity. The cornea (The cornea is an ectodermal structure, although, for convenience, it is considered as a dural extention), a nonvascular and transparent fibrous region of the eye, is in the exposed area of the eyeball, and it covers the anterior chamber (Fig. 12-2*A*).

The middle vascular tunic consists of the choroid, iris, ciliary muscle, and lens. The choroid contains an elastic connective tissue membrane that lines the internal surface of the sclera. The choroid is not only the source of the vascular supply to the sclera and outer retina but also contains **melanocytes** (pigment-producing cells). Normally, the choroid pigment melanocytes make the eyeball opaque by preventing stray light from entering the optic globe through the sclera. In the presence of pigment cell abnormalities related to **albinism** (with many grades of choroid pigment reduction due to many alleles), stray light that escapes absorption penetrates to the retina, making vision in bright light difficult and even painful (Box 12-2).

The iris and ciliary muscle are the connective tissue of the choroid. The radial (dilator) and circular (constrictor) fibers of the iris surround the **pupil**, an opening in the center of the iris. Working like a diaphragm and controlled by the autonomic nervous system, the iris regulates the amount of light that enters the eye by adjusting the pupil size. A contraction of the circular (constrictor) iris fibers in response to autonomic parasympathetic activity

BOX 12-2

Albinism

As an X-linked abnormality, albinism results in faulty melanin production in ectodermal derivatives so that the skin, iris, and choroid of the eye lack the pigment cells. The loss of ocular pigment cells impairs the absorption of stray light. Consequently, in bright light, the eye is flooded with stray light making vision difficult. Thus, the bright light is experienced as pain and leads to photophobia, in which the patient is fearful and avoids light. In addition, foveal underdevelopment and congenital nystagmus can occur.

decreases pupil size, reducing the amount of light entering the eye. On the other hand, a constriction of radial (dilator) fibers in response to autonomic sympathetic (T1–T3) activity enlarges the pupil, thus allowing greater amount of light to enter.

Ciliary muscle fibers, innervated by the parasympathetic projections of the oculomotor nerve (CN III), form a ring (sphincter) around the optic globe. These fibers contract to narrow the diameter of the optic globe, reducing the tension on the suspensory ligaments. This releases the tension on the lens capsule and allows the elastic lens to assume its natural spherical (round) shape. A denervated ciliary muscle results permanently in a more highly refracting lens. The increased refraction of light entering the pupil is necessary for producing a sharp image in near vision.

The lens, which consists of multiple layers of protein fibers, is enclosed in a transparent capsule of connective tissue. One of the common pathologic conditions of the lens is **cataract**, an age-induced painless production of nontransparent fibrous protein. It results in the clouding of the lens or its capsule, which degrades the quality of the focused image. The lens is held behind the pupil by suspensory ligaments that attach to the ciliary body. It is responsible for properly focusing images on the retina through the adequate refraction of light rays. Abnormalities in the lens structure affect its refraction capacity, resulting in impaired focusing. The ciliary muscle and its processes regulate the changes undertaken by the lens to accommodate for near vision.

Located in the posterior two-thirds of the eyeball, the nervous tunic (retina), the innermost layer of the eyeball, consists of 10 layers of cells. It contains the photoreceptor cells (**rods** and **cones**) that transduce the absorbed light energy into neural impulses and local potentials. Other retinal cells participate in the transmission of visual impulses to the cortex.

Retina

The cellular layer known as the retina, as a specialized growth of the brain, contains a complex arrangement of 10 layers of cells, including nerve cells, neuronal processes, and supporting cells (Fig. 12-3). The photoreceptors (cones and rods) form the most external cellular layer, whereas the ganglion cells constitute the proximal (internal) layer of cells in the retina. Light rays entering through the cornea, aqueous humor, pupil, lens, and vitreous humor first pass through the proximal layers of the ganglionic, amacrine, horizontal, bipolar, and other cellular components before striking the rods and cones. The electromagnetic energy in the light rays is absorbed by the photosensitive cells at the retinal level. Light rays that escape absorption at the retinal photosensor level are absorbed by the pigment cells of the surrounding choroid layer. In general, the outer segments of the photoreceptors absorb the photons (quantum of light) and convert them into electric signals, as graded potentials, which travel passively through synaptic transmission to the bipolar neurons and finally activate the ganglion cells, which process the signals as action potentials to the brain. The rods and cones are functionally and structurally different. They are sensitive to light rays of different wavelengths, mediate vision under different light conditions, and contain different visual pigments (Table 12-1).

Photoreceptors do not use action potentials. They respond to light energy in a graded fashion, and their photosensitive lamellae (identical to cilia) are continuously replaced. The absorbed electromagnetic energy of the light rays activates the rods and cones, which transduce energy into local potentials. By inhibiting and exciting the adjacent cells, the local potentials travel to the bipolar cells, which, by means of these potentials and the release of transmitters, influence the ganglion cell excitability. The ganglion cells are the retinal cells with voltage-gated sodium channels and are thus the first to generate action potentials. Ganglion cell axons converge at the **optic disk** (**papilla** or optic nerve head) to form the optic nerve. These axons pierce the eyeball and project to the **optic chiasm**, which also receives projections from the other eye.

Key Terms:

Blind spot	**Optic foramen**
Fovea centralis	**Papilledema**
Macula lutea	**Photopsin**
Opsin	**Rhodopsin**

The structure of the fundus (the retinal area seen with an ophthalmoscope) provides important clues about brain diseases. Of particular importance is **papilledema**, disc edema due to increased intracranial pressure in the brain (Box 12-3).

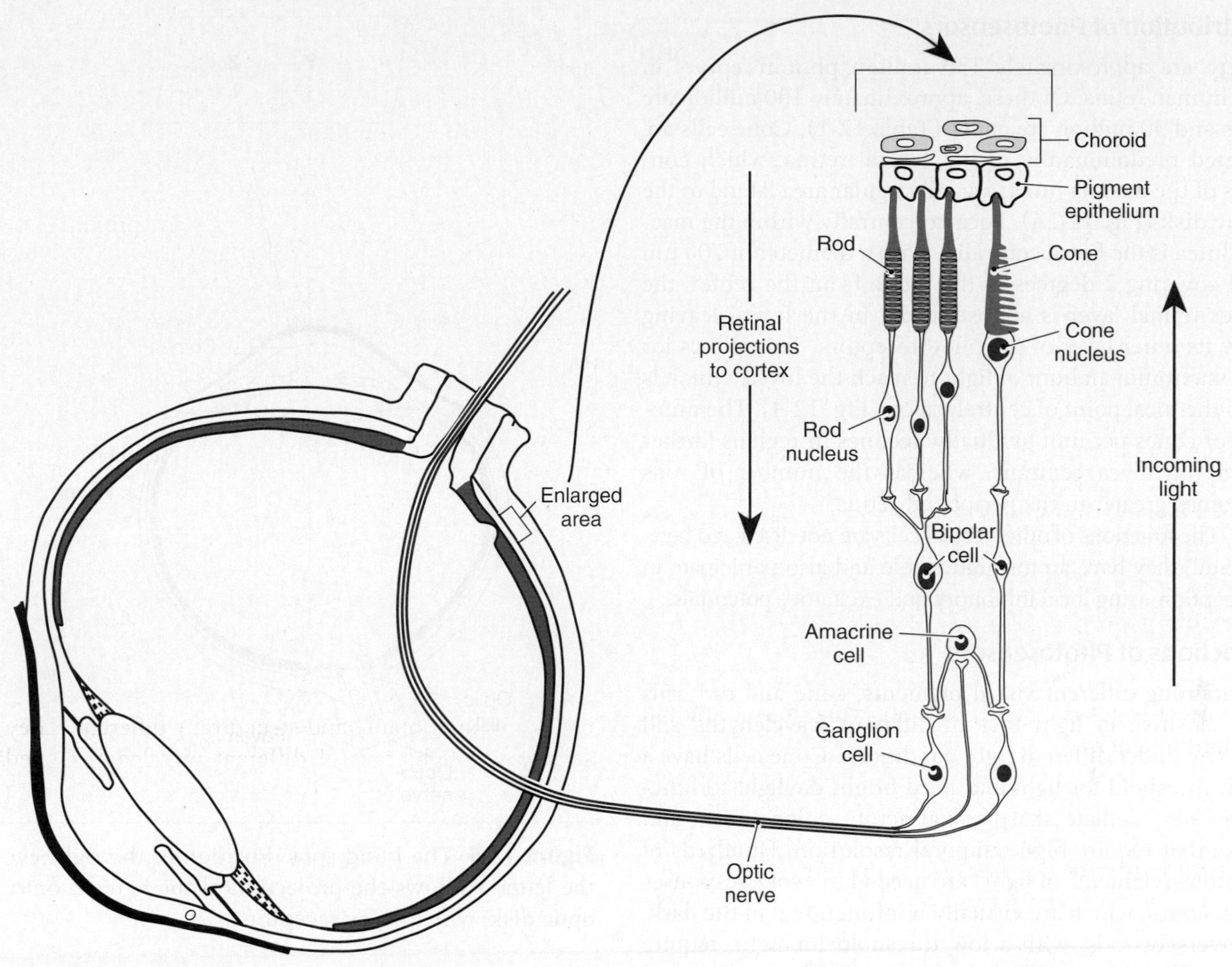

Figure 12-3 Cellular organization of the retina with its three layers of cells: photoreceptors (rods and cones), bipolar cells, and ganglion cells. Light rays enter and pass through all these layers to reach the cones and rods, which are activated to generate local potentials. Local potentials from the photosensors carrying the visual code travel back to the bipolar cells and ganglion cells.

Table 12-1

Functional Summary of Photoreceptors

Features	Cones	Rods
Number	30 million	100 million
Location	Fovea, central retina	Retina, except fovea
Functional	Bright light	Low-light conditions
Color processing	All colors shades	Only gray
Visual acuity	High	Low

BOX 12-3

Papilledema

A common pathology of the optic disk (the area of the ocular fundus at which the fibers from the retinal ganglion converge to form the optic nerve) is edema. The swelling of the disk results from the swelling of the connective tissues that surround the optic nerve axons at the disk. Visible through an ophthalmoscope, the swelling is marked by an elevated optic disk with poorly defined boundaries. The presence of the distorted disk provides clinically significant information about disease processes in the brain, such as hypertension and increased intracranial pressure.

Distribution of Photosensors

There are approximately 130 million photoreceptors in the human retina. Of these, approximately 100 million are rods and 30 million are cones (Table 12-1). Cone cells are located predominantly in the central retina, which consists of the **macula lutea**, a small circular area lateral to the optic disk (Fig. 12-2*A*). Located centrally within the macula lutea is the **fovea centralis**. With a diameter of 700 μm and covering 2 degrees of the retina from the center, the inner retinal layer is almost absent in the fovea, leaving only its outer layer of the photoreceptors. This allows for the maximum amount of light to reach the fovea, which is also the focal point of central vision (Fig. 12-4). The number of cones per unit gradually declines in regions farther from the fovea centralis, whereas the number of rods becomes greater in the peripheral retina.

The functions of other retinal cells are not discussed here. Overall, they have an integrative role and also participate in perception using local inhibitory and excitatory potentials.

Functions of Photosensors

Containing different visual pigments, cone and rod cells are sensitive to light rays of different wavelengths and operate under different light conditions. Cone cells have a high threshold for light and need bright daylight to function; they mediate sharp visual acuity, color vision, and tasks that require high temporal resolution. Hundreds of photons (elements of light) are needed to evoke responses from cones, which are virtually nonfunctional in the dark. Conversely, rods, with a low threshold for light, require only a few photons for their activation. They function in dim light and mediate night vision. The presence of fewer photons can evoke a maximal response from the rods. For this reason, rods are nonfunctional in bright daylight. With sensitivity to selective components of the color spectrum, rods differentiate black, white, and shades of gray; they also detect movement and identify shapes, but they cannot resolve details or mediate color vision. Rods and cones have specific patterns of connections to other nuclear layers of the retina. For example, because of poor spatial resolution, >20 rod cells converge on a single ganglion cell. Cone cells, which have a higher spatial resolution power, directly project to ganglion cells in a 1:1 ratio.

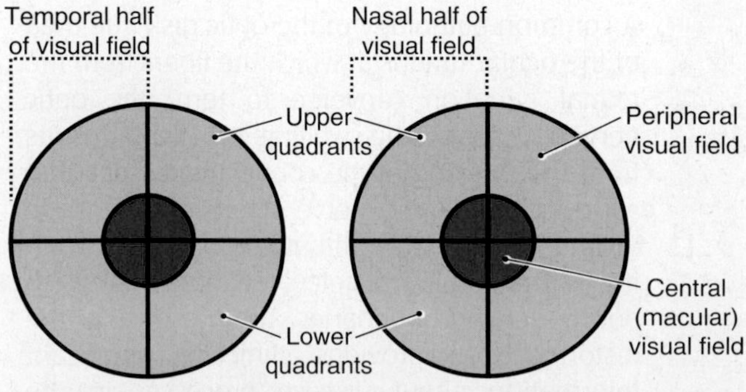

Figure 12-4 Central and peripheral visual fields and their divisions: temporal and nasal half-fields and upper and lower quadrants.

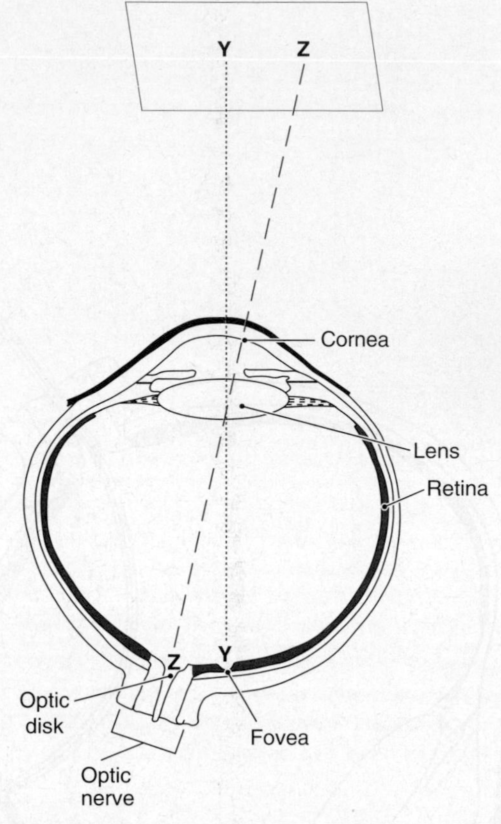

Figure 12-5 The blind spot. Fixation of the right eye on the letter Y allows the projection of the letter Z onto the optic disk, which lacks receptors.

Visual images are focused in the macula lutea for clarity of visual perception and color analysis. In the fovea centralis, the inner layer of the bipolar and ganglion cells is pushed apart and displaced laterally, giving the appearance of a depressed pit. This is because the fovea contains neither blood vessels nor many nerve fibers; it enables light rays to project directly on the photoreceptors and allows for the highest visual acuity and color perception.

The axons of the ganglion cells form the optic nerve, which travels the inner surface of the retina and converges at the optic disk (papilla) before exiting the retina (Figs. 12-3 and 12-5). Because it has no photoreceptors, the optic disk area is called the **blind spot**.

The object will briefly disappear as it is projected on the optic disk (e.g., the letter Z in Fig. 12-5).

VASCULAR SUPPLY OF THE RETINA

The cerebral part of the internal carotid artery as it passes the cranial dura gives off the ophthalmic artery, which passes through the **optic foramen** to enter the orbit. The ophthalmic artery branches into the **central retinal artery** and the

ciliary artery. The central retinal artery supplies the inner retinal layer. The ciliary artery, on the other hand, supplies the choroidal layer and the outer retinal layer. The retina, with its acute dependence on blood supply, is highly sensitive to vascular ischemia. Therefore, retinal dysfunction may indicate pathology involving the internal carotid artery.

RETINAL PHOTORECEPTOR FUNCTIONING

Photochemistry of rods and cones involves the absorption of electromagnetic energy in light by their visual pigments and their chemical decomposition and composition needed for converting the energy into neural impulses. Photopigments are colored proteins in the outer membranes that undergo structural changes on absorbing light and transmit local potentials to the bipolar cells, which in turn activate ganglion cells by means of neurotransmitters.

Located mostly in the peripheral retina, rods are sensitive to low-light conditions and mediate night vision. Structurally wide and containing a greater number of lamellae—analogous to cilia-containing photosegments—the rods have a greater photosensitivity but lack visual acuity. The absence of light triggers a series of neuronal events related to the decomposition and regeneration of pigments and membrane potentials. These biochemical events occurring to resynthesize the rhodopsin take 7 to 30 minutes. This is also the time needed for adapting to darkness.

The photochemical processing of cones is similar to that of rods, in which phototransduction (photopsin, the proteins found in the cone cells) involves the decomposition of the photopigment and its resynthesis. Because of sensitivity to different wavelengths (for color vision), cones contain three types of photopigments (proteins), which promote maximum absorption of light from different parts of the light spectrum accounting for the **trivalent color vision**. Three issues related to retinal neural coding are **spectral sensitivity**, **color vision**, and **dark adaptation**.

Spectral Sensitivity

In addition to being sensitive to different light conditions, rods and cones are sensitive to different light wavelengths. They have different visibility curves, known as scotopic (rods mediated) and photopic (cones mediated) vision. The rod-mediated visibility curve shows great sensitivity to light rays with wavelengths of 400 to 600 nm, with maximum sensitivity at 507 nm, in the blue-green range. The same eye adapted to light has a photopic visibility curve that covers wavelengths of 425 to 700 nm and maximum sensitivity at 555 nm, in the yellow-green range.

Color Vision

Cones in the human eye are sensitive to wavelengths ranging from 400 to 700 nm. In this spectrum, the colors change from blue to red after passing through green, yellow, and orange. There are three types of cones in the retina, and each has photosensitive pigments specialized for different wavelengths (blue cones, green cones, and red cones). Spectral differences make cones respond best to light of different wavelengths. Short-wavelength cones (S cones) are sensitive to blue and have a maximum absorption at 445 nm. Medium-wavelength cones (M cones) are sensitive to green and respond with a maximum absorption at 535 nm. Long-wavelength cones (L cones) are sensitive to red and respond with maximum absorption at 570 nm. **Trichromatic** color vision results from the combination of the activities of the blue, green, and red cones.

Dark Adaptation

Dark adaptation is the normal night vision possible within a few minutes after entering a darkened room. As noted, it normally takes 7 to 30 minutes for the eyes to adjust to a dark room. This is the time needed for the rhodopsin of rods to reconstitute. After one moves from bright daylight to a dark room, the cones initially remain sensitive to light and continue to process colors; thus, both cones and rods increase their sensitivity to light. If the low-light conditions persist, the cones, with their high threshold to light, gradually become nonfunctional. The rods, with their low threshold to light, then begin functioning. As the rods start adjusting to dim light, vision becomes achromatic. The only color that is still recognized is red, because rods remain insensitive to red light, which is processed exclusively by the rod-free fovea centralis. The inability to see at night after this normal period of dark adaptation from 7 to 30 minutes, is called night blindness (nyctalopia).

Key Terms:

Far point	**Meyer loop**
Focal length	**Near point**
Focal point	**Optic radiations**
Lens accommodation	

OPTICAL MECHANISM

The eye functions as an optical instrument. An adequate refraction of light rays ensures a properly focused image on the inner retina. Familiarity with the optical principle of refraction and the refractive properties of the lens is essential to understanding the mechanism of the eye.

Refraction

Light rays travel in straight lines and slow down when entering a transparent medium from a medium of greater density. If the light rays strike a surface with a different density at an angle, they bend; this is called refraction. If

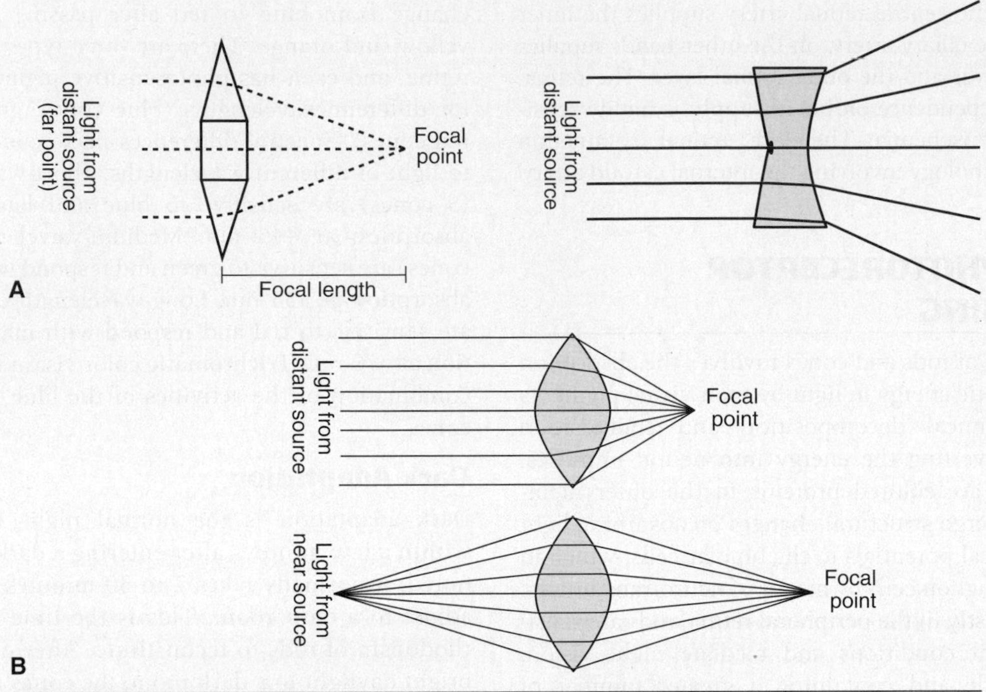

Figure 12-6 A. Refraction through convex and concave lenses. B. Two convex lenses possess similar refractive powers, but they have different focal lengths because the rays entering the upper lens are parallel, whereas rays entering the lower lens diverge.

the light rays strike this surface perpendicularly (i.e., not at an angle), they do not bend. The degree to which light rays bend depends on two factors: the **refractive index**† of the medium into which the waves enter and the **angle** at which the rays strike the surface.

Refractive power is measured in **diopter units**, and the total refractive power of the eye is 60 diopters. In the eye, refraction of light rays depends primarily on the curvature and optical density of the cornea and on the lens shape. The cornea contributes about 42 of the 60 diopters to the refraction. A simple example of refraction can be seen in a biconvex lens (Fig. 12-6*A*). In this lens, the top and bottom sections have an angulated shape, whereas the central section is rectangular. The angulated top section of the lens bends the striking waves downward, whereas the bottom angulated section of the lens bends the waves upward. The rectangular center portion of the lens (nonangulated and perpendicular to the wave front) permits light rays to pass through without deviation (refraction). The light rays converge at a common point (**focal point**) to form the focused image on the retina. The distance from the lens to the focal point is the **focal length**, and the point from which the rays originate is the **far point**.

† The refractive index of any transparent substance is the ratio of the velocity of light in air to the velocity of light in the second transparent substance. For example, a glass cube has a refractive index of 1.5: velocity of light through air (300,000 km/sec) divided by the velocity of light through glass (200,000 km/sec) = 1.5.

The action of the ciliary muscles increases the refractive power of a lens by about 12 diopters. This elasticity of the lens declines with age and leads to a gradual reduction in the ability to accommodate the lens, which is essential for near vision. This is called **presbyopia**; it begins around age 40 and it can pose a problem for reading, but reading glasses are helpful in overcoming this difficulty.

Lens Types

The two most common types of lenses are **convex** and **concave** (Fig. 12-6*A*). Each contributes differently to a refraction. A convex lens reduces focal length by adding greater convergence to bending light rays. Light rays striking the angled edges of the lens bend and converge to a common focus point beyond the lens, where they join the undeviating waves traveling through the center of the lens. In contrast, a concave lens, with its inward-angled edge, increases the focal length by diverging rays away from the centrally entering rays of the lens.

Optical Functioning of the Eye

Focusing an image on the retinas entails three processes: refraction of light rays by the lens, **pupillary aperture** control, and **ocular convergence**. Refraction of the rays leads to proper focusing of the image. The refractive power of a lens is controlled by its accommodation.

For all practical purposes, a distance of 20 ft (6 m) between the lens and the object is considered common for assessing visual acuity. Light rays originating from an object placed 20 ft or more away are parallel to each other. They must be bent adequately to converge on the fovea centralis. Light rays from an object closer than 20 ft are generally divergent (Fig. 12-6*B*). This divergence of rays is too great for the cornea and resting lens to focus the image on the retina. Therefore, greater refraction is required. Since the distance (focal length) between the center of the lens and the fovea centralis is fixed at 17 mm, the lens must assume different shapes to refract the parallel rays reflected from a distant object and the diverging rays from a near object. This is made possible with the regulation of the lens curvature (**lens accommodation**) by the action of the ciliary muscle. The curvature of a lens (as opposed to its flat surface) determines its refractive power. A lens with greater outward round curvature has more refractive power and acutely bends light rays toward the focus point.

If the refractive power of the lens is unchanged, the diverging rays from a near object will converge far behind the photosensors of the retina, resulting in an unfocused image. The process of accommodation keeps the image of a near object in sharp focus by modifying the lens's curvature. The power of a lens is defined in terms of the focal length. A lens with greater refracting power has a shorter focal length, whereas a lens with lower refractive power has a greater focal length.

The size of the pupillary aperture controls the amount of light entering the eyes. The pupillary aperture is controlled by sympathetic and parasympathetic innervation of the dilator (radial) and constrictor (circular) muscle fibers of the iris. In bright light, pupil constriction (regulated by parasympathetic activity) allows only a small amount of light to enter. In dim light, the sympathetically dilated pupil allows maximum light to enter the eye. Convergence is the inward turning of both eyes to keep an approaching object in focus. This movement also contributes to binocular vision, which results when the images of an object are projected on corresponding (homonymous) points in both retinas. This projection on homonymous retinal points ensures that the object will stay in focus.

Retinal Image Formation

The formation of an image on the retina is guided by one optical principle; the retinal image is a **reversed** and **inverted** form of what is seen in the visual field. The projected upside down image is also a mirror image of both the left and the right sides of an object. The correct interpretation of an upside down and reversed image is learned through a process that begins at birth and is mediated by the associational visual cortex.

CENTRAL VISUAL PATHWAYS

The central visual mechanism includes the pathway from the retina to the primary visual cortex, which is located on the midsagittal surface of the occipital lobe (Figs. 2-10 and 12-7). Two important characteristics of the central visual mechanism are, first, a point-to-point representation of the visual field from the retina through the lateral geniculate body to the primary visual cortex and, second, the projection from each eye to both cerebral hemispheres (binocular processing). Familiarity with the pathways carrying visual information and the crossing points of the visual fibers provides the basis for relating lesion sites with specific visual field defects (Fig. 12-7; Table 12-2).

The optic nerve (CN II) fibers from the retinal cells exit the orbital cavity through the optic foramina and enter the cranial cavity. Optic nerves from both eyes come together at the optic chiasm near the hypothalamus (see Figs. 2-8 and 2-11). The optic tract fibers from the optic chiasm travel caudally and laterally and terminate in the LGB, the thalamic visual relay center. The geniculocalcarine (optic radiation) fibers loop laterally and caudally in the temporal lobe, travel to the occipital cortex, and terminate in the superior and inferior opercula (lips) of the calcarine fissure, the primary visual cortex (Brodmann area 17), located on the midsagittal surface of the occipital lobe (Table 12-3).

Retinal Representation of Visual Fields

A large part of the visual field, the binocular area, is covered by both eyes (Fig. 12-1). Light rays from an object in the binocular visual field project to the corresponding portions of both retinas. However, for learning purposes and for keeping the path of visual projections precise and clear, the visual fields for each eye are depicted separately in Figure 12-7*A*.

The visual field, the area viewed by the eyes, has central and peripheral regions (Figs. 12-4 and 12-7). The central visual field is the small area in the center. This is projected onto the macula of the retina and is responsible for the sharpest vision, reading, and face/object recognition. The central field of vision is surrounded by a large peripheral visual field. The visual field for each eye is divided into two half fields: nasal and temporal halves. Each of these half fields is further divided into upper and lower quadrants (Fig. 12-4).

Retinal representation of the visual field for each eye is also divided into nasal and temporal halves, each of which contains upper and lower quadrants. The retinal representation of the visual field is in reversed and inverted form (Fig. 12-7*B*; Table 12-2). Light rays from the temporal half of the visual field project to the nasal half of the retina. Similarly, rays from the nasal half of the visual field fall on the temporal half of the retina. Light rays from the top of the object strike the lower retina, and rays from the bottom of the object strike the upper retina. Taking the projections for both eyes into consideration, light rays from an object in the right visual field fall on the nasal retina of the right eye and the temporal retina of the left eye. Light rays of an object from the left visual field strike the nasal half of the retina in the left eye and the temporal half of the retina in the right eye.

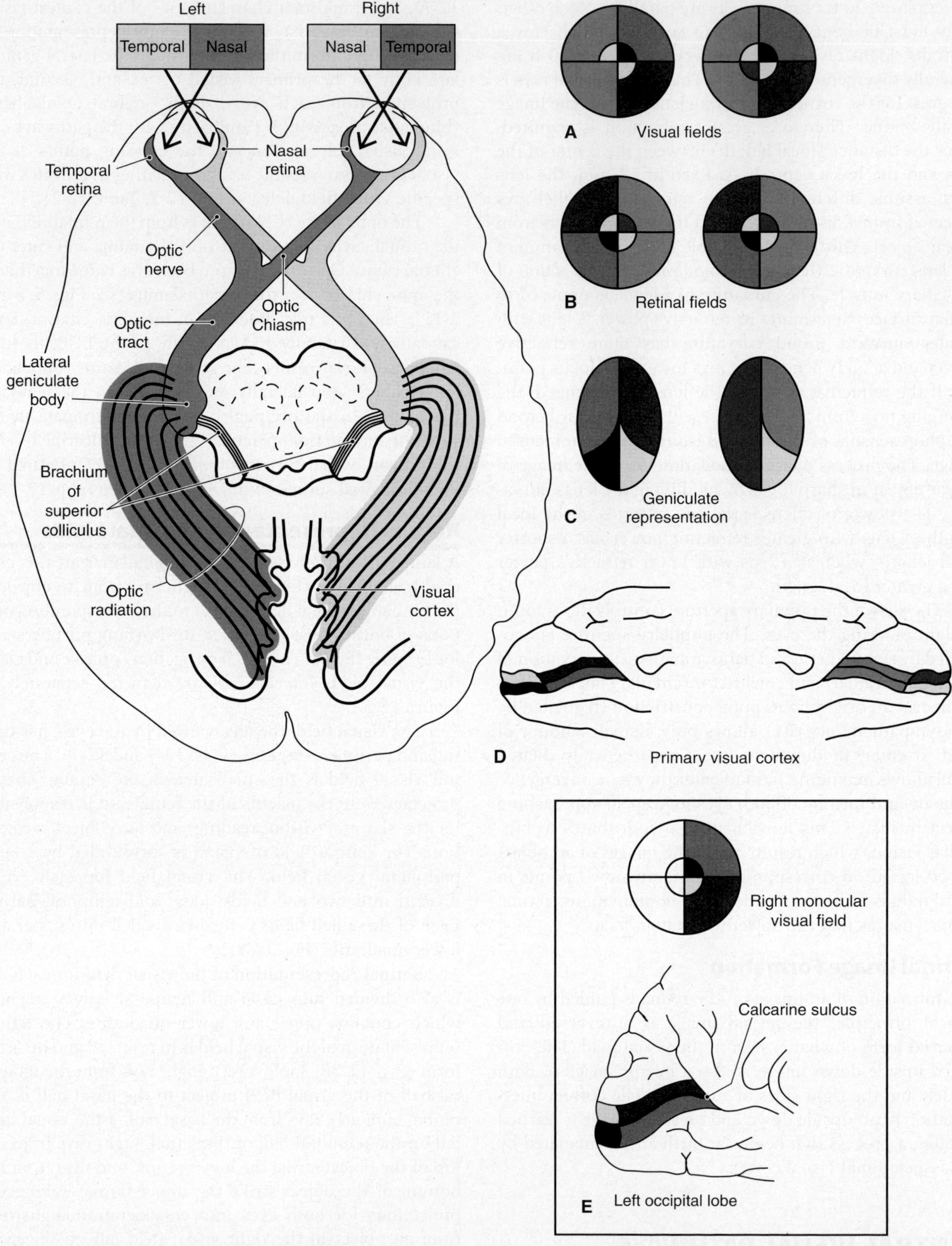

Figure 12-7 The visual pathways from the retina to the visual cortex in the occipital lobe and representation of the visual fields as processed along the optic pathway. A. The visual fields. B. The retinal fields. C. The geniculate representation. D. The cortex. E. The right monocular visual field as mapped on the left primary visual cortex in the occipital lobe.

Table 12-2

Rules Related to the Central Visual Mechanism

Rule	Description
1	Retinal image is a reversed and inverted form of visual field image
2	Nasal retinal fibers (representing temporal visual field) cross at optic chiasm and project to opposite cortex Temporal retinal fibers (representing nasal visual field) remain uncrossed and project to ipsilateral cortex
3	Geniculocortical fibers representing lower visual field quadrant pass dorsally (superior fibers) through cerebral white matter to reach visual cortex (upper lip of calcarine fissure) Geniculocalcarine fibers representing upper visual field quadrant pass ventrally (inferior fibers) and laterally through Meyer loop and project to visual cortex (lower lip of calcarine fissure)
4	Upper retinal fibers (representing lower visual field quadrant) terminate in upper visual cortex Lower retinal fibers (representing upper visual field quadrant) project to lower visual cortex
5	Peripheral visual field is represented rostrally along calcarine fissure Central (foveal) visual field is represented caudally along calcarine fissure and extends beyond to occipital pole cortex

Table 12-3

Panoramic View of Visual Processes

Process	Structures
Traveling light rays	Cornea Anterior cavity (aqueous humor) Lens Posterior cavity (vitreous humor) Retinal cells (ganglion, bipolar, rods, cones)
Retinal processing	Changes in membrane potential in rods and cones Bipolar cells (local potential) Ganglion cells (action potential) Optic nerve
Cortical processing	Optic chiasm Optic tract Lateral geniculate body Geniculocalcarine fibers Visual cortex

Retinal Representation to Optic Chiasm

Optic nerve fibers from the retinal ganglion cells enter the cranial cavity to reach the optic chiasm. Two rules account for the partial crossing of fibers at the chiasm. First, fibers from the nasal halves of the retinas (representing temporal visual fields for each eye) cross the midline to project to the opposite visual cortex. Second, fibers from the temporal half of each retina (representing nasal halves of the visual fields) remain uncrossed and project to the ipsilateral visual cortex. This accounts for projection of the right visual field to the left hemisphere and projection of the left visual field to the right hemisphere (Fig. 12-7; Table 12-2).

Retinal Representation to the Lateral Geniculate Body

Each optic tract (**postchiasmic fibers**) carries visual information from both eyes. The left optic tract mediates the right visual field for each eye. The left optic tract contains the projections from the temporal half of the left retina (nasal visual field for the left eye) and the nasal half of the right retina (temporal visual field for the right eye). Similarly, the right optic tract transmits the left visual field for each eye and includes the projections from the nasal half of the left retina (temporal visual field for the left eye) and temporal half of the right retina (nasal visual field for the right eye). Consistent with contralateral arrangement of sensory and motor organizations, the optic tract projects to the LGB of the thalamus.

Each LGB receives a point-to-point projection from the homonymous (left or right) halves of the field of both eyes (Fig. 12-7*C*). The visual information is distributed on both (lateral and medial) sides of the LGB. Fibers from the upper retinal quadrants (representing lower visual field quadrants) terminate in the medial portion of the LGB, whereas fibers from the lower retinal quadrants (representing upper visual field quadrants) project to the lateral portion of the LGB.

Retinal Representation to the Visual Cortex

Geniculocalcarine fibers, or **optic radiations**, constitute the last phase in the transmission of visual information to the visual cortex (Fig. 12-7*D*). They enter the retrolenticular portion of the posterior internal capsule on their way to the primary visual cortex (Fig. 12-7). They divide into dorsal and ventral bundles of fibers. The dorsal bundle of fibers, traveling straight to the cells in the visual cortex above the calcarine fissure, carries information from the upper retinal quadrants (representing the lower visual field quadrants). The ventral bundle of fibers forms the **Meyer loop**. These geniculocalcarine fibers first move rostrally and then make a lateral excursion around the inferior (temporal) horn of the lateral ventricle before traveling to the cells in the visual cortex below the calcarine fissure. These fibers mediate projections from the lower retinal quadrants (representing the upper visual field quadrants) (Table 12-2).

Primary Visual Cortex

The primary visual cortex (Brodmann area 17) is bilateral located on the midsagittal surface of the occipital lobe (Fig. 12-7; see Fig. 2-10). It is divided into two opercula (lips), which are separated by the calcarine fissure (see Fig. 2-10). Each visual cortex receives information from both eyes. The lower (inferior) lip of the visual cortex, on the lingual gyrus, receives projections from the lower portion of the retina (representing the upper quadrant in the visual field). The upper (superior) lip of the visual cortex receives projections from the upper retina (representing the lower quadrant in the visual field). The central visual field, representing the macular region of the retina, occupies a comparatively large area in the posterior part near the occipital pole, amounting to >50% of the primary visual cortex. The peripheral visual fields are represented in the anterior portions of the calcarine cortex (Fig. 12-7*E*; Table 12-2). The primary visual cortex is characterized by the wide cellular layer 4. It contains an extra band of myelinated fibers and is known to send cortical feedback projections to the LGB. This myelinated structure seems to be the site of large geniculocalcarine input.

VISUAL CORTEX DEVELOPMENT

In early development, visual pathways from both eyes compete for equal access to synaptic spaces in the visual cortex, in particular for the connectivity in layer 4. This competing input from both eyes is essential for normal vision and proper depth perception.

The critical period plays an important role in the development of normal axonal connections, when the axonal afferents from both eyes have equal access to the overlapping cortical regions and compete for the available synaptic spaces. This is measured in terms of the number of synapses. The connections that succeed during the critical period become permanent. If for some reason axons from one eye are not functional and do not properly connect during the critical period—from 5 to 6 years of age—they lose the claim for the synaptic spaces in the visual cortex. In this case, the axons from the other eye have exclusive control of all the available synaptic space in the brain

VISUAL REFLEXES

Visual reflexes are concerned with the changing of pupil size and lens curvature (lens accommodation). The ocular muscle fibers regulating these two reflexes are controlled by the parasympathetic fibers of the oculomotor nerve (CN III). Pupil dilation, on the other hand, is regulated by the sympathetic efferents (Fig. 12-8).

Key Terms:

Agnosia	**Hypermetropia**
Agraphia	**Miosis**
Alexia	**Mydriasis**
Astigmatism	**Myopia**
Hemianopia	**Ptosis**
Horner syndrome	

Pupillary Light Reflex

In the pupillary light reflex, the eyes react to bright light by constricting the pupils. The neural mechanism for these pupillary changes involves the **pretectal area**, the **Edinger–Westphal nucleus**, and fibers of the oculomotor nerve (Fig. 12-8*A*). The activated retinal ganglion cells send projections to the brain. These fibers leave the optic tract before the LGB and synapse on cells in the pretectal area. The pretectal area, a small unspecified area between the superior colliculi, bilaterally projects to the Edinger–Westphal (visceral) nucleus of the oculomotor (CN III) nerve. The preganglionic fibers from the Edinger–Westphal nucleus travel in the oculomotor nerve and innervate the ipsilateral **ciliary ganglion** in the orbit. The postganglionic fibers from the ciliary ganglion provide parasympathetic projections to the circular (constrictor) fibers of the iris. The constriction of the circular fibers narrows the aperture of the pupil, a condition called **miosis** (Fig. 12-9*A*).

Both pupils constrict in response to light entering one eye. The pupillary reaction in the eye exposed to light is the direct response, whereas the reflexive pupillary change in the other eye is the consensual response. In complete darkness, constriction of the radial (dilator) fibers of the iris results in pupil dilation, or **mydriasis** (Fig. 12-9*B*).

The pupil dilatory function involves both inhibition of the Edinger–Westphal nucleus and facilitation of sympathetic activity. Sympathetic projections exit from T1–T3 and travel in the cervical sympathetic chain to the **superior cervical ganglion (see Chapter 18)**, which sends postganglionic projections to the radial fibers of the iris muscle in the eyeball (Fig. 12-8*B*).

Clinically, oculomotor nerve (CN III) lesions alter the pupillary light reflex. Interrupted afferent projections from one eye affect the light reflex in both pupils. This reflex is tested by checking whether light projected into each eye elicits both direct and consensual responses. Presence of the consensual response without a direct pupil

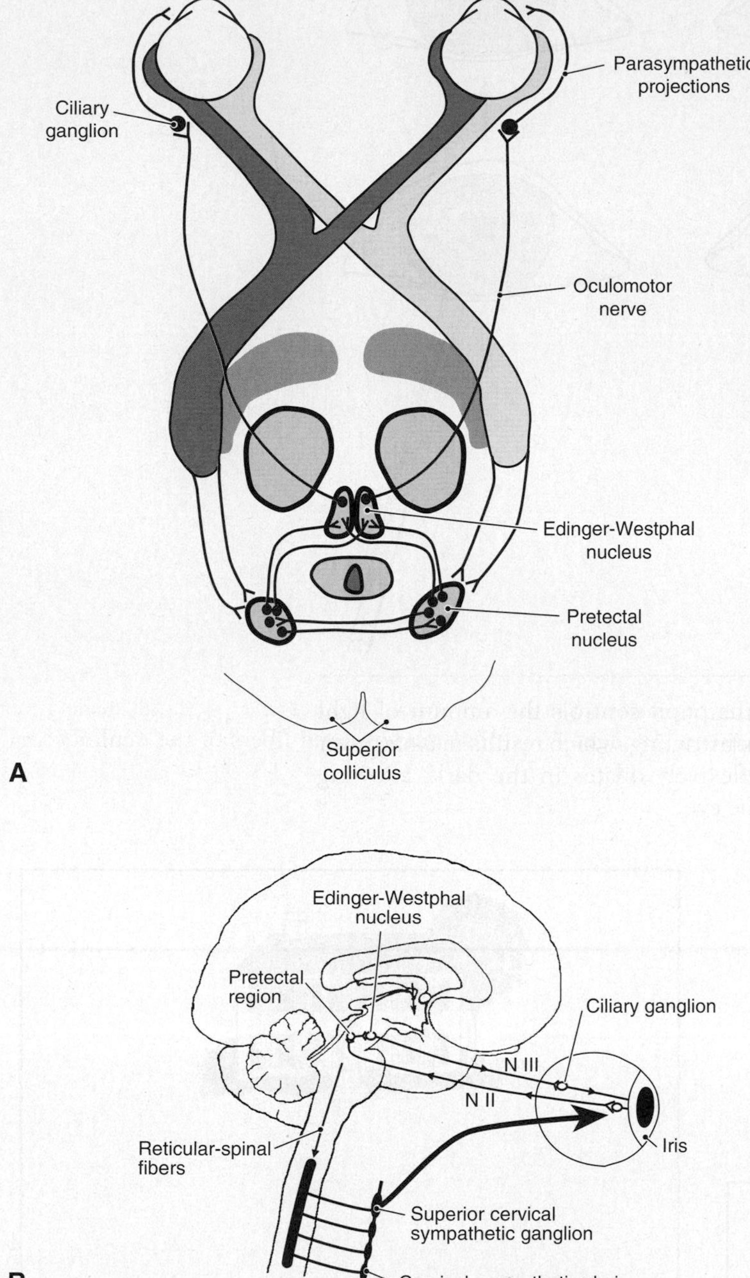

Figure 12-8 A. Parasympathetic innervation of the iris for pupil constriction in light. B. Sympathetic innervation of the eyeball for pupil dilation in dark. *N*, nerve.

response suggests a lesion involving the efferent projection from the Edinger–Westphal nucleus to the same eye. An interruption of the sympathetic fibers causes paralysis of the dilator fibers of the iris and results in a permanently constricted pupillary diameter (miosis). The resulting condition is part of **Horner syndrome**, which is characterized by an ipsilaterally constricted pupil (miosis), drooping eyelid (**ptosis**), and loss of facial sweating (**anhidrosis**).

Lens Accommodation Reflex

The accommodation (or near) reflex regulates the refractive power of the lens (Fig. 12-10*A*). The distance between the lens and the retina remains the same as an object is moved closer to the eyes. Keeping an object in focus requires increased refractive power of the lens, which occurs when the lens assumes a more rounded (spherical) form. This reflexive modification of the lens curvature is controlled by the contraction of the ciliary muscles through the suspensory ligaments. The parasympathetic contraction of the ciliary muscles reduces tension in the suspensory ligaments by pulling the ciliary processes forward. With no pulls from ligaments, the lens, because of its inherent elasticity, assumes a rounded form, thus acquiring greater refractive power. This refraction is needed for clearly viewing objects that are close (<20 ft) to the eye (Fig. 12-10*A*). The relaxed state of ciliary muscles

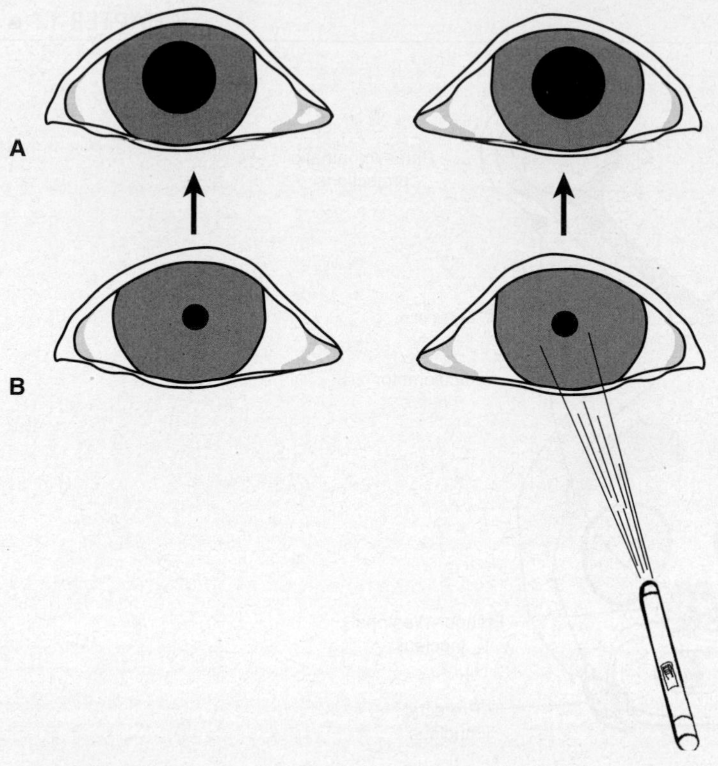

Figure 12-9 **A.** In light, the pupil controls the amount of light that enters by reflexively constricting, which results in a narrower opening. **B.** The pupil reflexively dilates in the dark, allowing maximum light to enter the eye.

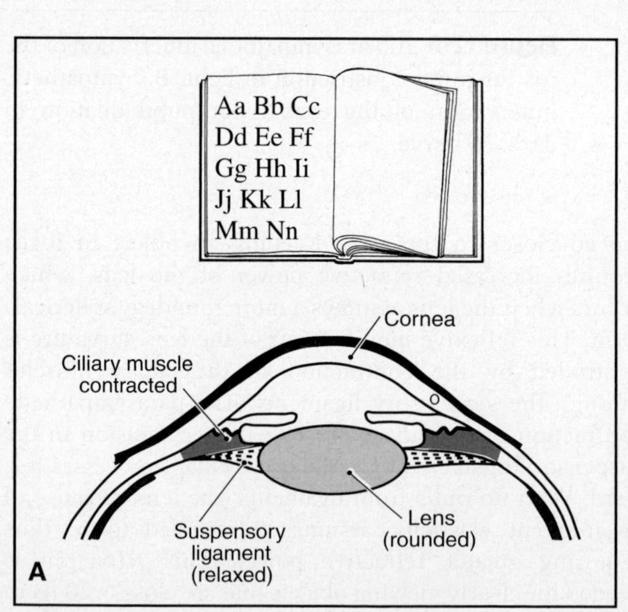

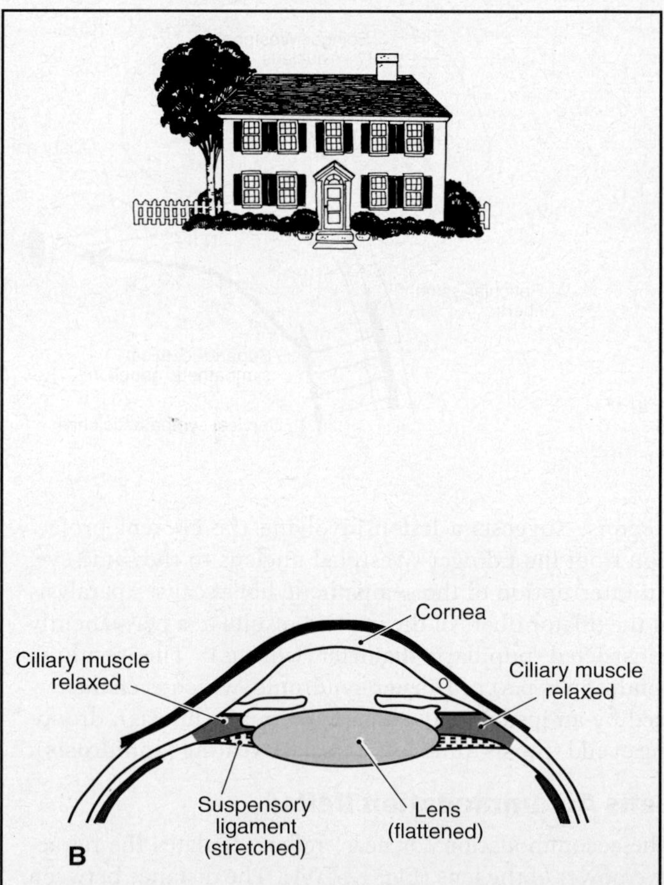

Figure 12-10 Lens accommodation (**A**) for near (<20 ft) objects and distant (**B**) (>20 ft) objects.

exerts tension on the suspensory ligaments that flatten the lens by pulling it. This reduces the refractive power, permitting far vision (Fig. 12-10*B*).

The neural mechanism of the accommodation reflex is different from the light reflex. It involves the primary visual cortex in addition to the LGB and the mesencephalic reflex center (Fig. 12-8*A*). As the image of an object moving closer begins to blur, the visual cortex sends projections to the superior colliculus, which mediates visual information to the pretectal area. The pretectal nuclei send crossed and uncrossed fibers to the Edinger–Westphal nucleus, which projects preganglionic parasympathetic fibers in the oculomotor nerve (CN III) to the ciliary ganglion. The postganglionic projections from the ciliary ganglion cause constriction of the ciliary muscle. Consequently, the lens, released from the tension of the suspensory ligaments, becomes round and acquires greater refractive power. The accommodation reflex has two additional components: eye convergence and pupillary constriction (discussed earlier). Children have greater ability to accommodate the lens than do adults; starting at about age 45, the lens gradually loses the flexibility to control the refractive power (presbyopia).

CLINICAL CORRELATES

Errors of Refraction

The refractive power of the eye is largely determined by the cornea and lens. In an **emmetropic** (normal) **eye**, there is a normal relationship between axial length and the eye's refractive power, so that light rays from objects beyond 20 ft can converge on the fovea without any lens accommodation (Fig. 12-11*A*). When the relationship between the refraction and the focal length is not optimal, parallel light rays from distant objects will converge either behind the retina or in front of it causing blurred vision and visual fatigue. There are three common types of refractive errors: **hypermetropia** (farsightedness), **myopia** (nearsightedness), and **astigmatism**.

Hypermetropia

The focal point in a hypermetropic or hyperopic eye falls behind the retina (Fig. 12-11*B*). Two factors contribute to this focusing error: the short axial length of the eyeball and the inadequate refractive power of the lens. Hypermetropic patients are farsighted (can see distant objects normally), because light rays from distant objects are parallel (less divergent) and are adequately refracted. The optical problem is in focusing near objects. Young hypermetropic patients may compensate for this refractive error by lens accommodation. Contracting the ciliary muscle removes tension from the suspensory ligaments and results in a convex lens with greater refractive power. However, after a limit, known as the **near point** of vision, the near objects can no longer be brought into focus. Furthermore, continuous use of accommodation may cause hypertrophy of the ciliary muscle. Hypermetropic error is corrected with a convex lens, which adds the greater refractive power needed to make the light rays converge on the retina (Fig. 12-11*B*).

Myopia

Because the focal point in a myopic eye falls in front of the retina (Fig. 12-11*C*), the subject cannot see distant objects well. The two factors that contribute to myopia are that the eyeball has a long axis and the lens has strong refractive power. Individuals with myopia are nearsighted, because light rays from near objects are divergent and thus require greater refraction and/or a longer axis for converging on the retina. Myopic errors of refraction may be corrected by placing a concave lens before the eye, which adds focal length by diverging the light rays (Fig. 12-11*C*).

Astigmatism

Astigmatism is a refractive error caused by irregular shape of the cornea, lens, or both (Fig. 12-11*D*). Horizontal corneal and/or lens diameters do not have the same refractive power as vertical diameters. Consequently, different portions of light rays passing through the lens focus at different depth points on or behind the retina. Astigmatic errors of refraction are corrected by a combined cylindrical and spherical lens, which can bring all light rays into focus at the same retinal point.

Disorders of Color Vision

Several forms of color blindness or confusion have been described in clinical populations. Three major kinds of color vision anomalies are **protanomaly**, **deuteranomaly**, and **tritanomaly**. A protanopic patient lacks red cones and sees only green and blue. A deuteranopic person lacks green cones and sees only red and blue. A tritanopic person lacks blue cones and sees only red and green. The degree of impairment varies from complete color blindness to partial impairment, marked by color confusion. This deficit can be acquired, though it is primarily inherited. Inherited color blindness occurs mostly in males, whose single X chromosome, from the mother, has the opsin for red and blue colors. The photopigment for blue color is on an autosome, and tritanomaly is rare. Color blindness is usually absent in women because at least one of their two X chromosomes is likely to have a normal gene for the cones.

Visual Acuity Assessment

Visual acuity refers to the ability to see details from a fixed distance. This is measured by use of a **Snellen chart**, which contains letters and numbers in a variety of sizes (Fig. 12-12). The chart specifies the distances, written as a fraction, from which the characters can be seen clearly by individuals with a normal visual acuity. The numerator is the distance (fixed at 20 ft) from which the visual acuity is

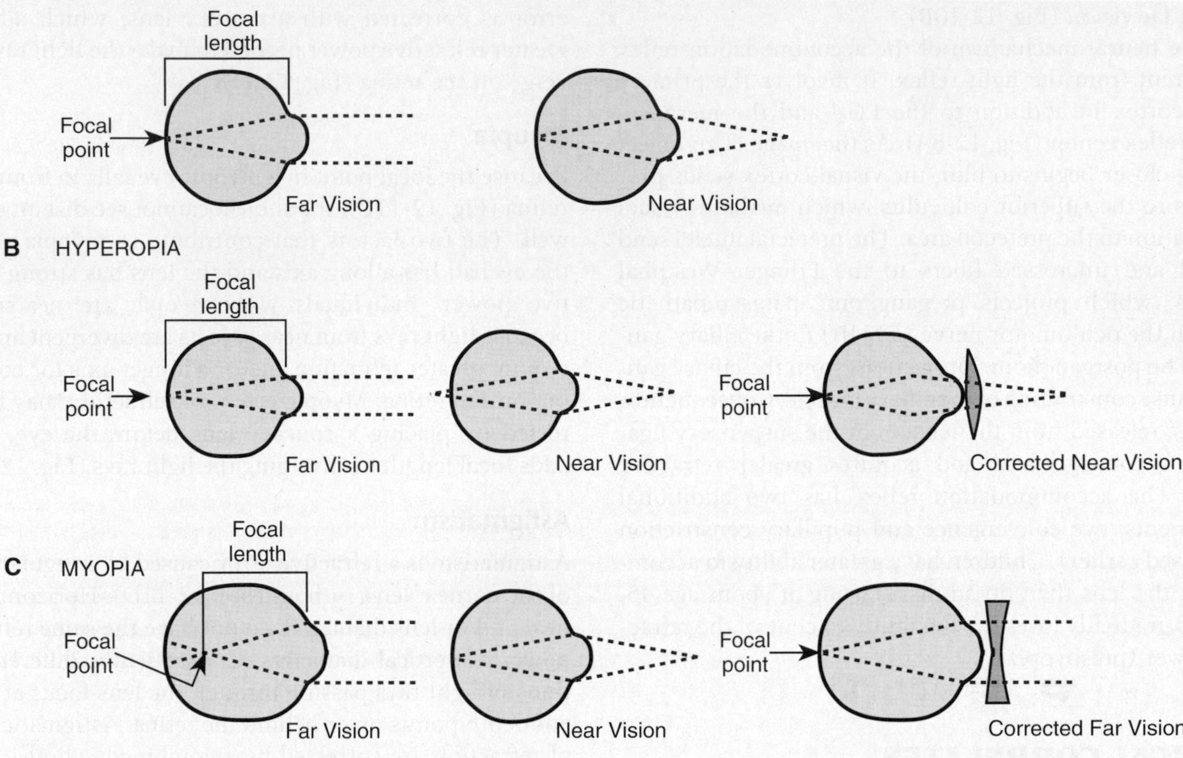

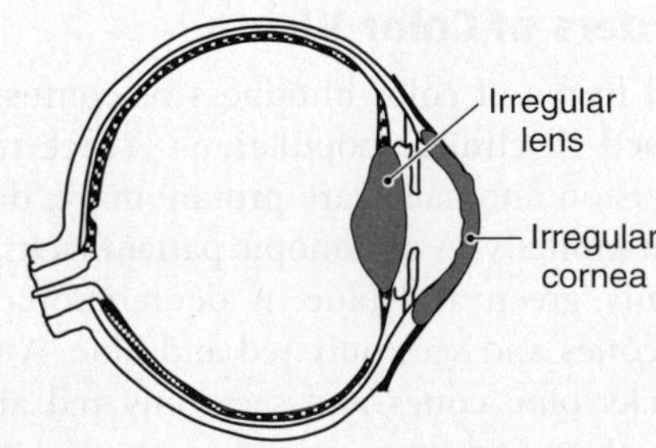

Figure 12-11 The normally refractive eye, common refractive errors, and their corrections. A. In a normal (emmetropic) eye, light rays from a near or far object are adequately refracted so that the rays converge directly on the retina, enabling formation of a clear image. B. In a farsighted (hypermetropic, hyperopic) eye, an image from a near point is focused behind the retina. The resulting condition can be corrected with convex lenses. C. In a nearsighted (myopic) eye, an image from a far point is focused in front of the retina. This refractive condition can be corrected with concave lenses. D. Refractive errors of astigmatism result from irregular curvatures of the cornea, lens, or both. Consequently, horizontal and vertical points from various visual fields are focused at two different focal points on the retina, resulting in distorted vision.

measured. The denominator is the distance from which a person with normal vision can read the letters/numbers of a specific size. For example, an acuity reading of 20/80 means that, although a person with normal vision could read that line at 80 ft, the individual being tested reads it at only 20 ft. The 20/20 reading is the normal acuity, while 20/400 is the worst acuity.

Visual Field Defects

A lesion at any point in the visual pathway results in the loss of a specific point in the visual field. The nature of the visual field loss depends on the point and extent of fiber interruption. The straightforward nature of the visual projections makes it easy to relate the locations of injury to specific patterns of field losses and vice versa. There are two

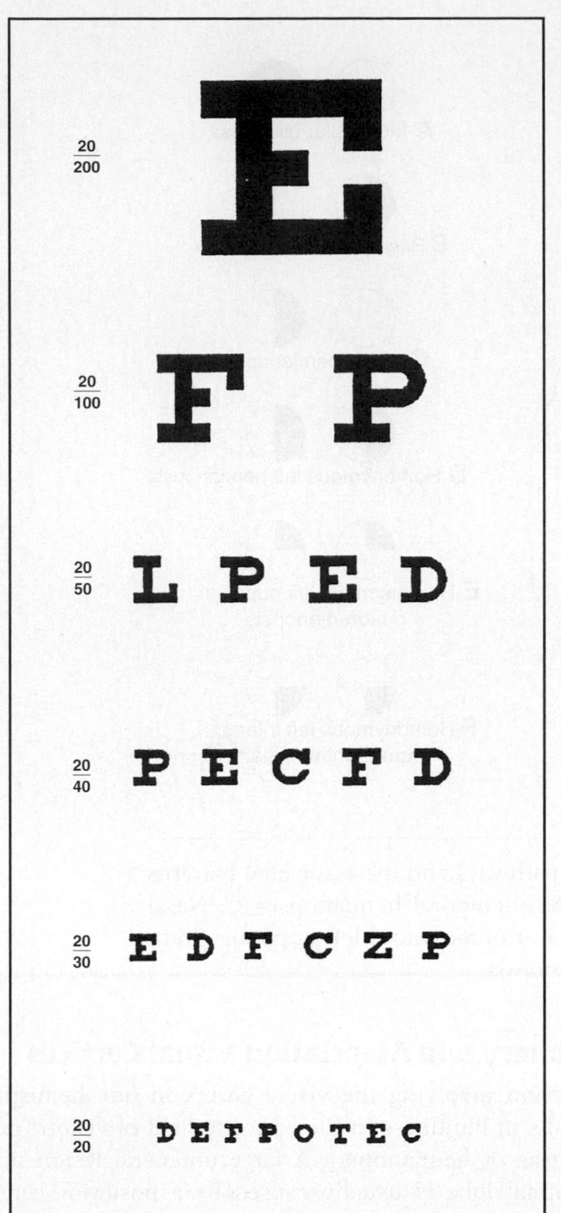

Figure 12-12 Snellen chart.

types of field defects: **homonymous** and **heteronymous**. Homonymous refers to similar visual field defects for each eye, either the right half of the visual fields or the left half of the visual fields for both eyes. Heteronymous refers to two different parts of the visual field being impaired, for example, the left half of the visual field for one eye and the right half of the visual field for the other; this is clinically known as **bitemporal hemianopia**. Injuries at selected points along the visual pathway result in predictable patterns of visual field defects (Fig. 12-13; Table 12-4).

Monocular Blindness

A complete severing of the optic (CN II) nerve at any point between the eyeball and the optic chiasm results in total blindness in that eye because none of the optic (CN II) nerve fibers from the retina is spared (Fig. 12-13*A*). However, the actual implications of **monocular blindness** are slightly different because of binocular vision. If one eye is blind or closed, the other eye is still capable of covering the entire visual field, except for a small, temporal crescent-shaped peripheral field for the blind eye (see Figure 12-1). Thus, even after severance of the optic (CN II) nerve, one is functionally blind only for this monocular portion of the field.

Bitemporal (Heteronymous) Hemianopia

Bitemporal hemianopia is loss of vision in the temporal visual fields. It is associated with pathology of the optic chiasm (Fig. 12-13*B*). A chiasmatic injury, usually induced by a tumor of the pituitary gland, interrupts fibers from both nasal retinas. It produces blindness in the temporal visual fields for both eyes, commonly called tunnel vision.

Nasal Hemianopia

Nasal hemianopia refers to loss of vision in the nasal field of only one eye. The associated pathology encroaches on the lateral edge of the optic chiasm and selectively interrupts the fibers from the ipsilateral temporal portion of the retina. The result is nasal hemianopia in the corresponding eye (Fig. 12-13*C*).

Homonymous Hemianopia

Homonymous hemianopia is loss of vision in homonymous—either right or left—fields for both eyes. An interruption of fibers at any point in the course of the optic tract, LGB, or geniculocalcarine fibers results in homonymous (same field in both eyes) visual field losses (Fig. 12-13*D*). For example, a lesion in the right optic tract interrupts visual fibers from the retinas of both eyes, resulting in a left visual field defect for both eyes.

Homonymous Left Superior Quadrantanopsia

Left superior **quadrantanopsia** is loss of vision in the superior left quadrants of the visual fields for both eyes. The geniculocalcarine fibers divide into the ventral (inferior) and dorsal (superior) fascicles while traveling to the visual cortex. The inferior fascicle of fibers carries information from the inferior retinal quadrants of the retina (representing the upper or superior quadrants in the visual fields); these fibers sweep around the inferior horn of the lateral ventricle in the temporal lobe in the Meyer loop. A temporal lobe lesion on the right side of the brain selectively interrupting the inferior fibers of the geniculocalcarine tract causes blindness in the left upper quadrants of the visual fields of both eyes (Fig. 12-13*E*).

Homonymous Left Inferior Quadrantanopsia

The inner (superior) fibers of the geniculocalcarine tract, carrying information from the superior or upper retinal quadrants, travel directly through the temporoparietal

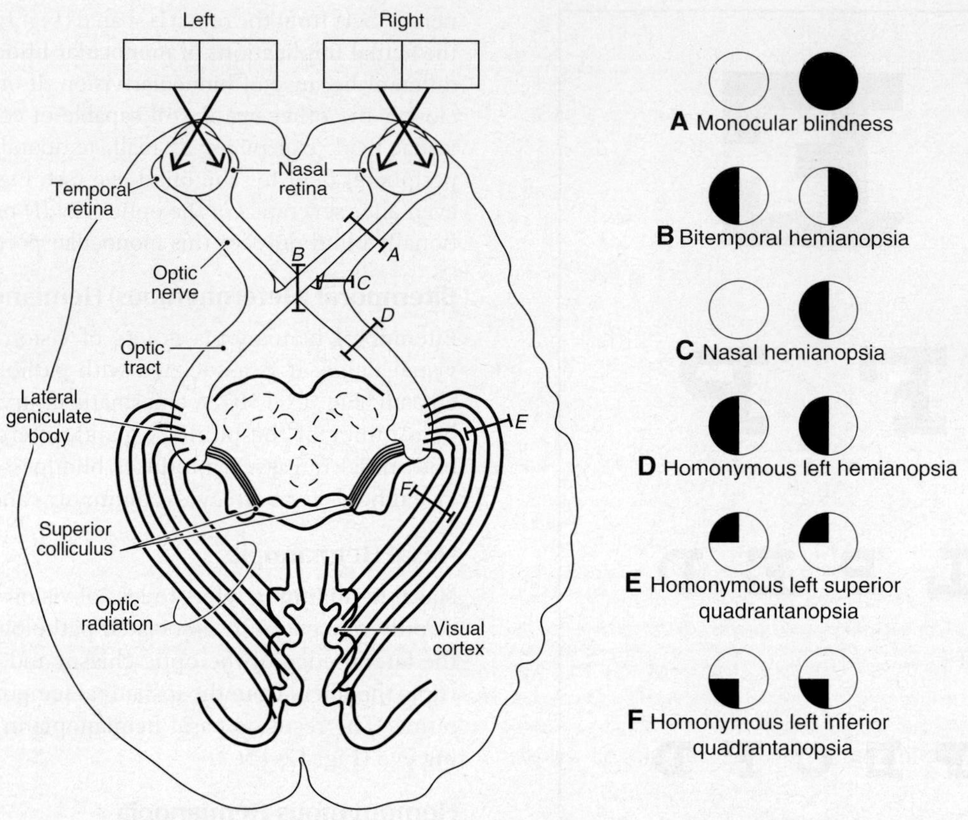

Figure 12-13 Common lesion sites in the visual pathways and the associated patterns of visual field losses: A. Monocular blindness, B. Bitemporal hemianopsia, C. Nasal hemianopsia, D. Homonymous left hemianopsia, E. Homonymous left upper quadrantanopsia, F. Homonymous left inferior quadrantanopsia.

substance. Therefore, a right-sided temporoparietal lobe lesion interrupts the geniculocalcarine tract inner (superior) fibers; this affects the transmission of visual information from the right upper retinal quadrants, resulting in vision loss in the left lower (inferior) visual field quadrants for both eyes (Fig. 12-13*F*).

Primary and Association Visual Cortices

A lesion involving the visual cortex in one hemisphere results in blindness in the opposite field of vision (hemianopsia or hemianopia). A large unilateral lesion in the occipital lobe is usually caused by a posterior cerebral

Table 12-4

Visual Field Loss and Associated Anatomic Sites

Lesion Site	Visual Field Loss
Optic nerve	Monocular blindness
Optic chiasm (usually secondary to a pituitary gland tumor)	Bitemporal hemianopsia (tunnel vision)
Lateral edge of optic chiasm, interrupting fibers from ipsilateral temporal retina	Nasal hemianopsia in one eye
Optic tract (postchiasmic or geniculocalcarine fibers)	Homonymous hemianopsia
Temporal lobe pathology interrupting inferior geniculocalcarine tract fibers	Upper (superior) quadrantanopsia
Temporoparietal lobe pathology interrupting superior geniculocalcarine tract fibers	Lower (inferior) quadrantanopsia

artery thrombosis. The central (macular) vision may be spared, which is attributed to the collateral circulation (anastomosis) from the middle cerebral artery branches. Bilateral visual cortical involvement results in cortical blindness, which is marked by blindness but with preserved ability to follow light.

The visual association cortex (Brodmann areas 18 and 19) wraps around the primary cortex on the medial and lateral surfaces and is reciprocally connected with the medial and inferior temporal lobe, the lateral parietal cortex, and the thalamic pulvinar. With afferents from the primary visual cortex, the dorsal visual association cortex deals with visually integrated motion, temporal, and spatial situations. The ventral association region, including the temporal fusiform gyrus, synthesizes and elaborates complex and cognitive aspects of information, such as recognition of objects (colors and shapes) and faces; this also contributes to visual memory, reading, and understanding written information. A lesion, depending on the region involved, would result in different degrees and types of visual agnosia, such as **apperceptive agnosia** (failure to recognize an object secondary to a perceptual deficit) and **associative agnosia** (failure to recognize an object or attach meaning with preserved perception). A bilateral lesion involving the association cortex (Brodmann areas 18 and 19) bilaterally and/or extending to the inferior temporal lobe areas (Brodmann areas 20, 21, and possibly 37) may result in **visual agnosia**, in which one cannot recognize an object or written name despite normal visual perception. A lesion in the association cortex, usually bilateral, can result in **prosopagnosia**, an impaired ability to recognize faces. A noted linguistic disorder associated with occipital lesions is **alexia without agraphia**, in which the patient cannot comprehend written information but can still write. The underlying pathology involves an infarct of the corpus callosum and infarct in the occipital cortex. (Higher visual cognitive functions are discussed in Chapter 19.)

Optic aphasia, another neurolinguistic syndrome associated with the occipital associative cortical lesion, refers to an impaired ability to name visually presented objects, although the semantic knowledge associated with object is retained. Such a patient cannot name an object presented visually, but he or she can name the actions associated with the object. A bilateral lesion at the junction of the parietooccipital region has also been associated with **Balint syndrome**, which is marked with the loss of voluntary control of eye movements while the reflexive movements are preserved.

Lesion localization

Rule 5: Symptoms Suggesting a Visual Pathway Lesion

- **Presenting Symptoms and Rationale.** Blindness in one eye suggests an optic nerve lesion anterior to the optic chiasm.
- The rationale is that each optic nerve receives fibers from both nasal and temporal regions of the retina of one eye.
- **Presenting Symptoms and Rationale**. Bitemporal hemianopia (one does not see things laterally in the visual fields) results from a lesion compressing or otherwise interrupting the crossing fibers (from the nasal retina of each eye) in the optic chiasm.
- The rationale is that the fibers mediating visual information from the temporal (outer) visual fields (received in the nasal part of the retina) cross the midline at the optic chiasm.
- **Presenting Symptoms and Rationale**. Homonymous hemianopia is associated with a lesion of the optic tract anywhere between the optic chiasm and the occipital lobe.
- The rationale is that the fibers from the both eyes representing the same (homo) visual fields (e.g., the temporal visual field of the left eye and the nasal visual field of the right eye) travel together in the optic tract.
- **Presenting Symptoms and Rationale**. Alexia (failure to comprehend written material), homonymous hemianopia, and **spared macular vision** are all associated with a lesion of the visual cortex (Brodmann area 17) and visual association areas (Brodmann areas 18 and 19). The rationale is that the involvement of the visual cortex receiving optic tract fibers accounts for contralateral hemianopia. Involvement of the bilateral primary and associational visual cortices, which are supplied by the posterior cerebral artery, results in **agnosia** and alexia.

CASE STUDIES FOR PROBLEM SOLVING

CASE ONE (12-1)

A 65-year-old man gradually began having visual difficulty. He could see things well if they were right in front of him but did not see them if they were to his left or right. He was worried about developing tunnel vision like his diabetic neighbor with retinal degeneration. His ophthalmologist found nothing wrong with his retina and found his visual acuity to be near-normal. However, the visual field examination revealed bitemporal hemianopia. A brain MRI study revealed a tumor in the lower anterior region of the hypothalamus.

Question: How can you relate the clinical symptoms to this hypothalamic tumor?

Case (12-1) Discussion: See discussion of case studies

(Continued)

CASE TWO (12-2) *(CONTINUED)*

A 60-year-old right-handed man was admitted to the hospital after suffering a stroke. After the first 3 weeks of acute and intensive care, he exhibited some visual problems and severe communicative deficit.

The neurologist noted that the sensorimotor functions were normal, but there was visual difficulty marked with upper right visual field defect (quadrantanopsia).

The attending SLP noted the following:

- Fluent verbal output that carried little meaning
- Moderate anomia
- Paraphasic (mostly unrelated) errors and perseverations
- Moderate reading and writing problems
- Normal hearing thresholds but difficulty in understanding others

A brain MRI study revealed an infarct in the left posterior superior temporal gyrus (Brodmann area 22) that extended to the inferior parietal lobe.

Question: How can you relate the clinical symptoms of aphasia and visual field deficit to left temporal lobe lesion?

Case (12-2) Discussion: See discussion of case studies

CASE THREE (12-3)

A 65-year-old man with a history of hypertension had a minor ischemic attack involving the brainstem. He lost consciousness for 15 minutes. He was taken to the hospital, where the attending neurologist noticed the following:

- Little lethargy but normal sensory and motor functions
- Normal communicative, cognitive and motor speech functions
- Asymmetry in pupil size; the left pupil was 2 to 3 mm larger in the dark

Question: How can you account for these clinical symptoms in light of a brainstem lesion?

Case (12-3) Discussion: See discussion of case studies

CASE FOUR (12-4)

A 55-year-old woman with a history of hypertension and cardiac problems woke up very confused and did not recognize the rooms and other locations in her house. She was taken to a neurologist who noted the following:

- Impaired left–right orientation
- Left spatial hemineglect
- Failure to draw objects
- Poor writing, marked by displaced and irregularly sized graphemes
- Inability to see people and objects on the left side with both eyes

The neurologist predicted that the patient had a temporal parietal lesion, which was confirmed with a brain MRI study.

Question: What side of the brain is involved? How can you explain the relationship between the visual field and cognitive deficit with a temporal parietal lesion?

Case (12-4) Discussion: See discussion of case studies

CASE FIVE (12-5)

A 70-year-old man complained of gradually losing his ability to see from his left eye; this posed a problem only when he drove and particularly when he needed to change lanes. After a few mishaps on the road, his alarmed wife took him to an ophthalmologist who noted the following:

- Complete blindness in the left eye
- Absence of direct pupillary light reflex but normal consensual reflex on the left side
- Normal direct light reflex but no consensual reflex in the right eye

An MRI revealed a large tumor of the left optic nerve anterior to the optic chiasm.

Question: How can you relate the visual field deficit with the diagnosed tumor?

Case (12-5) Discussion: See discussion of case studies

CASE SIX (12-6)

After dazzling graduate students with a Power Point presentation for an hour in a completely dark and silent room, the instructor turned the lights on to make sure that the students were still there and that they had not fallen asleep during his interesting presentation. This not only startled the students but also caused an instant constriction in their pupillary diameters.

Question: Why should students' pupil constrict? Can you explain the neural mechanism involved with the changes in pupillary apertures?

Case (12-6) Discussion: See discussion of case studies

SUMMARY

The visual system is concerned with image perception, which involves four events: (1) the lens and cornea of the eye refract light rays; (2) retinal photoreceptor cells then convert the electromagnetic energy of the light rays into changes in the membrane potential; (3) through integrating processing by other retinal neurons, the retinal ganglia cells transmit action potentials to the thalamus and the visual cortex; (4) Finally, visual images are perceived in the primary visual cortex and interpreted in the associational visual cortex. Optical disturbances affect image formation, whereas lesions interrupting visual fibers result in different but predictable visual field losses.

REVIEW QUESTIONS

1. Complete the following statements using the appropriate technical terms:

   A. An irregular ________ of the lens and/or the cornea causes a focusing disorder in which vertical and horizontal rays focus at two different retinal points; this leads to ________

   B. In ________ ________, the visual field area is simultaneously processed in both eyes.

   C. The retinal point at which light rays converge for focusing is called the ________ ________. The ________ ________ is the distance between the lens and this retinal focal point.

   D. The parasympathetically mediated response that the lens undergoes to keep a near object in focus is the ________ ________.

   E. The ________ ________ is the area through which the optic nerve (CN II) exits and arteries enter the eyeball; with no presence of photoreceptors at this point, it is also called the ________ ________.

   F. Change in diameter of the pupils in response to a projected light is called the ________ ________, which is mediated by the visceral fibers of the ________ nerve (________).

   G. The eye ball contains two types of fluids: ________ humor, a substance similar to CSF that is produced and drained in the posterior chamber of the anterior ocular cavity, and ________ humor in the posterior cavity that prevents the eyeball from collapsing.

   H. On exposure to light, the parasympathetic constriction of the circular fibers narrows the aperture of the pupil, a condition called ________; on the other hand in darkness, the sympathetic constriction of the radial (dilator) fibers of the iris results in pupil dilation, a condition called ________ .

   I. ________ is an optical condition in which the divergent light rays from a near (<20 ft away) object focus on the retina.

   J. ________ is an optical condition in which only the convergent rays from a far object focus on the retina.

   K. ________ ________ is the entire external area that is perceived in one eye.

   L. Containing only the cones, ________ is the retinal site responsible for sharp vision and color vision.

   M. ________ ________ represents one's ability to resolve the perceptual detains, and it is measured using a Snellen chart.

   N. As an eye disease and a common cause of blindness, ________ is marked by increased intraocular pressure and subsequent atrophy of the optic nerve.

2. Match the following conditions with corresponding description:

A. myopia	a. sympathetic constriction of radial fibers in dark
B. hypermetropia	b. parasympathetic constriction of circular fibers in response to light
C. astigmatism	c. autonomic regulation of lens refractive power
D. emmetropia	d. different refractivity at different retinal points due to unequal refractive surfaces
E. lens accommodation	e. adequately refracted image on the retina
F. pupil constriction	f. focusing of near object behind the retina
G. pupil dilation	g. focusing of converging rays from a far object in front of the retina

3. Below name each quarter and the side of the visual fields for each eye:

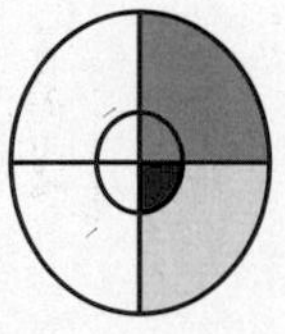
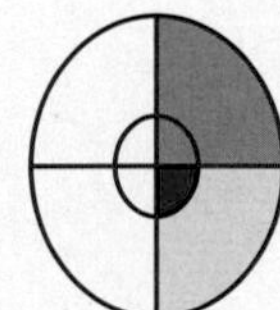

- Left Eye:
- Right Eye:

4. Name each of the visual field defects illustrated in the figure:

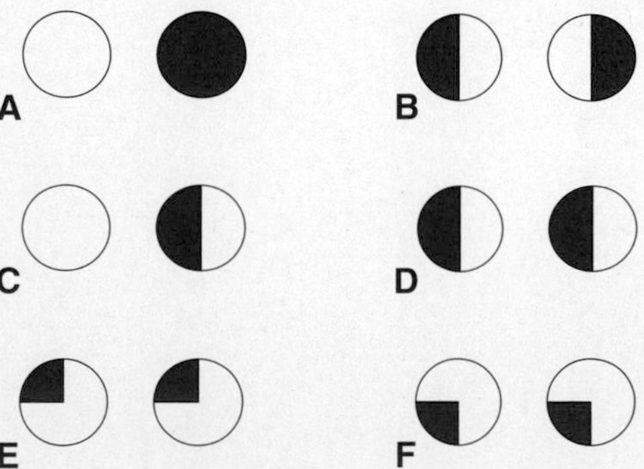

5. Match each of the following structures to its associated statement:

A. sclera	a. drains aqueous humor into the venous system
B. canal of Schlemm	b. outer tissue layer covering the eyeball
C. rods	c. transparent covering of the anterior eye chamber
D. cornea	d. containing melanocytes to make the eyeball opaque to stray light
E. choroids	e. regulation of the pupil size to control the light amount entering the eye
F. iris	f. smooth muscle fibers that reduce tension on the lens
G. lens	g. transparent structure that refracts light rays on retina
H. ciliary body	h. corresponds to the central retinal field
I. macula lutea	i. photoreceptors for visual acuity and color vision
J. cones	j. photoreceptors mediating night vision

6. What type of visual deficit results after a lesion affecting the Meyer loop?
7. What visual deficit results from a lesion in the dorsal/superior geniculocalcarine fibers?
8. List the light conditions in which rods and cones are respectively operational:

13

Motor System 1: Spinal Cord

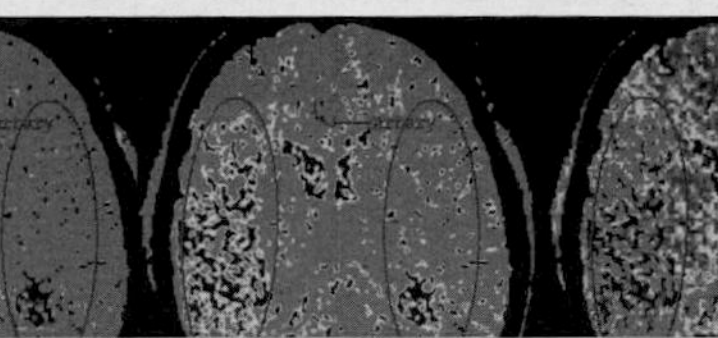

LEARNING OBJECTIVES

After studying this chapter, students should be able to:

- Describe the motor functions of the spinal cord
- Discuss the importance of the motor unit in movement
- Outline the functions of the major ascending and descending spinal tracts
- Explain the role of muscle spindles in reflexive motor functions
- Explain the physiology of basic spinal reflexes
- Discuss lower motor neuron syndrome
- Explain the rationale for the motor symptoms

HIERARCHY OF MOTOR FUNCTION

Motor activity is a hierarchically organized function under the control of reflex mechanisms and neural networks of volitional control in a rostral segment of the CNS (Fig. 13-1). From the lowest to the highest, these arbitrarily identified anatomic levels are the (1) spinal cord, (2) cerebellum, (3) basal ganglia, and (4) motor cortex. Each ascending level in the hierarchy makes a specific contribution to the final motor activity, which also is influenced in part by the activity of higher motor centers in the forebrain. For example, the midbrain systems modulate reflexes organized at the medullary or spinal level. The forebrain systems regulate the midbrain and spinal motor activity. Motor responses begin in the spinal cord as simple reflexes; the higher motor centers participate in the regulation of skilled and patterned movements. Neuronal impulses from higher levels also initiate, inhibit, or facilitate motor functions at the brainstem and spinal cord, thus partially regulating all motor behavior.

This cortical control provides a type of parallel processing with rostral domination of hierarchical motor organization and simultaneous control of the segmental output itself. Since a brief time period is involved in the conduction of afferent information, local (spinal) reflexes are activated first, and motor mechanisms at higher hierarchic levels are operational slightly later. The best example of reflexive movement is the body's response when one accidentally steps on a tack with barefoot. This triggers a leg-**withdrawal reflex**, which is already in progress before the forebrain is aware of the action or able to modify it. However, the higher motor systems can inhibit such a withdrawal reflex if the stimulus is expected and another response has been learned. For example, if someone has to pick up a hot cup, the withdrawal reflex can be inhibited while the hot cup is being moved to a supporting surface, even though the fingers are being burned.

The hierarchically defined motor functions and the nature of the specific contributions by each level are discussed in Chapters 13 to 16. The spinal cord is the first level in the regulation of sensorimotor functions. Stereotypical motor responses (reflexes), which are largely independent of voluntary motor control, are generated in the spinal cord and can be triggered by cortical and/or environmental stimuli.

SPINAL PREPARATION

Spinal cord functions are most easily demonstrated by a **spinal preparation**, which involves separating the cord from the controlling influence of the forebrain by cutting the cord. This separation allows for examination of spinal reflexes independent of the inhibitory or facilitatory influence exerted by higher motor centers. Immediately after the spinal cut, the flexor and extensor reflexes become inactive, but they gradually reemerge (Box 13-1).

INNERVATION PATTERN

The general motor function in the spinal cord and brainstem is organized ipsilateral to its output and reflex input. The spinal α-motor neurons and their axons (final common pathway) innervate the muscles ipsilaterally (Fig. 13-2). Consequently, lower motor neuron (LMN) signs in case of brainstem and spinal cord injuries are ipsilateral to the damage of the cell body or its axon.

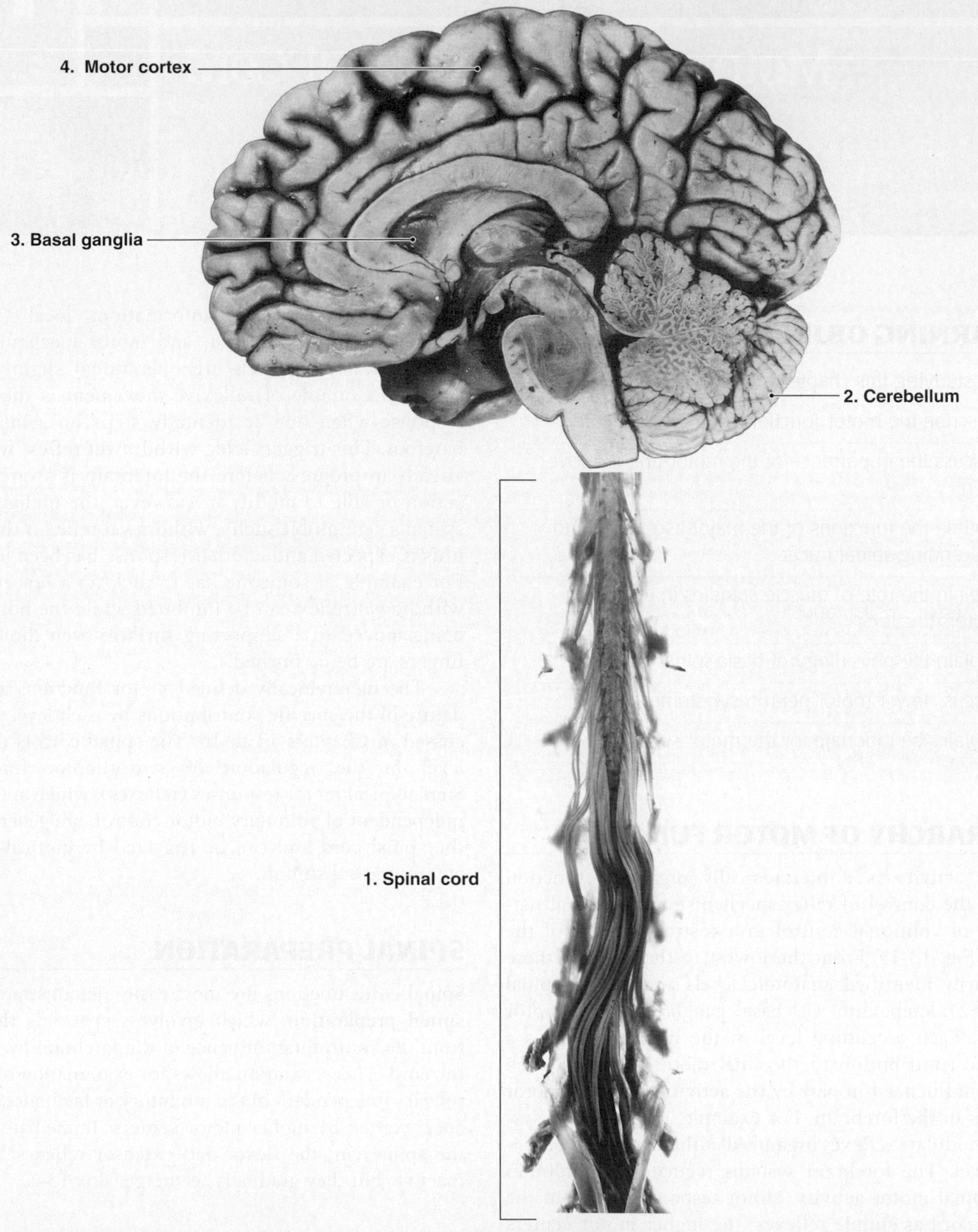

Figure 13-1 Four ascending levels of motor organization. 1. spinal cord; 2. cerebellum; 3. basal ganglia; and 4. cerebral motor cortex.

ANATOMICAL MARKINGS

Internal Anatomy

The spinal cord consists of an outer ring of white matter (ascending and descending fibers) and a butterfly-shaped central gray area (nerve cell bodies and a small unmyelinated network of fibers called neuropils) (Fig. 13-2). The dorsal horns contain the secondary sensory nerve cells that receive bodily sensory information through the dorsal root ganglia (DRG) fibers. The ventral horns contain motor (lower) nerve cells, which project through the anterior roots to activate muscles, glands, and joints.

BOX 13-1

Spinal Shock

As a syndrome caused by structural or functional interruption of ascending or descending fibers through one or more spinal segments, it is characterized by a loss of sensation from the segments below the lesion and the loss of descending influence on the lower motor neurons (LMNs) as well as spinal reflexes below the lesion site. Also associated are limb paralysis, loss of muscle tone, and reduced autonomic functions. There is notable recovery of functions within a week or so, marked with upper motor neuron symptoms of spastic muscles, increased tone, and hyperactive reflexes.

The degree of recovery of most spinal reflexes is highly variable depending on the severity of damage to the cord. Damaged axons may recover. More often, severed axons can grow collateral branches to and through the damaged area, depending on distance and the amount of scar tissue. If supranuclear controls are not reestablished, collateral branching of local stretch afferent axons gradually fill the emptied excitatory synapses on LMNs. As a result, muscle tone increases in strength from severely reduced and then to hyperactivity and spasticity.

The gray columns on each side of the cord are connected through the commissures, which consist of crossing fibers. The axonal processes of the motor neurons form the ventral nerve root fibers send motor impulses from the CNS to the muscles. After traveling through the pia mater, subarachnoid space, arachnoid membrane, dura mater, and intervertebral foramina, the fibers from both the dorsal and anterior roots merge to form a spinal nerve (also see Fig. 2-32).

After exiting the intervertebral foramina, the spinal nerve divides into dorsal and ventral rami. The dorsal ramus fibers of each spinal nerve are concerned with the muscles and skin in the posterior part of the body. The ventral ramus fibers of the spinal nerve supply anterior body parts, including the upper and lower limbs. Before projecting to target muscles and body parts, the ventral rami of the spinal nerves, except the nerves from T2 to T11, form a network of nerve fibers called plexuses (see Fig. 2-35). Rami of the nerves from T2 to T11 directly innervate body parts (see Chapter 2 for in-depth discussion of the external and internal anatomy of the spinal cord).

Segmental Organization

The spinal cord is anatomically and functionally organized in transverse segments extending from the cervical to the sacral region. This organization of the spinal cord indicates segmental sensorimotor innervation of the body (dermatomes and myotomes) with various distributional shapes and sizes (see Fig. 2-34). The dermatome (area

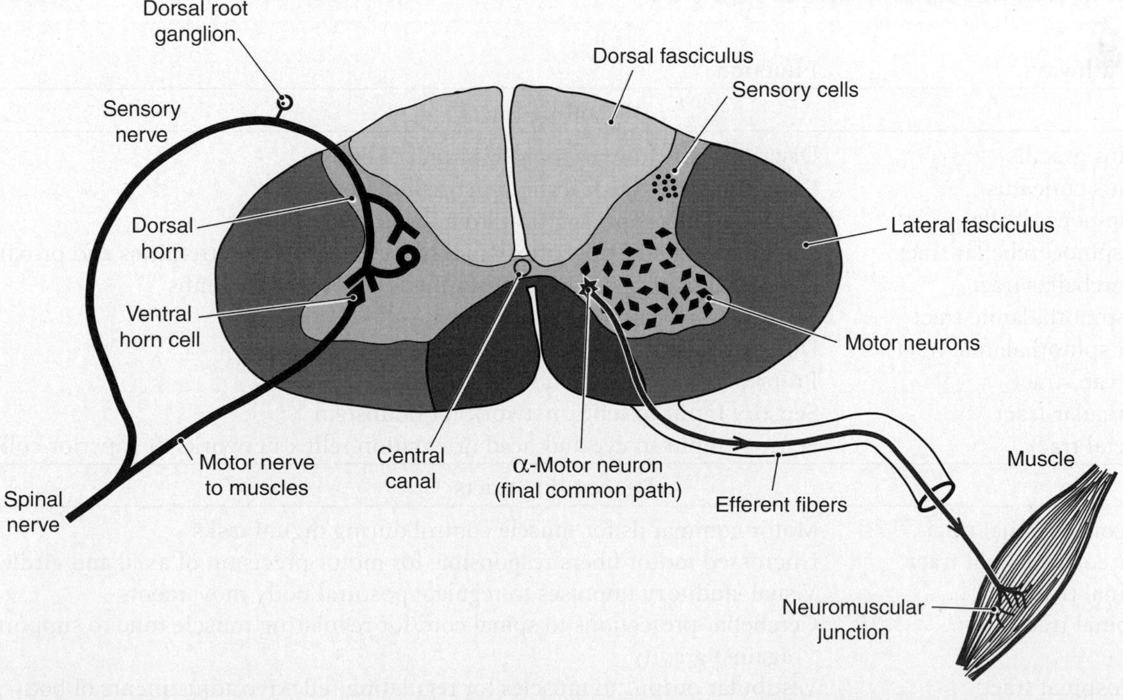

Figure 13-2 The final common pathway and the motor unit in a monosynaptic circuitry.

innervated by the afferent fibers of the neurons in a single DRG) and myotome (muscle or muscles innervated by the axons exiting the cord via a single ventral root) may overlap each other, but because of muscle migration during development, they are not always the same.

Key Terms :

Extrapyramidal tract
Motor unit
Muscular dystrophy
Myasthenia gravis
Myoneural junction

Motor Unit

The LMN and **motor unit** are two important components of spinal motor control circuitry (Fig. 13-2). The LMN cell body provides the output pathway via its axon, which travels through the ventral root and peripheral nerves to innervate a skeletal muscle, where it forms multiple axon branches to activate many muscle fibers. The LMN is also the final common pathway, because the efferent impulses from the motor cortex pass through this motor neuron before they can produce a muscle movement.

The motor unit consists of four components: **motor cell body**, efferent fibers, **motor end plate** (branching off the axonal fiber in **myoneural junction/neuromuscular junction**), and innervated muscle fibers. A motor unit can fire repeatedly, resulting in sustained shortening of the muscle fiber elements. Damage to the LMN cell or the beginning axon eliminates the entire function of a motor unit. Damage to one of the terminal axon branches weakens the unit projections. Generalized skeletal muscle disease (e.g., **muscular dystrophy**) or reduced nerve–muscle transmission/activity (e.g., **myasthenia gravis**) weakens or eliminates the unit's force generation and causes the denervated muscle to atrophy.

Motor units can be small or large, and a muscle can contain many motor units, depending on the nature of its motor control. For example, the small hand flexor muscle used for delicate and coordinated motor control can have 10 to 30 muscle fibers per motor unit, whereas large muscles like the quadriceps can have as many as 3,000 muscle fibers per motor unit.

TRACTS OF THE SPINAL CORD

The white matter of the spinal cord consists of three major bundles of longitudinal axons (fasciculi): **dorsal**, **lateral**, and **ventral columns** (Fig. 13-2). The tracts are difficult to pinpoint on a cross section of the spinal cord; however, their approximate locations are determined from clinical evidence. The dorsal fasciculus consists largely of ascending (sensory) fibers, whereas the lateral and anterior fasciculi contain both descending (motor) and ascending (sensory) fiber bundles (Table 13-1). General locations of the various sensorimotor spinal tracts are demonstrated in Figure 13-3.

Table 13-1

Ascending and Descending Spinal Pathways

Spinal Pathways	Function
	Ascending tracts
Fasciculus gracilis	Discriminative touch from lower half of body
Fasciculus cuneatus	Discriminative touch from upper half of body
Dorsal spinocerebellar tract	Unconscious proprioception from distal lower limbs
Ventral spinocerebellar tract	Unconscious proprioception from muscles of lower extremities and proximal limbs
Cuneocerebellar tract	Unconscious proprioceptive information from upper limbs
Lateral spinothalamic tract	Sensations of pain and temperature
Anterior spinothalamic tract	Diffuse touch; backup sensory system
Spinoolivary tract	Proprioceptive information from limbs
Spinoreticular tract	Sensory input to reflex networks of brainstem
Spinotectal tract	Sensory input to eye and head orientation reflex networks of superior colliculus
	Descending tracts
Lateral corticospinal tract	Motor commands for muscle control during digital tasks
Anterior corticospinal tract	Uncrossed motor fibers responsible for motor precision of axial and girdle muscles
Tectospinal tract	Visual–auditory impulses to regulate postural body movements
Rubrospinal tract	Cerebellar projections to spinal cord for regulating muscle tone to support body against gravity
Vestibulospinal tract	Vestibular output to muscles for regulating reflexive adjustments of body posture
Reticular descending tracts	Brainstem modulation of spinal reflex mechanism to regulate muscle preparedness

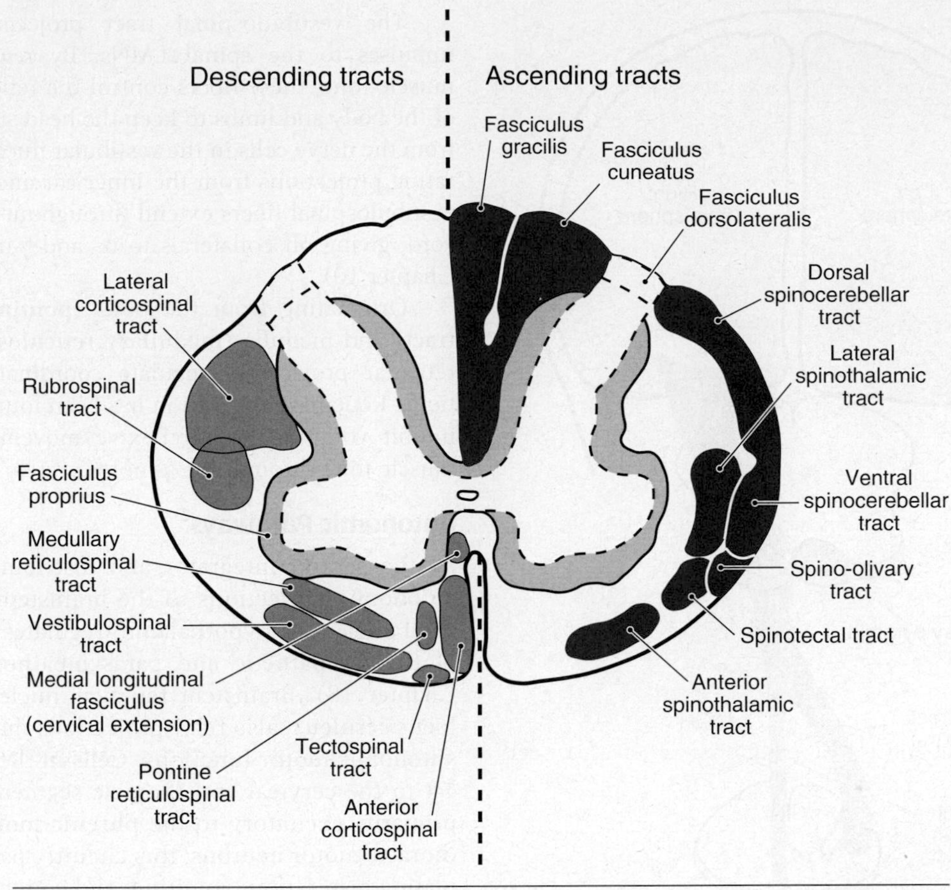

Figure 13-3 Ascending (*red*) and descending (*gray*) spinal pathways.

Descending Tracts

Corticospinal Tracts

Fibers of the corticospinal motor tract arise from pyramidal cells (the largest are **Betz cells**) in the cortex. Most of these cells are in the precentral gyrus (primary motor cortex, Brodmann area 4); however, some of these cells are in other areas of the brain, including the premotor cortex, primary somesthetic cortex (Brodmann areas 3, 1, 2), and supplementary motor cortex (Brodmann area 6). On their way to the spinal cord, the corticospinal fibers cross the midline at the caudal end of the medulla and form the **lateral corticospinal tract** in the spinal cord (see Chapter 16). There are two corticospinal tracts:

Lateral Corticospinal Tract

Lateral corticospinal fibers provide a mechanism by which the cerebral cortex intervenes in the control of skeletal muscles during delicate, skilled manipulation of the distal parts of the limbs, including the fingers and to some extent the toes and forearms. This tract contains long myelinated fibers and is the largest of the motor tracts. The corticospinal fibers cross the midline at the lower end of the medulla and enter with the spinal cord. Approximately 90% of the corticospinal fibers are known to cross the midline to form the **lateral corticospinal tract**. Its fibers synapse on the ventral horn α-motor neurons and regulate muscle activity. A lesion to the fibers of this tract causes profound weakness and loss of all individual digital manipulation skills.

Anterior Corticospinal Tract

The anterior corticospinal tract contains the 8% to 10% of the corticospinal fibers that do not cross the midline at the medulla oblongata. Instead, these fibers continue descending ipsilaterally (Fig. 13-4). These uncrossed fibers eventually cross the midline before synapsing on the ventral horn **α-motor neuron** and internuncial cells. These axons provide a mechanism through which the cerebral cortex regulates precision in the movements of axial and girdle muscles.

Extrapyramidal Tracts

The motor system is not exclusively a corticospinal system. Rather, its functional organization is highly complex, involving many **extrapyramidal** and autonomic pathways in the background that transmit information

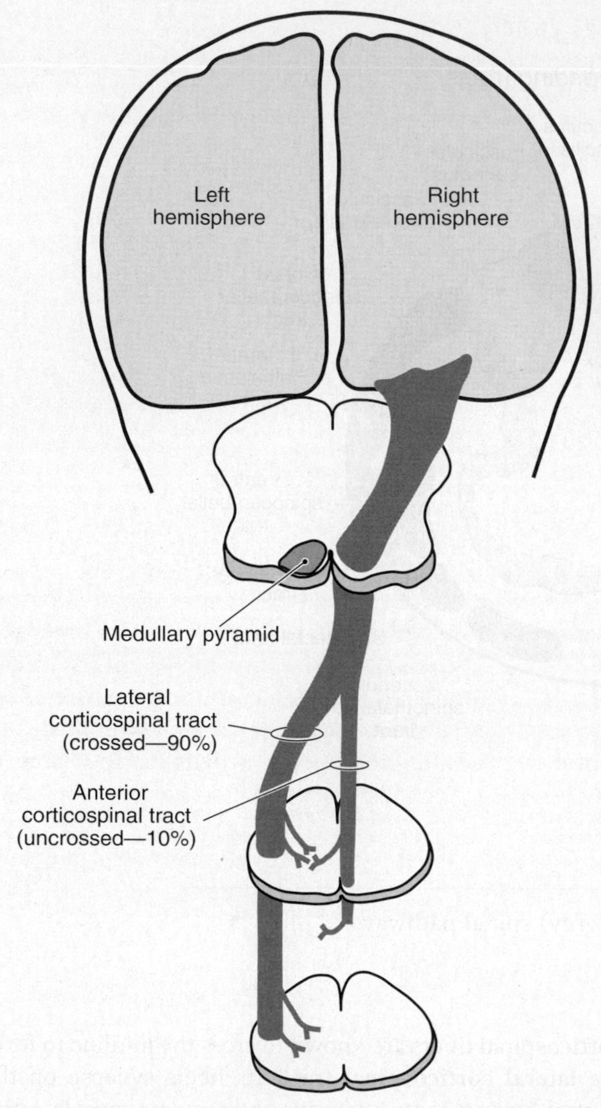

Figure 13-4 Corticospinal fibers predominantly project to the contralateral half of the body.

essential for smoothly coordinated motor function and upright, balanced posture. Some of the more notable extrapyramidal paths are the **tectospinal**, **rubrospinal**, and **vestibulospinal tracts**.

The tectospinal tract regulates neck and body twisting movements with extensor support for the startle (astonish) reflexes in response to visual and auditory stimuli. This powerful reflexive behavior involves the sudden turning of the head, neck, and/or body toward the stimulus. Originating from the superior colliculus, the tectospinal fibers descend to terminate in the ventral horn motor nuclei of the cervical and lower regions of the cord.

The rubrospinal tract transmits impulses from the red nucleus to the spinal LMN to regulate muscle tone for limb extension and posture in support of the body against gravity.

The vestibulospinal tract projects the vestibular impulses to the spinal LMNs. By regulating extensor muscle tone, these fibers control the reflexive adjustment of the body and limbs to keep the head stable. Originating from the nerve cells in the vestibular nucleus and incorporating projections from the inner ear and cerebellum, the vestibulospinal fibers extend throughout the length of the cord, giving off collaterals to α- and γ-motor nuclei (see Chapter 10).

Originating from the pons (**pontine reticulospinal tract**) and medulla (**medullary reticulospinal tract**), the reticular projections regulate coordinated motor functions. Reticular stimulation has been found to facilitate or inhibit voluntary and reflexive movements by altering muscle tone through the γ-motor system.

Autonomic Pathways

As the central integrator and distributor of important autonomic projections to the brainstem and spinal visceral nuclei, the hypothalamus regulates motor functions of the sympathetic and parasympathetic systems (see Chapter 18). Brainstem reticular nuclei, including the **locus ceruleus**, also relay projections that regulate spinal autonomic motor functions. Cells in the brainstem project to the cervical and thoracic segments, and they are primarily excitatory to the **phrenic motor neurons** and thoracic motor neurons; this circuitry participates in regulating respiration, vomiting, and coughing reflexes (see Chapter 18).

Ascending Tracts

The ascending fibers of the spinal cord transmit sensory information from various body parts (Fig. 13-3). The sensory impulses are pain, thermal sensation, touch, proprioception, and kinesthesia in addition to unconscious proprioception (see Chapter 11). Projections from the sensory cortex refine the cortical motor efferents to the spinal cord.

Key Terms :

α-motor neuron	**Phrenic nerve**
γ-motor neuron	**Renshaw cell**
Interneurons	

MOTOR NUCLEI OF THE SPINAL CORD

The spinal gray matter contains thousands of motor nerve cells, which are either **anterior motor neurons** or **interneurons (internuncial cells)**. The anterior motor neurons include α- and **γ-motor neurons** (Fig. 13-5). The efferent fibers of α- and γ-motor nerve cells form the ventral roots of spinal nerves that innervate skeletal muscles. These are called LMNs to distinguish them from the corticospinal neurons of the motor (and sensory) cortex, which are

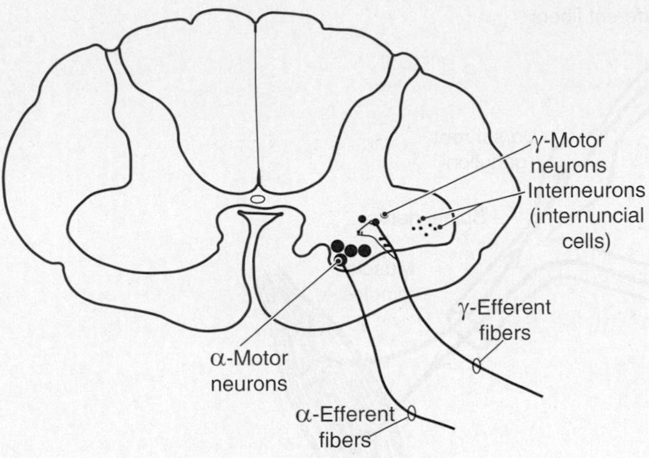

Figure 13-5 α-Cells, γ-cells, and internuncial cells in the anterior gray column of the spinal cord.

called upper motor neurons (UMN). The interneurons function as association cells interconnecting cell bodies within sensory and motor neuron pools. The dendritic and axonal projections of the internuncial cells connect adjacent spinal cord cells.

The cervical spinal cord gray matter also contains two specialized motor nuclei. One supplies the **phrenic nerve**, which innervates the diaphragm and participates in respiration (see Chapters 2 and 18). The other motor nucleus contributes to the spinal roots of the spinal accessory (CN XI) nerve, which regulates head and shoulder movements (see Chapter 17).

The α- and γ-motor neurons receive motor impulses directly from the motor centers in the forebrain and brainstem. The supraspinal projections to α- and γ-motor neurons, which initiate voluntary motor activities, are represented by balanced inhibitory (–) and excitatory (+) cortical outputs to the spinal motor neurons.

α-Motor Neurons

α-Motor neurons are the major spinal motor neurons. Their axons, which conduct rapidly and have a diameter of 9 to 16 μm, and conducting rapidly, pass through the ventral spinal root before innervating the **extrafusal fibers** of the skeletal muscles that are responsible for the voluntary and reflexive movements of the head, trunk, and extremities. On average, one α-neuron fiber innervates >200 muscle fibers. These motor neurons are also the final common pathway, because all efferent impulses from the CNS must pass through these cells before activating muscles.

γ-Motor Neurons

γ-Motor neurons, which lie alongside the α-cells in the spinal ventral horns, are smaller, half as numerous, and have smaller-diameter axonal processes. These neurons are slow impulse conductors. The primary role of γ-LMN neurons is to regulate the length of the spindle fibers and thus modulate the excitability of the annulospiral primary (Ia) endings. This regulates the stretch reflex muscle tone and allows the CNS to regulate its own state of excitability.

γ-Motor neurons are controlled by synaptic input from the brainstem reticular formation and the vestibular system. The γ-efferent fibers leave through the ventral nerve root and contract the end (contractile) portions of the intrafusal muscle fibers, stretching the central parts of the muscle spindles. On being stretched, the muscle spindles send a volley of afferent projections to the corresponding α-motor neurons, causing the reflexive contraction of the extrafusal fibers of the muscle.

Interneurons

As functionally specialized cells, the interneurons are diffusely present throughout the spinal cord and brain. There are approximately 30 times as many interneurons as motor neurons. With most being inhibitory, the interneuron cells serve as filters, integrating all sensory and motor functions of the CNS. The **Renshaw cell**, as an example of an interneuron, receives axonal collaterals from nearby motor neurons, inhibiting the activity of the same or related adjacent motor neurons. This recurrent inhibition by the Renshaw cell facilitates and sharpens the activity of the projecting motor neuron from which it receives the collaterals.

MOTOR FUNCTIONS OF THE SPINAL CORD

The first and basic motor function of the spinal cord is a reflexive motor response. A reflex response is a stereotyped and involuntary reaction in response to sensory stimulation. The neuronal circuitry for reflexes is present at each segmental level throughout the spinal cord. It consists primarily of muscle spindles, afferent fibers, α-motor neurons, efferent fibers, and muscle tissue (Fig. 13-6).

For the most part, reflex functions of the spinal cord are independent of cortical voluntary control, although they are influenced indirectly by descending impulses from the motor cortex and brainstem motor centers. The input from higher motor centers participates in providing a homeostatic state of motor control, resulting in smooth motor movements. If released from higher levels of motor control, as in the case of a lesion, the spinal cord reflexes become hyperactive.

Key Terms :

Extrafusal fibers	**Intrafusal fibers**
Golgi tendon organs	**Muscle spindles**

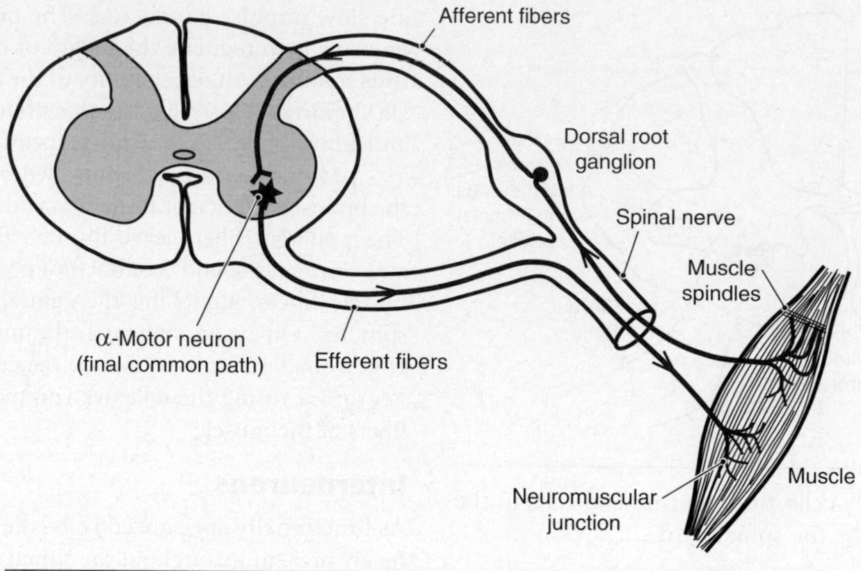

Figure 13-6 Neuronal circuitry for a spinal reflex.

Muscle Spindles and Motor Activity

There are two types of specialized receptors in muscles: **muscle spindles** and **Golgi tendon organs** (Fig. 13-7; Box 13-2). Muscle spindles detect the degree and rate of change in muscle length and help maintain muscle tone. Golgi tendon organs monitor muscle tension during muscle contraction and reflexively inhibit muscle contraction, permitting the muscle to stretch and thus prevent injury caused by excessive contraction; they do it by regulating the α-motor neuron activity through the circuitry of interneurons.

Muscle Spindles

As a complex sensorimotor organ, the muscle spindle is a small structure and consists of three to five specialized **intrafusal fibers** that are parallel to the surrounding extrafusal (striate) muscle fibers. The center of an intrafusal fiber is wrapped by a fast-conducting **annulospiral primary (Ia) sensory ending**. If stretched, it generates and sends impulses in the afferent fiber from the spindle. The afferent impulses travel to α-motor neurons in the spinal cord via fast-conducting type Ia nerve fibers with a velocity of approximately 100 m/second, causing the muscle to contract (Fig. 13-7*A*).

Muscles consist of extrafusal and **intrafusal** fibers. Extrafusal fibers that make up the large mass of the skeletal muscle are attached to bone by fibrous tissue extensions called tendons and are controlled by α-motor neurons. These striated muscles are composed of **myosin filaments**, which are responsible for the contractility (shortening) of the muscle. Intrafusal fibers, which contain muscle spindles, are attached to the extrafusal fibers and are controlled by γ-motor neurons. Both ends of the intrafusal fibers contract; but the central region, which is devoid of myosin filaments, does not contract.

The γ-motor neurons control both ends of the intrafusal fibers. A contraction of both ends of these fibers causes the central portion of the fiber to stretch passively. A similar stretch of the spindles can occur if the entire muscle (skeletal) mass is stretched. Whenever the central portion of the intrafusal fiber stretches, the annulospiral primary sensory endings become depolarized and discharge impulses, which travel in two types of sensory nerve fibers: **type Ia** (fast) fibers and **type II** (slow) fibers. Type Ia (primary) fibers originate from the central region of the spindles, whereas the type II (secondary) fibers innervate areas of the intrafusal fibers on each side of the primary ending.

As the spindles stretch, a surge of sensory input is directed to the α-motor neurons, which in turn reflexively contract the muscle mass to progressively decrease the muscle length. The contraction of the entire muscle mass halts the stretch and pacifies the spindles. With new muscle position and diminished spindle stretching, sensory input from the intrafusal fibers to the α-motor neurons stops.

Stretching the central portion of the intrafusal fibers themselves can induce a stretch reflex. This can be elicited either by activating γ-nerve impulses and contracting the ends of the intrafusal fibers or by lengthening the surrounding striate muscle through the alpha motor neurons. The former is illustrated by the classic knee-jerk (stretch or myotatic) reflex. When the patient's leg is in a relaxed state, a tap of the patellar tendon at the knee with a reflex hammer immediately stretches both the extrafusal and intrafusal fibers of the quadriceps muscle. After a brief

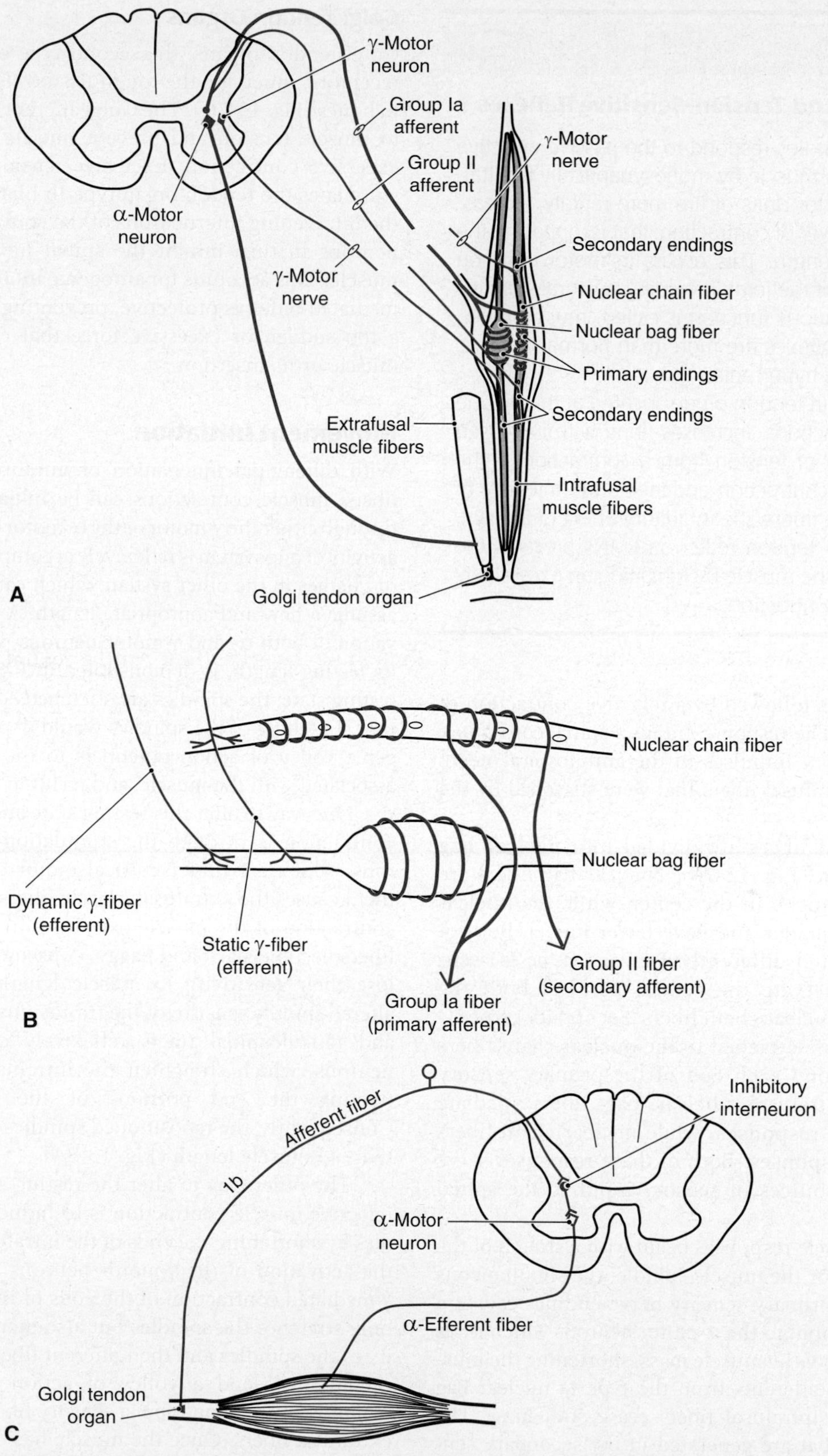

Figure 13-7 A. The relation of extrafusal and intrafusal muscle fibers to muscle stretch (muscle spindle) and tension (Golgi tendon) receptors. B. Nuclear bag and nuclear chain fibers. C. Golgi tendon organs, which mediate autogenic inhibition.

BOX 13-2

Length- and Tension-Sensitive Reflexes

Muscle spindles respond to the passive or active stretch of a muscle by monosynaptically facilitating the motor units of fire more rapidly, increasing the power of contraction, that is, opposing the muscle strength. This occurs in motor units on each side of the joint, providing postural stability. This continuous function is called "muscle tone." If stretch reflexes are more than normally active, it results in hypertonia.

The Golgi tendon organ, located at the muscle tendon junctions, increases firing with increased generation of tension from a contraction. If the force of a contraction endangers the integrity of the muscle fibers, the inhibitory effect of the synaptic Golgi tendon reflex on LMNs prevents the tearing of the muscle by inhibiting an excessively powerful contraction.

delay, the stretch is followed by a reflexive contraction of the same muscle. The response entails a spinal cord reflex triggered by sensory impulses in the annulospiral nerve endings of the intrafusal fibers that were stretched by the knee tap.

The intrafusal fibers are divided into **nuclear bag** and **nuclear chain** (Fig. 13-7*B*). Nuclear bag fibers are long with many nuclei in the center, while the nuclear chain fibers are smaller and have fewer nuclei. Both of these are innervated differently. Primary (type Ia) sensory endings innervate the central parts of both the nuclear bag and nuclear chain fibers. Secondary (type II) sensory endings are attached to the nuclear chain fibers only at sites beyond each end of the primary sensory endings. The intrafusal nuclear bag fibers mediate **dynamic sensory responses**, while nuclear chain fibers mediate **static responses**. Both of these responses serve as the constant sources of sensory input to the spinal motor neurons.

Dynamic muscle responses begin with a stretch of the muscle mass and/or the muscle spindle; the simultaneous distortion of the primary sensory nerve endings causes a surge of sensory input to the α-motor neurons which leads to the contraction of the muscle mass, shortening the muscle. The dynamic afferents from the type Ia nuclear bag fibers stop when intrafusal fibers cease stretching. The static responses that are generated in the secondary sensory endings of the nuclear chain fibers respond to stretching in proportion to the intensity of the stretch. The static sensory input from the intrafusal chain fibers maintains the muscle at the stretched position longer, from several minutes to hours.

Golgi Tendon Organs

Golgi tendon organs, the second type of sensory muscle receptors, innervate the tough tissues that attach muscles to bones (Fig. 13-7*C*). The Golgi afferent impulses respond to muscle tension and prevent muscle damage from an excessive contraction. Excessive tension in the muscles stimulates the tendon organ type Ib fibers, which activate the intervening interneurons of the spinal cord. The interneurons in turn inhibit the spinal motor nuclei to the muscle. This accounts for autogenic inhibition. The Golgi-mediated reflex is protective, preventing the generation of a too sudden or excessive force that could damage the muscle or its insertion.

Movement Initiation

With differential innervation of intrafusal and extrafusal fibers, muscle contractions can be initiated and modified through either the γ-motor or the α-motor systems. Increased activity of one system is reflexively accompanied by increased discharges in the other system, which causes the muscle to assume a new and appropriate length. A subthreshold activation of both α- and γ-motor neurons, with the muscle at its resting length, is demonstrated in Figure 13-8*A*. In the resting state, the spindles are stretched adequately. Any further stretching of the spindles would depolarize them, trigger a volley of action potentials to the α-motor neurons associated with the muscle, and result in a contraction.

One way to alter this resting state and initiate a muscle contraction is through the stimulation of α-motor neurons, which are under cortical motor control; activating them causes the extrafusal muscle fibers to contract. With contraction of the muscle extrafusal fibers, the intrafusal fibers become slack and baggy; consequently, the spindles lose their sensitivity to muscle length. To correct this altered spindle sensitivity, the rubrospinal, vestibulospinal, and reticulospinal tracts reflexively discharge γ-motor neurons, which straighten the intrafusal fibers by contracting the end portions of the intrafusal fibers. Consequently, the repositioned spindles regain their sensitivity to muscle length (Fig. 13-8*A*).

The other way to alter the resting state and initiate a reflexive muscle contraction is to induce tension to spindles by shortening the ends of the intrafusal fibers through the activation of the γ-motor neurons (Fig. 13-8*B*). The γ-mediated contraction of the ends of intrafusal fibers not only stretches the spindles but also increases the sensitivity of the spindles and their afferent fibers. The annulospiral endings send a volley of action potentials to the α-motor neurons on type Ia sensory fibers, shortening the extrafusal fibers. Once the muscle has contracted enough to decrease the stress on the center of the intrafusal fibers, the rate of the type Ia firing decreases, and the extrafusal fibers cease contracting. The new desired muscle length permits maintenance of equilibrium in which the activity in type Ia fibers is below threshold.

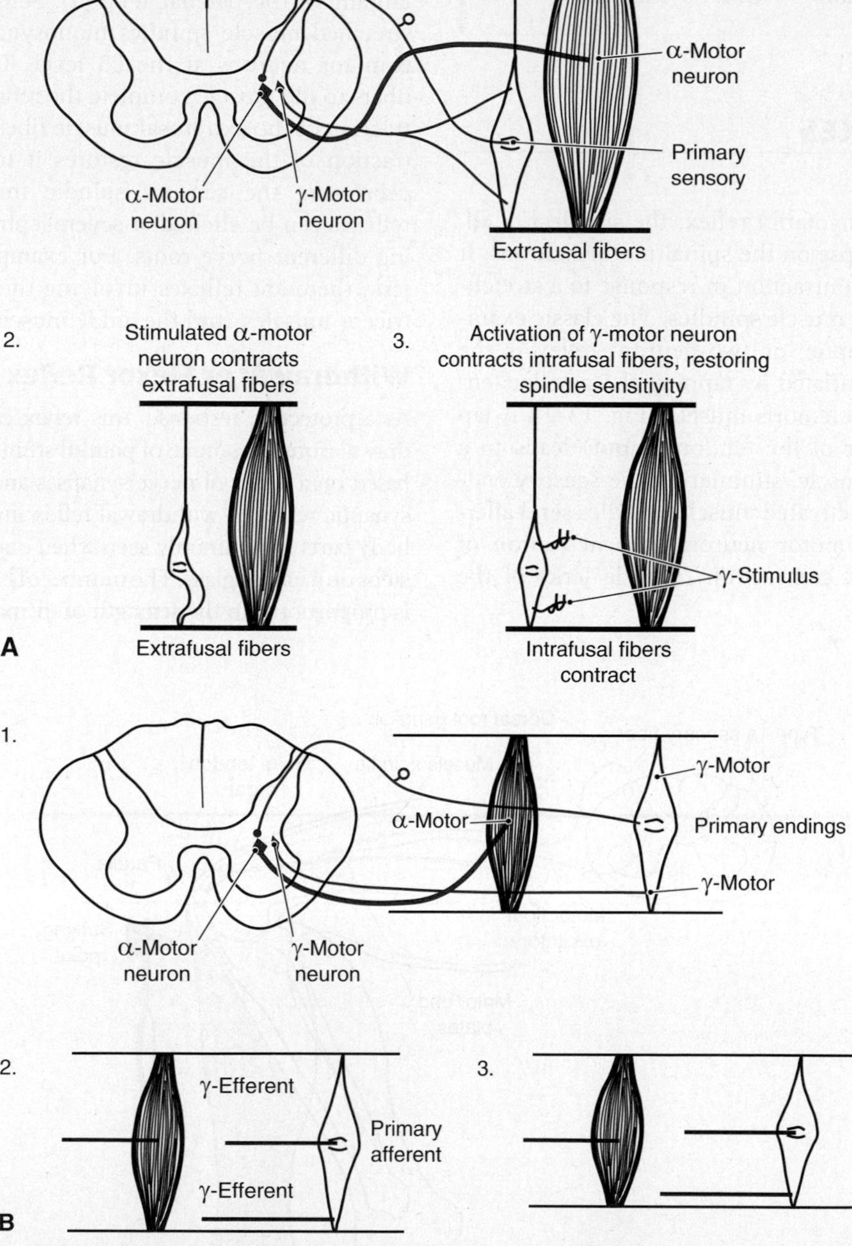

Figure 13-8 The α- and γ-motor neurons in movement initiation and the maintenance of sensitivity to stretch in the muscle spindles. A. α-mediated voluntary contraction of the extrafusal muscle fibers leaves intrafusal fibers and their spindles without sensitivity to stretch. This condition is corrected by the reticular and vestibulospinal projections to the γ-motor neurons, which contract intrafusal fibers and restore spindle stretch sensitivity. B. In γ-initiated movement, γ-cells activate intrafusal fiber ends, deforming the annulospiral endings of the spindle afferent fibers, which synaptically activate α-motor neurons, causing contraction of the extrafusal muscle cells.

Key Terms:

Crossed extensor reflex	**Stretch reflex**
LMN syndrome	**Withdrawal reflex**
Reciprocal inhibition	**UMN syndrome**

SPINAL REFLEXES

Stretch Reflex

The muscle stretch (myotatic) reflex, the simplest of all, involves a single synapse on the spinal motor neurons. It is a reflexive muscle contraction in response to a stretching/lengthening of the muscle spindles. The classic example of this monosynaptic, or two-neuron, reflex is the knee jerk, which is initiated by tapping the patellar tendon of the quadriceps femoris muscle (Fig. 13-9). A tap with a reflex hammer of the tendon (input) leads to a brief stretch of the muscle, stimulating the sensory endings of spindles. The activated muscle spindles send afferent projections to α-motor neurons, the activation of which causes a quick contraction (muscle jerk) of the same muscle (output).

The central point in stretch reflexes is that any stretched muscle invariably contracts after a brief delay. The principal receptors are the muscle spindles that respond to the stretching of the affected muscle (e.g., by tapping of the patellar tendon). Sensory inputs from the stretched muscle spindles monosynaptically activate the α-motor neurons at the L3 level. The α-motor efferent fibers to the muscle complete the reflex arc and cause contraction of the extrafusal muscle fibers. The reflexive contraction of the muscle restores it to a resting position, decreasing the sensory spindle impulses. Tendon-jerk reflexes can be elicited at several spinal segments, involving different nerve roots. For example, besides the knee jerk, there are reflexes involving the biceps muscles, the triceps muscles, and the ankle muscles (Table 13-2).

Withdrawal or Flexor Reflex

As a protective response, this reflex causes a limb to withdrawal from the source of painful stimuli. The limb flexion is based on a series of nerve synapses and is, therefore, a polysynaptic reflex. A withdrawal reflex involving one or several body parts is commonly seen when one touches a hot pan or steps on a nail or glass. The number of body parts that respond is proportional to the strength of the painful stimulus.

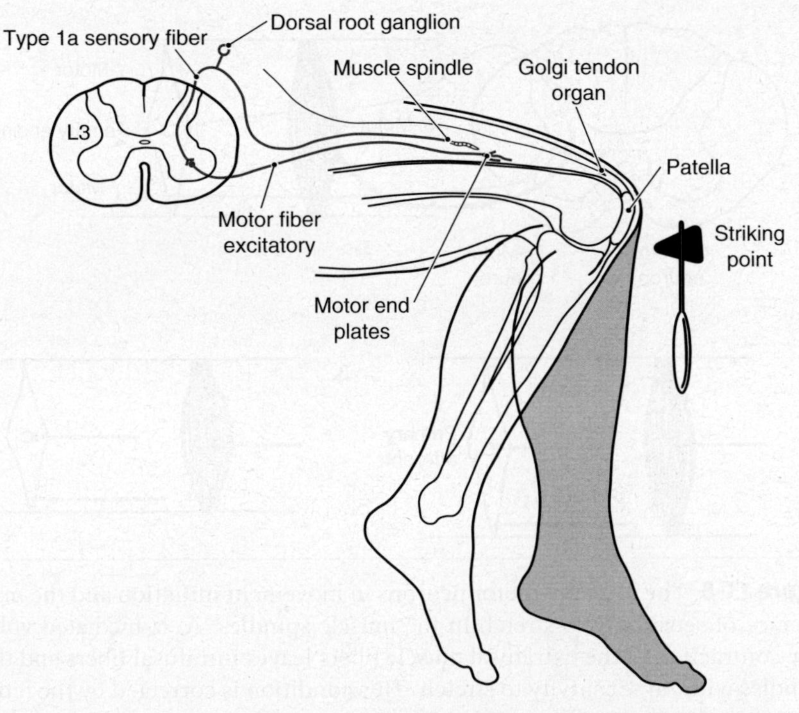

Figure 13-9 Neuronal circuitry for a stretch (patellar tendon) reflex. Tapping the patellar tendon briefly stretches extrafusal fibers of the quadriceps muscle and raises the tension of its muscle spindles. Spindles respond to muscle stretching by sending a volley of impulses directly to the α-motor neurons in the L3 segment of the spinal cord. L3 efferent fibers cause extrafusal fibers of the quadriceps to contract. This muscle contraction eliminates tension on the spindles.

Table 13-2

Muscle Stretch Reflexes

Roots	Reflexes
C5–C6	Biceps
C7–C8	Triceps
C8–T1	Finger flexors
L2–L4	Patellar-jerk reflex; Quadriceps
S1–S2	Ankle reflex; Achilles tendon

The neural mechanism of the limb-withdrawal reflex involves pain receptors in the skin, afferent pain fibers, substantia gelatinosa, interneurons, and α-motor neurons (Fig. 13-10). The afferent pain and temperature fibers from the skin enter the spinal cord through the dorsal root and terminate in the substantia gelatinosa, which sends collaterals to interneurons in the dorsal gray horns. Interneurons distribute signals to the appropriate α-motor neurons, initiating the limb-withdrawal response; the number of motor neurons recruited by pain fibers depends on the strength of the stimulus. The reflex continues for several seconds after the stimulus ceases. A withdrawal reflex generally begins even before one is aware of the painful stimulus because the afferent information triggers a spinal response before the ascending signal of pain reaches the forebrain.

An important clinical concept related to this reflex is **reciprocal inhibition**. It represents a neuronal arrangement in which the stimulation of one group of neurons causes inhibition of the motor neurons to the paired (antagonistic) muscle through the spinal interneurons. This neuronal arrangement is essential for smooth motor function. For example, in arm flexion, the interneurons activating the motor neurons for the biceps simultaneously inhibit the motor neurons for the paired triceps.

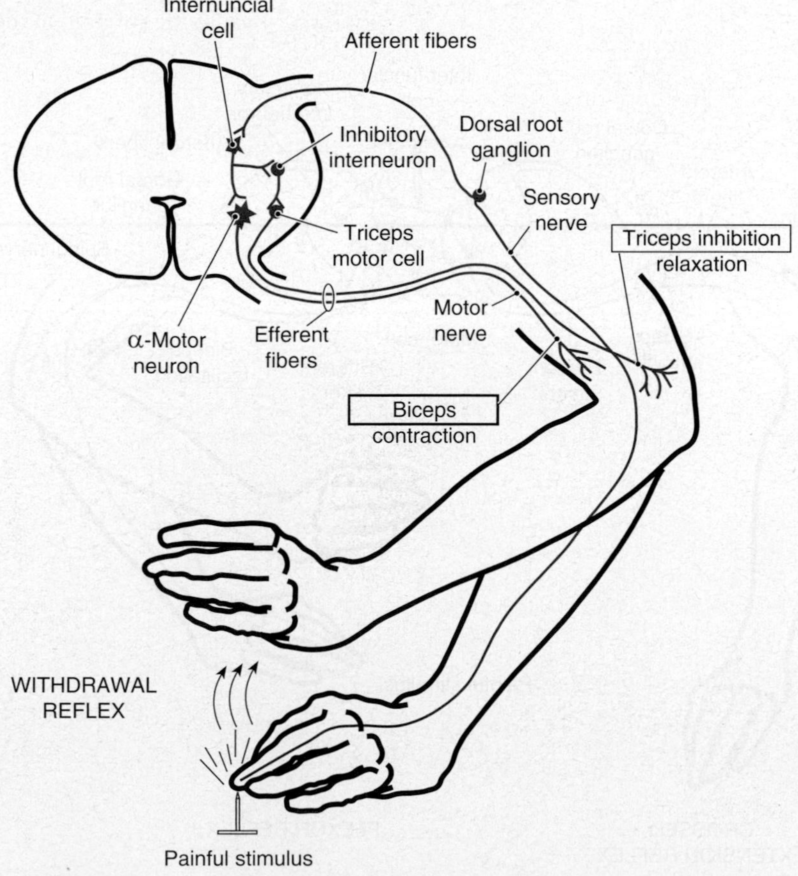

Figure 13-10 Neuronal circuitry for the withdrawal (flexor) reflex. The circuitry involves diverging interneuronal elements. This circuitry not only withdraws the limb but also inhibits the antagonistic muscle from contracting through reciprocal inhibition.

This antagonistic effect—wherein one muscle contracts while the paired muscle extends—exemplifies reciprocal inhibition; the paired muscle is inhibited from simultaneous contraction (Fig. 13-10). Anatomically, this involves interneurons that are inhibitory to α-motor neurons of the antagonistic muscle.

Crossed, or Intrasegmental, Extensor Reflex

The **crossed extensor reflex** involves the contralateral motor neurons for the antagonistic muscle. It is a complex movement pattern in which withdrawal of the limb (flexor response) on one side is accompanied by the extension of the opposite limb approximately 0.5 seconds after the flexor response (Fig. 13-11). This multisynaptic reflex system, which moves limbs on the opposite side of the body, is considered a genetically programmed protective behavior for survival because it moves the entire body away from the painful stimulus. Its neural mechanism involves the crossing of sensory information to the opposite side through polysynaptic circuits of interneurons recruiting the opposite limbs. The crossed limb extension follows the flexing action of the limb ipsilateral to the stimulus. Reverberating polysynaptic circuits in interneuronal pools thus sustains the complex withdrawal behavior for long periods, even after the reflex-triggering stimulus has ceased, which is necessary to keep the body protected until the brain takes over body control.

Spinal Regulation of Muscles for Respiration

Understanding the spinal control of the muscles of respiration is an important aspect of training for students in communicative disorders (Table 13-3). In addition to being vital for survival, respiration, with a patterned cycle of inhalation and exhalation, also regulates our speaking (see Chapter 18). The contraction of the diaphragm and external intercostal muscles increases the intrathoracic volume, triggering the process of inspiration. An increase in intra-abdominal pressure by the abdominal muscles and rib depression by internal intercostal muscles initiates exhalation. The motor nuclei from the anterior horns of the C3–C5 segments (predominantly from C4) form the phrenic nerve, which innervates the diaphragm, the primary muscle of inspiration. The efferents to the internal and external intercostals muscles exit from T1 to T12

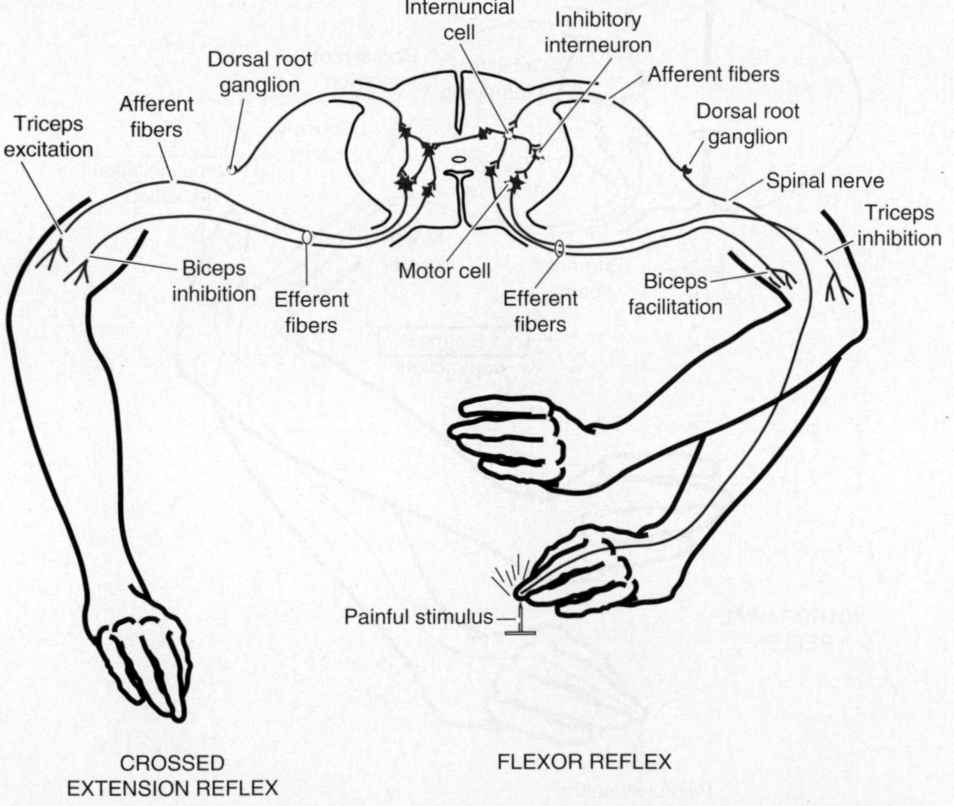

Figure 13-11 Neuronal circuitry for the crossed extensor reflex marked by the contraction of the muscle on one side accompanied by the extension of the opposing muscle or muscles. This reflex involves interneurons that diverge sensory information.

Table 13-3

Spinal Control of the Muscles of Respiration

Spinal Roots	Muscles	Functions
C3–C5	Diaphragm	Contracts to increase thoracic diameter for inspiration
T1–T12	External intercostals	Contract to raise ribs for inspiration
T1–T12	Internal intercostals	Assist in rib depression for forced expiration
T6–T12	Abdominal muscles Rectus abdominus Internal oblique External oblique Transversus abdominus	Increase intrathoracic pressure for forced expiration

spinal segments. The motor nuclei from segments T6 to T12 innervate the abdominal muscles (rectus abdominus, internal oblique, external oblique, and transversus abdominus). Spinal lesions involving these motor nuclei have different implications for respiration.

A patient with a spinal lesion above C4 has a complete paralysis of the respiratory muscles and may lose the ability to breathe (inhale), requiring artificial respiration for life support. A patient with a spinal injury below C4 will have paralysis of the lower intercostal muscles but not the diaphragm. With basic control of the diaphragm, this patient may inhale and quietly exhale because of muscle elasticity. Similarly, a patient with a thoracic lesion may be able to breathe quietly; however, he or she may have to learn to compensate to cough and exhale forcefully.

NEUROTRANSMITTERS

Four important neurotransmitters are released by the activity of brainstem projections to the spinal cord: acetylcholine, norepinephrine, serotonin, and epinephrine. Nonetheless, acetylcholine is the major chemical messenger of the PNS. Released by the efferent spinal fibers in the myoneural junction, acetylcholine regulates voluntary or reflexive motor movements. A diminished effect of acetylcholine, as seen in myasthenia gravis and other disorders, is associated with muscle weakness. Acetylcholine also regulates autonomic functions. Except for the sympathetic postganglionic cells, acetylcholine is the primary neurotransmitter of the autonomic nervous system, which controls major visceral functions (see Table 18-1).

The pontine reticular **nucleus ceruleus** and **lateral medullary reticular formation** transmit epinephrine and norepinephrine to the spinal cord. Their influence is thought to be inhibitory, enhancing the signal-to-noise ratio in the spinal sensorimotor conduction system. Located in the brainstem, the caudal reticular **raphe nuclei** send serotonin projections to the lower brainstem and spinal cord. By synapsing on spinal **enkephalin interneurons, these projections** provide some control over pain transmission.

CLINICAL CORRELATES

Trauma, tumors, infections, impaired blood circulation, and degenerative conditions are common causes of spinal cord lesions (Box 13-3). The testing of sensory and motor functions is the most reliable clinical method for determining the integrity of the spinal cord. The contraction of striate muscles during reflexes provides a clinician with important information about the complex internal mechanism of the entire motor system. Muscle reflexes are examined clinically on both sides of the body to determine whether muscular movements are symmetrical and the quality of movements is normal.

BOX 13-3

Ruptured Spinal Disc

The spinal disc is located between each of the vertebrae of the spine. Serving as shock absorbers, the discs keep the spine flexible. With increasing age, however, the discs become less flexible and lose elasticity. A disc can also be damaged by injury or by wear and tear and can bulge within or rupture through their connective tissue capsule. Neighboring spinal nerves can be compressed causing chronic pain in lower extremities. Compression of LMNS axons in the ventral roots can lead to muscle weakness.

Altered Reflexes

There are three patterns of altered reflexes: **hyperreflexia**, **hyporeflexia**, and **clonus reflex**. Reduced (hypoactive) or increased (hyperactive) quality of muscle reflexes indicates pathology in the nervous system. Spinal reflex functions are controlled via balanced excitatory (+) and inhibitory (–) supraspinal projections to the motor neurons. The corticospinal system is predominantly excitatory to motor neurons in the spinal cord. Loss of this system reduces recruitment of motor neurons and thus produces weakness. Spasticity in muscles is not instantly observed; rather, the muscle paresis is gradually converted over several weeks into spasticity, which includes hyperexcitability of many stretch reflexes (see the discussion of UMN syndrome in Chapter 16). In contrast to brisk (hyperactive) reflexes with interrupted supraspinal fibers, lesions involving spinal motor neurons and/or their efferent spinal fibers lead to reduced or absent muscle reflexes (hyporeflexia or areflexia, respectively). Clonus reflex is marked by a repeated contraction followed by relaxation of the muscle during a stretch reflex. Time delay in the afferent and efferent information secondary to reduced activation of α-motor neurons and spindles unloading contribute to this rhythmic muscle contraction and relaxation.

There are two types of spinal cord disorders: **segmental** and **longitudinal** (pathway specific). Segmental disturbance implies a lesion at a specific spinal level; below that level, sensory and motor functions are impaired. The severity of the deficit depends on the site and extent of the lesion. Longitudinal disturbance selectively affects specific nerve cells and their axons. The longitudinal involvement of axonal bundles may impair both sensory and motor systems.

Lower Motor Neuron Syndrome

The term LMN refers to a motor neuron and its axon in the brainstem (cranial nerves) or spinal cord (α-motor neurons). An LMN cell body provides the output pathway to peripheral function via its axon, which traverses the ventral root and peripheral nerves to innervate a skeletal muscle. LMN lesions of either the spinal cell bodies in the ventral horn (e.g., poliomyelitis, amyotrophic lateral sclerosis, vascular damage, and spinal cord tumor) or of the axon (in the ventral root or peripheral nerve) result in **denervation** of the **skeletal muscle fibers**, which leads to muscle weakness and loss of control.

Small lesions can result in the loss of one or several motor units. Large lesions or peripheral nerve destruction can result in complete muscle weakness and total flaccidity; this is called the **LMN syndrome** (Fig. 13-12; see Table 16-1). In LMN syndrome, muscle fibers are disconnected from motor efferents and thus cannot receive descending cortical impulses and reflexive sensory input. Deprived of their trophic efferents, the affected muscle fibers gradually degenerate. Clinical signs of LMN include flaccid paralysis, absent reflexes, muscular fibrillation, and eventual severe atrophy (wasting) of the muscle involved; these signs occur unilateral to the lesion and involve only selected muscles.

With no projections of motor impulses from the motor neuron, the muscle fibers are completely paralyzed for both reflexes and voluntary motor movements; this paralysis is characterized by flaccid muscle tone. Denervated muscle fibers pass through several stages: a brief period of hyperexcitability and spontaneous firing (**fibrillation**), followed by silence of firing and shrinking of the muscle (**atrophy**). If they are not reinnervated

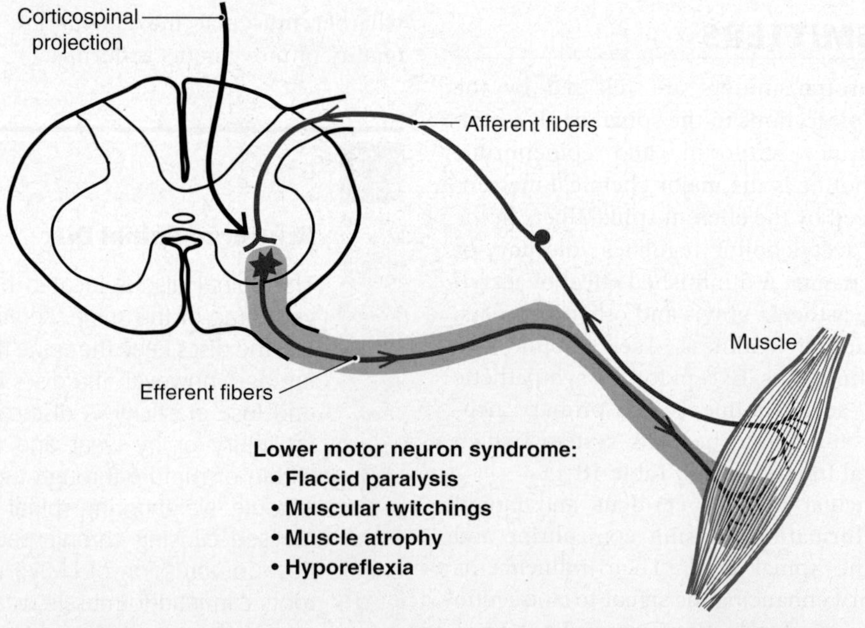

Figure 13-12 Injury to the motor unit (lower motor neuron syndrome).

within 6 months or so, the denervated skeletal muscle cells die and are replaced permanently by scar tissue. This is more severe than reduced muscle mass from disuse, which often is seen in **UMN syndrome**.

If the LMN cell survives, the normal membrane potential eventually is restored, and the unit returns to its normal condition, except for when the motor system excites the cell body past threshold. Destruction of the LMN cell body or its axon results in denervation of the muscle fibers or motor unit. Destroyed LMN cell bodies are not replaced. However, destroyed LMN axons (PNS) may regenerate, and if they are directed properly past scar tissue and through their former peripheral nerve path, they can reinnervate to their former muscle fiber targets (see Chapter 5). Skilled peripheral nerve surgery, inhibition of scar tissue formation, and efforts to maintain denervated muscle fibers until reinnervation occurs are all necessary for the success of reinnervation.

Common Spinal Syndromes

Complete Spinal Transection

Vertebral dislocations, myelitis (inflammation of the spinal cord), and tumors can cause spinal transection. Immediately after the transection, all sensory and motor functions are lost bilaterally below the lesion but are spared above the lesion (Fig. 13-13; see "Lesion Localization" later in this Chapter). The body region affected depends on the spinal

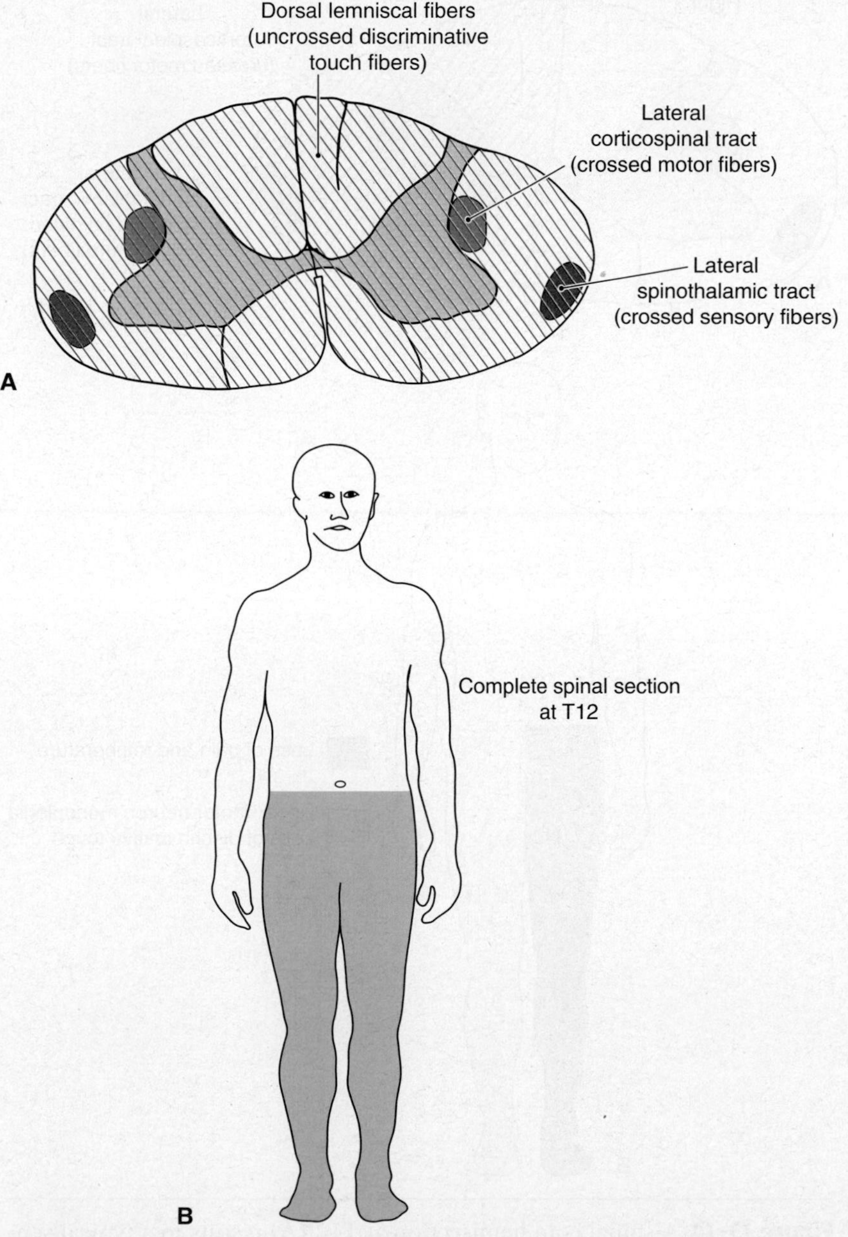

Figure 13-13 Complete transection of the thoracic spinal cord (A), resulting in bilateral paralysis and sensory loss below the level of the lesion with spared functions above the level of lesion (B).

level of the lesion. Spinal shock can abolish sensorimotor functions and persists for weeks. After a while, the reflex activity gradually returns at levels below the lesion. However, within a few weeks after the interruption of the corticospinal tract, the patient exhibits UMN syndrome (see Chapter 16), which includes loss of delicate capabilities of the forearm and fingers, hyperactive stretch reflexes, and Babinski sign. Also present are the clonic movements, in which a passively moved limb muscle exhibits repeated contraction and relaxation.

Brown–Séquard Syndrome: Spinal Hemisection

Lateral hemisection of the spinal cord produces the following three clinical conditions; understanding them requires knowledge of the locations and crossing points of the sensorimotor pathways (Fig. 13-14, also see Chapter 11).

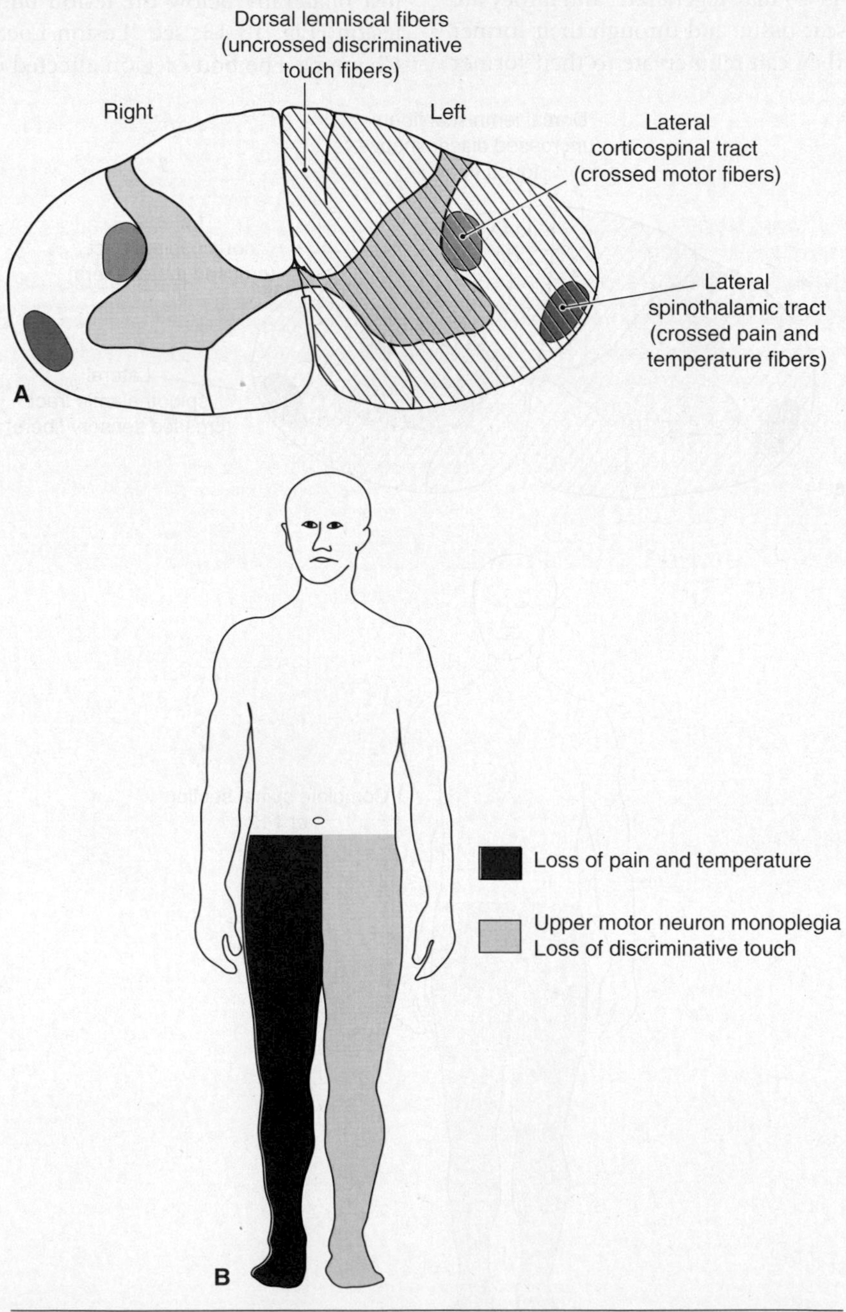

Figure 13-14 A spinal cord hemisection at T12 (A) results in a typical sensorimotor deficit pattern characterized by ipsilateral paralysis, ipsilateral sensory loss (discriminative sensation), and contralateral pain and temperature loss (B).

- **Signs of a lesion in the corticospinal tract on the ipsilateral half of the body.** In the case of a right-sided lesion at C4, there is spastic paralysis in the right arm and leg (UMN symptoms). The Babinski sign presence is abnormal; it is marked by the extension of the big toe in response to scraping to the sole of the foot (Fig. 16-5).
- **Ipsilateral discriminative sensory loss.** Destruction of the dorsal lemniscal column, which contains tactile and proprioceptive axons ascending ipsilaterally to relay to the contralateral forebrain, results in loss of vibratory and discriminative sensation in the ipsilateral half of the body. The ascending dorsal lemniscal fibers cross the midline in the caudal medulla (see Chapter 11).
- **Contralateral pain and temperature sensation loss.** With fibers of the lateral spinal thalamic tract crossing immediately after entering the spinal cord, an interruption at the right C4 level affects pain and temperature from the left (contralateral) side of the body below the level of the lesion (see Chapter 11).

Syringomyelia

Syringomyelia is a developmental condition marked by a cyst or cavity within the central portion of the spinal cord. It is characterized by two clinical symptoms: bilateral loss of pain and temperature sensation from selected limbs and impaired motor control (see Fig. 11-12). With the degeneration of the central (gray) region, the crossing of sensory (pain and touch) fibers is interrupted, which results in a bilateral pattern of pain and temperature loss (see Fig. 11-12). If the cyst extends into the spinal motor nuclei in the involved segments, bilateral signs of LMN syndrome in the involved muscles include flaccid paralysis, hyporeflexia, and hypotonia.

Subacute Combined Degeneration

Subacute combined degeneration is associated with pernicious anemia (when the number of red blood cells and the amount of hemoglobin in blood is less than normal), which results from malabsorption of vitamin B_{12}. The bilateral subacute degeneration of the spinal cord mostly involves the fibers in the dorsal lemniscal column and corticospinal tract. Involvement of the dorsal column fibers results in bilateral loss of position and vibratory sense, whereas the interruption of the corticospinal fibers produces a weakness of limbs bilaterally. The presence of paresthesia (numbness and tingling) indicates peripheral nerve involvement. As the disease progresses to the cerebral cortex, higher mental functions are affected.

Lesion Localization

Rule 6: Symptoms Suggesting a Complete Spinal Cord Lesion

Presenting Symptoms. Paralysis and sensory loss bilaterally below the level of the lesion with spared functions above indicate a complete spinal cord transectional injury.

Rationale. The spinal cord contains all ascending (sensory) and descending (motor) fibers. A complete lesion would affect the transmission of these functions below the lesion point and spare such functions above the lesion point. Impaired bowel and bladder control and autonomic reflexes are commonly seen in a spinal cord injury.

Rule 7: Symptoms Suggesting a Spinal Hemisection

Presenting Symptoms. Ipsilateral loss of position and vibratory sensation below the level of the lesion, ipsilateral body paralysis, and contralateral loss of pain and temperature indicate a spinal hemisection (Brown–Séquard syndrome).

Rationale. The reasons for this rule are the following:

1. Transection of the dorsal column (fasciculus gracilis and fasciculus cuneatus) results in the loss of position and vibration sense along with discriminative touch on the side of the lesion.
2. Involvement of the fibers of the corticospinal tract below its decussation produces spastic hemiplegia on the side of the lesion.
3. Because the fibers mediating pain and temperature cross the midline after entering the spinal cord, their interruption results in loss of pain and temperature sensation on the opposite side.
4. Impaired bowel and bladder control is commonly seen in spinal cord injury.

Rule 8: Symptoms Suggesting a Peripheral or Central Lesion

Presenting Symptoms. Paralysis and sensory (pain and temperature) loss affecting the same single limb suggest a lesion either in the peripheral nerve or in the cortex.

Rationale. The descending and ascending sensory fibers supplying a single limb are together only in the peripheral (nerve, plexus) area or in the somatosensory cortical area.

CASE STUDIES FOR PROBLEM SOLVING

CASE ONE (13-1)

A 20-year-old athletic female student had been experiencing progressive weakness in her right leg for the past 2 months, which made playing sports difficult. One day she woke up with pain in her right leg. She realized that she had no control of her right leg and could not walk. She was taken to the ER, where she presented with the following:

- No voluntary movement in the right leg
- Diminished tone in the leg muscles
- Absent knee jerk and Achilles (calf muscle contraction) reflexes
- Largely intact sensation

A clinical analysis of the CSF withdrawn through spinal tap was normal as there were no increased white blood cells indicating any infection. A spinal MRI study revealed a small growth in the anterior horns of the L4 regions on the right.

Question: How can you explain these clinical signs?

Case (13-1) Discussion: See discussion of case studies

CASE TWO (13-2)

A 30-year-old window-washer fell from her ladder and injured her back at the T11–T12 level. She had bilateral flaccid paralysis of the legs and was rushed to the hospital, where she was observed for a few days. In an examination completed a few weeks later, she demonstrated the following symptoms:

- Spastic paralysis in the left leg
- Positive Babinski sign in the left leg
- Loss of position sense (proprioception) and discriminative touch in the left leg
- Loss of pain and temperature in the right foot

A spinal MRI study revealed a crushed appearance of the cord at T11–T12 on the left.

Question: How can you relate these symptoms to a crushed cord at the T11–T12 level?

Case (13-2) Discussion: See discussion of case studies

CASE THREE (13-3)

A 16-year-old gymnast lost control of her body while exercising and fell flat on her back. Unconscious for several minutes, she was rushed to a nearby hospital. After she awoke, she was unable to move. A neurologic examination revealed the following:

- Flaccid paralysis of both lower limbs
- No deep tendon reflexes in either leg
- Loss of touch, pain, and temperature sensation below the midthoracic (T6–T7) region
- No bladder or bowel control

A spinal MRI study revealed a complete spinal section at the midthoracic level. The patient's clinical picture changed within a week, and she began to exhibit these signs:

- Hyperreflexia in both lower limbs
- Spastic paralysis of both lower limbs
- Impaired control of bowel and bladder functions
- Some return of touch and pressure sensation in the lower limbs

Question: How can you account for this clinical picture by relating the symptoms to a complete midthoracic spinal section?

Case (13-3) Discussion: See discussion of case studies

CASE FOUR (13-4)

A 45-year-old man was taken to a neurologist with a complaint of a progressively worsening weakness of both lower limbs for the past 2 months. The neurologist noted the following:

- Paralysis (flaccid) in both lower limbs and fasciculation in the muscles
- Reduced reflexes involving both limbs
- Loss of pain and temperature involving both extremities
- Impaired bladder function

A spinal MRI study revealed a large intraspinal, centrally placed tumor at the level of the conus medullaris.

Question: How can you relate these symptoms to the lesion site?

Case (13-4) Discussion: See discussion of case studies

(Continued)

CASE FIVE (13-5) (CONTINUED)

A 54-year-old man was involved in a head-on automobile accident and began experiencing difficulty breathing; he was taken to the emergency room, where the following signs and symptoms were noted:

- Paralysis of both right upper and lower limbs
- Loss of discriminative sensation from the right half of the body
- Profound breathing problem marked with inability to inhale
- No difficulty in exhaling
- Unintelligible speech marked with weakly articulated one-word utterances

A spinal MRI study revealed a partial spinal lesion on the right involving C3–C5. The attending neurologists concluded that the partial lesion had affected the epicritic system, corticospinal tract fibers, and phrenic nerve.

Question: How can you relate these clinical symptoms to the lesion site?

Case (13-5) Discussion: See discussion of case studies

SUMMARY

Motor function is hierarchically organized at four arbitrarily identified neuraxial levels, with the spinal cord being the lowest. Motor nuclei of the spinal cord are the final common pathway for both spinal reflex and cortical projections to muscle fibers. The spinal cord is crucial for reflex muscle contractions and voluntary movements. The environmentally triggered reflex responses regulated by the spinal cord include the stretch (myotatic) reflex, withdrawal (flexor) reflex, and crossed extensor reflex. Even though these reflexes are independent of voluntary motor control, intact cortical projections to the spinal cord are important in their regulation. Constantly relayed sensory information, which is vital to coordinated motor activity, is integrated at every level of the nervous system. Spinal lesions that interrupt both cortical and spinal reflex projections to limb muscles result in LMN syndrome, which is marked by flaccid paralysis of selected muscles, absent reflexes, and atrophy of muscle fibers.

REVIEW QUESTIONS

1. Complete the following statements using the appropriate technical terms:
   A. The ________ is the wasting away of muscle tissue secondary to damage to the ________ neurons and/or subsequent loss of nerve supply (denervation).
   B. The ________ reflex involves the withdrawal of a limb in response to painful stimuli with the simultaneous extension of the limb on the opposite side.
   C. Located in specialized ________ fibers of skeletal muscle, the ________ are sensitive to changes in muscle length.
   D. The ________ junction is the area of synaptic connection between an axon terminal and single skeletal muscle fiber, and it is also the site in which the acetylcholine is released.
   E. Using selective inhibitory and excitatory circuits, the ________ ensures that when one muscle is contracting, its paired (agonist) muscle is relaxed.
   F. A ________ reflex refers to skeletal muscle contraction resulting from passive or active stretching of the same muscle.
   G. Withdrawal of a limb by the flexions of multiple joints in response to a painful stimulus is a ________.
   H. The ________ muscles are under voluntary control.
   I. As part of the LMN syndrome, ________ is marked by reduced or absent reflexes in a hypotonic muscle.
   J. The degeneration of lateral and posterior spinal columns secondary to vitamin B_{12} deficiency (pernicious anemia) is known as ________ degeneration of spinal cord.
   K. As part of the UMN syndrome, ________ is characterized by brisk reflexes in addition to increased muscle tone.
2. Name the parts of a motor unit.
3. List five clinical characteristics of LMN syndrome.
4. List the location of the spinal motor neuron innervating the following muscles of respiration:
   A. Diaphragm
   B. Internal and external intercostals
   C. Abdominal muscles
5. Match each of the following clinical concepts with its associated information:

A. complete spinal transection	a. degenerating α-motor neurons
B. spinal hemisection	b. denervated unused muscle fibers
C. syringomyelia	c. bilateral spinal (dorsal column and corticospinal tract) degeneration due to pernicious anemia
D. subacute combined degeneration	d. interrupted crossing of the pain and temperature fibers in the anterior commissure
E. muscle atrophy	e. loss of sensorimotor functions ipsilaterally and pain and temperature contralaterally
F. fasciculation	f. total bilateral loss of sensorimotor functions below the lesion site

14

Motor System 2: Cerebellum

LEARNING OBJECTIVES

After studying this chapter, students should be able to:

- Discuss the importance of the cerebellum in skilled motor activity
- Outline the functions of major cerebellar structures
- List cerebellar afferent and efferent projections
- Describe the neuronal circuitry of a cerebellar functional unit
- Discuss the major symptoms of cerebellar dysfunctioning
- Outline diseases and pathologies of the cerebellum

The primary level planning of a movement sequence involves the premotor cortex (lateral surface) and the supplementary motor cortex (midsagittal surface). The fine details of this plan are managed by the motor cortex. However, ongoing modifications to the motor plan require participation of the cerebellum, a structure that functions as an error-control device and coordinates all relevant input and output systems during movement, particularly rapid, alternating, and sequential movements. The more precise and skilled activity, the greater cerebellar functional participation, either normal or abnormal, becomes evident. The need for the cerebellum would be minimal if there were no sequential and rapid movements.

CEREBELLAR ROLE IN MOVEMENT

In its regulation of movement, the cerebellum participates in motor planning, and it constantly monitors all cortical motor output to muscles by receiving input from the motor cortex, brainstem reticular reflex networks, and spinal cord (information on body and limb position and joint movement). The cerebellum compares the efferent commands against the intended movements with the sensory information received in terms of anticipated and ongoing motor programs. It considers targeted movement in relation to body position, muscle preparedness, muscle tone, body equilibrium, distance, and duration. If any sensorimotor discrepancy is detected between body position and cortical motor impulses, the cerebellum sends corrective outputs in two directions: motor cortex and spinal cord.

Ascending feedback, related to what is going on and what modifications have to be made in terms of limb preparation, travels to the motor cortex via the red nucleus and ventrolateral (VL) thalamus. Descending feedback (via the rubrospinal tract and reticulospinal tract) to the lower motor neurons modulates muscle tone and reflexes at each moment during the ongoing movement (see Chapter 13). The ascending output is informational; it is used by the thalamus and cortex for modifying the next movement. In the case of sensorimotor discrepancy, the cerebellum can increase or decrease the rate of movement and stop movements at any time.

Most importantly, the cerebellum is vital to the control of rapid muscular activities, such as speaking, running, typing, playing the piano, and dancing; these activities require the highest level of constantly changing muscle synergy and movement range and velocity. The cerebellum contributes specifically to muscle synergy, muscle tone, movement range, velocity, and strength and maintenance of body equilibrium by contributing both built-in and learned modifications to the motor plan. Muscle synergy refers to the coordination and smoothness in time and space of the ongoing movement, essential for fine and skilled movements. Transitions and alterations in trajectory are smoothed out by the anticipatory checking of momentum and damping of oscillations. Muscle tonal regulation involves maintaining constant tension in healthy muscles and ensuring that the muscles are prepared. Equilibrium maintains the stable posture that is needed for executing motor movements.

The cerebellum is not concerned with the conscious appreciation of sensations and cognitive processing. Rather, it participates in motor learning, motor memory, and movement execution by automatically regulating and integrating information with sensorimotor mechanisms without reaching conscious awareness. In the case of cerebellar malfunctioning, a cortically controlled movement results in hitting the target, but its trajectory becomes erratic.

INNERVATION PATTERN

The relevant cerebellar sensorimotor organization is ipsilateral to both the input source (muscle spindles) and the output (LMN) target (Fig. 14-4). This is in contrast to the contralateral forebrain motor mechanism (see Chapter 16). Thus, the clinical signs are located ipsilateral to a lateralized cerebellar lesions because of a double crossing of the pathways.

Key Terms :

Archicerebellum
Dentate nucleus
Emboliform nucleus
Fastigial nucleus
Globose nucleus
Neocerebellum
Paleocerebellum
Reticulospinal tract
Rubrospinal tract
Tentorium cerebelli
Vestibulocerebellum

CEREBELLAR ANATOMY

The cerebellum, located dorsal to the junction of the pons and medulla (see Figs. 2-9 and 2-30), occupies most of the posterior fossa under the tentorium cerebelli. It consists of the cerebellar cortex, two hemispheres, the internal white substance, four pairs of nuclei embedded within the cerebellar white matter, and three cerebellar peduncles. The cerebellar surface is folded into small folia to accommodate its large size (see Fig. 2-27). Each cerebellar hemisphere is divided into three transverse lobes: anterior, posterior, and flocculonodular (Fig. 14-1*A*; see Figs. 2-28 and 2-29). Longitudinally, the cerebellum is divided into **median** (vermal), **paramedian** (paravermal), and **lateral** hemispheres (Fig. 14-1*B*).

Four large embedded nuclei listed from lateral to medial, are the **dentate nucleus**, **emboliform nucleus**, **globose nucleus**, and **fastigial nucleus** (Fig. 14-2). The dentate, the largest of the group, has a convoluted appearance in cross section. Most fibers traveling through the superior cerebellar peduncle originate from the dentate nucleus; this pathway

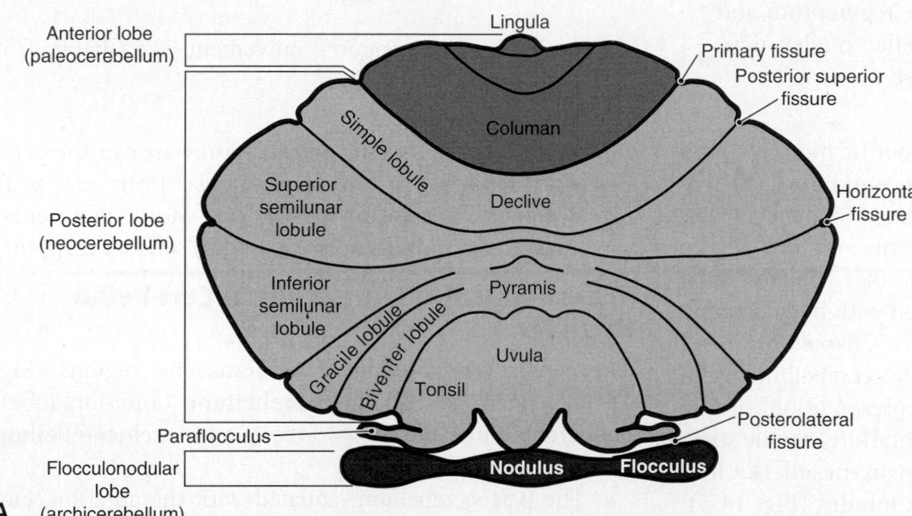

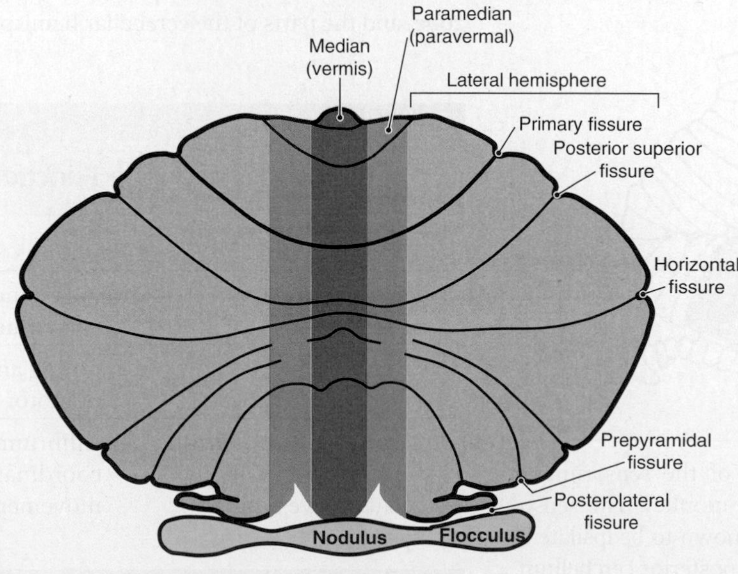

Figure 14-1 The cerebellum. A. Horizontal divisions of the cerebellum into archicerebellum (flocculonodular) lobe, the anterior lobe, and the posterior lobe (neocerebellum). B. Longitudinal divisions of the cerebellum into the vermal, paravermal, and lateral cortices.

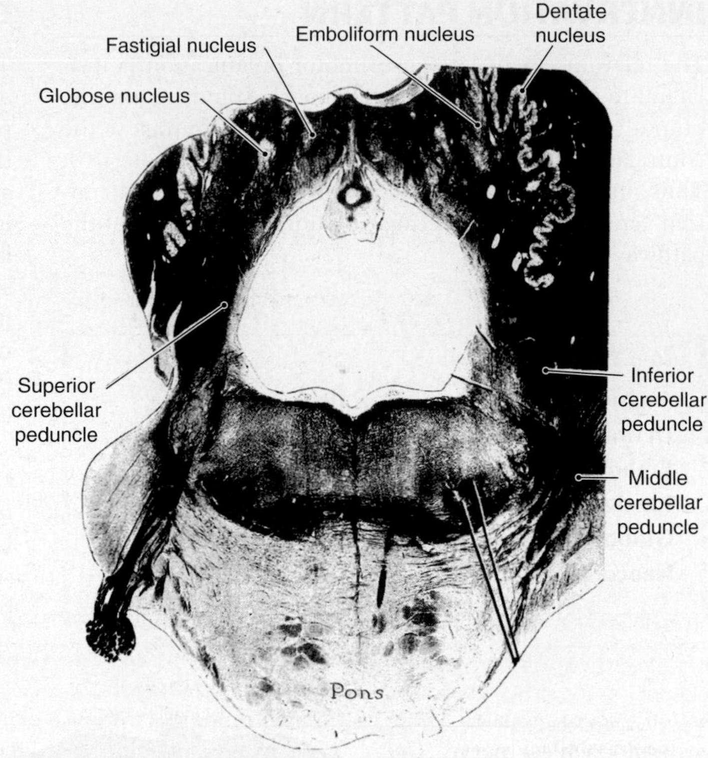

Figure 14-2 A section of the pontine tegmentum and cerebellum showing the deep cerebellar nuclei: dentate, emboliform, fastigial, and globose.

participates in the planning and coordination of limb movements, along with the motor cortex and basal ganglia. Emboliform and globose nuclei are related to spinocerebellar (unconscious proprioception) afferents and regulate the movements of ipsilateral extremities (see Chapter 11), whereas the fastigial nucleus, concerned with body posture, is related with the vestibular system (see Chapter 10).

Similar to the cerebral cortex, the cerebellum has a well-defined sensory and motor representation of the body. It has two sensory body representations: tactile stimulation activates potentials ipsilaterally in the anterior lobule and bilaterally in the paramedian lobules (Fig. 14-3).

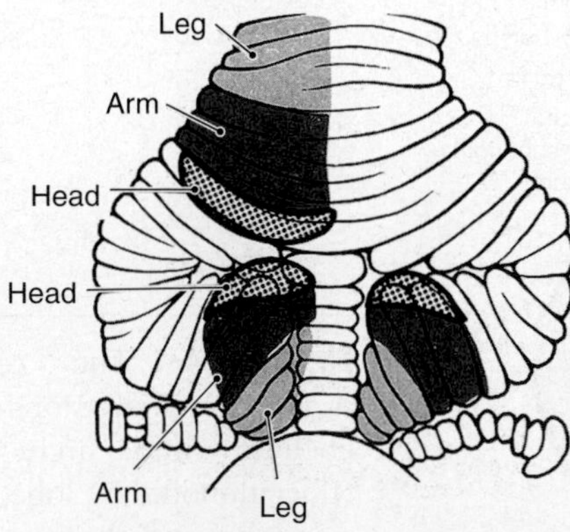

Figure 14-3 Somatotopic localization of the sensorimotor functions in the cerebellar cortex of a monkey. The sensorimotor representation of the body is known to be ipsilateral in the anterior lobe and bilateral in the posterior cerebellum.

An activation of a specific sensorimotor area in the cerebral cortex evokes a similar response from the same somatotopic region in the cerebellum. Motor representation tends to overlap the area covered by sensory mapping.

Transverse and Longitudinal Cerebellar Regions

The cerebellum contains three transverse regions (Fig. 14-1A; Table 14-1): **paleocerebellum** (anterior lobe), **neocerebellum** (posterior lobe), and **archicerebellum** (flocculonodular lobe).

The paleocerebellum, equated with the anterior cerebellar lobe, includes the superior vermis, the **paravermal zone**, and the parts of the cerebellar hemispheres. It receives

Table 14-1

Cerebellar Lobes and their Functions

Cerebellar Lobe	Functions
Paleocerebellum (anterior lobe)	Muscle tone, body posture, and equilibrium
Neocerebellum (posterior lobe)	Planning and coordination of motor movements
Archicerebellum (floccular nodular lobe) Closely related to vestibular system	Equilibrium and coordination of eye movements

impulses from proprioceptive stretch receptors (spindles) in the muscles of the arms, legs, trunk, and face. It is most concerned with muscle tone and walking posture. The cerebellar projections through the reticulospinal, rubrospinal (red nucleus to spinal cord), and vestibulospinal tracts modify muscle tone (see Chapter 13).

The neocerebellum (posterior lobe), developmentally newer and the largest part of the cerebellum, includes the remaining lateral region of the cerebellar hemisphere. Located between the primary and the posterolateral fissures, the neocerebellum receives crossed afferents from the contralateral sensorimotor cortex. The afferent fibers make up most of the crossed middle cerebellar peduncle. After the necessary sensorimotor integration processing, the neocerebellum projects to the contralateral motor cortex and spinal cord by way of the dentate nucleus and red nucleus; this underscores the ipsilaterality of the innervation pattern. It is concerned with the planning and coordination of the cortically directed skilled, movements, such as speaking, writing, and dancing.

The archicerebellum (or **vestibulocerebellum**), the oldest part of the cerebellum, includes the **nodulus** and paired **flocculi**. Related to the vestibular component of the vestibulocochlear nerve (CN VIII), it receives vestibular projections. The flocculi- and nodulus-containing lobe regulates muscle tone via the vestibulospinal tract (see Chapters 10 to 13) and is concerned with equilibrium and eye movements.

There are three longitudinal cerebellar regions (Fig. 14-1*B*): **vermal**, **paravermal**, and lateral hemispheres. The most medial region is the tree-like vermis, which contributes to body posture by regulating axial muscles (see Fig. 2.28). On either side of the vermis is the paravermal region, which is associated with the regulation of movements of ipsilateral extremities. The remainder of the cerebellar hemisphere forms the lateral zone, which, along with the red nucleus and motor cortex regulates or adjusts skilled movements of the ipsilateral extremities.

Cerebellar Peduncles

The inferior peduncle (restiform body), middle peduncle (brachium pontis), and superior cerebellar (brachium conjunctivum) peduncles connect the cerebellum to the brainstem (Fig. 14-4; see Figs. 2-29 and 2-30). All afferent and efferent fibers traveling to and from the cerebellum pass through these three bundles (Table 14-2). Fibers that travel through the inferior and middle cerebellar peduncles are largely afferent, mediating all sensorimotor input to the cerebellum. Fibers of the superior cerebellar peduncle are largely efferent transmitting cerebellar output to the brainstem and on to the thalamus, motor cortex, and spinal cord.

Afferent Pathways

With a 40:1 ratio of afferent to efferent fibers, the cerebellum receives inputs from the spinal cord, brainstem, and motor cortex (Fig. 14-4). The inferior cerebellar peduncle is an important afferent pathway through which ascending inputs from the distal limbs gain rapid entry to the ipsilateral cerebellum. The fiber bundles that enter through the inferior cerebellar peduncle are the **vestibulocerebellar** (information from the cristae of the semicircular ducts related to equilibrium), **dorsal spinocerebellar** (information related to unconscious proprioception from the muscle spindles and brainstem reticulation), **olivocerebellar** (information related to intended motor movement from the contralateral motor cortex), and **cuneocerebellar** (information related to proprioception from the stretch receptors of the upper limbs and neck) **tracts**.

Fibers entering the cerebellum via the middle cerebellar peduncle contain massive afferents from the cerebral motor cortex that synapse in the ipsilateral pontine nuclei. Forming the largest of the tracts to the cerebellum, the middle cerebellar fibers enter the cerebellum as the mossy fibers. The pontine nuclei, with inputs from the tectum (superior and inferior colliculi), also mediate visual and auditory information, which provide directional context for ongoing movement.

Efferent Pathways

The cerebellar efferents arise from three deep cerebellar nuclei—the dentate, emboliform, and globose—and course through the superior cerebellar peduncle (Fig. 14-4). Although the superior cerebellar peduncle also contains some afferents to the cerebellum from the proximate parts of the limbs, it is largely efferent. Carrying cerebellar efferents to the brainstem, thalamus, and motor cortex, the fibers of the superior cerebellar peduncle decussate at the level of the inferior colliculus (Fig. 14-4; see Fig. 3-15); some of the crossed fibers terminate in the contralateral red nucleus, although most continue and project to the thalamus on their way to the motor cortex. The cerebellar efferent fibers from the red nucleus also project to the spinal cord (contralateral γ-motor neurons), motor cortex, reticular formation (cranial nerves and vital brainstem centers), and vestibular nuclear complex (posture maintenance).

CEREBELLAR CORTEX

Structure

The cerebellar cortex is uniform in all areas and consists of three cellular (**molecular**, **Purkinje**, and **granular**) layers (Fig. 14-5). The molecular layer, the most external layer, is composed of parallel fibers (axons) running in a medial–lateral direction and synapsing with each successive **Purkinje cell** dendrite, much like telephone wires running through cross pieces of successive telephone poles. The middle layer is the Purkinje cell layer, which consists of a thin row of large nerve cells. Purkinje cell axons penetrate the granular cell layer, and most of these fibers terminate in deep cerebellar nuclei. All impulses leaving the

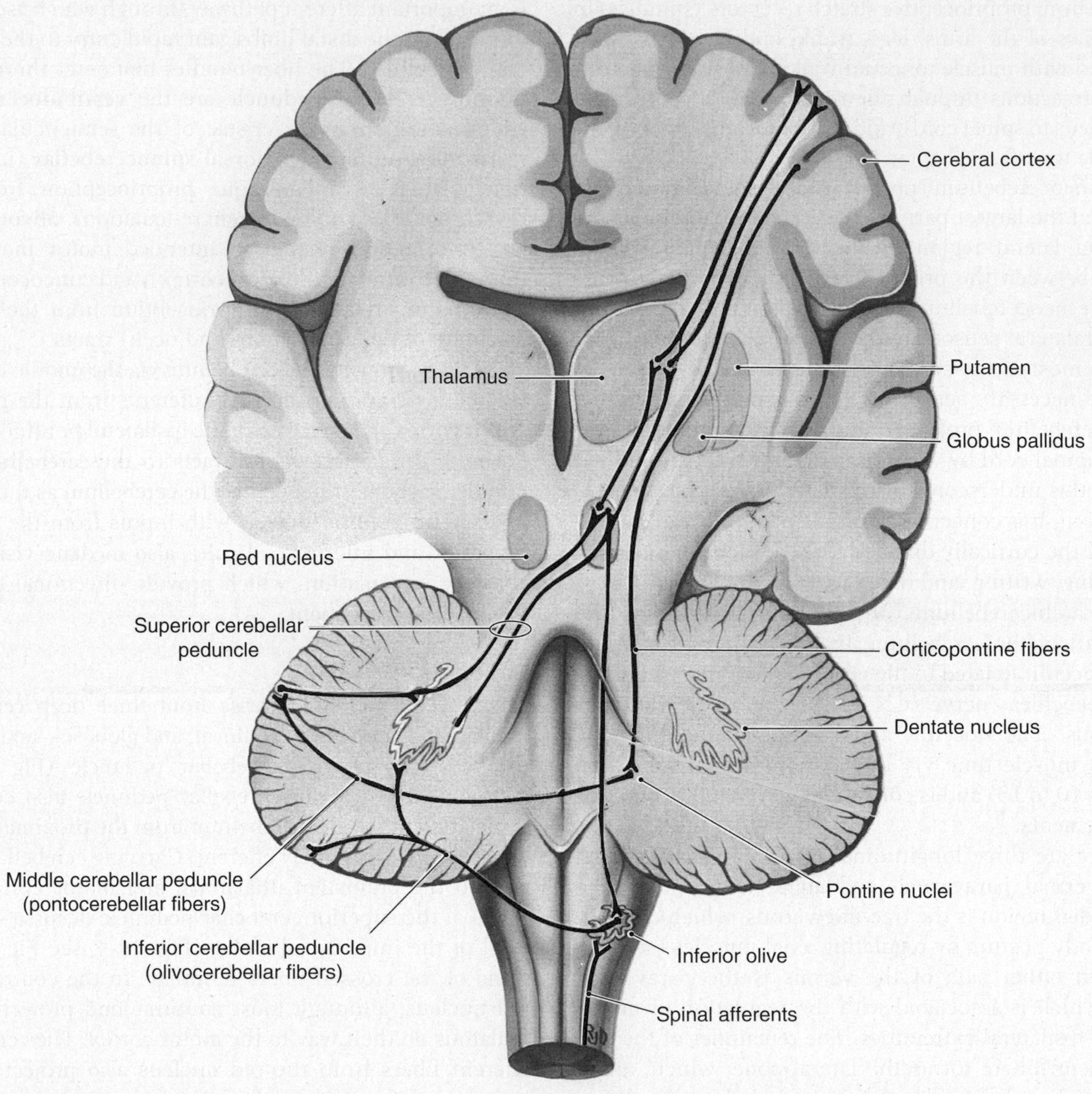

Figure 14-4 The principal afferent and efferent cerebellar projections traveling through the inferior, middle, and superior cerebellar peduncles. The olivocerebellar fibers traveling through the inferior cerebellar peduncle transmit brainstem and spinal projections to the cerebellum. Traveling through the middle cerebellar peduncle, the corticopontine and pontocerebellar fibers form the major cerebellar afferent system. Efferent fibers of the superior cerebellar peduncle ascend to contralateral motor cortex and descend to the brainstem reticular nuclei and spinal cord after decussating in the mesencephalon.

cerebellar cortex pass through a Purkinje axon. Granular cells have short dendrites that synapse onto the mossy fiber axons. The granular cells also project to the molecular layer and provide extensive axonal parallel fibers that synapse on the dendritic spines of the Purkinje cells.

> ***Key Terms :***
>
> **Climbing fibers** **Mossy fibers**
> **Deep nuclei**

Circuitry of a Cerebellar Functional Unit*

The microcircuitry of the cerebellum follows a uniform functional and anatomic pattern in all areas of the cerebellum: archicerebellum, paleocerebellum, and neocerebellum. All input axons, with branches to both the **deep nuclei** and cerebellar cortex, mediate excitatory (+) information to the outer cellular layer. Besides facilitating the

*This section is based on Guyton (1976).

Table 14-2

Afferent and Efferent Cerebellar Connections

Cerebellar Peduncle	Afferent Fibers	Efferent Fibers	Function
Inferior	Spinal cord, reticular formation, olivary nucleus, and stretch receptors of the upper limbs		Mediates sensorimotor information from the spinal cord and brainstem.
	Vestibular projections travel through juxtarestiform body.	Fastigiovestibular fibers	Mediates vestibular information.
Middle	Cerebral cortex via the pontine nuclei		Relays ongoing sensorimotor information from opposite cerebral hemispheres.
Superior		Projections from the dentate, emboliform, and globose cerebellar nuclei	Transmits cerebellar outputs to the brainstem, then to the thalamus, motor cortex, and spinal cord.
		Spinocerebellar feedback	Mediates ongoing movements.

deep nuclie, they also excite a stripe of Purkinje cell dendrites. Axons of the Purkinje cells, on the other hand, also project to inhibit (–) the activity of the deep cerebellar nuclei, which serve as the final cerebellar output. These neuronal circuits process all of the afferent information and form the outgoing cerebellar feedback essential for regulating muscle synergy and tone.

The neuronal circuitry of a functional unit consists of cerebellar-cortical cellular layers, deep nuclei, and afferent and efferent fibers (Fig. 14-6). There are millions of functional units, each with identical neuronal circuitry. All afferents to the cerebellum travel via either the **climbing** or **mossy fibers**. Climbing fibers, the most directly related to the cerebellar Purkinje cells, include all olivocerebellar projections (inferior cerebellar peduncle) to the cerebellar cortex. Highly developed in primates and humans, the **cortico-olivary cerebellar projections** of the climbing fibers provide the motor and premotor cortexes with a

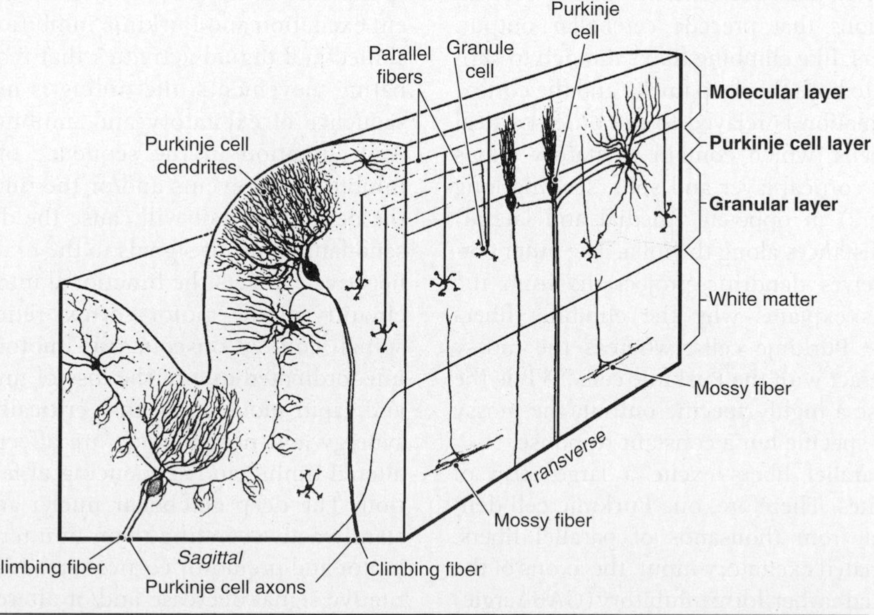

Figure 14-5 The cerebral cortex in transverse and sagittal planes showing the arrangement of the cellular layer and fibers.

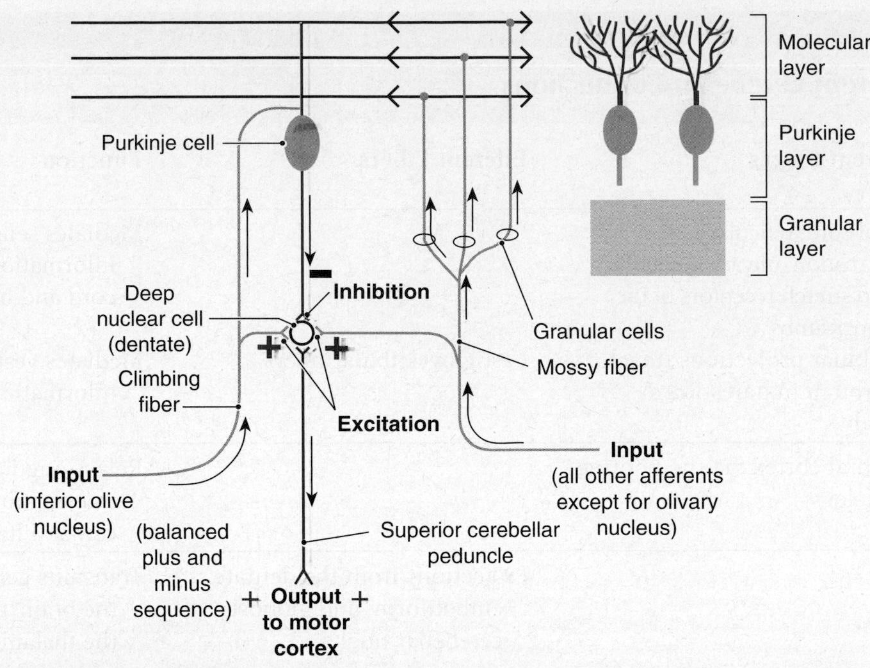

Figure 14-6 A cerebellar functional unit.

means of determining the activity status of the cerebellar region at any moment, an important aspect for regulating muscle synergy. The climbing fibers are extremely powerful and excitatory to the Purkinje cells and to deep nuclei cells. After sending excitatory **collaterals** to these cells (Fig. 14-6), the climbing fibers travel to the cerebellar cortex, where they synapse on the dendrites of Purkinje cells, which fire their inhibitory (GABAergic) synapses to the deep cerebellar nuclei.

Mossy fibers, which make up all other sources of afferent projections to the cerebellum, are related most directly to the sensory input systems concerned with the correlations and modulations that precede cerebellar output. First, the mossy fibers, like climbing fibers, branch to supply excitatory input to both the deep nuclei and the cortex. In the cortex, information is relayed to the outer cortical layer by granular cells, which contain excitatory axons that enter the outer cortical layer and split, sending long axons (parallel fibers) in opposite (medial and lateral) directions for long distances along the folia. The outer cortical layer also receives dendritic projections from the Purkinje cells. This explains why the climbing fibers directly activate the Purkinje cells, whereas the mossy fibers indirectly interact with the Purkinje cells. While the climbing fibers cause a highly specific output, the mossy fibers provide a less specific but a constant response.

The cortical parallel fibers excite a large strip of Purkinje cell dendrites. Therefore, one Purkinje cell dendrite receives input from thousands of parallel fibers. Mediating the summated excitatory input, the axons of the Purkinje cells, as noted earlier, form inhibitory (GABAergic) projections to the deep cerebellar nuclei, which are also bombarded by the prior excitatory inputs from both the climbing and mossy afferent fibers. The deep nuclei fire, depending on the relative timing and strength of the ascending and descending inputs, to provide cerebellar output. The cerebellar cortex also contains an elaborate series of inhibitory feedback circuits that regulate the general excitability of the cortex and prevent it from a general cerebellar seizure state.

Nature of Output

Under normal physiologic conditions, the cerebellar output to the cortex, basal ganglia, reticular formation, and spinal cord is excitatory, continuously balanced by afferent excitation and Purkinje inhibition of deep nuclei. For skilled and digital activities that require rapid and alternating movements, the timing is most important in the sequence of excitatory and inhibitory neuronal events. Any alteration in the sequence of excitatory (+) and inhibitory (–) events and/or the timing interval between the neuronal event will cause the deep cerebellar nuclei send faulty output signals to the brainstem. This, in turn, negatively affects the functional integrity of the neuronal circuitry of the motor cortex, reticular formation, and spinal cord. Consequently, motor functions become uncoordinated due to the loss of muscle synergy. Skilled and rapid movements that critically depend on muscle synergy and normal tone are affected most strongly by altered timing and sequencing of facilitation and inhibition. The deep cerebellar nuclei are known to be constantly active sending them uninterrupted signals to the motor and premotor cortical areas (Fig. 14-7). Any quantitative signal decrease and/or altered signal sequence in cerebellar output disrupts the cerebellar feedback that is essential for well-coordinated activity.

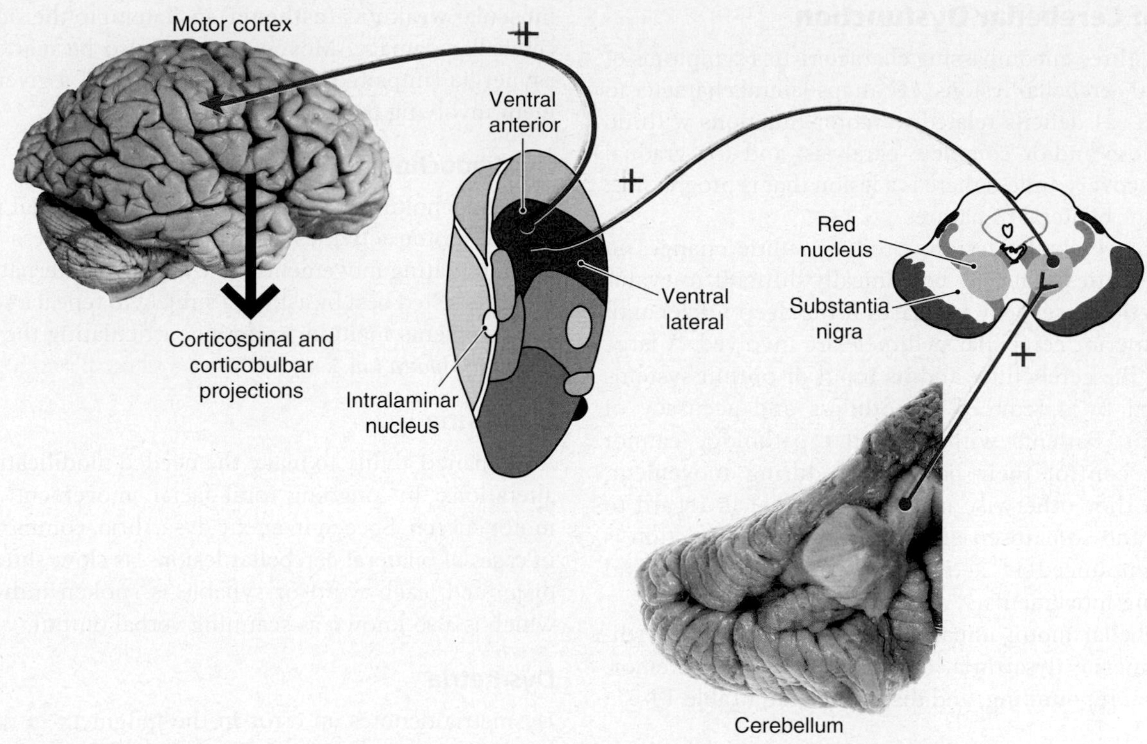

Figure 14-7 The principles of the cerebellar efferents to the motor cortex.

MOTOR LEARNING

The cerebellum has also been implicated with motor learning, which relates to its unique reorganizational ability. Motor learning begins with a conscious control of movement and gradually ends with the skill acquisition that no longer requires a conscious regulation of the tactile motor activities. What supports the role of the cerebellum in motor learning is that the patients with cerebellar pathology are known to lose movement automaticity and they revert back to the stage of conscious controlling of tactile motor patterns. This acquisition of skilled learning is related to increased and complex activity involving the climbing fibers. Once the motor skill is learned and tactile movements do not require voluntary control, the axonal activity in the climbing fibers is minimal and becomes random on achieving the motor automatism.

CLINICAL CORRELATES

The neocerebellar cortical region is essential for the learning of precision in sequential movements. It is not clear, though, whether the synaptic connectivity is necessary in the cerebellum alone, or somewhere else, or both. Smaller unilateral cerebellar lesions can be compensated by retraining. However, unless they occur in young children, massive and bilateral cerebellar lesions result in lack of adaptation and cause long-term effects.

Vision, which plays an important role in equilibrium, cannot compensate for cerebellar abnormality. In fact, vision helps differentiate between the disturbances of the cerebellum and dorsal column–medial lemniscal ascending system (see Chapter 11). For example, in the Romberg test, used to evaluate proprioception, a subject stands with arms extended in front, feet together, and eyes closed. If one of the arms drifts downward and/or the patient begins to tilt to one side because of unsteadiness, it can be caused by proprioceptive (cerebellar input or output) or vestibular abnormality. However, if the patient's eyes are open and the arm drifts or unsteadiness persists, the abnormality is in the cerebellum, not in the dorsal column–medial lemniscal system, since vision does not compensate for cerebellar malfunctioning.

Further distinction between vestibular and cerebellar abnormalities requires additional clinical observations, because lesions involving both systems produce unsteadiness and a tendency to fall to one side. The caloric test in each ear and vertigo testing can help determine the underlying cause.

Key Terms :

Asynergia	**Dysmetria**
Ataxia	**Friedreich ataxia**
Dysdiadochokinesia	**Intention tremor**
Dysarthria	**Rebounding**

Signs of Cerebellar Dysfunction

There are three encompassing characteristics symptoms of lateralized cerebellar lesions: (1) an ipsilateral character to the signs; (2) deficits related to motor functions with no sensory loss and/or complete paralysis; and (3) gradual natural recovery, unless there is a lesion that is progressive, massive, or bilateral in nature.

Minor cerebellar lesions produce subtle changes in motor activities that may be clinically difficult to evaluate. Functional severity increases if the deep nuclei and/or the superior cerebellar peduncle are involved. A large lesion in the cerebellum and its input or output systems is marked by a reduced smoothness and accuracy of movement. Patients with cerebellar pathology cannot precisely control their body parts during movement, although they otherwise may seem normal in regard to strength and somatosensation. Cerebellar dysfunction is most pronounced in activities that require rapid and alternating movements.

Cerebellar motor impairments include **ataxia**, **dysdiadochokinesia**, dysarthria, **dysmetria**, **intention tremor**, hypotonia, **rebounding**, and disequilibrium (Table 14-3).

Ataxia

Ataxia is lack of order and coordination in muscle activities. Uncoordinated motor activities are clumsy and decomposed into segments—for example, while walking and turning, a patient stops before making a turn and then turns in slow motion (**bradykinesia**). The subject then resumes walking awkwardly and slowly. There is mild muscular weakness (**asthenia**) ipsilateral to the side of the cerebellar damage. Movement may also be marked with **asynergia** (impaired direction and force of a given movement involving paired muscles).

Table 14-3

Clinical Signs of Cerebellar system

Ataxia	Clumsy and incoordinated movements
Dysarthria	Disjoined speech movements with reduced intelligibility
Dysmetria	Overshooting and undershooting of movements due to impaired judgment about the target distance
Intention tremor	Characteristic tremor movements that are present during an action and disappear during rest
Hypotonia	Reduced muscle tone (tension) makes muscle easily tired
Rebounding	Inability to predict, stop, or dampen movements
Disequilibrium	Impaired balance

Dysdiadochokinesia

Dysdiadochokinesia is a failure in the sequential progression of motor activities displayed by clumsiness in rapid and alternating movements. The ability to alternate movements is tested best by asking a subject to repeat a sequence of movements including tapping, articulating the syllabic sequence /*pa ta ka*/.

Dysarthria

An impaired ability to make the needed modifications and alterations in ongoing oral–facial movement impairs motor speech. Speech in ataxic dysarthria, commonly seen in cases of bilateral cerebellar lesions, is slow, slurred, and disjointed; each word or syllable is spoken individually, which is also known as scanning verbal output.

Dysmetria

Dysmetria denotes an error in the judgment of the range or the distance to the target movement. Examples of dysmetric error are the movements that fall short of the target (undershooting) and extend past it (overshooting) when touching a mark.

Intention Tremor

Intention tremor results from impaired ability to dampen accessory movements during a skilled movement sequence. Evident during a movement, the tremor becomes more severe as the target is approached—as demand for the function of the cerebellum becomes more important. Perhaps a better term for this clinical phenomenon is motion tremor, as the tremor disappears during rest. Intention tremor is different from resting tremor, which is a characteristic of Parkinson disease in which the patient exhibits a pill-rolling tremor only while resting (see Chapter 15).

Hypotonia

Tone is the slight tension that is constantly present in the muscle and easily detected during passive manipulation of the limbs. The functional cerebellum is trained via the γ-efferent influence on the stretch reflex to continuously optimize the motor tone of each muscle contributing to a movement. In hypotonia, normal muscle tension (resistance to passive stretch) is decreased and the muscle becomes floppy. Hypotonia ipsilateral to the side of cerebellar dysfunction is accompanied by asthenia, a condition in which the muscles are likely to tire quickly.

Rebounding

Rebounding reflects impaired motor tone adjustment as well as a loss of rapid and precise corrective response, as the patient loses the ability to predict, stop, or dampen movement. For example, if a flexed arm is held back and suddenly let go, a person with cerebellar pathology cannot detect the sudden limb release. The hand movement does not stop, and the patient is likely to strike his or her own face.

Disequilibrium

Impaired vestibular processing in the cerebellum results in disequilibrium that predominantly affects the legs. The gait is unsteady, and the body wavers toward the side of the lesion like people who are drunk.

Cerebellar dysfunction is tested by tandem gait, the finger-to-nose test, alternating movements, hopping, limb rebounding, and diadochokinetic movements. As with many other cerebral degenerative conditions, there is no treatment for degenerative cerebellar lesions.

Cerebellar Pathologies

Cerebrovascular Accident

The vertebrobasilar artery serves as the source of blood to all three cerebellar arteries: posterior inferior cerebellar, anterior inferior cerebellar, and superior cerebellar; each covering a specific cerebellar region (see Chapter 7). Thromboembolic or hemorrhagic involvement of the vertebrobasilar artery system interrupts blood circulation to the cerebellum. The posterior inferior cerebellar artery not only supplies the inferior surface of the cerebellum and the flocculonodular lobe but also supplies the inferior cerebellar peduncle and dorsal and lateral surfaces of the medulla. The cerebrovascular accident involving this artery produces symptoms related to damage of the vestibular and cochlear nuclei, spinocerebellar tracts, and various cranial nerves, such as the spinal tracts of the trigeminal, facial, glossopharyngeal, and vagus nerves (see Fig. 7-1)

Toxicity

Toxicity consequent to chronic alcoholism may cause progressive subacute cerebellar degeneration. Occurring mostly in late middle age, it is characterized by gross cerebellar atrophy and the loss of cellular elements in the anterior lobe, most crucially the Purkinje cells. The most significant symptom is a wavering (wide-based shuffling) gait similar to that of an intoxicated person. In half of the cases, the disturbance is limited to the lower extremities. In other cases, there is incoordination, dysmetria, and dyskinesia in the upper extremities as well. Speech becomes monotonous, slurred, or explosive, which disappears as the blood alcohol level attenuates with time. However, the remaining cerebellar deficits, once established, may not improve even with proper nutrition and vitamin treatment.

Progressive Cerebellar Degeneration

Many types of ataxias result from cerebellar degeneration. **Friedreich ataxia**, the most common progressive degenerative hereditary syndrome, is an autosomal recessive genetic condition characterized by combined sensory and motor dysfunctions. Most commonly affected are the cerebellar afferent (olivocerebellar or spinocerebellar) and efferent (dentatorubral) pathways. Usually appearing between ages 10 and 20 years, it is characterized by ataxia (incoordination), progressive imbalance (unsteadiness in walking), dysarthria, tremor, and weakness, loss of proprioception, nystagmus, dysmetria, and scanning speech.

CASE STUDIES FOR PROBLEM SOLVING

CASE ONE (14-1)

A 19-year-old man on the college basketball team began experiencing weakness in his legs; his movements were clumsy when he was playing and running. He was taken to the family physician, who noted the following signs:

- Broad-based gait
- Unsteadiness in walking
- Weakness in the lower limbs and loss of delicate movements
- Loss of proprioception and discriminative touch from both lower limbs
- Positive Romberg sign (the patient could not stand straight with his eyes closed)
- Release of primitive reflexes, such as positive Babinski sign

A brain MRI study revealed no pathologic changes in the spinal cord involving the dorsal and lateral funiculi at the lumbar level. Friedreich ataxia was suspected.

Question: How can you explain these symptoms?

Case (14-1) Discussion: See discussion of case studies

CASE TWO (14-2)

An 18-year-old male complained of headaches, nausea, and vomiting for the several months. He was first treated with aspirin. He returned to the hospital as his condition worsened, and he exhibited the following:

- Drowsiness
- Ataxia
- Spells of falling down
- Marked dysarthric speech

A brain MRI study confirmed a cerebellar tumor.

Question: How can you explain these symptoms?

Case (14-2) Discussion: See discussion of case studies

(Continued)

CASE THREE (14-3) *(CONTINUED)*

The speech quality of a 52-year-old speech language pathology professor with a drinking problem had deteriorated gradually. She denied any drinking problem and thought that it was nothing but fatigue from speaking in long classes. This provoked complaints from her students, who found her to be unintelligible particularly articulating complex technical terms. She was seen by a neurologist who noted the following:

- Disorientation and confusion
- Subdued personality
- Wide-based gait pattern
- Unstable posture with impaired balance
- Poor performance on finger-to-nose-test
- Moderately unintelligible speech

An SLP consultation revealed the following:

- Irregular alternate motion rate
- Vowel prolongation
- Distorted consonants
- Loudness variations
- Irregular articulatory breakdown (slowly articulated and periodically overexaggerated articulation)
- Amnesia for recent information but with preserved old memories
- Word-finding deficit

A brain MRI study revealed areas of atrophy in the orbital frontal region as well as in the area located dorsal to the brainstem.

Question: How can you account for the professor's somatosensory symptoms and speech-related disorders in light of the MRI findings?

Case (14-3) Discussion: See discussion of case studies

SUMMARY

The cerebellum does not initiate motor movements, nor does it alter sensation. It functions as a servomechanism, constantly monitoring body motor activities and comparing intended movements (planned by the motor and premotor cortex) against the updated sensory information it receives. By detecting discrepancies between sensory and motor states, it regulates the quality of motor movements generated elsewhere in the motor cortex or spinal cord. With its ability to make alterations for precision and smoothness during ongoing movement, the cerebellum is essential for learning and executing skilled movements. It contributes to muscle synergy, tone, and equilibrium. Signs of cerebellar dysfunction include hypotonia, ataxia, dysmetria, intention tremor, dysdiadochokinesia, dysarthria, and disequilibrium. Patients with cerebellar pathology lack the ability to control and regulate motor functions. Small lesions of the cerebellar cortex may cause minimal impairments. However, massive cerebellar damage involving the deep nuclei or the superior cerebellar peduncle can cause permanent and lasting deficits unless it occurs at a very young age. Cerebellar impairments do not affect reasoning, thinking, memory, or the comprehension of language.

REVIEW QUESTIONS

1. Complete the following statements using the appropriate technical terms:

   A. ________ is the muscle weakness caused by cerebellar dysfunctioning.

   B. ________ is the impaired ability to coordinate muscular activity during voluntary movement subsequent to a cerebellar pathology.

   C. ________ is a disorder of motor speech that results from central or peripheral disturbances and affects motor control of the articulators.

   D. ________ is the decomposed motor activity marked with the loss of speed and skill in a movement.

   E. As an error in the judgment of a movement's range and distance to the target, ________ is another cerebellar motor disorder.

   F. The ________ is the jerky motor action present during the performance of a targeted movement subsequent to a cerebellar pathology.

   G. ________ represents a reduced tone and lessened resistance to passive movement.

   H. As a disorder of impaired motor tone adjustment and the loss of rapid and precise corrective response, ________ refers to an inability to predict, stop, or dampen a movement.

2. Match each of the following statements with its associated neurological condition:

A. incoordination of muscular activity	a. ataxia
B. impaired control of distance and speed	b. dysmetria
C. impaired ability for controlling alternating movements	c. asthenia
D. muscle weakness	d. dysdiadochokinesia
E. inability to dampen accessory movements during voluntary movement	e. Rebounding
F. impaired ability to predict and stop movements	f. intention tremor

3. A lateralized cerebellar lesion is likely to cause motor dysfunctions marked by intention tremor, ataxia, asynergia, and dysdiodochokinesia; these dysfunctions would affect which half (ipsi- or contra-) of the body?
4. Name the most recently developed cerebellar lobe and describe its function.
5. What part of the cerebellum is likely to cause truncal ataxia, unsteadiness, and postural abnormality?
6. List four clinical signs of cerebellar pathology.
7. Name a common cerebellar degenerative disease.
8. Why is it that a person with cerebellar lesion demonstrates unsteadiness and arm drifting even with the eyes open?

15 Motor System 3: Basal Ganglia

LEARNING OBJECTIVES

After studying this chapter, students should be able to:

- Describe the role of the basal ganglia in movement
- Outline the anatomical structures of the basal ganglia and discuss their functions
- Describe the neuronal circuitry of the basal ganglia
- Outline the afferent and efferent projections of the basal ganglia circuits
- Describe the integrated inhibitory or excitatory influence of the afferent and efferent projections of the circuits
- Explain the clinical signs of basal ganglia impairments
- Outline the role played by primary neurotransmitters in the basal ganglia circuitry
- Discuss common neurologic conditions associated with the basal ganglia circuitry dysfunction.

The vertically organized hierarchical motor system (see Fig. 13-1), which also serves speech and other visceral motor activities, is regulated by motor inputs from various sources. Direct motor pathways, originating in the primary motor cortex (Brodmann area 4) and adjacent somatosensory regions, descend in the pyramidal (corticonuclear and corticospinal) tract to the motor neurons in the brainstem and spinal cord. Indirect cortical motor projections are to the basal ganglia (BG). In addition to cortical input, the brainstem and spinal motor neurons also receive projections from extrapyramidal sources that include the BG, cerebellum (see Chapter 14), vestibular nuclear complex (see Chapter 10), and reticular formation. Together these inputs refine the cortical motor directives to the lower motor neurons (LMNs) in the brainstem (see Chapter 17) and spinal cord (see Chapter 13).

BASAL GANGLIA MOTOR FUNCTIONS

As an encompassing circuit, the BG nuclei do not initiate motor activity; rather, they regulate cortically initiated motor activity including speech, by modifying it. Current understanding of the BG functioning is based on observations of movement disorders that result from the pathologies in their circuitry. Under normal physiologic conditions, the BG nuclei refine cortically generated movements by suppressing competing movements extraneous to precise and target motor activity. The BG nuclei also help adjust associated automatic motor movements (arm swinging during locomotion, follow-through during throwing, facial expressions, and basic emotional vocalization) and participate in learned reflex control, which relates to the automatic aspects of skilled motor activity after overlearning and adds grace to motor movements.

In general, the circuitry of the BG provides species-specific learned motor control and built-in reflex control patterns as a component of highly skilled movement sequences (Figs. 15-1 and 15-2). The motor cortex is very much involved in the early acquisition of all skilled movements. With practice, many aspects of learned movements later become motor automatisms and require some regulating role by the BG. One less-discussed aspect of BG nuclei is their role in higher mental functions. With greater axonal connections to the temporal and frontal cortex than those to the areas concerned with motor functions, the BG nuclei are also involved with memory, emotions, and cognitive and linguistic functions (Bhatnagar and Mandybur, 2006).

The BG nuclei do not directly control spinal motor neuronal activity. Instead, they use multiple parallel or serial channels to modify cortical motor activity within a period of approximately 100 ms, the estimated time difference between the activation of the cortical motor nuclei and the response by the target spinal motor nuclei. The BG nuclei primarily project their modifying ascending input to the cortical motor areas on the ipsilateral side by way of the thalamus; secondarily, they project their descending input to the contralateral brainstem reticular reflex network (Box 15-1).

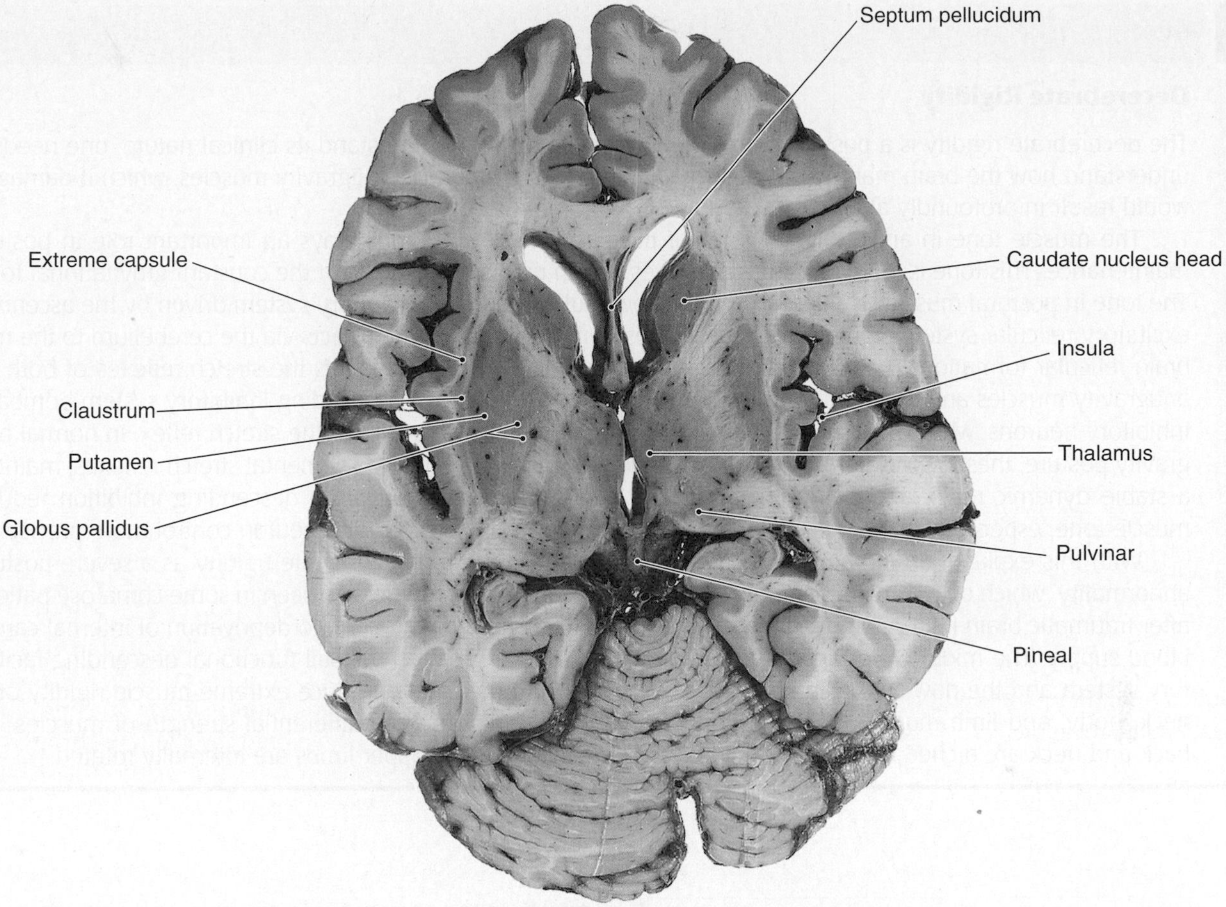

Septum pellucidum
Extreme capsule
Caudate nucleus head
Insula
Claustrum
Putamen
Thalamus
Globus pallidus
Pulvinar
Pineal

Figure 15-1 A view of basal ganglia nuclei on a horizontal section of the brain.

External capsule
Fornix
Claustrum
Thalamus
Extreme capsule
Putamen
Globus pallidus
Substantia nigra

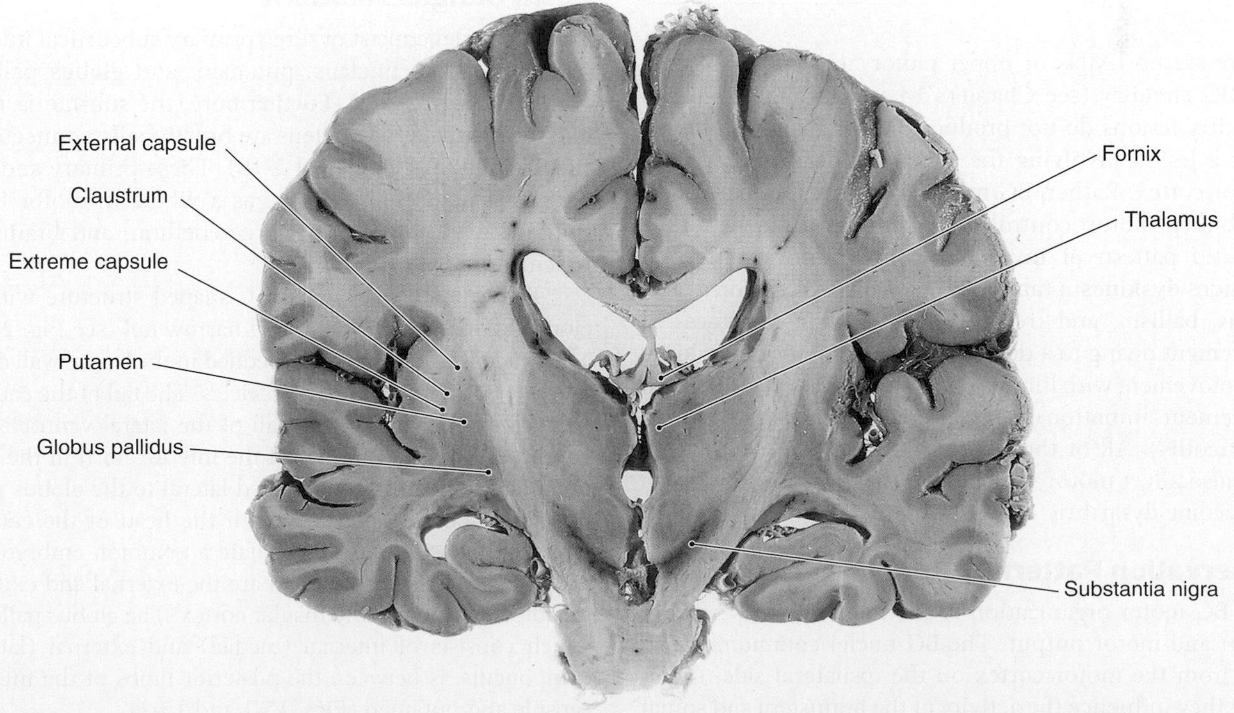

Figure 15-2 A view of basal ganglia on a coronal section of the brain at the midthalamic level.

BOX 15-1

Decerebrate Rigidity

The decerebrate rigidity is a postural tonal abnormality. In order to understand its clinical nature, one needs to understand how the brain maintains the normal postural state involving antigravity muscles, which if damaged, would result in profoundly altered muscle tone.

The muscle tone in antigravity muscles of the back, neck, and limbs plays an important role in postural maintenance. This tone is driven by stretch reflexes, which oppose the effects of the constant gravitational force. The tone in postural muscles is maintained by a powerful descending excitatory system driven by the ascending excitatory reticular system along with the active vestibular system, which projects via the cerebellum to the midbrain reticular formation. The descending excitation from this system facilitates the stretch reflexes of both the antigravity muscles and their antagonists. Coming from the forebrain, a descending inhibitory system bombards inhibitory neurons, which act on the same lower motor neuron components of the stretch reflex. In normal antigravity posture, these two systems (excitatory and inhibitory), in addition to segmental stretch reflexes, maintain a stable dynamic reflex antigravity tonic support. During fine movements, the descending inhibition reduces muscle tone, especially in distal flexor muscles making excitatory upper motor neuron control more precise.

With this explanation in background, it is easy to understand the decerebrate rigidity as a severe postural abnormality, which occurs in patients with a significant midbrain lesion. It is also seen in some comatose patients after traumatic brain injury and in patients with bilateral forebrain damage due to deprivation of internal carotid blood supply. The midbrain lesion causes a massive imbalance between the still functional descending facilitatory system and the now-absent inhibitory system that can immediately produce extreme muscle rigidity of all neck, body, and limb muscles. The consequent rigid posture results from differential strength of muscles: the back and neck are arched backward, the limbs are extended and the upper limbs are internally rotated.

Key Terms :

Akinesia **Dyskinesia**
Bradykinesia **Hypokinesia**

There are no LMNs or upper motor neurons (UMNs) in the BG circuitry (see Chapters 13 and 16); therefore, BG circuitry lesions do not produce the paralysis that is seen after a lesion involving the spinal cord and the primary motor cortex. Rather, BG nuclei lesions result in a loss of inhibitory motor control, and thus, patients exhibit a released pattern of involuntary motor movements that includes **dyskinesia** (abnormal movements of chorea, athetosis, ballism, and tremor), **bradykinesia** (slowness of movement owing to a decrease in spontaneity), **hypokinesia** (movement with limited excursion), **akinesia** (impaired movement initiation), and altered posture in **dystonia** (**torticollis**). All of these cannot be inhibited voluntarily and also affect motor speech quality and cause the speech to become dysarthric.

Innervation Pattern

The BG motor organization is contralateral to its sensory input and motor output. The BG nuclei communicate to and from the motor cortex on the ipsilateral side; therefore, they influence the activity of the brainstem and spinal nuclei on the opposite side. Consequently, the effects of a BG lesion are evident on the side of the body contralateral to the lesion (Fig. 15-3).

Basal Ganglia Anatomy

The BG nuclei consist of three primary subcortical nuclear masses: caudate nucleus, putamen, and globus pallidus (Figs. 15-1 and 15-2). Furthermore, the substantia nigra and the subthalamic nucleus are functionally connected to the BG (see Figs. 3-17 and 3-18). These primary and secondary structures participate as a whole in motor functions with the motor cortex, cerebellum, and brainstem reticular formation.

The caudate nucleus is a C-shaped structure with an elongated mass, large head, and narrow tail (see Fig. 2-17). The head of the caudate is embedded in the lateral wall of the anterior horn of the lateral ventricles. The tail of the caudate nucleus extends along the wall of the lateral ventricle and continues along the surface of the inferior horn in the temporal lobe. The putamen, located lateral to the globus pallidus, is connected anteriorly with the head of the caudate nucleus; this is because they share a common embryologic origin. Lateral to the putamen are the external and extreme capsules, claustrum, and insular cortex. The globus pallidus, which consists of internal (medial) and external (lateral) components, is between the posterior limbs of the internal capsule and putamen (Figs. 15-1 and 15-2).

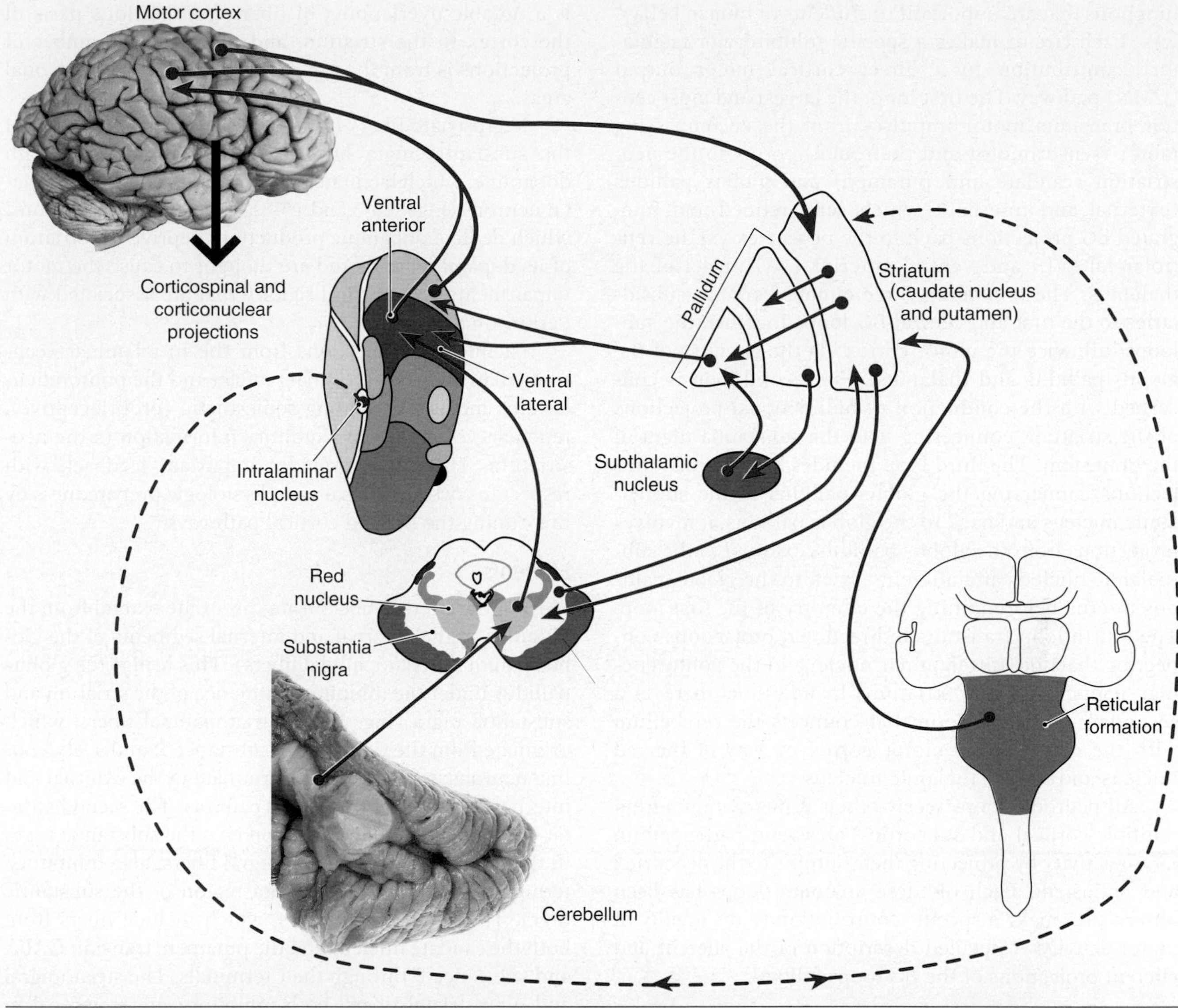

Figure 15-3 The components of the basal ganglia and their afferent and efferent projections. The major basal ganglia loops are as follows: 1. cortex → striatum → globus pallidus → thalamus (VL and VA nuclei) → cortex; 2. striatum → substantia nigra → striatum; 3. globus pallidus → subthalamic nucleus → globus pallidus; 4. thalamus (intralaminar nuclei) → striatum; 5. cerebellum → red nucleus → thalamus (ventrolateral and ventral anterior) → motor cortex. *Arrows* mark projections to targets.

Basal Ganglia Circuitry

The anatomy and physiology of the BG nuclei can be understood best if the nuclei are viewed as a series of interconnected (inhibitory or facilitatory), parallel-running loops with each loop processing corticostriatal information differently to modulate cortically generated efferents (Fig. 15-3). As a rule, cortical and brainstem afferents to the BG enter the striatum, whereas the integrated efferents of the BG leave through the globus pallidus and project to the cortex via the thalamus. The BG nuclei also receive reticular afferents from the thalamus (centromedianum nucleus) and send bidirectional projections to and from the substantia nigra and brainstem reticular reflex networks. The primary projections of the BG involve the central route of sensorimotor cortex → striatum → globus pallidus external → globus pallidus internal → thalamus (ventrolateral and ventral anterior nuclei) → primary motor cortex (Fig. 15-3).

There are four major loops or circuits of the BG; these circuits influence motor speech and cognitive functions that are important to students of human behaviors. Each circuit makes a specific inhibitory or facilitatory contribution to a direct cortical motor output (UMN) pathway. The first loop, the largest and most central, transmits motor impulses from the encompassing motor (sensorimotor and prefrontal) cortex to the neostriatum (caudate and putamen) and globus pallidus (external and internal), which send refined and integrated BG projections back to the neocortex via the ventrolateral (VL) and ventral anterior (VA) nuclei of the thalamus. The remaining three circuits serve as subsidiaries to the first and central BG loop. Together, the subloops influence the motor cortex via the circuitry of the globus pallidus and thalamus. The second loop is concerned with the conduction of bidirectional projections of the striatum, connecting it to the substantia nigra in the brainstem. The third loop includes bidirectional projections connecting the globus pallidus to the subthalamic nucleus and back to the globus pallidus; it involves projections from the globus pallidus, external to the subthalamic nucleus and afferents, back to the globus pallidus interna before joining the circuitry of the first loop. The fourth loop transmits bidirectional projections connecting thalamic intralaminar nuclei and the pontoreticular region with the striatum. In addition, there is a secondary (non-BG) loop that connects the cerebellum with the contralateral motor cortex by way of the red nucleus and the VL thalamic nucleus.

All neuronal loops receive their primary inputs from multiple cortical and subcortical areas and participate in motor activity by projecting their outputs to the neocortex and brainstem. Each of these anatomic loops has been observed to make a specific contribution to the quality of motor activity. A detailed description of the afferent and efferent projections of the BG loops follows.

Striatum

The striatum, made up of the caudate nucleus and putamen, uses GABAergic projections to inhibit the activity of the globus pallidus and substantia nigra.

Afferents

The striatum receives input from the cortex (corticostriate fibers), substantia nigra (nigrostriate fibers), thalamus (thalamostriate fibers), and brainstem reticular formation (reticulostriate fibers) (Fig. 15-3). The glutamate-carrying corticostriate fibers, which are excitatory, project from all parts of the primary and associational (premotor and supplementary) motor cortical areas to the caudate nucleus and the putamen. The corticostriate connections are reciprocal, and there is no greater representation of the cortex in one area of the striatum than another. Most of these projections from the cortex enter the caudate nucleus and putamen through the internal capsule, but some enter from the external capsule. There is a notable overlapping of fibers from various parts of the cortex to the striatum, and the greatest number of projections is from the prefrontal and other associational areas.

Nigrostriate fibers from the **pars compacta** region of the substantia nigra have axonal terminals filled with dopamine, which facilitates some but mostly inhibits striatal neurons (Figs. 15-3 and 15-6). Substantia nigra lesions, which deplete dopamine production, deprive the striatum of its dopamine input and are thought to cause the motor impairments, tremor, and rigidity that are associated with Parkinson disease.

Facilitatory projections from the intralaminar (centromedian and parafascicular) nuclei and the pontoreticular area mediate ascending somesthetic (proprioceptive), reticular, vestibular, and auditory information to the neostriatum. This input provides important feedback with respect to cortical arousal and physiologic preparedness by fine-tuning the BG and cortical pathways.

Efferents

Most of the efferent fibers from the striate extend from the putamen to the external and internal segments of the globus pallidus (striatopallidal fibers). This brings the globus pallidus under the inhibitory influence of the striatum and substantia nigra (Fig. 15-3). Striatopallidal fibers, which originate from the GABAergic, substance P, and acetylcholine neurons in the striatum, terminate in the external and internal segments of the globus pallidus. The second striatal GABAergic efferent projection is to the substantia nigra in the mesencephalon. Striatonigral fibers, also inhibitory, terminate in the **pars reticulata** region of the substantia nigra. The striatonigral fibers, which include fibers from both the caudate nucleus and the putamen, transmit GABA and substance P through their terminals. The striatonigral and nigrostriatal fibers, both inhibitory, are reciprocal in organization.

Globus Pallidus

The wedge-shaped globus pallidus, serving as the striatal and BG output to the thalamus, consists of external and internal components (Figs. 15-1 and 15-2).

Afferents

Afferents entering the globus pallidus arise from the striatum and the subthalamic nucleus. All striatal afferents to the globus pallidus are GABAergic and thus inhibitory; more importantly, its own neurons are GABAergic and thus inhibitory. Its afferents from the subthalamic nucleus are glutamatergic and, therefore, facilitatory.

Efferents

As the output nucleus of the BG, the globus pallidus projects to the thalamus via the pallidothalamic fiber bundles (Fig. 15-4). The major BG output to the

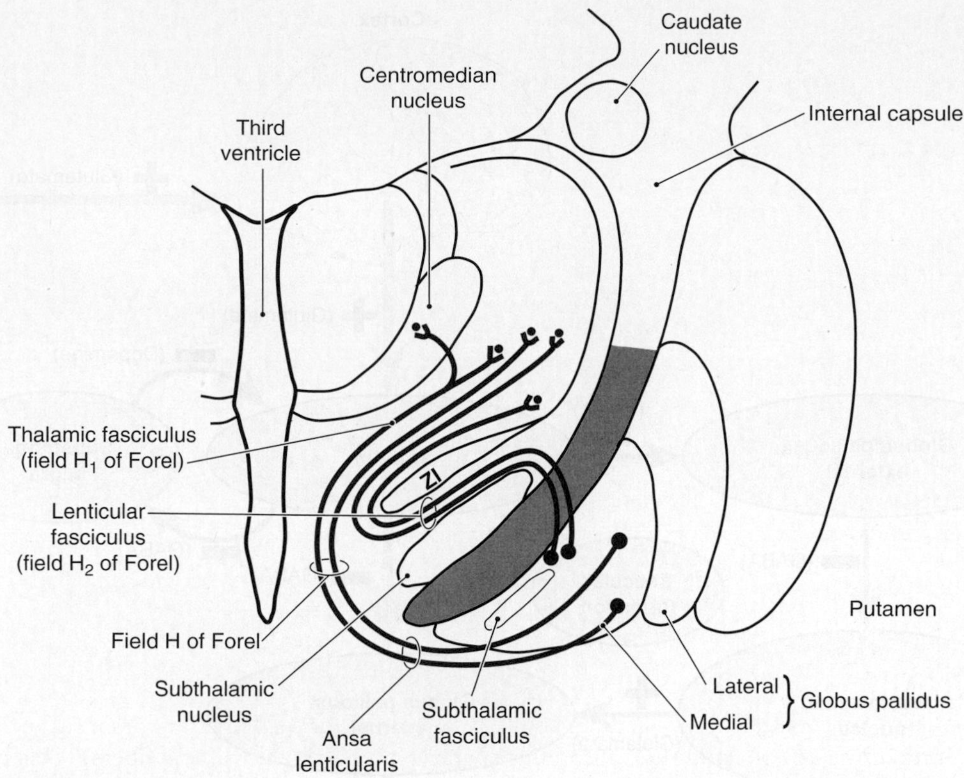

Figure 15-4 Origin and course of the pallidothalamic (ansa lenticularis and lenticular fasciculus) projections. The fibers of the ansa lenticularis travel around the internal capsule and enter the prerubral field (field H of Forel). The fibers of the lenticular fasciculus leave the inner globus pallidus and course through field H_2 of Forel and join the fibers of the ansa lenticularis to form the thalamic fasciculus (field H_1 of Forel).

thalamus, which is GABAergic and inhibitory, arises from the internal segment of the globus pallidus and terminates in the VL and VA nuclei of the thalamus (see Chapter 6). These pallidal projections are transmitted through two fasciculi: **ansa lenticularis** and **lenticular fasciculus** (Fig. 15-4).

Three anatomic structures that pertain to the pallidothalamic fibers can be confusing: field H of Forel (prerubral area), field H_1 of Forel, and field H_2 of Forel. These three fields of H are where the pallidothalamic fibers cross the internal capsule, turn laterally to move upward, and enter the thalamus. Fibers of the ansa lenticularis loop around the internal capsule and enter field H of Forel (prerubral field) in the subthalamic region. They turn rostrally and laterally, forming part of the thalamic fasciculus, in field H_1 of Forel. Conversely, the lenticular fasciculus fibers pass through the internal capsule and appear as field H_2 of Forel. The lenticular fasciculus fibers join the ansa lenticularis fibers at field H_1 of Forel and merge to form the **thalamic fasciculus**. The thalamic fasciculus fibers terminate in the VL nucleus of the thalamus, which projects to the motor cortex. The VL and VA thalamic nuclei also receive cerebello cortical projections from the contralateral dentate nucleus of the cerebellum. Thus, at the thalamic level, the cerebellocortical projections intermingle with the BG projections to the cortex.

The fibers from the external region of the globus pallidus also send inhibitory (GABAergic) projections to the subthalamic nucleus (Figs. 15-3 and 15-6), which sends its facilitatory (Glutamate) projections to the inner region of the globus pallidus. In addition, descending BG output also travels to the reticular reflex network in the midbrain tegmentum (Fig. 15-3). Interruption of these projections to the subthalamus and reticular network has been associated with disorders of associated movements, such as arm swinging during locomotion and follow-through during throwing.

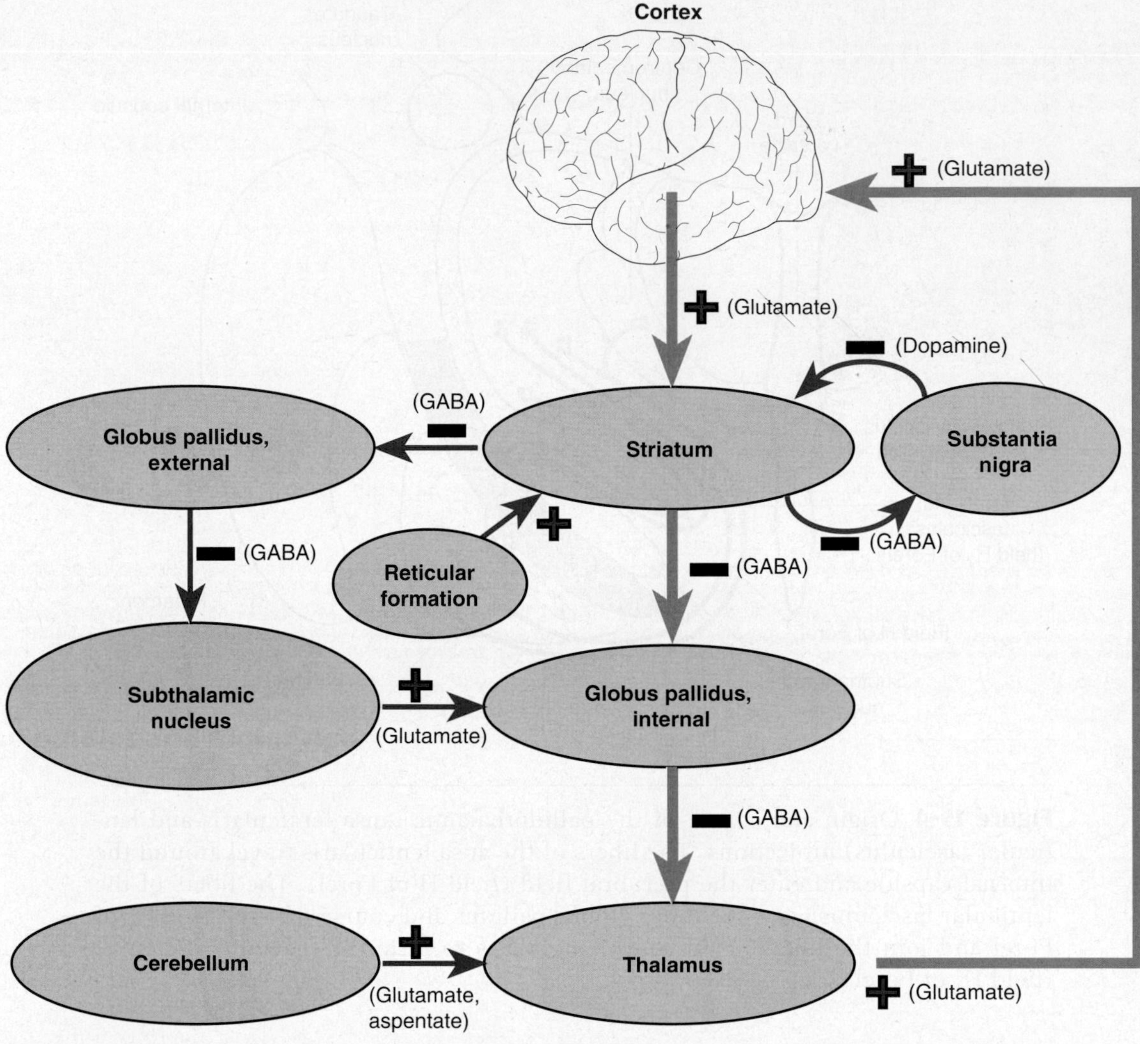

Figure 15-5 The inhibitory and excitatory basal ganglia loops along with their probable neurotransmitters.

Subthalamic Nucleus

The subthalamic nucleus, a lens-shaped structure, is located next to the inner surface of the internal capsule and above the medial part of the substantia nigra (see Figs. 3-18 and 3-23). Anatomically linked with the globus pallidus of the BG, its dysfunction is associated with ballism on the side opposite of the lesion.

Afferents

The BG enkephalin and GABAergic (inhibitory) afferents to the subthalamic nucleus emerge from the external segment of the globus pallidus (Fig. 15-3). Additional excitatory and inhibitory projections come from the motor cortex and the substantia nigra.

Efferents

Subthalamic efferents include glutamatergic (facilitatory) projections, primarily to the internal globus pallidus (Fig. 15-3). With its integrated facilitatory efferent projections to the inner pallidal region, the subthalamic nucleus can modulate all output from the striatal system. An important clinical point about this circuitry is that the globus pallidus and subthalamic nucleus have been chosen as the optimal site for the neurosurgical treatment of tremor and rigidity in Parkinson disease; the primary goal of the pallidotomy (lesion placement in the pallidus) and inducing a functional lesion through the stimulation of the subthalamus is to attenuate the inhibitory output from the globus pallidus with a net facilitatory effect on the cortical motor movement.

Substantia Nigra

The substantia nigra, a mesencephalic horizontal band of neurons, consists of the **pars compacta** and **pars reticulata** regions. The pars compacta region is packed with dark-pigmented neuromelanin-containing cells that produce

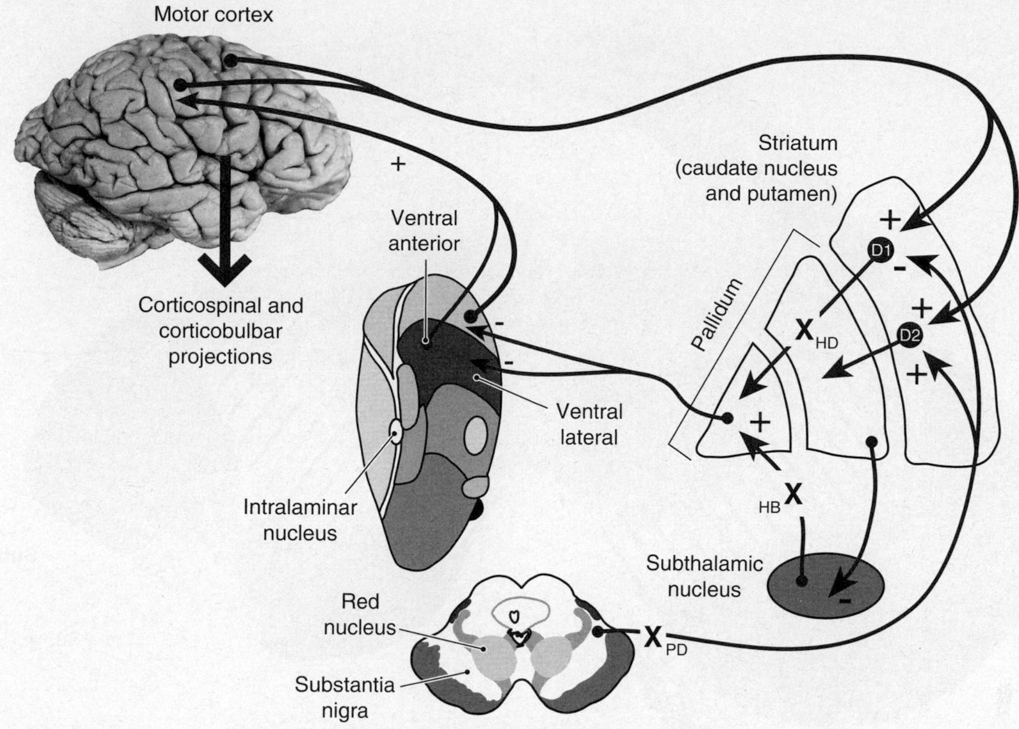

Figure 15-6 A schematic illustration of anatomic-chemical disconnectivity involving the pathways underlying basal ganglia diseases like Parkinson (PD) with two dopaminergic receptors in the striatal neurons: D1(direct) and D2 (indirect). The D1 receptors (incorporating GABA and substance p) are facilitatory to cortical motor movement. The D2 receptors (incorporating GABA and enkephalin neurotransmitters) have a net inhibitory impact on the cortical motor movement (as their facilitation of the globus pallidus is inhibitory to thalamus). The loss of nigrastriatal projections in PD not only impedes the facilitation of D1 receptors but also disinhibits D2 receptors. This disconnectivity results in reduced (bradykinesic/akinesic) movements of PD. Subthalamic stimulation and pallidotomy improves the movement quality by reducing inhibitory GP output to the thalamus. Also depicted are the lesion sites associated with Huntington chorea and hemiballism.

dopamine or dopamine precursors. Degeneration of the neuromelanin-containing cells in the substantia nigra has been associated with Parkinson disease (Fig. 15-7).

Afferents

The major input to the substantia nigra comes from the striatum via the striatonigral fibers; these GABAergic striatal projections inhibit the functioning of neurons in the substantia nigra (Figs. 15-3 and 15-6). The substantia nigra also receives some secondary projections from the subthalamic nucleus and pontoreticular formation.

Efferents

The substantia nigra projects back to the striatum through its terminals, which contain dopamine. Dopamine inhibits most of the striatal functioning (Fig. 15-3). The substantia nigra's afferent and efferent projections involve different neurotransmitters, though both are inhibitory. The projections from the substantia nigra are also to the brainstem reticular formation.

Physiology of Basal Ganglia Circuitry

The physiology of the BG is discussed in terms of its ascending feedback to the motor cortex. The BG nuclei influence the activity of the motor cortex by facilitating, inhibiting, or disinhibiting (release from inhibition) other components of its circuitry and their projections using the neurotransmitters that are facilitatory or inhibitory, such as glutamate, dopamine, GABA, acetylcholine, enkephalin, and substance P. The circuitry modulation regulates the net inhibitory output of the BG to the thalamus, which contains intrinsically facilitatory output to the motor cortex (Fig. 15-6).

In a normal physiologic state, the neostriatum receives largely facilitatory (+) afferents from the motor (premotor, motor, and supplementary motor) and association cortical areas, the thalamic intralaminar centromedian nucleus,

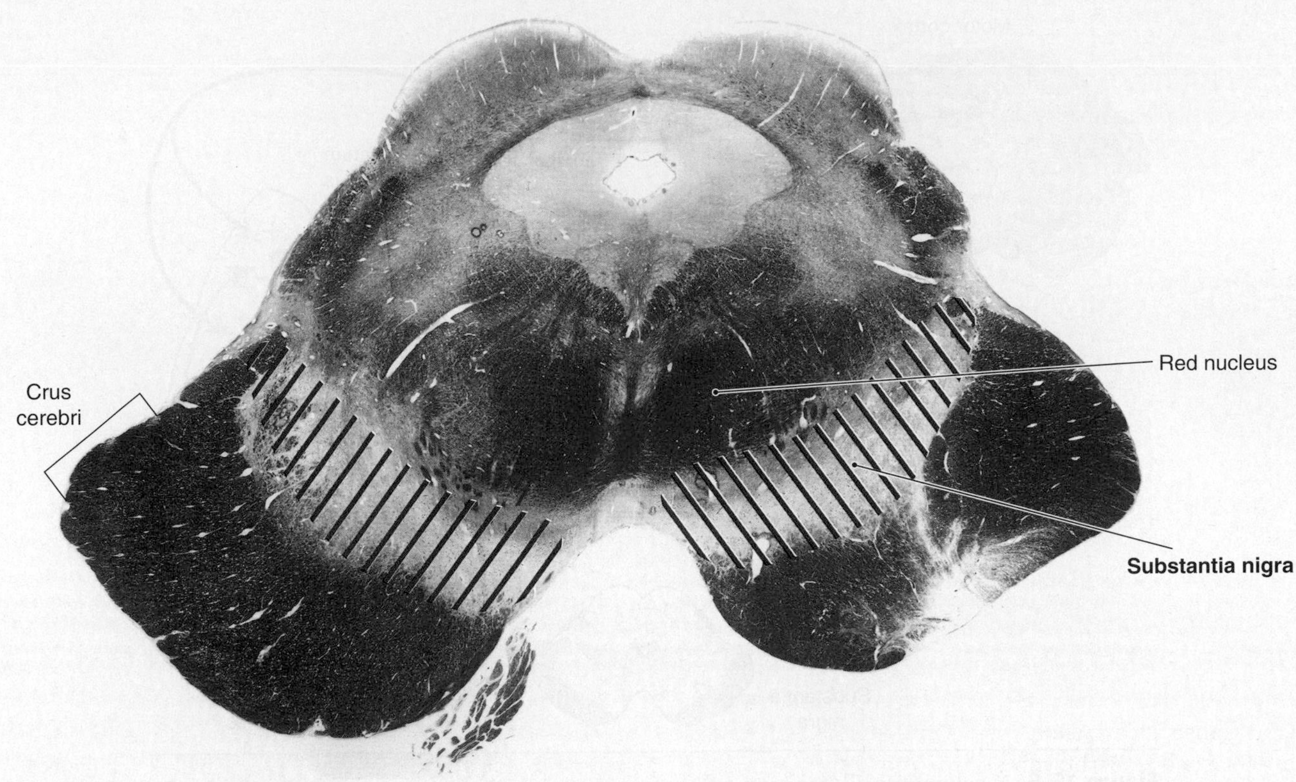

Figure 15-7 Schematic illustration of a degenerative lesion in the substantia nigra.

and the pontoreticular formation. These afferents are glutamatergic. Neostriatal influence on both segments of the globus pallidus (external and internal), subthalamic nucleus, substantia nigra, and thalamocortical system is inhibitory (–). Neostriatum uses two different connections to influence the internal and external divisions of the globus pallidus (Fig. 15-5).These pathways (loops) have opposite effects on the thalamocortical motor system. The "direct" connections (loop) originate from the striatal neurons containing GABA and substance P. Increased activity in these neurons leads to inhibition of the globus pallidus internal, thus with net facilitatory effect on the thalamocortical system and motor cortex. Different striatal neurons containing GABA and enkephalin form the "indirect" pathway (loop). This indirect pathway, passing through the subthalamic nucleus acts, is a disinhibitory to the external globus pallidus and facilitatory to the internal globus pallidus with a net inhibitory effect on thalamocortical projections resulting in a decreased activation of the motor cortex. Similarly, an increased activation of the subthalamus (such as through stimulation) results in a reduced inhibitory output from the globus pallidus, with a net facilitating effect on movement (Fig. 15-6).

The nigrostriatal projections render additional complexity to the BG circuitry. The dopaminergic projections from the substantia nigra (pars compacta), largely inhibitory to most of the striatum, differently influence the neurons with dopaminergic receptors (D1—direct and D2—indirect). The dopaminergic nigrostriatal projections facilitate the striatal neurons (GABA and substance P) with D1 dopamine receptors, but the nigrostriatal efferents inhibit the striatal neurons (GABA and enkephalin) with D2 receptors with indirect path. In normal physiologic condition, the activity of both of these dopaminergic pathways activates the thalamus and thalamocortical system (Fig. 15-4).

The globus pallidus external, which receives inhibitory GABAergic projections from the striatum, is further disinhibitory to the globus pallidus internal and to the subthalamic nucleus; the subthalamic nucleus, in turn, facilitates the internal globus pallidus using glutamatergic impulses. The globus pallidus, integrating all the extrinsic and intrinsic impulses of the BG circuitry, is net inhibitory to the thalamus, which integrates the inhibitory BG output with corrective and facilitatory cerebellar (aspartate) output and sends glutamatergic projections with net intrinsic facilitation of the motor cortex (Fig. 15-6).

The functional quality of the striatal activity depends on the effectiveness of the balance provided by the inhibitory dopaminergic projections and the facilitatory afferents from the cortex, reticular formation, and centromedian nucleus. An imbalance in the facilitatory and inhibitory circuits disinhibits the BG output, resulting in an altered cortical activation associated with a variety of movement disorders, such as bradykinesia, akinesia, dystonia, chorea, ballism, and tremor.

Basal Ganglia Neurotransmitters

The function of the BG depends on a balanced interaction involving the major neurotransmitters: glutamate, dopamine, acetylcholine, GABA, enkephalin, and substance P. All of these neurotransmitters, except glutamate and acetylcholine, are inhibitory and are vital to the regulation of motor movements. Dopaminergic neurons from the substantia nigra project to the striatum (caudate nucleus and putamen) and inhibit facilitatory cholinergic (acetylcholine) as well as inhibitory GABAergic neurons, which project intrinsically to the globus pallidus, subthalamus, and the substantia nigra in the BG. Terminals with substance P, enkephalin, and GABA project to the globus pallidus and substantia nigra. Enkephalin projections to the surrounding structures, such as the thalamus, primarily participate in controlling pain and may inhibit movements. Further, the serotonin projections from the midbrain to the striatum participate in the metabolic activity of the BG by regulating the striatal GABAergic neurons. Impairment within a neurotransmitter system results in specific movement disorders, such as Parkinson disease and Huntington chorea (Box 15-2).

CLINICAL CORRELATES

In addition to serving personality, cognitive, and language functions (a lesser known function), the BG nuclei serve an important role in refining motor activity. The involvement of various neurotransmitters differentially affects the quality of motor functions. BG diseases result in a loss of precision and inhibitory control, which leads to an inappropriate release of patterned motor behavior, involving dyskinesia (involuntary movements, such as tremor at rest, chorea, athetosis, dystonia, and ballism), bradykinesia (slow movement), hypokinesia (movements with limited range), and disturbance of posture (Table 15-1).

The involuntary movements of dyskinesia interrupt the phasic motor activities of the speech musculature (dysarthria) or the limbs. At this time, only limited chemical and surgical treatment is available for BG disorders; the goal of such treatments is to restore the optimal inhibitory function of the BG largely by obliterating the pathologic component of the circuitry or by mimicking or inhibiting the neurotransmitters. While supplementing dopamine secretion with L-dopa (Sinemet) has been used with limited success, adrenal-medulla transplant has not proven to be the treatment of choice in United States; the deep brain stimulation (DBS) of the subcortical (subthalamus or globus pallidus) structures appears to be the most promising avenue of treatment at this point.

DBS has become more effective and accessible in the treatment of movement disorders, especially Parkinson disease, essential tremors, and generalized dystonia. The surgical placement of a lesion (stereotaxy) in the brain as a treatment for movement disorders has been available for over 50 years, but only recently have technological advances allowed for reversible perturbation of specific nuclear sites within the brain with deep stimulation. The technique requires precision guidance of a narrow stimulating electrode that is permanently implanted with a pacemaker-like

BOX 15-2

A Continuum of Dopaminergic Abnormality

Schizophrenia (characterized by disorganized thoughts and confused language) and Parkinson disease (characterized by bradykinesia, rigidity, and tremor) are related to two opposite ends of dopaminergic activity. Excessive functional activity in the mesocortical dopaminergic projections and/or oversensitivity involving certain dopaminergic receptors are two possible causes of schizophrenia. On the other hand, underactive mesostriatal dopaminergic projections secondary to the degeneration in the substantia nigra leads to akinesia, rigidity, and tremor of Parkinson syndrome.

This neurotransmitter continuum is well figured in the treatment that is provided in both conditions. Schizophrenia is treated with antipsychotic drugs (like Haldol and Chlorpromazine), which reduce the dopaminergic activity in the neurons of the ventral tegmental area by blocking the dopamine receptors in the projected areas of nucleus accumbens, amygdala, hippocampal gyrus, and the prefrontal cortex. One of the side effects of the dopamine blockers is that their long-term use induces movement disorders. Conversely, augmenting dopamine in the treatment of Parkinson (e.g., with L-dopa) has the long-term risk of adversely affecting the thought processes and causing symptoms typical of schizophrenia.

Tardive dyskinesia is another drug side effect; it is marked with involuntary movements localized in the facial muscles. It is caused by a long-term use of antipsychotic medications that are used to treat behavioral, personality, and thought abnormalities. The facial movements persist even after the medications are discontinued.

Table 15-1

Movement Disorders and Diseases

Lesion Site	Involuntary Movements	Pathological Conditions
Globus pallidus and corpus striatum (putamen)	Athetosis: constant slow twisting movements in muscles of upper extremities	Toxicity, striatal degeneration, and hypoxia owing to carbon monoxide poisoning
Subthalamic nucleus	Ballism: wild swinging movements that usually involve one side of body	Stroke or denervation
Striatum (primarily caudate nucleus)	Chorea: rhythmic and quick involuntary movements of the muscles in proximal extremities	Huntington chorea
Substantia nigra (dopaminergic deficiency owing to degenerative changes in substantia nigra)	Dyskinesia: sustained accessory movements with a desired motor act Akinesia: difficulty in initiating a movement Bradykinesia: slowness of movement Hypokinesia: quick movements of smaller range Tremor: rhythmic pill-rolling movements of fingers at rest accompanied by akinesia and rigidity	Parkinson disease

programmable battery pack. This treatment is used mainly when medications fail to control symptoms adequately. Effectiveness can range from improved gait and increased movement to nearly 100% of tremor relief depending on what structure/site is selected (Bhatnagar and Mandybur, 2006). The philosophy underlying the DBS is to use an externally applied current to create a reversible functional lesion in the subthalamus with a goal to reduce the inhibitory BG output from the globus pallidus with facilitatory impact on the thalamocortical system, which in turn attenuates akinesia and associated movement disorders.

Key Terms :

Athetosis
Ballism
Chorea
Dystonia
Myoclonus
Tremor
Torticollis

Signs of Basal Ganglia Dysfunction

Athetosis

Athetosis refers to the slow, involuntary twisting of predominantly mostly upper limb and speech muscles accompanied by varying degrees of hypertonia in between movements. Athetosis of the buccofacial muscles causes speech to become dysarthric. These movements occur in a sequence so that they blend together to form a continuous action. Athetotic movements commonly occur after a lesion involving the globus pallidus that affects its descending projections to the brainstem reticular network and ascending projections to the cortex.

Ballism

Ballism, the most violent form of dyskinesia, is characterized by forceful, swinging, jerky, and sudden movements of the arms and legs. It may also involve the neck musculature. The swinging movements involve one side of the body (hemiballism) and are usually associated with a destructive lesion in the subthalamic nucleus contralateral to the side with the dyskinesia. These ballistic movements are known to result from a loss of the facilitatory output from the subthalamic nucleus to the globus pallidus, which in turn sends more net inhibitory projections to the thalamus and to the motor cortex.

Chorea

Chorea is a series of brief, rhythmic, and jerky yet graceful involuntary movements involving multiple muscles. The choreic movements occur predominantly in the upper distal extremities and muscles of the face, tongue, and pharynx, which affect speech and swallowing. The affected muscles are in a hypotonic stage when not in contraction.

Two common BG diseases associated with chorea are **Sydenham** and **Huntington**. Sydenham chorea is a postinfectious condition that usually appears in childhood several months after a streptococcal infection with subsequent rheumatic fever. The clinical characteristics (purposeless involuntary contractions of the muscles in the upper limbs, hypotonia, and emotional lability) become apparent between ages 5 and 13 years. Improvement occurs over weeks or months, and exacerbations of the disease can occur without recurrence of infection.

Huntington chorea, a more common clinical condition of adult onset, is inherited through an autosomal-dominant gene. This progressive neurologic condition is additionally characterized by cognitive deficits (dementia), dysarthric speech, and altered personality. It is associated with degenerative changes in the caudate nucleus and frontal and parietal lobes.

Tremor

Tremor, the most common form of dyskinesia, consists of constantly alternating motor activity in one or more parts of the body. The tremor, which results from the alternate contraction of opposing muscles, occurs in a rhythmic sequence of 4 to 6 contractions per second. Clinically, tremors are divided between resting and action types. Resting tremor, associated with Parkinson disease, results from the degenerative changes in the substantia nigra and also involves akinesia and rigidity. Intentional, or action, tremor is associated with cerebellar lesions and is evident during voluntary movements.

Electrically, tremor results from a low-threshold discharging system. This is supported by clinical observations demonstrating the elimination of abnormal discharges, either by a lesion or through therapeutic DBS. Common symptoms associated with resting tremor include a masked face, infrequent blinking, slow movement, disturbed equilibrium, stooped posture, impaired speech, and impaired swallowing. Dyskinetic movements disappear in sleep when the brainstem reticular activating system is suppressed. Anxiety exaggerates dyskinetic movements.

Dystonia

The most common form of dystonia is **spasmodic torticollis**, which is marked with lateral fixation of the neck; consequently, the head is drawn to the affected site in a manner that the chin points to the other side. Another example of dystonia is **musculorum deformans**, a condition marked by the sustained involuntary movements of the axial and limb muscles.

Myoclonus

Consisting of muscle contractions that are isolated and repetitive, myoclonus can be a significant problem if its presence interrupts the phasic movements of speech muscles. The etiology for the myoclonic movement is unknown. Tics, the other form of dyskinesia, are the habitual contraction of certain muscles that look like stereotypical actions, such as throat clearing, sniffing, pursing the lips, and excessive blinking. They can be voluntarily suppressed but eventually are released. They are primary characteristics of (Gilles de la) Tourette syndrome, a condition caused by hypersensitive dopaminergic receptors in the BG.

Basal Ganglia Diseases

BG pathologies result in a series of neurological conditions, each of which is marked with differential patterns of involuntary movements. A few common diseases are discussed below (Table 15-2).

Parkinson Disease

Parkinson disease (PD), the best-understood BG disease, was first described by James Parkinson in 1817 as a "progressive condition marked with involuntary tremulous motion with rigidity and reduced muscular power, with a propensity to bend forward (stooped posture), and to pass from a walking to a running phase." The primary symptoms of PD are tremor at rest, **cogwheel** rigidity (stiff muscles with cogwheel-like jerks to the use of constant pressure for bending the limb), bradykinesia (slowed

Table 15-2

Common Basal Ganglia Diseases

Diseases	Causative Etiology
Parkinson disease	Degeneration of the secretory cells in substantia nigra leading to dopamine deficiency
Huntington chorea	Striatal degeneration
Wilson disease	Hepatolenticular degeneration subsequent to impaired copper metabolism
Progressive supranuclear palsy	Movement disorder caused by cellular death in the brainstem
Tardive dyskinesia	Involuntary movements of the oral facial muscles subsequent to a long-term use of psychotropic (dopaminergic antagonistic) medications

execution of body movements), loss of postural reflexes like arm swings, paucity of facial expression, and micrographia (smaller writing).

The additional clinical signs are akinesia (slow beginning or inability to initiate a movement), shuffling (short and quick) gait, and expressionless face. Diagnosed on clinical grounds, the onset of its symptoms occurs between 40 and 70 years of age, and it equally affects men and women.

Parkinsonian symptoms relate to pathologic changes in the dopamine-producing nerve cells in the pars compacta region of the substantia nigra (Fig. 15-7). Degeneration of these cells causes dopamine deficiency, and approximately 80% of the cells die off before clinical symptoms become significant. The dopaminergic neurons in the substantia nigra project to the striatal neurons, which have two types of dopamine receptors (Fig. 15-6): D1 (direct pathway) and D2 (indirect pathway). Both of these receptors respond differently to dopaminergic projections from the substantia nigra. The nigrostriatal projections facilitate (+) neurons with D1 but inhibit (–) neurons with D2 receptors. In normal conditions, the neurons with D1 receptors (with GABAergic and substance P projections) have net facilitatory effect on cortical motor activity movement; this relates to their inhibition of the GPi, which in turn promotes the intrinsically facilitatory output from the thalamus to the motor cortex. The net effect of GABAergic and enkephalin projections from neurons from D2 (indirect pathway) receptors is inhibiting to movement. The activation of the indirect (D2) pathway facilitates the GPi inhibitory activity, thus extending its inhibition of the thalamus and to the cortical motor nuclei (Fig. 15-4). With the loss of nigral dopaminergic neurons, dopaminergic deficiency in the nigrostriatal fibers has a different impact on neurons with D1 and D2 receptors. This nigrostriatal dopaminergic loss causes a decreased facilitation of the D1 striatal neurons and disinhibition (decreased inhibition) of D2 striatal neurons. Thus, the altered outputs decreased inhibition of the globus pallidus by neurons with D1 receptors and altered disinhibition of D2 results in Parkinson symptoms of reduced movement (akinesia) and tremor.

L-Dopa (Sinemet), a biosynthetic precursor of dopamine capable of crossing the blood–brain barrier (see Chapter 7), has been used to treat patients with dopamine deficiency. This drug increases dopamine synthesis in the surviving substantia nigra cells and avails it to the striatum. However, L-dopa is found to control some symptoms for only a few years. This biochemical understanding of the BG has been in some ways the basis for using stereotactic surgery, which involves placing permanent electrolytic lesions for alleviating Parkinsonian symptoms by targeting a selective structure, such as the inner globus pallidus or subthalamic nucleus. The net effect of the induced lesion has been to block or reduce the inhibitory BG output to the thalamus and brainstem structures, subsequently reducing the bradykinesia and facilitating involuntary movements.

Recently, DBS has been the choice treatment for Parkinson disease. The stimulation induces a functional lesion to interrupt the negative outflow from the globus pallidus. Stimulation of the subthalamic nucleus has resulted in improved motor performance in Parkinson patients; however, its impact on language processing has not been dramatic. This may be related to the reduced inhibitory output of the internal globus pallidus and its facilitatory regulation of cortical motor activity by the theory just explained.

Intralaminar centromedianum nucleus stimulation has also rendered an inhibitory and dampening effect on cortical motor movements. Furthermore, it has also yielded a facilitatory influence on the processing of language and other higher mental functions (Bhatnagar and Mandybur, 2005). This improved performance may have resulted from the activation of the reticularly synchronized response of the cortical mechanism.

Huntington Chorea

Huntington disease (HD), another well-understood disease of the BG, was described by George Huntington in 1872. Huntington, his father, and his grandfather observed the same symptoms in members of successive generations of the same families. HD has four characteristics: hereditary transmission, adult onset, chorea, and gradual cognitive deficits (dementia). It is inherited as an autosomal-dominant disease in which each offspring of an affected parent has a 50% chance of inheriting and developing the disorder (see Chapter 20). Affecting equally both men and women around the third decade, the first signs of the disease to appear are forgetfulness, personality changes, and clumsiness in motor movements. The choreiform movements gradually increase. The cognitive deficits lead to the subcortical type of dementia. Speech becomes dysarthric and gradually deteriorates into muteness.

Patients exhibit nonspecific atrophy in the caudate nucleus and prefrontal and parietal lobes (Fig. 15-8). In HD, the involvement of the caudate nucleus leads to degeneration of intrinsic striatal cholinergic and striatonigral GABAergic neurons. The loss of enzymes that biosynthesize acetylcholine and GABA contribute to further loss of GABA inhibition of the globus pallidus. In addition, the loss of striatonigral inhibition leads to the disinhibition of dopaminergic cells in the substantia nigra. Involuntary movements are caused by an imbalance from lesions anywhere along the dopaminergic–cholinergic–GABAergic loop. There is no cure for the condition; haloperidol (a dopamine antagonist) has usually been used to control behavioral abnormalities.

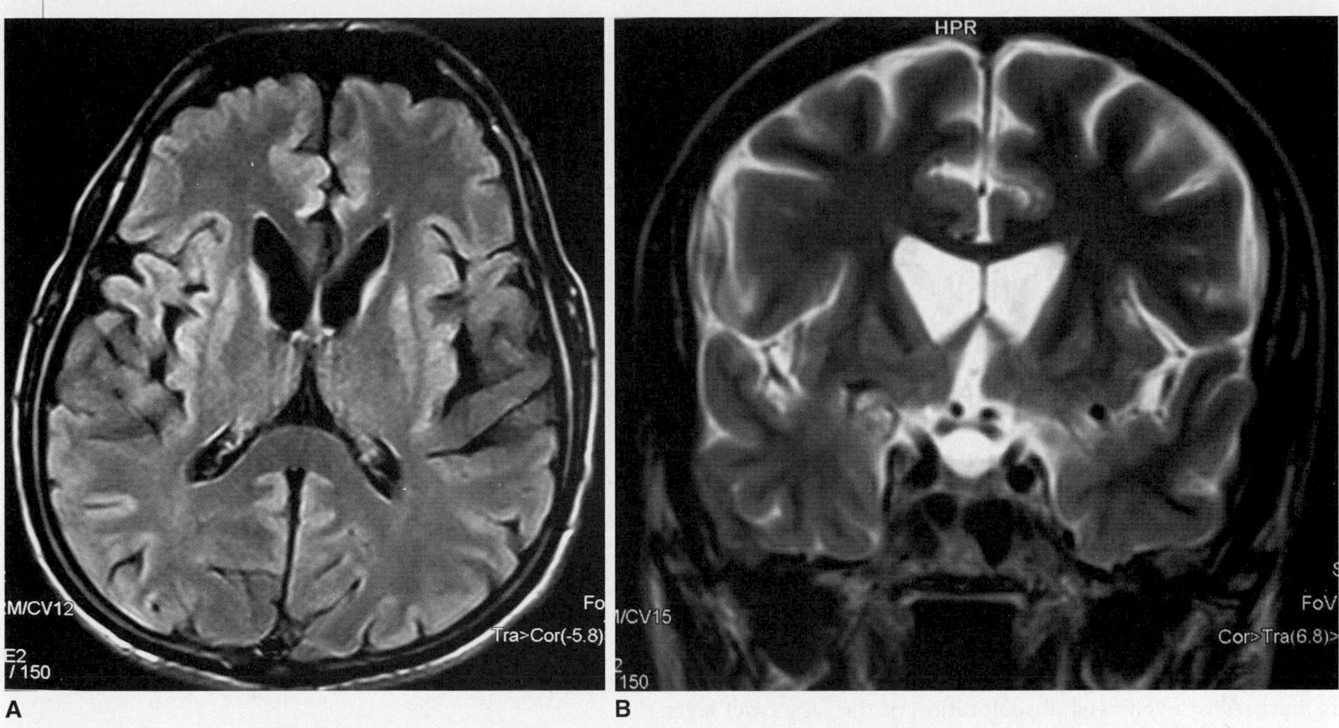

Figure 15-8 T2 axial (A) and coronal (B) MRI studies showing the caudate degeneration and dilated ventricles in a patient with Huntington disease.

Wilson Disease (Hepatolenticular Degeneration)

Wilson disease (WD) is a progressive disease of early life, with the onset of clinical manifestations between 10 and 25 years of age. It results from a disorder of copper metabolism, leading to the degeneration of internal brain regions, particularly the BG, and to cirrhosis (damage to and degeneration of hepatic cells) of the liver. It is clinically characterized by increased muscular rigidity, tremor, dysarthric speech, and progressive dementia. Corneal pigmentation (Kayser–Fleischer ring) is perhaps the most important diagnostic attribute of Wilson disease (Fig. 15-9). It is an autosomal-recessive disease (see Chapter 20).

Progressive Supranuclear Palsy

Progressive supranuclear palsy (PSP), a slowly progressive degenerative condition of the brain cells, is often confused with other neurodegenerative diseases, such as Parkinson, as it mimics Parkinson symptoms of gait difficulty, movement disorder, imbalance, and rigidity. However, it differs from Parkinson disease as there is no tremor, and it does not respond to treatment given to patients with Parkinson. Early clinical symptoms include lack of balance, bradykinesia (decreased spontaneity in movement initiation), impaired gait control, and supranuclear gaze palsy, or loss of voluntary eye movements. This usually begins with impaired downgaze, then upgaze, and horizontal gaze late in the course. The inability to look down, together with the neck extension, makes it hard for the patient to walk down steps. The patient often has an eyes-wide-open expression with a look of perpetual surprise. Additional symptoms may include facial grimaces, dysarthria, and dysphagia. PSP patients also exhibit personality changes, losing interest in activities they liked before and socially withdrawn. Some patients develop cognitive impairments (forgetfulness, slow thinking, and inattention). There is an accumulation of tau protein, a feature also of frontotemporal dementia and Pick disease. At present, there is no known treatment for the disease. PSP patients may show minimal response to L-dopa (as in Sinemet), the drug that is used to treat Parkinsonism. Botulinum toxin injections have been used to treat the involuntary eyelid closure.

Basal Ganglia and Higher Mental Disorders

Traditionally, the functions of the BG nuclei were implicated exclusively with the refinement of cortically generated motor movement; this view was based on the BG projections to the cortical motor neural circuitry. Recently, however, the BG connectivity, BG excitability, and the temporal relationship between the cortical neuronal event and

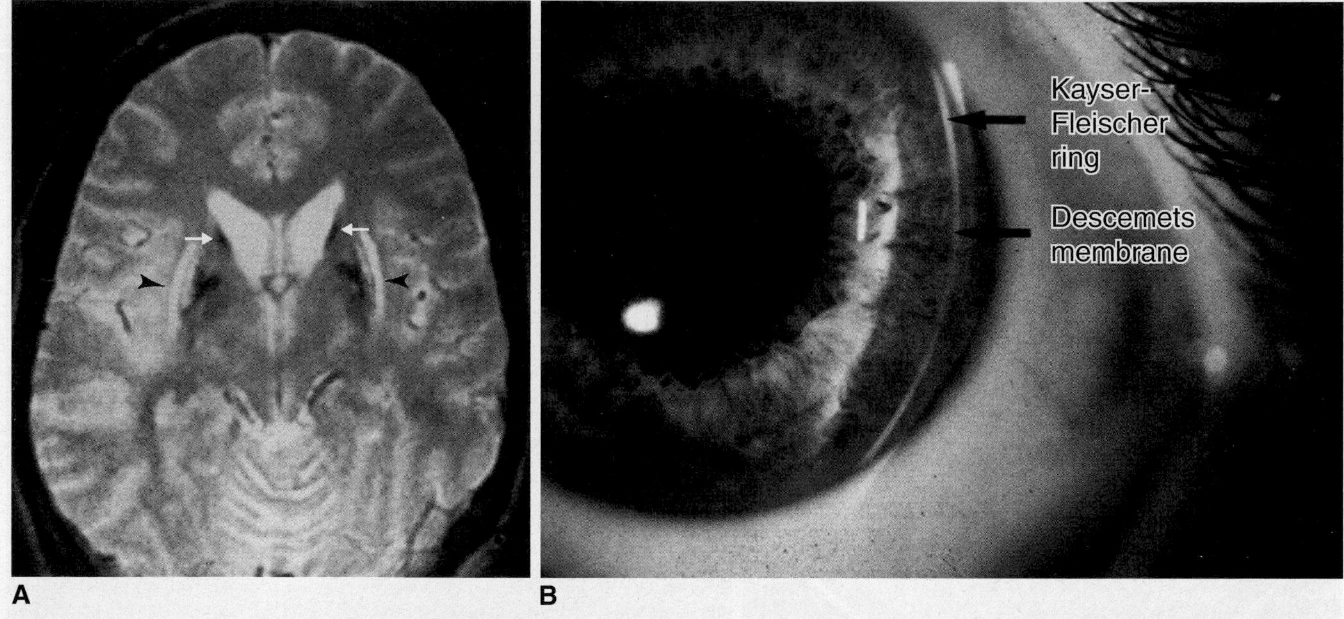

Figure 15-9 A. MRI study showing copper accumulation in the basal ganglia. B. Note the Kayser–Fleischer ring, which is marked by a yellowish discoloration of the Descemet layer.

function have revealed that the BG nuclei have additional roles in emotions, personality, and cognition (Bhatnagar and Mandybur, 2006). Research has determined that a substantial amount of the BG connectivity is to the orbital, dorsolateral, and medial prefrontal regions (Brodmann areas 9, 12, 46, and 47) and to the inferior temporal region (Middleton and Strick, 2000).

The prefrontal cortex is involved with cognition (planning, organizing, sequencing goal-oriented movements, learning, regulating attention, and solving problems), motivation, emotion, and personality, and the striatum is concerned with cortically mediated higher functions (Paxinos and Mai, 2004). The dorsolateral striatum receives projections from the entire frontal cortex, whereas the ventromedial striatum is connected to the orbital (emotional) and medial (motivational) prefrontal lobe and the limbic motor (cingulate) region. Striatal cellular activity has been associated with movement selection and initiation, repetitive and overlearned movements, working memory, and the development of reward-based behavior. Caudate pathology has been associated with an acquired deficit in memory related to delayed tasks and sequential movement learning in humans and nonhuman primates (Levy et al., 1997).

The clinically confirmed presence of cognitive disorders, seen in virtually all patients with Huntington chorea and Wilson disease and in some of those with Parkinson disease, has further provided support for the cognitively relevant neural circuitry in the striatum and the reciprocally connected pars reticulata region of the substantia nigra.

Basal Ganglia and Psychiatric Disorders

The BG-based movement disorders are also known to have psychiatric concomitants. There is a high incidence of depression in patients with Parkinson disease; similarly, patients with Huntington chorea exhibit a high suicide rate along with obvious personality and mood disorders. Research has revealed important analogies between the neurotransmitter dysfunctions in movement disorders and psychiatric illnesses, such as schizophrenia and depression, and in Tourette syndrome and dopaminergic receptors. Furthermore, a wide range of motor disorders, such as rigidity, dystonias, and TD, are known to result from the use of neuroleptic medications, which are used for behavioral modification and for treating psychiatric conditions, particularly schizophrenia and mood disorders. The neuroleptic drugs cause dysfunction of the striatal dopaminergic system by either blocking or changing the sensitivity of dopaminergic receptors, which results in dyskinesias. The presence of the psychiatric condition can negatively affect the treatment rendered to improve the motor speech quality.

The discovery of the Huntington gene, which is localized to chromosome 4, has revealed how molecular genetics is involved with the mind–body relationship. This gene encodes the protein huntingtin, which gradually accumulates and damages dopaminergic receptors. Identification of the gene has contributed to the development of a genetic test to diagnose Huntington disease prenatally or before symptoms appear.

CASE STUDIES FOR PROBLEM SOLVING

CASE ONE (15-1)

A 60-year-old woman suddenly developed partial paralysis (weakness) in her left leg while sitting in the same posture for sewing. Within 24 hours, the paralytic attack was replaced by involuntary movements in her leg and arm. She was admitted to the hospital. On testing, she exhibited the following signs:

- Wild swinging movements of the left arm and leg that gradually became more intense
- Flaccid muscle tone particularly in between the movements
- Dysarthria with altered speech quality and reduced loudness

A brain MRI study revealed a subcortical infarct in the right subthalamic nucleus. The swinging movements gradually became more intense. Several weeks of conservative therapy did not decrease the movements, so an electrolytic lesion was stereotactically placed in the right subthalamic nucleus, relieving the dyskinesia. She could then walk and eventually feed herself, and there were no complications. Her speech with reduced loudness also improved.

Question: How can you relate the infarct of the subthalamic nucleus with the BG mechanism?

Case (15-1) Discussion: See discussion of case studies

CASE TWO (15-2)

A 64-year-old college dean saw his physician after he gradually began experiencing muscle rigidity and mild involuntary movements, primarily in his right hand, and some difficulty with articulatory precision when speaking. He also was easily tired, and the impairment affected his ability to work. Examination revealed the following:

- Tense face without much expression
- Impaired ability to initiate a movement
- Periodic passive rigidity during the bending of arms
- Subtle not easily visible tremor in both hands with more in the right hand
- Awkward gait, resembling shuffling
- Mild dysarthria (his words were imprecise and were uttered quickly, mostly in sentence-end positions)
- Slightly stooped posture

A brain MRI study revealed changes bilaterally in the lower brainstem. The attending physician suspected this to be a case of akinesia and tremor associated with the degeneration of neurons in the substantia nigra.

Question: How can you explain these clinical symptoms in light of bilateral degenerative changes in the lower midbrain?

Case (15-2) Discussion: See discussion of case studies

CASE THREE (15-3)

A 37-year-old teacher began to experience weakness and uncontrollable clumsiness in his movements. He also exhibited dysarthric speech, some confusion, and mild cognitive impairments. This also changed his personality, and he was gradually becoming socially reclusive. His wife took him to their family doctor, who made the following observations:

- Postural imbalance
- Mild weakness of the upper and lower limbs
- Hypotonia and hyporeflexia
- Choreic movements involving the shoulders, head, and tongue
- Dysarthric speech marked by jumbled articulation
- Family history of similar condition; his father and uncle died young with similar symptoms, including dementia

A brain MRI study revealed wider anterior horns of the lateral ventricles, indicating the degeneration of the caudate head. Some degenerative changes were also noted in the basal region of the prefrontal lobe. The physician suspected this to be a case of a BG condition of dominant inheritance.

Question: What clinical characteristics helped the physician make this diagnosis?

Case (15-3) Discussion: See discussion of case studies

(Continued)

CASE FOUR (15-4) (*CONTINUED*)

A 35-year-old male politician became concerned about his gradually worsening speaking ability, which was becoming detrimental to his public image. He also noted subtle shaking movements involving both arms. He consulted a neurologist who noted the following:

- Very mild involuntary arrhythmic movements of the hands
- Rigidity in limb muscles
- Rigidity in both legs with an unsteady gait
- Amnesia for recent events
- Short attention span
- Presence of pigmentation at the sclerocornea junction (Kayser–Fleischer rings)
- Unintelligible speech subsequent to phonemic deletion and sound distortions
- A consultation with an SLP revealed the following:
- Irregular articulatory breakdown
- Voice stoppages
- Loudness variations
- Prolonged intervals
- Vowel prolongation
- Consonant distortion
- Confused language
- Anomia

A brain MRI study revealed degenerative changes bilaterally in the BG. Laboratory testing also confirmed cirrhosis (dysfunction) of the liver. The attending neurologist diagnosed it as a case of hepatolenticular degeneration, an autosomal-recessive condition of impaired copper metabolism.

Question: How can you relate these speech, language, and motor symptoms to the underlying disease process?

Case (15-4) Discussion: See discussion of case studies

CASE FIVE (15-5)

On his first week of work at an academic hospital, a 28-year-old SLP visited the neuro floor. After introducing himself, he told the senior resident of his interest in neurogenic disorders of communication. The resident, who herself had an interest in the brain–behavior relationship, welcomed him and said that he would find it very stimulating to work there, as patients on that floor exhibited a variety of disorders. She said, for example, that there were currently three patients with 2 to 4 year long histories of "relapse and remission" of sensorimotor symptoms. There were two patients with acute cortical insult, who had been exhibiting a rapid, though differential, rate of natural restitution. A new patient admitted that morning had the "Kayser– Fleischer" ring in her cornea. One 35-year-old man suffered a contrecoup cortical pathology. There was one patient with peripheral demyelination who also exhibited an ascending pattern of sensorimotor deficit that began with weakness and tingling in the toes, fingers, and legs and spread to the upper limbs; his symptomatology would not last more than 4 to 6 weeks. There was one patient in isolation with a bacterial infection involving meninges. There was a patient with a myoneural junction problem who looked better after rest. There was another young patient whose caudate was shrunken; he demonstrated dysarthria and impaired cognition. Last, but not least, there was an elderly patient with gait and balance problems who had lost control on eye movement; he was originally confused with mild dementia and Parkinson syndrome. "Anyway," the resident concluded, "I don't want to overwhelm you on your first visit. Feel free to ask me if you have any questions."

Question: The neurologist presented important clinically circumlocuting symptoms without naming the neurological conditions. While the final diagnosis is not based on these symptoms alone, these clinical statements are still very revealing. The SLP needs to relate the reported descriptions with the corresponding diseases. Can you help the SLP identify the suggested syndromes?

Case (15-5) Discussion. See discussion of case studies

SUMMARY

The BG nuclei are a series of interconnected anatomic loops that are functionally contiguous with the thalamus and neocortex. The interconnected loops are the sites of reverberating circuits of electrical currents and neurotransmitter transmission sustaining and modulating motor activity. The subthalamic nuclei and rostral brainstem also tie into the circuit, contributing to its stability. Lesions in one or more components of the system result in dyskinesias of varying types. Ballism is the only dyskinesia known to be produced by a single and focal lesion in the subthalamic nucleus. The rest of the dyskinesias seem to be associated with diffuse lesions in different parts of the system. The neurotransmitter dopamine is deficient in Parkinsonism owing to the degeneration of the substantia nigra dopaminergic cells that project to the striatum. Dopamine-replacement therapy and surgical intervention have been helpful in relieving Parkinsonian tremors, but neither is a cure. In recent years, electrical stimulating through chronically implanted electrodes in the subcortical and thalamic nuclei has been found to control some forms of dyskinesia, such as Parkinson disease. Most of the BG disorders also cause significant cognitive and emotional deficits.

REVIEW QUESTIONS

1. Complete the following statements using the appropriate technical terms:

   A. ________ refers to a loss of motor power of voluntary movements secondary to basal ganglia pathology.

   B. ________ is the slow writhing (undergoing constant flexion and extension) movements of the limb.

   C. ________ refers to the acquired wild flinging movements involving one side of the body secondary to a lesion in the subthalamic nucleus.

   D. Located within the white matter of the brain, the ________ include a group of nuclei that refine the cortically generated motor movements.

   E. As a clinical symptom Parkinson disease, ________ marks the slowness in the initiation of voluntary motor movements.

   F. The ________ refers to irregular, spasmodic, involuntary movements of the limbs or facial muscles, which are commonly seen in patients with Huntington disease.

   G. Emerging subsequent to lesions in the brainstem reticular formation above the vestibular nucleus, the ________ is marked by the sustained stiffness in the extensor limb muscles.

   H. Developing as a complication of neuroleptic medications, the ________ dyskinesia is marked by involuntary and deforming movements involving the facial muscles.

   I. ________, a repetitive movement secondary to alternate contraction of opposing muscles, is associated with the pathologies of basal ganglia circuitry.

   J. The ________ rigidity is marked by stiffness and tremor so that the muscle responds with intermittent spasms (ratchety feeling) to a constant limb bending.

   K. ________ stands for the inability to perform a voluntary movement because of the presence of abnormal and involuntary movements in basal ganglia diseases.

2. List four major basal ganglia nuclei.

3. Name the midbrain structure with the dopaminergic projections to the striatum.

4. Match each of the following diseases with associated description:

A. Huntington chorea	a. tremor in young age after streptococcal infection and rheumatic fever
B. Parkinson disease	b. disease of gene mutation marked with chorea and dementia
C. Wilson disease	c. degenerative disease initially marked with balance disorders, loss of ocular movement, dysarthria, and dysphagia
D. progressive supranuclear palsy	d. progressive motor disease with dysarthria and dementia secondary to impaired copper metabolism
E. Sydenham chorea	e. motor disorder marked with tremor and rigidity subsequent to dopaminergic cell loss

5. Match each of the following definitions with its associated statement:

A. sudden and forceful movements	a. athetosis
B. pill-rolling movements of fingers during rest	b. chorea
C. rhythmic, quick, involuntary movements of proximal muscles	c. ballism
D. difficulty in performing voluntary movements	d. dyskinesia
E. slow twisting movements in the muscles of the upper extremities	e. tremor

6. Loss of which neurotransmitter is associated with Parkinson disease?

7. What structure and neurotransmitter are implicated with Huntington chorea?

8. What basal ganglia structure is associated with hemiballism?

9. What structure first receives net summative basal ganglia output from the globus pallidus?

10. The presence of the Kayser–Fleischer ring at the edge of the cornea is suggestive of what disease?

11. Name four signs of basal ganglia dysfunction.

12. What mental disorder has been associated with increased dopaminergic projections to the forebrain?

16 Motor System 4: Motor Cortex

LEARNING OBJECTIVES

After studying this chapter, students should be able to:

- Discuss the role of the motor cortex and surrounding areas in movement
- Outline the anatomic organization of the primary motor cortex
- Describe the functions of the corticospinal and corticonuclear (corticobulbar) pathways
- Discuss the bilateral cortical innervation of speech-related muscles
- Explain the pathophysiology of the upper motor neuron syndrome
- Differentiate between upper and lower motor neuron syndromes
- Explain the pathophysiology of spasticity
- Discuss the pathophysiology of pseudobulbar palsy and its effects on speech muscles
- Explain the intact emotional responsiveness in pseudobulbar palsy
- Discuss the pathophysiology of alternating hemiplegia and its clinical symptoms

Up to this point, motor functions have been discussed in relation to the spinal cord (see Chapter 13), cerebellum (see Chapter 14), and basal ganglia (see Chapter 15). These structures represent organizational levels that do not initiate volitional motor movements on their own but instead act on efferent motor information that originates in the cerebral cortex and/or sensory information from various parts of the body and the environment.

The efferent impulses from the primary motor cortex (PMC) activate spinal and brainstem motor (LMNs) neurons and induce contraction of specific muscles. The cortical motor projections regulate a series of movements that are complex, discrete, precise, and skilled, such as finger tapping, dancing, running, and speaking. In addition to activating the LMNs in the brainstem and spinal cord, the PMC participates in the cognitive planning of purposeful motor activity in conjunction with afferents from the premotor (PreMC), prefrontal, sensory, and associational cortices. This planning includes the integration of sensory information regarding what and where the object is, calculation of the extent of muscle movements, determination of body parts that must be recruited, and generation of efferent signals for regulating specific muscles. The cerebral motor cortex executes movements with constant and updated feedback to and from the adjacent cortical and subcortical areas.

ANATOMY OF MOTOR CORTEX

The PMC is in the precentral gyrus of the frontal lobe (Fig. 16-1*A*), which is rostral to the central sulcus. The PMC contains large **Betz cells**, which are unique to this cortical area and are important in voluntary motor movement. A low intensity of electric stimulation can evoke motor acts from this cortical area. The functional organization of the PMC can be represented in terms of the body limbs (homunculus) superimposed on the motor cortical region. The face, speech muscles, and head are shown in the lower third of the motor cortex near the Sylvian fissure, the arms and trunk are in the upper motor cortical region, and the legs and toes are in the midsagittal area (Fig. 16-1*A*,*B*). In comparison, the face and mouth occupy a disproportionately large cortical area in the motor cortex caudal to the premotor area. The disproportionately large representation of the face and mouth in the human PMC corresponds to the importance of the elaborate apparatus required for speech, an important point for professionals in human behaviors to remember.

The motor neural impulses that travel in the pyramidal tract originate from the three cortical regions (Fig. 16-2): PMC, PreMC, and primary sensory cortex (PSC). In humans, 25% to 30% of the pyramidal tract fibers are known to arise from the PMC. Of those, only 2% come from the large Betz cells. Located in the layer V, the Betz cells are pyramidal cells whose long axons extend to the lower limbs and thus require large cell bodies for metabolic support. There are relatively few large motor cells

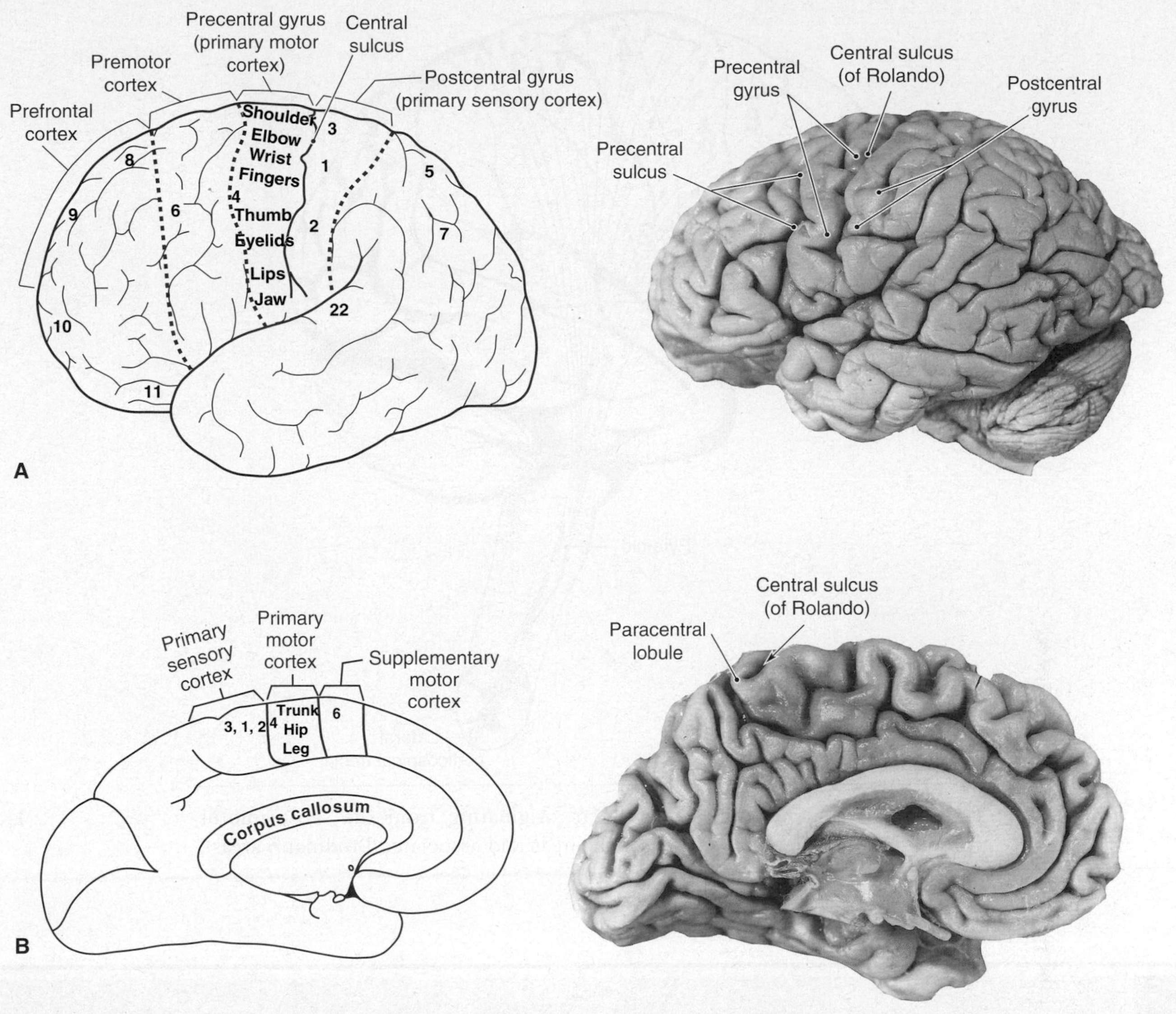

Figure 16-1 The human body representation in the primary motor cortex and important Brodmann areas on the lateral (A) and medial (B) brain surfaces.

because humans have a much greater need for the shorter cortical projections to the cranial nerve nuclei (**cortico-nuclear/corticobulbar projections**) and upper limb levels in the cord (**corticospinal projections**). Therefore, the small neurons in the motor cortex give rise to the remaining pyramidal fibers. Approximately 30% of the remaining descending motor fibers arise from the PreMC, which extends midsagittally within the interhemispheric fissure as the supplementary motor cortex (Fig. 16-1*B*). The remaining 40% of the motor fibers arise from the PSC (Brodmann areas 3, 1, 2) in the parietal lobe and the adjacent somatosensory association cortex (Brodmann areas 5 and 7) (Figs. 16-1 and 16-2). Most of the efferents from the cortex project to the contralateral limbs (Box 16-1). Substantial bilateral projections, however, are known to exist, particularly from the supplementary cortical area.

The motor cortex circuitry is organized into columns of neurons arranged vertically from the surface into the depth of the cortex. Each single column provides circuitry responsible for directing a group of muscles. Thus, the simultaneous and sequential organization of movement patterns, but not the individual muscles, is considered to be organized in the motor cortex. Direct control from the cortex allows higher primates, including humans, to control individual and grouped proximal and distal muscles for performing specific movements.

This cortical motor system integrity is maintained and enhanced by the thalamocortical excitatory loop, which itself is modulated by the intrinsic inhibitory basal ganglia functions and excitatory afferents from the cerebellum (see Chapters 14 and 15). To maintain the precision, accuracy, smoothness, and sequential nature of the motor

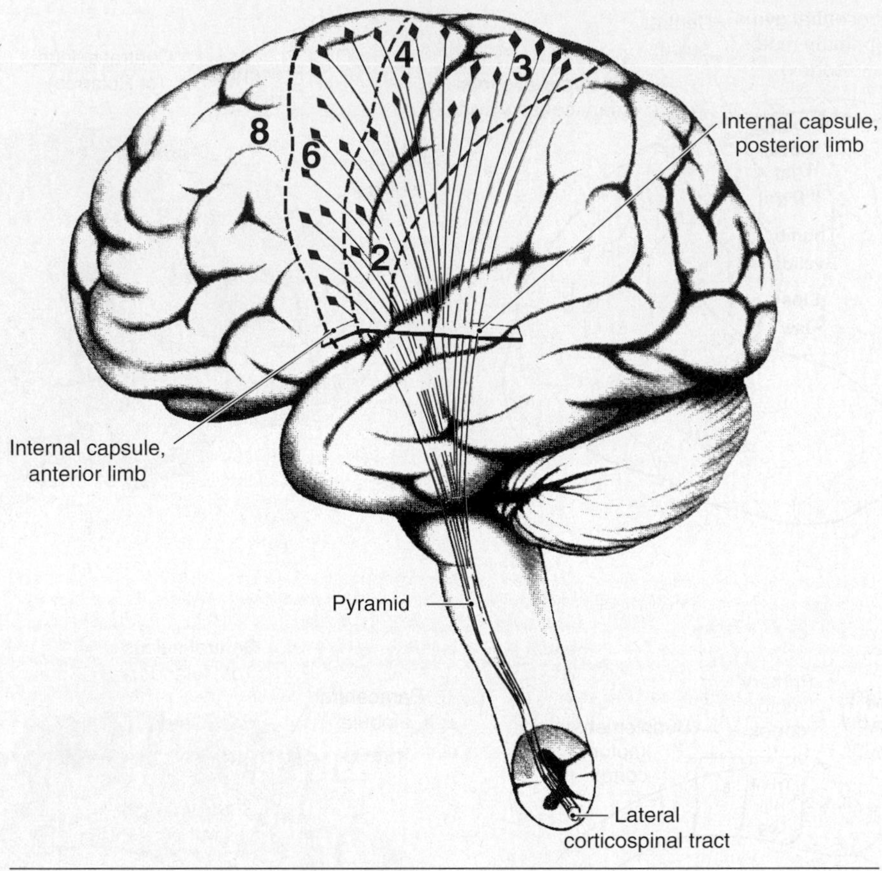

Figure 16-2 The pyramidal tract fibers originating from the sensorimotor (premotor, motor, and sensory) cortical areas and associated Brodmann areas.

BOX 16-1

Muscle Tone

Muscle tone is defined by a "steady state of contraction which resists a force in the direction of passive stretch" such as gravitational pull or pull of flexor force from the opposite side of a joint. This is based on normal levels of excitability of the muscle spindle IA **stretch** afferent monosynaptic stretch reflexes, which function to resist muscle fiber stretch in muscles on both sides of a joint. If the UMN innervation of a motor unit is lost, excitability of the stretch reflex is reduced (reduced descending facilitation). Immediate weakness from reduced muscle tone results. With the passage of weeks or months, excitability of the reflex increases above normal through hyperreflexia of the stretch reflex (hypertonia) and often, then to extreme hyperexcitability generating stiffness, especially in antigravity muscles (spasticity). This increase in stretch reflex excitability is now believed to be produced by collateral sprouting of stretch afferent terminals at the spinal level, replacing the lost UMN synapses and thus abnormally increasing the power of the stretch reflex.

Spasticity refers to an increased muscle tone (hypertonic and hyperreflexive) and is best illustrated by a "clasp-knife" resistance in which, during a passive movement, the limb initially moves freely and is followed by a resistance. This resistance though melts away in face of a continued force. Clinically it is associated with a lesion involving the upper motor neurons and their descending projections. Another abnormality associated with increased muscle tone is muscle rigidity, which is marked by the presence of a constant resistance throughout the passive limb movement (lead-pipe pattern). It implies an extrapyramidal lesion involving the basal ganglia structures (see Chapter 15). Parkinson patients exhibit "cogwheel rigidity," a different pattern of rigidity in which the muscle responds with jerks (ratchety feeling) to a constant limb bending.

activity, the PMC depends on constant feedback from the adjacent cortical and subcortical regions. The cortical input includes afferents from the PreMC (Brodmann area 6), which, with input from the prefrontal cortex (Brodmann areas 8 and 10), is concerned with setting up a motor plan of a skilled movement pattern involving specific limbs. As the site of reasoning, thinking, and planning, the prefrontal cortex, with afferents from the occipital, parietal, and temporal lobes, adds the quality of judgment and foresightedness to motor movements. The supplementary motor cortex (Brodmann area 6) regulates planning and the implementation of bilateral aspects of movements. Projections from the somesthetic cortex modulate sensory feedback, whereas fibers from the association somesthetic cortex (Brodmann areas 5 and 7) regulate higher-order spatial aspects of the movement plan.

Much highly skilled movement is learned through a background of species-specific, built-in capabilities. The sensory feedback aspects of the sensorimotor cortex and corticospinal projections to the spinal cord contribute to the process of motor learning. Once a skilled movement pattern is well learned, these feedback systems are usually not required unless a deterrent to the movement is encountered.

Innervation Pattern

The motor cortex is organized contralateral to output and input. The short (corticonuclear/corticobulbar) and long (corticospinal) efferent projections from the motor cortex cross the midline to innervate contralateral cranial nerve and spinal output motor nuclei. Consequently, a lesion of the motor fibers above the point of decussation (caudal medulla for long fibers and multiple brainstem points for short fibers) produces clinical signs contralateral to the site of damage (Fig. 16-3; see Fig. 1-1). In the case of a lesion below the decussation point, clinical signs of the spinal upper motor neurons (UMNs) and lower motor neurons (LMNs) are ipsilateral to the locus of the damage.

Key Terms:

Abdominal reflex	**Crossed hemiplegia**
Alternating hemiplegia	**Spastic hemiplegia**
Babinski reflex	**Spasticity**
Clasp-knife rigidity	**Upper motor neuron syndrome**
Cremasteric reflex	

TERMS RELATED TO MOTOR FUNCTION

Common clinical terms associated with cortical motor dysfunctions are paralysis, UMN syndrome, LMN syndrome, and spasticity. Clinical terms related to paralysis (loss of voluntary muscle movement) are **monoplegia**, **hemiplegia**, **triplegia**, and **quadriplegia**.

The term "UMN" is used in reference to the cortical motor neurons and their axons before they synapse on the spinal motor neurons. The UMNs are also called pyramidal neurons because their descending axons pass through the pyramids in the medulla. A lesion in the UMN system is associated with specific symptoms of delayed muscle spasticity, increased tone and hyper reflexes, and paralysis. Spasticity refers to increased muscle tone and resistance to passive manipulation of the muscle (Box 16-2). The term "LMN" is used in reference to the motor neurons located in the brainstem and spinal cord that directly project to the skeletal muscles. Damage to the LMNs is associated with symptoms of flaccid paralysis, decreased tone and reflexes, and muscle atrophy (see Chapter 13).

Monoplegia is the paralysis of a single limb, hemiplegia is the paralysis of one side of the body involving both upper and lower limbs, paraplegia involves the paralysis of both lower limbs, and quadriplegia refers to the paralysis of all four (two upper and two lower) limbs.

DESCENDING PATHWAYS

Originating from the (internal pyramidal) layer V of the motor cortex, the descending efferents to the LMNs travel on one of two pathways, either the corticospinal tract or the corticonuclear tract (Fig. 16-3). The corticospinal tract, which contains merely 30% of the motor fibers, mediates voluntary movements of the skeletal muscles through the spinal α-motor neurons (LMNs). Containing the remaining approximately 70% of the motor fibers that are also short, the corticonuclear/corticobulbar tract controls the facial, oral, and associated muscles through activation of cranial nerve nuclei in the brainstem. Virtually all efferent fibers in both tracts cross the midline before synapsing on their respective LMNs.

Corticospinal Tract

The corticospinal fibers arise from the upper two-thirds of the PMC (precentral gyrus), PreMC, and SMC. These fibers travel through the corona radiata and then descend, in a compact bundle, through the posterior limb of the internal capsule of the forebrain (see Fig. 2-38). Later, they run through the midbrain pes pedunculi. These descending fibers separate into several longitudinal but diffuse fascicles as they pass between the masses of neurons in the ventral pons, mingling with the pontine nuclei (Fig. 16-3*A*). Some fibers terminate in the pontine nuclei and project to the cerebellum, while the rest continue to the medulla to form the pyramid (source of the term: the pyramidal tract) before crossing at the caudal end of the medulla. After crossing, the motor fibers descend into the lateral corticospinal tract of the spinal cord (Figs. 16-2 and 16-3*A*), named after the location of

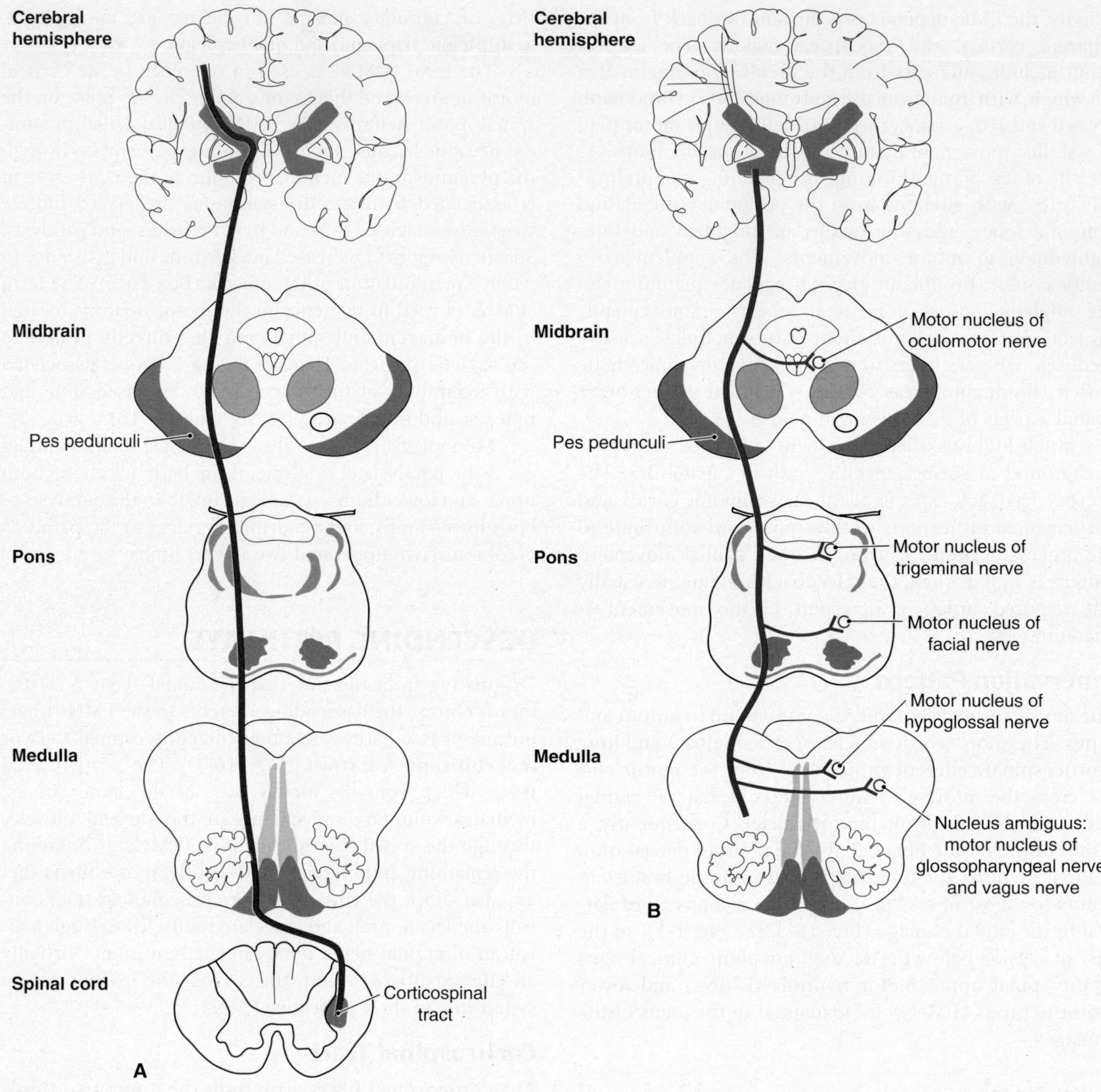

Figure 16-3 Origin and course of the pyramidal fibers. A. Corticospinal fibers projecting to the spinal motor nuclei. B. Corticonuclear/corticobulbar fibers projecting to the motor nuclei of the cranial nerves. Some cranial nerve nuclei receive motor commands from the contralateral motor cortex; the motor nuclei for the upper face, larynx, and jaw receive bilateral projections.

these fibers in the lateral funiculus of the spinal cord. Through the fibers of the lateral corticospinal tract, the motor cortex participates in digital control of the skeletal muscles of the distal limbs (fingers and toes) required for fine manipulative skills (Box 16-3).

An uncrossed smaller fasciculus of motor fibers (anterior corticospinal tract) descends into the ventral funiculus of the spinal cord, which eventually crosses the midline before synapsing on the α-motor neurons (see Fig. 13-5). The anterior corticospinal tract fibers control the proximal axial and girdle muscles, which provide the postural platform required for skilled digital movements.

The UMN fibers of the lateral corticospinal tract terminate on the interneurons and α-motor neurons in the spinal anterior gray horns to initiate movements. Some of the fibers also terminate on γ-motor neurons, providing

BOX 16-2

Contralaterality of Upper Motor Neuron Symptoms

The UMN system is primarily a crossed (decussated) system. The giant pyramidal neurons of the motor cortex project their axons through the brainstem to provide precise control of skeletal motor functions at all spinal levels on the opposite side of the body. The axons of these cortical neurons pass caudally through the posterior internal capsule, the cerebral peduncle, the medullary pyramids, and then abruptly cross to the opposite side of the CNS and descend in the lateral white column of the spinal cord to reach the motor (lower motor) neurons at all spinal levels. The innervation pattern is more complicated for UMN axons targeting cranial nerve skeletal motor nuclei (corticobulbar UMN axons). Collectively called the corticonuclear/corticobulbar tract fibers, they leave the pyramidal system just rostral to each target nucleus, cross to the opposite side and innervate LMNs of the cranial nerves V, VI, VII, IX, X, and XII. LMNs of *upper* face muscles (CN VII) and of swallowing and vocal muscles (CNs IX and X) receive UMN control from both sides of the cortex. Thus, a unilateral cortical lesion is less likely to produce a profound impact on motor speech functions.

UMN axons reach the XIth nerve nucleus in the upper cervical cord. These cross the midline in the pyramidal decussation (the caudal medulla) to reach the LMNs of the XIth nerve which innervates the motor units of the trapezius or the sternocleidomastoid muscles. Eye movement control involves UMN innervation of nuclei in the roof of the midbrain and these nuclei control, in bilaterally coordinated fashion, the LMNs of cranial nerves III, IV, and VI.

Any damage to the motor fibers before the decussation point would result in weakness and paresis in the body contralateral to the site of lesion; any lesion below the decussation would cause limb weakness ipsilateral to the lesion site. Since the LMNs in the brainstem and spinal cord receive only the crossed efferents, their involvement invariably affects the muscles ipsilateral to the lesion site.

a means for the motor cortex to modulate the stretch reflex. This ensures an appropriate level of tone in the muscles in which the α-motor neurons are influenced to provide the motor control. Some fibers also synapse on the sensory cells in the dorsal gray horns through which the cortex modulates somesthetic feedback data, which consist largely of messages noting deviations from what the premotor cortex planned and the motor cortex actuated. On its way to the spinal motor neurons, the corticospinal tract also emits multiple collaterals to the basal ganglia, thalamus, brainstem reticular formation, and pontine nuclei. The axonal processes of the LMNs exit at all levels of the spinal cord, terminating in the skeletal muscles.

BOX 16-3

Sensorimotor Involvement without Cortical Dysfunctions

A lesion in the posterior part of the internal capsules results in a UMN lesion, which interrupts the integrity of corticospinal and/or corticobulbar axons. Therefore, their functions, affecting the opposite side of the head and body (hemiparesis or weakness of muscles involved in fine manipulative skills), are lost but other cortical functions may be spared. Clinically what would differentiate an internal capsule lesion from a cortical region lesion is that there are no cognitive or linguistic symptoms associated with the internal capsule lesions.

Corticonuclear/Corticobulbar Tract

The corticonuclear fibers, similar to the fibers of the corticospinal tract, control skilled and fine movements. However, the corticonuclear fibers exclusively control the skeletal muscles of the head and face through the motor nuclei of the trigeminal (CN V), facial (CN VII), glossopharyngeal (CN IX), vagus (CN X), spinal accessory (CN XI), and hypoglossal (CN XII) nerves. The corticonuclear fibers arise from the lower third of the motor cortex and adjacent area (Fig. 16-1) and travel through the genu of the internal capsule and pes pedunculi. Unlike the corticospinal fibers, the corticonuclear projections to the cranial nerve nuclei do not cross the midline at a single point; rather, they do so at multiple points before synapsing on the cranial LMNs (Fig. 16-3*B*).

The corticonuclear projection to some cranial nerves is contralateral, whereas the regulation of some cranial nerve LMNs is bilateral (see innervation pattern in

Chapter 17; Fig. 17-8). The corticonuclear fibers from the left motor cortex innervate both the left and right motor nuclei of some of the cranial nerves. Similarly, projections from the right motor cortex control the functioning of some cranial nerve nuclei on both sides. The pontine gaze center controls the ocular cranial nerves on both sides (see Fig. 17-6 and Chapter 17).

An important clinical point about the corticonuclear system is that since the muscles of the jaw, larynx, and upper face receive projections from the bilateral motor cortices, a unilateral cortical lesion does not profoundly impair the function of some cranial nerves (facial [CN VII], trigeminal [CN V], and vagus [CN X]) and spares the vital functions of mastication, phonation, and speech. The functions of such cranial nerves, however, are severely affected in the case of a bilateral cortical pathology (pseudobulbar palsy) or after a bilateral LMN lesion (Table 16-1).

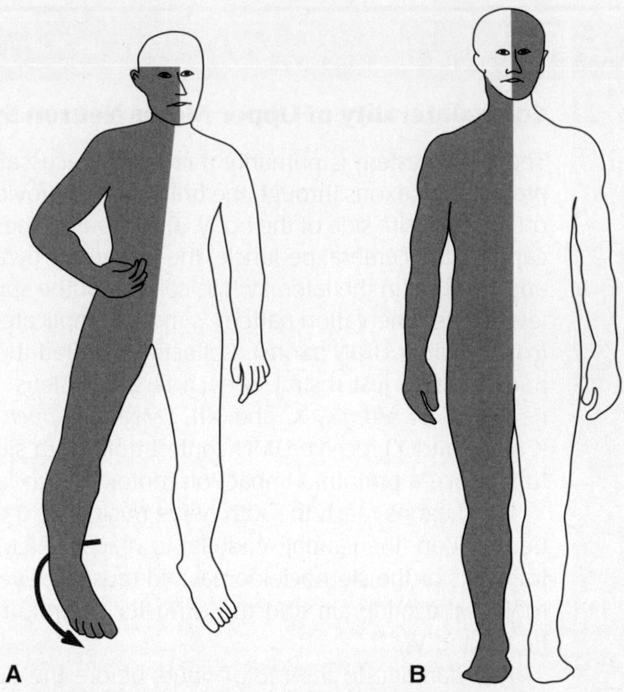

Figure 16-4 A. Diagrammatic illustration of right spastic hemiplegia. B. Left alternating hemiplegia (left facial palsy and right-sided hemiplegia in addition and hemianesthesia).

CLINICAL CORRELATES

Differential Involvement of the Arm and Leg after Cerebral Lesion

There is a close relationship between vascular functioning and clinical anatomy. Cerebral injuries affect the contralateral limbs, and the upper limbs are more involved than the lower limbs. This is clinically crucial because the lateral cortical surface, with motor representation for the upper limb and face, is served by the middle cerebral artery, whereas the midsagittal extension of the motor cortex, with representation for the leg and toes, is served by the anterior cerebral artery (see Chapter 7).

Spastic Hemiplegia

Lesions of the corticospinal tract (UMNs) at various neuraxial locations usually produce symptoms concomitant with the contralateral hemiplegia and spasticity. **Spastic hemiplegia** is a state of paralysis with hypertonia, hyperreflexia, and clasp-knife rigidity. Typical posture of spastic hemiplegia consists of a flexed upper arm, thumb, and fingers with the neck bent toward the affected side (Fig. 16-4*A*). While walking, the subject usually circumvents the affected leg. The clinical symptoms appearing immediately after an acute pyramidal tract lesion first include profound weakness and flaccidity in contralateral distal muscles and a loss of delicate and manipulative skills; also present are the loss of **abdominal** and **cremasteric reflexes**, positive **Babinski reflex**, and flaccid tone in the affected muscles. The muscle tone not only returns in 1 to 4 weeks but also increases and the muscle becomes spastic.

Table 16-1

Effects of Corticonuclear/corticobulbar System Lesions

Unilateral Lesion	Bilateral (Pseudobulbar Palsy) Lesions
Variable degrees of contralateral paresis in oral structures Jaw and tongue deviation away (contralateral) from the lesion site Greater motor difficulty with unilaterally innervated structures like the lower face and tongue than the upper (eyes and forehead) structures	Profound effect on facial expression, speaking, swallowing, and phonating

The gradual emergence of spasticity is related to the outgrowth of local stretch afferents, which fill the depopulated synapses on the α-motor neurons after a cortical lesion. This growth may subsequently promote increased afferents on type Ia fibers from the muscle spindles, causing greater activation of the motor neurons. This axonal outgrowth takes considerable time, explaining the span of several weeks that it takes for spasticity to appear.

The spasticity is most evident during a passive limb extension. This is mostly present in antigravity muscles, such as the proximal flexors in the upper extremity and extensors in the lower extremity. Spasticity is also speed dependent; the resistance is stronger if the affected limb is moved rapidly. Furthermore, it is present only in the muscles that are no longer under voluntary control. If pressure is persistently applied, the muscle resistance may suddenly disappear. This is called **clasp-knife** rigidity pattern, which is different from the jerky **cogwheel** rigidity seen in patients with Parkinson disease (see Chapter 15).

Involvement of the corticonuclear fibers also results in the paralysis of the facial, lingual, palatal, and laryngeal muscles. Nonetheless, extreme levels of hypertonia and clasp-knife rigidity are rarely seen in lesions restricted to the corticonuclear system. Furthermore, corticonuclear damage does not usually produce the same level of spasticity as that which develops in the distal limbs after a corticospinal tract lesion.

Common causes of spastic motor dysfunctions are cerebrovascular accidents, tumors, and degenerative diseases of the nervous system. None of these causes respects the anatomic boundaries; therefore, the clinical pictures evolving from these conditions are usually mixed and may also implicate extrapyramidal structures.

Pseudobulbar Palsy

Pseudobulbar (supranuclear) **palsy** results from a bilateral involvement of the corticonuclear pathways and is associated with a bilateral spastic paralysis of the speech musculature. It causes a supranuclear paralysis of the cranial nerves (Box 16-4). The patient has difficulty controlling facial muscles for delicate and discrete motor control, such as in speech; however, there is little spasticity in facial and neck muscles.

A clinically critical characteristic of pseudobulbar palsy is that the facial emotional response pattern remains intact. When the patient attempts to move the facial muscles in voluntary motor activities, they respond poorly. However, the patient's facial muscles respond strongly to an emotional stimulus. The pathways activated during a true emotional response are not as fully understood as the pathways that control voluntary actions. The emotional responses involve some limbic afferents. When the cranial nerve motor nuclei are activated through the intact emotional pathways, the facial response is actually exaggerated; when asked to show the teeth or perform a voluntary smile, the patient may assume the appearance of a "Greek mask of tragedy," with forceful contraction of the same muscles that otherwise appear to be weak. Often exaggerated emotional responses are accompanied by excessive laughter, sobbing, or choking; these acts may pose a hazard to the patient in eating.

BOX 16-4

Nuclear/Bulbar and Pseudobulbar Palsies

"Bulb" refers to the medullary region of the brainstem. Bulbar palsy results from injuries to the LMNs in the brainstem. The motor nuclei located in the brainstem relate to the efferent mechanisms of the cranial nerve. The Nuclear/bulbar palsy, characterized by paralysis (and muscle wasting) of the bulbar muscles, includes difficulty in swallowing (dysphagia), phonating, articulating sounds and words, and maintaining proper balance in the oral–nasal cavities (dysarthria). It is a unilateral motor condition, and it involves the motor nuclei on one site of the brain. It is never caused by a lesion in the cortical motor area (UMNs). The cranial nerves that are most affected in nuclear/bulbar palsy are the vagus (CN X), facial (CN VII), and hypoglossal nerves (CN XII). Degenerative conditions, stroke, and neoplasm are the etiologies that are commonly associated with bulbar palsy.

Pseudobulbar (supranuclear) palsy results from a bilateral involvement of the corticonuclear/corticobulbar pathways and is associated with a bilateral paresis (somewhat spastic) of the speech musculature. It is also known as the supranuclear paralysis of the cranial nerves. The patient has difficulty controlling facial muscles for delicate and discrete motor control, such as phonation, articulation, swallowing, and resonance. Since many speech-related cranial nerves receive corticobulbar projections from both sides of the motor cortex, their functions in pseudobulbar palsy are profoundly affected. Despite the buccofacial weakness, the facial emotional responses remain intact. The patient exhibits uncontrolled expression of emotions (crying or laughing) in response to minimal emotional information. The emotional expression is not considered under the motor cortex; rather, a limbic involvement in its control is suspected.

Alternating Hemiplegia

Brainstem lesions produce **alternating or crossed hemiplegia**; mostly the lesions involve small arteries that supply the pons and medulla (Box 16-5; also see Chapter 7). A lesion on one side of the brainstem affects the ipsilateral cranial nerve motor nuclei and/or nerves (motor units) extending to

BOX 16-5

Alternating Hemiplegia

Brainstem lesions, depending on their extent, result in a different pattern of paralysis, called "alternating hemiplegia," which is marked by cranial nerve dysfunctions ipsilateral to the lesion site and hemiparesis always contralateral to the lesion site. Unilateral damage to the motor nucleus of the vagus nerve (CN X, lower motor neuron [LMN]) produces flaccid paralysis of the pharyngeal and/or laryngeal muscles, resulting in a weak and hoarse voice and swallowing difficulty. Unilateral involvement of the motor nucleus of the facial nerve (CN VII; LMN) causes facial asymmetry and affects eating and articulation; damage to the motor nucleus of the hypoglossal nerve (CN XII; LMN) would produce unilateral (ipsilateral) flaccid paralysis and denervation atrophy of the intrinsic and extrinsic tongue muscles, resulting in eating and speaking disturbances. However, if the lesion extends to the lateral brainstem, it would also cause hemianesthesia and hemiplegia in contralateral limbs. This contralaterality results from the interruption of the long ascending (somesthetic) and descending (motor) fibers, which are yet uncrossed. Since cranial nerve involvement impairs the LMNs, the resulting symptoms are flaccid paralysis, absent reflexes, muscular fibrillation, and eventual atrophy of the involved muscle. However, the involvement of the long motor fibers produces the upper motor neuron syndrome, which is marked by hemiplegia, spasticity, and the presence of Babinski sign.

the target facial muscles on the same side. This leads to LMN signs unilateral to the side of the lesion. The lesion also interrupts the unilateral uncrossed corticospinal fibers, which descend to cross the midline in the caudal medulla (Fig. 16-4*B*). Thus, a brainstem lesion, interrupting both LMN and UMN systems, results in an alternating pattern of symptoms: ipsilateral pharyngeal, lingual, facial, and/or ocular palsy (LMN) and contralateral spastic hemiplegia (UMN).

Upper Motor Neuron Syndrome

Interruption of the descending motor (corticospinal and corticonuclear) tracts have two clinically important components: the UMN (central nuclei and fibers) and the LMN (spinal and cranial nuclei and peripheral fibers). The UMNs relate to the cell bodies in the motor cortex and descending axons before their synapse on the cranial or spinal motor (LMN) neurons. The LMNs are the cell bodies in the anterior gray column in the spinal cord or cranial motor nuclei in the brainstem (see Chapters 13 and 17). The LMNs provide the output pathway to peripheral functions via their axons and innervate muscle fibers. The difference between the locations of the UMNs and LMNs has important clinical implications (Fig. 16-5; Table 16-2).

Table 16-2

Clinical Characteristics of Upper and Lower Motor Neuron Syndromes

Characteristic	Upper Motor Neuron Syndrome	Lower Motor Neuron Syndrome
Lesion site	Cortical motor neurons and their axons before synapses on spinal/cranial motor nuclei	Spinal/cranial motor neurons and their axons
Paralysis	Paralysis (spastic) or weakness	Paralysis (flaccid) or weakness
Muscle tone	Increased tone	Decreased tone
Muscle atrophy	Not present	Present due to unused muscles
Denervation	No twitching or fasciculation	Fibrillations and fasciculations
Reflexes	Hyperreflexia	Hyporeflexia
Abnormal reflexes	Babinski	No abnormal reflexes
Limb involved	Multiple muscles/limbs examples are monoplegia or hemiplegia, or quadriplegia	A single limb or selected muscles

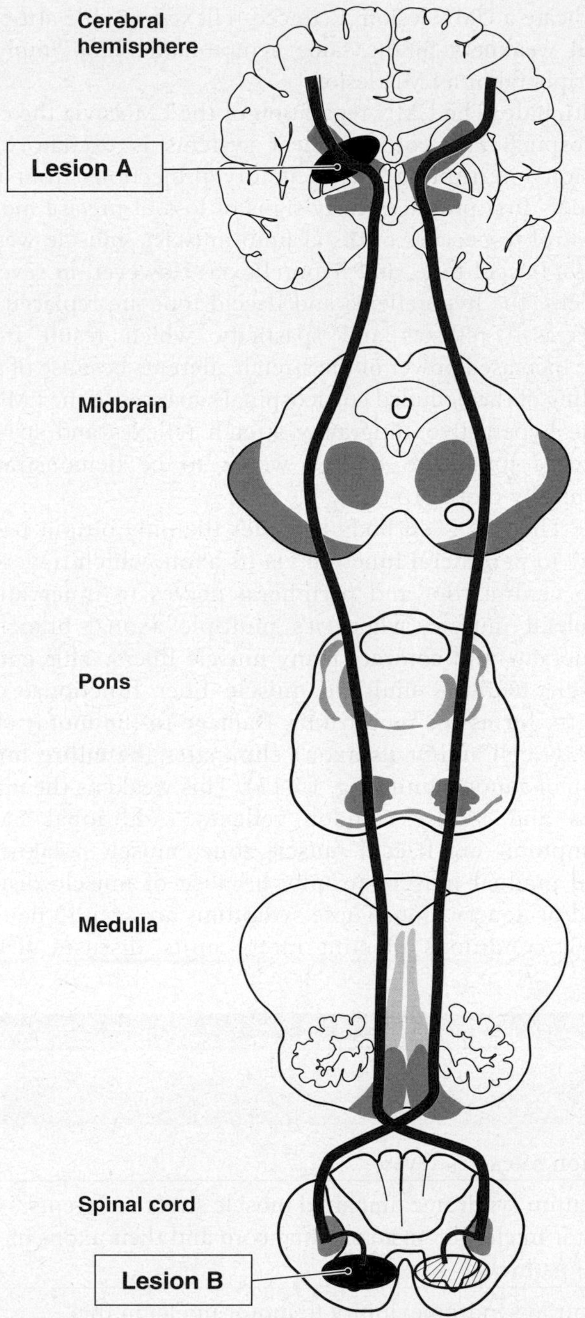

Figure 16-5 Lesion sites implicated in upper and lower motor neuron syndromes. Each site results in a different set of clinical symptoms. Lesion A (UMN lesion) results in a contralateral hemiplegia (flexed arm and extended leg), increased muscle tone (spastic), hyperactive reflexes, no muscle atrophy, and positive Babinski sign. Lesion B (spinal LMN lesion) causes ipsilateral paralysis in specific muscles, reduced/absent muscle tone (flaccid), hypoactive or absent reflexes, and muscular atrophy.

Lesions of the descending corticospinal fibers result in UMN syndrome (Fig. 16-5, Lesion A), which has the following clinical characteristics:

- Loss of voluntary movements in the affected muscles. With the loss of the pyramidal motor system, there is no cortical motor control on limb muscles. The muscles are paralyzed and the patient loses precise and delicate motor control of the distal limb muscles used in fine manipulative skills, along with the facial muscles used for speech, and facial expression.
- Paralyzed muscles are initially flaccid, but there is increased muscle tone (spastic hemiplegia) after several weeks. This is largely the result of collateral sprouting (scrambled wiring) of the type Ia (annulospiral) endings to the spinal motor neurons, which fill depopulated or denuded corticospinal synapses.
- Contralateral spinal reflexes are hyperactive (Table 16-2). There is some wasting of muscles, but the paralyzed muscles do not atrophy, because there is no denervation of the muscles, whose motor control in reflexes is preserved.
- Muscle tone profoundly increases, and that contributes to the muscle spasticity. The muscle with increased tone responds with clasp-knife rigidity to any passive stretch.
- Altered Reflexes. The plantar reflex, also called the Babinski reflex, is present, which represents a corticospinal abnormality. Normally the big toe flexes when the lateral margin of the sole is firmly stroked. This toe dorsiflexes in case of Babinski sign (Fig. 16-6*B*). A positive

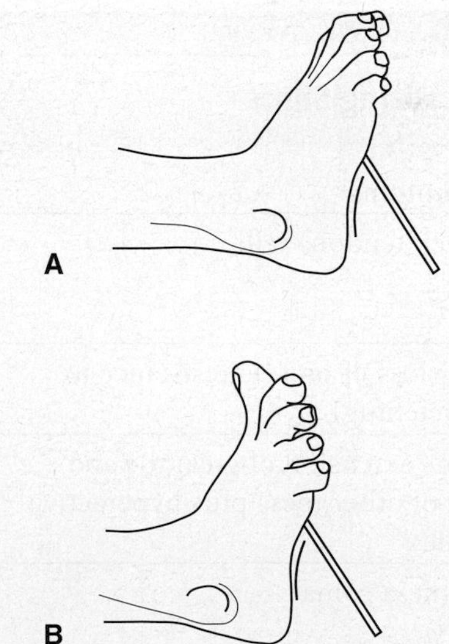

Figure 16-6 Upper motor neuron symptoms. A. Normal motor response. B. The Babinski sign in adults indicates dysfunctioning of the corticospinal system.

Babinski sign in a child is not an indication of disorder. Before maturation of the corticospinal system, during the first 5 to 7 years of development, earlier (or primitive) reflexes are pronounced; these include the protective flexor-withdrawal reflex. As the developing corticospinal system begins to dominate, Babinski and other primitive reflexes disappear.

The abdominal and cremasteric reflexes are two other reflexes that are lost in UMN syndrome. There is no abdominal muscle contraction in response to stroking the skin over the abdominal quadrant and no testicle elevation in response to stroking up the inner thigh (Table 16-3).

There is always some recovery from spastic paralysis, and it may result in varying degrees of flexion in the upper extremity and hyperextension in the lower limbs (Fig. 16-4). In general, gross motor movements recover, with proximal muscles displaying the greatest recovery.

No treatment is available to alleviate UMN symptoms other than minimizing the damage by reducing cerebral edema and by enhancing the blood supply to the damaged tissue. Future treatment is concerned with finding a way to get UMN axons to grow past the damage and reinnervate former targets, an extremely challenging task.

Lesion Localization

Rule 9: Symptoms Suggestive of a UMN or an LMN Lesion

Presenting Symptoms. Increased reflexes, hemiplegia, and spastic tone in a symptomatic (sensorimotor) limb indicate a UMN lesion. Reduced reflexes, muscle atrophy, and weakness in the same symptomatic limb imply a peripheral or a LMN lesion.

Rationale. The UMN regulation of the LMNs via the corticospinal and corticonuclear systems is excitatory. A lesion interrupting the excitatory projections from the UMNs first produces early signs of loss of precise motor control, especially of distal limb muscles, muscle weakness, flaccid tone, and hyporeflexia. However, in several weeks, the hyporeflexia and flaccid tone are replaced by increased reflexes and spasticity, which result from the increased power of the stretch afferents because of the filling of the denuded corticospinal synapses to the LMNs. The hyperactive antigravity stretch reflexes and spastic muscle tone take 1 to 4 weeks to be demonstrated clinically (Table 16-3).

The LMN cell body provides the only output pathway to peripheral function via its axon, which traverses the ventral root and peripheral nerves to innervate a skeletal muscle, where it's multiple axonal branches innervate and contract many muscle fibers. This entire single neuron– multiple muscle fiber functional circuitry forms the motor unit. Damage to the motor unit (LMN cell and/or its axon) eliminates the entire function of a motor unit (Fig. 13-13). This weakens the muscles and reduces tendon reflexes. Additional LMN symptoms are flaccid muscle tone, muscle weakness, and gradual muscle atrophy because of muscle disuse and/or denervation. These symptoms are seen in neurologic conditions affecting motor units, diseases of the

Table 16-3

Lesion-Localizing Signs

Clinical Symptoms	Implicated Lesion Sites
Reduced (deep tendon) reflex	Lower motor neuron syndrome: impaired muscle stretch afferents involving motor nuclei (brainstem/spinal cord and their axons in the peripheral pathway)
Flaccid tone (loss of muscle resistance to passive stretching)	Lower motor neuron syndrome: injury to motor nuclei in the brainstem or spinal cord
Babinski sign (extension of great toe and abduction of other toes) plus hyperactive (brisk) reflex	Upper motor neuron syndrome: damage to motor neurons in the motor cortex or interruption in the descending fibers
Unconsciousness/coma	Diffuse massive cortical, subcortical, or brainstem dysfunction or bilateral affection of the ascending reticular projections
Tremor (at rest) and cogwheel rigidity	Parkinson disease with degeneration of dopaminergic neurons in the brainstem
Progressively severe exacerbation and remission of sensorimotor functions	Multiple sclerosis, demyelination in the brain and spinal cord
Involuntary movements (chorea and/or tremor)	Basal ganglia circuitry dysfunction

skeletal muscles (e.g., muscular dystrophy), and reduced nerve–muscle transmission (e.g., myasthenia gravis).

Rule 10: Symptoms Suggestive of a Brainstem Lesion

Presenting Symptoms. Motor and sensory losses of the extremities on one side with contralateral cranial nerve signs imply a brainstem lesion. An altered level of consciousness can also be associated with such a lesion. An extension of this rule is that no lesion lower than the mid-pons can impair the function of the facial muscles.

Rationale. A lesion anywhere in the neuraxis can interrupt the long ascending and descending fibers, causing sensory loss and paralysis. However, the presence of cranial nerve symptoms suggests a bulbar location of the lesion since cranial nuclei are located in only the brainstem. In alternating hemiplegia, the involved cranial nerves receive projections that have already crossed the midline, thus are contralateral, whereas the involved descending corticospinal fibers have not yet crossed the midline. Thus, a brainstem involvement would result in crossed or alternating symptoms, where the spastic hemiplegia (UMN symptom) involves the body contralateral to the lesion, and the cranial nerve signs (LMN symptom) occur on the side of the brainstem lesion. Common cranial nerve symptoms are dysarthria (laryngeal, pharyngeal, facial, or glossal dysfunctions) and dysphagia. A lesion extending to the brainstem reticular formation can affect attention and consciousness, which otherwise require bilateral cortical lesions.

The locations of the cranial nerve nuclei can further be used for identifying the lesion location. For example, the motor nucleus supplying the muscles of facial expression is located at the middle pons, thus, lesions below the mid-pons will not impair facial functions.

CASE STUDIES FOR PROBLEM SOLVING

CASE ONE (16-1)

A 47-year-old woman had a stroke while sleeping. When she awoke, she could not move her left arm and leg. She could talk, but her speech was slurred and unintelligible. She was rushed to the ER of a hospital, and on testing, she presented with

- Weakness in the left upper and lower limbs (hemiplegia)
- Drooping lower left face
- Distorted smile with the mouth pulled to the normal (right) side
- Intact upper facial functions (frowning and eye closing)
- Loss of proprioceptive and pain sensation on left side of the body
- Hyperactive deep tendon reflexes, including a positive Babinski sign on the left side.
- Dysarthria (imprecise and weak articulatory movements and breathy voice)

A brain MRI study revealed an infarct in the posterior region of the right internal capsule.

Question: How can you relate this lesion site with her UMN symptoms?

Case (16-1) Discussion: See the discussion of case studies

CASE TWO (16-2)

A 61-year-old man had a stroke while confined to a hospital for heart disease. He suddenly felt that he had no control of his left arm and leg and could not move his mouth. He was seen by a physician, who observed the following:

- Weakness in the right half of the face
- Inability to close his right eye and a widened palpebral fissure
- A weak bite on the right side
- No pain or touch sensation in the right half of his face
- Spastic paralysis of the left upper and lower limbs
- Left-sided Babinski sign

A brain MRI study revealed a massive infarct in the right ventrolateral pons.

Question: How is it that there was sensorimotor loss of the right face and right masticator muscles and yet left hemiplegia? Can you account for the discrepancy in the clinical features observed?

Case (16-2) Discussion: See the discussion of case studies

(Continued)

CASE THREE (16-3) (*CONTINUED*)

A 55-year-old man had a stroke while sleeping; he woke up and noted that he had no control of his right limbs and did not speak well. He was taken to the emergency room and was seen by a neurologist who noted the following:

- Right hemiplegia: paralysis of the right lower and upper limbs
- Right hemianesthesia: loss of touch and pain in right lower and upper limbs
- Drooping right lower face
- When smiling the weakened right side of the face moved to the left
- Intact upper right facial functions, such as wrinkling
- Weakened tongue deviating to right
- Some dysarthria with imprecise articulation
- Nonfluent, effortful, and halting verbal output containing two- to three-word utterances

A brain MRI study revealed a large infarct in Brodmann area 4, extending to parts of areas 3, 1, 2 and area 44 in the left hemisphere. The patient was seen again 3 weeks later and exhibited the following additional symptoms:

- Hyperactive deep tendon reflexes
- Spasticity in limb muscles
- Positive Babinski sign

Question: How can you relate these symptoms to the cortical lesion evident on MRI?

Case (16-3) Discussion: See the discussion of case studies

CASE FOUR (16-4)

A 65-year-old man suffered a stroke while sleeping and woke up to find that he could not use his right limbs and had problems speaking. He was taken to the hospital where the physician noted the following:

- Dysarthric speech subsequent to a left-sided lingual paralysis
- Swallowing difficulty owing to weakness of the pharyngeal muscles
- Loss of pain and temperature on the left side of the face
- Loss of pain and temperature on the right half of the body
- Paralysis of the right limbs
- No sign of aphasia or cognitive impairment

A brain MRI study revealed an infarct in the left brainstem.

Question: What lesion location in the brainstem can account for these symptoms?

Case (16-4) Discussion: See the discussion of case studies

SUMMARY

The multiple motor cortices control voluntary manipulative and delicate motor movements and initiate motor performance. Descending cortical motor projections to the motor neurons travel via the corticonuclear and the corticospinal tracts, collectively called the pyramidal tract. These tracts control cranial and spinal motor neurons (LMN), respectively. Activity at the motor cortex is influenced by extensive feedback channels from the cerebellum, brainstem, thalamus, and basal ganglia.

A lesion interrupting the excitatory projections from the motor cortex results in a specific loss of delicate motor control. It also results in muscle weakness, flaccid tone, hyporeflexia, and loss of reflexes. However, in several weeks, the hyporeflexia and flaccid tone are replaced by increased reflexes (hyperreflexia) and spastic tone in muscles.

REVIEW QUESTIONS

1. Complete the following statements using the appropriate technical terms:

   A. Dorsal flexion of the great toe and fanning of other toes on the stroking of the sole are indicative of ________ pathology, and is called the ________.

   B. ________ is the representation of the body in the sensorimotor cortex.

   C. The ________ of the descending and ascending fiber tracts accounts for the ________ sensorimotor organization in the brain.

   D. The ________ include the motor cells in the primary motor cortex and their descending axonal fibers.

   E. The motor neural fibers that travel in the pyramidal tract arise from three cortical regions: ________, ________, and ________.

F. Interruption of the descending corticospinal tract results in contralateral ________ hemiplegia.

G. Bilateral involvement of the corticonuclear fibers results in ________, which has a profound impact on motor speech and facial expression.

H. The primary motor cortex is located in the ________, the Brodmann area 4.

I. Efferents from the motor cortex travel descend in two tracts: ________ and ________.

2. List two clinical signs of alternating hemiplegia.
3. What motor function that is important to SLPs is profoundly affected in pseudobulbar palsy?
4. Match each of the following conditions with its associated lesion site:

A. muscle atrophy and flaccidity — a. LMN
B. loss of stretch reflex — b. UMN
C. spasticity and hypertonia — c. cerebellum
D. fasciculation — d. basal ganglia
E. positive Babinski sign
F. ataxia and asynergia
G. tremor and chorea
H. spastic hemiplegia

5. Name four clinical signs of UMN syndrome.
6. Why does a lesion at the internal capsule cause greater motor deficits than in the primary motor cortex?
7. Is the presence of the Babinski sign in children considered abnormal?
8. Name the descending motor pathway that innervates cranial nerve nuclei.
9. From what layer of the cerebral cortex do the descending motor fibers originate?
10. Name the muscle spasticity in which initially there is resistance to any muscle stretch, which suddenly discontinues.
11. Name the lesion site that is associated with clasp-knife reflex.

17 Synopsis of Cranial Nerves

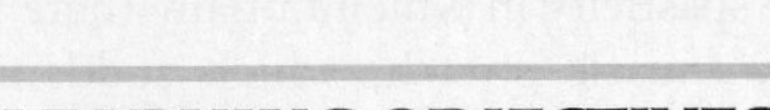

LEARNING OBJECTIVES

After studying this chapter, students should be able to:

- Relate the nerve numbers to the names of cranial nerves
- Follow the functional classification of cranial nerves
- Identify the locations of the brainstem attachments of cranial nerves
- Explain the clinical implications of the bilateral/unilateral innervation of motor nerve nuclei
- Discuss the branchial and somatic bases of muscles
- Identify functional components for each cranial nerve
- Relate cranial nerve nuclei and their projections to specific sensorimotor functions
- Explain idiosyncratic distribution and innervational properties of cranial nerves
- Discuss clinical symptoms associated with disorders of cranial nerves and nuclei
- Perform an oral–facial examination in accordance with the pertinent functional components of cranial nerves
- Differentiate between upper and lower motor neuron symptoms of the cranial nerves

EVOLUTIONARY BASE OF CRANIAL NERVES

The cranial nerves (CNs) in humans represent an evolutionary modification of a basic organizational pattern of the vertebrate CNS, which consisted of 40 bilaterally symmetrical repeating segments, each with a dorsal and a ventral horn. Each CNS segment innervates the corresponding head or body region by means of the afferent (dorsal) and efferent (ventral) nerve roots on each side. The peripheral processes of the ganglion cells in the dorsal root innervate the tissue of the body segment as receptor endings with its central axons traveling to the dorsal horns of the corresponding CNS segment. The efferent fibers from the ventral horn innervate the skeletal muscles.

Early in evolutionary development, additional (intermediate) roots of efferent fibers emerged between the dorsal and the ventral roots. These roots, present in only the rostral 15 segments of the CNS, extended from the head to the C5 segment. The efferent axons leaving the **intermediate roots** innervated muscle related to gill opening and closing for filtering food and absorbing oxygen from the water. In mammals, these gill-related muscles evolved into many of the muscles of the head and face and are modified for other visceral purposes, such as phonation and speech, the area of most concern to students of human communication. The cranial nerves are the evolutionary remnants of the intermediate nerve roots (Box 17-1).

The stable arrangement of afferent and efferent neurons for cranial nerves continues in the brainstem. The peripherally located afferent neurons of the cranial nerves are homologous to the spinal dorsal root ganglia and have names such as **semilunar ganglion** (trigeminal nerve [CN V]), **geniculate ganglion** (facial nerve [CN VII]), and the **superior** and **inferior ganglia** (vagus nerve [CN X]). The efferent neurons of the cranial nerves, whether related to gill muscles or somite muscles, contain both alpha- and gamma-motor neurons and lie within the nuclei of the brainstem.

The first two cranial nerves (olfactory [CN I] and optic [CN II]) are part of the forebrain; the other 10 cranial nerves are attached to the brainstem (Fig. 17-1). Some cranial nerves serve only sensory functions; others serve only motor functions. Many of the nerves are mixed, serving both sensory and motor functions. Furthermore, cranial nerves have evolved specialized functions, not required at the spinal level, such as vision, audition, gustation, and olfaction. Thus, the cranial nerves have a more complex organization than the spinal nerves.

Key Terms :

Branchial arch	**Postganglionic neuron**
General	**Preganglionic neuron**
Somatic	**Visceral**
Special	

BOX 17-1

Evolutionary Basis of the Cranial Nerves

The cranial nerves are the result of an evolutionary modification of the basic organizational pattern of the vertebrate CNS. In mammals, the ancient gill-related muscles have evolved into many of the skeletal muscles of the head and face, which were later modified for the visceral purposes of swallowing, phonation, and speech. The "gill muscle" innervating cranial nerves are V (motor branch), VII (facial), IX (glossopharyngeal), and X (vagus). This explains not only the differential evolutionary basis for the muscles now used for motor speech, but also why the head and face muscles are classified differently as visceral special.

FUNCTIONAL CLASSIFICATION OF CRANIAL NERVES

Spinal nerves serve only general motor and general sensory functions, involving both somatic (skeletal) and visceral (internal organ) muscles, and are classified into four functional components (Table 17-1). Besides serving general motor and general sensory functions, cranial nerves also use special receptors and neurons to serve special functions. The general and special functional components of the cranial nerves can be further classified by their innervation (somatic muscles or visceral structures) and type of information (sensory [afferent] or motor [efferent]). The somatic component of the cranial nerves with special functions contains only afferent fibers, whereas the visceral component contains both afferent and efferent fibers (see Chapter 1). Thus there are seven functional types of cranial nerves, discussed in the following sections (Tables 17-2 and 17-3; Box 17-2).

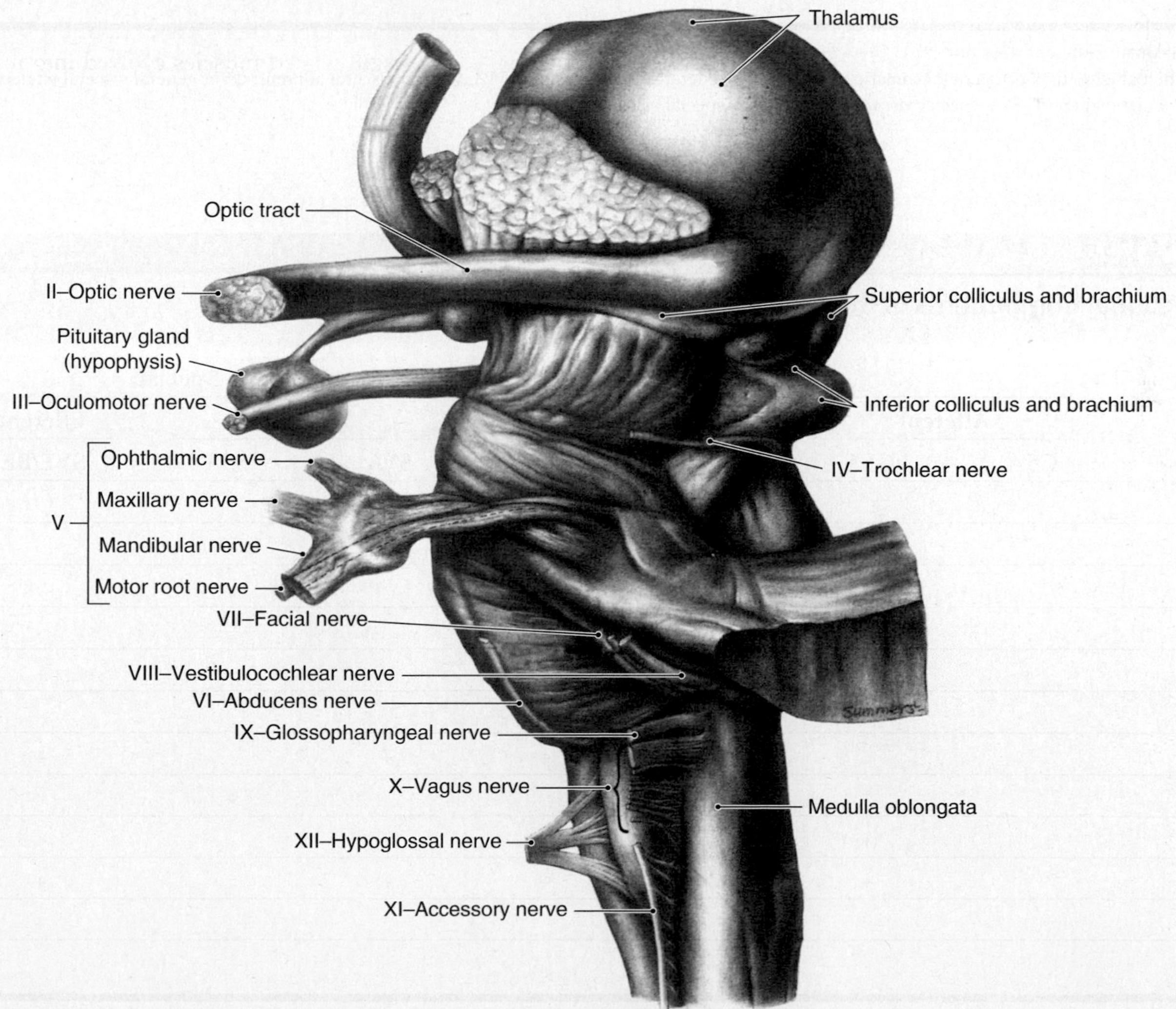

Figure 17-1 Cranial nerve roots and other structures on the lateral surface of the brainstem.

Table 17-1

Functional Components of the Nervous System

General		Special	
Somatic	Visceral	Somatic	Visceral
GSE: controls muscles derived from somites (e.g., skeletal, extraocular, glossal)	GVE: sends preganglionic axons to peripheral parasympathetic ganglia, which regulate autonomic functions of smooth muscles, cardiac muscles, glands	SSE[a]	SVE/BE: controls gill-related muscles of face, pharynx, larynx, and neck (evolved from branchial arches)
GSA: mediates somesthetic input (pain, temperature, touch) from somatic muscles, skin, ligaments, and joints	GVA: mediates sensations of pain, temperature, tissue stretch, and pressure from visceral organs	SSA: conducts special sensory mechanism of vision from retina and audition and equilibrium from inner ear; includes spindle afferents and Golgi tendon organ afferents	SVA: mediates information from specialized receptors related to taste from tongue and pharynx, olfaction from nasal mucosa

[a]Special somatic efferent does not exist.
BE, branchial efferent; *GSA*, general somatic afferent; *GSE*, general somatic efferent; *GVA*, general visceral afferent; *GVE*, general visceral efferent; *SSA*, special somatic afferent; *SVA*, special visceral afferent; *SVE*, special visceral efferent.

Table 17-2

Functional Components of the Cranial Nerves

	General				Special[a]		
	Afferent		Efferent		Afferent		Efferent
Nerve	GSA	GVA	GSE	GVE	SVA	SSA	SVE/BE
I					+		
II						+	
III			+	+			
IV			+				
V	+						+
VI			+				
VII				+	+		+
VIII						+	
IX		+		+	+		+
X		+		+	+		+
XI							+
XII			+				

[a]Special somatic efferent does not exist.
BE, branchial efferent; *GSA*, general somatic afferent; *GSE*, general somatic efferent; *GVA*, general visceral afferent; *GVE*, general visceral efferent; *SSA*, special somatic afferent; *SVA*, special visceral afferent; *SVE*, special visceral efferent.

Table 17-3

Summary of the Functional Components of the Cranial Nerves

Cranial Nerve (Number)	Classification	Cell Nuclei	Function
Olfactory (I)	SVA	First order: neuroepithelial olfactory cells in nasal mucosa Second order: olfactory bulb	Smell
Optic (II)	SSA	Ganglion cells in retina	Vision
Oculomotor (III)	GSE	Oculomotor nucleus in upper midbrain tegmentum	Eye movements: controls all eye muscles except lateral rectus (CN VI) and superior oblique (CN IV) muscles Regulates eyelid elevation (levator palpebrae superioris)
	GVE	Edinger–Westphal nucleus in midbrain tegmentum Preganglionic parasympathetic projections to ciliary ganglion	Reflexive constriction of pupil and accommodation of lens for near vision
Trochlear (IV)	GSE	Trochlear nucleus in midbrain tegmentum	Eye movements: innervates contralateral superior oblique muscles
Trigeminal (V)	GSA	First order: trigeminal (semilunar) ganglion Second order: primary sensory (pons), descending spinal nucleus (pons, medulla, and upper cervical levels)	Receives pain and touch sensations from skin and muscles in face, orbit, nose, mouth, forehead, teeth, meninges, anterior two-thirds of tongue, external auditory meatus, and external surface of tympanic membrane
		Mesencephalic nucleus (midbrain)	Proprioception from jaw
	SVE/BE	Trigeminal motor nucleus in pons	Innervates muscles of mastication (masseter internal and external pterygoid and temporal), mylohyoid, anterior belly of digastric, tensor velum palatini, and tensor tympani muscles
Abducens (VI)	GSE	Abducens nucleus in tegmentum of pons	Eye movements: innervates ipsilateral lateral rectus muscle
Facial (VII)	GVE	Superior salivatory nucleus: preganglionic parasympathetic to ganglia associated with oral, lacrimal, and nasal glands	Parasympathetic regulation of secretion from nasal, palatal, lacrimal, submaxillary, and sublingual glands and mucous membrane of nasopharynx
	SVA	First order: geniculate ganglion Second order: nucleus solitarius	Mediates gustatory sensation from taste buds in anterior two-thirds of tongue
	SVE/BE	Facial motor complex in lateral pons	Innervates muscles of facial expression and platysma, extrinsic and intrinsic ear muscles, and stapedius muscle

(continued)

Table 17-3

Summary of the Functional Components of the Cranial Nerves *(Continued)*

Cranial Nerve (Number)	Classification	Cell Nuclei	Function
Vestibulocochlear (VIII)	SSA	First order: superior and inferior vestibular ganglia Second order: vestibular nuclei in medulla and pons	Maintains equilibrium and head orientation in space
	SSA	First order: spiral ganglion Second order: cochlear nuclei in medulla	Mediates audition
Glossopharyngeal (IX)	GVA	First order: inferior ganglion Second order: nucleus solitarius	Mediates general sensation from palate, posterior third of tongue, oral pharynx, middle ear, eustachian tube (ear ache), and carotid sinus
	GVE	Inferior salivatory nucleus: preganglionic to otic ganglion	Parasympathetic regulation of secretion from parotid gland and oral pharyngeal mucosal glands
	SVA	First order: inferior ganglion Second order: nucleus solitarius	Mediates taste sensation from posterior third of tongue and oral pharynx
	SVE/BE	Nucleus ambiguus	Contributes to swallowing by controlling stylopharyngeus muscle
Vagus (X)	GVA	First order: inferior ganglion Second order: nucleus solitarius	Receives general sensation from pharynx, larynx, thorax, abdomen, carotid body, and aortic body Regulates nausea, oxygen intake, and lung inflation
	GVE	Dorsal motor nucleus: preganglionic parasympathetic innervation	Innervates glands and muscles in heart, blood vessels, trachea, bronchi, esophagus, stomach, and intestine
	SVA	First order: inferior ganglion Second order: nucleus solitarius	Mediates taste sensation from sensory buds in epiglottis and pharynx, and laryngeal pharynx
	SVE/BE	Nucleus ambiguus	Controls muscles of larynx, pharynx, soft palate for phonation, deglutition, and resonance
Spinal accessory (XI)	SVE/BE	Spinal accessory nucleus in C1–C5 ventral horns	Controls head and shoulders by innervating trapezius and sternocleidomastoid muscles
Hypoglossal (XII)	GSE	Hypoglossal nucleus in medulla	Controls tongue movement by regulating intrinsic and most extrinsic muscles

BE, branchial efferent; *GSA*, general somatic afferent; *GSE*, general somatic efferent; *GVA*, general visceral afferent; *GVE*, general visceral efferent; *SSA*, special somatic afferent; *SVA*, special visceral afferent; *SVE*, special visceral efferent.

BOX 17-2

Multiple Cranial Nerve Functions

Spinal nerves serve general motor and general sensory functions for somatic (voluntary) and visceral (internal organ) muscles resulting in four functional components (general somatic efferent, general visceral efferent, general somatic afferent, and general visceral afferent). What adds to the functional complexity of the cranial nerves is that they not only serve the four general sensory and motor functions, but also regulate three special sensory functions including vision, audition, olfaction, gustation, and speech. Examples of this functional categorization are as follows: **general somatic efferent**: hypoglossal (CN XII), oculomotor (CN III), trochlear (CN IV), and abducens (CN VI) nerves; **general visceral efferent**: oculomotor [CN III], facial [CN VII], glossopharyngeal [CN IX], and vagus [CN X] nerves; **special visceral efferent**: trigeminal nerve (CN V), facial nerve (CN VII, glossopharyngeal nerve (CN IX), the vagus nerve (CN X), and the accessory nerve (CN XI); **general somatic afferent:** trigeminal (CN V) sensory nerve; **general visceral efferent:** glossopharyngeal nerve (CN IX) and the vagus nerve (CN X); **special somatic afferent:** optic nerve [CN II] and vestibulocochlear nerve [CN VIII]; **special visceral afferent:** olfactory nerve (CN I), facial nerve (CN VII), glossopharyngeal nerve (CN IX), and vagus nerve (CN X).

Efferent

General Somatic Efferent

The general somatic efferent (GSE) nuclei innervate the skeletal muscles derived from somites. This category includes the innervation of the ocular muscles (oculomotor [CN III], trochlear [CN IV], and abducens [CN VI]) and lingual muscles (hypoglossal [CN XII]).

General Visceral Efferent

The general visceral efferent (GVE) nuclei regulate the autonomic (parasympathetic) innervation of smooth muscles and glands. As the source of preganglionic parasympathetic projections, the GVE nuclei include the Edinger–Westphal nucleus (oculomotor [CN III]), **superior salivatory** nucleus (facial [CN VII]), **inferior salivary** nucleus (glossopharyngeal [CN IX]), and **dorsal motor nucleus** (vagus [CN X]). These nerves are responsible for pupillary constriction; gland secretion; and the regulation of the muscles of the heart, trachea, bronchi, esophagus, and lower viscera.

Special Visceral or Branchial Efferent

The special visceral efferent (SVE), or branchial efferent (BE), nuclei control the muscles of the face, pharynx, larynx, and some neck muscles, which evolve from the **branchial arches** (Fig. 17-2). This functional component consists of the motor nucleus of the trigeminal nerve (CN V), the motor nucleus of the facial nerve (CN VII), the nucleus ambiguus of the glossopharyngeal nerve (CN IX), the vagus nerve (CN X), and the motor nuclei of the accessory nerve (CN XI) in the C1–C5 segments. They control the muscles of expression, mastication, phonation, deglutition, head turning, and shoulder elevation.

Afferent

General Somatic Afferent

The general somatic afferent (GSA) nuclei mediate somesthetic input, including pain, pressure, temperature, and touch sensations, from the skin and somatic muscles in the head, neck, and face. This functional category primarily includes the trigeminal (CN V) sensory nuclei (**chief sensory nucleus** and **spinal descending nucleus**).

General Visceral Afferent

The general visceral afferent (GVA) nuclei serve general sensation, including pain and temperature, from the visceral structures of the pharynx, palate, larynx, aorta, and abdomen. This functional category includes the glossopharyngeal nerve (CN IX) and the vagus nerve (CN X).

Special Somatic Afferent

The special somatic afferent (SSA) nuclei regulate special senses, such as vision (optic [CN II]) and audition and equilibrium (vestibulocochlear [CN VIII]). This functional component includes proprioception and stretch afferents from muscle spindles.

Special Visceral Afferent

Special visceral afferent (SVA) nuclei mediate taste (gustation) and smell (olfaction). This functional component includes the olfactory nerve (CN I), facial nerve (CN VII), glossopharyngeal nerve (CN IX), and vagus nerve (CN X).

BRANCHIAL ORIGIN OF SPEECH-RELATED MUSCLES

The classification of speech and the related muscles of phonation, mastication, deglutition, articulation, head turning, and shoulder elevation as SVE can be confusing, as these muscles are structurally identical to other skeletal muscles derived from the somites that are classified as somatic (Table 17-4; Box 17-3). The reason for their classification as visceral (SVE) is that they are derived from

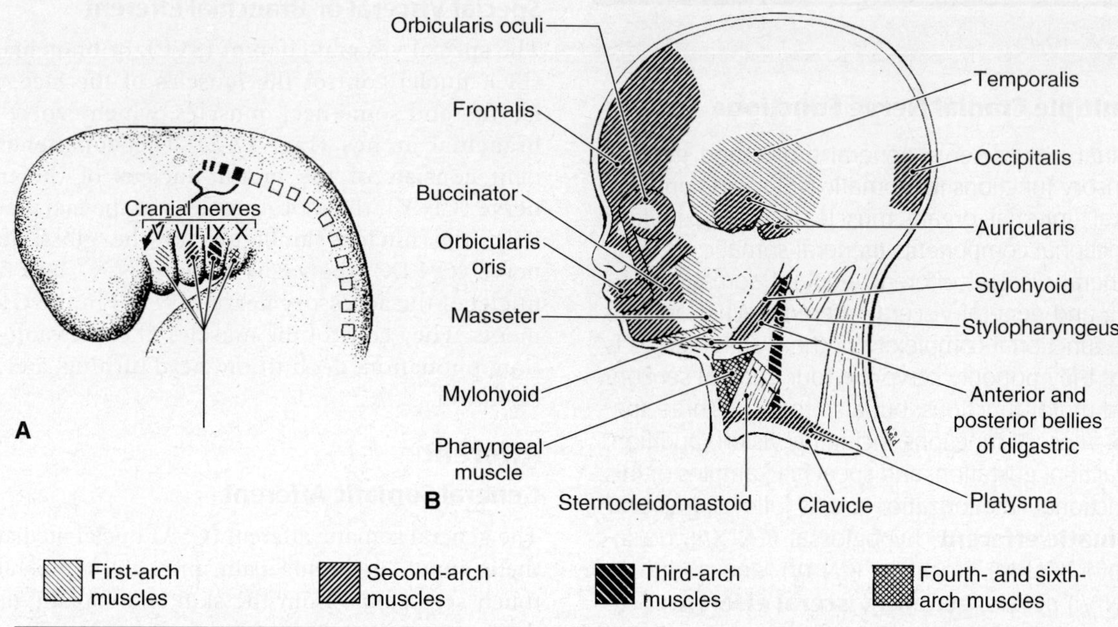

Figure 17-2 Lateral view of a 4-week-old embryo. A. Arches and the cranial nerves derived from each branchial arch. B. Major muscles derived from each arch.

the **branchial arches** and gill-related structures of the embryo. To minimize the categorical confusion, these muscles are also identified as **branchial efferent** in this chapter.

Early in human embryonic development, six branchial arches emerge (Fig. 17-2). The first four arches are well marked, the fifth arch disappears during development, and the sixth arch is present but not obvious. Each branchial arch relates to specific groups of muscles (Table 17-4): the muscles of mastication (trigeminal nerve [CN V]) relate to the **first branchial arch**, the muscles of facial expression (facial nerve [CN VII]) relate to the

Table 17-4

Branchial Arches, Associated Cranial Nerves, and Derived Muscles

Branchial Arch[a]	Cranial Nerve (Number)	Muscles
First (mandibular)	Trigeminal (V)	Of mastication: temporalis, masseter medial, and lateral pterygoid Additional: mylohyoid, anterior belly of digastric, tensor tympani, and tensor veli palatini
Second	Facial (VII)	Of facial expression: buccinator, auricularis, frontalis, platysma, orbicularis oris, and orbicularis oculi Additional: stapedius, stylohyoid, and posterior belly of digastric
Third	Glossopharyngeal (IX)	Stylopharyngeus
Fourth and sixth	Superior laryngeal and recurrent laryngeal branches of vagus (X)	Pharyngeal and laryngeal: cricothyroid, levator veli palatini, constrictors of pharynx, and intrinsic muscles of larynx
Unnumbered gill structures	Spinal accessory nuclei in C1–C5	Sternocleidomastoid and trapezius muscles

[a]The fifth branchial arch is not developed in human embryo.

BOX 17-3

Confusion Related to Speech Muscles

The classification of the muscles of speech (used for phonation, mastication, deglutition, articulation, head turning, and shoulder elevation) as the "special visceral efferent" is often confusing for students of communicative disorders. These muscles are under voluntary control and are similar to other skeletal muscles, which are classified as somatic efferent. The unique classification of these muscles is based on their derivation from the branchial arches of the embryo. On the other hand, the skeletal muscles are derived from the somites, thus are classified as "somatic."

second branchial arch, and the **stylopharyngeus muscles** (glossopharyngeal nerve [CN IX]) relate to the **third branchial arch**. The remaining pharyngeal muscles (vagus nerve [CN X]) are derived from the **fourth branchial arch**, and the laryngeal muscles (vagus nerve [CN X]) are derived from the **sixth branchial arch**.

The spinal accessory nerve [CN XI], also branchial in origin, is related to a series of unnumbered gill structures that extended down to the C5 segment in mammals. The lower motor neurons (LMNs) exiting the C1–C5 segments form the spinal accessory nerve and innervate the neck muscles.

CRANIAL NERVES AND THE AUTONOMIC NERVOUS SYSTEM

The parasympathetic efferents of the autonomic nervous system (ANS) exit the CNS from the craniosacral region (brainstem area and spinal segments S2–S4) (see Chapters 2 and 18). Therefore, the cranial nerves have only parasympathetic function of the ANS via the innervation of the postganglionic neurons that are located in the peripheral ganglia. These functions, classified as GVE, are carried out by the preganglionic LMNs in the Edinger–Westphal nucleus (oculomotor [CN III]), superior salivatory nucleus (facial [CN VII]), inferior salivatory nucleus (glossopharyngeal [CN IX]), and the dorsal vagal nucleus (vagus [CN X]).

CRANIAL NERVE NUCLEI

Most of the cranial nerve nuclei are located in the ventricular floor of the brainstem (Figs. 17-3 and 17-4). Depending on what functions they serve, some nuclei are connected to several related nerves. Note that the cranial nerves take a fixed path and exit through specific foramina in the skull (Fig. 17-5).

Midbrain

There are three cranial nerve motor nuclei in the adult midbrain tegmentum: **Edinger–Westphal nucleus** (oculomotor [CN III]), **oculomotor nucleus** (CN III), and **trochlear nucleus** (CN IV). The Edinger–Westphal nucleus contains preganglionic parasympathetic efferents to innervate the **ciliary muscle** and the sphincter (constrictor) fibers of the pupil. The oculomotor nucleus contains the LMNs that control most of the muscles of the eye. The trochlear nucleus contains the LMNs that innervate the **superior oblique**, one of the muscles of the eye.

Pons

Six major cranial nerve nuclei lie in the pontine tegmentum. There are three sensory nuclei of the trigeminal nerve (CN V): the **primary sensory** nucleus, **spinal trigeminal** nucleus, and **mesencephalic** nucleus. The first two nuclei join to form the sensory branch of the trigeminal nerve (CN V). The mesencephalic nucleus contains (proprioceptive) afferents from spindles (in the muscles of mastication) and regulates the jaw reflex. Located adjacent to the trigeminal sensory complex is the **trigeminal motor nucleus**, which innervates the muscles of mastication and other associated muscles. The **abducens motor nucleus** (CN VI), with LMNs, innervates the **lateral rectus muscle** of the eye. Located below the abducens nucleus is the **facial motor nucleus** (CN VII) that contains LMNs to innervate the muscles of facial expressions (Fig. 17-4).

Medulla

There are nine major nuclei in the medulla. The **cochlear** and **vestibular nuclear complexes** (not shown in Fig. 17-4) are laterally located at the junction of the pons and medulla (see Chapters 9 and 10). At the rostral medulla is the salivary nucleus (shared by the facial [CN VII], glossopharyngeal [CN IX], and vagus [CN X] nerves), a motor nucleus responsible for controlling secretion from various glands. The dorsal motor nucleus of the vagus nerve (CN X) controls autonomic motor activity of various visceral organs. Medial to the dorsal motor nucleus is the **hypoglossal nucleus** (CN XII), whose LMNs innervate extrinsic and intrinsic muscles of the tongue. The nucleus solitarius, a visceral sensory nucleus responsible for taste, nausea, heart rate, respiration, and blood pressure, is shared by the facial (CN VII) and glossopharyngeal (CN IX) nerves. It receives the taste and gustatory input from the facial (CN VII; intermedius), vagus (CN X), and glossopharyngeal nerves (CN IX). Located between the **inferior olivary nucleus** and the **spinal**

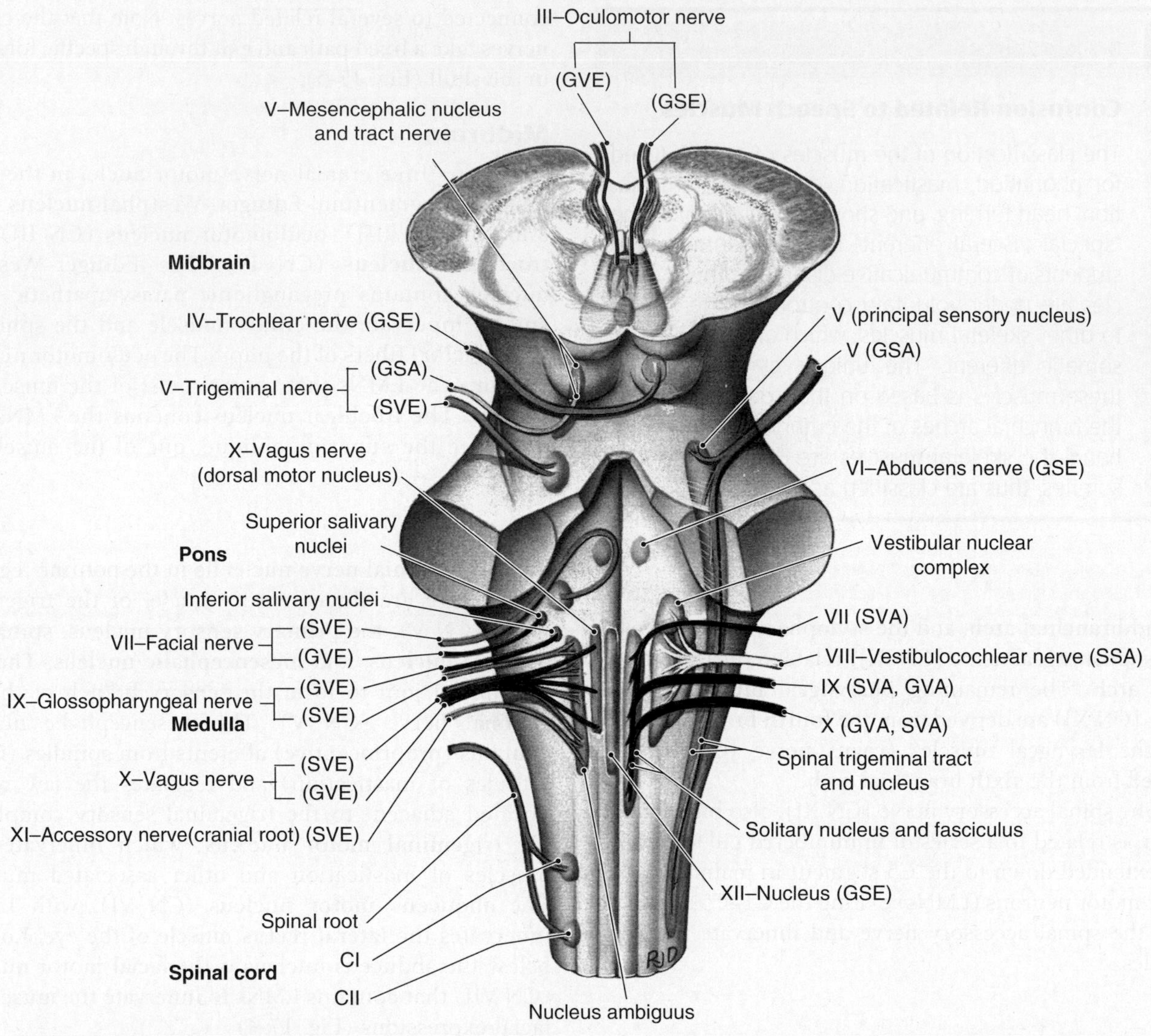

Figure 17-3 Intramedullary cranial nerves, their nuclei of origin, and their functional classifications. *GSA*, general somatic afferent; *GSE*, general somatic efferent; *GVA*, general visceral afferent; *GVE*, general visceral efferent; *SSA*, special somatic afferent; *SVA*, special visceral afferent; *SVE*, special visceral efferent.

trigeminal nucleus, the **nucleus ambiguus**, also shared by the glossopharyngeal (CN IX) and vagus (CN X) nerves, controls the movements of the laryngeal and pharyngeal muscles. The only cranial nerve nuclei outside the brainstem are the ones that relate to the accessory nerve (CN XI), and these are located in the upper cervical (C1–C5) segments.

PATHWAYS

Motor or Efferent Pathways

The cranial nerve nuclei receive their motor projections from the **corticonuclear fibers** (Fig. 17-6). Corticonuclear fibers arise from the motor cells (UMNs) in the lower part of the precentral cortex and descend through the genu of the internal capsule to synapse on the motor cranial nerve nuclei (LMN) in the brainstem. Before synapsing on the cranial nerve motor nuclei, most corticonuclear fibers cross the midline at different brainstem locations. However, a substantial bilateral cortical innervation of the cranial motor nuclei exists for the muscles of the face, jaw, larynx, and pharynx (see Chapter 16).

Cortical damage interrupts the corticonuclear (corticobulbar) projections, resulting in UMN symptoms of increased deep tendon reflexes and contralateral paralysis (see Chapter 16). The many unusual (such as bilateral) corticonuclear fibers in the brainstem protect cranial nerve motor functions from damage; therefore, cortical lesions do not result in profound spasticity and weakness in the cranial muscles. Lesions of the brainstem cranial motor nuclei and their axons (nerves) produce LMN

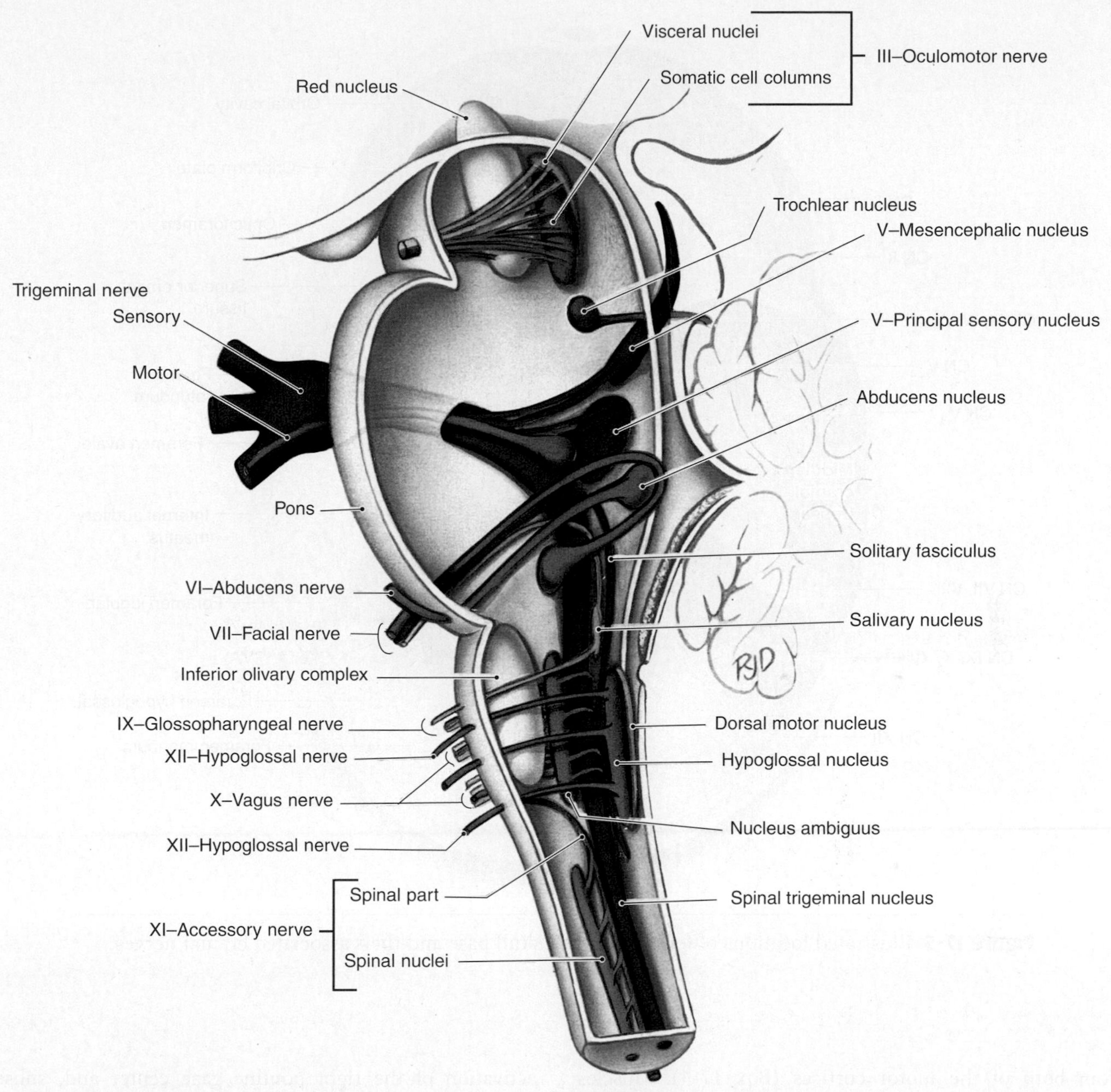

Figure 17-4 Midsagittal brainstem view of the intramedullar nuclei of all the cranial nerves except the vestibulocochlear nerve/nuclei.

syndrome, which is characterized by flaccid tone, muscle paralysis, absent reflexes, fibrillations (single denervated fiber), fasciculation (spontaneous firing of motor units), and atrophy of the muscles (see Chapters 13 and 16).

Sensory or Afferent Pathways

Most of the sensory pathways of the cranial nerves consist of three-order nuclei and their fibers (Fig. 17-7; see also Chapter 11). The cell bodies of the first-order fibers are outside the CNS. The second-order fibers, with cell bodies in the gray matter of the brainstem, cross the midline and terminate in the thalamus. The third-order fibers, with cell bodies in the ventral posterior medial (VPM) nucleus of the thalamus, project to the lower region of the sensory cortex in the parietal lobe. Smell, audition, and vision are exceptions to the sensory organization of three-order cells and fibers.

INNERVATION PATTERN

The corticonuclear regulation of several branchial motor nuclei is largely bilateral (Fig. 17-8; Table 17-5). The nuclei of such cranial nerves receive corticonuclear input

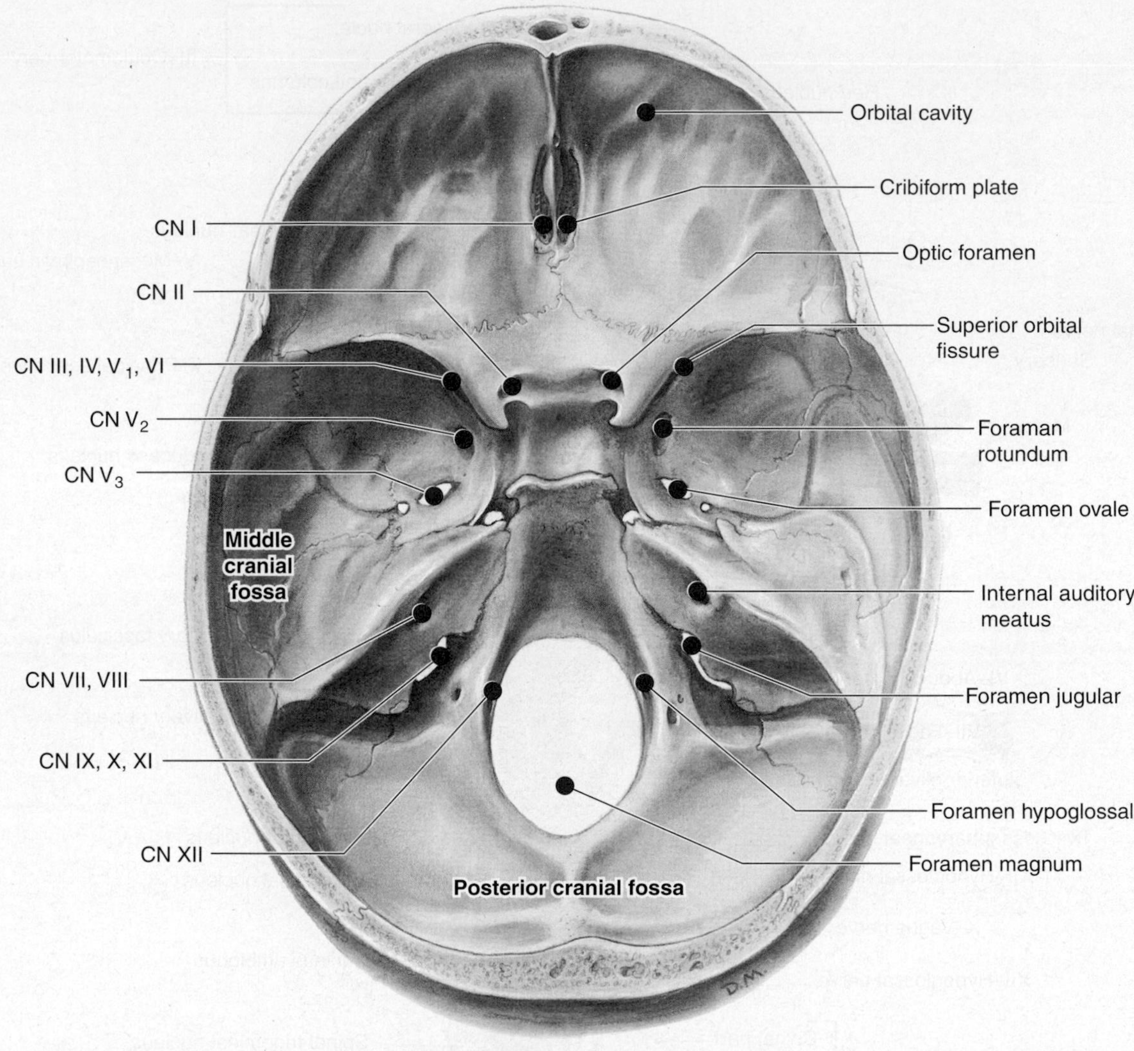

Figure 17-5 Illustrated locations of foramina in the skull base and their associated cranial nerves.

from both of the motor cortices (Box 17-4). Muscles receiving only contralateral innervation are the lower facial muscles (facial nerve [CN VII]), sternocleidomastoid and trapezius muscles (spinal accessory [CN XI]), tongue muscles (hypoglossal [CN XII]), and ocular muscles (oculomotor [CN III], trochlear [CN IV], and abducens [CN VI]). The presence of many collateral corticonuclear fibers further provides protection from spasticity in the cranial muscles in the case of pyramidal (UMN) lesions.

The pyramidal tract provides minor cortical regulation of eye movement (oculomotor [CN III], trochlear [CN IV], and abducens [CN VI]). For the innervation of ocular muscles, a corticonuclear projection to the midbrain **conjugate gaze center** coordinates the movement of the eyes as a unit. For example, activation of the left frontal cortex leads to activation of the right pontine gaze center and, subsequently, to activation of the right abducens (lateral rectus) and left oculomotor nucleus (medial rectus). This results in contraction of the right lateral rectus and left medial rectus muscles, causing both eyes to turn to the right.

SENSORIMOTOR FUNCTIONS OF CRANIAL NERVES

Olfactory Nerve

The olfactory system consists of the afferent neuron in the olfactory **mucosal membrane**, the olfactory bulb, the olfactory tract, part of the temporal cortex, and a limited region of the inferior fronto-orbital cortex. The cortical olfactory area, located on the basomedial surface of the

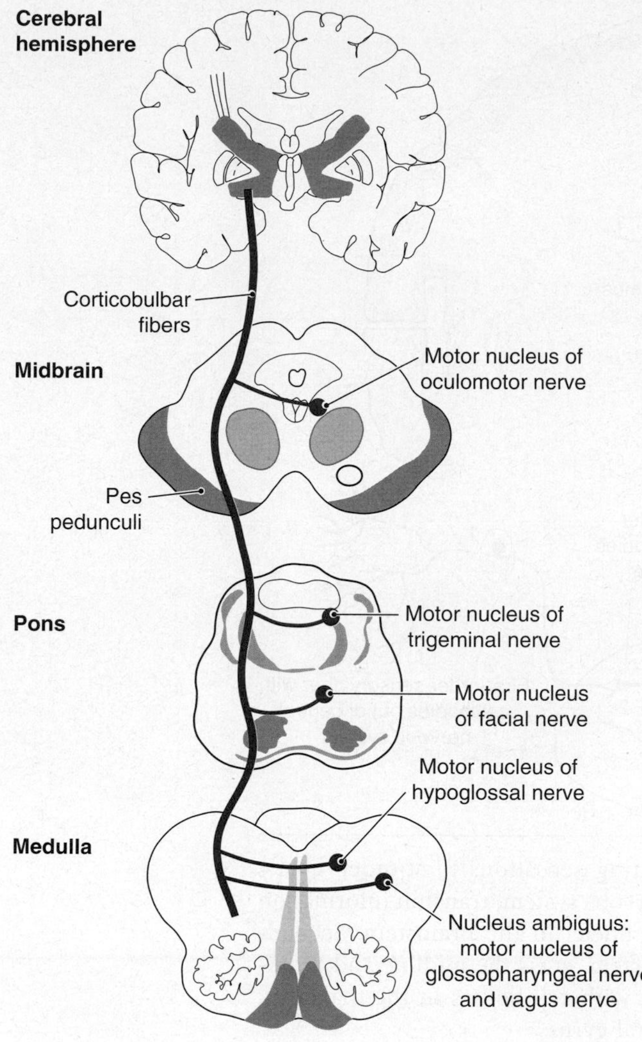

Figure 17-6 Corticonuclear (corticobulbar) fibers projecting to the contralateral motor nuclei of the oculomotor, trigeminal, vagal, and hypoglossal nerves in the brainstem.

cerebral hemisphere, includes the uncus, periamygdaloid nucleus, anterior hippocampal gyrus, and parts of the temporal lobe.

Special Visceral Afferent

The SVA begins with neurosensory cells that transduce odor molecules and are embedded in the **olfactory epithelium** in the roof of the nasal cavity, which is approximately 2 cm^2 (Fig. 17-9A; Table 17-6). The other function of the highly vascularized mucosa membrane is to warm and humidify the incoming air. Also found in the epithelium are the sensory endings of the trigeminal nerve (CN V), which respond to noxious sensation, such as concentrated ammonia. The unmyelinated axons of the olfactory neurons that group together to form the olfactory nerve (CN I) pass through the foramina in the **ethmoid cribriform plate**, terminating on the **mitral** and other cells in the olfactory bulbs on the basal surface of the frontal lobe. The axonal projection from the mitral and associated cells form the olfactory tract, which travels caudally to the **olfactory trigone** area and divides into subtracts or bundles (**striae**) of fibers (Fig. 17-9*B*).

The intermediate stria terminates in the trigone area and the **anterior perforated substance** anterior to the optic chiasm (Fig. 17-9*B*). Some fibers terminate in the subcallosal area and are associated with the limbic lobe functions (see Figs. 2-10 and 2-14). Other fibers cross the midline through the anterior commissure and connect with the opposite olfactory bulb. However, the majority of the fibers (lateral stria) terminate in the vicinity of the medial temporal lobe of the (primary) olfactory area, called the **pyriform cortex** (Fig. 17-9*B*). This area includes the cortex of the uncus, the amygdaloid nucleus, and the anterior part of the parahippocampal gyrus and it mediates olfactory awareness. Various projections from the primary olfactory cortex to the neocortex and limbic region help integrate smell with the emotional brain and serve many vegetative functions. These extrinsic olfactory connections include projections to the orbitofrontal cortex and the hypothalamus, which integrate olfaction with personality and feeding behavior.

Clinical Correlates and Assessment

The olfactory receptor cells are unique as they are the only mammalian neurons that are replaced with new cells in 30 to 60 days. At approximately 60 to 65 years of age, humans gradually begin to lose acuity of the sense of smell. As part of normal aging, this is largely caused by ongoing degeneration of olfactory sensory cells, which can also be subsequent to a brain degenerative disease, such as Parkinson and Alzheimer. Anterior fossa skull fracture, seen in traumatic brain injury (TBI), also affects smell sensation and can cause a CSF leakage from the subarachnoid space that runs through the nose (CSF rhinorrhea), which can also provide a path for a bacterial infection.

A lesion that interrupts the olfactory fibers or the primary olfactory cells results in **anosmia**, a condition in which the ability to smell is partially or fully impaired. Two associated conditions are **hyposmia** (decreased olfactory sensation) and **hyperosmia** (abnormally acute sense of smell). An irritating lesion involving the olfactory cortex can cause **uncinate fits**, which are marked by imaginary odor, and involuntary movements of the lips and tongue in addition to other temporal lobe symptoms. One common complaint of patients with anosmia is their loss of taste, which is mostly related to impaired olfaction. Olfactory loss may involve the neural mechanism of olfaction unilaterally or bilaterally. Bilateral lesions, however, have a drastic impact on olfactory function.

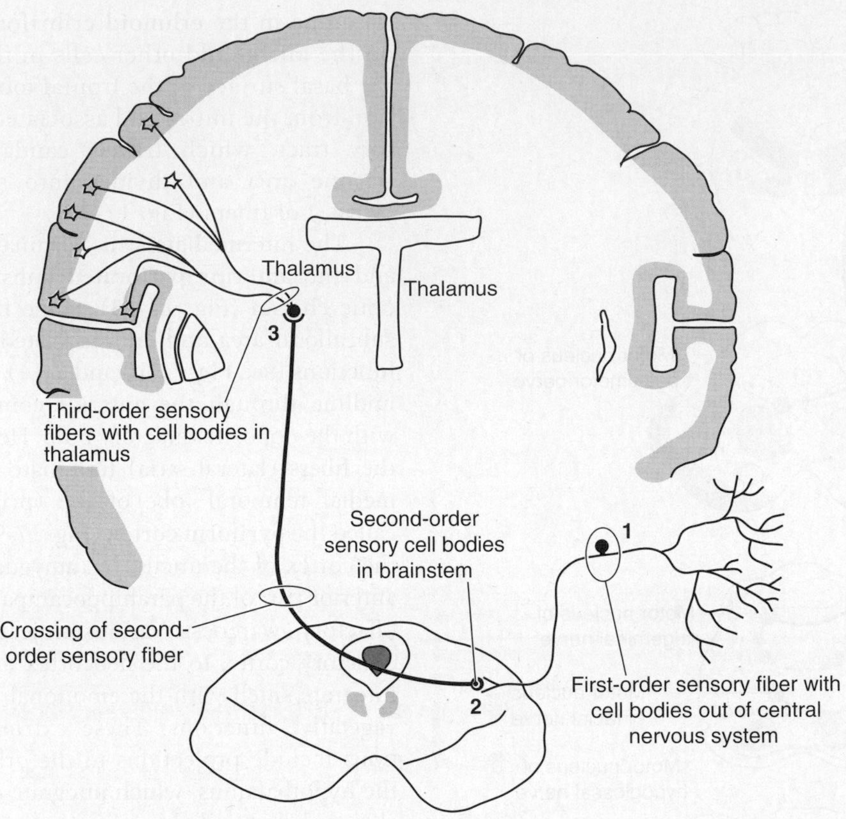

Figure 17-7 Cranial nerve fibers mediating sensation. First-order fibers, with cell bodies external to the central nervous system, transmit information from the periphery to the second-order nuclei in the brainstem. Second-order fibers, with cell bodies in the brainstem, cross the midline and terminate in the thalamus. Third-order fibers, with cell bodies in the thalamus, project to the lower parts of the postcentral gyrus.

Olfactory nerve function is tested by asking the patient to identify various odors, such as coffee, using one nostril at one time.

Optic Nerve

Special Somatic Afferent

Light rays entering the eye are bent (refracted) by the curvature of the cornea and lens and converge on rods and cones in the retina (Table 17-7; see Chapter 12). The rods that populate the peripheral regions of the retina are sensitive to white light and movement; they are needed for night vision. The cones populate mostly the central retinal region (fovea) and mediate color vision.

The photoreceptor cells transduce light energy into local potentials. These potentials travel to the bipolar cells, which, by means of local potentials and neurotransmitters, affect the excitability of the ganglion, whose axonal processes transmit the action potentials through the optic nerve, optic chiasm, and optic tract. Ganglion cell fibers from the nasal half of the retina cross the midline at the optic chiasm; ganglion cell axons from the temporal retina do not cross through the chiasm. Optic tract fibers, which are formed by the postchiasmatic fibers, travel posteriorly around the pes pedunculi and terminate in the lateral geniculate body, the thalamic relay center for vision. Geniculocalcarine projections, also called optic radiations, travel to the visual cortex in the occipital lobe. The primary visual cortex, which is located in the upper and lower banks of the calcarine fissure, receives projections from both eyes.

Clinical Correlates and Assessment

Injury to any part of the visual pathway results in selected visual field loss. The area and type of loss depend on the site and extent of the lesion. A lesion of the entire optic nerve would lead to a complete blindness in one eye. Cerebrovascular accidents and neuritis, an inflammation of the optic nerve, are common causes of optic nerve disorders. Common visual field defects are bitemporal hemianopsia, homonymous hemianopsia, homonymous

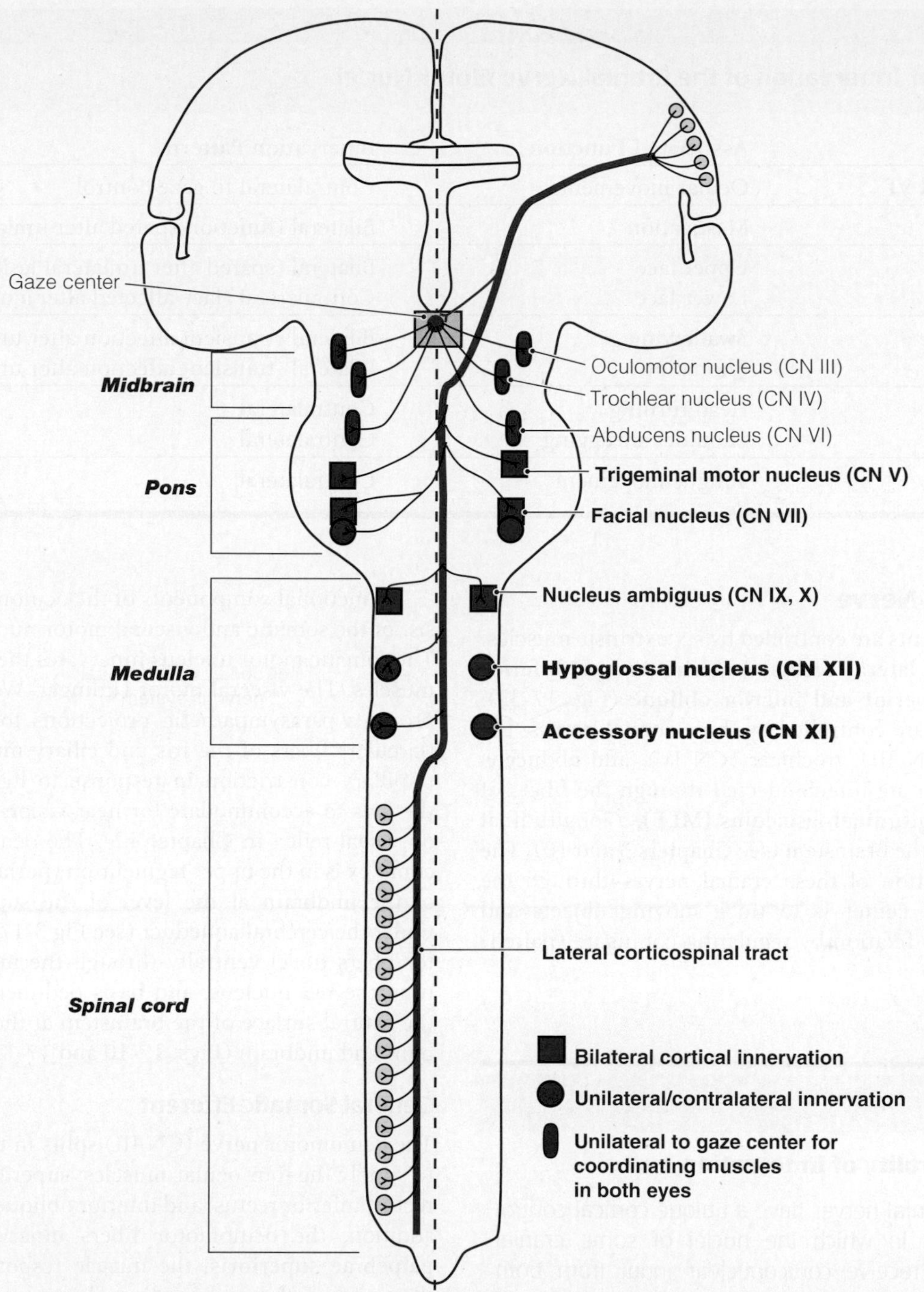

Figure 17-8 Neuronal pattern of unilateral and bilateral innervation of the cranial nerve nuclei.

superior quadrantanopia, and homonymous inferior quadrantanopsia (see Fig. 12-13).

Visual field loss can be informally tested by having the patient close one eye and fix the other eye on a point straight ahead. The clinician then moves his or her index finger, with arm outstretched, from the periphery to the midline from all directions (left, right, up, and down) and the patient is asked to report the point at which the finger is seen. Any difference in clarity and delay in seeing can be a clue to a visual field defect.

> ***Key Terms:***
>
> **Accommodation**
> **Anosmia**
> **Ophthalmoplegia**
> **Ptosis**
> **Strabismus**

Table 17-5

Supranuclear Innervation of the Cranial Nerve Motor Nuclei

Cranial Nerve	Associated Function	Innervation Pattern
CN III, IV, and VI	Ocular movements	Contralateral to gaze control
CN V	Mastication	Bilateral (function spared after unilateral lesions)
CN VII	Upper face Lower face	Bilateral (spared after unilateral lesions) Contralateral (face affected after a unilateral lesion)
CN IX and X	Swallowing Phonation	Bilateral (transient affection after unilateral lesions) Bilateral (transient affection after unilateral lesions)
CN XI	Head turning Shoulder shrugging	Contralateral Contralateral
CN XII	Tongue movement	Contralateral

Oculomotor Nerve

Ocular movements are controlled by six extrinsic muscles: **medial rectus**, **lateral rectus**, **superior rectus**, **inferior rectus**, and **superior and inferior oblique** (Fig. 17-32). These muscles are controlled by three cranial nerves: the oculomotor (CN III), trochlear (CN IV), and abducens (CN VI), which are interconnected through the fibers of the **medial longitudinal fasciculus (MLF)**, a longitudinal fiber bundle in the brainstem (see Chapters 3 and 10). The combined function of these cranial nerves through the brainstem gaze center is to track moving objects and maintain visual fixation by regulating conjugate (paired) eye movements.

BOX 17-4

Bilaterality of Innervation

The cranial nerves have a unique cortical control pattern, in which the nuclei of some cranial nerves receive corticonuclear input from both sides of the motor cortex. This bilaterality of innervation ensures that a unilateral cortical lesion would not profoundly impair the function of the facial (CN VII; upper face), trigeminal (CN V), vagus (CN X), and glossopharyngeal (CN IX) nerves. The function of these cranial nerves is severely affected only in the case of bilateral cortical destruction or after a LMN (final common path) lesion as seen in pseudobulbar palsy. Another important clinical concept that needs to be remembered is that the **LMN** damage results in ipsilateral signs and the **UMN** damage causes contralateral clinical signs.

Functional components of the oculomotor nerve consist of the somatic and visceral motor nuclei (Table 17-8). The somatic motor nucleus innervates the extrinsic ocular muscles. The visceral motor (Edinger–Westphal) nucleus provides parasympathetic projections to the constrictor (circular) fibers of the iris and ciliary muscle, regulating pupillary constriction in response to light and enabling the lens to accommodate for near vision (see the section on visual reflex in Chapter 12). The oculomotor nuclear complex is in the upper tegmentum (**periaqueductal gray**) of the midbrain at the level of the superior colliculus under the cerebral aqueduct (see Fig 3-17). The oculomotor fibers travel ventrally through the midbrain tegmentum, the red nucleus, and basis pedunculi, exiting from the ventral surface of the brainstem at the junction of the pons and midbrain (Figs. 17-10 and 17-11; see Fig. 3-16).

General Somatic Efferent

The oculomotor nerve (CN III) splits in the orbital cavity to supply the four ocular muscles: superior rectus, medial rectus, inferior rectus, and inferior oblique (Fig. 17-11). In addition, the oculomotor fibers innervate the **levator palpebrae superioris**, the muscle responsible for lifting the upper eyelid and implicated in **ptosis** (upper eyelid paralysis). Each muscle makes an individual contribution to the total eye movement: the superior rectus moves the eyeball upward and inward, the medial rectus adducts the eyeball medially, and the inferior rectus moves the eyeball downward and inward. The inferior oblique and the superior rectus contribute to upward gazing and rotating the eye upward and outward (Table 17-12). These ocular muscles do not work alone; they require synergistic participation from all of the muscles of the eye. For example, looking to the left entails contraction of the lateral rectus of the left eye and the medial rectus of the right eye, with simultaneous relaxation of their opposite muscles, which is coordinated by the brainstem gaze center.

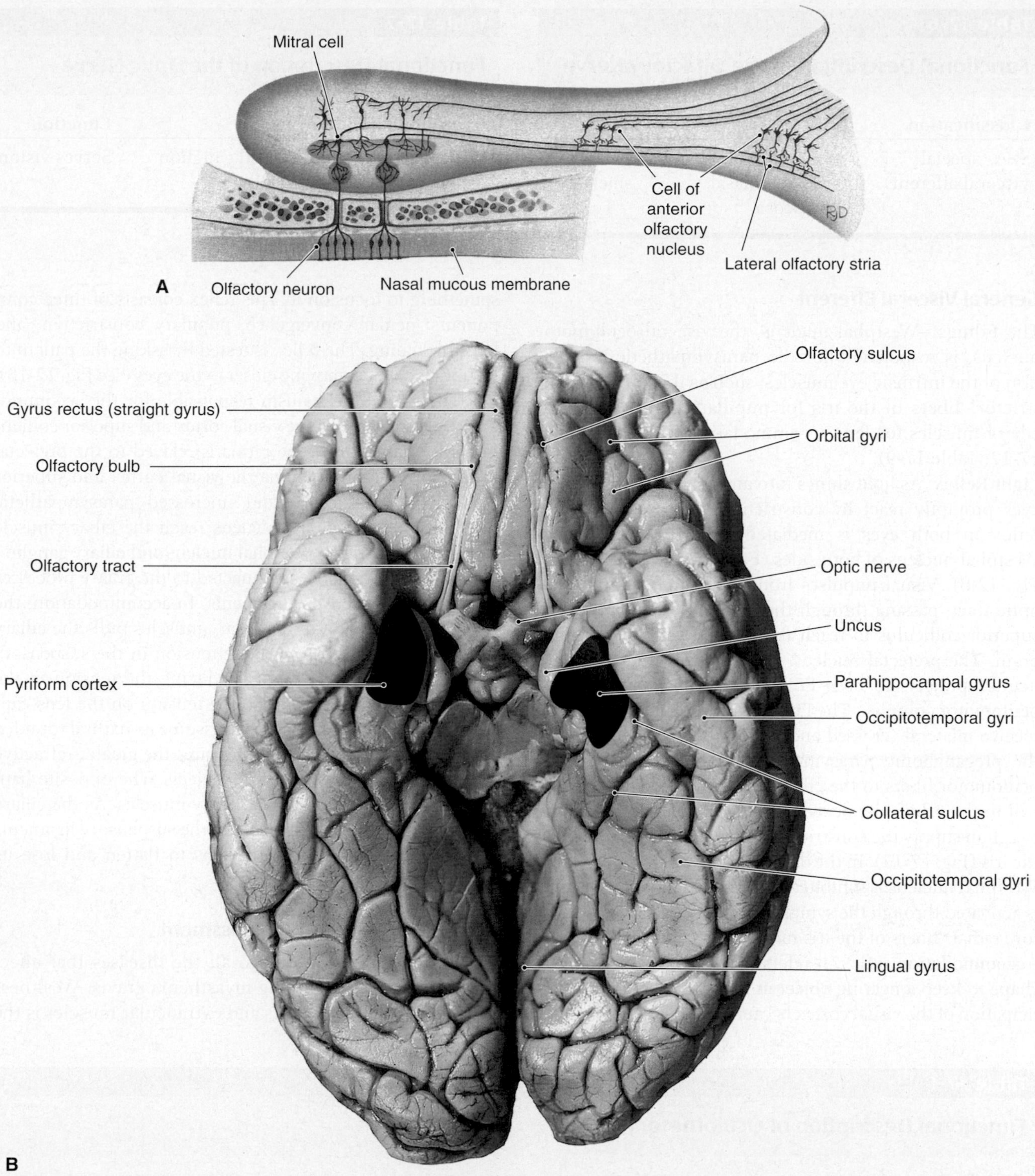

Figure 17-9 A. Olfactory neurons in the nasal mucosa, bulb, and centrally projecting fibers. B. A view of the olfactory structures on the ventral surface of the frontal lobe from the bulb to the anterior perforated substance, primary olfactory (pyriform) cortex, and associated structures on the ventral surface of the temporal and frontal lobes.

Table 17-6

Functional Description of the Olfactory Nerve

Classification	Nuclei	Function
SVA (special visceral afferent)	Neuroepithelial cells in nasal mucosa	Regulates smell

Table 17-7

Functional Description of the Optic Nerve

Classification	Nuclei	Function
SSA (special somatic afferent)	Retinal ganglion cells	Serves vision

General Visceral Efferent

The Edinger–Westphal nucleus, the visceral oculomotor nucleus, is responsible for the parasympathetic innervation of the intrinsic eye muscles, such as the circular (constrictor) fibers of the iris for pupillary constriction and ciliary muscles for lens accommodation (Figs. 17-10 and 17-12; Table 17-9).

Light Reflex. As light shines into an eye, the pupils in both eyes promptly react by constricting. The pupillary light reflex in both eyes is mediated through the Edinger–Westphal nucleus of both sides (Fig. 17-12; Table 17-9; see Fig. 12-8). Visual impulses from the retina travel via the optic tract, passing through the LGB and brachium of the superior colliculus to reach the pretectal area in the midbrain. The pretectal nucleus, anterior to the superior colliculus, projects to both Edinger–Westphal nuclei in the oculomotor complex. The Edinger–Westphal nuclei, which receive bilateral (crossed and uncrossed) projections, send the preganglionic parasympathetic projections along the oculomotor fibers to the ciliary ganglion lateral to the eyeball in the orbit. The postganglionic fibers from the ciliary ganglion supply the constrictor (circular) pupillary fibers of the iris (Fig. 17-12). In the dark, the activity of the Edinger–Westphal nucleus is inhibited, and the dilation of the pupils is activated through the sympathetic projections to the dilator (radial) fibers of the iris muscle (see Chapter 12).

Accommodation reflex. It refers to adjustments in the lens shape to keep a nearing object in focus. It involves the participation of the visual cortex because an organism has to see something to focus on it. This reflex consists of three components: ocular convergence, pupillary constriction, and lens thickening. The reflex is tested by asking the patient to focus on an object moving closer to the eyes (see Fig. 12-10).

The neural mechanism responsible for the accommodation reflex involves the visual cortex and superior colliculus. Information from the retina is relayed to the pretectal nucleus in the midbrain via the visual cortex and superior colliculus. The crossed and uncrossed parasympathetic fibers from the pretectal nucleus reach the ciliary muscle through the Edinger–Westphal nucleus and ciliary ganglion (Fig. 17-12). The lens is connected to the ciliary processes through the suspensory ligaments. In accommodation, the reflexive contraction of the ciliary muscles pulls the ciliary processes forward, reducing the tension in the suspensory ligaments (zonules of Zinn). Reducing the tension in the suspensory ligaments releases the tension on the lens capsule and allows the elastic lens to assume its natural rounded shape; consequently, the lens acquires the greater refractive power needed for viewing near objects. The opposite happens during relaxation of the ciliary muscles. As the ciliary muscles relax, they put tension on the suspensory ligaments and lens capsule, causing the lens to flatten and lose its refractive power.

Clinical Correlates and Assessment

Ocular muscles are prone to all the diseases that affect skeletal muscles, including myasthenia gravis. Weakness of the palpebrae superioris and extraocular muscles is the

Table 17-8

Functional Description of Oculomotor Nerve

Classification	Nuclei	Function
GSE (general somatic efferent)	Oculomotor (lower motor neuron) nucleus in midbrain	Responsible for eye movement; regulates the activity of all ocular muscles except superior oblique and lateral rectus; regulates levator palpebrae superioris (lid elevation)
GVE (general visceral efferent)	Edinger–Westphal nucleus in midbrain tegmentum Preganglionic parasympathetic projections to ciliary ganglion	Responsible for reflexive constriction of pupil and lens accommodation for near vision

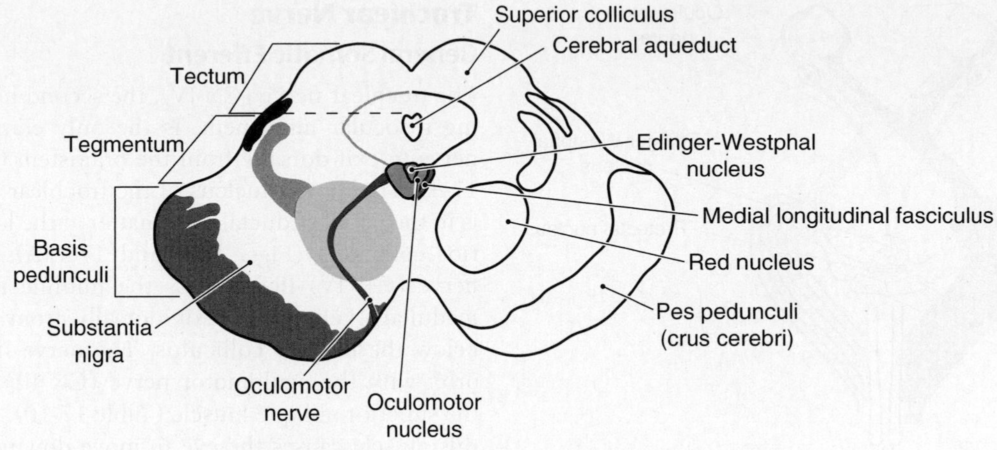

Figure 17-10 Section at the superior colliculus level showing the oculomotor nucleus and its fibers traveling through the midbrain tegmentum.

first clinical sign of this disease. Other conditions that can also affect the oculomotor nerve (CN III) functioning are inflammation, nerve compression because of tumor, and TBI.

A lesion that affects the nucleus and/or oculomotor nerve (CN III) may result in weakness/paralysis of three recti, inferior oblique, and palpebrae superioris muscles. This also causes the paralysis of the pupillary sphincter muscle and the ciliary muscle leaving the pupil dilated and lens flat.

Depending on the site and extent of lesion, this oculomotor nerve dysfunctioning results in the following symptoms: **ophthalmoplegia** (external and internal) and **ptosis.**

External ophthalmoplegia. With the paralysis of the extrinsic ocular muscles, the affected eye deviates to the lateral side (**lateral strabismus**). The eye deviates not only laterally but also ventrally because of the unopposed action of the intact superior oblique (trochlear nerve [CN IV]) and lateral rectus muscles (abducens nerve [CN VI]). Failure to direct both eyes toward an object (**strabismus**) in the direction opposite to the paralyzed side results in double vision (diplopia). A patient with left oculomotor nerve palsy is likely to have double vision when looking either straight or to the right (Fig. 17-13).

Ptosis. With paralysis of the palpebrae superioris, the affected upper eyelid droops. A patient with ptosis may compensate for the eyelid paralysis by using the frontalis muscle (facial cranial nerve [CN VII]) to raise the eyelid (Fig. 17-13*B*).

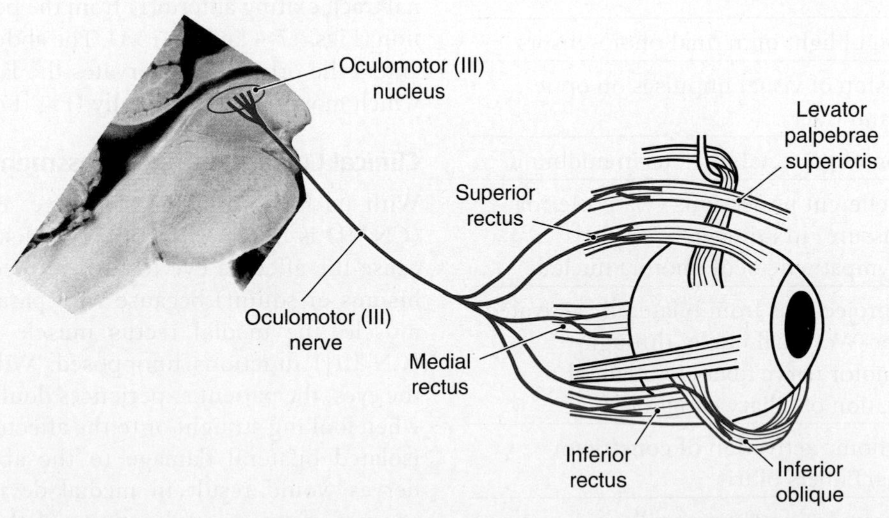

Figure 17-11 Oculomotor nucleus, course of its nerve fibers, and innervated ocular muscles.

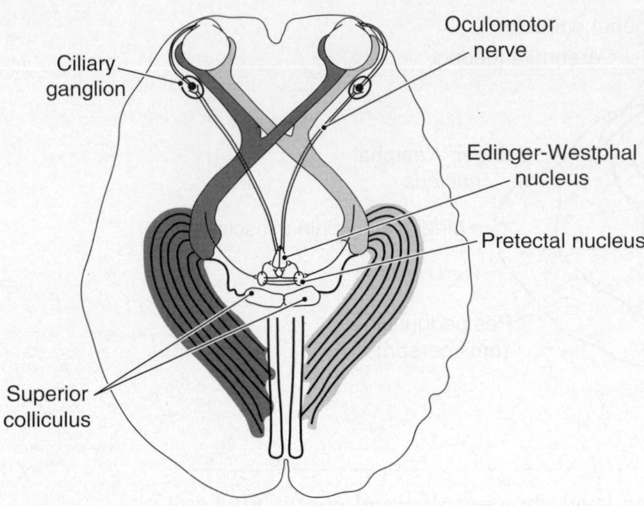

Figure 17-12 Pathway serving the visual reflexes. Retinal–tectal axons (*red*) leave the ipsilateral optic tract to synapse in the pretectal nucleus and related nuclei, which are interconnected through the posterior commissure (*red*). The direct light reflex is pupil constriction to light in the ipsilateral eye, and the consensual light reflex is pupil constriction in the contralateral eye.

Internal ophthalmoplegia. With interruption of the parasympathetic projections to the constrictors of the iris, the pupil is permanently dilated (**mydriasis**) because of unopposed activity of the dilator pupillae with sympathetic innervation (Fig. 17-13*C*).

Table 17-9

Neuronal Events of the Pupillary Light Reflex

Step	Event
1	Projection of light on retinal photosensors
2	Transmission of visual impulses on optic nerve and tract
3	Activation of pretectal nucleus in midbrain
4	Bilateral efferent projections (via posterior commissure) to Edinger–Westphal (parasympathetic oculomotor) nucleus
5	Efferent projections from bilaterally activated Edinger–Westphal nuclei through oculomotor nerve fibers to bilateral innervation of ciliary ganglion
6	Postganglionic activation of constrictor (circular) fibers of iris
7	Bilateral parasympathetic pupillary constriction

Trochlear Nerve

General Somatic Efferent

The trochlear nerve (CN IV), the second nerve contributing to ocular movement, is the only cranial and motor nerve to exit dorsally from the brainstem (Figs. 17-3 and 17-4). The motor nucleus of the trochlear nerve (CN IV) is in the periaqueductal gray matter at the level of the inferior colliculus (Figs. 17-3 and 17-14A). The trochlear nerve (CN IV) fibers cross the midline in the anterior medullary velum and exit dorsally from the brainstem below the inferior colliculus. The nerve fibers enter the orbit with the oculomotor nerve (CN III) and innervate the superior oblique muscle (Table 17-10). Contraction of this muscle causes the eye to move downward and laterally (Fig. 17-14B).

Clinical Correlates and Assessment

Denervation, compression, peripheral neuropathy can interrupt trochlear nerve (CN IV) projection, which causes the weakness or paralysis of the superior oblique muscle. This results in diplopia particularly when looking downward and inward, causing misalignment of the eyes. The eye is fixed with an upward medial gaze because the actions of the inferior oblique, superior and medial recti muscles (oculomotor nerve [CN III]) are unopposed; the patient often reports difficulty in walking down stairs.

Abducens Nerve

General Somatic Efferent

The abducens nerve (CN VI) is the third nerve to contribute to ocular movements (Tables 17-11 and 17-12). The abducens motor nucleus is in the dorsal tegmentum of the pons within a loop formed by the facial nerve (CN VII) (Fig. 17-4). Fibers of the abducens nerve (CN VI) pass through the pontine tegmentum and pierce the corticospinal tract, exiting anteriorly from the pontomedullary junction (Figs. 17-4 and 17-15*A*). The abducens nerve (CN VI) enters the orbit and innervates the lateral rectus muscle, which moves the eye laterally (Fig. 17-15*B*).

Clinical Correlates and Assessment

With its long intracranial course, the abducens nerve (CN VI) is highly susceptible to disruption. Its injuries cause the affected eye to turn in medially (**medial strabismus** or squint) because with paralyzed lateral rectus muscle, the medial rectus muscle (oculomotor nerve [CN III]) functions unopposed. With misalignment of the eyes, the patient experiences double vision (diplopia) when looking straight or to the affected side (Fig. 17-16). Isolated bilateral damage to the abducens nuclei and nerves would result in medial deviation of both eyes because of unopposed activity of the both medial recti muscles, which are controlled by the oculomotor nerve (CN III).

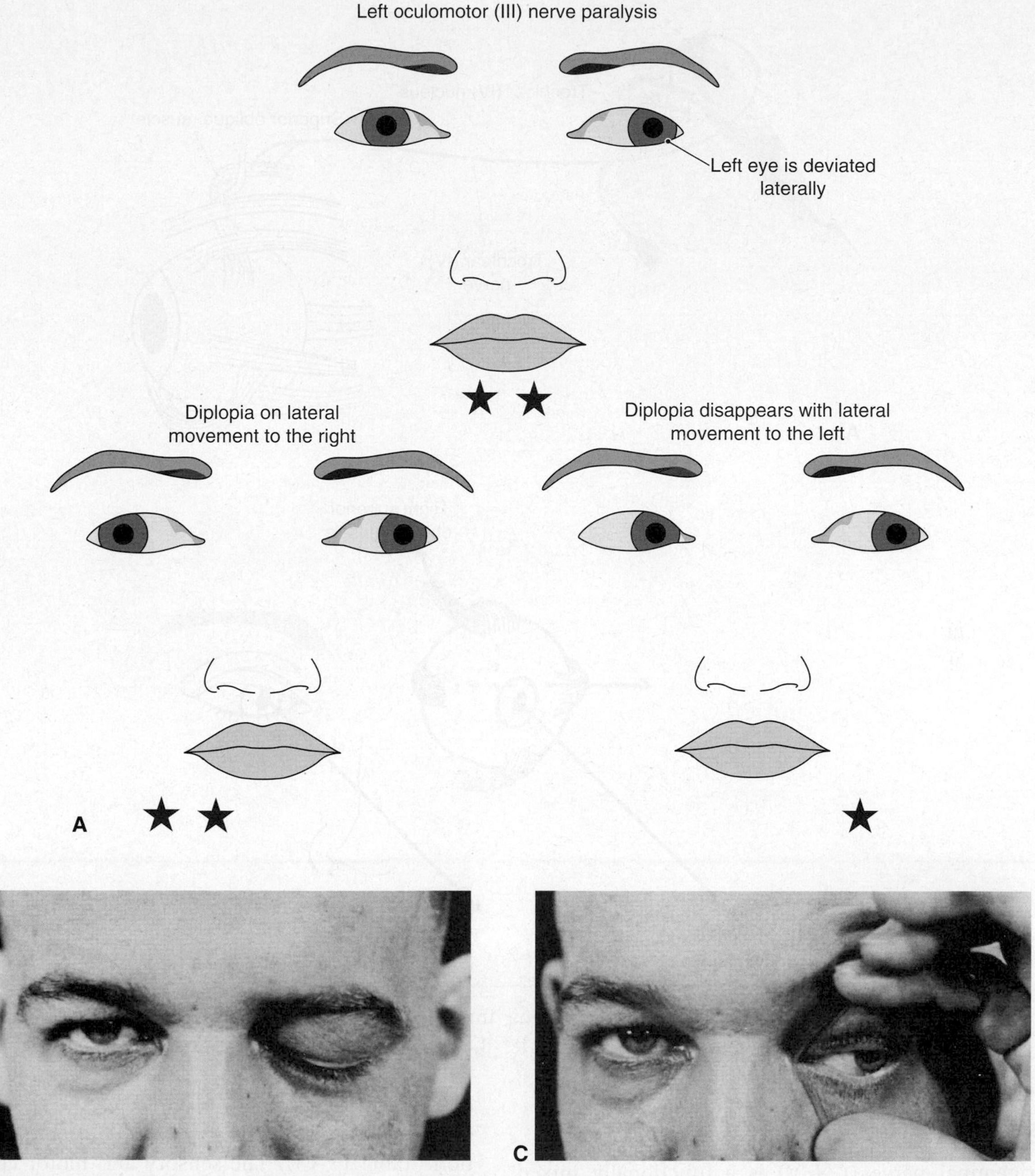

Figure 17-13 A. Double vision caused by oculomotor nerve paralysis. In left oculomotor paralysis, the eye moves laterally, making the eyes disconjugate (lateral strabismus). When looking straight ahead **(top)** or when looking to the right, the patient sees two images **(bottom left)**. However, a left movement of the right eye allows the eyes to conjugate **(bottom right)**; hence the diplopia disappears. **B.** Ptosis (eyelid drop) in the left eye. **C.** A manual elevation of the paralyzed lid with dilated and left deviated pupil.

The MLF is an important brainstem tract with inputs from the vestibular complex and neck muscles. It projects bilaterally to the motor nuclei of the ocular cranial nerves: oculomotor (CN III), trochlear (CN IV), and abducens (CN VI) (see Chapter 10). It coordinates the movements of the eye muscles for gaze control and coordinates head position with eye movements. Lesions involving the MLF severely affect gaze control.

Ocular movements are best tested by asking the patient to follow the vertical and horizontal finger/light movement. Impaired gaze movements that contribute to double vision are slow, jerky, and unconjugated.

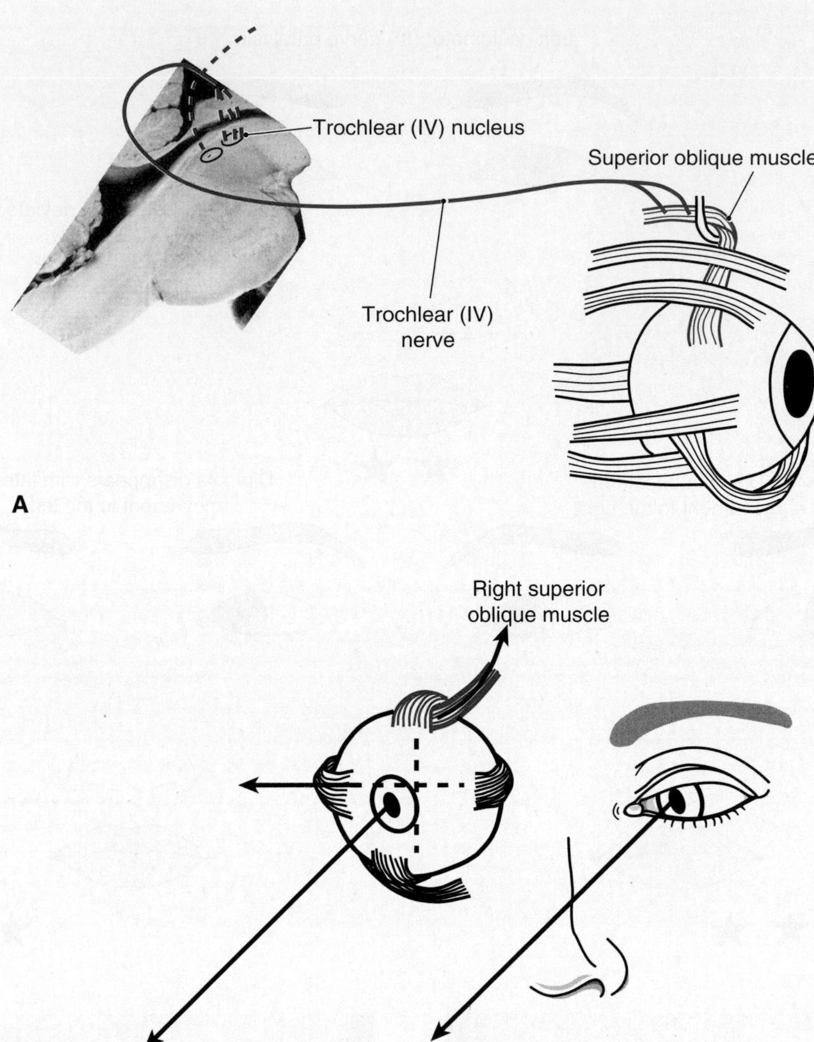

Figure 17-14 A. Trochlear nucleus, intramedullary course of the cranial nerve, and the innervated muscle. B. The functioning of the superior oblique muscle.

Trigeminal Nerve

The trigeminal nerve (CN V) is a functionally mixed nerve. As the principal sensory nerve for the head, face, orbit, and oral cavity, it mediates the sensations of pain, temperature, and discriminative touch (see Chapter 11). It has a small motor component that supplies the jaw muscles along with other muscles and controls mastication (Table 17-13). The sensory and motor components together form the pathway for the jaw-jerk reflex. It also mediates SSA (kinesthetic and proprioceptive awareness) information, which is responsible for stretch receptor feedback for the masticators.

Table 17-10

Functional Description of the Trochlear Nerve

Classification	Nuclei	Function
GSE (general somatic efferent)	Trochlear (lower motor neuron) nucleus in midbrain	Responsible for downward and outward eye movement by innervation of the contralateral skeletal muscle (superior oblique)

Table 17-11

Functional Description of the Abducens Nerve

Classification	Nuclei	Function
GSE (general somatic efferent)	Abducens (lower motor neuron) nucleus in tegmentum of pons	Responsible for lateral eye movements (abduction of eyeball) by innervation of skeletal muscle (lateral rectus)

Table 17-12

Cranial Nerves, Innervated Eye Muscles, and Their Functions

Cranial Nerve (Number)	Muscle	Functions
Oculomotor (III)	Inferior oblique	Elevates eyeball upward and outward
	Inferior rectus	Depresses eyeball downward and inward
	Medial rectus	Adducts eyeball medially and inward
	Superior rectus	Elevates eyeball upward and inward
	Levator palpebrae superioris	Elevates upper eyelid
Trochlear (IV)	Superior oblique (contralateral)	Rotates eyeball downward and outward
Abducens (VI)	Lateral rectus	Abducts eyeball laterally and outward

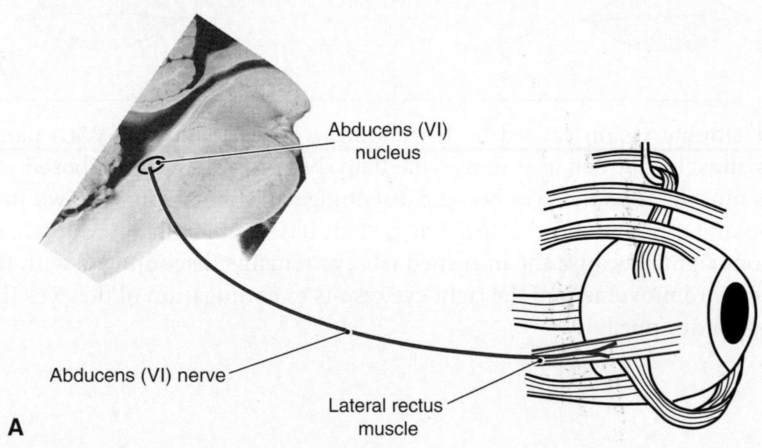

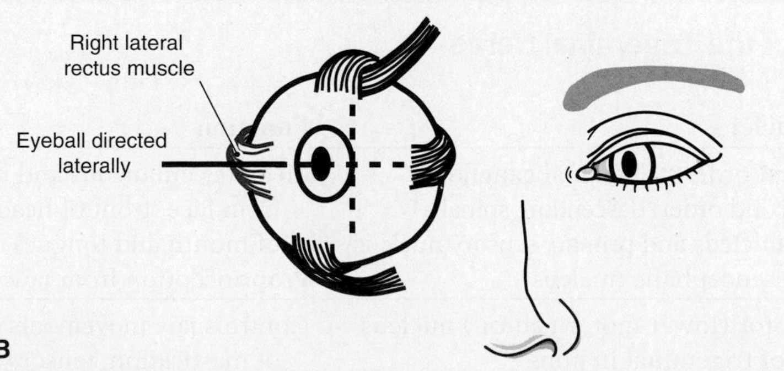

Figure 17-15 A. Abducens nucleus, intramedullary course of the cranial nerve, and the lateral rectus muscle. B. Lateral eye movement as regulated by the lateral rectus muscle.

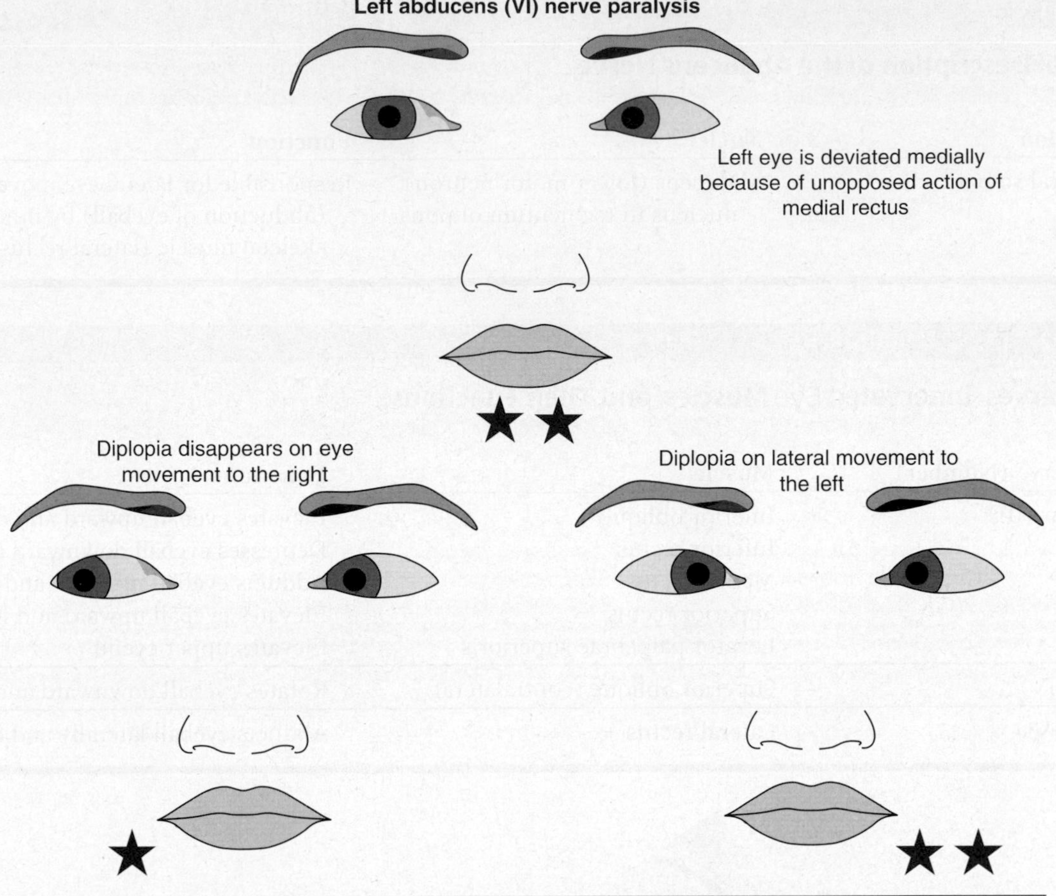

Figure 17-16 Double vision caused by left abducens nerve paralysis. With paralysis of left lateral rectus muscle, the left eye moves medially because of the unopposed action of the medial rectus muscle; thus the eyes become disconjugate. The patient sees two images (diplopia) when looking straight ahead (**top**). The patient has double vision even when looking to the left (**bottom right**) because the in-turned left eye remains disconjugate with the right eye. However, rightward movement of the right eye results in conjugation of the eyes (**bottom left**); thus the diplopia disappears.

Table 17-13

Functional Description of the Trigeminal Nerve

Classification	Nuclei	Function
GSA (general somatic afferent)	First order: trigeminal ganglion Second order: descending spinal nucleus and primary sensory nucleus Mesencephalic nucleus	Mediates cutaneous and proprioceptive sensation from face, front of head, and oral cavity (mucosa of mouth and tongue) Proprioception from jaw muscles
SVE (special visceral efferent)/BE (branchial efferent)	Motor (lower motor neuron) nucleus of trigeminal in pons	Controls jaw movements by innervation of muscles of mastication, tensor veli palatini, tensor tympani, and anterior belly of digastric muscle

General Somatic Afferent

The trigeminal nerve (CN V) is responsible for cutaneous (touch, pain, and temperature) and proprioceptive (awareness of posture and muscle movement) sensations from the face, head, oral and nasal cavities, sinuses, teeth, anterior two-thirds of the tongue, anterior half of the pinna, external auditory meatus, and external surface of the tympanic membrane. The sensory function of the trigeminal nerve (CN V) is organized along three neurons (Fig. 11-9; see Chapter 11): the **semilunar** or **trigeminal ganglion** (first-order nerve cell) that is located external to the pons, **trigeminal complex** (second-order nerve cell), and ventral posteromedial thalamic nucleus (third-order nerve cell).

The trigeminal nuclear complex, consisting of the **chief sensory nucleus**, **descending spinal nucleus**, and **mesencephalic nucleus**, is located in the lateral tegmentum of the pons. Each of these sensory nuclei mediates different modalities of sensation (see Chapter 11). The chief sensory nucleus mediates discriminative sensation from the head and face. The descending spinal nucleus is primarily involved with pain and temperature and secondarily with diffuse touch. The descending spinal nucleus and its tract also receive GSA projections from the facial (CN VII), glossopharyngeal (CN IX), and vagus (CN X) nerves. The mesencephalic nucleus contains the neurons that mediate proprioceptive sensation from the jaw muscles (of mastication).

The trigeminal nerve has three sensory branches: **ophthalmic**, **maxillary**, and **mandibular** (Fig. 17-17). These nerves project sensory information from the entire face and part of the head to the semilunar ganglion (first-order sensory nucleus). The ophthalmic nerve mediates the sensations of touch, pain, temperature, and proprioception from the skin of the forehead, anterior scalp, vertex, eyeball, upper eyelid, cornea, conjunctivum, anterior and

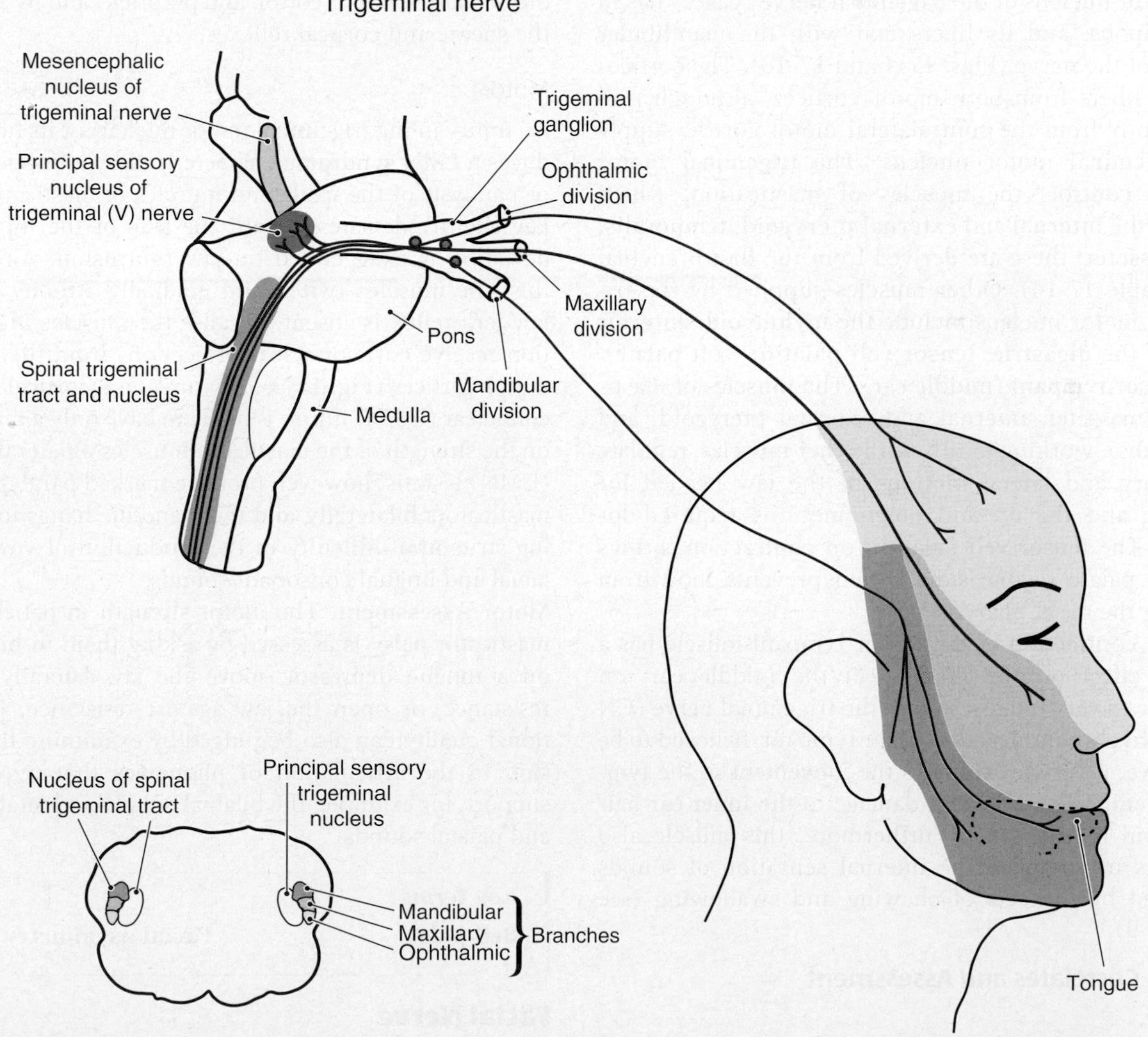

Figure 17-17 The trigeminal nuclear complex in the brainstem and the divisions of the trigeminal nerve.

lateral surfaces of the nose, frontal and nasal sinuses, and tentorium cerebelli.

The maxillary nerve mediates sensation from the skin of the temples, posterior portion of the nose, upper cheeks, lower eyelids, and upper lips. Additional innervated oral structures include the upper gum, teeth (molar and premolar), mucosal membrane, and soft and hard palates. The maxillary nerve also receives sensations from the nasal cavity, maxillary sinus, and dura mater in the medial cranial fossa.

The mandibular nerve, the largest of the trigeminal branches, mediates sensations from the skin on the sides of the scalp, the mucosal membrane of the lower gum, the mouth, and the meninges of the anterior and middle cranial fossae. Additional structures innervated by the trigeminal nerve (CN V) include the anterior half of the pinna, external auditory meatus, external surface of the tympanic membrane, and the mucosa of the anterior two-thirds of the tongue.

Special Visceral Efferent/Branchial Efferent

The motor nucleus of the trigeminal nerve (CN V) lies in the midpons, and its fibers exit with the mandibular branch of the nerve (Figs. 17-4 and 17-18). The corticonuclear fibers from both motor cortices, although predominantly from the contralateral motor cortex, supply the trigeminal motor nucleus. The trigeminal motor nucleus controls the muscles of mastication, which include the **internal** and **external pterygoid**, **temporalis**, and **masseter**; these are derived from the first branchial arch (Table 17-14). Other muscles supplied by the trigeminal motor nucleus include the **mylohyoid**, **anterior belly of the digastric**, **tensor veli palatini** (soft palate), and **tensor tympani** (middle ear). The muscles of mastication (masseter, internal and external pterygoid, and temporalis), working jointly with other muscles, regulate the rotary and lateral motions of the jaw needed for chewing and the up and down motions required for speech. The tensor veli palatini, on contraction, brings the soft palate to one side, which prevents food from entering the nasal pharynx.

The contraction of the tensor tympani muscle has a pulling effect on the malleus in the middle ear; on exposure to very intense sound, the trigeminal nerve (CN V) reflexively contracts the tensor tympani. Believed to be protective, this reflex restricts the movement of the tympanic membrane to prevent damage to the inner ear hair cells from loud sounds. Furthermore, this muscle also contracts to attenuate the internal sensation of sounds generated by the acts of chewing and swallowing (see Chapter 9).

Clinical Correlates and Assessment

Sensory

The distribution of the trigeminal branches on the head, face, and oral cavity is well differentiated. Damage to any peripheral branch/branches would result in an ipsilateral loss of sensation in the area of distribution for the nerve, which includes the face, rostral tongue, teeth and gingiva, and the cavities of the nose, orbit, and mouth. The sneezing and blinking reflexes are also lost because of the interrupted innervation of the nasal mucosa and exterior surface of the eye (Table 17-20).

The most common trigeminal pathology is **trigeminal neuralgia** (pain), or **tic douloureux** (Box 17-5). It is marked by an excruciating chronic pain of unknown cause, usually in the territory of the ophthalmic or mandibular branch. This pain, often described as burning or stabbing, can be elicited by the slightest tactile stimulus in the trigger zones of the trigeminal distribution. The recurrent stabbing pain of trigeminal neuralgia has often been surgically treated by transecting the involved nerve branch or by sectioning the sensory nerve root.

Sensory Assessment. The affected branch of the nerve and the related modality (touch, pain, temperature) of sensation can be determined by clinical testing with various sensory stimuli (cotton and pinprick) and by assessing the sneeze and corneal reflexes.

Motor

An injury in the trigeminal motor nucleus or its fibers produces a LMN syndrome characterized by a flaccid paresis or paralysis of the ipsilateral muscles of mastication. The jaw slightly deviates toward the side of the injury; this deviation is exaggerated on jaw protrusion. Along with this, the muscles twitch and gradually atrophy, and the jaw-jerk reflex is absent. Because the muscles of mastication receive corticonuclear projections from the bilateral motor cortices (Fig. 17-8), any unilateral cortical or corticonuclear (UMN) injury is likely to have only a mild effect on the strength of the masticator muscles. Bilateral cortical (UMN) lesions, however, produce marked paralysis of the masticators bilaterally, and the mandible hangs low, causing structural difficulty in the production of vowels and labial and lingual consonant sounds.

Motor Assessment. The motor strength in patients with masticator palsy is assessed by asking them to bite down on a tongue depressor, move the jaw laterally against resistance, or open the jaw against resistance. Its functional quality can also be judged by examining the precision in the articulation of phonemes that require jaw support, for example, the bilabial, and labiodental, dental, and palatal sounds.

Key Terms :

Bell palsy **Facial asymmetry**

Facial Nerve

The facial nerve (CN VII), a functionally mixed nerve, is primarily a motor nerve for the muscles of facial expression

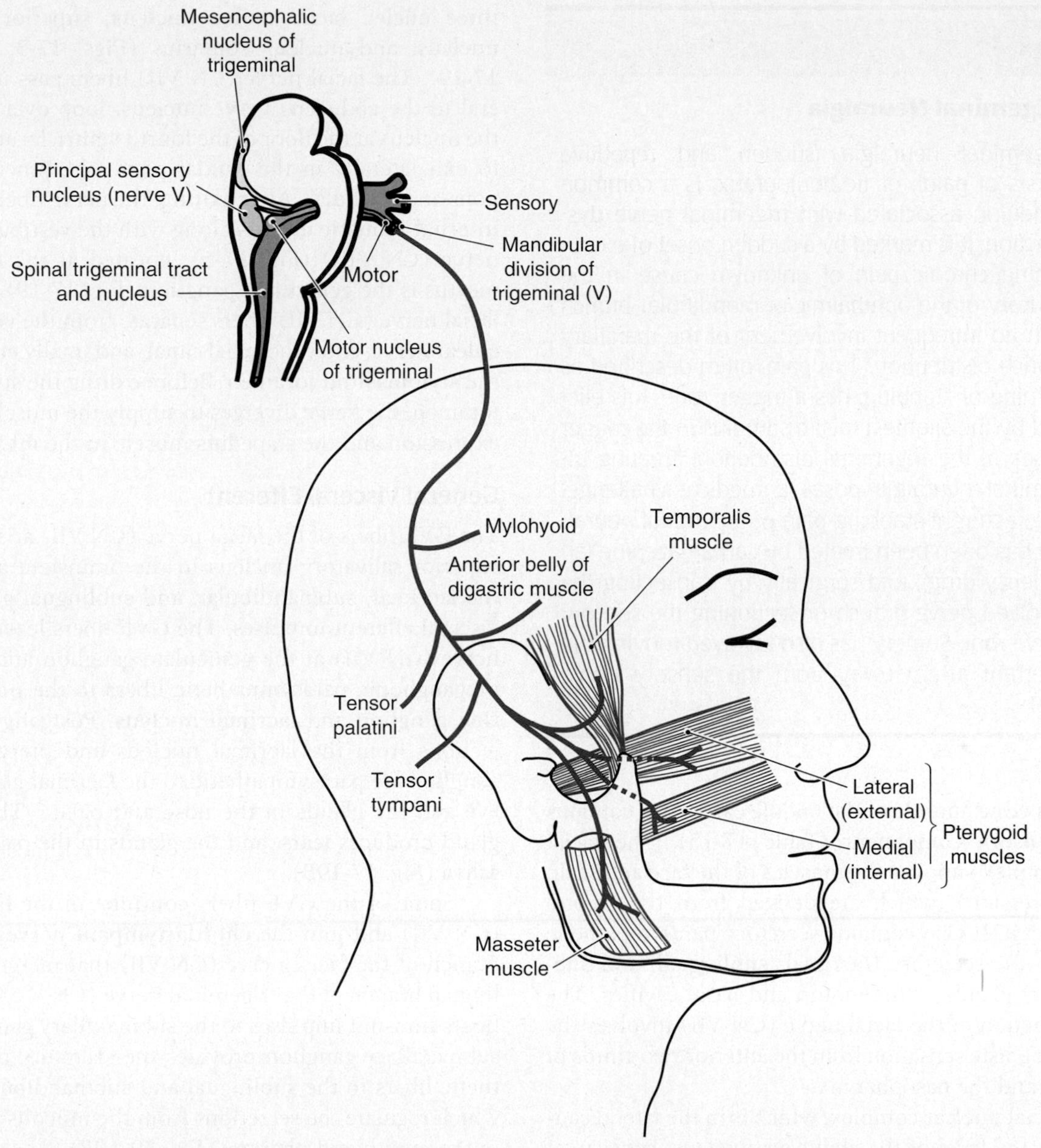

Figure 17-18 The motor branch of the trigeminal nerve, its nucleus, and the innervated muscles.

Table 17-14

Muscles of Mastication and Their Functions

Muscle	Function
Lateral and external pterygoid	Depresses and protrudes mandible toward opposite side; regulates movement side to side
Masseter	Elevates, closes, and slightly protrudes mandible
Medial and internal pterygoid	Elevates and assists in mandible protrusion
Temporalis	Elevates and retracts mandible

BOX 17-5

Trigeminal Neuralgia

Trigeminal neuralgia (sudden and repetitive bursts of pain), or tic douloureux, is a common condition associated with trigeminal nerve dysfunction. It is marked by a sudden onset of excruciating chronic pain of unknown cause in the territory of the ophthalmic or mandibular branch with an infrequent involvement of the maxillary branch distribution. This pain, often described as burning or stabbing, has a trigger zone. It is elicited by the slightest tactile stimulus in the trigger zones of the trigeminal distribution. Treating trigeminal neuralgia poses a medical challenge. The recurrent stabbing pain of trigeminal neuralgia has often been treated by carbamazepine (an epilepsy drug), and surgically by transecting the involved nerve branch or sectioning the sensory nerve root. Surgery has also involved moving the aberrant artery away from the sensory nerve root.

and the stapedius muscle of the middle ear; it also contains a small sensory component (Table 17-15). The facial nuclear complex supplies the muscles of the face and scalp (facial expression), which are derived from the second branchial arch. It also contains secretory parasympathetic efferents to the secretory (**lacrimal, sublingual, and submandibular**) glands in the mouth and nasal cavities. The sensory function of the facial nerve (CN VII) involves the mediation of taste sensation from the anterior two-thirds of the tongue and the nasopharynx.

The facial nuclear complex, which is in the lateral caudal pons at the level of the abducens nucleus, consists of three nuclei: **facial motor nucleus**, superior salivatory nucleus, and nucleus solitarius (Figs. 17-3, 17-4, and 17-19). The facial nerve (CN VII) fibers pass upward lateral to the abducens nerve nucleus, loop over the top of the nucleus at the floor of the fourth ventricle, and descend to exit laterally in the caudal pons (the junction of the pons and medulla). After exiting, the nerve fibers enter the **internal acoustic meatus** along with the vestibulocochlear nerve (CN VIII) (Fig. 17-5). Located at the end of the meatus is the **geniculate ganglion** (Fig. 17-19), where the facial nerve (CN VII) fibers separate from the vestibulocochlear nerve, enter the facial canal, and finally emerge from the **stylomastoid foramen**. Before exiting the stylomastoid foramen, the nerve diverges to supply the muscles of facial expression and the stapedius muscle in the middle ear.

General Visceral Efferent

The GVE fibers of the facial nerve (CN VII) arise from the superior salivatory nucleus in the brainstem and supply the lacrimal, submandibular, and sublingual glands with visceral efferent impulses. The GVE fibers leave the facial nerve (CN VII) at the geniculate ganglion and carry the preganglionic parasympathetic fibers to the **pterygopalatine ganglion** and **lacrimal nucleus**. Postganglionic projections from the lacrimal nucleus and pterygopalatine ganglion are parasympathetic to the lacrimal glands in the eye and the glands in the nose and palate. The lacrimal gland produces tears, and the glands in the palate secrete saliva (Fig. 17-19*B*).

Some of the GVE fibers continue in the facial nerve (CN VII) and join the **chorda tympani nerve**, a sensory branch of the facial nerve (CN VII) that merges with the lingual branch of the trigeminal nerve (CN V). These GVE fibers transmit impulses to the submaxillary ganglion. The submaxillary ganglion provides the secretory parasympathetic fibers to the sublingual and submandibular glands, which regulate the secretions from the mucous membrane in the mouth and pharynx (Fig. 19-19*B*).

Table 17-15

Functional Description of the Facial Nerve

Classification	Nuclei	Function
GVE (general visceral efferent)	Superior salivatory nucleus: preganglionic parasympathetic to pterygopalatine, submandibular, and sublingual ganglia associated with glands	Regulates secretions from lacrimal gland and mucosal glands of nasopharynx and salivary secretion from sublingual and submaxillary glands
SVA (special visceral afferent)	First order: geniculate ganglion Second order: nucleus solitarius	Mediates taste sensations from anterior two-thirds mucosa of tongue and palate
SVE (special visceral efferent)/BE (branchial efferent)	Motor (lower motor neuron) nucleus in lateral pons	Innervates muscles of facial expression, scalp muscles, and stapedius muscle of the middle ear

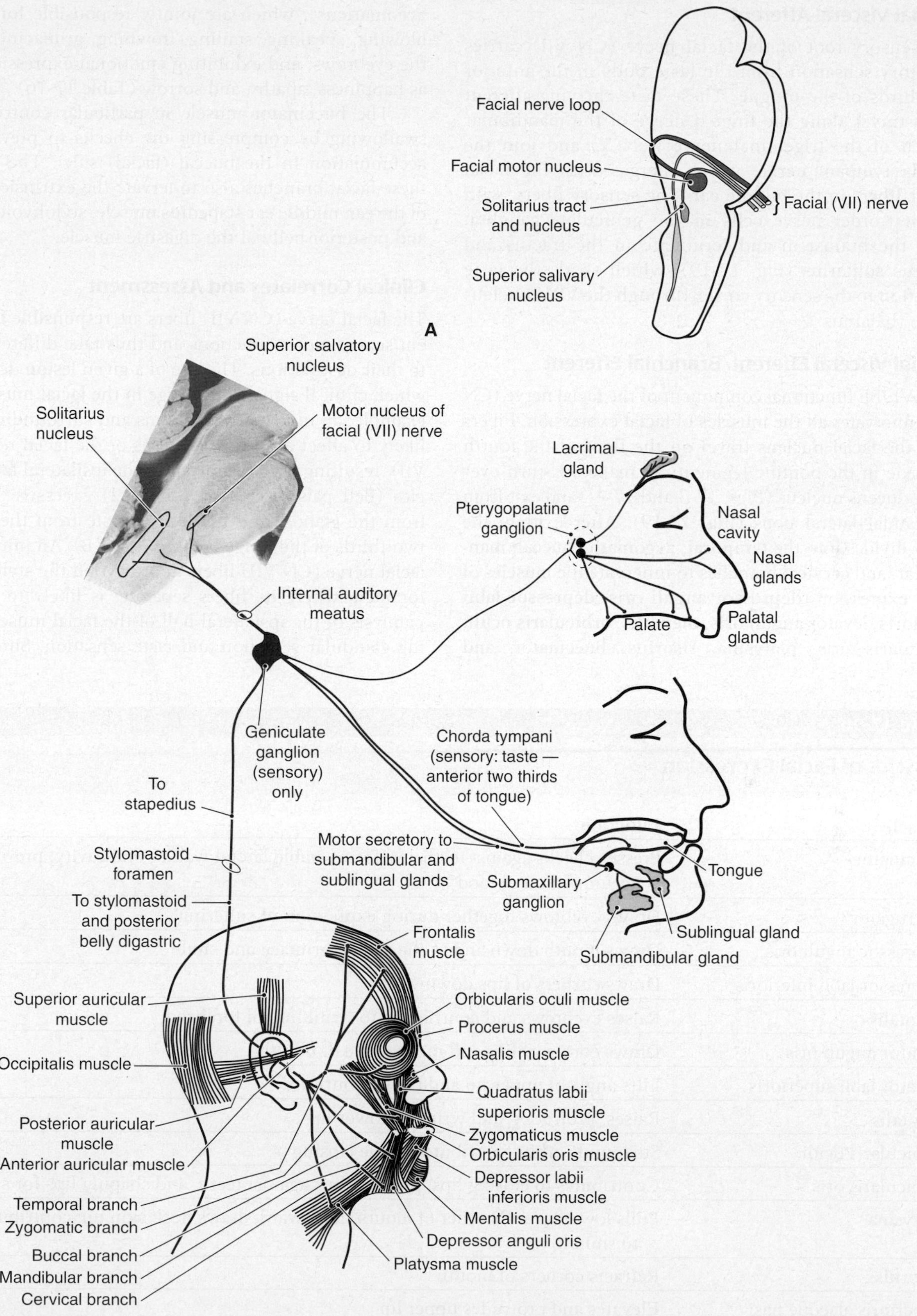

Figure 17-19 A. The facial nuclear complex in the brainstem. B. Sensorimotor branches of the facial nerve, and innervated structures (glands, oral pharynx, and muscles).

Special Visceral Afferent

The sensory root of the facial nerve (CN VII) carries gustatory sensation from the taste buds in the anterior two-thirds of the tongue. These taste-carrying afferent fibers travel along the lingual nerve of the mandibular branch of the trigeminal nerve (CN V) and join the chorda tympani nerve, which merges with the facial motor fibers in the middle ear. The sensory fibers, with the first-order nerve cells in the geniculate ganglion enter the brainstem and terminate in the tractus and nucleus solitarius (Fig. 17-19), which sends the taste sensation to the sensory cortex through the VPM nucleus of the thalamus.

Special Visceral Efferent/Branchial Efferent

The SVE/BE functional component of the facial nerve (CN VII) innervates all the muscles of facial expression. Fibers from the facial nucleus travel on the floor of the fourth ventricle in the pontine tegmentum, make a U-turn over the abducens nucleus (Figs. 17-3 and 17-4), and exit from the caudal–lateral pons (Fig. 17-19). After exiting, the nerve divides into the **temporal**, **zygomatic**, **buccal**, **mandibular**, and **cervical** branches to innervate the muscles of facial expression (**depressor anguli oris**, **depressor labii inferioris**, **levator anguli oris**, **mentalis**, **orbicularis oculi**, **orbicularis oris**, **platysma**, **risorius**, **buccinator**, and **zygomaticus**), which are jointly responsible for kissing, blowing, speaking, smiling, frowning, grimacing, raising the eyebrows, and exhibiting emotional expressions such as happiness, apathy, and sorrow (Table 17-16).

The buccinator muscle in particular contributes to swallowing by compressing the cheeks to prevent food accumulation in the buccal (facial) sulci. The fibers of these facial branches also innervate the extrinsic muscles of the ear, middle ear stapedius muscle, stylohyoid muscle, and posterior belly of the digastric muscle.

Clinical Correlates and Assessment

The facial nerve (CN VII) fibers are responsible for different sensorimotor functions and thus take different routes to their destinations. The site of a given lesion determines which clinical signs will emerge in the facial muscles. For example, an injury near the pons and surrounding area is likely to affect all three functions of the facial nerve (CN VII), resulting in (1) paralysis of the ipsilateral facial muscles (Bell palsy; see Fig. 1-17), (2) excessive secretion from the glands, and (3) loss of taste from the anterior two-thirds of the tongue (Fig. 17-19*A,B*). An injury in the facial nerve (CN VII) fibers at or beyond the stylomastoid foramen, where its fibers separate, is likely to result in paralysis of the ipsilateral half of the facial muscles, sparing glandular secretion and taste sensation. Similarly, an

Table 17-16

Muscles of Facial Expression

Muscle	Function
Buccinator	Presses cheeks against teeth and forms stable lateral wall to oral cavity; prevents accumulation of food
Corrugator	Draws eyebrows together during expression of suffering
Depressor anguli oris	Draws mouth down and to the side in grimace and smile
Depressor labii inferioris	Draws corners of lips downward
Frontalis	Raises eyebrows and contributes to wrinkling of forehead.
Levator anguli oris	Draws corner of lips and raises angle of mouth
Levator labii superioris	Lifts angle of upper lip and turns it outward
Mentalis	Raises, protrudes, and wrinkles lower lip
Orbicularis oculi	Surrounds orbit; contributes to eye closing
Orbicularis oris	Contributes to closing lips, pressing lips against teeth, and shaping lips for speech
Platysma	Pulls lower lip and corner of mouth downward; draws neck skin up; contributes to smiling
Risorius	Retracts corners of mouth
Superioris alaeque nasi	Elevates and protrudes upper lip
Zygomaticus major	Functions as a sling with depressor anguli oris; draws angle of mouth up and to side
Zygomaticus minor	Raises upper lip, contributing to a broad smile

injury to the chorda tympany fibers before they merge with the facial motor root would affect only taste sensation from the anterior two-thirds of the tongue and secretion from sublingual and submandibular glands.

Involvement of the GVE fibers to the pterygopalatine ganglion may cause secretory dysfunctions of the glands in the eye and palate. However, the secretion disorder alone is not clinically significant. For example, in the case of an UMN lesion, the contribution of the sublingual gland is small; there is never a complaint of oral dryness since the parotid glands are functional. In case of a LMN syndrome of the facial nerve, the lesion can take out the ipsilateral sublingual gland if the lesion is proximal to the superior salivary nucleus. However, the effect remains ipsilateral and is minimally noted since the parotids and the sublingual gland on the other side continue working.

Interruption of the efferents to the middle ear causes paralysis of the stapedius muscle (working jointly with the tensor tympani); impaired control of stapedius results in **hyperacusia**, a condition in which there is a heightened sensitivity to sounds so that normal sounds seem very loud; this may lead to aversive reactions to normal sounds. The stapedius muscle, when functioning properly, reflexively dampens the ear drum and constricts ossicular movements, a reflex function that protects the delicate organ of Corti from extreme movement (see Chapter 9).

Differential Cortical Innervation

The corticonuclear fibers differentially innervate the upper and lower face muscles (Fig. 17-20; Boxes 17-6 and 17-7). The motor nucleus that controls the lower half of the face receives projections from the contralateral motor cortex alone. However, the facial nerve nucleus controlling the upper facial muscles (frontalis and orbicularis) receives corticonuclear projections from both motor cortices (bilateral innervation), although it receives more from the contralateral motor cortex. This scheme of motor innervation has clinical implications for UMN (supranuclear and pseudobulbar) and LMN (internuclear) syndromes.

A dysfunction in the unilateral motor cortex (UMN) affects the muscles in the contralateral lower half of the face (Fig. 17-20*A*). The upper facial muscles are spared in the case of a contralateral cortical lesion. The patient is able to wrinkle the forehead and close the eye, because these muscles continue to receive partial projections from the ipsilateral motor cortex. Complete destruction of either the facial nucleus (LMN), which involves the nuclear regions for both the upper and the lower face, or a bilateral cortical lesion is necessary to cause paralysis of all the upper and lower muscles in the face (Fig. 17-20*B*); both of the conditions produce disastrous effects on the articulation of labial and labiodental sounds. Bilateral corticonuclear (UMN) lesions, also known as pseudobulbar palsy, produce bilateral facial palsy and result in profound impairments of motor speech (see Chapter 16). Patients lose delicate and discrete motor control, and muscles become paralyzed.

In the case of a facial paralysis with bilateral cortical motor involvement, the face becomes impassive, and it lacks any facial expression; the lips are parted at rest and remain so during a smile and/or speech attempts. The eyes cannot be closed tightly. Further, the patient cannot blow out the cheeks or attempt to blow out the cheeks without popping them, a sign of facial weakness.

An interesting clinical observation in the case of facial paralysis from a bilateral supranuclear lesion (pseudobulbar palsy) in the motor cortex (UMN) is the preservation of emotional expression while the facial muscles are paralyzed for voluntary control. The paralyzed facial muscles continue to respond involuntarily to genuine emotional stimuli and states (see Chapter 16). One explanation is that pathways mediating preserved emotional expression differ from the ones originating in the motor cortex. Emotional pathways consist of extrapyramidal integrated prefrontal, limbic, basal ganglia, and hypothalamic projections to the brainstem premotor reticular generator that controls the muscles of facial expression.

A condition commonly associated with facial nerve (CN VII) dysfunctioning is Bell palsy, a LMN syndrome. It is characterized by a paresis or paralysis of all unilateral upper and lower facial muscles (Fig. 17-20*B*; see Fig. 1-17). The muscles of the lower face sag, the fold around the lip and nose (nasolabial fold) flattens, and the palpebral fissure widens (see Fig. 1-17). The patient is unable to wrinkle the forehead, close the eye, show the teeth, or purse the lips on the side of the lesion (Box 17-8). Additional symptoms include impairments of sublingual and submandibular salivary secretion, hyperacusis, and loss of taste from the anterior two-thirds of the tongue.

The motor functions of the facial nerve (CN VII) are tested by asking the patient to smile, part the lips, show the teeth, puff out the cheeks, pucker the lips, and express emotions, while the examiner looks for signs of facial asymmetry. A careful examination of speech (labial and labiodental) sounds also provides information about the nerve integrity. Sugar, salt, and vinegar are used to assess taste from the tongue.

Vestibulocochlear Nerve

The vestibulocochlear nerve (CN VIII) consists of vestibular and acoustic branches (Table 17-17; see Chapters 9 and 10). Both branches are laterally attached to the brainstem at the junction of the medulla and pons (Figs. 17-1 and 17-3). The vestibular division mediates head position (equilibrium) in space, whereas the acoustic branch serves hearing.

Special Somatic Afferent

Vestibular Nerve

The vestibular system is a reflexive sensorimotor system that controls equilibrium, including regulation of neck position. In addition, the vestibular apparatus helps humans coordinate head and body movements and retain a stable visual fixation point in space during body and

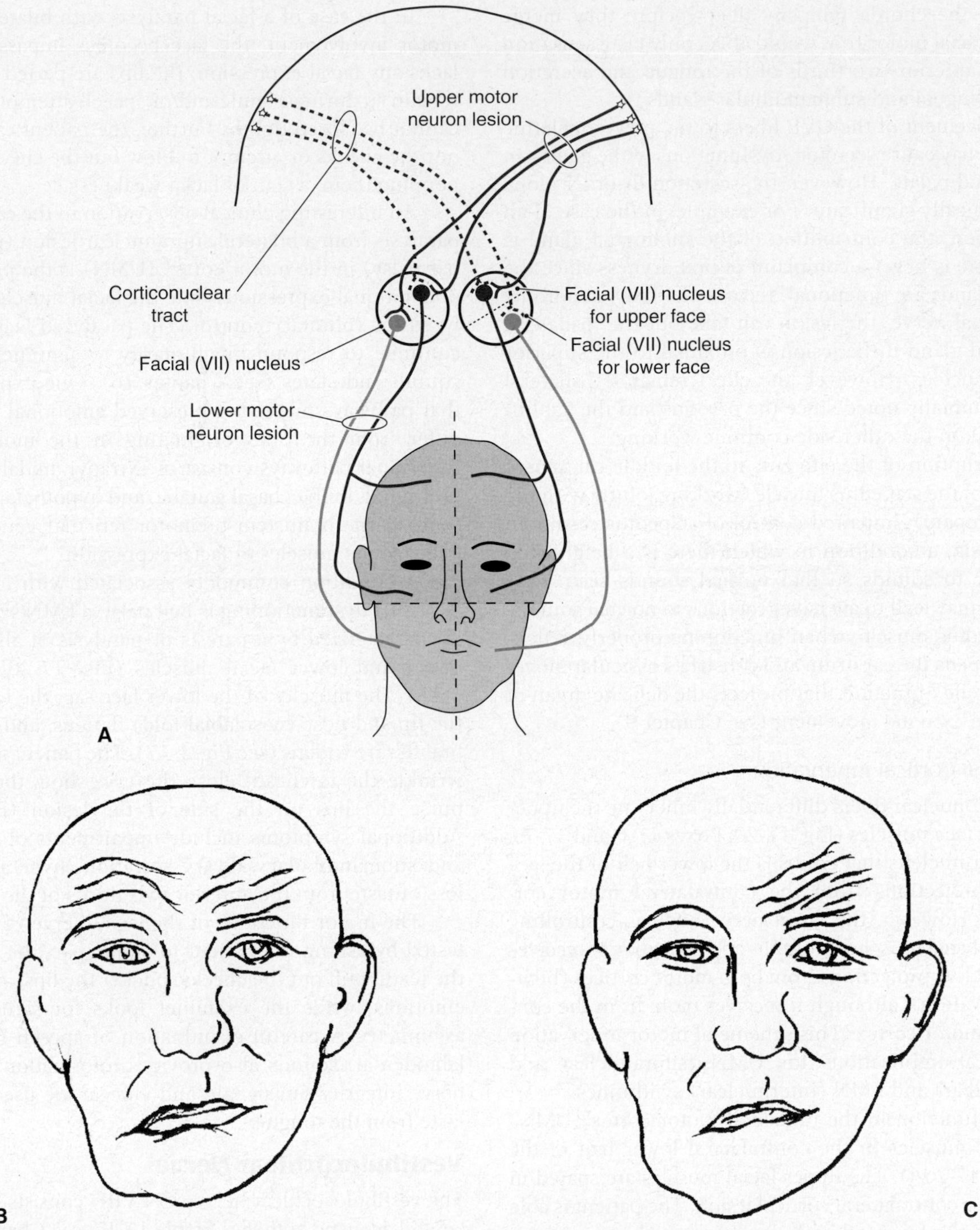

Figure 17-20 A. Distribution of the facial nerve fibers carrying unilateral and bilateral projections from the cortex. The upper portion of the face receives bilateral cortical projections, and the lower half of the face receives efferent commands from the contralateral motor cortex only. This differential neuronal organization for the facial muscles accounts for different patterns of facial paralysis after UMN and LMN lesions. B. In UMN syndrome, the patient exhibits only lower facial palsy (loss of the nasolabial fold and sagging of the lower mouth) and has preserved strength in the frontalis and ocular muscles. C. In LMN syndrome (Bell palsy), the entire side of the face is paralyzed.

BOX 17-6

Facial Innervation

The cortical motor control of the facial muscles is complex. The facial nerve motor nucleus that controls the lower half of the face receives projections from the contralateral motor cortex alone (unilateral innervation), whereas the facial motor nucleus innervating the upper facial muscles (frontalis and orbicularis) receives corticonuclear projections from both motor cortices (bilateral innervation). This innervation scheme has differential clinical implications for UMN (supranuclear) and LMN (internuclear) lesions. A unilateral motor cortex lesion (UMN) affects only the muscles in the contralateral lower face, and the patient is still able to wrinkle the forehead and close the eye, because these muscles continue to receive minor ipsilateral projections. Bilateral corticonuclear (UMN) lesions produce bilateral facial palsy and produce profound impairments of facial function and motor speech.

BOX 17-7

Neuraxial Lesions and Cranial Nerves

With idiosyncrasies of cranial nerves innervation, the impact of a lesion varies depending on its neuraxial site: the upper motor or lower motor neuron.

In general the LMN lesions cause a paralysis of the facial or swallowing muscles only on one side. Muscle wasting, areflexia, and fasciculations are common LMN features. Fasciculations can easily be visualized in muscles with large motor units. Bilateral LMN lesions have a profound effect on the facial and swallowing muscles. The face becomes largely impassive (devoid of any expressions) and the patient is unable to tightly close both eyes. The LMN involvement does not affect sensation. In case of the UMN pathology, the lesion must be bilateral before it will cause a profound and complete bilateral paralysis of the facial, lingual, and pharyngeal muscles. A unilateral UMN lesion largely affects the lower face and one-half of the tongue.

BOX 17-8

Bell Palsy

Also called facial nerve palsy, it involves blockade or destruction of the facial nucleus, facial nerve within the temporal bone (facial canal), or damage after the nerve leaves the facial foramen but before its many branches to the facial and scalp muscles. It is marked with unilateral paresis or paralysis of both the upper and lower facial muscles. Without motor control of the facial muscles, the face appears asymmetrical. The paralyzed side of the face is pulled toward the unaffected side. Food and saliva accumulate in the affected side of the mouth and the corner of the mouth droops. This asymmetry becomes most visible as the patient attempts to smile or attempts to show teeth; the lower portion of the face pulls toward the unaffected side, resulting in a transverse shape of the lips and mouth opening. Furthermore, the corneal reflex (afferent through trigeminal and efferent through the facial nerve) is absent on the side of the lesion, but the corneal sensation remains intact. Additional symptoms may include the impairments of sublingual and submandibular salivary secretion, hyperacusis, and loss of taste from the anterior two-thirds of the tongue on the affected site.

Degenerative inflammatory injury or infection, generally demyelinating type, of the facial nerve (CN VII) are the common causes of the palsy. If there is merely a nerve conduction block, the subjects completely recover within a few weeks. This recovery may take 4 to 5 months if the nerve involved undergoes the Wallerian degeneration followed by regeneration from the most distal part.

head movements. The vestibular branch of the vestibulocochlear nerve (CN VIII) originates from the vestibular (superior and inferior) ganglia equivalent of the dorsal root ganglia (DRG) neurons in the internal auditory meatus. The distal fibers of the vestibular ganglia innervate the hair cells in the cristae of the semicircular canals, saccule, and utricle. Their proximal axons make up the vestibular nerve and project impulses from the hair cells to the vestibular complex in the floor of the medulla's fourth ventricle (see Fig. 10-4). The vestibular nuclei send ascending projections to the flocculonodular lobe of the cerebellum, reticular formation, MLF, and motor nuclei of other cranial and spinal nerves (see Chapter 10). The descending projections from the vestibular nuclei to the spinal cord coordinate the limbs for standing balance. The importance of the vestibular system becomes evident in

Table 17-17

Functional Description of the Vestibulocochlear Nerve

Classification	Nuclei	Function
SSA (special somatic afferent)	First order: superior and inferior vestibular ganglia Second order: vestibular nuclei in caudal pons	Maintains equilibrium and head orientation in space
SSA (special somatic afferent)	First order: spiral ganglia Second order: cochlear nuclei in caudal pons	Mediates audition

patients whose body equilibrium is impaired by vestibular dysfunctioning, as in Ménière disease or because of a vestibulocochlear schwannoma.

Auditory Nerve

The acoustic fibers of the vestibulocochlear nerve (CN VIII), which serve hearing, originate in the spiral ganglia (equivalent to dorsal root ganglion neuron); the peripheral processes of the cells in the spiral ganglia innervate the hair cells in the organ of Corti in the inner ear. The proximal axons of the spiral ganglion, the primary cell bodies of the auditory nerve, mediate auditory impulses to the cochlear nuclei in the rostrolateral medulla (see Fig. 9-5). Some of the auditory fibers from the cochlear nuclei ascend ipsilaterally, whereas several others cross the midline through the trapezoid bodies. Most of the crossed auditory fibers terminate in the superior olivary nucleus, although some bypass it and ascend to the midbrain.

Besides transmitting the information, the function of the superior olivary nucleus is to compare the timing of the auditory signals received from the two ears, which provides the basis for judging sound source direction. The projections from the superior olivary nucleus form the lateral lemniscus, which ascends to the inferior colliculus of the midbrain. The fibers from the inferior colliculus travel through the brachium of the inferior colliculus to the medial geniculate body of the thalamus. The auditory fibers from the thalamus pass posterior to the internal capsule, then project to the primary auditory cortex in the temporal lobe (see Fig. 9-6). The auditory nerve has two important characteristics: first, its crossed and uncrossed fibers result in bilateral projections to the cortex; second, throughout its projections to the brain, a spatial tonotopic representation in tract fibers of various frequencies is discretely maintained.

Clinical Correlates and Assessment

Injuries to the vestibulocochlear nerve and nuclei are associated with disturbances of equilibrium and audition. Symptoms of vestibular nerve dysfunctioning are impaired equilibrium, vertigo or dizziness (the sensation of moving around in space), and nystagmus (rhythmic movement of the eye in which the eye moves slowly away from the center and then returns rapidly).

Auditory symptoms include a range of hearing impairments, which include conductive, sensorineural, and mixed. The exact nature of a hearing impairment depends on the site of the lesion. Damage to the peripheral auditory mechanism, involving the tympanic membrane and/or middle ear ossicles, results in a conductive type of hearing loss, which may not be very disabling. Damage to the **labyrinthine systems** (organ of Corti), spiral ganglia, cochlear nerve, and cochlear nuclei results in sensorineural impairment, which can seriously affect communicative ability. For example, if the cochlear nerve is damaged, hearing impairment in the affected ear may be permanent and profound. However, in the case of a brainstem lesion (central auditory pathways), impairment is only partial because of the bilaterality of auditory projections to the cortex. An important symptom of sensorineural hearing loss is tinnitus, a sensation of ringing, buzzing, or other noises in the absence of any external sounds (see Chapters 9 and 10).

Glossopharyngeal Nerve

The glossopharyngeal nerve (CN IX) and vagus nerve (CN X) share similar anatomy and many functions, although they follow different peripheral pathways. The glossopharyngeal nerve serves both sensory and motor functions (Table 17-18). The sensorimotor nucleus complex of the nerve consists of the inferior salivatory nucleus, **nucleus ambiguus**, and nucleus solitarius (Figs. 17-21 and 17-22); the latter two nuclei are shared with the vagus nerve (CN X). After exiting laterally from the medulla, posterior to the inferior olivary nucleus, the nerve fibers leave the skull through the **jugular foramen** (Fig. 17-5; see Figs. 2-49 and 2-50). At the opening of the foramen are two DRG of the glossopharyngeal nerve (CN IX): superior and inferior ganglion. The superior ganglion contains stretch afferent cell bodies innervating stylopharyngeus muscle spindles; the inferior ganglion contains GVA (cutaneous) and SVA (taste) DRG cell bodies of glossopharyngeal nerve (CN IX).

Table 17-18

Functional Description of the Glossopharyngeal Nerve

Classification	Nuclei	Function
GVA (general visceral afferent)	First order: inferior ganglion Second order: nucleus solitarius	Mediates gag and respiratory reflexes by regulating visceral sensation (pain and pressure) from oral pharynx mucosa, soft palate, palatal arch, posterior third of tongue mucosa, eustachian tube, middle ear cavity, and carotid sinus
GVE (general visceral efferent)	Inferior salivatory nucleus with preganglionic parasympathetic projections	Regulates salivatory secretion from parotid gland and mucous secretion from oral pharynx
SVA (special visceral afferent)	First order: inferior ganglion Second order: nucleus solitarius	Transmits taste sensation from posterior third of tongue, oral pharynx, and epiglottis
SVE (special visceral efferent)/BE (branchial efferent)	Nucleus ambiguus (lower motor neuron)	Contributes to swallowing reflex by activating stylopharyngeus and upper pharyngeal constrictor fibers

General Visceral Afferent

GVA fibers, which are primarily concerned with the initiation of reflexes, mediate the touch, pain, tension, and temperature sensations from intraoral visceral structures including the upper pharynx, tonsils, eustachian tube, middle ear cavity, soft palate, and mucosa of the posterior third of the tongue. With the primary sensory cell bodies in the inferior ganglion near the jugular foramina, the central processes from the inferior ganglion project to the nucleus solitarius in the medulla

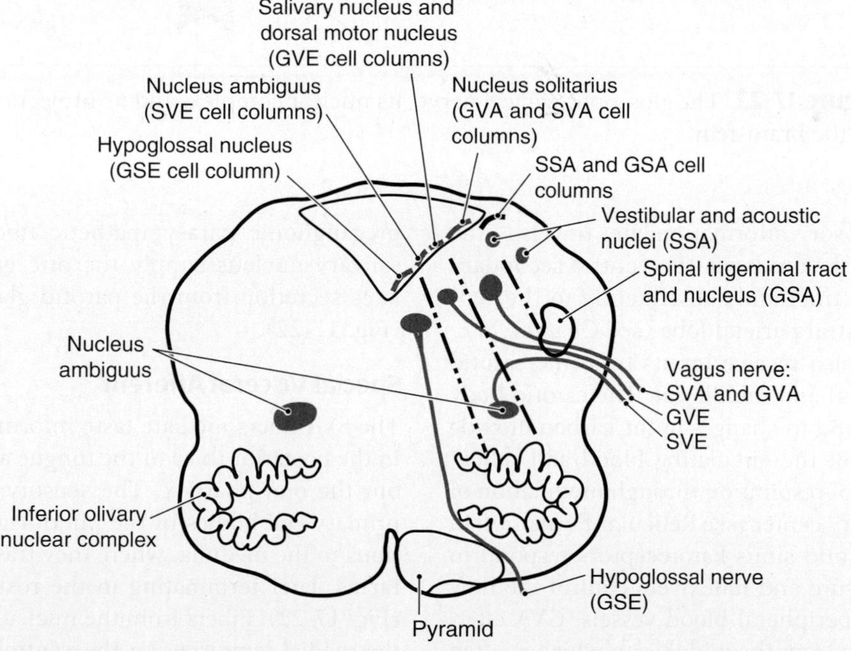

Figure 17-21 Cross section of the medulla showing the locations of the nuclei: hypoglossal nucleus (general somatic efferent [GSE]), nucleus ambiguus (special visceral efferent [SVE]/branchial efferent [BE]), salivary nucleus and dorsal motor nucleus (general visceral efferent [GVE]), nucleus solitarius (general visceral afferent [GVA] and special visceral afferent [SVA]), vestibular and acoustic nuclei (special somatic afferent [SSA]), and trigeminal nucleus (general somatic afferent [GSA]). Many of these nuclei are shared by the glossopharyngeal and vagus nerves.

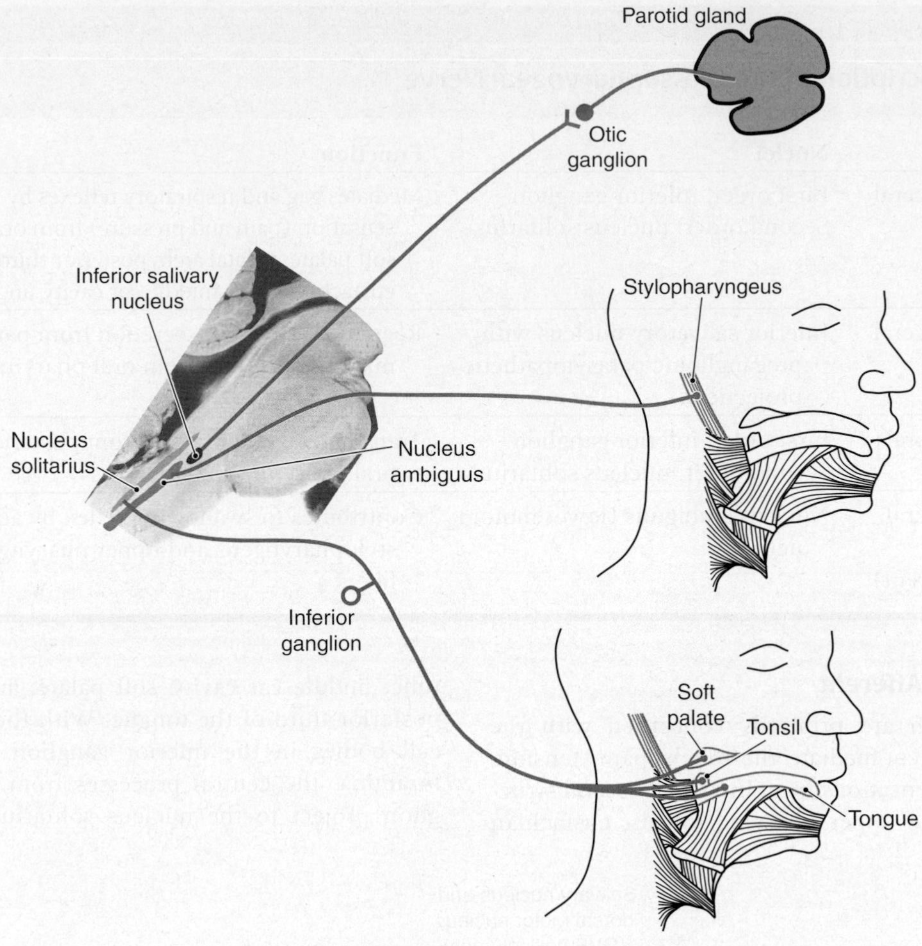

Figure 17-22 The glossopharyngeal nerve, its nuclear complex, and its projections to the brainstem.

(Fig. 17-22). This sensory information later travels to the VPM nucleus of the thalamus via the ventral secondary ascending trigeminal tract and subsequently to the sensory cortex in the rostral parietal lobe (see Chapter 11).

The GVA fibers also receive inputs from the carotid body (chemoreceptors) and middle ear. The carotid body chemoreceptors respond to changes in the carbon dioxide and oxygen content of the circulating blood and reflexively control the rate of respiration through modulation of the reticular respiratory center (see Reticular Formation in Chapter 18). The carotid sinus baroreceptors respond to increased blood pressure and reflexively control the flow of blood by dilating peripheral blood vessels. GVA afferents also mediate pain from the middle ear, which is often seen in the case of infection.

General Visceral Efferent

The GVE system is concerned with the autonomic control of visceral body structures including glands and cardiac muscles. The inferior salivatory nucleus mediates parasympathetic projections to the parotid gland. The preganglionic parasympathetic fibers from the inferior salivary nucleus supply the otic ganglion, which regulates secretion from the parotid gland in the oral cavity (Fig. 17-22).

Special Visceral Afferent

The SVA fibers mediate taste information from taste buds in the posterior third of the tongue and scattered throughout the oral pharynx. The sensory processes, with their primary cell bodies in the inferior ganglion, send projections to the medulla, where they travel in the **tractus solitarius**, later terminating in the rostral nucleus solitarius (Fig. 17-22). Fibers from the nucleus solitarius proceed in the medial lemniscus to the ventral posterior nucleus of the thalamus and then to the tongue area in the primary sensory cortex (Fig. 2-6).

Special Visceral Efferent/Branchial Efferent

The SVE/BE projections of the glossopharyngeal nerve contribute to swallowing by innervating the stylopharyngeus, a branchial or special visceral muscle derived from the third branchial arch (Fig. 17-2). The BE fibers of the glossopharyngeal nerve (CN IX) originate in the rostral region of the nucleus ambiguus, a column of motor nuclei also shared by the vagus nerve (CN X). The nucleus ambiguus, dorsolateral to the inferior olivary nucleus (Fig. 17-21), receives UMN input from both sides of the motor cortex (corticonuclear tracts), with contralateral input being stronger. The fibers from the nucleus ambiguus exit the lateral medulla, supplying the ipsilateral stylopharyngeus muscle, which plays an important role in swallowing (Fig. 17-22).

Clinical Correlates and Assessment

Because of the overlapping of nuclei and their proximity to other cranial nerves and nuclei, a lesion selectively affecting the glossopharyngeal nerve (CN IX) or its nuclei is rare. Nevertheless, a discrete lesion would result in partial paresis of the unilateral stylopharyngeal muscle, impairing ipsilateral pharyngeal elevation in deglutition. An additional symptom is loss of general and taste sensation from the ipsilateral posterior third of the tongue. Impaired cutaneous sensation from the posterior tongue would cause a loss of the gag reflex (Table 17-20). Furthermore, poor control of the parotid gland leads to excessive oral secretion. The symptoms are particularly pronounced after bilateral damage of the nerve. Dysfunctions of the glossopharyngeal nerve (CN IX) are usually assessed with the functions of the vagus nerve.

Vagus Nerve

The vagus nerve (CN X), with a more extensive distribution than any other cranial nerve, is 90% sensory and 10% motor (Table 17-19). From the perspective of students and professionals in communicative disorders, by far the most important function of the vagus nerve (CN X) is its control of the muscles used for phonation and swallowing (deglutition). The vagus nerve (CN X) innervates the cardiac muscles and smooth muscles of the esophagus, stomach, and intestine, and the branchial muscles of the pharynx and larynx. This nerve mediates sensations of pain, touch, and pressure from mucosa of the pharynx, inferior surface of the epiglottis, the trachea, bronchi, esophagus, and stomach. It also mediates general somesthetic (pain) input (GSA) and special stretch afferent feedback (SSA) from the pharyngeal and laryngeal muscles.

The vagal nuclear complex is in the ventricular floor of the medulla oblongata. It consists of the dorsal motor nucleus, nucleus ambiguus, and nucleus solitarius (Fig. 17-21). The nucleus ambiguus receives UMN input from both sides of the cortex, but with a stronger contralateral projection. The vagus nerve (CN X) exits the brainstem from the lateral medulla between the inferior olivary nucleus and the inferior cerebellar peduncle (see Figures 2-49 and 2-51); after passing through the jugular foramen (Fig. 17-5), it distributes its sensorimotor branches peripherally (Figs. 17-1 and 17-3).

General Visceral Afferent

The GVA sensation is involved with the regulation of cardiovascular, respiratory, and gastrointestinal functions. The GVA component mediates general sensation, including touch, pain, tension, and temperature, from receptors in the walls of the viscera: pharynx, larynx, thorax, abdomen, heart, bronchi, carotid sinus (baroreceptors; detect

Table 17-19

Functional Description of the Vagus Nerve

Classification	Nuclei	Function
GVA (general visceral afferent)	First order: inferior ganglion Second order: nucleus solitarius	Receives general sensation from muscles of pharynx, larynx, thorax, carotid body, and abdomen Regulates nausea, oxygen intake, and lung inflation (respiratory reflex)
GVE (general visceral efferent)	Dorsal motor nucleus with preganglionic projections to visceral plexuses	Innervates glands, cardiac muscles, and muscles of heart, trachea, bronchi, esophagus, stomach, and intestine
SVA (special visceral afferent)	First order: inferior ganglion Second order: nucleus solitarius	Mediates taste sensation from mucosa of posterior pharynx, larynx, and epiglottis
SVE (special visceral efferent)/BE (branchial efferent)	Nucleus ambiguus (lower motor neuron)	Controls muscles of larynx, pharynx, and soft palate for phonation, swallowing, resonance, and for opening respiratory pathway

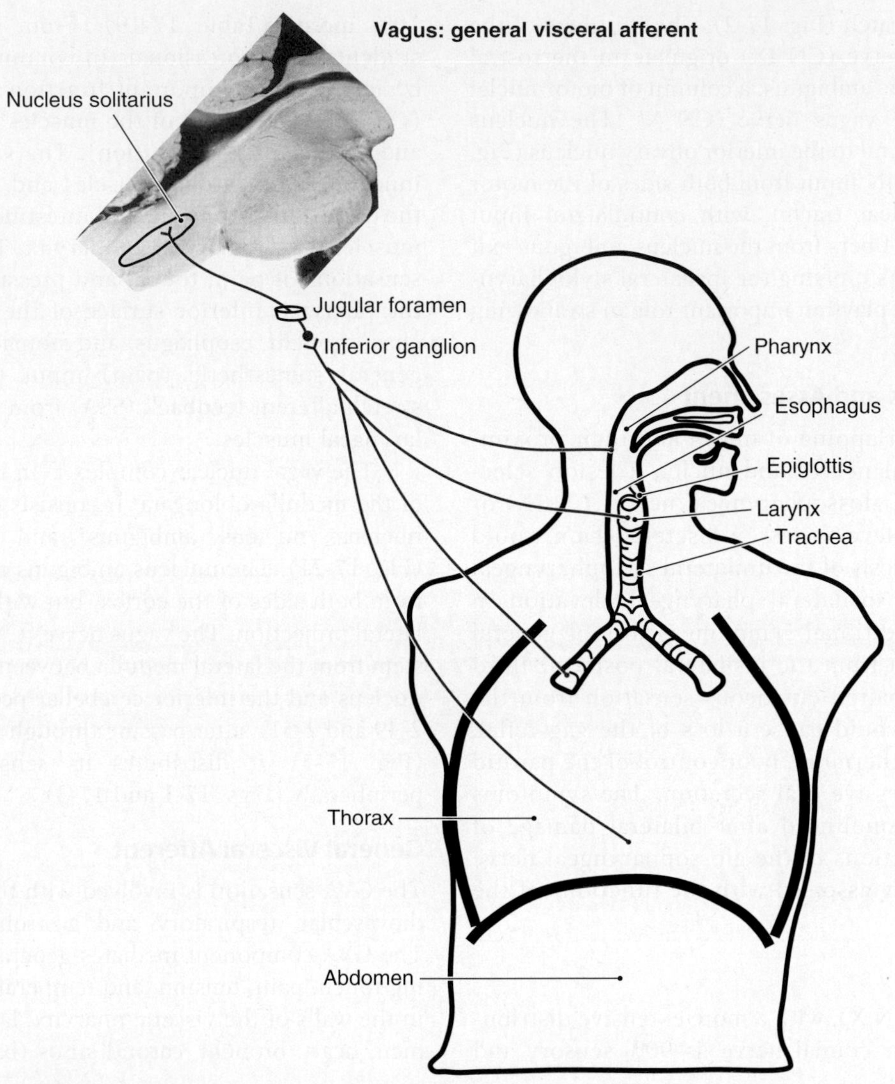

Figure 17-23 The nucleus solitarius with its general visceral afferent fibers, which mediate the general sensation from the muscles of the pharynx, larynx, thorax, and abdomen.

pressure changes), and esophagus (Fig. 17-23). The primary cell bodies of these sensory fibers are in the inferior ganglion (equivalent of the DRG), which is in the jugular foramen (Fig. 17-5). The inferior ganglion projects to the tractus and nucleus solitarius. The nucleus solitarius projects into many medullary reflex networks through the medial lemniscus and to the VPM nucleus of the thalamus on the way to the parietal superior opercular part of the sensory cortex in the Sylvian sulcus.

General Visceral Efferent

As part of the ANS, the GVE fibers parasympathetically innervate the viscera, including the cardiac muscles and the smooth muscles of the trachea, bronchi, esophagus, stomach, and intestines. The dorsal motor nucleus, which is located laterally in the ventricular floor, receives afferents from the hypothalamus, brainstem reflex network, and solitary tract. The long fibers leaving the dorsal motor nucleus send preganglionic projections to distal ganglia in the walls of the alimentary canal and digestive organs, including the trachea, bronchi, heart, esophagus, stomach, and intestines. The short postganglionic fibers regulate the functions of these structures (Fig. 17-24). The parasympathetic autonomic innervation of the rectum, bladder, and genitals is supplied by the S2–S4 spinal segments (see Chapter 18).

Special Visceral Afferent

The SVA fibers mediate taste sensation from the pharyngeal area. The sensory fibers from the base of the tongue,

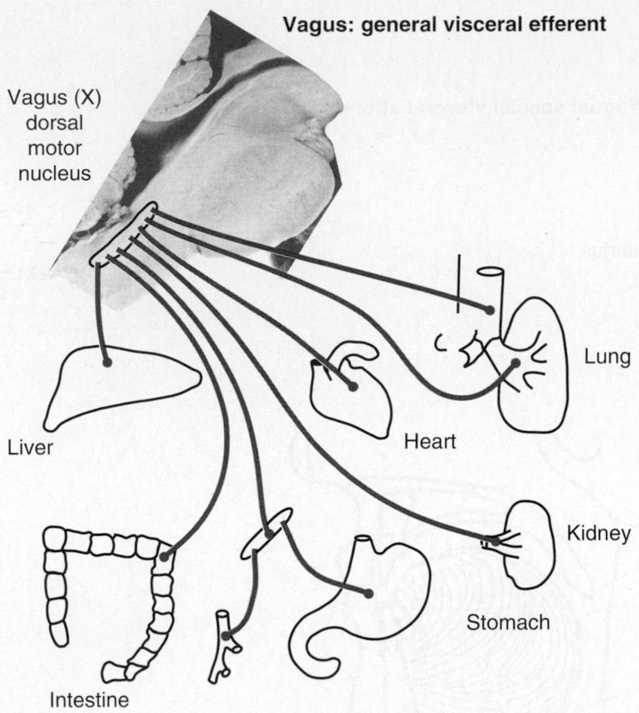

Figure 17-24 The dorsal motor nucleus of the vagus nerve in the medulla and its general visceral efferent nuclei projections to the smooth muscle fibers of the heart, trachea, bronchi, esophagus, stomach, and intestine. Red lines, preganglionic parasympathetic fibers, which innervate the postganglionic cells in the small ganglion near the target structures.

epiglottis, larynx, and pharynx have their cell bodies in the inferior ganglion (equivalent to the DRG); they project to the tractus and nucleus solitarius in the medulla oblongata (Fig. 17-25). The fibers from the nucleus solitarius ascend in the medial lemniscus to the VPM nucleus of the thalamus, from which fibers project to the sensory cortex in the parietal lobe. The primary (inferior ganglia) and secondary (solitarius) nuclei are shared by the glossopharyngeal nerve (CN IX), and they both serve similar SVA and GVA functions.

Special Visceral Efferent/Branchial Efferent

SVE/BE projections of the vagus nerve (CN X) innervate muscles that are important to students of communicative disorders: those of the larynx, pharynx, and the upper part of the esophagus (Fig. 17-26). These motor fibers of CN X originate from the posterior two-thirds of the nucleus ambiguus (one-third of the nucleus is related to the glossopharyngeal nerve [CN IX]), which is known to receive corticonuclear projections from both sides of the cortex. The efferent fibers supply the branchial muscles of the pharynx, the muscles of the soft palate (except for the tensor palatini, which is served by the trigeminal nerve [CN V]), the intrinsic muscles of the larynx, and the upper area of the esophagus.

The pharyngeal branch of the nerve supplies the three constrictor muscles (superior, middle, and inferior) of the pharynx and all soft palate muscles (palatoglossus and levator palati), except for the tensor palatini (trigeminal nerve [CN V]). The superior laryngeal branch of the vagus divides into internal and external laryngeal branches. The external branch of the superior laryngeal nerve controls the cricothyroid muscle, an internal laryngeal muscle. The internal branch is sensory to the mucous membrane as far down as the vocal cords and adjacent area.

The recurrent laryngeal branch of the vagus nerve (CN X) takes different routes on the two sides. It curves around the subclavian artery before emerging on the right side but curves around the aortic arch on the left side. The recurrent laryngeal nerve fibers innervate the intrinsic muscles of the larynx and epiglottis and, therefore, play an important role in phonation (Fig. 17-26). While these branches provide motor control to the larynx, some of the recurrent laryngeal fibers are responsible for sensory innervation of the mucous membrane inferior to the vocal cords.

The nucleus ambiguus also receives afferent projections from the tractus solitarius, which contains stretch afferent feedback from the muscles innervated by the glossopharyngeal (CN IX) and vagus nerves (stretch reflexes). These afferent and efferent projections form the reticular neuronal circuitry that enables reflexes such as gagging, coughing, vomiting, and swallowing (Table 17-20).

Clinical Correlates and Assessment

The medulla oblongata, the site of many reticular networks, vital reflex centers, and several cranial nuclei, is an important anatomic structure. Reflexes required for survival—such as swallowing, gagging, coughing, sneezing, vomiting, breathing, and cardiac rate—require the normal functioning of output nuclei (e.g., from nucleus ambiguus, dorsal vagus nucleus, and hypoglossal nuclei) and input association nuclei (especially the nucleus solitarius). Vagus nerve (CN X) fibers participate in almost all of these functions. Most of the networks that organize and control these vital reflexes involve many regions of the reticular formation in the medulla, with hierarchical control from the higher CNS. Consequently, medullary lesions, especially large ones that damage both sides of the medullary reticular area, can damage parts of these networks and their input and/or output nuclei, often with lethal consequences (see Chapter 18).

For students of communicative disorders, the functions of the nucleus ambiguus are essential (Fig. 17-27*A*). A unilateral lesion of the nerve fibers and/or nucleus ambiguus is likely to result in ipsilateral paresis or

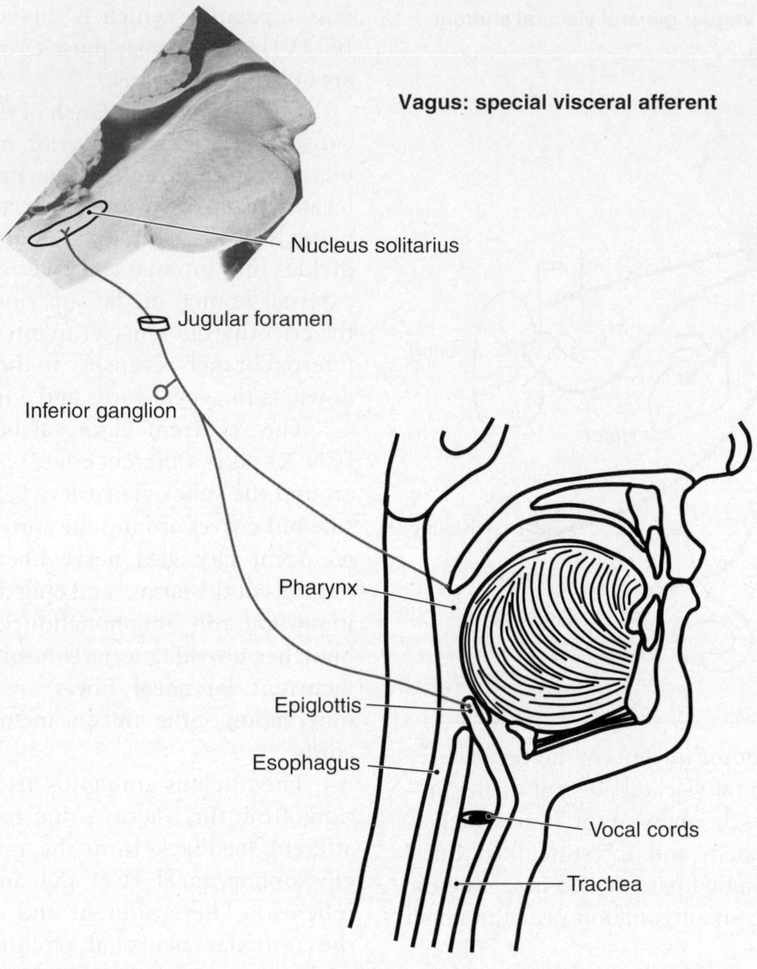

Figure 17-25 The nucleus solitarius and special visceral fibers from the muscles of the larynx, pharynx, epiglottis, and palate.

paralysis of the soft palate, pharynx, and larynx. Injuries specifically to the pharyngeal branch of the vagus nerve (CN X) cause paralysis of the pharynx and the soft palate, leading to swallowing difficulty. With unilateral paralysis of the levator muscle of the soft palate, the soft palate lowers on the affected side, and the uvula is pulled to the unaffected side (Fig. 17-27*B*). With bilateral soft palate paralysis, despite symmetry, the soft palate hangs lower than its normal curvature (Fig. 17-27*C*). Recurrent laryngeal nerve disorders lead to paralysis of the vocal folds. Unilateral LMN paralysis of the vocal folds causes breathy voice, diplophonia, and hoarseness but only minimally affects the ability to phonate. Vocal cord paralysis may also cause choking and pulmonary aspiration. Bilateral injury to the recurrent laryngeal nerve, however, produces inspiratory stridor and aphonia. It can also be life threatening if the paralyzed vocal cords impair airflow.

Unilateral central (UMN) lesions in the brainstem involving the corticonuclear fibers cause harsh voice quality. However, such lesions do not produce severe phonatory and swallowing symptoms because the nucleus ambiguus receives UMN input from both sides of the cortex (Fig. 17-8). Bilateral central (UMN) lesions will produce profound phonatory and swallowing problems.

With vagus nerve injuries, many autonomic functions and visceral reflexes are impaired, such as coronary circulation, heart rate, and relaxation and contraction of tracheal and bronchial muscles. Altered autonomic reflexes include vomiting, coughing, sneezing, sucking, hiccupping, and yawning. An injury to the sensory nuclear complex of CN X would lead to anesthesia of the larynx, pharynx, and associated structures and to loss of taste sensation from the pharyngeal and epiglottic areas. Because the glossopharyngeal nerve (CN IX), vagus nerve (CN X), and spinal accessory nerve (CN XI) all pass through the jugular foramen, peripheral lesions involving the vagus nerve alone are uncommon.

Assessment. Loss of vagus nerve functions is tested by visual examination of the soft palate during rest and action

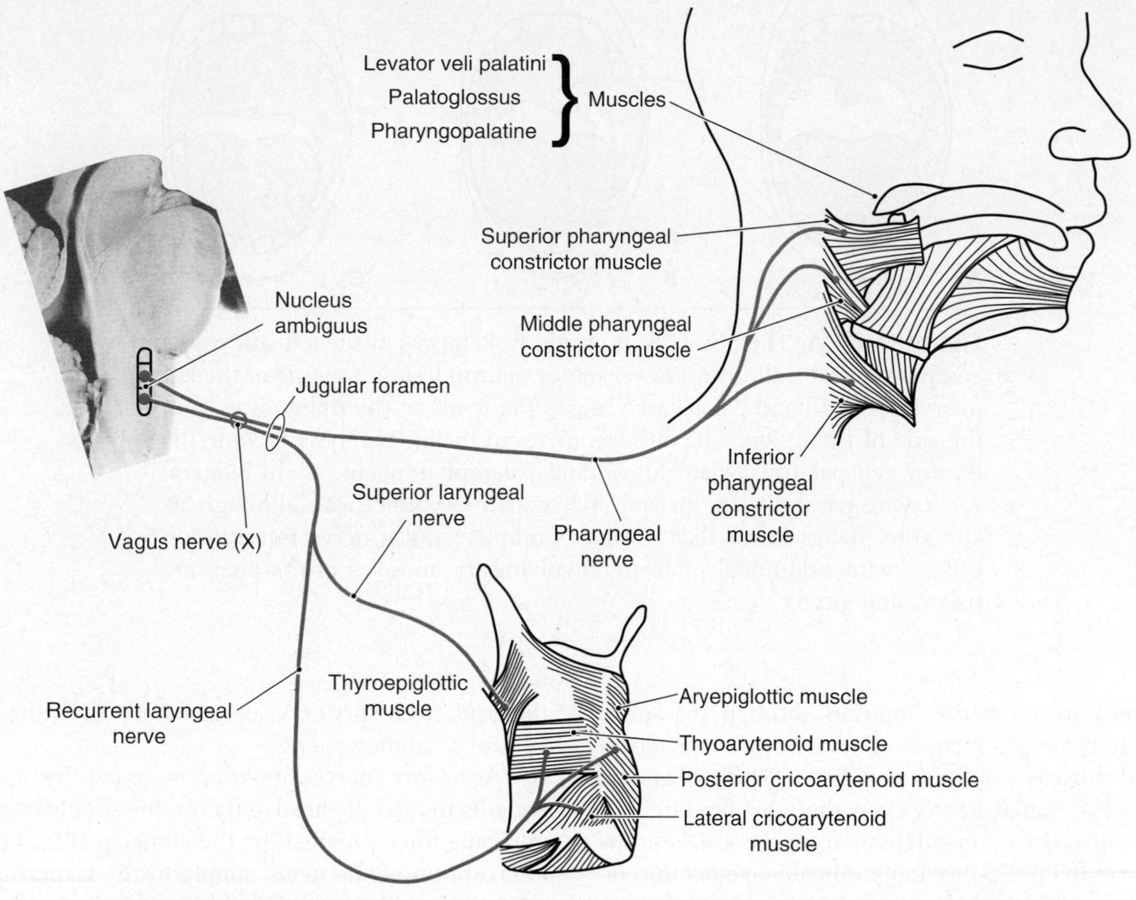

Figure 17-26 The vagus nucleus ambiguus with its special visceral efferent fiber/branchial efferent projections to the branchial muscles of the larynx and pharynx.

(phonation of "ah"), visual inspection of pharyngeal cavity, and assessment of quality in phonation (breathy, horse, altered voicing, and diplophonia) and swallowing (coughing after food consumption, choking on food, multiple efforts in moving the bolus through the pharynx, and pain sensation during swallow) tasks.

Spinal Accessory Nerve

Special Visceral Efferent/Branchial Efferent

The spinal accessory nerve (CN XI) is a branchiomeric motor nerve that receives projections primarily from the contralateral motor cortex (Table 17-21). The corticospinal

Table 17-20

Common Cranial Nerve–Mediated Reflexes

Reflexes	Reflexive Activity	Initiating Stimulus
Pupillary	Pupillary constriction (CN III efferent fibers)	Shining light in eye (CN II afferent fibers)
Corneal	Eye blink (CN VII efferent fibers)	Touching cornea (CN V afferent fibers)
Gag	Involuntary effort to vomit (CN X efferent fibers)	Pharyngeal touch (CN IX and X afferent fibers)
Sneeze	Involuntary contraction of muscles of expiration (CN X efferent fibers)	Nasal mucous membrane irritation (CN V afferent fibers)

CN, cranial nerve.

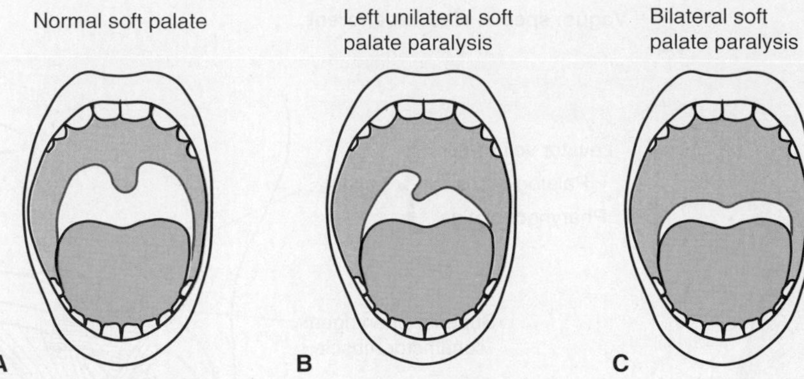

Figure 17-27 A. The normal soft palate. B. Paralysis of the left soft palate and pharyngeal wall from a lower motor neuron lesion. Sagging of the left pharyngeal wall and palatal arch moves the uvula to the right, away from the side of the lesion. The muscles involved in this paralysis include the levator veli palatini, palatoglossal, and palatopharyngeus. C. In bilateral soft palate paralysis, the palatal arch remains symmetrical, although its curvature hangs lower than normal. Complete vagus nerve interruption causes many additional problems involving the muscles of the pharynx, palate, and larynx.

projections transmit nerve impulses through the spinal roots of the nerve. As mentioned earlier, the remnants of gill-related muscles continue to C1–C5. These fibers are classified as a cranial nerve, even though they originate from the spinal cord. The efferents from the LMNs in the ventral horns in C1–C5 fuse longitudinally to enter the cranial cavity through the foramen magnum and leave the cranium via the jugular foramen (Figs. 17-3 and 17-5). They follow the vagus nerve (CN X), and the efferent fibers innervate two neck muscles: the **trapezius** and **sternocleidomastoid** (Fig. 17-28). The trapezius muscle tilts the head back and to the side and contributes to shrugging. The sternocleidomastoid muscle pulls the mastoid process and the clavicle closer together on one side, rotating the head and jaw to the opposite side.

Clinical Correlates and Assessment

The trapezius and sternocleidomastoid muscles, combined with other adjacent neck muscles, contribute to tilt, forward and backward extension, and lateral rotation of the head. Accessory nerve dysfunctions affect the ability to control head movements.

Accessory nerve function is tested by asking the patients to turn the head and raise the shoulder against an opposing force provided by the clinician (Fig. 17-29). An interruption of the nerve supply to the trapezius muscle results in a dropped shoulder that cannot be raised. Damage to the sternocleidomastoid restricts head turning to the side away from the lesion. Paralysis of these muscles may also indirectly affect speech resonance.

Hypoglossal Nerve

General Somatic Efferent

The hypoglossal nerve (CN XII) is a motor nerve (Table 17-22). The nerve fibers originate from the hypoglossal nucleus in the ventricular floor of the fourth ventricle close to the midline in the medulla (Figs. 17-1 and 17-3). The hypoglossal nucleus receives its direct corticonuclear input from the contralateral motor cortex (Fig. 17-8). The efferent fibers from the hypoglossal nucleus travel ventrally,

Table 17-21

Functional Description of the Spinal Accessory Nerve

Classification	Nuclei	Function
SVE (special visceral) efferent)/BE (branchial efferent)	Spinal accessory nucleus in C1–C5 ventral horns of spinal cord	Controls head position by controlling trapezius and sternocleidomastoid muscles

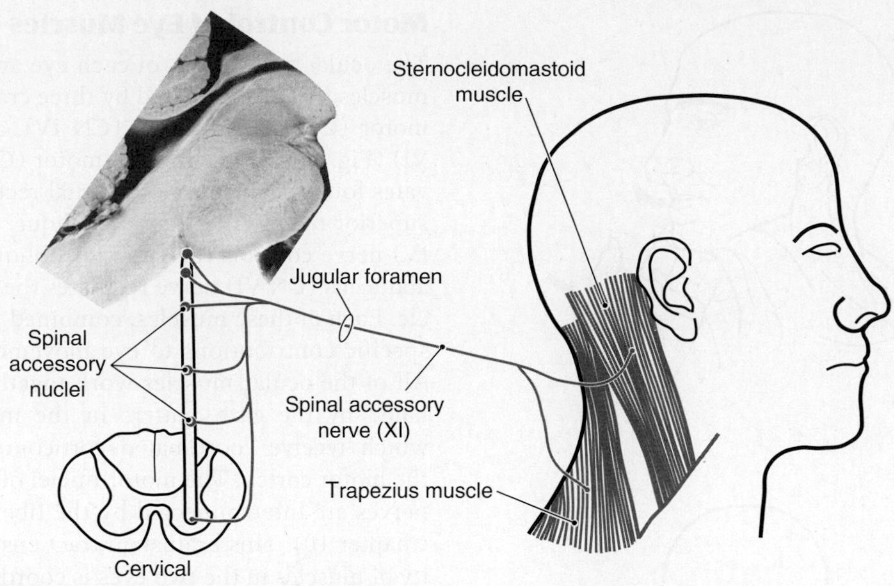

Figure 17-28 Origin of the spinal and cranial fibers of the spinal accessory nerve and distribution to the muscles in the neck.

pass through the medullary substance medial to the inferior olivary nucleus, and exit lateral to the pyramidal tract (Fig. 17-21).

The hypoglossal nerve (CN XII), which controls tongue movement, innervates all ipsilateral intrinsic and most extrinsic (genioglossal, styloglossus, and hyoglossus) tongue muscles except the palatoglossal, a vagus nerve (CN X)-controlled muscle (Fig. 17-30; Table 17-23). The afferent projections from the nucleus solitarius and trigeminal sensory nuclei are functionally linked with efferent hypoglossal fibers. This forms the neuronal circuitry for eating, sucking, and chewing reflexes.

Clinical Correlates and Assessment

Unilateral damage to the hypoglossal nucleus or interruption of nerve projections results in LMN symptoms. Consequently, the ipsilateral half of the tongue is paralyzed and it becomes flaccid and wrinkled. With no voluntary control or reflexes, the paralyzed half of the tongue eventually atrophies, which is characterized by loss of contour and corrugation of the edge. This weakness and muscle atrophy contribute to dysarthria and chewing difficulty, in which the patient has problems with formation and control of the bolus that is essential for normal swallowing. On palpation, the affected side of the tongue appears flaccid (soft) and wrinkled. On protrusion, the tongue deviates to the side of the lesion because of the unopposed protrusion of the normal half (genioglossal muscle) of the tongue (Fig. 17-31*A*). Bilateral LMN damage to the nucleus or nerve is likely to cause severe difficulty in swallowing, eating, and speaking (Fig. 17-31*B*).

After a unilateral supranuclear lesion, the loss of UMN influence on the contralateral hypoglossal nucleus results in significant loss of skill in using the affected half of the tongue during articulation, swallowing, and eating. However, the presence of some aberrant corticonuclear fibers may somewhat limit the effect of the loss. Initially, on protrusion, the affected and weakened tongue deviates to the paralyzed side away from the hemisphere with a supranuclear (UMN) lesion. However, with recovery over time, the tongue may no longer deviate on protrusion, but the nerve function still may not be normal.

Assessment. The hypoglossal nerve function is tested by asking the patient to protrude, retract, raise, and move the tongue laterally and by examining the quality of lingual and dental sounds.

FUNCTION-BASED CRANIAL NERVE COMBINATIONS

There are two important aspects of cranial nerve functions. The first is multiple innervations, in which two or more cranial nerves innervate the same anatomic structure. For example, several cranial nerves combine to serve eye movement, sensory innervation of the tongue, and soft palate and pharyngeal movements. The second is that some cranial motor (branchial) nuclei nerves receive corticonuclear projections from both motor cortices, although the contralateral projection is stronger. This has significant clinical implications for preserved motor speech functions after a unilateral lesion.

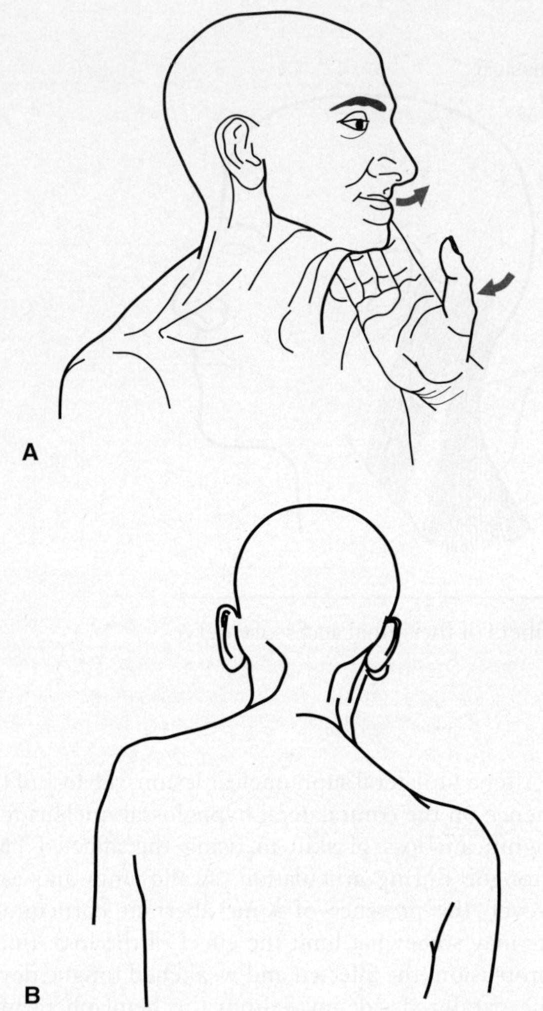

Figure 17-29 Paralysis of the spinal accessory nerve. A. The sternocleidomastoid muscle pulls the mastoid process and clavicle closer together on one side, rotating the head and jaw to the opposite side. Paralysis of the sternocleidomastoid muscle restricts movement of the jaw and neck, thus limiting the head movement opposite the side of damage. B. With paralysis of the trapezius muscle, the ipsilateral shoulder sags because of the loss of the normal contour between the neck and shoulder.

Motor Control of Eye Muscles

The ocular movements of each eye are controlled by six muscles that are regulated by three cranial nerves: oculomotor (CN III), trochlear (CN IV), and abducens (CN VI) (Fig. 17-32*A*). The oculomotor (CN III) nerve innervates four ocular muscles: medial rectus, inferior rectus, superior rectus, and inferior oblique. The trochlear (CN IV) nerve controls the superior oblique muscle, and the abducens (CN VI) nerve regulates the lateral rectus muscle. Each of these muscles, combined with others, makes specific contributions to eye movements (Fig. 17-32*B*). All of the ocular muscles work together and are coordinated by the gaze centers in the midbrain and pons, which receive coordinated corticonuclear signals from the motor cortex. The motor nuclei of these three cranial nerves are interconnected by the fibers of the MLF (see Chapter 10). This brainstem tract ensures that the activity of muscles in the two eyes is coordinated and that the eyes move in the same direction concurrently with head movement.

The midbrain conjugate gaze control center coordinates the movement of both eyes together. For example, activation of the left frontal cortex (premotor area) leads to activation of the right pontine gaze center and then to activation of the right abducens (lateral rectus) and left oculomotor nucleus (medial rectus). This results in contraction of the right lateral rectus and left medial rectus muscles to ensure a smooth turn of both eyes toward the right. The activation of the right frontal cortex (premotor area) would lead to activation of the left pontine gaze and cause the contraction of the left lateral rectus and right medial rectus muscle.

Sensory Nerve Supply to Tongue

The tongue displays a distinctive pattern in which three cranial nerves innervate general (cutaneous) and special (taste) sensations from its anterior and posterior regions (Fig. 17-33). The general sensations of pain, touch, and proprioception from the anterior two-thirds of the tongue are carried in the lingual branch of the trigeminal nerve (CN V). General sensations from the posterior third of the

Table 17-22

Functional Description of the Hypoglossal Nerve

Classification	Nuclei	Function
GSE (general somatic efferent)	Hypoglossal nucleus (lower motor neuron) in medulla	Controls motor movements of tongue by regulating intrinsic and extrinsic glossal muscles

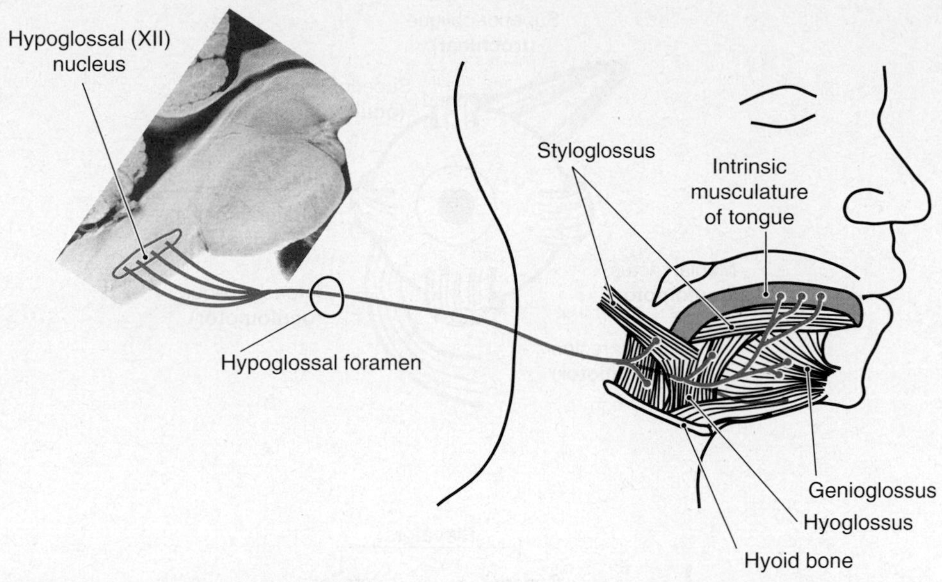

Figure 17-30 The hypoglossal nucleus in the medulla, the intramedullary course of the nerve, and the distribution of the nerve fibers to the glossal muscles.

Table 17-23

Muscles of the Tongue

Muscle	Function
Extrinsic muscles	
Genioglossus (CN XII)	Raises hyoid bone and protrudes and retracts tongue
Hyoglossus (CN XII)	Retracts tongue and lowers its side
Palatoglossus (CN X)	Narrows fauces and elevates back of tongue
Styloglossus (CN XII)	Retracts and elevates tongue
Intrinsic muscles	
Superior longitudinal	Shortens and curls tip of tongue upward
Inferior longitudinal	Shortens and curls tip of tongue downward
Transverse	Elongates and narrows and raises sides of tongue
Verticalis	Flattens and broadens tongue

CN, cranial nerve.

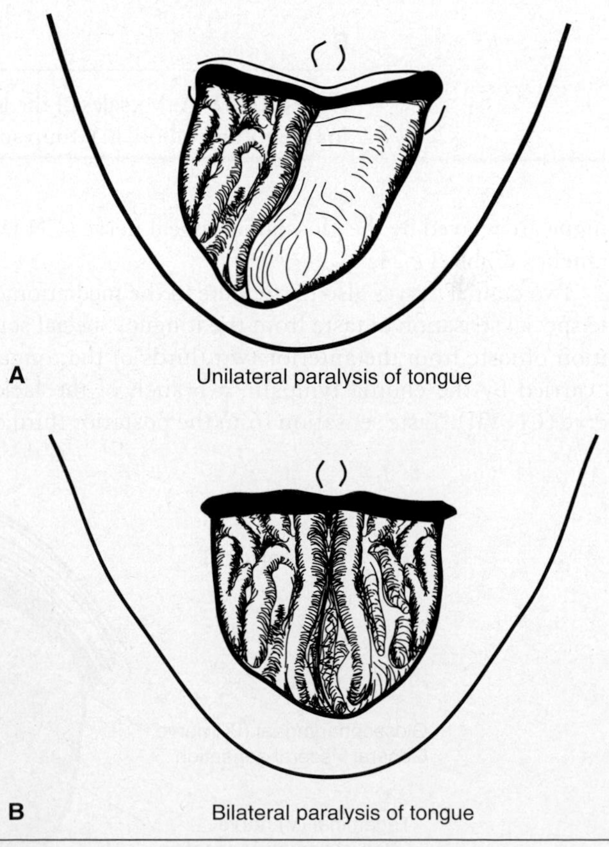

Figure 17-31 Paralysis of the right half of the tongue. **A.** The loss of bulk is evident; and on protrusion, the tongue deviates to the side of weakness. **B.** Bilateral palsy of the tongue is characterized by general atrophy.

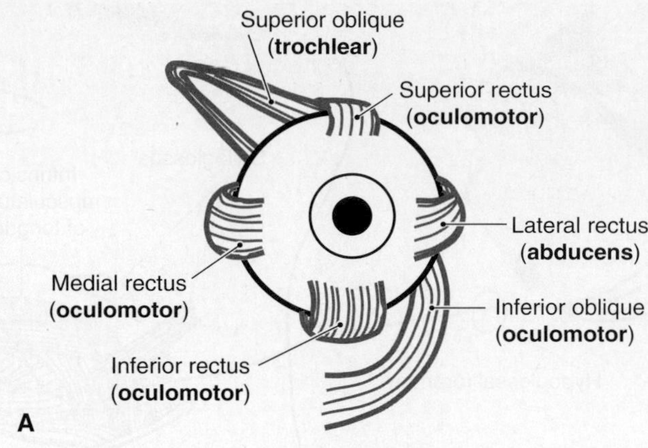

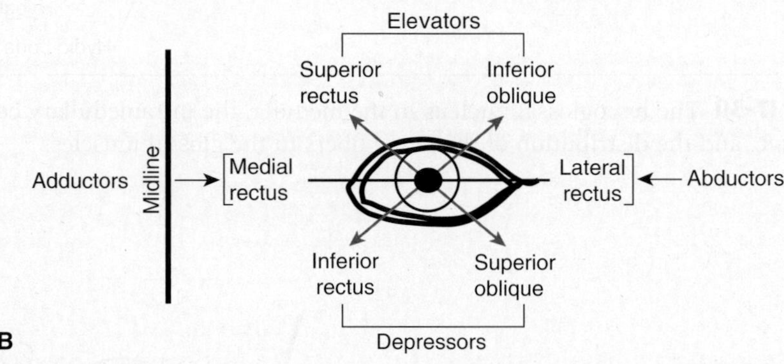

Figure 17-32 A. Muscles of the left eye and the cranial nerves responsible for their innervation. B. Group actions of the ocular muscles of the left eye.

tongue are relayed by the glossopharyngeal nerve (CN IX) branches (Table 17-24).

Two cranial nerves also participate in the mediation of the special sensation of taste from the tongue. Special sensation of taste from the anterior two-thirds of the tongue is carried by the chorda tympani, a branch of the facial nerve (CN VII). Taste sensation from the posterior third of the tongue is carried by the fibers of the glossopharyngeal nerve (CN IX).

Motor Nerve Supply to the Soft Palate and Pharynx

The soft palate and tube-shaped pharyngeal cavity are important in swallowing and speech resonance. The soft palate seals

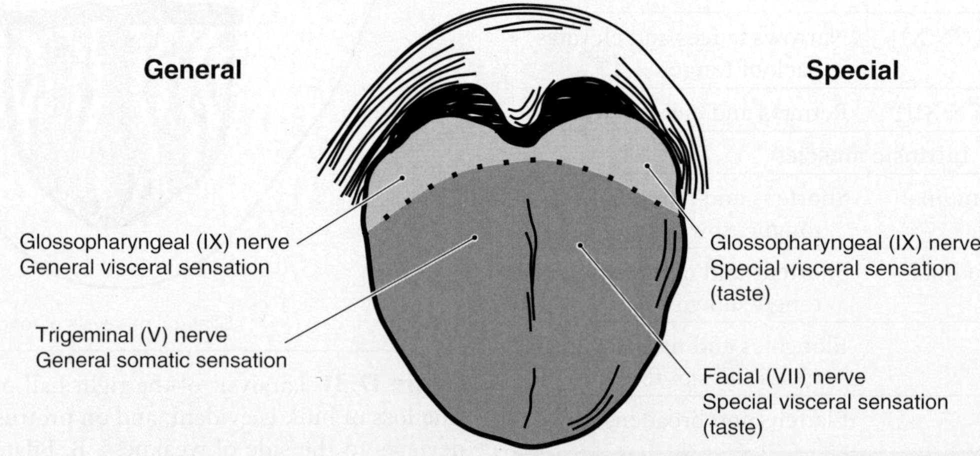

Figure 17-33 General and special sensory innervation of tongue.

Table 17-24

Sensory Innervation of the Tongue

Cranial Nerves (Number)	General Sensation (GSA)	General Visceral (GVA)	Taste Sensation (SVA)	Tongue Region
Lingual branch of trigeminal nerve (V)	+			Anterior two-thirds of tongue
Glossopharyngeal nerve (IX)			+	Taste buds in mucosa of posterior third of tongue
Chorda tympani of facial nerve (VII)			+	Taste buds in mucosa of anterior two-thirds of tongue
Glossopharyngeal nerve (IX)		+		Posterior third of tongue

GSA, general somatic afferent; *GVA*, general visceral afferent; *SVA*, special visceral afferent.

the nasopharynx to prevent the entrance of food during swallowing. It also regulates speech nasality. The circular constrictor (superior, middle, and inferior) muscles of the pharynx perform squeezing actions on the bolus, and vertical muscles (stylopharyngeus, palatopharyngeus, and salpingopharyngeus) elevate the larynx during swallowing. The motor innervation of the muscles of the soft palate and pharyngeal cavity is supplied by the pharyngeal branches of the vagus nerve (CN X), except for the tensor veli palatini (trigeminal [CN V]) and stylopharyngeus (glossopharyngeal [CN IX]) (Fig. 17-34).

Sensory Innervation of the Soft Palate and Pharynx

The glossopharyngeal nerve (CN IX) and vagus nerve (CN X) are responsible for general sensation from the pharynx, a visceral structure. The vagus alone carries the general sensation from the larynx, another visceral structure. However, a branch of the facial nerve (CN VII) complex (pterygopalatine nerve) mediates general sensation (GVA) and taste (SVA) from the nasopharynx and soft palate.

CLINICAL CORRELATES

Upper and Lower Motor Neuron Syndromes

Lesions involving the UMNs and LMNs affect the function of buccofacial muscles differently. Interruption in corticonuclear projections from the motor cortex to the cranial nerve motor nuclei on the opposite side results in UMN syndrome, which is characterized by a loss of discrete and delicate motor control, muscle weakness, and brisk reflexes, but has a milder effect on buccofacial muscles. This milder effect is related to a substantial number of collateral corticonuclear fibers that probably provide safety

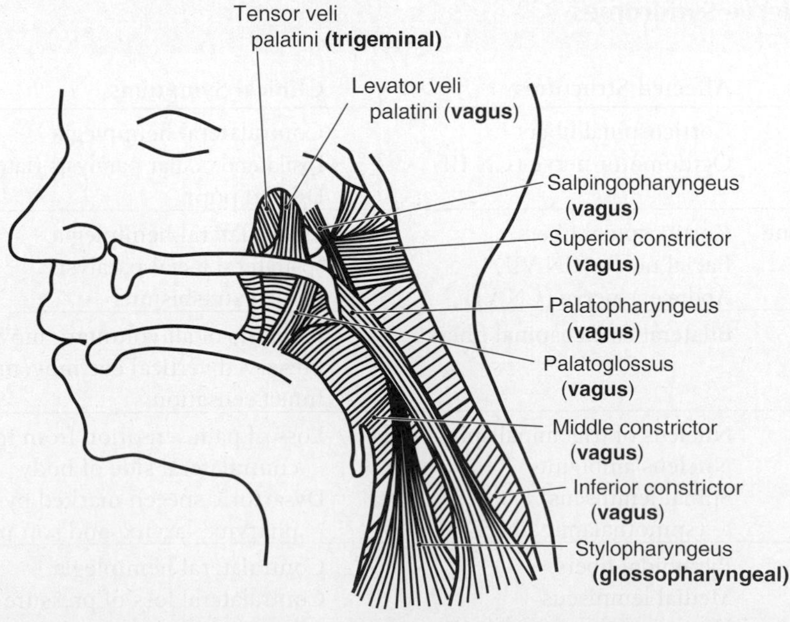

Figure 17-34 Nerve supply to the muscles of the soft palate and pharynx.

from damage for cranial nerve functions. The involvement of the corticonuclear fibers, after they have separated from the major pyramidal tract, does not result in any more than a minimal spasticity in cranial muscles.

Bilateral involvement of UMN (pseudobulbar palsy), which profoundly affects cranial muscle function and motor speech, is characterized by hypertonia and loss of discrete motor control, again with little or no spasticity in the cranial muscles.

LMN lesions affect the motor cranial nuclei (final common pathways) and their projections and produce the LMN symptoms, which include flaccid paralysis of the selected muscles alone, absent or reduced reflexes, muscular fibrillations and twitching, and muscle atrophy. The muscular twitching results from spontaneous firing of an α-LMN cell body or its axons, resulting in an entire motor unit firing at the same time. If the LMN cell body dies, the innervating terminals (neuromuscular junctions) degenerate, and fasciculation ceases. When deprived of efferent impulses (reflexive or voluntary) from the LMN cell body, the muscle fibers eventually atrophy and degenerate. LMN lesions greatly affect the functioning of the ipsilateral buccofacial, glossal, laryngeal, and neck muscles.

Key Terms :

Dejerine syndrome	**Wallenberg syndrome**
Locked-in syndrome	**Weber syndrome**
Millard-Gubler syndrome	

Common Cranial Nerve Syndromes

Cranial nerve nuclei are packed in a small area of the brainstem (Fig. 17-3; Table 17-25). Their compact location and close proximity to both crossed and uncrossed ascending and descending fibers makes them susceptible to even small brainstem lesions, vascular being the most common. Brainstem hemorrhagic lesions produce selected established neurologic syndromes: **Weber**, **Millard–Gubler**, **locked-in**, **medial medullary**, and **Wallenberg**. Most of these syndromes also involve the disorders of motor speech functions.

Weber Syndrome (Medial Midbrain Lesion)

Weber syndrome is associated with a ventral medial midbrain lesion that affects the oculomotor nerve (CN III) fibers along with descending corticospinal (pes peduncle) fibers (Fig. 17-35). Clinically, it is marked with contralateral hemiplegia (with the interruption of the descending motor fibers) and ipsilateral ocular paralysis (with the involvement of the oculomotor [CN III] nerve). With the paralysis of all the extraocular muscles except the lateral rectus (abducens [CN VI] nerve) and superior oblique (trochlear [CN IV] nerve), the patient displays ptosis (impaired ability to raise the upper eyelid), pupil dilation (parasympathetic CN III paralysis), and lateral deviation (strabismus) of the ipsilateral eye (secondary to the unopposed activity of the lateral rectus muscle).

Millard–Gubler Syndrome (Lower Pons Lesion)

In Millard–Gubler syndrome, a basal pontine lesion affects the facial nerve (CN VII) motor nucleus and the descending motor fibers (Fig. 17-36A). This lower medial pontine lesion results in alternating symptoms (see Chapter 16), which are marked by contralateral hemiplegia (secondary to interrupted corticospinal fibers) and

Table 17-25

Brainstem Cranial Nerve Syndromes

Syndrome	Affected Structures	Clinical Symptoms
Weber syndrome (midbrain lesion)	Corticospinal fibers Oculomotor nerve (CN III)	Contralateral hemiplegia Ipsilateral ocular paralysis (lateral strabismus) Dilated pupil
Millard-Gubler syndrome (lower pons lesion)	Corticospinal fibers Facial nerve (CN VII) Abducens nerve (CN VI)	Contralateral hemiplegia Ipsilateral facial paralysis Medial strasbismus
Locked-in syndrome (bilateral basal pons lesion)	Bilateral corticospinal fibers	Paralysis of all voluntary movements (quadriplegia) Preserved vertical eye movements Intact sensation
Wallenberg syndrome (lateral medullary lesion)	Nucleus of trigeminal spinal tract Nucleus ambiguus Spinal lemniscus (spinothalamic fibers)	Loss of pain sensation from ipsilateral face and contralateral side of body Dysarthric speech marked by paralysis of muscles of pharynx, larynx, and soft palate
Dejerine syndrome (medial medullary lesion)	Pyramidal fibers Medial lemniscus Hypoglossal nerve (CN XII)	Contralateral hemiplegia Contralateral loss of pressure and vibration (medial lemniscus) Dysarthria owing to ipsilateral lingual paralysis

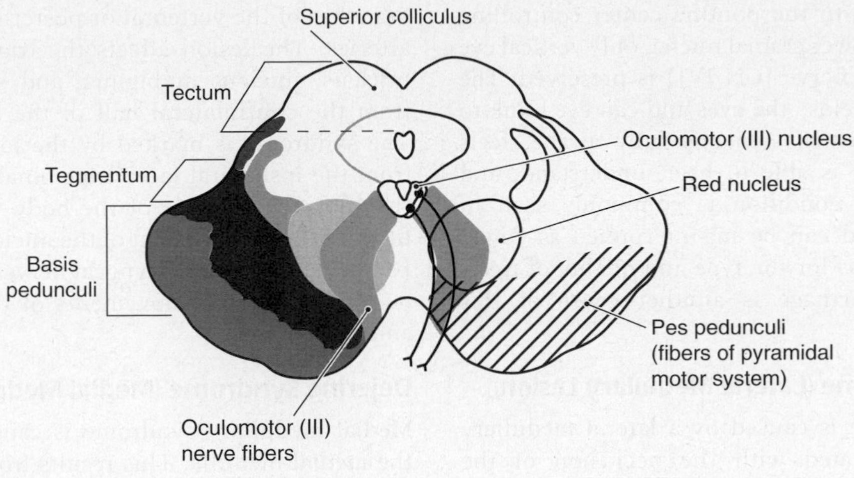

Figure 17-35 A lesion in the midbrain involving the descending corticospinal fibers and the oculomotor nerve.

ipsilateral facial paralysis due to the affection of the facial nucleus/nerve. If not spared, the abducens (CN VI) involvement would result in medial strabismus. The facial palsy affects motor speech. This syndrome is usually caused by the occlusion of the pontine branches of the basilar artery (see Figs. 7-1 and 7-2).

Locked-In Syndrome (Bilateral Basal Pons Lesion)

Locked-in syndrome is associated with a bilateral ventral pontine lesion, which interrupts all the descending corticospinal fibers (Fig. 17-36B). It is clinically characterized by quadriplegia (paralysis of all voluntary movements) and loss of all motor speech functions. With

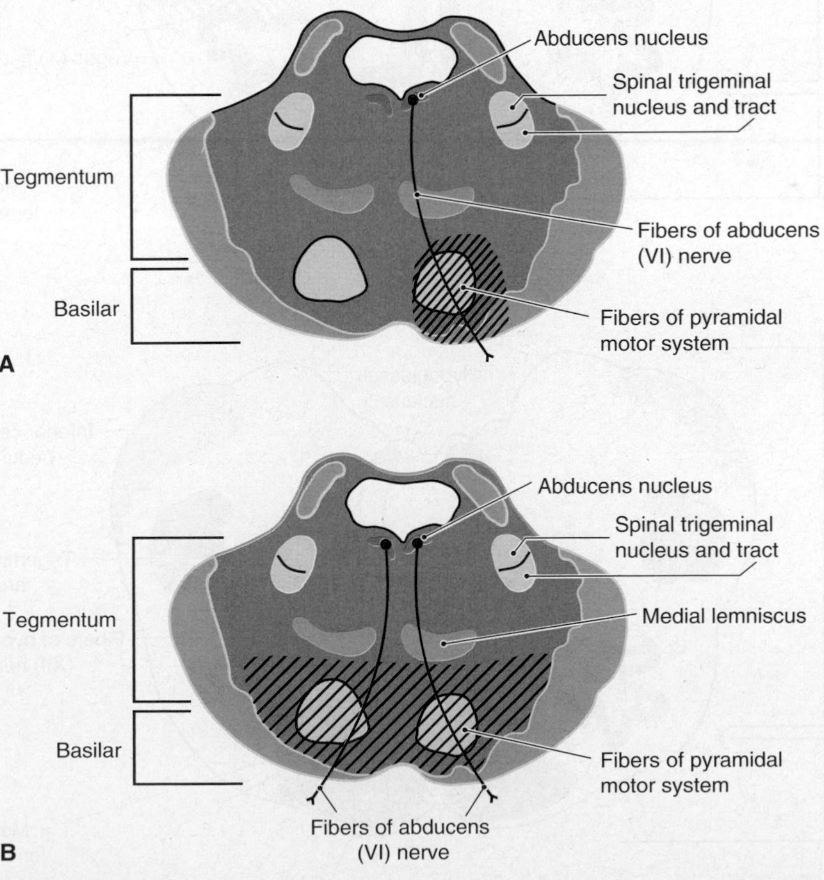

Figure 17-36 Pontine cranial nerve syndromes. A. A basal pontine lesion involving the descending corticospinal fibers and the abducens nerve fibers. B. A bilateral pontine lesion associated with locked-in syndrome.

interruption of fibers to the pontine center controlling horizontal gaze and lower cranial nuclei, only vertical eye movement (trochlear nerve [CN IV]) is preserved. The patient can open and close the eyes and can eye blink to communicate. The patient remains fully awake, feels somatosensation, and is able to hear, understand, and reason. This clinical condition is commonly seen in patients with TBI and can be misinterpreted as coma, which has implications for the type and quality of treatment. Pontine hemorrhage is another cause of this syndrome.

Wallenberg Syndrome (Lateral Medullary Lesion)

Wallenberg syndrome is caused by a lateral medullary lesion and is associated with the occlusion of the branches of the vertebral or posterior inferior cerebellar arteries. The lesion affects the trigeminal spinal tract/nucleus, nucleus ambiguus, and spinothalamic fibers from the contralateral half of the body (Fig. 17-37*A*). The syndrome is marked by the loss of pain sensation from the ipsilateral face (trigeminal nerve [CN V]) and the contralateral side of the body (spinothalamic tract fibers). The involvement of the nucleus ambiguus (vagus [CN X] and glossopharyngeal nerves [CN IX]) limits the motor and speech movements of the pharynx, larynx, and soft palate.

Dejerine Syndrome (Medial Medullary Lesion)

Medial medullary syndrome is caused by an infarct in the medial medulla. This results from a hemorrhagic or

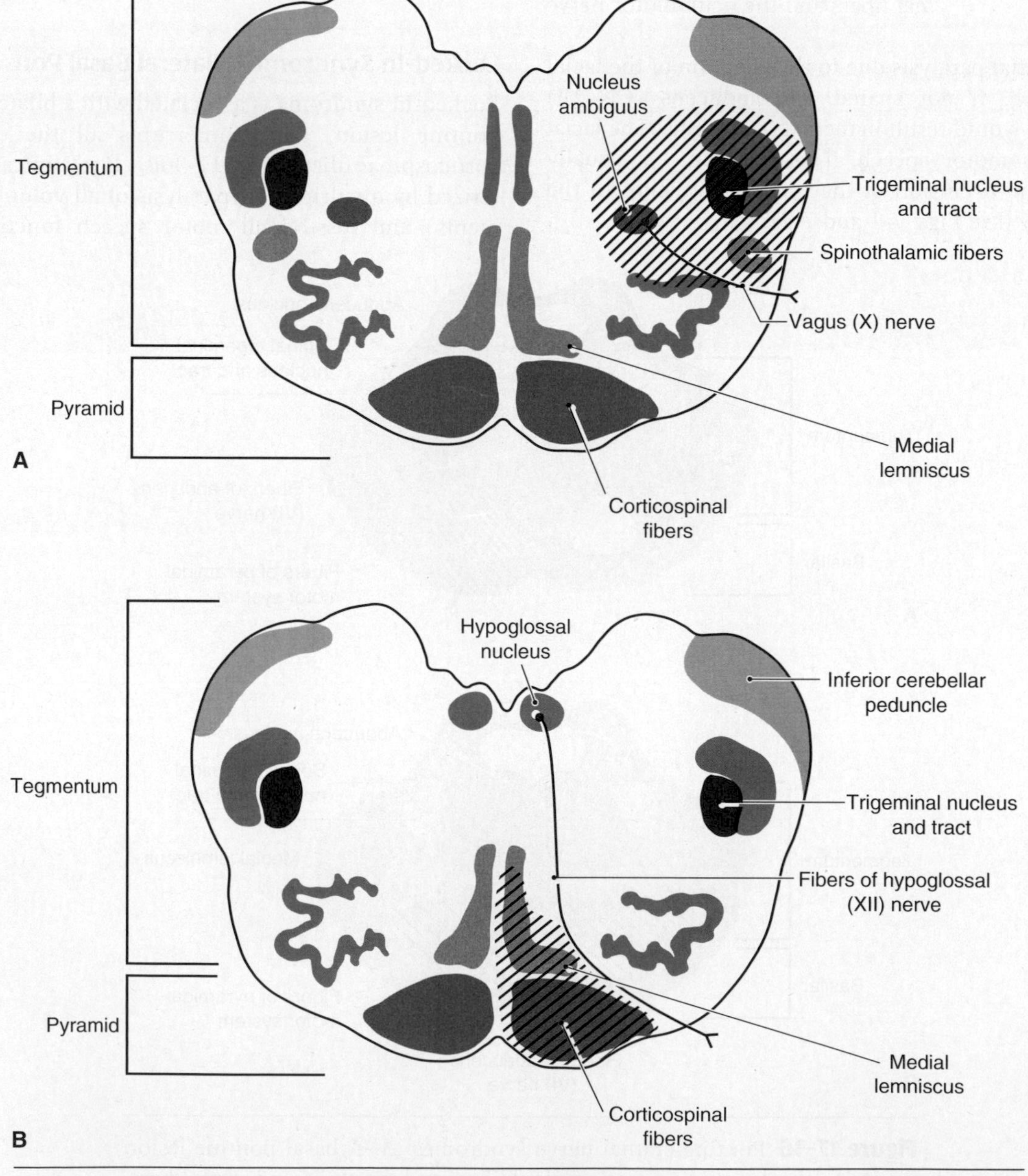

Figure 17-37 A. A lesion producing lateral medullary syndrome. B. A lesion producing medial medullary syndrome.

thrombotic involvement of the anterior spinal artery branches or the medullary branches of the vertebral artery. The lesion affects the descending pyramidal fibers, ascending sensory fibers in the medial lemniscus, and hypoglossal nerve (CN XII) fibers (Fig. 17-37*B*), and it causes contralateral loss of strength (hemiplegia with the involvement of the pyramidal tract fibers), contralateral loss of proprioception and vibration (with the involvement of the medial lemniscus), and ipsilateral lingual paralysis (involvement of the hypoglossal nerve). The lingual paralysis has significant speech-related implications.

CASE STUDIES FOR PROBLEM SOLVING

CASE ONE (17-1)

A 60-year-old man had several lacunar strokes bilaterally in the region of the internal capsule and basal ganglia, as demonstrated on MRI studies. The bilateral UMN lesions to the corticonuclear fibers affected multiple cranial nerves and caused sensorimotor dysfunctions in the extremities. Neurologic examination revealed the following abnormalities:

- Mild cognitive decline (impaired ability to learn new information and a short-term memory deficit)
- Stiff gait with slow, short steps
- Hyperactive muscle stretch reflexes and bilateral Babinski signs
- Impaired control of the facial muscles, with inability to show his teeth, pucker his lips, or wrinkle his forehead
- Difficulty controlling excessive laughter and sobbing
- Difficulty protruding the tongue
- Difficulty chewing and swallowing; food accumulating laterally in his mouth
- Failure of the soft palate to rise bilaterally on phonation

Question: Can you account for this clinical picture (loss of control for the muscles of facial expression, mastication, and deglutition) based on these multiple subcortical lesions? What cranial nerves were affected?

Case (17-1) Discussion: See discussion of case studies

CASE TWO (17-2)

A 63-year-old man had a stroke while sleeping and woke up in confusion and panic. He was taken to the emergency room where the examining physician noticed the following:

- Complete left-side facial paralysis
- Inability to move the left eye laterally (medial strabismus)
- Hearing loss in the left ear
- Absence of pain and touch sensation on the left side of the face
- Some weakness in jaw movement

A brain MRI study revealed an infarct in the left superior tegmentum of the pons that affected the lower motor neuron nuclei within the brainstem.

Question: How can you account for these cranial nerve–related sensorimotor symptoms on the left side and the absence of paralysis in the muscles of the extremities?

Case (17-2) Discussion: See discussion of case studies

CASE THREE (17-3)

A 35-year-old SLP on her day off decided to shadow her neurologist father, who examined a 45-year-old man with complaint of a pain from the neck and difficulty in both raising his arm and turning his head. As the neurologist continued with his exam, the SLP also noted the following important signs:

- Lowered right side of the palate
- Absence of gag reflex
- Presence of coughing reflex after fluid intake
- Weak phonation, diplophonia, and breathy voice
- Nasal speech
- Absence of soft palate elevation on the right during the sustained phonation of "ah"
- Some nasal regurgitation of fluid

On her father's request, the SLP performed a quick language assessment and found that language and cognitive functions were nearly intact.

The patient's MRI revealed a tumor at the base of the brain that appeared to be in the vicinity of the jugular foramen.

Question: The neurologist father asked the SLP daughter to explain how this localized tumor cold cause these speech and swallowing problems and what cranial nerves are affected by the tumor?

Case (17-3) discussion: See discussion of case studies

(Continued)

CASE FOUR (17-4) *(CONTINUED)*

A 60-year-old priest was taken to the emergency room for sensorimotor problems that developed abruptly while speaking to the members of his church during a Sunday mass. The attending physician noted the following:

- Dysarthric speech
- Lowered left side of the palate
- Dysphagia
- Sensation loss on the left side of the face
- Difficulty balancing, with falling to the left
- Left-sided facial paralysis
- Weakness in the right leg and arm

An informal SLP consultation revealed only 55% speech intelligibility. The speech was marked with imprecise articulation, hypernasality, and breathiness.

A brain MRI study revealed an infarct in the left caudal lateral ventral pons and medulla.

Question: How can you explain these symptoms of the left face, speech unintelligibility, and the paralysis of the right half of the body?

Case (17-4) Discussion: See discussion of case studies

CASE FIVE (17-5)

A 39-year-old woman suffered a stroke while sleeping. When she woke, she was unable to speak and control her right limbs (arm and leg). She was taken to the emergency room where the examining neurologist noted the following:

- Adducted (drawn toward the median plane) left eye with inability to move it laterally
- Paralysis of the left face with drooling from the left of mouth
- Slowly uttered unintelligible speech
- Weakened tongue deviating to the left
- Loss of pain sensation on the entire left face
- Profoundly impaired hearing in the right ear
- Right hemiplegia
- Loss of pain and temperature on right half of the body

A speech–language pathologist consultation revealed:

- Poorly articulated speech which was judged to be only 60% intelligible
- Slurred articulation, imprecise consonants, phonemic omissions, and vowel prolongations
- Breathy voice
- Swallowing difficulty on food of all consistencies
- No sign of aphasia or cognitive impairment

An MRI study revealed a large infarct in the right rostral medulla.

Question: How can you explain the symptoms in relation to the right medullary lesion?

Case (17-5) Discussion: See discussion of case studies

CASE SIX (17-6)

A 39-year-old woman suffered a stroke while sleeping. When she woke, she was unable to speak and control her right limbs (arm and leg). She was taken to the emergency room where the examining neurologist noted the following:

- Adducted (drawn toward the median plane) left eye with inability to move it laterally
- Paralysis of the left face with drooling from the left of mouth
- Slowly uttered unintelligible speech
- Weakened tongue deviating to the left
- Loss of pain sensation on the entire left face
- Profoundly impaired hearing in the right ear
- Right hemiplegia
- Loss of pain and temperature on right half of the body

A speech–language pathologist consultation revealed:

- Poorly articulated speech which was judged to be only 60% intelligible
- Slurred articulation, imprecise consonants, phonemic omissions, and vowel prolongations
- Breathy voice
- Swallowing difficulty on food of all consistencies
- No sign of aphasia or cognitive impairment

An MRI study revealed a large infarct in the right rostral medulla.

Question: How can you explain the symptoms in relation to the right medullary lesion?

Case (17-5) Discussion: See discussion of case studies

(Continued)

CASE SEVEN (17-7) *(CONTINUED)*

A 55-year-old speech-language pathologist professor woke up in the middle of the night to use the bathroom. Before returning to bed, she glanced in the mirror on the door and was shocked to see a profound asymmetry in her face. She first thought that her husband had played a trick by placing a "fun house" mirror in the bathroom but then noted that it was the same old mirror. Since she did not have any sensorimotor symptoms in hands or legs and was thinking clearly, she herself drove to the emergency room, where the attending physician noted the following:

- The mouth on right was lower with dripping saliva
- No motor control on her entire right face
- Inability to close her right eye
- Speech was slow, slurred, and quite unintelligible
- No sign of aphasia or amnesia
- No hemiplegia or hemianesthesia

A CT study revealed no vascular abnormality.

Question: How can you explain these selected facial symptoms?

Case (17-7) Discussion: See discussion of case studies

CASE EIGHT (17-8)

A 52-year-old communicatively impaired woman, diagnosed with a brainstem (medullary) stroke, was seen by a consulting SLP who noted the following:

- Moderately unintelligible speech marked with slurred articulation, articulatory breakdown, hypernasality, impaired phonation, and intermittent breathiness
- Inability to protrude the tongue
- Difficulty with swallowing and food aspiration
- No other sensorimotor impairment
- No sign of language or cognitive disorder

The attending SLP suspected the involvement of selected cranial nerves.

Question: How can you explain these symptoms and relate them to a brainstem stroke?

Case (17-8) Discussion: See discussion of case studies

CASE NINE (17-9)

A 60-year-old man developed gradually worsening ringing and decreased hearing in his left ear. He began to hold the telephone to his right ear instead of the left. Shortly before consulting his physician, he began to walk with a stiffly extended right leg, tending to scrape the toe of the right foot. He was also somewhat clumsy with his right hand. Examination by the physician revealed the following signs:

- Mild right-sided weakness of the hand and lower limb
- Increased muscle stretch reflexes (deep tendon reflexes) and Babinski sign on the right
- Tendency to stagger and fall to the left while walking (a sign of cerebellar or vestibular injury)****
- Decreased sensitivity to temperature and pinprick on the left side of the face
- Normal light touch sensation
- Absence of left corneal reflex
- Mild left-sided weakness when wrinkling his forehead, forcibly closing his eye, and retracting the corner of his mouth
- Loss of hearing in the left ear, with lateralization of the tuning fork to the right ear on the Weber test and severely diminished air–bone conduction on the left

A brain MRI study revealed an egg-shaped mass in the left cerebellopontine angle that was expanding the internal auditory meatus of the temporal bone, compressing the left cerebellar hemisphere from below, and indenting the pons and upper medulla on the left side.

Question: Can you account for the cranial nerve symptoms? How can a tumor mass at the cerebellopontine account for the spastic (UMN) weakness of the right side of the body (the side opposite the lesion) and the tendency to fall to the left side (ipsilateral to the lesion)? How does cranial nerve injury explain the sensory findings on the face and facial weakness? Does the hearing loss indicate disease of the middle ear or of the stato-acoustic vestibulocochlear (CN VIII) nerve? If it is nerve injury, would you expect any other abnormality of function of the vestibulocochlear nerve?

Case (17-9) Discussion: See discussion of case studies

SUMMARY

The human cranial nerves are the result of evolutionary modifications to a basic vertebrate pattern of CNS organization, constructed of approximately 40 bilaterally symmetrical repeating segments. During development, the first two nerves (olfactory [CN I] and optic [CN II]) became elaborated as the forebrain and involve the thalamus before reaching the cortex. The remaining 10 cranial nerves originate from the brainstem and innervate the muscles of the head, neck, face, larynx, tongue, and pharynx. These muscles serve speech, resonance, swallowing, facial expression, chewing, and phonation. Besides serving special senses such as vision, audition, smell, and taste, the cranial nerves regulate autonomic secretive functions of glands in the oral, nasal, and orbital cavities.

Some cranial nerves mediate only sensation, whereas others exclusively serve motor functions. Some cranial nerves serve only a single functional component, whereas others contain fibers to serve two or more functional components. Several motor cranial nuclei receive corticonuclear projections from both sides of the motor cortex. This bilaterality of projection has important clinical implications for the motor speech processes.

REVIEW QUESTIONS

1. Complete the following statements using the appropriate technical terms:

A. A lesion that interrupts olfactory fibers causes ________, in which the ability to ________ is partly or fully impaired.

B. ________ is an optical condition in which an object is seen as being two.

C. In ________ the internal and/or external ocular muscles are paralyzed.

D. Bilateral involvement of the corticonuclear fibers results in ________ ________.

E. Denervated muscles become hypotonic and paralyzed, which eventually ________.

F. ________ ________ refers to the paralysis of the face subsequent to a unilateral involvement of the facial nerve or nucleus.

G. In ________ ________, the pupils react to light by constricting, whereas in ________ reflex, the lens undergoes refractive changes in order to keep a moving object in focus.

H. In ________, one experiences pain sensation along the course of the nerve.

I. The ________ ________ causes severe motor speech disorder because it has an impact on both the unilaterally and/or bilaterally innervated speech muscles.

J. Often confused with coma, the patients with ________ ________ are quadriplegic and can only communicate using the preserved vertical eye movement.

K. Often caused by the virus-induced dysfunctioning of the VII cranial nerve, ________ ________ results in paralysis involving one-half of the face.

L. ________ results in selected double vision subsequent to errors in improperly focused visual axes in misaligned eyes.

2. Match each of the following classification types with its associated function:

A. GSA — a. pain and temperature
B. GSE — b. vision and audition
C. SSA — c. eye movements
D. SVA — d. speech, phonation, and swallowing
E. SVE/BE — e. taste and smell
F. GVA — f. organ content
G. GVE — g. autonomic activities

3. Match each of the following branchial arches with its associated motor cranial nerve:

A. first — a. glossopharyngeal nerve
B. second — b. vagus nerve
C. third — c. facial nerve
D. fourth and sixth — d. trigeminal nerve

4. A 45-year-old woman experiences decreased hearing in the right ear, the entire right side of her face is paralyzed, and she has no reflex to touch in the cornea of the right eye. What cranial nerves are suspected to be damaged?

5. Clinical symptoms displayed by a stroke patient included left ptosis, pupil unresponsiveness to light with dilated left pupil, and laterally deviated left eye. Name the cranial nerve that is involved in this case.

6. Which cranial nerve is involved in tic douloureux?

7. What cranial nerve is involved with Bell palsy?

8. Why is pseudobulbar palsy so detrimental to speech and other facial functions?

9. What cranial nerves provide the afferent and efferent paths for the pupillary light reflex?

10. A lesion at what neuraxial region might produce right facial symptoms and left hemiplegia?
11. What communication mode can be used with a patient who has locked-in syndrome?
12. Involvement of what primary cranial nerve is associated with abnormal phonation, resonance, and dysphagia?
13. In case of left hypoglossal nerve dysfunction, the weakened half of the tongue will deviate to which side on protrusion?
14. A left lower motor neuron lesion involving the vagus and trigeminal nerves lowers the ipsilateral palate. Will this result in the deviation of the uvula toward the right (normal) or the left (paralyzed) side of the palate?
15. How many cranial nerves are involved with ocular movements?

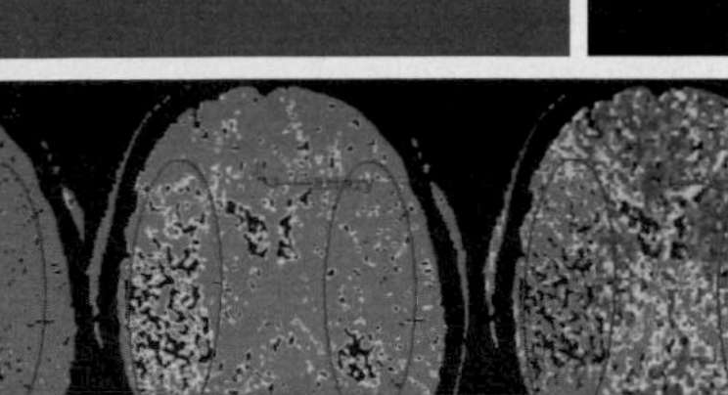

18 Axial–Limbic Brain: Autonomic Nervous System, Limbic System, Hypothalamus, and Reticular Formation

LEARNING OBJECTIVES

After studying this chapter, students should be able to:

- Describe the structural and functional organization of the autonomic nervous system
- Discuss the opposing functions of the sympathetic and parasympathetic systems
- Explain the central neural mechanism that controls the autonomic nervous system
- Describe the anatomic and functional organization of the limbic system
- Discuss the functions of the cingulate gyrus, amygdala, septum, and hippocampus
- Describe the anatomic and functional organization of the hypothalamus
- Discuss the autonomic and endocrinic functions of the hypothalamus
- Outline the functions of common hormones
- Explain the anatomic organization of the reticular formation
- Discuss the functions of the reticular formation, including cortical arousal, attention, swallowing, and respiration

The autonomic nervous system (ANS), limbic lobe, hypothalamus, and reticular formation (RF) are functionally and anatomically integrated and are identified as the limbic–axial brain. As early-developing parts of the brain, these structures control basic physiologic functions and behaviors at the unconscious level. Together, the four components of the limbic–axial brain control all visceral and somatic activities vital to sustaining body functions.

The ANS regulates the functions of the heart, lungs, and blood vessels as well as the organs of the digestive, reproductive, and urogenital systems. As a transitional structure, the limbic lobe (central unit of the limbic system) connects the thinking (neocortical) brain to the nonthinking and older (subcortical) axial brain. It regulates drives, moods, motivation, and visceral activities that relate to the emotional aspects of sensorimotor behaviors and learning. The hypothalamus, a visceral–somatic and metabolic control system, which is also functionally related to the limbic system, controls activity of the ANS and regulates instinctual behaviors including copulation, defecation, urination, alimentation, and aggression. In addition, the hypothalamus contains selective centers that control respiration, blood pressure, pulse rate, temperature, electrolyte balance, fluid balance, food intake, metabolism, diurnal (repeating daily) rhythms, and endocrine production. Furthermore, the hypothalamus contributes to the internal emotional state of well-being and pleasure. The brainstem RF influences brain activity by regulating the alerting mechanism. As the integrator of the sensory and motor mechanisms, the RF participates in the generation of well-coordinated motor functions, such as speech, eye–body coordinated movements, swallowing, and respiration. It also participates in regulating blood pressure rate, respiration, cortical arousal, and sleep and awake states.

All four components of the limbic–axial brain are connected by a system of complex fiber bundles. Though not central to language and speech, their collective influence on higher mental functions is through their regulation of brain homeostasis. In order to expose students to the functional organization of the axial brain, only the basic functions and physiology of these related systems are discussed.

Key Terms :

Celiac
Craniosacral system
Enteric system
Gray communicating ramus
Inferior cervical
Middle cervical
Paravertebral ganglia
Piloerector
Prevertebral ganglia
Superior cervical
Superior mesenteric
Thoracolumbar system
White communicating ramus

AUTONOMIC NERVOUS SYSTEM

The ANS involuntarily regulates visceral body functions by controlling the cardiac muscles, smooth muscles, and glands. This brings together all vital body functions, including the cardiovascular, pulmonary, digestive, urinary, and reproductive systems, maintaining body homeostasis. The ANS is integrated tightly with automatic and volitional sensorimotor behaviors.

The ANS is composed of the sympathetic and parasympathetic systems (Table 18-1; Box 18-1). The sympathetic system mobilizes the vital organs for discharging energy, as in cases of danger, whereas the parasympathetic system is responsible for the restitution of metabolic energy, and thus promotes relaxation and growth. Most of the smooth muscles, glands, and cardiac muscles are under the influence of both divisions. Each system renders its influence, which is often antagonistic (opposite) to the effects of the other system (Table 18-2). Exceptions are the **piloerector** (erection of hair) **muscles** and **sweat glands**, which are regulated solely by the sympathetic system with no innervation from the parasympathetic system. Parasympathetic projections, which selectively innervate the gastrointestinal system, are also grouped under the **enteric system**.

Anatomic Organization

Unlike **somatic motor system impulses**, efferents of the ANS do not directly innervate the visceral organs. Instead, the ANS efferents travel to the target structures via the secondary (peripheral) ganglia, which are located in the peripheral nervous system (PNS). Thus, the efferents of the ANS are made of two neurons in tandem (Fig. 18-1). The cell body of the first neuron for each system is within the central neuraxis (brainstem and spinal cord) and is called the **preganglionic autonomic neuron**. Traveling from the cell body, preganglionic fibers project to a peripheral ganglion, the postganglionic autonomic neuron. Postganglionic fibers regulate the activity of the specific visceral organs and glands. The postganglionic neuron of the sympathetic system is located bilaterally along the spinal cord, whereas that of the parasympathetic system is near the target organ (Box 18-2).

Visceral Efferent System

The ANS is largely a motor system, although it also has a sensory component in which afferent fibers carry sensory information from the visceral structures to the central nervous system (CNS). Its motor fibers project neural impulses to the visceral organs through the sympathetic and parasympathetic channels of the ANS (Table 18-1). These two systems must work together to maintain optimal functioning of the visceral structures, such as the smooth muscles, glands (lacrimal, salivary, and sweat), cardiac muscles, blood vessels, and gastrointestinal system (Table 18-2). The location of the postganglionic cells is different for the two systems. The postganglionic cells are closer to the spinal column in the sympathetic system, whereas the postganglionic cells are farther from the neuraxis and closer to or within the target organs in the parasympathetic system (Box 18-2).

Sympathetic System

The sympathetic nervous system is also called the thoracolumbar system because the preganglionic cell bodies are located in the **intermediate–lateral** gray matter between the sensory and motor columns in the thoracic and upper lumbar segments of the spinal cord (Fig. 18-2). These cell bodies give rise to preganglionic efferent fibers. Efferent fibers of the preganglionic cells leave through the ventral spinal roots of the thoracic and lumbar segments and travel through the **white communicating ramus** of each spinal nerve (Fig. 18-3). They are white because most of the fibers are myelinated. These fibers terminate on the postganglionic neurons in the sympathetic chain or on other postganglionic sympathetic neurons in the abdomen around the aorta. The postganglionic neurons in the sympathetic chain are also known as the **paravertebral ganglia** and the postganglionic sympathetic neurons close to the large abdominal arteries are called **prevertebral ganglia**. The prevertebral ganglia surround the visceral branches of the aorta and include the **celiac**, **superior mesenteric**, and **inferior mesenteric ganglia** (Fig. 18-2). The sympathetic ganglionic chain extends from the base of the skull to the coccyx along the anterolateral area of the vertebral column.

The cervical portion of the sympathetic trunk contains three specific ganglia that are formed by a fusion of the original eight segmental ganglia: **superior**, **middle**,

Table 18-1

Sympathetic and Parasympathetic Systems

Structure	Sympathetic	Parasympathetic
General function	Expenditure of metabolic energy	Restoration of metabolic energy
Preganglionic cells	Thoracic and lumbar cord	Brainstem and sacral segments of cord
Postganglionic cells	Sympathetic chain; near vertebral column	Near target organs
Distribution	Scattered throughout body; projections render widespread influence on multiple visceral organs	Localized projections activate specific effectors

BOX 18-1

Divisions of the Autonomic Nervous System

The autonomic nervous system (ANS) consists of two divisions: sympathetic and parasympathetic. The sympathetic system mobilizes the vital organs for discharging energy, as in cases of danger, whereas the parasympathetic system is responsible for the restitution of metabolic energy and thus promotes relaxation and growth. The enteric nervous system, a subdivision of the parasympathetic system, controls gastrointestinal functions. Some anatomists consider the enteric system to be a separate division of the ANS, which regulates visceral organ functions such as digestion, intestinal motility, and bladder emptying.

The functions of the sympathetic and parasympathetic systems can be understood best by examining a common anxiety causing life experience and reviewing the reactive bodily changes associated with each division. Think about a mother driving during rush hour on an icy road with poor visibility who is getting late to pick her son up from the day care that closes in 15 minutes. Her car slides into other lane but with her presence of mind manages to avoid a head-on collision but is shaken up. The possibility of a near-fatal accident will trigger anxiety and bodily responses marked with rapid heartbeats, dilated pupils, pale skin (because of decreased blood circulation), and profuse perspiration. These visceral responses that represent body energy expenditures were regulated by the sympathetic division of the ANS.

Later, after she is safely home, the woman's internal system is no longer agitated. The anxiety-causing environmental stimuli are no longer present, and she feels relaxed. Her heartbeat and body temperature return to normal levels, pupils are no longer dilated, and blood circulation to the skin and visceral organs is restored. This visceral reaction is regulated by the parasympathetic division of the ANS.

Table 18-2

Differential Effects of the Sympathetic and Parasympathetic Systems on Glands and Muscles

Structure	Sympathetic System	Parasympathetic System
Glands		
Nasal	Decreased secretion	Increased secretion
Lacrimal	Decreased secretion	Increased secretion
Intestinal	Decreased secretion	Increased secretion
Gastric	Decreased secretion	Increased secretion
Sweat	Increased secretion	No known effect
Smooth muscles		
Iris	Pupil dilation	Pupil constriction
Ciliary	Relaxation for far vision	Contraction for near vision
Urinary bladder	Relaxation	Contraction
Anal sphincter	Constriction	Dilation
Digestive tract	Reduced activity	Increased activity
Bronchi	Dilation	Constriction
Lungs	Vasodilation	Vasoconstriction
Skin	Sweating and piloerection	None
Cardiac muscles	Increased rate and force of heartbeat; vasodilation	Decreased activity; vasoconstriction
Blood vessels	Vasoconstriction in viscera and skin; vasodilation in skeletal muscle and heart	None
Genitals	Vasoconstriction	Vasodilation

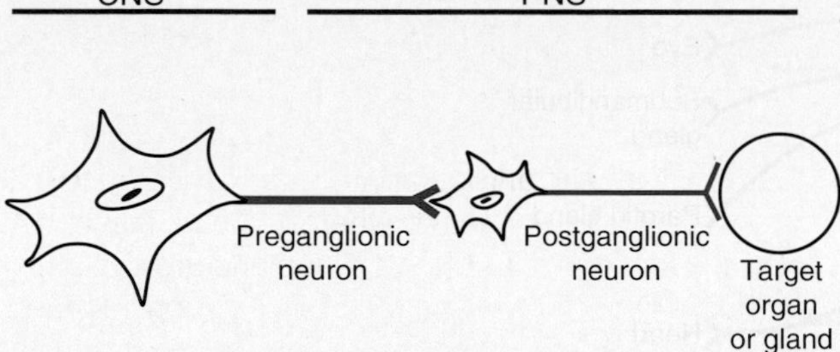

Figure 18-1 Two-neuron organization of the peripheral nervous system (PNS): preganglionic and postganglionic. CNS, central nervous system.

and **inferior cervical** (Fig. 18-2). The cervical sympathetic ganglia innervate the smooth muscles and glands in the head and upper limbs. Postganglionic fibers from the 11 thoracic ganglia innervate the heart, lungs, and thoracic and abdominal viscera. Postganglionic fibers from the lumbar ganglia are distributed via the spinal nerves and innervate the upper abdominal viscera, intestines, bladder, and genitals. Some of the unmyelinated sympathetic postganglionic fibers rejoin the spinal nerves via the **gray communicating ramus** (Fig. 18-3). They travel with the spinal nerves but separate from them before innervating blood vessels, smooth muscles, and sweat glands.

The sympathetic system, which mobilizes metabolic energy for expenditure, plays an important role in stressful situations in which a person's heart rate accelerates, arterial pressure rises, blood sugar level increases, and blood flow diverts from the visceral structures to the skeletal muscles (Tables 18-2 and 18-3).

BOX 18-2

Locations of the Peripheral Sympathetic and Parasympathetic Ganglia

The location of the peripheral ganglia differs in the two divisions of the autonomic nervous system. With short preganglionic and long postganglionic fibers, the sympathetic ganglion is located near the neuraxis. With long preganglionic and short postganglionic fibers, the parasympathetic ganglion is located closer to or within the innervated organ. These autonomic ganglia contain internuncial neurons that enhance the differential reflex functions. The ganglia also include large numbers of "postganglionic" neurons that spread the autonomic reflex functions to all parts of the body and to the blood vessels of the central nervous system via unmyelinated axons.

Parasympathetic System

The parasympathetic system restores the spent metabolic energy. This system is also known as the **craniosacral system** because the cell bodies giving rise to preganglionic fibers are in the brainstem and sacral region of the spinal cord. The parasympathetic efferent fibers innervate the visceral structures in the head, neck, thorax, much of the abdominal cavity, and pelvic organs (Fig. 18-4; Table 18-4). The cranial section of the parasympathetic system includes the following four cranial nerves (CNs): oculomotor (CN III), facial (CN VII), glossopharyngeal (CN IX), and vagus (CN X). The Edinger–Westphal nucleus, the visceral component of the oculomotor complex in the midbrain (see Chapter 17), sends preganglionic fibers to the postganglionic neurons in the ciliary ganglion. The postganglionic fibers from the ciliary ganglion innervate the sphincter of the iris and smooth muscle of the ciliary body. The facial preganglionic parasympathetic fibers supply the pterygopalatine and submandibular ganglia; the postganglionic fibers innervate the lacrimal glands and their blood vessels as well as the mucous membrane glands. Postganglionic fibers of the facial cranial nerve (CN VII) also innervate the submandibular and sublingual salivary glands and the mucous membranes in the floor of the mouth. Postganglionic fibers from the **otic** ganglion of the glossopharyngeal nerve activate the parotid gland.

The largest source of preganglionic parasympathetic fibers is from the vagus nerve (CN X), which supplies practically all of the thoracic and abdominal viscera except for the pelvis. The vagus nerve (CN X) supplies the parasympathetic ganglia in the heart, bronchial musculature, stomach, large and small intestines, liver, pancreas, and kidneys. In the intestinal system, short postganglionic fibers terminate in the smooth muscle and glands and serve motor and secretory functions. The sacral parasympathetic postganglionic fibers supply the urinary bladder, colon, rectum, accessory reproductive organs, and intestinal viscera that is not innervated by the vagus nerve (CN X).

The parasympathetic system dominates during periods of relaxation because it reduces the activity of various organs and conserves metabolic energy. Common parasympathetic activities include decreasing heart rate, lowering blood pressure, constricting pupils, and increasing digestion.

Visceral Afferent System

Sensory fibers from the thoracic, abdominal, and pelvic viscera travel through sympathetic nerves, ultimately reaching the sympathetic chain. They enter the T1–L2 region of the cord via the white communicating rami.

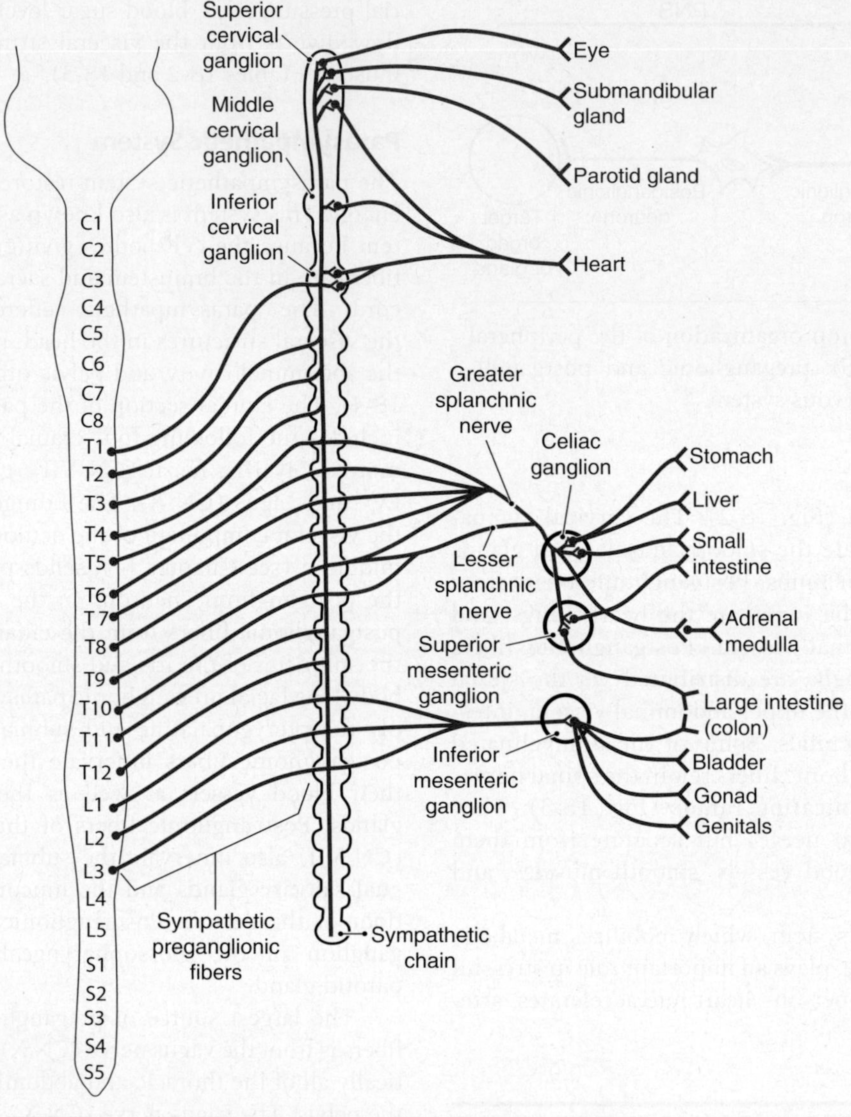

Figure 18-2 The sympathetic autonomic nervous system.

From there they ascend into the dorsal lemniscus and anterolateral systems. The visceral afferent fibers of the vagus nerve (CN X), which has cell bodies in the inferior (nodose) ganglion, are distributed peripherally in the heart, lungs, and other viscera. Fibers from the bladder, rectum, and accessory genital organs travel through the splanchnic nerves and enter the spinal cord through the S2–S4 nerves.

Afferent visceral fibers are important for visceral and viscerosomatic reflexes mediated through the spinal cord, brainstem, and hypothalamus. For example, sacral visceral afferents from stretch receptors of the urinary bladder control the bladder reflex and sensations that occur with bladder distension. The nucleus of the solitary tract in the medulla receives stimuli from the walls of the digestive tract, respiratory tract, and heart as well as its vascular trunks. These projections mediate respiratory and cardiovascular reflexes regulated by the medulla and hypothalamus.

Most autonomic sensory reactions remain subconscious but cause visceral pain, distress, nausea, hunger, and other less well-localized visceral sensations. A constant stream of visceral impulses allows for the general feeling of either internal well-being or malaise. Almost all visceral abdominal pain is projected in the sympathetic system. Intense visceral pain from internal organs is often felt on the skin in an area supplied by the somatic fibers arising from the same cord segment; this is known as referred pain (see Chapter 11).

Neurotransmitters

Acetylcholine is the main neurotransmitter for the preganglionic and postganglionic fibers of the parasympathetic system and the preganglionic fibers of the sympathetic

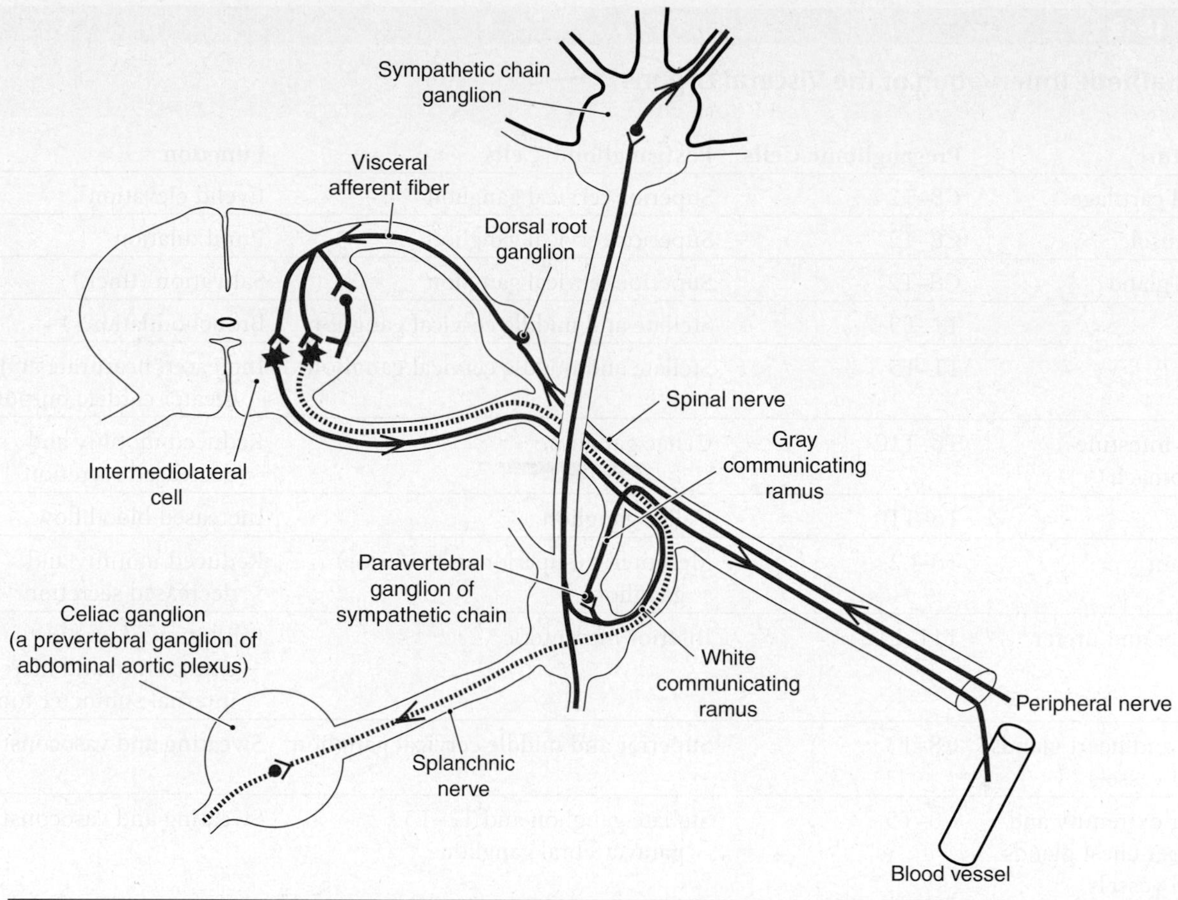

Figure 18-3 The sympathetic reflex arc.

system. The postganglionic sympathetic nerves secrete norepinephrine as a transmitter (Table 18-5).

Central Autonomic Pathways

The hypothalamus centrally controls the ANS. The hypothalamic regulation of the ANS is mediated in part by a series of synaptic relays from the neocortex, limbic system, diencephalon, brainstem, and spinal cord. Activation of the anterior hypothalamus stimulates the parasympathetic system, whereas activation of the posterolateral hypothalamus stimulates the sympathetic system. Hypothalamic impulses are transmitted to the midbrain via a descending component of the **medial forebrain bundle**, the **mamillotegmental tract**, and through other descending projections. Continuing from the midbrain, hypothalamic impulses are relayed caudally through synaptic relays in the brainstem RF, which in turn conveys the impulses to visceral motor nuclei of the brainstem and spinal cord.

Clinical Correlates

Interruptions of the autonomic regulation of visceral functions are characterized by impaired control of blood pressure, respiration, cardiovascular activity, gland secretion, sexual activity, bladder incontinence, and urinary retention. In the case of disturbance in the sympathetic system, unopposed parasympathetic control of visceral structures results in symptoms indicating the restoration of metabolic energy in activities, such as decreased heart rate, lowered blood pressure, constriction of the pupils, and increased digestion. The reverse is true in cases of parasympathetic disturbance, in which unopposed activity of the sympathetic system results in expenditure of metabolic energy (e.g., acceleration of the heart rate, elevation of arterial pressure, and increased blood flow to the skeletal muscles) (Tables 18-3 and 18-4).

Summary of the Autonomic Nervous System

The ANS regulates visceral functions and maintains homeostasis by regulating vital body systems, including the cardiovascular, pulmonary, digestive, urinary, and reproductive systems. The ANS uses its sympathetic and parasympathetic systems—functionally antagonistic components—to render opposite effects on the activities of visceral organs. For instance, sympathetic neurons expand metabolic energy by dilating the pupils, accelerating the heartbeat, inhibiting intestinal movements, and contracting the rectal sphincters. Conversely, the parasympathetic

Table 18-3

Sympathetic Innervation of the Visceral Organs

Structure	Preganglionic Cells	Postganglionic Cells	Function
Eyelid cartilage	C8–T2	Superior cervical ganglion	Eyelid elevation
Iris muscle	C8–T2	Superior cervical ganglion	Pupil dilation
Saliva gland	C8–T2	Superior cervical ganglion	Salivation (thick)
Lungs	T1–T5	Stellate and middle cervical ganglion	Bronchodilation
Heart	T1–T5	Stellate and middle cervical ganglion	Increased heart rate and greater cardiac output
Small intestine (stomach)	T6–T10	Celiac ganglion	Reduced motility and decreased secretion
Liver	T6–T10	Celiac ganglion	Increased blood flow
Column	T8–L2	Mesenteric (superior and inferior) ganglion	Reduced motility and decreased secretion
Bladder and ureter	T11–L12	Inferior mesenteric	Inhibition of ureter contraction and increased internal sphincter tone
Neck and heart glands and vessels	C8–T3	Superior and middle cervical ganglion	Sweating and vasoconstriction
Upper extremity and upper chest glands and vessels	C8–T5	Stellate ganglion and T2–T5 paravertebral ganglion	Sweating and vasoconstriction
Lower chest and abdominal glands and vessels	T6–L2	T6–L2 paravertebral ganglion	Sweating and vasoconstriction
Lower extremity gland and vessels	T10–L2	L1–S4 paravertebral ganglion	Sweating and vasoconstriction

neurons constrict the pupils, slow the heart, increase peristaltic movement, and relax the sphincters. The parasympathetic system is concerned with **anabolic** activities, such as the restoration and conservation of energy. The sacral parasympathetics activate the excretion of intestinal and urinary wastes.

LIMBIC SYSTEM

The limbic system regulates emotion, motivation, learning, and memory. Limbic projections to the forebrain contribute to emotions and provide motivation for behaviors that are fundamental to survival (feeding, mating, aggression, and flight). With connections to the prefrontal lobe and hippocampus, the limbic structures also participate in memory and learning. Most understanding of limbic behaviors and their impairments, such as **Klüver–Bucy syndrome**, is based primarily on animal experiments. Humans with dementias, carbon monoxide poisoning, and temporal lobe seizures may exhibit similar behaviors found in animals with impaired limbic systems.

Key Terms :

Amygdala
Cingulate gyrus
Fornix
Klüver–Bucy syndrome
Hippocampus
Mammillary body
Mamillothalamic tract
Mamillotegmental tract
Medial forebrain bundle
Septum
Stria medullaris
Stria terminalis

Anatomic Structures

As a regulator of emotion and motivation, the limbic system (visceral brain) refers to closely related functional structures of the limbic lobe, diencephalon, septum, and

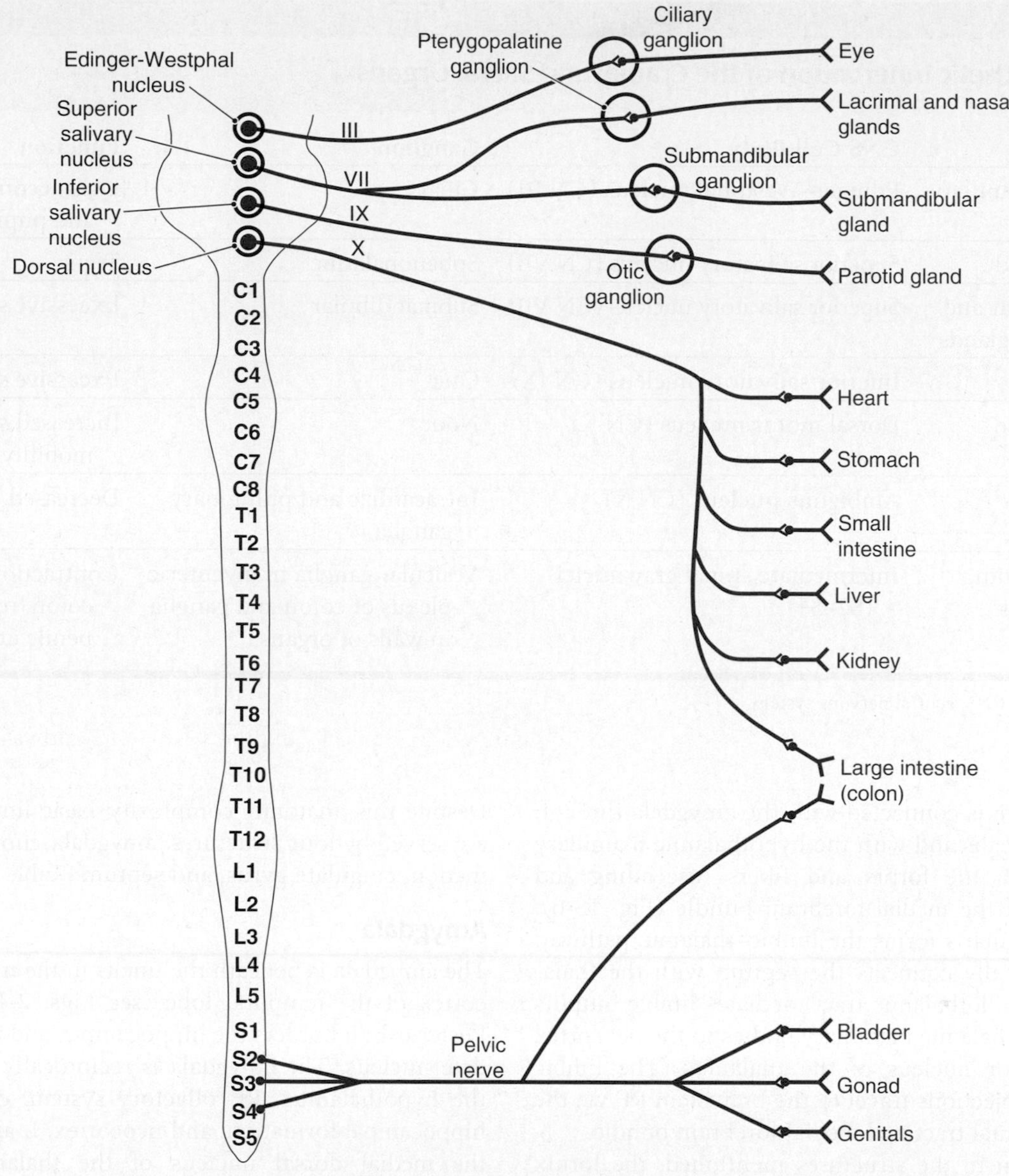

Figure 18-4 The parasympathetic autonomic nervous system.

midbrain. The limbic lobe includes the subcallosal gyrus, cingulate gyrus, isthmus, parahippocampal gyrus, hippocampus, olfactory cortex, uncus, and amygdala (Figs. 18-5 and 18-6). The limbic lobe derives its strength through its connections to intra- and interlimbic structures (Fig. 18-7). The septal area, located at the rostral diencephalon, forms the septo-hypothalamus–midbrain continuum (Fig. 18-5). It is essential for completing the limbic system's bidirectional circuitry, connecting the limbic lobe to the hypothalamus, thalamus, and midbrain. The fornix, a large C-shaped bundle of bidirectional fibers, serves as the main circuitry connecting the limbic lobe to the diencephalon and visceral centers of the hypothalamus (Box 18-3).

The key limbic structures are connected by an extensive network of afferent and efferent fibers. These interconnecting fibers account for the limbic influence on virtually all cortical, brainstem, as well as visceral functions and the regulation of emotions and motivation. Not all limbic connections are completely understood. Major inputs to the limbic lobe are from the neocortex, olfactory bulb, thalamus, hypothalamus, septum, and RF. The limbic output goes to the neocortex, hypothalamus, thalamus, and RF. Projections to the prefrontal lobe in the neocortex regulate affective aspects of emotion, such as moods and feelings. Projections to the hypothalamus and RF regulate ANS activities and motor aspects of emotions, such as fear, flight, and sex. Major ascending and descending pathways of the limbic system include the **medial forebrain bundle**, **stria medullaris**, **stria terminalis**, mamillothalamic tract, mamillotegmental tract, fornix, and medial longitudinal fasciculus (Fig. 18-7).

Table 18-4

Parasympathetic Innervation of the Cranial and Sacral Organs

Structure	CNS Cell Body	Ganglion	Function
Ciliary and pupillary muscles	Edinger–Westphal nucleus (CN III)	Ciliary	Lens accommodation and pupil constriction
Lacrimal gland	Superior salivatory nucleus (CN VII)	Sphenopalatine	Tears
Submandibular and sublingual glands	Superior salivatory nucleus (CN VII)	Submandibular	Excessive saliva (thin)
Parotid gland	Inferior salivatory nucleus (CN IX)	Otic	Excessive saliva (thin)
Small intestine	Dorsal motor nucleus (CN X)	None	Increased secretion and mobility
Heart	Ambiguus nucleus (CN X)	Intracardiac and pulmonary ganglia	Decreased heart rate
Column, rectum, and genitals	Intermediate spinal gray nuclei (S2–S4)	Vesicular ganglia in myenteric plexus of colon and ganglia in walls of organs	Contraction of bladder, colon, rectum, and penile erection

CN, cranial nerve; CNS, central nervous system.

The septum is connected with the amygdala through the stria terminalis and with the hypothalamic mamillary bodies through the fornix and fibers (ascending and descending) of the medial forebrain bundle (Fig. 18-6). The stria medullaris forms the limbic–thalamic pathway, which reciprocally connects the septum with the thalamus. The mamillothalamic tract mediates limbic outputs from the hypothalamic mamillary bodies to the neocortex via the anterior nucleus of the thalamus. The limbic descending projections travel to the brainstem RF via the mamillotegmental tract and medial forebrain bundle.

In addition to the structures mentioned, the fornix and cingulum are two important pathways that interconnect the major limbic structures. The cingulum, a massive fiber bundle, circulates limbic information from the cingulate gyrus to the parahippocampal gyrus and then to the hippocampus. Forming the major link between the forebrain and midbrain, the fornix connects the hypothalamus with both the hippocampus and the olfactory cortex. Despite this anatomic complexity, basic limbic functions are served by four structures: amygdala, hippocampal formation, cingulate gyrus, and septum (Table 18-6).

Table 18-5

Sympathetic and Parasympathetic Neurotransmitters

Structure	Sympathetic	Parasympathetic
Preganglionic cells	Acetylcholine	Acetylcholine
Postganglionic cells	Norepinephrine	Acetylcholine

Amygdala

The amygdala is beneath the uncus in the medial anterior cortex of the temporal lobe (see Figs. 2-16 and 3-30). Posteriorly, it borders the hippocampus and tail of the caudate nucleus. The amygdala is reciprocally connected to the hypothalamus, RF, olfactory system, orbital region, hippocampal formation, and neocortex. It also projects to the medial dorsal nucleus of the thalamus, septum, cingulate gyrus, and prefrontal region (Fig. 18-6). Along with bidirectional projections to the prefrontal orbital cortex and hypothalamus, the amygdala directly controls drive and motivation associated with visceral brain activities and the accompanying internal feelings.

Stimulation-based investigations of amygdaloid function in animals suggest that its activation with high-threshold stimulation can produce all the behaviors that are elicited from the hypothalamus—for example, defecation, micturition, pupillary dilation, hair erection, pituitary hormone secretion, blood pressure and heart rate changes, and gastrointestinal motility and secretion. Other behaviors are associated with sexual activities: erection, copulatory movements, ejaculation, ovulation, uterine activity, and premature labor. Rage, escape, punishment, and fear also are associated with the amygdala. Stimulation of the amygdala results in motor activities such as head movements, circling, dystonic movements, licking, chewing, swallowing, and vomiting. Combined stimulation of

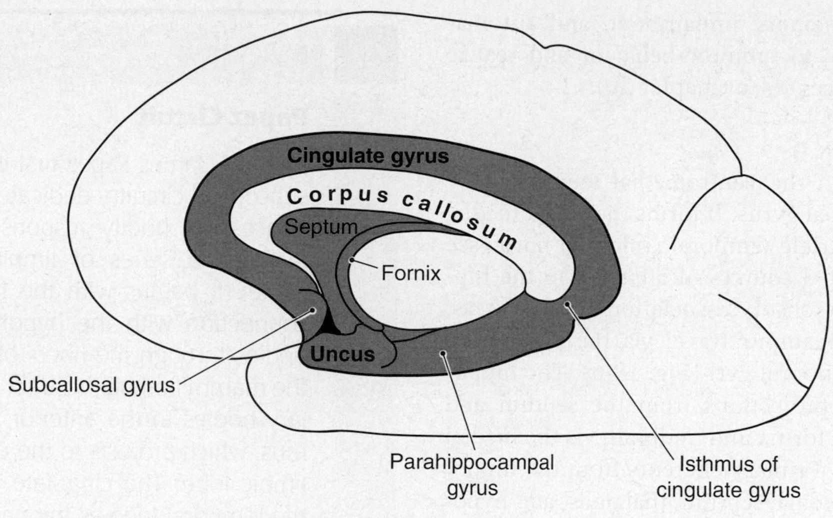

Figure 18-5 Midsagittal view showing the limbic structures.

the amygdala and hypothalamus facilitates the rage reaction, and amygdala stimulation may increase or decrease hypothalamic-induced rage.

Clinically, a bilateral ablation of the amygdala and surrounding temporal tissues is associated with Klüver–Bucy syndrome, which is characterized by indiscriminate eating, oral exploration, fearlessness, psychic blindness, and inappropriate hypersexuality. Complex partial seizures, which emanate from the amygdala and surrounding temporal lobe structures, are characterized by automatic

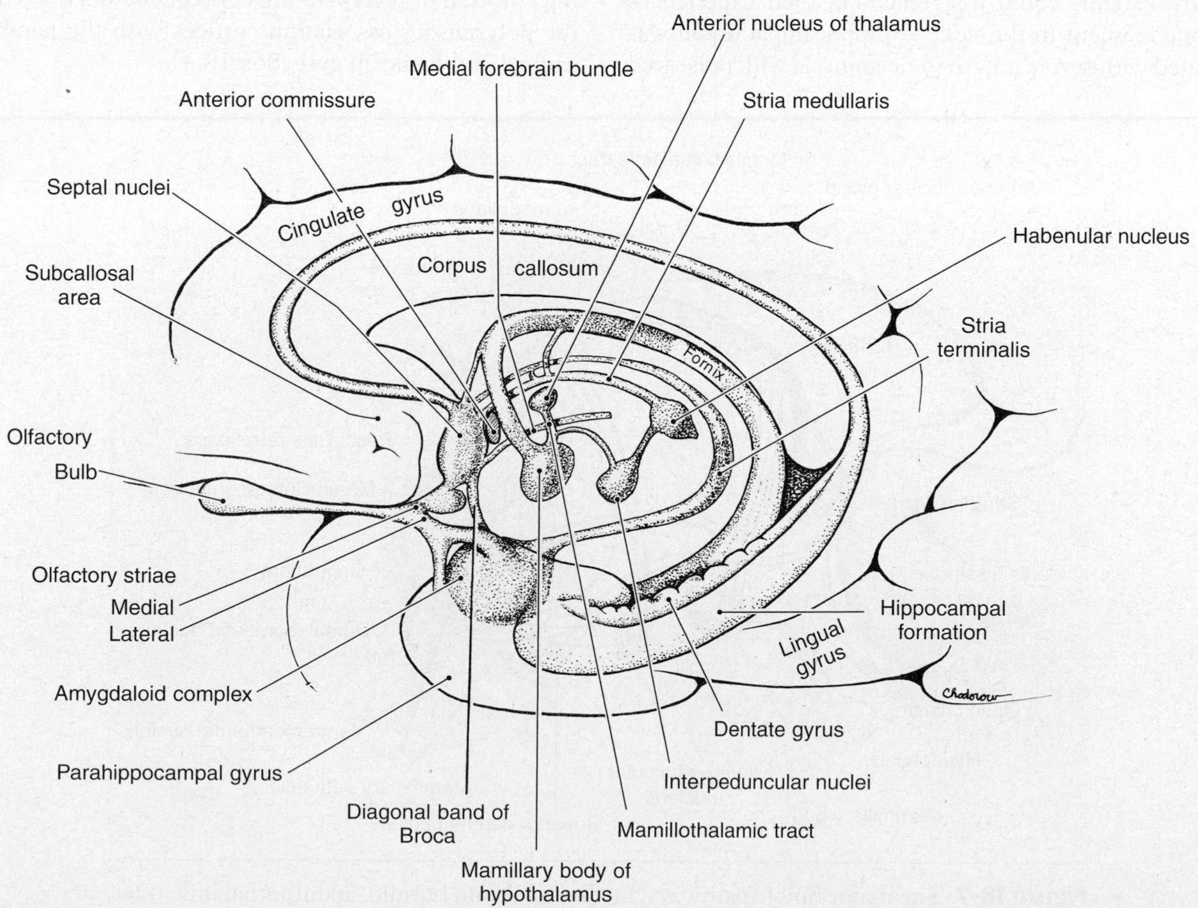

Figure 18-6 Medial view of the major limbic structures and their connections.

aggressive behavior, memory impairment, and automatisms (impaired ability to monitor behavior and realize subsequent consequences) (see Chapter 20).

Hippocampus

The hippocampus is in the ventromedial temporal lobe beneath the hippocampal gyrus. It forms the ventromedial wall of the lateral ventricle temporal (inferior) horn (see Fig. 3-30). The principal sources of afferents to the hippocampus are the polysensory association cortical areas. Impulses to the hippocampus travel via the parahippocampal and occipitotemporal gyri (Fig. 18-6). The hippocampus also receives projections from the septum and hypothalamus through fornix and midbrain via the medial forebrain fiber bundle. Primary efferents from the hippocampus are to the amygdala, septum, thalamus, and hypothalamus. Hippocampal stimulation and ablation implicate endocrine and autonomic functions that are generated in the hypothalamus. However, the hippocampus is best known for its involvement with memory and learning.

Clinically, the hippocampus has been implicated with memory and new learning. In the early 1950s, drastic and persistent anterograde memory deficits were noted to have occurred after radical bilateral ablations of the hippocampal formation that extended posteriorly in the region of the caudal parahippocampal and fusiform (occipitotemporal) gyri. Patients could not remember their experiences from one moment to the next. A hippocampal lesion was associated with severe anterograde amnesia with preserved retrograde memories. The patients consistently lost newly acquired data but retained memory of events that preceded the lesion. Clinical and experimental findings suggest that the anterograde memory deficit may be the result of the interruption of reverberating cortical circuits that connect the polysensory association cortices with the parahippocampal and fusiform gyri (Box 18-4).

BOX 18-3

Papez Circuit

In 1937, James Papez first described the specific subcortical circuitry dedicated to emotional experience and bodily responses to it. The circuit includes a series of limbic and hypothalamic nuclei. It begins with the hippocampus and its connection with the hypothalamic mammillary bodies through the fibers of fornix. The fibers of the mammillothalamic tract connect the mammillary bodies to the anterior nucleus of the thalamus, which projects to the cingulate gyrus of the limbic lobe. The cingulate gyrus continues into the temporal lobe as the parahippocampal gyrus and completes the circuit by merging with the adjacent hippocampus. This entire system is surrounded by higher-order, six-layered neocortex of the temporal and frontal lobes.

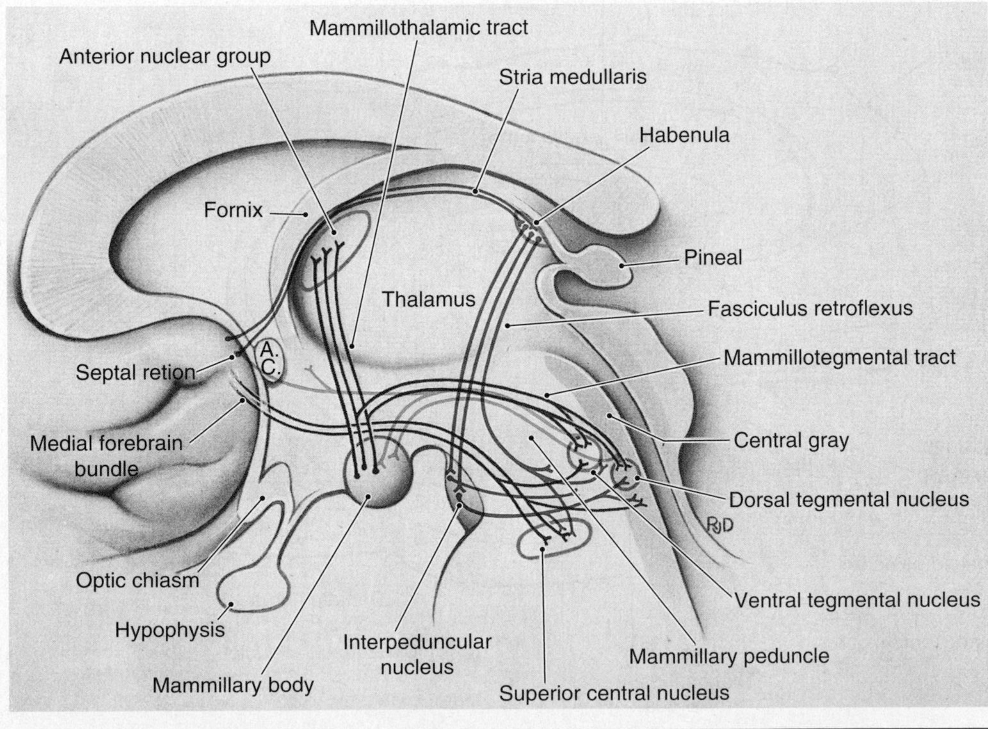

Figure 18-7 The major limbic pathways: medial forebrain bundle, mamillothalamic tract, mamillotegmental tract, and stria medullaris. AC, anterior commissure.

Table 18-6

Limbic Structures and Their Functions

Structure	Afferents	Efferents	Functions
Amygdala	Hypothalamus, reticular formation, olfactory system, orbital region, hippocampal formation, and neocortex limbic cortex	Thalamus, septum, cingulate, hypothalamus, and prefrontal cortex	Aggression, mating, stress-mediated responses, memory, feeding, and drinking
Hippocampus	Neocortex, limbic cortex, olfactory area, hypothalamus, and septal area	Amygdala, septum, hypothalamus, and thalamus	Memory and learning
Septal nuclei	Hippocampus, amygdala, and hypothalamus	Hippocampus, amygdala, and hypothalamus	Hormonal secretion, behavioral reaction, and memory facilitation
Cingulate gyrus	Hypothalamic mamillary bodies and anterior thalamic nucleus	Hypothalamic mamillary bodies and anterior thalamic nucleus	Anxiety and altered behavior (panic and compulsion)

Cingulate Gyrus

Located above the corpus callosum, the cingulate gyrus receives projections from the hypothalamic mamillary bodies by way of the mamillothalamic tract and the anterior thalamic nucleus (Figs. 18-5 and 18-6; also see Fig. 2-10 and Chapter 6). The cingulate gyrus projects to the hypothalamic mamillary bodies via the fornix fibers that arise in the entorhinal cortex (part of the hippocampus and uncus forming the lateral olfactory area). Clinically, this cingulate–limbic circuit has been associated with anxiety and obsessive–compulsive behaviors.

Septum

The septum consists of two parts. Dorsally, it consists of a midline fibrous sheet attached to the corpus callosum (Figs. 18-5 and 18-6; see Fig. 2-11). Ventrally, it consists

BOX 18-4

Memory Disorders

Although the exact location of memory storage in the brain is elusive, clinical evidence has implicated the hippocampus and its connections with short-term memory and the consolidation of new information. This evidence has come from observations on individuals with seizure, stroke, and trauma involving the temporal lobes. The best-described case of memory loss with hippocampal lesions came from the observations of Penfield in one of his patients (HM) in whom a bilateral surgical removal of the hippocampus resulted in permanent anterograde amnesia. This hippocampal dysfunction also occurs if an arterial occlusion causes an infarct in one side of the hippocampal formation, which later is followed by an infarct in the hippocampal formation on the other side. Even ischemic attacks can deprive the hippocampus of oxygen, affecting transiently its ability to remember new information. The transient amnesia has been seen in patients with unconsciousness due to traumatic brain injuries as well as in patients with cardiac arrest. Additional structures that have been implicated with memory are the hypothalamic mammillary bodies and their projections to the thalamus (mammillothalamic tract, which is seen in subjects with nutritional deficiency [Wernicke–Korsakoff syndrome]). Profound amnesia has also been seen after a bilateral lesion involving the mediodorsal nuclei of the thalamus, which is connected with the executive prefrontal lobe. Degenerative changes in the brain as well as impaired cholinergic projections from the basal forebrain to bilateral hippocampi have been associated with the progressive memory deficits in patients with Alzheimer syndrome. Associational areas of the neocortex are involved in long-term memory functions. Access to this storage can involve the function of the hippocampal system. In addition, the cerebellar cortex is suggested to be involved in motor skill learning and motor memory.

of a collection of nuclei. In conjunction with the diencephalon, and brainstem, and a major component of the axial brain, the septum forms the septo-hypothalamus–midbrain continuum. The fornix provides a vital portal entry connecting the limbic lobe to the diencephalon and brainstem. It is also involved actively in processing autonomic, visceral, endocrine, sensorimotor, reproductive, neurotransmitter, emotional, and motivational functions.

Clinical Correlates

Clinical symptoms that appear after limbic system lesions involve emotions and motivation. They are characterized by uninhibited instinctual acts, altered sexual behavior, excessive fear, aggression, and disturbances in circadian rhythm. Limbic dysfunctions also have substantial implications for memory and learning (Table 18-6).

Summary of the Limbic System

Anatomically, limbic structures form the inner brain neural circuitry that connects the cortex to the diencephalon and midbrain structures. Functionally, they regulate all visceral, endocrine, and sensorimotor functions. With rich interconnections, the limbic system forms the neural mechanism responsible for motivational drive and emotions.

HYPOTHALAMUS

Consisting of only 4 g of gray matter and occupying a small area in the anterior region of the diencephalon beneath the thalamus, the hypothalamus has an importance that greatly exceeds its size. Interconnected with the forebrain, brainstem, and spinal cord, the hypothalamus is the central structure for controlling autonomic and visceral behaviors, such as vasodilation, body homeostasis (internal body environment), anger, reproduction, hunger, and thirst. With its projections to the limbic lobe, it provides the substrates for regulating motivation and emotions. The neurosecretory cells of the hypothalamus regulate the production and circulation of hormones by the pituitary gland.

Key Terms:

Adipsia	**Polydipsia**
Adrenocorticotropic hormone	**Polyuria**
	Prolactin hormone
Gonadotropin	**Thyrotropin**
Growth hormone	**Vasopressin**
Hyperthermia	**Vasopressin hormone**
Poikilothermic state	

Anatomic Structures

The hypothalamus is exposed fully on the medial surface of the brain and is located symmetrically along the lateral walls of the third ventricle (see Figs. 2-11, 2-12, and 6-1). Dorsally delineated by the hypothalamic sulcus, the hypothalamus extends from the optic chiasm to the posterior border of the mamillary bodies. The anterior commissure identifies its rostral limit, whereas caudally it extends to the central gray matter in the midbrain tegmentum.

On the midsagittal surface, the hypothalamus is divided into the **anterior**, **tuberal**, and **posterior regions** (Fig. 18-8). The anterior hypothalamus is above the optic chiasm. The tuberal region is enclosed by the optic chiasm, optic tract, and mamillary bodies. The posterior hypothalamic region includes the mamillary bodies and the nuclei above them. The principal hypothalamic nuclei are **preoptic**, **supraoptic**, **ventromedial**, **dorsomedial**, **paraventricular**, **anterior**, **posterior**, and **mamillary body** (Fig. 18-8).

As the stalk of the pituitary gland, the infundibulum comes from the floor of the third ventricle. The infundibulum is the transitional structure between the CNS and peripheral endocrine system and it serves as the interface between the brain and pituitary gland. The median eminence of the hypothalamus (**tuber cinereum**) is just caudal to the infundibulum. Above this tuberal level are the ventromedial and dorsomedial hypothalamic nuclei.

The hypothalamus is connected to the cerebral cortex, thalamus, and midbrain with extensive afferent and efferent fiber tracts. Afferents to the hypothalamus come primarily from the limbic region of the forebrain, brainstem, and spinal cord. The bidirectional connections of the hypothalamus to the brainstem and spinal cord regulate visceral and autonomic functions. The major fiber bundles that interconnect the hypothalamus with other neuraxial structures are the medial forebrain bundle, stria terminalis, fornix, and mamillothalamic, mamillotegmental, and dorsal longitudinal fasciculi (Figs. 18-7 and 18-9).

Afferents

The medial forebrain bundle, which primarily connects the midbrain tegmentum to hypothalamus and limbic structures, also channels the forebrain input to the hypothalamus and is the major bidirectional tract formed by the cells in the olfactory region, septum, and amygdala. This pathway mediates information basic to the emotional drives. Other important input for emotional drives comes from the amygdala, which is connected to the hypothalamus via the stria terminalis (Fig. 18-6). The bidirectional fibers of the fornix curve around the thalamus and connect to the hypothalamic mamillary bodies with the hippocampus via the septum. The bidirectional fibers of the mamillothalamic tract connect the mamillary bodies to

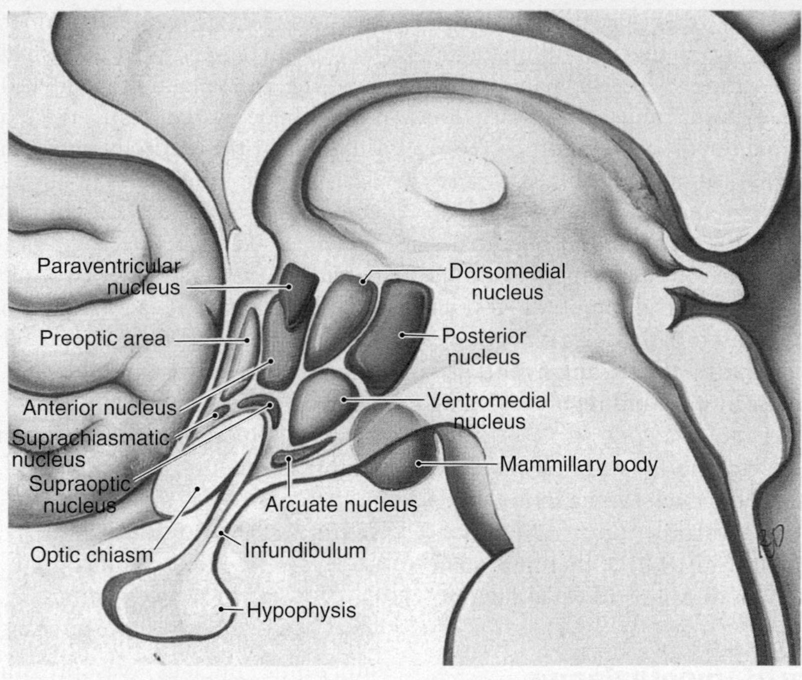

Figure 18-8 Midsagittal view of the hypothalamic nuclei.

the anterior nucleus of the thalamus, which projects to the cingulate gyrus of the limbic lobe (Fig. 18-7). The brainstem and reticular input to the hypothalamus enter by way of the mamillary bodies, dorsal longitudinal fasciculus (connecting the periventricular hypothalamic zone with the central gray of the midbrain), and medial forebrain bundle (Figs. 18-7 and 18-9).

Efferents

Efferents of the hypothalamus project to the forebrain limbic structures (septum, hippocampal formation, and amygdala). Projections also reach the brainstem reticular region, which includes the periaqueductal gray matter, by way of bidirectional fibers in the tracts previously described under afferents. The efferent hypothalamic

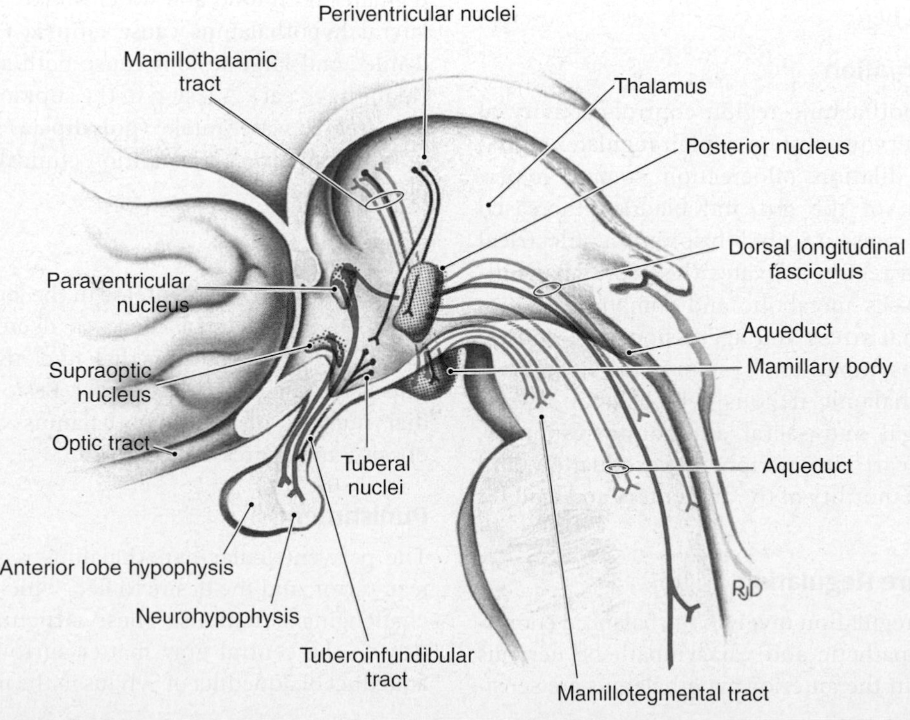

Figure 18-9 The major hypothalamic primarily efferent pathways.

projections to the limbic lobe travel via the septum to the hippocampus and by way of the mamillothalamic tract to the cingulate gyrus (Fig. 18-9). The mamillothalamic fibers connect the hypothalamus to the anterior thalamic nucleus (see Chapter 6), which in turn connects to the cingulate gyrus, another limbic structure. Hypothalamic projections to the amygdaloid nucleus travel primarily via the stria terminalis and hypothalamus-amygdaloid fibers. The multisynaptic outputs travel through the fibers of the dorsal longitudinal tract to the sympathetic and parasympathetic preganglionic cranial and spinal cells. Because of this, the hypothalamus controls the autonomic system and regulates eating and drinking.

Additional projections to the lower brainstem and spinal preganglionic autonomic nuclei come from the RF, which in turn receives hypothalamic input via fibers of the mamillotegmental tract (Fig. 18-9). Other important neural projections of the hypothalamus travel to the posterior pituitary gland.

Functional Circuitry of Hypothalamus

Most understanding of hypothalamic functions is based on the electrical stimulation of the hypothalamus and/or observations of impaired functions after lesions induced in the hypothalamus of animals. In addition to regulating autonomic (sympathetic and parasympathetic) functions, the hypothalamus has specific centers for controlling eating, drinking, reproduction, aggression, and biologic body rhythms. The hypothalamus also contributes to blood electrolyte balance and temperature control. Most important, it controls endocrine-monitored behaviors through the secretion of hormones. Only a few hypothalamic functions are discussed here.

Autonomic Innervation

The posterior hypothalamic region controls activity of the sympathetic nervous system, which regulates activities such as pupil dilation, piloerection, somatic hyperactivity, inhibition of the gut and bladder, increased heart rate, blood pressure, and respiration. Electrical stimulation of this region activates thoracolumbar outflow, which increases metabolic and somatic activities typical of emotional stress and aggression. The control center for the parasympathetic system is in the anterior and medial hypothalamic regions, which, upon activation, increase vagal and sacral autonomic responses, such as reduced heart rate, peripheral vasodilation, and increased tone and motility of the alimentary and bladder walls.

Body Temperature Regulation

Body temperature regulation involves the balanced coordination of the sympathetic and parasympathetic nervous systems. Neurons in the anterior hypothalamus are sensitive to increases in blood temperature. They react to an increase in temperature by dissipating excess heat through sweating (a sympathetic activity) and by inhibiting the sympathetic system, causing cutaneous blood vessels to dilate. The posterior hypothalamus, however, preserves heat by inhibiting the sympathetic system in constricting cutaneous vessels and stopping sweat secretion. This is accompanied by shivering (a somatic activity) and decreased visceral activity. An anterior hypothalamic lesion impairs the heat dissipation mechanism and results in **hyperthermia**, whereas a posterior hypothalamic lesion impairs the pathways responsible for both heat conservation and dissipation, resulting in a **poikilothermic state** in which body temperature is governed by environmental temperature.

Water Intake Regulation

Adequate water input and output, essential for normal body activity, is regulated by **vasopressin**, an antidiuretic (urine volume reduction) hormone. Synthesized in the supraoptic nucleus, vasopressin is released into the bloodstream per physiologic circumstances by way of the posterior pituitary gland. Vasopressin production is controlled by blood osmotic pressure and hydration. A rise in blood osmotic pressure or a reduction in circulating vascular volume increases vasopressin production, causing fluid retention. A dehydrated state activates the supraoptic hypothalamic vasopressin system. Vasopressin is resynthesized and stored in the posterior pituitary gland after water balance is reestablished.

Activation of the anterior hypothalamus causes increased water intake. In fact, the anterior hypothalamus regulates both food and water intake. Small lesions in the lateral hypothalamus cause **adipsia** (a lack of desire to drink), and large lesions cause both adipsia and **aphagia** (inability to eat). A lesion in the supraoptic nucleus results in increased water intake (**polydipsia**) and increased urine output (**polyuria**), a condition clinically known as diabetes insipidus.

Feeding

The feeding (phagic) center is in the lateral hypothalamus. A lesion in this area causes a decreased desire to eat (anorexia). The ventromedial nucleus of the hypothalamus is the site of a satiety center. Lesions of the ventromedial nucleus of the hypothalamus cause hyperphagia, obesity, and aggressive behavior.

Punishment

The periventricular hypothalamus regulates feelings like fear, terror, and the desire to flee, which are engendered by challenging situations. These structures extend posteriorly to the central gray matter surrounding the cerebral aqueduct or aqueduct of Sylvius in the midbrain. Prolonged stimulation in these areas may cause death. By varying the electrical parameters, stimulation of the ventromedial hypothalamus may elicit fear, rage, and aggression. Stimulation of the more rostral midline preoptic area elicits the fear and anxiety that are associated with escape. In generating these behaviors, the cerebral cortex, in conjunction with various environmental inputs, must recruit somatic and hypothalamic visceral systems. Together they control the expression of pleasure or displeasure associated with the behavior.

Hypothalamic Regulation of the Pituitary Gland (Hypophysis)

Nicknamed the master gland, the pituitary gland forms the central endocrine system and works with the nervous system to maintain body homeostasis. The pituitary gland controls the functioning of other glands and tissues in the body by secreting hormones and chemical messengers. The pituitary gland consists of a large anterior lobe (**adenohypophysis**) and small posterior lobe (**neurohypophysis**) (Fig. 18-9).

The release of hormones produced in the neurosecretory hypothalamic cells stimulates the adenohypophysis to secrete the following hormones: **growth hormone**, **thyrotropin**, **adrenocorticotropin**, **gonadotropin**, and **prolactin**. The releasing hormones are transported into the anterior lobe of the pituitary gland through the hypothalamic hypophyseal portal (blood) circulation (Fig. 18-10; Table 18-7).

Thyrotropic hormones stimulate and regulate thyroid gland hormone secretion. Adrenocorticotropin regulates steroid secretion by the adrenal cortex. Gonadotropin

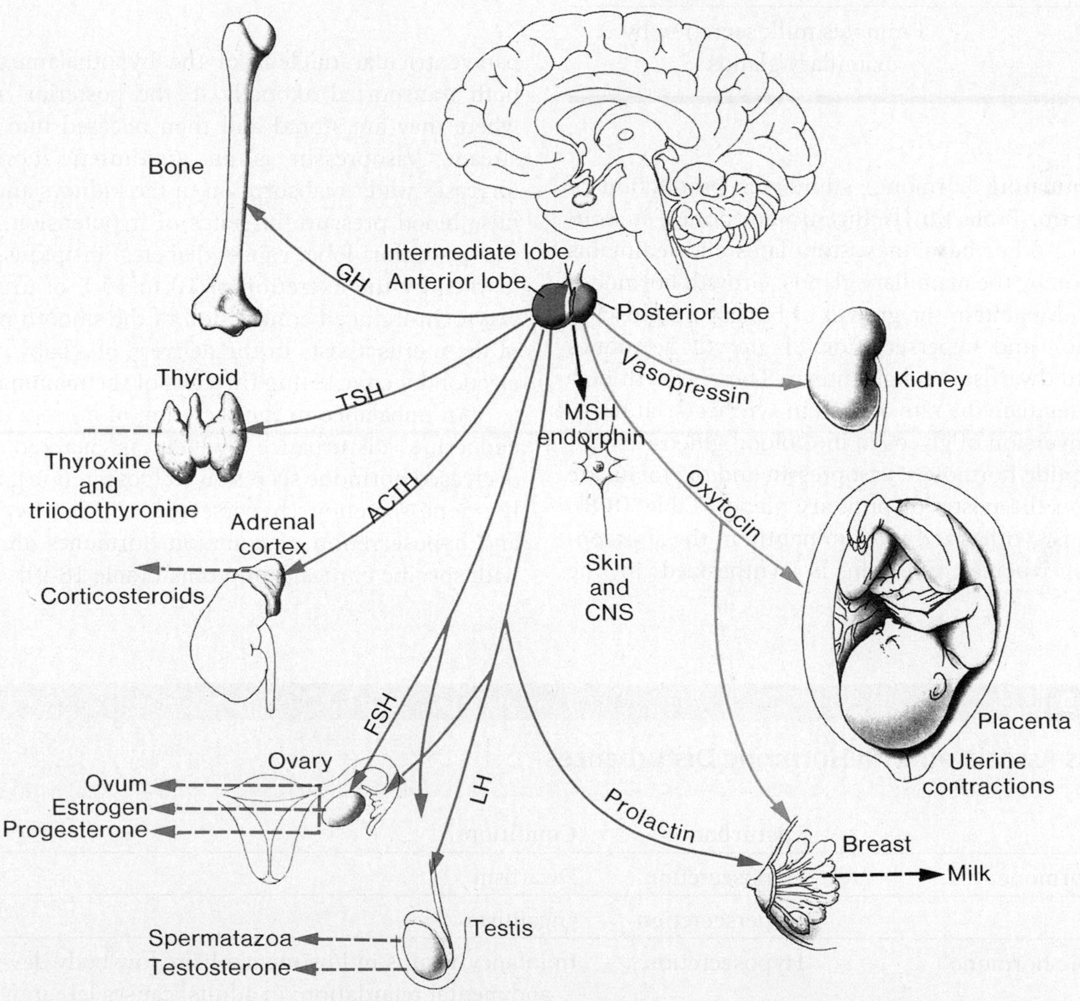

Figure 18-10 Commonly secreted pituitary hormones in the adenohypophysis and neurohypophysis. Hormones of the anterior pituitary gland, or adenohypophysis, are growth hormone (GH), thyrotropin, adrenocorticotropic hormone (ACTH), gonadotropin, and prolactin. The posterior pituitary lobe, or neurohypophysis, contains vasopressin and oxytocin. CNS, central nervous system; FSH, follicle-stimulating hormone; LH, luteinizing hormone; MSH, melanocyte-stimulating hormone; TSH, thyroid-stimulating hormone.

Table 18-7

Anterior Pituitary Gland Hormones and Their Functions

Hormones	Primary Function
Growth hormone	Controls general body growth.
Thyroid-stimulating hormone (thyrotropic)	Controls thyroid hormone secretions
Adrenocorticotropic hormone	Controls secretion of adrenal cortex hormones
Gonadotropic hormone	Initiates sperm production in males; promotes development of ova in females
Prolactin	Promotes milk secretion by mamillary glands

Table 18-8

Posterior Pituitary Gland Hormones and Their Functions

Hormones	Primary Function
Oxytocin	Stimulates uterine contraction and mamillary gland alveoli, causing milk secretion
Vasopressin	Decreases urine volume and raises blood pressure by constricting arterial lumen, particularly during hemorrhage

(follicle-stimulating hormone) stimulates production of ova and sperm. Prolactin (lactogenic hormone), in conjunction with other hormones, stimulates and maintains milk secretion by the mamillary glands. Growth hormones stimulate and maintain the growth of bones and muscles. Hyposecretion and hypersecretion of growth hormones are related to dwarfism and gigantism. These growth hormones also regulate the rate of protein synthesis, fat burning, and conversion of glycogen into blood glucose.

Two peptide hormones, vasopressin and oxytocin, are released from the posterior pituitary gland (Table 18-8). Vasopressin is synthesized predominantly in the supraoptic nucleus, whereas oxytocin is synthesized in the paraventricular nucleus of the hypothalamus. They are both transported axonally to the posterior hypophysis, where they are stored and then released into the bloodstream. Vasopressin is an antidiuretic hormone that increases water reabsorption in the kidneys and is used to raise blood pressure in states of hypotension. Lesions of the posterior lobe cause diabetes insipidus, which is marked by the excretion of 10 to 15 L of urine per day. Oxytocin-induced contraction of the smooth muscle cells of the uterus assists in the delivery of a baby and in milk ejection by contracting the cells of the mammary gland.

An imbalance in the secretion of hormones results in endocrine disturbance, which is marked either by decreased hormone secretion (hyposecretion) or increased hormone secretion (hypersecretion). The hypersecretion and hyposecretion of common hormones are associated with specific clinical symptoms (Table 18-9).

Table 18-9

Disorders Associated with Hormone Disturbances

Hormone	Disturbance	Condition
Growth hormone	Hyposecretion	Dwarfism
	Hypersecretion	Gigantism
Thyrotropic hormone	Hyposecretion	In infancy, results in low metabolism, low body development, and mental retardation; in adults, causes lethargy, excessive sleeping, and slow mental activity
	Hypersecretion	Increased metabolic rate increases hunger and food intake
Adrenocorticotropic hormone	Hyposecretion	Impaired synthesis of glucose and loss of sodium in urine
	Hypersecretion	Decreased immune response and excessive fat deposits
Gonadotropic hormone		Impaired sexual functions
Vasopressin		Water imbalance

Neurotransmitters and Behaviors

Neurotransmitters play an important role in the regulation of behaviors mediated by the hypothalamus. The interaction of vasopressin with noradrenergic synapses influences memory consolidation. Norepinephrine released in the hypothalamus may block visceral drives, such as eating, drinking, and sexual behavior. This suggests that while norepinephrine activates the neocortex, it inhibits the competing visceral drives. Excessive production of norepinephrine causes manic psychosis, whereas insufficient production of it leads to depression. Stimulation of dopamine projections to the hypothalamic area enhances eating and fighting drives. A bilateral hypothalamic lesion that impairs the dopaminergic systems reduces these drives.

Clinical Correlates

Clinical symptoms that commonly result from hypothalamic dysfunction are characterized by disturbances of food intake, water balance, libido, menstruation, and temperature control. Also, pituitary hormone changes can affect body growth, the ability to reproduce, and milk secretion.

Summary of the Hypothalamus

The hypothalamus is the central structure for controlling autonomic and visceral behaviors. It is the central generator of motivational and emotional motor behaviors and controls visceral functions, such as vasodilation, body homeostasis (internal body environment), reproduction, hunger, and water and food intake. Its neurosecretory cells regulate pituitary gland hormone production and release.

RETICULAR FORMATION

Key Terms :

Involuntary respiratory center
Reticular activating system
Voluntary respiratory control center

The RF consists of a group of neurons that are interconnected by a complex web of parallel and serial running neuronal circuits. Composing most of the brainstem (medulla, pons, and midbrain), it is also functionally wired to nuclei in the thalamus and spinal cord (see Fig. 2-23). With their central location, the neuronal circuits of the RF converge or diverge to inhibit, facilitate, modify, and regulate all cortical functions; they also integrate all sensorimotor stimuli with internally generated thoughts, emotions, and cognition. The RF is also responsible for maintaining the homeostatic state of the brain, which is essential for regulating visceral, sensorimotor, and neuroendocrine activities such as sleep, blood pressure, posture, and movement. The RF also regulates emotions, mood, and cognition. Furthermore, it energizes the **reticular activating system (RAS)**, which controls the brain's arousal and consciousness. A single lesion of the RAS can produce complex illnesses, and altered states of arousal, or permanent unconsciousness, such as coma, stupor, insomnia, headaches, depression, and forgetfulness. Descending reticular fibers regulate the quality of motor movement and muscle tone. They also inhibit sensory inputs at the spinal level. Finally, for students of communicative disorders, two important functions of the RF are its regulation of respiration and swallowing.

Anatomic Structures

The reticular circuitry is characterized by a web of multiple parallel and serial running circuits that can diverge or converge. This organization of circuitry allows for reticular cells to influence over 25,000 to 30,000 neurons in the brainstem. This architectural property also enables the reticular cells to amplify a weak impulse and to disseminate that amplified signal to thousands of other nuclei. The RF can consolidate and integrate impulses from thousands of neurons to a single neuronal circuit. It can also channel and screen information and respond to the amount of information rather than to the details.

The reticular cells are arranged longitudinally in transverse modules and project to overlapping dendrites, which generally lack dendritic shafts. The dendritic processes look like radiating spokes of a wheel. Each dendrite shaft receives input from different combinations of axons throughout the neuraxis. The axons, the efferent component of the reticular cells, are long (Golgi type I) and tend to bifurcate and project in opposite directions to distant structures. Projections run caudally to the spinal cord and rostrally throughout the brainstem, diencephalon, limbic structures, basal ganglia, and cortex.

The brainstem reticular cells are arranged in three broad longitudinal columns: **median**, **medial**, and **lateral** (Fig. 18-11). The median reticular cell column contains the midline nucleus raphe, which forms a continuous cellular column in the brainstem and consists of regions that provide projections to the brain and spinal cord. The medial cell column consists of a central group of reticular nuclei, including the gigantocellular reticular nucleus, whereas the lateral cell column contains small to intermediate-size nuclei.

Afferents

Overlapping afferents, some of which are inhibitory and others facilitatory, converge on a given reticular neuron. Reticular afferents consist of collaterals from the ascending and descending spinal tracts (pain, proprioception, tactile, temperature, and vibration), cranial nerve nuclei, cerebellum, midbrain, thalamus, subthalamus, hypothalamus, striatum, limbic lobe, and various cortical areas.

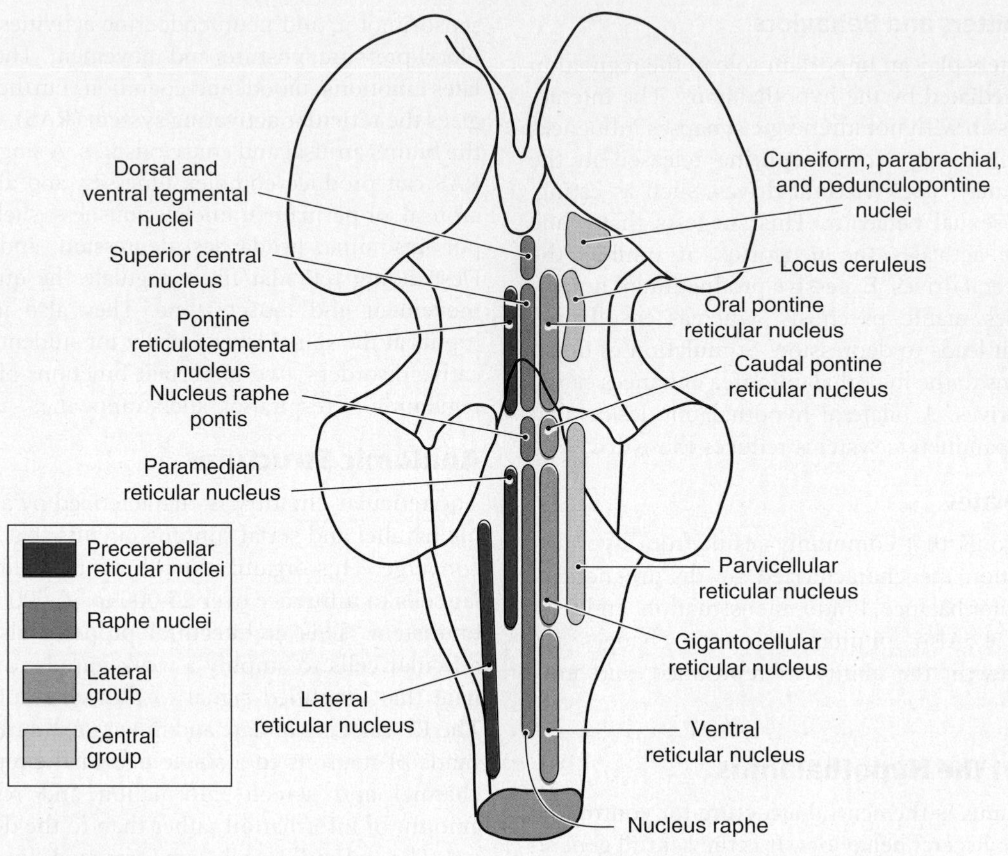

Figure 18-11 A diagrammatic illustration of reticular columns and nuclei.

Efferents

Through its direct and indirect projections to the cortical and subcortical regions, the RF influences all nervous system functions. It sends projections to somatic and autonomic nuclei in general, autonomic and somatic motor nuclei of cranial nerves in the brainstem, and interneuronal pools in the spinal cord. Direct and indirect reticular projections also travel to the cerebellum, red nucleus, substantia nigra, midbrain tectum, subthalamic nuclei, thalamus, hypothalamus, limbic lobe (septum, hippocampus, amygdala, and cingulate gyrus), and the forebrain.

Functional Considerations

Within the diffuse reticular core of nuclei in the brainstem, specific nuclear cell aggregates form closed-loop circuits and serve as the reticular centers for regulating various sensorimotor, visceral, and cortical activating functions. Reticular centers may combine to form reticular networks that help regulate complex sensorimotor and visceral behaviors, such as eating, swallowing, vomiting, coughing, sneezing, copulation, and fighting.

Examining all of the unifying functions of the RF is beyond the scope of this chapter. However, to provide a simpler way to describe these functions, the reticular functions have been divided into three types: cortical arousal, sensorimotor elaboration, and visceral integrated activity.

Regulation of Cortical Arousal

The activation and regulation of cortical arousal are perhaps the best-known functions of the RF. The serotonergic, cholinergic, and catecholaminergic cells of the ascending RAS and their projections from the brainstem to the neocortex and limbic structures collectively contribute to cortical arousal (Box 18-5; see Fig. 2-23). The RAS is indiscriminate to variations between sensory input and its modality; rather it responds best to stimulus intensity and novelty.

Clinically, cortical electrical activity is the best indicator of cortical arousal and brain functions. Various patterns

BOX 18-5

Reticular Serotonin and Depression

Low levels of serotonin in the brain are associated with mental illness, such as depression and obsessive–compulsive disorder. Selective serotonin reuptake inhibiting drugs, such as Prozac, Celexa, and Zoloft, target depression control by increasing serotonin and by preventing its cellular reuptake.

of the brain's electrical activity are known to relate to different mental states of arousal. For example, if a person is relaxed with closed eyes, the usual electrical activity observed is the α-rhythm (see Chapter 20). Opening the eyes or exposing the individual to other sensory stimuli causes the α-rhythm to change to a high-frequency, low-amplitude (electroencephalographic [EEG] activation) wave pattern. This electrical activity reflects changes in the arousal or alertness of the cerebral cortex and is related to functions of the reticular system.

Terms that are related to clinically altered consciousness or awareness are drowsiness (impaired awareness associated with sleep), **minimally conscious state**, **acute confusional state**, **stupor** (impaired consciousness in which the patient can be transiently aroused by stimulation), and **coma** (a state of profound unconsciousness). Consciousness level is a clinically important concept since neurolinguistic patients with brain damage exhibit various levels of altered consciousness, which relates to their ability to use language and cognitive skills.

As an active state of mind, sleep is related to the states of arousal and consciousness and is involved directly with the functioning of the RAS. In general, there are two sleeping states: deep sleep or non–rapid-eye movement (NREM) and paradoxical or rapid-eye movement (REM) sleep. NREM sleep has several substages, representing progressively deeper states of unconsciousness, which are characterized by slower and higher-amplitude EEG patterns. EEG recordings of deep sleep are characterized by slow-frequency waves of large amplitude from which one can recover with full restoration of awareness and cognitive functions (see Chapter 20).

Deep sleep is interrupted periodically by REM sleep, in which the individual is as physically relaxed as in deep sleep but displays the EEG pattern characteristic of being awake. This is associated with the dream state. REM sleep also is characterized by variations in heart rate, blood pressure, and respiration. Being awake is accompanied by a low-voltage and fast-frequency desynchronized wave form. Electrical stimulation of the RF can change EEG patterns of deep sleep to the pattern of wakefulness, indicating that the RAS may regulate levels of cortical arousal and wakefulness.

The median raphe nucleus (serotonergic) and locus ceruleus (noradrenergic) are two important reticular neurotransmitter nuclei concerned with sleep (Fig. 18-11). Their alternating actions trigger NREM and REM sleep phases. The median raphe nucleus generates the high-amplitude, slow waves of deep sleep. A lesion of the raphe nucleus causes constant wakefulness or insomnia. Conversely, the nucleus locus ceruleus generates REM sleep. If the locus ceruleus is damaged, REM does not occur.

Most coma or altered consciousness-causing lesions are in the midbrain, hypothalamic, and thalamic junctions. The lesion can result from traumatic injury, vascular occlusion, tumors, or encephalitis. Impairment of the brainstem RF may be a major causative factor, especially at the midbrain level. Arousal, a state of awareness or wakefulness, is also related to attention, the central-most attribute of cognition besides memory. The attention allows focusing on a particular modality-specific stimulus, and is an essential skill for new learning.

Central to the neural circuitry of arousal and its integration with attention are the diffuse cortical projections of the medial reticular formation (MRF) by way of thalamic nuclei, such as the intralaminar centromedian and reticular thalamus. Documenting the driving force of this mechanism, Magoun (1963) noted that the centromedian stimulation with afferents from the MRF induced a global cortical activation, exemplifying the electroencephalic pattern of one being fully awake and alert. The reticular activation not only tunes the physiology for cognitive functions but also promotes learning by facilitating information flow to the brain and by opening the neuronal gates.

Stimulation of the centromedian nucleus with an externally applied current has been found to enhance the processing of virtually all language (verbal and nonverbal) functions in neurologically impaired patients. This performance enhancement was measured in terms of response latencies and reduced number of errors (Bhatnagar and Mandybur, 2005) and speech fluency (Andy and Bhatnagar, 1992; Bhatnagar and Buckingham, 2011). This reticular–thalamic neuronal circuitry interacts with the prefrontal lobe and drives the brain's intentional–attentional mechanisms, which allow focusing on selective modality processing in the tactile, visual, or auditory mode. Reactive attention, on the other hand, involves simple environmental (visual, auditory, and painful) stimuli that initiate bodily reactions such as removing oneself from the path of danger or recognizing a friendly face. Behavior triggered by visual recognition involves the participation of the parietal association cortex.

Regulation of Sensory Functions

The reticulospinal projections also modulate the quantity and quality of sensory information and employ a gating mechanism that screens information at both the spinal and thalamic levels. The brainstem collateral terminals of the primary sensory fibers are under direct reticular influence. The RF affects sensory impulse transmission in presynaptic and postsynaptic terminals.

Reticular nuclei send input to brain structures that process specialized and general sensory input, such as the cochlear and vestibular nuclei, tectal and pretectal structures, geniculate nuclei, and thalamic nuclei. These direct reticular projections influence information processing by either accentuating or attenuating the sensory (audition, vision, olfaction, pain, temperature, and tactile) stimuli. There is a reticular pain-monitoring and pain-control system at the midbrain level and the posterior diencephalic RF, especially in the tegmental and periaqueductal regions.

Integrated Motor Functions

Integrated motor functions include unconscious activities that are vital to survival and are controlled by the brainstem reticular nuclei. The RF uses convergent multimodal input and diffuse divergent output to control the vital centers of the brainstem that regulate cardiac activity, respiration, and swallowing. The reticular modulation of the lower motor neuron and resultant altered muscle tone are discussed in Chapter 15.

Cardiovascular Activity

The reticular nuclei regulating vasomotor functions of the heart extend from the rostral medulla to the mid-pons. These nuclei receive extensive projections from peripheral receptors and are in part controlled by the hypothalamus. They project information via fibers of the vagus nerve (CN X). Stimulation of the lateral reticular pressor center increases heart rate and causes vasoconstriction. However, stimulation of the depressor center in the lower medulla decreases heart rate and causes vasodilation. Most spinal nerves and some cranial nerves, when stimulated, raise arterial pressure by exciting the pressor region and inhibiting the depressor region. Lesions of the medullary center for cardiovascular control can cause cardiac irregularities and blood pressure changes, both of which are life threatening.

Respiration

Though the primary function of respiration is to maintain the proper level of oxygen in body tissue and remove carbon dioxide through the regulated cycles of inhalation and exhalation, respiration is also the most basic process underlying speech. Changes in the concentration of oxygen or carbon dioxide render an immediate effect on respiratory activity. For example, the higher concentration of carbon dioxide in blood, which is detected by chemoreceptors located in the carotid and aortic bodies, stimulates the respiratory center through inspiratory and expiratory signals to the respiratory muscles.

The primary muscles of respiration are the diaphragm, internal and external intercostals, and abdominal muscles. The contraction of the diaphragm and external intercostal muscles increases the intrathoracic volume but decreases the pleural cavity pressure, thus prompting the inspirational phase, in which air is forced into the pleural cavity according to the Boyle law. Expiration is a passive process controlled by the elasticity of the lungs and the walls of the abdomen and chest. However, forced expiration, as during coughing and defecating, requires muscle contraction from the abdominals and internal intercostals.

Neural Control of Respiration

The neural control of respiration is complex and it involves two control mechanisms: voluntary and autonomic. The nuclei forming the **voluntary respiratory control center** are in the motor cortex. The **autonomic brainstem respiratory center** is formed by several groups of scattered neurons in the pontomedullary RF, with each nucleus making specific contribution to the breathing process (Fig. 18-12; Box 18-6).

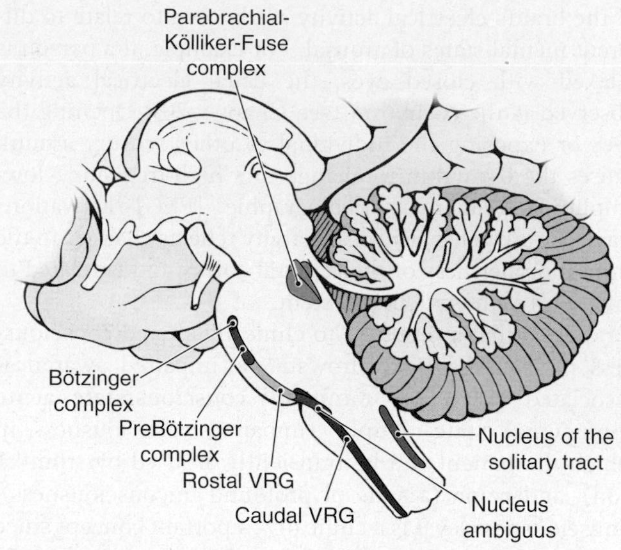

Figure 18-12 Nuclei associated with the autonomic (pontine and medullary) respiratory centers in the brainstem.

Voluntary Respiration Control

Located in the motor cortex, the voluntary respiratory center controls temporary increases and decreases in the rate and depth of breathing owing to different motor activities. Projections from the motor cortex descend through the internal capsule (diencephalon), pes peduncle (midbrain), and pyramidal fibers (medulla) before innervating the spinal motor neurons in the cervical, thoracic, and lumbar regions of the spinal cord, which control the activity of the muscles of respiration.

Automatic Respiration Control

The autonomic respiration controlling center is located in the brainstem. It consists of a group of reticular nuclei

BOX 18-6

Brainstem in Respiratory Function

Acting as a pacemaker, the brainstem respiratory centers regulate the depth, rhythm, and duration of breathing. Thus, brainstem lesions, commonly seen in traumatic brain injuries, can cause respiratory dysfunction. Furthermore, vagus nerve (CN X) dysfunctions, anesthetic drugs, and barbiturates can depress the activity of the respiratory pacemaker cells, causing apnea.

that are scattered in the pontomedullary region. Among others, this brainstem respiratory network includes the medial and lateral parabrachial nuclei, Bötzinger and pre-Bötzinger nuclear complex, ventral respiratory group of nuclei, and the nuclei of the solitary tract (Fig. 18-12). Together they serve as the central pattern generator and regulator for breathing. As a reflexive and autonomic activity of timed inspiration and expiration phases, breathing is initiated by inputs from the chemoreceptors, located in the carotid body and aorta, and pulmonary mechanoreceptors that are present in the lungs. The chemoreceptors respond to reduced levels of oxygen (hypoxia) and increased levels of carbon dioxide (hypercapnia) in the blood. Their insensitivity can lead to syndromes like sudden infant death or congenital central hypoventilation. The pulmonary mechanoreceptors respond to lung dilation. The afferents from the chemoreceptors and pulmonary mechanoreceptors ascend through the vagus (CN X) and glossopharyngeal (CN IX) nerves to the brainstem reticular network.

The descending signals from the respiratory network to the spinal (cervical and thoracic) motor neurons initiate reflexive breathing and control respiratory activity. Efferent projections from C3–C5 (predominantly from C4) form the phrenic nerve, which causes contraction of the diaphragm, the main muscle of respiration (see Chapter 2). Contraction of the diaphragm increases the intrathoracic volume, which begins the cycle of inspiration. Efferent projections from the thoracic regions lead to the contraction of the internal intercostals and abdominal muscles that regulates the forced expiration.

There are four components of the reflexive respiration: regulation of respiratory rhythm, regulations of inspiratory–expiratory phases, and phase switching between inspiration and expiration. The ventral respiratory nuclei of the medulla project to the spinal motor neurons for controlling the expiratory (caudal nuclei) and inspiratory (rostral nuclei) muscles. The lateral parabrachial nuclei are responsible for regulating inspiratory phase of breathing; they do so by limiting the duration of the inspiration phase in the lungs. Based on physical activity and bodily needs, the strong signals from the lateral parabrachial nuclei temporarily would shorten the filling phase of the lungs. However, weaker signals would lengthen the inspirational phase, resulting in excessive filling of the lungs. By limiting the duration of inspiration, these nuclei also contribute to the duration of expiration, which primarily is controlled by the Bötzinger nuclear complex. The medial parabrachial nuclei are responsible for switching the cyclic phases between expiration and inspiration. The pre-Bötzinger nuclear complex sets the rhythm of the breathing cycle (Benarroch, 2007).

Muscles of Respiration

The most important function of the spinal cord for motor speech is its control of the muscles that regulate respiration, a patterned cycle of inhalation and exhalation that not only is vital for survival but also contributes to loudness, an important motor speech process (Table 18-10).

Respiration involves over 15 muscles, the four major groups of which are the diaphragm, abdominals, external intercostals, and internal intercostals. The sternocleidomastoid and scalenus are two additionally important accessory muscles. The motor nuclei from the anterior horns of the C3–C5 (with predominance from C4 through the phrenic nerve) innervate the diaphragm. The efferents to the internal and external intercostals exit from T1–T12. The abdominal muscles receive efferents from the motor nuclei of T6–T12. The diaphragm and external intercostals are the primary muscles of inspiration, whereas the abdominal and internal intercostals participate in forced expiration (Table 18-10).

During the inspiratory phase, contraction of the diaphragm and external intercostals increases the intrathoracic volume, which lowers the pressure within the lungs and thoracic cavity. The reduced intrathoracic pressure forces air (inhalation) into the lungs. Exhalation, on the other hand, is initiated by an increase in intra-abdominal pressure and a decrease in intrathoracic volume caused by the abdominal and internal intercostal muscles. In quiet inspiration, the diaphragm and external intercostals actively participate, whereas quiet exhalation does not require active muscular activity because the elastic recoil

Table 18-10

Motor Innervation of the Muscles of Respiration

Spinal Roots	Muscles	Functions
C3–C5, mainly C4	Diaphragm	Increases intrathoracic volume for inspiration
T1–T12	External intercostals	Increases intrathoracic volume by raising ribs for inspiration
T1–T12	Internal intercostals	Decreases intrathoracic volume by depressing ribs for expiration
T6–T12	Abdominal muscles	Increases intrathoracic pressure for expiration

of the lungs restores intrathoracic volume to the resting level. However, forced inspiration (during exercise) and expiration (while blowing out a candle or coughing) requires active muscle contraction.

Clinical Correlates

A patient with a complete spinal lesion above C3 has complete paralysis of all respiratory muscles and is likely to lose the ability to breathe spontaneously. Such a patient will require artificial respiration/tracheostomy for survival. Patients with a spinal injury below C4 but above T12 display varying degrees of paralysis of all primary respiratory muscles except the diaphragm. With intact control over the diaphragm, such a patient may continue to inhale and quietly exhale because of the elastic recoil of lungs. With full control of diaphragm, inspiration is not a problem; however, with reduced or impaired control over the abdominal and internal intercostal muscles, such a patient would not be able to undertake the forced exhalation needed for coughing, bowel movements, and blowing. In the case of any lesion below T12, the patient's control of respiratory muscles is likely to remain intact (Box 18-7).

Swallowing

The physiology of swallowing has recently become an important clinical issue in communicative disorders because many clinicians are involved with diagnosing and managing disorders of deglutition. As with respiration, the specialized reticular nuclei regulate the swallowing acts by integrating the functions of the following cranial nerves: trigeminal (CN V), facial (CN VII), glossopharyngeal (CN IX), vagus (CN X), and hypoglossal (CN XII). Swallowing is a reflexive action instigated by the sensory and motor components of these cranial nerves along with reticular participation.

Swallowing has two stages: **voluntary** and **involuntary**. The voluntary stage consists of masticating a bolus and moving it into the pharyngeal cavity. The involuntary or reflexive stage involves the passage of the bolus through the pharynx and esophagus. The voluntary stage covers the act of chewing, bolus formation, and bolus movement in the oral cavity. It ends as the upward and backward motion of the tongue forces the bolus against the palate. As the bolus presses against the palate to enter the pharynx, the involuntary stage begins through sensory projections from the posterior palate to the reticular swallowing center in the lower pons and upper medulla.

The reticular swallowing center directs projections to the adjacent respiratory center and subsequently to the nuclei of trigeminal (CN V), facial (CN VII), glossopharyngeal (CN IX), vagus (CN X), and hypoglossal (CN XII) nerves, which initiate a series of reflexive motor actions to ensure proper breathing management while the bolus passes through the pharynx. Major reflexive actions include the upward movement of the palate to close the nasopharynx, backward and downward movement of the epiglottis to seal off the glottis, raising of the larynx to close the airway, and enlarging the esophageal opening to allow entrance of the bolus. As the bolus passes the pharyngeal phase, the reticular respiratory center regulates the reopening of the respiratory passageway.

Brainstem lesions interrupting the afferent and efferent projections of the RF also alter the integrity of the swallowing reflex and cause aspiration. Common disturbances of swallowing seen in neurogenic patients are poor mastication, delayed swallowing reflex, reduced peristalsis of the bolus through the pharynx, and aspiration.

Vomiting

The reticular nuclei that regulate vomiting are in the medulla. They receive inputs from the oropharynx and gastrointestinal tract. Noxious impulses mediating irritations of the intestinal tract and oropharynx initiate reflexive vomiting. Projections from the vomiting center in the medulla descend through the fibers of the glossopharyngeal (CN IX) and vagus nervea (CN X) and coordinate the contraction of the abdominal, diaphragmatic, and intercostal muscles. The oropharyngeal musculature, which facilitates vomiting, works with all of these muscles.

Coughing

Afferents mediating irritation from laryngeal and tracheal lining tissues initiate the coughing reflex via the vagus nerve (CN X) and solitary tract nuclei. As with the vomiting reflex, the diaphragmatic, abdominal, and intercostal muscles are involved; however, they contract alternately, not simultaneously.

BOX 18-7

Spinal Lesions Affecting and the Muscles of Respiration

A complete spinal transection above C3 causes a complete paralysis of all respiratory muscles; patients with such a lesion lose the ability to spontaneously breathe and require immediately artificial respiration/tracheostomy for survival. Patients with a spinal injury below C4 but above T12 exhibit varying degrees of paralysis of all respiratory muscles except the diaphragm. With intact control over the diaphragm, these patients can inhale and quietly exhale because of the elastic recoil of lungs, but they cannot undertake activity related to forced expiration. Since respiration is the foundation of the phonation and speech intelligibility, a knowledge of spinal innervation of the respirators is important.

Autonomic Functions

The RF contributes to the autonomic system through its **reticulobulbar** and **reticulospinal** fiber projections. Input to the reticular autonomic regulatory system comes from limbic and diencephalic structures of the forebrain, which include the orbitofrontal cortex, cingulate gyrus, amygdala, hippocampus, hypothalamus, and the medial, anterior, and dorsal groups of the thalamic nuclei. Reticular projections regulate hypothalamic centers specializing in endocrine production and release, temperature, food and fluid intake, sexual activity, diurnal body rhythms, blood electrolyte balance, visceral and autonomic functions, emotional states, and learning.

Biologic Rhythms

A self-regulated internal clock, a characteristic of all living systems, determines the turnover rates of macromolecules, annual seasonal variations, and daily environmental changes in the body. Biologic rhythms govern reproductive cycles and development, division, and death of cells. Many rhythms depend on an intact hypothalamus with its multiple connections, including those from the RF. The RF is also indirectly involved in neural control of the pineal gland, a structure that participates in regulating circadian rhythms (repetitive cycles or biorhythm).

Self-Awareness

Deep cellular layers of the superior colliculus receive multimodal inputs that outline the space around the body. This input stems from overlapping visual, auditory, and somatic stimuli, representing various temporal and spatial reference points surrounding the body. These stimuli form a three-dimensional body image in the midbrain RF. The RF projects this image to nonspecific and specific thalamic nuclei and thus enables humans to have conscious self-awareness. The thalamus in turn relays information to the neocortex for further in-depth analysis.

Head and Eye Movement

The RF regulates the rotation of the head and eyes. Through fibers of the medial longitudinal fasciculus, the RF mediates impulses connecting various participating cranial and cervical muscles that control head and eye movements (see Chapter 10).

Reticular Neurotransmitters

The RF uses a variety of neurotransmitters to communicate with the brain, spinal cord, and neighboring reticular regions. These neurotransmitters are synthesized by a specialized population of cells (see Chapter 5). A monoamine imbalance can generate somatic and psychic symptoms such as excitement, agitation, depression, anxiety, and insomnia. Overabundance of norepinephrine can lead to the somatic symptoms of rapid heart rate, increased blood pressure, dry mouth, and cessation of intestinal peristalsis, whereas low levels of serotonin are associated with depression and anxiety.

Serotonin

Electrical discharge firing rates of serotonin and noradrenergic neurons fluctuate with sleep and wakefulness. Therefore, they participate in the general activity level of the CNS. Serotonin is thought to be concerned with overall levels of arousal and slow-wave sleep as well as severe depression (Box 18-5). In the treatment of depression, antidepressant drugs appear to enhance the concentration of serotonin at the synapse by reducing its uptake. Serotonin is also an important contributor to the descending pain-control system.

Norepinephrine

The **locus ceruleus** is the major noradrenergic reticular nucleus. Its noradrenergic projections have a profound influence on brain function and are known to regulate brain tone by inhibiting background activity, thus enhancing the signal-to-noise ratio in the brain. Behaviorally, the locus ceruleus contributes to the generation of REM sleep (see Chapter 20). Along with other noradrenergic neurons, the locus ceruleus is also thought to mediate attention and vigilance. Depression can be treated with drugs that enhance the transmission of norepinephrine at the synapse.

Dopamine

Dopamine projections to the cortex and limbic structures seem to influence cognitive functions and motivation. Cocaine and amphetamine, drugs that enhance the action of dopamine, induce syndromes resembling paranoid schizophrenia. Drugs of substance abuse cause dopamine release in the nucleus accumbens, suggesting that this mesolimbic projection may be associated with a sense of pleasure. Thorazine and related drugs used in the treatment of schizophrenia block dopamine receptors, which suggests that the mesolimbic and mesocortical dopaminergic systems may be involved in this psychotic disorder.

Enkephalins

Enkephalins in the RF contribute to pain suppression. As a subgroup of the endorphin opiates, they are primarily present in the PNS. They form local neuronal circuits found in the gastrointestinal system, which respond to opiates by reducing gastrointestinal motility. Abdominal pain (colic) often responds best to opiates.

Substance P

Substance P has a slow and long-lasting inhibitory effect on neuronal firing. It attenuates pain and is present in the RF and spinal dorsal root ganglia. Fibers of the opiate-like enkephalin cells form axoaxonic synapses with substance P fibers.

This connectivity is thought to control the pain that may occur with movement disorders, such as Parkinson disease.

γ-Aminobutyric Acid

y-Aminobutyric acid (GABA), the most prevalent inhibitory transmitter, dominates in local circuit neurons. It is produced from the decarboxylation of glutamate. GABA serves as the inhibitory neurotransmitter from the Purkinje cells to the deep cerebellar nuclei, from the striatum to the globus pallidus and substantia nigra, and from the globus pallidus and substantia nigra to the thalamus.

Tranquilizers, such as diazepam (Valium), bind to GABA receptors and increase the effects of the transmitter released at GABA synapses. Abnormal movements, as seen in Huntington chorea, are caused by the loss of GABA neurons in the caudate and putamen. This elevates the ratio of dopamine to acetylcholine, producing abnormal movements. However, a reduced ratio of dopamine to acetylcholine causes the abnormal motor movements of Parkinsonism (see Chapter 15).

Summary of the Reticular Formation

A diffuse core of nuclei in the brainstem, the RF serves as a fine-tuner of cortical functions. With extensive dendrites and axons, it regulates sensorimotor, visceral, and cognitive functions. An important function of the RF is to regulate cortical arousal, which is measured by various patterns of brain electrical activity. It also regulates functions such as sleep and awake states.

Clinical symptoms that may occur after lesions of the RF are irregularities in sleep, blood pressure, pulse rate, respiration, vigilance, and states of consciousness. Motor dysfunctions may include tremors and altered muscle tone, ranging from hypertonic rigidity to flaccidity. Speech and swallowing disorders may occur after lesions in the caudal brainstem RF.

CLINICAL CORRELATES

CASE STUDIES FOR PROBLEM SOLVING

CASE ONE (18-1)

A 55-year-old schoolteacher consulted his physician for what he thought was a strange feeling of nervousness, which resulted in embarrassment and frequent episodes of bladder incontinence. Other sensorimotor functions were normal. A spinal MRI study revealed a tumor in the sacral region of the spinal cord.

Question: How does sacral lesion cause bladder incontinence?

Case (18-1) Discussion: See discussion of case studies

CASE TWO (18-2)

A 45-year-old unpaid politician consulted his physician about his visual problem subsequent to the asymmetrical pupil sizes. On examination, he exhibited right pupil constriction (miosis). Additional signs included ptosis of the right upper eyelid and an inability to perspire on the forehead. The attending physician suspected Horner syndrome, an autonomic nervous system impairment, and a spinal MRI study confirmed an infarct in the right cervical sympathetic chain.

Question: How does a cervical sympathetic chain lesion cause these symptoms?

Case (18-2) Discussion: See discussion of case studies

CASE THREE (18-3)

A 25-year-old woman was very slim and had a history of poor appetite, weight loss, and episodes of high fever. She had lost interest in sex and her menses were irregular. She drank large quantities of water but considered her behavior to be normal. Her physician suspected it to be a case of anorexia subsequent to a lower diencephalic lesion.

Question: How can a lower diencephalic lesion cause these symptoms?

Case (18-3) Discussion: See discussion of case studies

CASE FOUR (18-4)

A 35-year-old man had a history of temporal lobe seizures. During his seizure attacks, he would become violent, throwing objects at people. He frequently harmed his wife and abused his children. Strangely, he retained no memory of his actions.

Question: How did seizure activity in the temporal (limbic) lobe affect memory?

Case (18-4) Discussion: See discussion of case studies

(Continued)

CASE FIVE (18-5) *(CONTINUED)*

A 25-year-old automobile salesperson was in a head-on car collision in which his forehead slammed against the dashboard and he was unconscious for 3 days. When he recovered, he had no memory of the accident or the events preceding it. According to his wife, he became a totally different person after regaining consciousness. He lost energy, did not want to do anything, and had no ambition. Physically, his actions were slow and he was not very clear in his thinking. With faulty reasoning, he could not think abstractly or make decisions. He also lost interest in grooming and hygiene.

Question: How can you account for the loss of consciousness, memory loss, and personality changes in this patient after traumatic accident?

Case (18-5) Discussion: See discussion of case studies

CASE SIX (18-6)

On his first day of work at a hospital, a rookie speech–language pathologist met a neurologist who informally began discussing a 20-year-old traumatic brain injury patient whom she had seen that morning. The patient had no apparent cognitive or communicative impairments but presented with an excessive perspiration, irregular sleep–wake cycle, and altered sexual behavior with no reported libido. His speech was a little slurred as he spoke with a mouth full of saliva. "This is a classical case of a lesion in the lower diencephalon," she stated before rushing off to a call on her pager.

Question: How can you explain the occurrence and relatedness of symptoms?

Case (18-6) Discussion: See discussion of case studies

CASE SEVEN (18-7)

A 19-year-old man with traumatic brain injury caused by a car accident was referred for a speech–language–cognitive assessment. The attending speech–language pathologist SLP noted the following:

- Mild retrograde amnesia
- Profound anterograde amnesia
- Agitated behavior
- Uninhibited expression of sexuality
- Inappropriate and vulgar language

Question: How can you relate these symptoms to the associated damaged structure?

Case (18-7) Discussion: See discussion of case studies

SUMMARY OF THE AXIAL BRAIN

The ANS, limbic lobe, hypothalamus, and RF are functionally integrated structures with nebulous anatomic borders. Working together, they influence the vital automatic and unconscious bodily functions that are indispensable for reproduction and survival. The system's interwoven cellular networks modulate visceral, somatic, autonomic, endocrine, alimentary, vascular, respiratory, and sexual behaviors. Each of these systems is represented by specialized overlapping cellular networks that extend throughout the septum, hypothalamus, and brainstem RF.

By using sympathetic and parasympathetic projections, the ANS controls visceral functions, regulating body homeostasis and the functioning of the cardiovascular, pulmonary, digestive, urinary, and reproductive systems. The integrated activity of the limbic system regulates the emotional and motivational aspects of behavior fundamental to survival, such as feeding, mating, aggression, and flight.

The hypothalamus, as the central regulator of the ANS and endocrine functions, controls visceral functions, including vasodilation, body homeostasis, reproduction, hunger, and the intake of water and food. The neurosecretory cells of the hypothalamus regulate pituitary gland hormone production and endocrine body functions.

By integrating stimuli with internally generated thoughts, feelings, and emotions, the RF regulates the homeostatic state of the brain essential for controlling sleep and vigilance. It also controls metabolic, respiratory, visceral, sensorimotor, neuroendocrine, emotional, and cognitive activities. A single lesion of the reticular system may generate complex illnesses characterized by a variety of symptoms, including insomnia, headaches, depression, tremors, aggression, and forgetfulness.

REVIEW QUESTIONS

1. Complete the following statements using the appropriate technical terms:
   A. The activation and regulation of cortical arousal are perhaps the best known functions of the ________.
   B. As a subdivision of the nervous system, the ________ regulates the activities of the heart, blood vessels, and lungs.
   C. Resulting from a hypothalamic lesion, ________ is marked by the absence of thirst.
   D. ________ represents a long-term memory disturbance which is marked by impaired recall of past memories and failure to remember new details.

E. ________ is an impaired ability to swallow.

F. In ________, a reduced exchange of oxygen and carbon dioxide causes the brain cells to die secondary to ________.

G. As part of the three-layered cortex, the ________ is related to the registration and consolidation of memory.

H. Functionally related to the limbic system, the ________ regulates visceral, somatic, and metabolic systems.

I. Associated with the bitemporal pathology, the ________ syndrome is marked by psychic blindness, increased oral tendency, and abnormal sexual behavior.

J. Representing a natural rhythm, the ________ rhythm occurs once each 24 hours.

K. As part of the limbic lobe, the ________ has been linked with anxiety and obsessive behaviors.

L. Consisting of multiple polysynaptic descending and ascending connections, the ________ not only controls autonomic functions (e.g., respiration, blood pressure, and thermoregulation), but also regulates behavioral states such as alertness, cortical arousal, and sleep.

M. The antidiuretic hormone named ________ causes water retention in the body.

N. A complex neuronal circuitry in the mammalian forebrain involving the hippocampus, fornix, mammillary body, anterior thalamic nuclei, cingulate gyrus, and parahippocampal, the ________ is dedicated to experiences of and responses to emotion.

2. Match each of the following structures with its associated function:

A. sympathetic system	a. control of the heart, lungs, blood vessels, and the organs of the digestive, reproductive, and urogenital systems
B. parasympathetic systems	b. energy expenditure during fight, freight, and flight experience
C. hypothalamus	c. energy restoration
D. limbic lobe	d. regulation of autonomic and endocrinic function
E. reticular formation	e. control of motivation, moods, and emotional drive
F. autonomic nervous system	f. maintenance of cortical arousal and brainstem-mediated visceral activities

3. Name the core structures of the limbic lobe.

4. Name three primary functions of the limbic lobe.

5. Which part of the axial–limbic brain has dedicated circuitries for the water intake, food intake, body temperature, and endocrinic secretion?

6. Match each of the hormones with its associated dysfunction:

A. growth hormone	a. dwarfism/gigantism
B. thyroid-stimulating hormone	b. reduced milk secretion
C. gonadotropic hormone	c. impaired sexual function
D. adrenocorticotropic hormone	d. low body development, low metabolism, and slow mental activity
E. prolactin	e. impaired glucose synthesis

7. Which structure of the axial–limbic brain regulates cortical arousal, cardiovascular activity, respiration, swallowing, vomiting, and coughing?

8. Why is it that a lesion in the brainstem is so damaging?

9. Match each of the activities by matching it with the associated autonomic system:

A. decreased lacrimal secretion	a. sympathetic system
B. decreased intestinal secretion	b. parasympathetic system
C. decreased gastric secretion	
D. reduced digestive tract activity	
E. increased lacrimal secretion	
F. increased intestinal secretion	
G. increased sweat secretion	
H. pupil constriction	

10. Match the following pathways with the structures it connects:

A. fornix	a. hypothalamus and the midbrain (tegmental) region
B. mammillothalamic tract	b. hypothalamus (mammillary bodies) with the hippocampus
C. stria medullaris	c. hypothalamus (mammillary body) to the thalamus
D. stria terminalis	d. septum with habenula thalamic nucleus
E. medial forebrain bundle	e. hypothalamus and amygdala

11. At what area of the neuraxis are the autonomic respiratory centers located?

12. Which reticular nucleus with role in respiration receives projections from the chemoreceptors of the carotid body?

19

Cerebral Cortex: Higher Mental Functions**

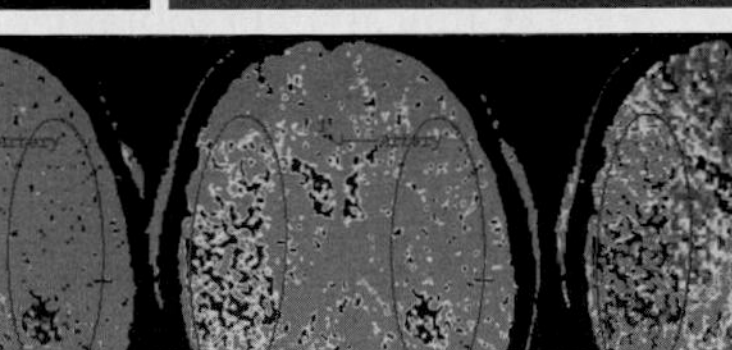

LEARNING OBJECTIVES

After studying this chapter, students should be able to:

- Describe the functional importance of the primary and associational cortical areas
- Discuss major mental functions of the brain
- Describe the relationship between cerebral dominance and handedness
- Describe the neurologic diagnosis of behavioral deficits
- Describe the linguistic characteristics of major aphasia types
- Discuss the neurology of apraxias
- Outline the neurology of reading and writing
- Describe the neurology of motor speech disorders
- Discuss the neurology of cognition with reference to dementia and traumatic brain injuries
- Solve related clinical problems

Key Terms :

Abulia	**Akinetic mutism**
Acalculia	**Anosognosia**
Agnosia	**Frontal lobe syndrome**
Agraphia	

Chapters 1 to 18 focus on the structural organization of the nervous system and the sensorimotor functions that are organized bilaterally in the brain. The true uniqueness of the human brain, however, lies in its ability to serve the higher mental functions, such as reasoning, memory, language, speech, calculations, praxis, and recognition of objects (gnosis). These functions are asymmetrically organized in the cerebral hemispheres. Cerebral dominance, or the specialization of one cerebral hemisphere in specific functions, relates to the unique cytoarchitectural organization of the brain.

As the site of higher mental functions, the cerebral cortex, a massive, convoluted structure makes up an area of about 2.5 ft^2 and contains as many as 20 plus billion neurons. The brain is divided into four primary lobes: frontal, parietal, temporal, and occipital. Each lobe has a relatively constant cortical anatomy, which is divided by sulci or fissures into discrete gyri (see Figs. 2-4 and 2-5).

METHODS OF STUDY

Neurology is the study of diseases that affect the nervous system. Classically, neurology depended on observations of behavior gathered during the medical examination of stroke patients, then laboriously correlated with brain lesions seen at autopsy.

Currently, brain imaging modalities permit the simultaneous visualization of brain structure and examination of associated behavior. Computed tomography (CT), magnetic resonance imaging (MRI), positron-emission tomography (PET), and single photon emission computed tomography (SPECT) are commonly used neuroimaging methods (see Chapter 20). The diagnostic brain imaging techniques of functional MRI, PET, and SPECT can also be used to study cognitive functions in normal human subjects. These techniques allow for visualizing the brain areas that are active during specific neurolinguistic activities and identifying the networks of interrelated brain regions. Our knowledge of brain structure and function has advanced much more rapidly since the introduction of these imaging techniques.

Another area of advancement in brain localization is electrical stimulation. The electroencephalogram is an electrical study of neuronal firing patterns in the brain. Computer-assisted techniques such as brain electrical activity mapping increase the anatomic accuracy of the electroencephalogram but are still less precise in anatomic localization than are CT and MRI. Electrical stimulation of the awake patient, used as a guide for excision of epileptic foci in the brain, has further delineated areas of the brain that are important for language and speech (Bhatnagar et al., 2000; Ojemann et al., 1989). Most recently, transcranial magnetic stimulation has been used to activate brain regions noninvasively.

**Written by Haward Kirshner, MD. Dept of Neurology. Vanderbilt College of Medicine.

FUNCTIONAL LOCALIZATION IN THE BRAIN

Clinical data obtained from imaging studies and from patients undergoing surgical ablation of brain structures for epilepsy or brain tumor have helped reveal the functional regional anatomy of the brain in terms of the four major lobes and their cortical gyri. These gyri, or parts of them, operate as modules dedicated to specific cognitive or behavioral functions. The modules act somewhat like the brain centers that 19th-century physicians described, but they are organized not as individual centers but as parts of interacting networks, interconnecting modules in different regions or lobes of the brain. The cortical modules also connect with subcortical centers, such as the basal ganglia and other deep brain structures. The emerging understanding of the major functions of the four lobes of each hemisphere of the brain is summarized briefly here.

In general, the cortex of the brain is divided into primary motor areas, primary sensory areas (for vision, hearing, touch, smell, and possibly taste), and association areas (see also Chapter 2). The association cortex is divided into unimodal association cortices, such as the visual and auditory association cortices, and heteromodal association cortices. The heteromodal cortical areas include the parietal cortex, a sensory association area for interaction between the senses, and the prefrontal cortex, which provides the executive function for the entire brain. Executive function refers to the processes that decide which of the many incoming sensory stimuli should receive attention and in what order and what responses or motor outputs should be activated, and in which order. These heteromodal association cortices represent the areas of largest expansion of the brain from apes to humans, and they are critically important in making possible the extraordinary cognitive and behavioral capabilities that our species, *Homo sapiens*, has attained.

Frontal Lobe

The posterior limit of the frontal lobe, on the lateral surface of the brain, is the precentral gyrus, which contains motor cells of the primary motor cortex (Brodmann area 4). This cortical strip carries a map of the contralateral side of the body (homunculus), with cells programmed to produce contractions of specific muscles or specific movements (see Fig. 2-6). The motor homunculus has its face and lips in the most inferior part of the gyrus, just above the sylvian fissure; the hand and arm are above that, and the leg and foot extend over the superior part of the gyrus and continue downward on the medial aspect of the hemisphere. Stimulation of cells in the motor cortex produces specific movements of contralateral parts of the body. The large size of the cortical representation of the thumb, fingers, and hand compared to the arm reflects the importance of fine finger movements. Similarly, the large space reserved for the mouth and lips indicates the importance of speech.

Anterior to the primary motor cortex is the premotor cortex, which is involved in the initiation and planning of skilled motor movements. Just anterior to the face area of the motor strip is the cortical Broca area (Brodmann area 44 and possibly 45), thought to program patterned movements of the vocal apparatus to produce phonemes and words. Damage to this area results in Broca aphasia, a syndrome of nonfluent speech, in the presence of at least partially preserved comprehension (to be discussed later in the chapter). Brodmann area 8, in the superior frontal lobe, is involved in movement of the eyes and head to the contralateral side. The supplementary motor cortex is on the medial side of the hemisphere, anterior to the leg area of the primary motor cortex. Stimulation of this area produces complex postures or patterned movements. Lesions in this area also disrupt the initiation of speech.

Another function of the dorsolateral frontal lobe, the frontal heteromodal association cortex of the brain, is critically related to executive functions, as described earlier (Goldman-Rakic, 1996). The dorsolateral frontal lobe is also important for working memory, also called immediate memory or attention span.

Functions of the prefrontal cortex anterior to the premotor area and the orbitofrontal cortex are quite complex and are incompletely understood. Lesions of the frontal cortex may produce disinhibition of speech and other behaviors, known as the **frontal lobe syndrome**. Patients with lesions of the orbitofrontal cortex may have normal intelligence and memory, but families may state that the individuals have totally changed personality, marked by short temper, irritability, poor impulse control, sociopathic (antisocial) personality, and a general tendency to act out. Blumer and Benson (1975) refer to this behavior as **pseudopsychopathic**, in that it resembles the behavior of a sociopathic personality.

Such syndromes are frequently seen after frontal head injuries. The lateral frontal convexities also are involved in the initiation of behavior. Bilateral lesions of this area tend to produce a reduction or cessation of behavior, often referred to as **akinetic mutism** or **abulia**. Patients may sit and stare passively, not speak, or may respond only in a whisper or after a delay. This type of frontal lobe syndrome is called **pseudo depressed**. In general, frontal lobe syndromes resemble psychiatric disorders because they involve profound alterations of behavior and personality, yet the basic cognitive functions, such as memory, language, visuospatial functioning, and elementary motor, and sensory functions remain intact.

On the medial surface of the frontal lobe lies the cingulum, or cingulate gyrus. This gyrus is a part of the limbic system, or **Papez circuit**, of projections from the hippocampus via the septum and fornix to the mamillary bodies and then to the anterior thalamic nuclei. Projections then go to the cingulate gyrus and back to the hippocampus. This circuit is important for memory and for elementary limbic functions, such as motivation and drive (see Chapter 16). The cingulate gyrus is also important for the experience of pain.

Parietal Lobe

The parietal lobe consists of a superior and inferior parietal lobule. The anterior part of the parietal lobe contains Brodmann areas 3, 1, and 2, which are devoted to sensory function. In the inferior parietal lobule are Brodmann areas 39 and 40, the angular and supramarginal gyri. The inferior parietal lobule in the left hemisphere is tied to language function, especially reading and naming, to calculations and arithmetic, and to telling left from right. This region is the second part of the heteromodal association cortex, along with the dorsolateral frontal lobe. The parietal association cortex may be thought of as a center for the association of information from different sensory modalities, such as vision, hearing, and touch.

Gerstmann (1930) associated four deficits with lesions of the left inferior parietal lobule: **agraphia**, **acalculia**, right–left confusion, and finger agnosia (loss of the ability to know which finger is which). The inferior parietal lobule in the right hemisphere is involved with the body schema. Right inferior parietal lobe lesions produce neglect of the left side of the body. The superior parts of the parietal cortex are devoted to visuospatial and constructional functions and higher-level cortical sensory functions, such as stereognosis (recognition of palpated shapes) and graphesthesia (ability to recognize letters or numbers drawn on the skin).

Lesions of the right parietal lobe produce important neurobehavioral deficits, including left-side neglect, denial of the presence of a motor deficit (**anosognosia**), and dressing apraxia (inability to place garments correctly in relation to body parts). Other spatial and topographical dysfunctions associated with right parietal lobe lesions are difficulty finding one's way around and an inability to draw or read a map. Constructional tasks, such as copying figures, drawing a clock or house, and bisecting a line, may reveal difficulty with spatial relationships or neglect of the left side of space. Although speech and language are relatively well preserved in patients with right parietal lesions, the emotional intonation of speech may be lacking, as may the ability to comprehend emotional tone in the speech of others. Patients with strokes or other pathology in the right parietal region may fail to grasp sarcasm or humor. They also may fail to respect the proper turn-taking of a normal conversation, or they respond to questions asked of the patient in the next bed.

Some researchers consider this aspect of language the pragmatics of communication, as opposed to semantics (meanings) or syntax (grammar). Such deficits mean, in effect, that the patient may understand what is said, but not how it is said. In other words, the patient understands only the literal meaning of the words and not the emotional, humorous, ironic, or sarcastic meanings that reflect the tone in which the words are spoken. Such "paralinguistic" deficits are disabling to patients in the social world and affect communication even when speech and language functions are preserved. Emotional indifference often characterizes the mood of these patients; they may be undisturbed by left-sided paralysis or by the impending loss of ability to work. These right hemisphere deficits, expressed over time, change the personality of affected individuals. Families often have more difficulty accepting a change in personality after a stroke or brain injury than they do in accepting handicaps, such as the inability to speak or understand language, seen after left hemisphere injuries.

Temporal Lobe

The superior temporal gyrus of each hemisphere contains the primary auditory cortex (Brodmann areas 41 and 42), which lies buried within the sylvian fissure (see Fig. 9-8). Lesions of the primary auditory cortex on both sides cause cortical deafness. Such patients are rarely totally deaf and often hear some pure tones. In some patients, bilateral superior temporal damage results in **pure word deafness** (inability to understand spoken words, with preserved pure tone hearing and recognition of nonverbal sounds). Another bitemporal syndrome is auditory agnosia, or the inability to recognize nonverbal sounds. Finally, phonagnosia refers to the inability to recognize familiar voices.

The left superior temporal gyrus contains the Wernicke area, which is critical to the comprehension of spoken language. There may be a language comprehension area in the inferior temporal gyrus and adjacent fusiform gyrus, as identified by electrical stimulation (the basal temporal language area, BTLA). It is interesting that surgical ablation of this area usually does not cause lasting aphasia. Therefore, the BTLA may be part of a network involved in understanding language but may not be a necessary component to the functioning of the language comprehension system.

The right temporal lobe is a silent, or noneloquent, area of the brain because surgical resection of this area produces only very subtle deficits. Acute lesions of the right temporal lobe, however, can produce syndromes of acute confusion and delusional (false belief) thinking, or delirium. Appreciation of rhythm and musical qualities may be affected by right temporal lesions, along with deficits in nonverbal memory. In general, the medial temporal areas, such as the hippocampus, together with their connections to the thalamus, septal area, and cingulate gyrus of the medial frontal lobes, are most clearly related to memory. Bilateral lesions produce lasting loss of new learning and recent memory. Unilateral left medial temporal lesions produce disorders of verbal memory, whereas unilateral right temporal lesions produce nonverbal memory loss.

Occipital Lobe

The most posterior, medial poles of the occipital lobes are the primary visual cortices (Brodmann area 17). Damage to this cortex on one side produces a contralateral hemianopic visual field defect in both eyes. Damage to both sides may produce cortical blindness. Some patients with cortical blindness are unaware of their blindness and confabulate descriptions of objects and scenes they claim to see (Anton syndrome). In recent years, emphasis has been placed on a dorsal visual pathway through the parietal lobe, involved with spatial aspects of visual perception, seeing where something is, as opposed to a ventral visual pathway through the temporal lobe, involved in identifying what one sees. Areas adjacent to the primary visual area (Brodmann areas 18 and 19) are called the visual association cortex and are thought to contribute to complex visual analysis. Lesions of these areas on both sides produce a complex visual syndrome called visual **agnosia**.

DISORDERS OF CORTICAL FUNCTIONS

Cerebral Dominance and Functional Specialization

Since Broca's observations in 1861, it has been known that in most humans the left hemisphere is at least relatively dominant for language. Virtually 99% of right-handed people and most left-handed people have left hemisphere dominance for language (Rasmussen and Milner, 1977). Handedness has some correlation to cerebral dominance, so left-handed individuals are more likely than right-handed people to have right hemisphere language dominance. However, most left-handers still become aphasic if the left hemisphere is damaged, and only a few become aphasic if the right hemisphere is damaged. Some left-handed individuals appear to have mixed dominance, such as having speech expression in the left hemisphere and comprehension in the right hemisphere.

The right hemisphere, often called the minor hemisphere, serves many nonlanguage functions. As discussed with reference to the parietal lobes, right hemisphere functions include visuospatial and constructional tasks, knowledge of maps and topography, dressing, emotional feeling and processing, production of emotional intonation of speech, and music appreciation.

Cerebral dominance may have structural correlates. Geschwind and Levitsky (1968) reported that right-handed people have a longer planum temporale in the left hemisphere than in the right (see Fig. 9-10). Similar asymmetries have been described in newborn infants and in illiterate people, suggesting that these anatomic asymmetries are genetically programmed, not acquired through use. Cerebral asymmetries also have been reaffirmed using CT and MRI studies. The relationship of such asymmetries to language dominance holds true in groups, but it is not sufficiently definite to be predictive of dominance in individual patients.

Speech and Language Disorders

Speech and language disorders have long held great interest for students of the nervous system. First, the ability to communicate verbally sets humans apart from other animal species. Second, language disorders were the first behavioral or cognitive impairments to be correlated with disease processes involving specific areas of the brain, ever since, they have served as an important source of knowledge about the correlation of brain structure with behavior.

Motor Speech Disorders

Motor speech disorders consist of abnormal speech articulation in the absence of any language disorder. Abnormal motor speech control, or dysarthria, can involve abnormal strength or place of articulation, abnormal timing or speed of articulatory movement, or abnormal voicing. Dysarthric patients can comprehend both spoken and written language, and their speech output, if comprehensible, can be transcribed into normal language. Darley et al. (1975), in a comprehensive study of dysarthric speech at the Mayo Clinic and later reaffirmed by Duffy (2005), divide these neurogenic dysarthrias into six types: **flaccid**, **spastic**, **ataxic**, **hypokinetic**, **hyperkinetic**, and **mixed**.

Flaccid dysarthria results from lesions of the bulbar muscles, neuromuscular junction, cranial nerves, and anterior horn cells of the brainstem nuclei and is characterized by hypernasal, breathy speech with imprecisely articulated consonants. Spastic dysarthria is seen in patients with bilateral lesions of the motor cortex or corticobulbar tracts. Speech characteristics involve harsh, strain-and-strangle speech, with a slow speaking rate, low pitch, and imprecisely articulated consonants. A variant of spastic dysarthria is unilateral upper motor neuron dysarthria, resulting from a unilateral lesion, such as a stroke. The same characteristics pertain but are less severe.

Ataxic dysarthria, seen in cerebellar disorders, involves irregular cadence or prosody of speech with long pauses and sudden explosions of sound, abnormal and sometimes excessively equal stress on specific syllables, and imprecisely articulated consonants. This pattern is sometimes called scanning speech. Some patients simply speak in a very slow pattern, similar to an exaggerated regional drawl. Hypokinetic dysarthria, classically seen in Parkinson disease, is associated with decreased and monotonous loudness and pitch, occasional rushes of syllables, occasional pauses, and some imprecisely articulated consonants. Hyperkinetic dysarthria, seen in chorea and related movement disorders, including Huntington chorea, is characterized by variable rate, excessive variation in loudness and timing, and distorted vowels. In dystonia, this form of dysarthria can also involve harsh strain-and-strangle speech, with imprecisely articulated consonants.

Mixed dysarthria can involve combinations of any of the other five types. Common examples include **amyotrophic lateral sclerosis** (ALS), in which spastic and flaccid elements coexist, and multiple sclerosis, in which spastic and ataxic characteristics predominate. In practice, there is considerable overlap among the categories of dysarthria.

Apraxia of Speech

Apraxia of speech is difficult to separate from aphasia. Speech apraxia entails abnormal articulation of sequences of phonemes, usually with inconsistent error patterns from one attempt to the next, in contrast to the consistent misarticulation of the dysarthrias. Apraxia of speech is an inability to program sequences of sounds, especially consonants. Consonants are more often substituted than distorted. Apraxia of speech is most obvious with polysyllabic words. Difficulty with initial consonants is common, and speech takes on a hesitant, groping quality. A patient may attempt to say a word like *catastrophe* five times and produce five different errors or may achieve the correct pronunciation once or twice. Apraxia of speech is only rarely seen without aphasia. More commonly, apraxia of speech is part of an aphasic deficit, particularly Broca aphasia.

Key Terms:

Agraphesthesia	**Isolation syndrome**
Agraphia	**Transcortical motor aphasia**
Alexia	
Apraxia	**Transcortical sensory aphasia**
Broca aphasia	
Conduction aphasia	**Wernicke aphasia**

Aphasia

Aphasia is an acquired disorder of language functions secondary to brain disease (Alexander and Benson, 1992). This definition excludes developmental or congenital language problems (dysphasia), motor speech or articulation disorders (dysarthria, dysphonia, and pure apraxia of speech), and impaired thought processes (especially abnormal language expression in schizophrenia, bipolar affective disorder, and other psychoses). Language deficits in dementia are a more complex issue, as these often combine focal language disorders resembling aphasia with more general cognitive loss.

Broca Aphasia

The French physician Paul Broca first described Broca aphasia in 1861. It is characterized by nonfluent, often halting, dysarthric, and ungrammatical speech in which meaning is conveyed largely by information-carrying items, such as nouns and verbs, leaving out the minor structural words (Table 19-1). Naming is also deficient, but the patient can often pronounce the first letter or phoneme (tip-of-the-tongue phenomenon). Auditory comprehension often seems relatively normal, although deficits may occur in comprehension of multistep commands or in sentences with complex grammatical structure.

Those with Broca aphasia tend to have difficulty comprehending complex syntax, just as they have difficulty producing such syntax. For example, a person with Broca aphasia might have difficulty with a sentence such as "The book Bill gave to Betty was thick." The patient might understand that a book was given but not specify who gave and who received the book. Deficits in comprehension can virtually always be detected on standard language batteries. Repetition in Broca aphasia is usually halting and reduced in fluency. Reading is often more severely affected than auditory comprehension.

Patients exhibit writing deficits, not only because most of these individuals have right hemiparesis (paralysis of right arm and leg), forcing them to write with the nondominant left hand, but because of the damage to the left frontal lobe. Patients with Broca aphasia have awkward handwriting and spell poorly; many cannot write even single words or short phrases. This agraphia of Broca aphasia greatly exceeds the difficulty normal persons have in writing with the left, or nondominant hand. If forced to use the nondominant hand because of a fracture of the right arm or writer's cramp, normal people learn to write quite successfully.

Lesions of Broca aphasia involve the left frontal region. Broca identified the area as the posterior part of the inferior frontal gyrus, although both of his patients had much more extensive lesions. Mohr et al. (1978) found that

Table 19-1

Language Features of Common Types of Aphasia

Feature	Broca	Wernicke	Global	Conduction	Anomia
Spontaneous speech	Nonfluent	Fluent and paraphasic	Nonfluent	Fluent	Fluent with pauses
Naming	Impaired	Paraphasic	Poor	Variable	Most impaired
Comprehension	Mildly impaired	Poor	Poor	Intact	Intact
Repetition	Impaired	Impaired	Impaired	Impaired	Intact
Reading	May be impaired	Impaired	Poor	May be intact	Intact
Writing	Impaired	Impaired	Poor	May be intact	Intact

patients with lesions in or near Broca area exhibit an excellent recovery within weeks, whereas patients with lasting expressive deficits, such as Broca's original patients, have more extensive lesions involving most of the frontal and parietal lobes. Patients with lasting nonfluent aphasia also nearly always have damage to subcortical structures, particularly the subcallosal fasciculus and periventricular white matter (Naeser et al., 1989).

Aphemia, a variant of Broca aphasia, is a rare syndrome of muteness or nonfluent speech with good language comprehension and preserved writing. Because there is very little true language disturbance, aphemia may not be a true aphasia; it is most closely related, and even perhaps identical with, the equally rare syndrome of pure apraxia of speech (see above).

Wernicke Aphasia

Carl Wernicke described an aphasia syndrome in 1874. In contrast to those with Broca aphasia, patients with Wernicke aphasia speak fluently and effortlessly, although their meaning is obscured by the paucity of meaningful nouns and verbs, overabundance of stock phrases and idioms, and the presence of numerous verbal paraphasic errors (Table 19-1). Neologisms are usually present in severe cases, transforming the speech of these patients into jargon. In milder cases, many paraphasic substitutions and idioms take the sentences in directions not intended by the speaker. Naming in Wernicke aphasia is paraphasic, often with bizarre substitutions. Auditory comprehension may be so severely impaired that the patient cannot answer simple yes-or-no questions. Repetition is also paraphasic, and reading comprehension usually mirrors the poor language comprehension seen in auditory testing. In some cases, either auditory comprehension or reading may be less affected than the other (Kirshner et al., 1989), and this spared language modality can be used to communicate with the patient.

Writing is also abnormal in Wernicke aphasia. Unlike patients with Broca aphasia, most of those with Wernicke aphasia have no hemiparesis, and they can grip a pen and write without difficulty. The content of the writing, however, shows the same abnormality as the speech and is characterized by abnormal spelling patterns. Thus, writing samples may be a good way to detect mild Wernicke aphasia, especially in patients with slowly developing syndromes related to brain tumors.

Lesions associated with Wernicke aphasia generally involve the posterior two-thirds of the left superior temporal gyrus, although in some cases they extend into other parts of the temporal lobe and into the inferior parietal lobule. Lesions that damage most of the traditional Wernicke area are especially well correlated with lasting impairments of comprehension, whereas those involving primarily the inferior parietal lobule may be more associated with reading and writing disorders. As patients with Wernicke aphasia recover, their deficits often evolve into the milder syndromes of conduction or anomic aphasia.

A variant of Wernicke aphasia is pure word deafness, selective loss of auditory comprehension, and repetition with preserved naming, reading, and writing. Many patients have mildly paraphasic speech. The syndrome classically results from bilateral temporal lobe lesions, which disconnect the auditory cortices from the left temporal Wernicke area. Cases resembling pure word deafness have been reported with unilateral, left temporal lobe lesions, thus overlapping Wernicke aphasia with spared reading comprehension.

Global Aphasia

Global aphasia may be thought of as the sum of the deficits of Broca and Wernicke aphasias (Table 19-1). Patients with global aphasia are nonfluent or mute, and they exhibit impaired comprehension. All elements of language—speech, naming, comprehension, repetition, reading, and writing—are severely impaired. Syndromes of less severe but equally generalized impairments of language are called **mixed aphasia**. Lesions associated with global aphasia involve much of the left middle cerebral artery territory of the frontal, temporal, and parietal lobes. Large lesions of the subcortical white matter and basal ganglia result in a similar syndrome. As the patient with global aphasia recovers, the deficit profile often evolves toward Broca aphasia.

Conduction Aphasia

Although conduction aphasia occurs in <10% of aphasia cases, it demonstrates important lessons about language. In this syndrome, repetition is the most severely affected language modality (Table 19-1). Spontaneous speech is fluent, often with many literal paraphasic errors. The patient is aware of these errors and makes efforts at self-correction. Naming is variable, but auditory comprehension is usually normal. The patient understands well but cannot repeat what was said. Reading aloud may show similar deficits to repetition, as may writing to dictation.

Wernicke originally postulated a lesion disconnecting the auditory word association area (Wernicke area) in the left temporal lobe from Broca area in the left frontal lobe. Two general locations of lesion have been reported in conduction aphasia: the left superior temporal region, with incomplete damage to Wernicke area, and the inferior parietal lobule, especially the supramarginal gyrus. Benson et al. (1973) and Damasio and Damasio (1980) noted that patients with conduction aphasia secondary to parietal lobe lesions often have associated limb apraxia, whereas those with temporal lobe lesions do not. The supramarginal gyrus area may be important to the generation of phonemes in response to repetition or naming (Demonet et al., 1992; Hickok and Poeppel, 2000). An alternative explanation for conduction aphasia is a short-term memory deficit specific to auditory verbal material (Shallice and Warrington, 1977).

Anomic Aphasia

Also called amnesic or amnestic aphasia, anomic aphasia refers to syndromes in which naming is the most severe deficit. The patient speaks fluently, with some word-finding pauses and circumlocutions. Repetition, auditory comprehension, reading, and writing are intact. Many patients show no other abnormalities on neurologic examination. The lesions producing anomic aphasia are more variable than those underlying the other aphasic syndromes discussed thus far. Some authors have emphasized lesions of the angular gyrus, although lesions there often produce other deficits, including alexia, constructional impairment, and the four elements of Gerstmann syndrome.

Anomic aphasia also is seen in conditions without clearly localized lesions, as in confusional states and dementing disorders, such as Alzheimer disease (AD). An aphasia test battery given to a patient with early AD will often give a score consistent with anomic aphasia. According to some sources, left frontal lobe lesions disproportionally affect naming of actions (verbs), whereas left temporal lesions are more associated with the misnaming of objects (nouns).

Transcortical Aphasias

The next three aphasic syndromes discussed here are transcortical aphasias. The responsible lesions affect not the primary language cortex or the circuit from Wernicke to Broca area but rather other areas of the brain that project to the language cortex. Specific lesions are quite variable, including cortical damage in the frontal, temporal, and parietal areas and subcortical white matter. Table 19-2 lists key features of the three transcortical aphasia syndromes.

In **transcortical motor aphasia**, the patient speaks little, much as in Broca aphasia. In response to questions, the patient may either remain mute or may give a one- or two-word answer, often in a whisper or after a delay. As in Broca aphasia, the patient utters the most important, meaningful words of a sentence, often communicating adequately. Unlike the patient with Broca aphasia, however, a patient with transcortical motor aphasia can repeat normally. Auditory comprehension tends to be preserved, whereas naming, reading, and writing are more variable. Lesions associated with this syndrome usually involve the left frontal lobe, anterior to, superior to, or beneath Broca area. The most common location is the frontal cortex within the territory of the left anterior cerebral artery.

Transcortical sensory aphasia is a Wernicke-like syndrome in which speech is fluent but paraphasic and auditory comprehension is severely impaired. Unlike the patient with Wernicke aphasia, however, the patient with transcortical sensory aphasia can repeat phrases and sentences without difficulty. Naming is typically paraphasic, and reading comprehension and writing are impaired, similar to Wernicke aphasia. Lesions of the left posterior temporo-occipital lobe have been described, and the syndrome also occurs in patients with AD, though more so in moderate stages of the disease.

The final transcortical aphasic syndrome is **mixed transcortical aphasia** (syndrome of the isolation of the speech area). This syndrome is the transcortical equivalent of global aphasia. The patient cannot speak fluently, comprehend spoken language, follow commands, name objects, read, or write. It is surprising, however, that these patients can repeat fluently, and some are even echolalic. A patient reported by Geschwind et al. (1968) could even learn lyrics of popular new songs only after her illness, indicating that some memory storage of words was possible. **Isolation syndrome** is just another name for mixed transcortical aphasia, or the syndrome of isolation of the speech area. The perisylvian language cortex in this syndrome is intact but not connected to other cortical areas necessary for propositional speech or comprehension. It usually indicates extensive cortical damage to both cerebral hemispheres, sparing the perisylvian cortex, as in watershed infarctions seen in states of hypotension, hypoxia, carbon monoxide poisoning, or bilateral carotid artery occlusion.

Subcortical Aphasias

Subcortical aphasias are defined by the lesion localization rather than by the characteristics of the aphasia. Although

Table 19-2

Language Features of Transcortical Aphasias

Feature	Isolation	Transcortical Motor	Transcortical Sensory
Speech	Nonfluent and echolalic	Nonfluent	Fluent and echolalic
Naming	Impaired	Impaired	Impaired
Comprehension	Impaired	Intact	Impaired
Repetition	Intact	Intact	Intact
Reading	Impaired	May be spared	Impaired
Writing	Impaired	Impaired	Impaired

aphasia usually reflects dysfunction of the language cortex, subcortical lesions can disrupt connections to the language cortex. The most common subcortical aphasia syndrome, often called the **anterior subcortical aphasia syndrome**, is seen in patients with lesions involving the head of the caudate nucleus, anterior limb of the internal capsule, and anterior putamen. Speech is usually dysarthric and nonfluent, with mild deficits of repetition and comprehension. Lesions of the dominant thalamus produce fluent aphasia with paraphasic errors but with relatively spared auditory comprehension. Thalamic aphasia can also produce a dichotomy between relatively intact speech when the patient is awake and paraphasic speech when the patient is drowsy. The thalamus may play a role in activating the language cortex; thus, thalamic lesions may result in putting the language areas to sleep. Subcortical lesions also can involve the temporal isthmus, cutting off connections to Wernicke area and producing severe disturbance of comprehension. Delineation of the precise neuroanatomy of the subcortical aphasia syndromes is an active area of research.

Alexia: Neurology of Reading

Disordered reading and writing are important aspects of most aphasia syndromes. In some syndromes, however, reading and writing are affected out of proportion to the deficits in spoken language and auditory comprehension. The French physician Joseph J. Déjérine delineated the two classical **alexia syndromes**, with and without agraphia, more than 100 years ago.

Alexia with Agraphia

Alexia with agraphia is acquired illiteracy: the patient becomes unable to read or write (Table 19-3). Although spoken language is relatively intact, most patients have a fluent, paraphasic speech pattern. Auditory comprehension and naming are often impaired to some degree. The syndrome results from lesions in the left inferior parietal lobule, including the supramarginal and angular gyri. As such, the syndrome overlaps with Wernicke aphasia, and some cases may evolve as a stage in the recovery of acute Wernicke aphasia.

Alexia without Agraphia

Pure alexia without agraphia (pure alexia or word blindness) can be thought of as a linguistic blindfold in which the inability to read is an isolated deficit (Table 19-3). These patients have normal spontaneous speech, repetition, and auditory comprehension; in fact, most patients can comprehend words spelled aloud, indicating that their spelling is not disturbed. There is often some naming difficulty, particularly for colors. Writing is intact, and one of the most intriguing aspects of the syndrome is that a patient may write a phrase or sentence but shortly afterward may be unable to read it. The inability to read is often complete at first, then improves such that the patient can spell out words letter by letter. Most of these patients have reduced short-term memory and right hemianopsia.

The lesion is almost always a stroke in the territory of the left posterior cerebral artery, which supplies the medial occipital and medial temporal lobes and the splenium of the corpus callosum. Déjérine's explanation was that the left occipital lesion caused right hemianopsia, and the lesion of the corpus callosum prevented visual information from being transmitted from the intact right occipital lobe to the left hemisphere language centers. Thus, the patient can see in the left visual field but cannot decode written language. This model of the pure alexia syndrome is a good example of a disconnection syndrome (see Box 2-7).

Aphasic Alexia

Aphasic alexia occurs in association with aphasic disturbances. Benson (1977) uses the term **third alexia** to characterize the reading disorder of Broca aphasia. In this classification, the first and second alexias are the classical syndromes of alexia with and without agraphia. Benson notes that most patients with Broca aphasia have more difficulty with reading than with auditory comprehension.

Neurolinguists have developed a different classification of reading disorders based on the mechanisms of the

Table 19-3

Language Features of Alexias

Feature	Alexia with Agraphia	Pure Alexia
Spontaneous speech	Mildly paraphasic	Intact
Naming	Often impaired	Normal except for colors
Comprehension	May be mildly impaired	Intact
Repetition	Intact	Intact
Reading	Poor	Poor; letter reading may be spared
Writing	Poor	Intact

disorder itself rather than on the pattern of associated language disorders or location of the responsible lesions. **Deep dyslexia** implies a defect in the basic reading process or the conversion of printed graphemes to spoken phonemes. The characteristics of the reading disorder in deep dyslexia include the inability to read nonwords, semantic and visual errors in reading words (*boat* for *schooner* or *perform* for *perfume*), and marked effects of word class and word imageability on reading performance. Nouns and verbs generally are read better than adjectives, adverbs, and prepositions; likewise, concrete nouns, which have referents that can be visualized, are more likely to be read correctly than abstract nouns. These patients appear to read more by direct recognition of familiar words (access of the semantic system directly from orthography, or spelling) than by conversion of the grapheme into a phoneme, and then processing it into the semantic system. Most deep dyslexic patients have large left hemisphere lesions and significant aphasia of mixed or Broca type.

A second alexia syndrome is **phonologic dyslexia**, which is similar to deep dyslexia except that the reading of single content words may be nearly normal and semantic errors are rare. Reading of nonwords is difficult, as in deep dyslexia. In this syndrome, patients may be able to read aloud not only by recognition of the words' meanings but also by a process of conversion of words to phonemes (lexical–phonologic route). However, conversion of individual graphemes to phonemes is still defective.

Another seemingly opposite type of dyslexia is **surface dyslexia**. This syndrome occurs in patients who can read phonetically by grapheme-to-phoneme conversion but cannot recognize words directly. In this syndrome, words of irregular spelling, such as *yacht* or *colonel*, are particularly difficult to read. Surface dyslexia is a rare syndrome that has been reported in patients with anterior left hemisphere lesions and in primary progressive aphasia.

A fourth neurolinguistic alexia syndrome, **letter-by-letter reading**, is synonymous with the syndrome of pure alexia without agraphia discussed earlier, in which patients have recovered enough reading ability to read letters and to spell words aloud letter by letter.

Agraphia: Neurology of Writing

Writing, a basic element of language, often is disrupted in aphasic syndromes. The classical syndrome of **pure agraphia** affects patients with minimal or no aphasic deficits other than the inability to write. Pure agraphia is a rare syndrome. The diagnosis of pure agraphia requires that the failure to write not be explainable by simple motor deficit (hemiparesis), apraxia (discussed later), or visuospatial difficulties. Lesions of pure agraphia are usually found in the left superior frontal region, although left parietal lesions have been reported to cause pure agraphia as well.

Agraphia is divided into phonologic and lexical types, corresponding to the process of writing by producing a whole word from the semantic meaning (lexical pathway) or by production of the phoneme and then derivation of the corresponding graphemes (phonologic pathway). A patient with phonologic agraphia can write common words from dictation but cannot write dictated nonword phonemes. Such a patient's spontaneous writing contains semantic errors or words of similar meaning but dissimilar spelling to the target word. There is also a preference for concrete over abstract nouns as well as both nouns and verbs over prepositions, adjectives, and adverbs. Phonologic agraphia thus bears a close resemblance to the pattern of deep dyslexia, but the two deficits do not necessarily affect the same patient.

In the other type of agraphia, **lexical agraphia**, the patient can write nonwords from dictation but cannot write irregularly spelled words and is confused by words of the same sound but different spelling (homophones). The clinical syndromes of phonologic and lexical agraphia are still in an investigational stage in terms of correlations with lesion localizations, other aphasia phenomena, and practical use in rehabilitative therapy.

Apraxia: Neurology of Learned Movement

Apraxia is a disorder of learned motor acts not caused by paralysis, incoordination, sensory deficit, or lack of understanding of the desired movement. In practical terms, apraxia is an inability to carry out skilled motor acts to command when it can be demonstrated that the patient understands the command and can perform the same motor act in a different context (Geschwind, 1975; Kirshner, 1992). Liepmann (1920), a German physician, described three types of apraxia: **ideomotor**, **ideational**, and **limb kinetic**.

It is important to differentiate several diverse motor phenomena that are commonly confused with the principal varieties of apraxia. These are constructional, dressing, oculomotor, and gait apraxia. **Constructional apraxia**, which is characterized by visuospatial difficulties, is associated with right hemispheric lesions. These patients may be unable to construct or copy a drawing of simple items (e.g., a clock or house). In most instances, this deficit is related to neglect of the left side of space or failure to appreciate the spatial relations of items, not to a motor planning deficit. In **dressing apraxia**, which is associated with right hemisphere lesions, the patients have difficulty with the spatial perception of a garment in relation to the body, again a visuospatial deficit, not a true motor apraxic deficit. **Oculomotor apraxia** refers to a difficulty with voluntary direction of the eyes in gaze and is associated with damage to the brainstem mechanism for control of eye movements. **Gait apraxia** refers to an inability to walk that is not clearly explained by primary motor weakness, ataxia, or sensory loss. There is no easy way to demonstrate that the same sequential actions can be performed normally in a different context; therefore, it is unclear whether this gait disorder is a true apraxia. Perhaps even more problematic is apraxia of speech (discussed earlier). Whether apraxia of speech is a true apraxia is debated by aphasiologists.

Ideomotor Apraxia

Ideomotor apraxia refers to the failure to carry out a motor act in response to a verbal command when the patient understands the command and has the motor capacity to perform the same motor act under a different context. By Liepmann's (1920) model, the idea of the movement, decoded in Wernicke area, is disconnected from its execution in the premotor cortex of the frontal lobe. Ideomotor apraxia often accompanies aphasia in patients with left hemisphere lesions (Geschwind, 1975). In published series, only a small percentage of patients with ideomotor apraxia have right-sided lesions. A high percentage of patients with aphasia and left hemisphere lesions have ideomotor apraxia, whereas a much smaller percentage of nonaphasic patients with left hemisphere lesions demonstrate such apraxia (DeRenzi et al., 1980). Patients with ideomotor aphasia typically fail to carry out the test act to verbal command and perform only slightly better in imitation of the examiner; however, they carry out the act almost normally if given the actual object.

According to the anatomic model of Liepmann (1920), later modified by Geschwind (1975), a lesion in the left temporal lobe, which also causes aphasia, prevents information regarding the desired act from reaching the left premotor area. Thus, ideomotor apraxia may be part of the deficit in Wernicke aphasia, but the impairment of comprehension makes it questionable whether the patient has understood the command.

In conduction aphasia and Broca aphasia, there may be associated ideomotor apraxia that interferes with the carrying out of commands with limbs on either side of the body. Such apraxic deficits may create the mistaken impression that the patient has a comprehension deficit; asking the patient yes-or-no questions or simple pointing commands can be used to establish normal comprehension. Finally, lesions of the corpus callosum can prevent motor information from reaching the right hemisphere motor area. This callosal apraxia affects movement of the left limbs only. The existence of callosal apraxia implies that the left hemisphere is dominant not only for speech but also for learned motor acts, because the right hemisphere cannot program the skilled movement independently.

This association of aphasia and apraxia may reflect the underlying symbolic nature of both speech and gestural expression, or it may simply reflect the anatomic contiguity of centers for speech–language function and those for learned motor acts. The association between apraxia and aphasia explains why most aphasia patients cannot learn complex linguistic gestural systems, such as American Sign Language.

Ideational Apraxia

Ideational apraxia is an even more complex phenomenon than ideomotor apraxia. Heilman (2000) proposes the term *conceptual apraxia* as a similar form of apraxia. There are two competing definitions of ideational apraxia. First, some authors use it to mean apraxia for real objects. Ochipa et al. (1989) describe a patient who could name objects but not demonstrate their uses, as if he had lost the concepts of their purposes (apraxia for tool use). The second definition of ideational apraxia is loss of the ability to carry out a multistep activity, although each individual step may be performed appropriately. For example, a patient may not be able to fill, light, and smoke a pipe or assemble a coffee percolator and make coffee. This type of apraxia may reflect a motor planning difficulty, as seen in frontal lobe lesions. It also may simply be a more sensitive test for apraxia than single motor commands. However defined, ideational apraxia also is associated with left hemisphere lesions, more often temporoparietal lesions associated with severe aphasia. Both ideomotor and ideational apraxia can occur in AD.

Limb-Kinetic Apraxia

The third of Liepmann's types of apraxia is limb-kinetic apraxia, a deficit of fine motor acts involving only one limb. Patients with mild pyramidal tract lesions may not be weak in gross limb movements but may have difficulty with rapid or fine movements of the fingers. Such apraxia may be a sign of a partial corticospinal tract lesion with mild weakness. Heilman et al. (2000) refer to this type of apraxia as a loss of deftness. A left hemisphere lesion may be associated with limb-kinetic apraxia of both hands, whereas a right hemisphere lesion is usually associated with limb-kinetic apraxia of the left hand only.

Agnosia: Neurology of Recognition

Agnosias are disorders of recognition. Most affect a single sensory system (visual, auditory, or tactile agnosia), whereas others involve selected classes of items within a modality (prosopagnosia, or agnosia for faces). In each case, the patient must be shown to have normal primary sensory perception, normal ability to name the item once it is recognized, and no general cognitive deterioration or dementia. For example, a patient with visual agnosia may fail to recognize a key ring by sight but is able to identify and name it from the sound of the keys jingling or from the feel of the keys in his or her hand. Each sensory modality carries a somewhat arbitrary division between primary sensory cortical deficits and agnosia. Most agnosias require bilateral cortical lesions, cutting off input from the sensory modality to the left hemisphere language centers.

In the visual system, bilateral occipital lesions may cause cortical blindness. More partial lesions, however, may permit primary visual perception of the elements of an object or picture, such that the patient can even draw lines or angles representing the item but cannot identify the item. Shown a bicycle, the patient may report two circles and identify it as eyeglasses. Prosopagnosia, or failure to identify faces, is a subtype of visual agnosia in which patients cannot recognize family members or friends, though they can describe features, such as hair color, a mustache or beard, or accessories (e.g., hats or glasses). Frequently, the prosopagnostic patient identifies the person by voice or gait pattern. Oliver Sacks (1998) described prosopagnosia, or perhaps a more profound visual agnosia, in *The Man Who Mistook His Wife for a Hat*.

Auditory agnosias also overlap with the syndrome of cortical deafness, resulting from bilateral lesions of the temporal cortex. Some patients with bilateral temporal lobe lesions have preserved pure tone hearing but cannot understand spoken language or repeat. As discussed earlier, this deficit is referred to as pure word deafness. Geschwind (1970) postulates that pure word deafness results from a bilateral disconnection of the input from the primary auditory cortex (Heschl gyrus) to the left hemisphere Wernicke area. More rarely, patients show preserved auditory comprehension but impaired nonverbal auditory recognition, for example, identification of animal sounds or the characteristic sounds associated with objects such as bells and whistles. This deficit is called auditory nonverbal agnosia. A last bitemporal syndrome is phonagnosia, or inability to recognize familiar voices.

In the tactile modality, parietal lesions often disrupt the identification of objects by feel, a deficit called **astereognosis**. A related deficit, **agraphesthesia**, is the inability to recognize letters or numbers drawn on their hands. If the patient can describe the sensory characteristics of an object but not identify it, this can also qualify as tactile agnosia. Rare patients with bilateral parietal lesions have no ability to recognize objects by touch on either side.

Key Terms:

Alzheimer disease	**Dialysis dementia**
Creutzfeldt–Jakob syndrome	**Pick disease**
	Viral encephalitis

Dementia: Neurology of Cognition

Dementia is defined as a gradual deterioration of previously intact cognitive functions secondary to diffuse rather than focal brain disease. The *Diagnostic and Statistical Manual of Mental Disorders,* 4th edition (DSM-IV), commonly used by psychiatrists, defines dementia in terms of memory loss and at least one additional cognitive function, such as language, visuospatial functioning, apraxia, or executive function. Although the pattern of cognitive deterioration varies, memory loss is usually the first symptom, and other deficits follow. Tests of language function frequently show deficient naming, although fluency of spontaneous speech and repetition remain normal. In later stages, reading, writing, and auditory comprehension begin to deteriorate. Patients may evolve from an initial deficit of anomic aphasia to a pattern resembling Wernicke or transcortical sensory aphasia. Other cortical deficits, such as apraxia and acalculia, are frequently present.

In contrast to the common pattern of language dissolution in dementing illness, typical of AD, there is a less common pattern, in which focal deficits predominate early in the illness. For example, cases of primary progressive aphasia have apparently focal aphasic deficits that gradually progress over years. Such patients resemble stroke survivors, in having a focal deficit such as a nonfluent aphasia. Some patients fail to show memory loss or other cognitive deficits for years after onset. Mesulam (1982) first called this syndrome primary progressive aphasia, but more recent studies have placed this presentation within a broader category of frontotemporal dementia (discussed later in this chapter). The primary progressive aphasia syndrome is also divided into nonfluent and fluent forms; one of the latter is a syndrome called semantic dementia in which the patient not only cannot think of names but does not understand the meaning of words. In most series, nonfluent aphasia in dementia usually indicates a pathology other than typical AD, whereas the pathology of semantic dementia and fluent progressive aphasia is more variable (Mesulam, 2000, 2003).

Dementia can be caused by any of a multitude of diseases, which can be classed into three major groups of conditions: **systemic diseases**, primarily involving organ systems outside the central nervous system; **neurologic diseases**, marked by degeneration of other systems than the higher cortical functions; and diseases presenting primarily with loss of cognitive faculties.

Dementias Secondary to Systemic Diseases

Most of the dementia-causing systemic diseases are listed in Table 19-4. Because most of these conditions are treatable, identifying them is essential. For many metabolic disorders, such as disturbances of electrolytes (hyponatremia), failure of the liver or kidneys, and calcium disturbances, patients present with an acute confusional state or delirium rather than chronic dementia. Toxic disorders include the effects of chemicals, heavy metals, alcohol, and drugs. Chronic alcohol ingestion coupled with poor nutrition may cause symptoms of thiamine deficiency, Wernicke–Korsakoff syndrome. Technically, this syndrome is a pure amnesia (loss of memory) rather than a dementia, but there is evidence that chronic alcohol abusers may develop a true dementia as well. Among toxins, prescribed drugs are among the most common treatable causes of dementia. Sedative effects of multiple medications may combine to cause chronic mental impairment. A few drugs cause confusional states when used alone—for example, the anticholinergic effects of drugs, such as tricyclic antidepressants, antihistamines, and neuroleptics, may produce anticholinergic encephalopathy. A nutritional cause of dementia is vitamin B_{12} deficiency. Recently, vitamin D deficiency has also been reported to cause memory loss.

Infections are a relatively infrequent but important cause of dementia. The most treatable cause is infectious meningitis. Viral encephalitis is a more acute syndrome that may leave dementia in its wake. Dementia is also an aspect of AIDS. Although some patients have secondary infections and tumors affecting the nervous system, the HIV itself appears to cause chronic encephalitis, resulting in dementia (**AIDS dementia complex**). Multiple strokes also can cause dementia, and vascular cognitive impairment

Table 19-4

Systemic Diseases Associated with Dementia

Metabolic disorders
Low sodium, low calcium, high calcium, and aluminum
Renal, hepatic, and pulmonary failure
Dialysis dementia
Nutritional
Vitamin B_1 and B_{12} deficiency and pellagra
Endocrine
Hypothyroidism, hyperthyroidism, Cushing, and hyperparathyroidism
Toxic
Heavy metals and organic compounds
Drugs, polypharmacy, and alcoholism
Infections
Neurosyphilis
Chronic meningitis: bacterial, fungal, and tuberculous
Parasitic diseases
Sequelae of viral encephalitis
Subacute sclerosing panencephalitis
Progressive multifocal leukoencephalopathy
Creutzfeldt–Jakob disease
AIDS dementia complex
Vascular diseases
Multi-infarct dementia and Binswanger disease
Multiple cholesterol emboli
Collagen vascular diseases and vasculitis
Arteriovenous malformations
Neoplasms
Brain tumor and increased intracranial pressure
Multiple metastatic tumors
Neoplastic meningitis
Chemotherapy and radiation toxicity
Limbic encephalitis

often is mixed with AD, representing the second most common cause of dementia after AD itself.

Neurologic Diseases Associated with Dementia

The second group of dementias involves neurologic diseases that lead to cognitive deterioration. Normal pressure hydrocephalus and basal ganglia diseases are the most common examples. Normal pressure hydrocephalus is characterized by the gradual onset of mental slowing and then frank dementia, gait difficulty, and urinary incontinence. Brain imaging studies show dilation of the cerebral ventricles out of proportion to the degree of brain atrophy. Some patients respond dramatically to shunting procedures, in which spinal fluid is rerouted from the cerebral ventricles into the abdomen, and experience return of mental function and improved gait and urinary continence.

Most other neurologic diseases associated with dementia fall under the heading of neurodegenerative diseases, in which specific populations of neurons deteriorate. Several diseases that affect the basal ganglia also produce a pattern of subcortical dementia. The most common is Parkinson disease, which is characterized by bradykinesia (slowed movement), rigidity, resting tremor, mask-like or expressionless face, and dysarthric speech. Patients exhibit slowed mental processes. A variant of Parkinson disease is Lewy body dementia in which subtle motor manifestations of Parkinson disease accompany a dementing illness, often with prominent visual hallucinations and confusion. At autopsy, the Lewy bodies are present not only in the substantia nigra but in the cortex. The family of Parkinson-plus disorders—corticobasal degeneration, progressive supranuclear palsy, and multisystem atrophy—are also associated with dementia. Other diseases that combine a movement disorder with a dementing illness are Huntington disease and Wilson disease.

Another neurologic disease not considered primarily a dementia is multiple sclerosis. Recent studies that have included neuropsychological test batteries have found that most patients with chronic multiple sclerosis have significant cognitive impairments. There is some suggestion from recent studies that multiple sclerosis plaques in the deep periventricular white matter, seen frequently on brain MRI studies of these patients, may correlate better with cognitive and mood disturbances than with physical disability.

Primary Degenerative Dementias

A few diseases primarily cause slowly progressive dementia. AD is the most common, accounting for 50% to 60% of most series of autopsied cases of dementia. The disease is defined by the presence of senile plaques in the neuropil of the cerebral cortex and neurofibrillary tangles (silver-staining strands) in the neurons of the cerebral cortex, hippocampus, and nucleus basalis of Meynert. The disease is not truly diffuse, but rather a multifocal disorder with a predilection for specific structures. The hippocampus and adjacent structures are critical for memory storage and retrieval. The nucleus of Meynert has cholinergic projections to wide areas of the cerebral cortex. The pathology of AD is difficult to separate from that of normal aging of the brain, and recent studies have found that nearly 50% of people > 80 years meet the clinical criteria for dementia (Evans et al., 1989). Careful examination and testing for treatable factors, as discussed earlier, are therefore essential for diagnosing AD. Although many drug therapies are being tested in AD, the ultimate cause of the neuronal degeneration and curative or disease-modifying treatment remains to be discovered. Genetic defects have been found to underlie some early-onset cases of AD, and a gene for apolipoprotein E4 appears to increase the likelihood of development of the sporadic disease.

Recently, drugs that block acetylcholinesterase have been found to improve memory in patients with AD. These agents likely improve the cholinergic transmission of the nucleus of Meynert, which is thought to be involved in memory. The drugs tacrine (Cognex), donepezil (Aricept), rivastigmine (Exelon), and galantamine (Razadyne) are the first agents to show clear benefit to patients with AD. Another U.S. Food and Drug Administration (FDA)–approved drug, memantine (Namenda), has been shown effective in patients with moderate to severe AD. This drug blocks the N-methyl-D-aspartate subtype of the glutamate receptor in the brain. Overstimulation of neurons by glutamate may increase nerve cell death in AD, though the precise mechanism of how this drug brings about clinical benefit is unclear. Other promising therapies are in the experimental pipeline. Many involve attempts to reduce amyloid deposition in the senile plaques and blood vessels. Various vaccines and enzyme inhibitors are in clinical trials, though some disappointing results have delayed the goal of a disease-modifying treatment for AD. Other recent clinical trials have been disappointing in regard to antioxidants, such as vitamin E, and nonsteroidal anti-inflammatory drugs. Estrogen hormones, previously thought to be protective against cognitive decline in older women, have been shown to be associated with dementia. Healthy diet, exercise, and treatment of vascular risk factors, such as hypertension and elevated lipids, may be the most effective ways to prevent dementia in normal people.

Pick disease is a dementing disease that has a predilection for the frontal and temporal lobes, often beginning unilaterally. The findings include silver-staining intraneuronal inclusions called Pick bodies but few or none of the senile plaques and neurofibrillary tangles seen in AD. Pick disease may be clinically indistinguishable from AD, but many cases present with focal frontal lobe syndromes or isolated aphasia before progressing to general dementia. Pick disease now is considered to be part of a family of diseases called frontotemporal dementia, in which there is selective degeneration of the frontal and temporal lobes on one or both sides of the brain. Patients may present with progressive aphasia, usually of the nonfluent type, or with behavioral disturbances similar to those discussed for frontal lobe syndromes. Semantic dementia is another syndrome of progressive, fluent aphasia with anomia, that often reflects FTD. Finally, a logopenic variant of progressive aphasia has been described, with a main deficit of anomia, and this variety of PPA appears most often related to AD. Two genetic variants of FTD have been described: one involving mutations of the tau gene on chromosome 17 and the other, with ubiquitin staining, involving a progranulin mutation of the TAR-DNA–binding protein (TDP-43), a major component of the ubiquitinated inclusions in these cases. A minority of patients with FTD also develop motor neuron disease.

The syndrome of primary progressive aphasia, especially the nonfluent type, is rarely secondary to AD but can be considered a part of the spectrum of frontotemporal dementia. Disorders underlying this syndrome include Pick disease, nonspecific neuronal loss and gliosis, and corticobasal degeneration. Some familial cases of frontotemporal dementia are associated with a gene defect on chromosome 17.

Creutzfeldt–Jakob disease is a rapidly progressive syndrome characterized by mood changes, dementia, seizures, myoclonus, and exaggerated startle responses. The course progresses from first symptoms to death in 6 to 12 months or less. The disease is rare, occurring in approximately one per 1 million people per year worldwide. Creutzfeldt–Jakob disease is interesting because it was found to be transmitted by inoculation of tissues via contaminated surgical instruments, corneal transplants, and pituitary extracts. A proteinaceous infectious particle is thought to be the cause of the disease, not a DNA-containing virus. Early changes on MRI studies and a new spinal fluid test called the 14-3-3 protein can be helpful in diagnosis. A variant of this disease is bovine spongiform encephalopathy, or mad cow disease, which has been transmitted by beef from infected cattle.

Traumatic Brain Injury

Traumatic brain injury (TBI) is a major cause of death and disability, particularly in young people. An acute blow to the head may cause instantaneous loss of consciousness and a brief period of retrograde amnesia, such that the patient does not remember the blow that caused the loss of consciousness. The term *cerebral concussion* implies a head injury with a brief loss of consciousness and brief retrograde amnesia but no other evidence of structural disruption of the brain. A great deal of research has concentrated on these minor head injuries and the resultant postconcussive syndrome. Such patients have normal brain imaging studies, including skull radiographs, CT scans, MRI studies, and electroencephalograms. Patients frequently complain of headaches, poor concentration and memory, insomnia, irritability, mood swings, and sometimes vertigo or dizziness. The damage caused by repeated concussions is a major concern in competitive athletics, and recent guidelines have been promoted to avoid such repetitive injuries.

More severe brain injuries may initially cause coma and evidence of contusion or bruising of the brain, shear hemorrhages into the brain tissue, or pooling of blood in the subdural or extradural space. Such patients are more severely impaired than patients with concussive injuries, and they frequently have motor deficits as well as impaired cognition. These patients commonly require prolonged rehabilitation, first in inpatient and later outpatient settings. Impaired memory and attention are common accompaniments, as are frontal lobe syndromes, such as impulsive or agitated behavior. These patients are typically uninhibited and inappropriate in their behavior, and they frequently call attention to themselves on rehabilitation units. In terms of language, high-level impairments are frequently found, especially in the organization of discourse. Occasionally, aphasias similar to those seen in stroke patients develop after TBI, especially in patients with localized damage to the left cerebral hemisphere from subdural hematomas, intracerebral hemorrhages, or contusions.

CLINICAL CORRELATES

CASE STUDIES FOR PROBLEM SOLVING

CASE ONE (19-1)

This 51-year-old woman, previously healthy except for smoking and postmenopausal hormone-replacement therapy, underwent an elective total knee-replacement surgery. The evening after the surgery, she was noted to be somewhat confused, but no other specific symptoms were noted. There was a question of an irregular heart rhythm postoperatively, but she was in normal sinus rhythm at the time of evaluation. She went to sleep uneventfully. She apparently had a stroke during sleep. The next morning, her family reported she was speaking gibberish. She did not have any facial droop, arm or leg weakness, or numbness. The attending neurologist requested speech–language assessment. The consulting speech–language pathologist noted the following:

- Fluently spoken speech
- Paraphasic substitutions and meaningless jargon utterances
- Poor repetition
- Impaired auditory comprehension
- Poor processing of written language
- Substantial naming difficulty

A brain MRI study showed an acute infarction in the left temporal lobe (Fig. 19-1). The frontal and parietal lobes were not affected.

Question: Can you identify the aphasia type and relate it with the lesion site. Also comment on the nature of the underlying cause?

Case (19-1) Discussion: See discussion of case studies

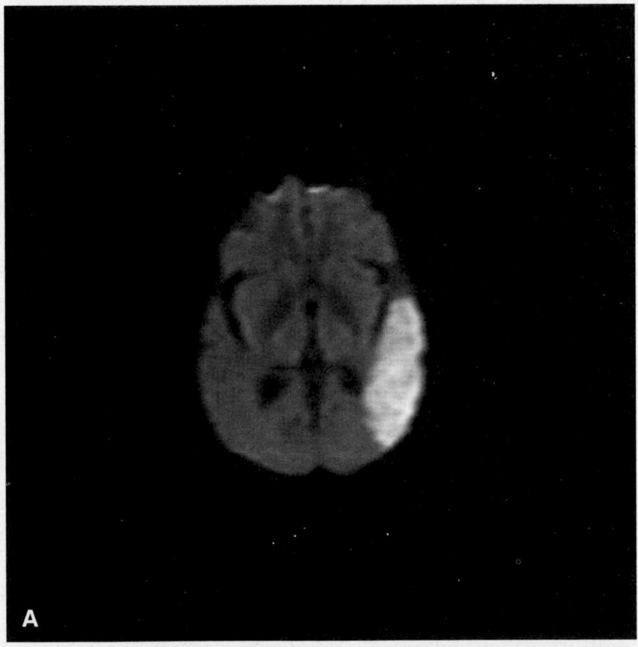

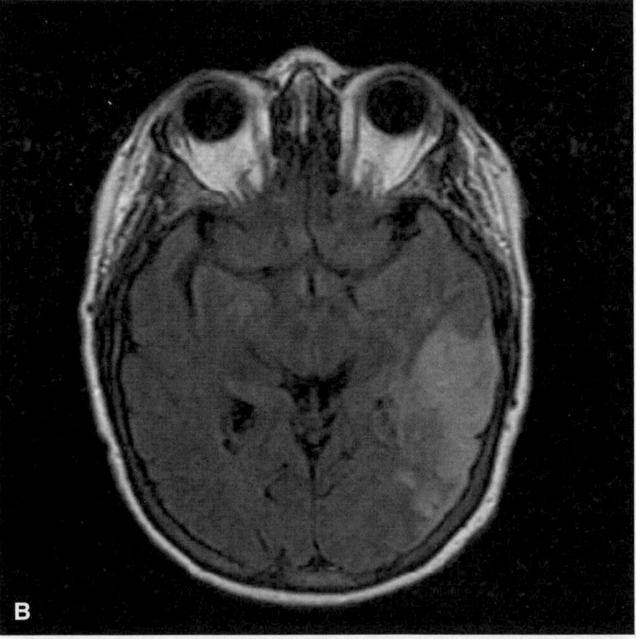

Figure 19-1 A. An acute left temporal lobe infarct is shown on a diffusion-weighted MRI image. B. Verification of the infarct on fluid-attenuated inversion recovery imaging (FLARE), which is essentially a T2-weighted image with the cerebrospinal fluid signal subtracted.

(Continued)

CASE TWO (19-2) *(CONTINUED)*

A 72-year-old man with a prior history of hypertension, hyperlipidemia (elevated cholesterol), and obstructive sleep apnea developed the abrupt onset of difficulty seeing out in the right visual field. He was noted to have confusion and mild memory difficulty. He was taken to the emergency room and was examined by a neurologist who noted the following:

- Well oriented and able to speak fluently
- No ability to name colors
- Complete inability to read
- Mild short-term memory difficulty
- No motor or sensory deficits
- A faint carotid bruit

A brain MRI study showed an infarction in the left occipital lobe, within the territory of the left posterior cerebral artery (Fig. 19-2). Magnetic resonance angiography showed reduced filling of branches of the left posterior cerebral artery.

Question: Can you explain what type of aphasia is usually associated with the lesion noted in the MRI study?

Case (19-2) Discussion: See discussion of case studies

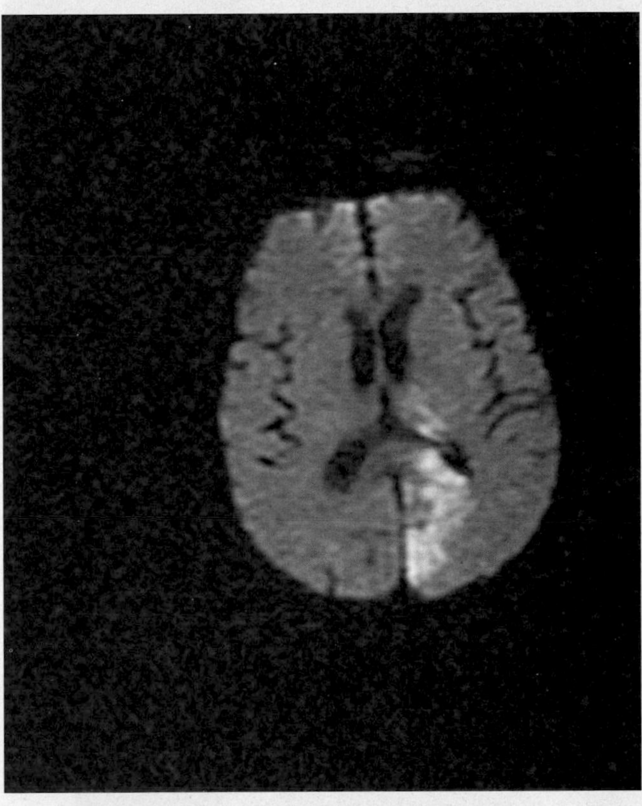

Figure 19-2 Axial diffusion–weighted MRI study showing an acute infarction in the left occipital lobe, extending into the splenium of the corpus callosum, the thalamus, and the medial temporal region.

CASE THREE (19-3)

A 47-year-old HIV-positive man with an acute onset of dysarthria was taken to the ER, where he presented with the following symptoms:

- Speech marked by slowness of articulation, explosive and overarticulated syllabic stress, loudness, and pitch breaks as well as prolonged intervals between sounds
- Difficulty with swallowing
- Impaired balance with a tendency of falling to the left
- Left ptosis and a smaller pupil on the left than the right
- Left facial numbness
- Weakness of the left palate
- Numbness of the right side of the body
- Ataxia of the left limbs and the trunk
- No language or cognitive impairments

A brainstem MRI study revealed an infarction in the left lateral medulla (Fig. 19-3).

Question: Can you explain how a left medullary lesion could relate to the observed clinical signs?

Case (19-3) Discussion: See discussion of case studies

(Continued)

CASE THREE (19-3) *(CONTINUED)*

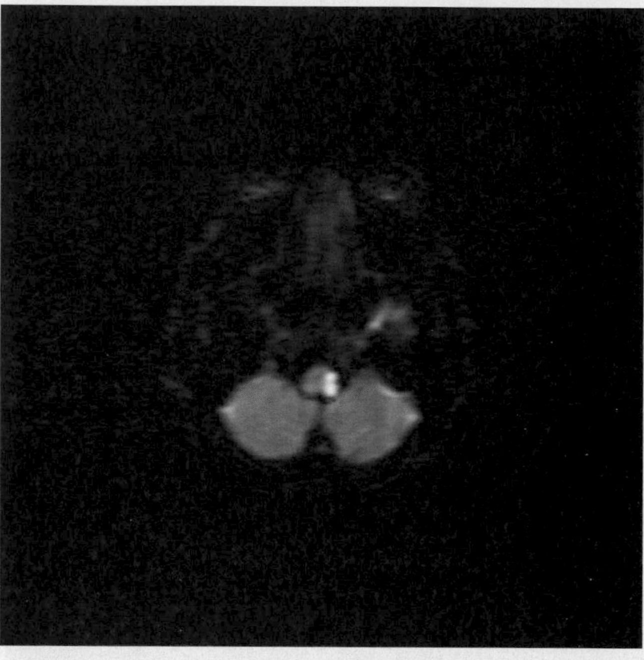

Figure 19-3 Axial diffusion–weighted MRI study showing a left lateral medullary infarction after the occlusion of the left vertebral artery.

CASE FOUR (19-4)

A 63-year-old woman had to stop working as a secretary because of increasing difficulty in thinking of words and signs of nonfluent verbal output. Neurologic examination showed a healthy-appearing woman with nonfluent speech, poor naming, and relatively preserved comprehension. She had no other neurologic deficits. A brain MRI study showed severe atrophy of the left temporal lobe (Fig. 19-4).

Question: Can you explain the type of aphasia that is usually associated with the lesion site revealed in the MRI study?

Case (19-4) Discussion: See discussion of case studies

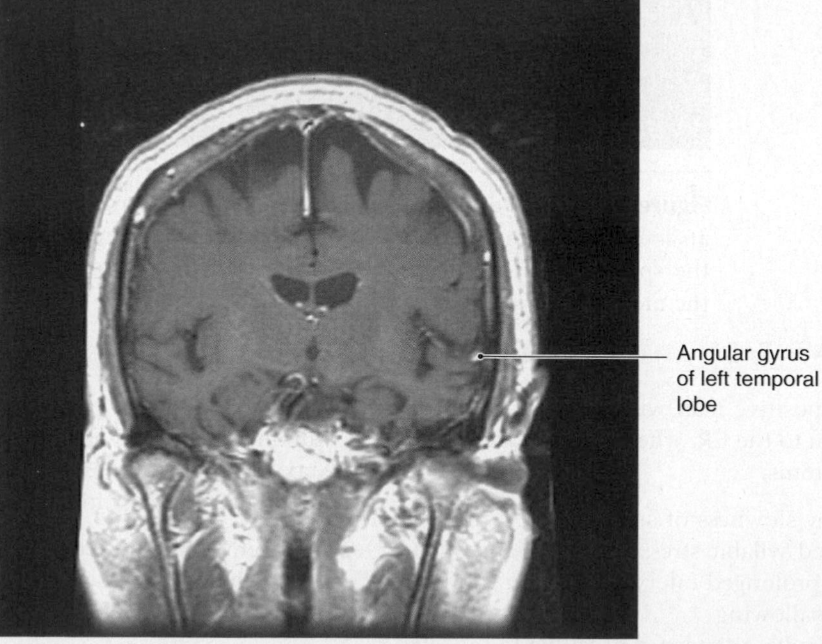

Figure 19-4 Coronal brain MRI study showing left temporal lobe atrophy with some frontal atrophy.

(Continued)

CASE FIVE (19-5) (*CONTINUED*)

A 76-year-old woman presents with acute confusion, memory loss, difficulty thinking of names, inability to calculate, draw, and copy (constructional apraxia), with a very mild and subtle comprehension problem. She also exhibited mild right face and arm weakness. MRI showed patchy areas of acute infarction in the left inferior parietal region (Fig. 19-5*A*), and magnetic resonance angiography (Fig. 19-5*B*) disclosed critical stenosis of the left internal carotid artery. She was recommended for the removal of the carotid plaque, and her motor and linguistic performances improved after carotid endarterectomy.

Question: Did this patient have aphasia or a dementia, or a focal lesion? How could the endarterectomy improve her functional ability?

Case (19-5) Discussion: See discussion of case studies

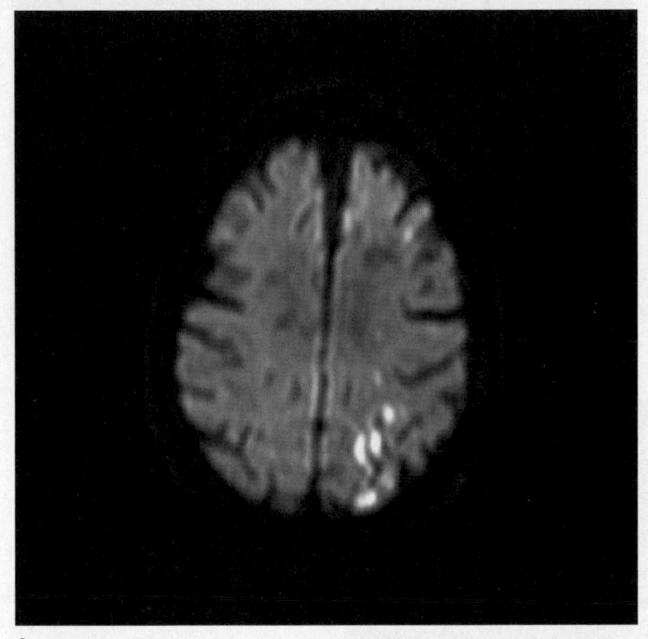

A

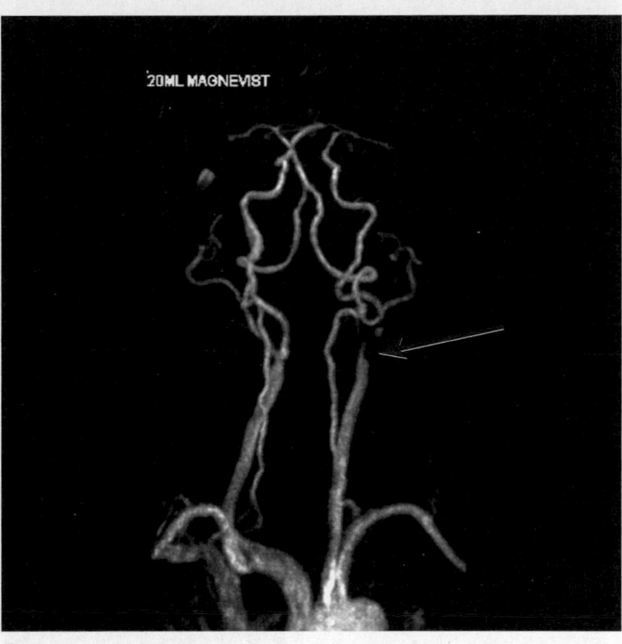

B

Figure 19-5 A. Multiple small areas of acute infarction in the "watershed" area of the left parietal lobe on a diffusion-weighted MR image. B. An illustration of the left internal carotid artery occlusion on a magnetic resonance angiography.

CASE SIX (19-6)

An 82-year-old man had a history of a stroke in the right anterior cerebral artery territory in 1999, secondary to atrial fibrillation, leaving him with a residual left leg weakness. In 2010, he presented with confusion and impaired memory, without any obvious, new focal deficit. MRI disclosed the old right ACA territory infarction (Fig. 19-6*A*), but also an "old" infarction in the left frontal region (Fig. 19-6*B*), and an acute infarction in the right temporal–parietal region (Fig. 19-6*C*).

Question: Can strokes cause a generalized cognitive deficit marked with dementia?

Case (19-6) Discussion: See discussion of case studies

(*Continued*)

CASE SIX (19-6) *(CONTINUED)*

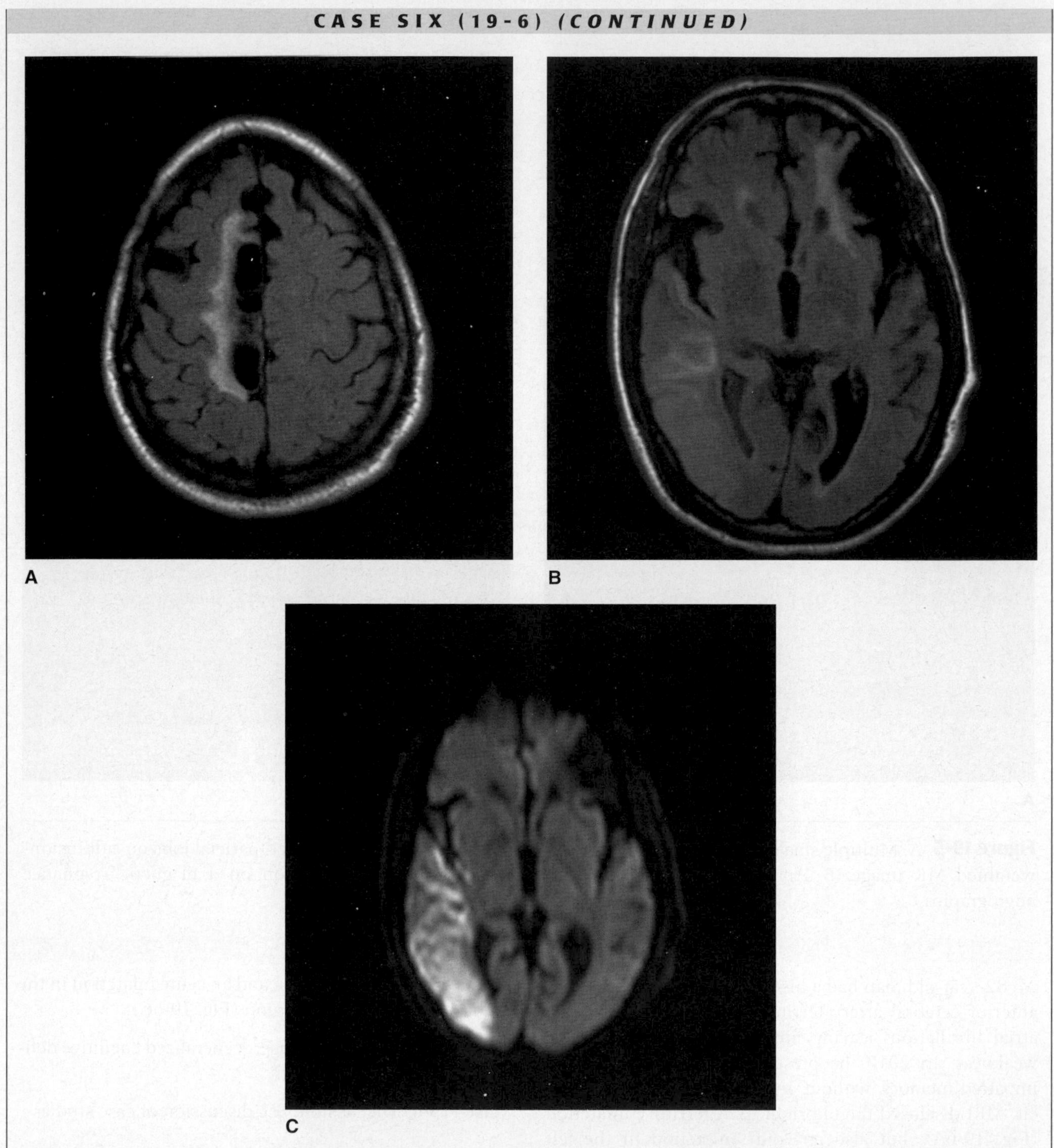

Figure 19-6 An old infarct in the right medial frontal lobe within the territory of the anterior cerebral artery (A) on a fluid-attenuated inversion recovery imaging (FLAIR) MRI. An old left frontal infarction (B) on a FLAIR MRI. Diffusion-weighted MR image of an acute right infarct (C) in the temporal–parietal.

SUMMARY

This chapter discusses the functional organization of the human cerebral cortex and the principal syndromes of abnormal cortical functioning that result from brain diseases. The emphasis is on speech and language disorders, including related disorders, such as apraxia, agnosia, dementia, and TBI. These topics constitute the part of neurology increasingly known as behavioral neurology or cognitive neuroscience.

REVIEW QUESTIONS

1. Complete the following statements using the appropriate technical terms:

   A. As a common accompaniment of aphasia,________ is an acquired inability to perform simple mathematical problems.

   B. As a common accompaniment of aphasia,________ is an acquired inability to express through writing.

   C. Impaired ability to read and comprehend written information secondary to brain damage is called_____.

   D. As a common accompaniment of aphasia, _____ is the impaired ability to perform skilled movements on command.

   E. ________is a progressive and persistent loss of cognitive functions, which are mostly caused by degenerative brain diseases.

   F. A disorder of motor speech that results from central and/or peripheral lesions and affects muscular control of the articulators is________.

   G. ________ are the new words or phrases of the patient's own making often seen in acute aphasia mostly by patients with________.

   H. An inappropriate selection of related or unrelated words by subjects with aphasia is an example of ________.

   I. ________ is a disorder of recognition, which can involve one or multiple modalities (visual, auditory, or tactile).

   J. ________ is the failure to recognize familiar faces.

   K. ________ is a nondominant parietal symptoms in which the patients tend to deny the presence of paralysis.

   L. The cerebral dominance may have a structural basis, which relates to the size of the________.

   M. The________ involves carotid infusion of sodium amytal, and it is used to assess the cerebral dominance.

   N. Related to traumatic brain injuries, ________ refers to a bruising of the brain marked by torn brain tissues; on the other hand, there is no visible bruising of the brain in________.

2. Match each of the following brain regions with its associated function:

A. superior parietal lobule	a. visual agnosia
B. nondominant inferior parietal lobe	b. musical function and nonverbal memory
C. dominant inferior parietal lobe	c. language comprehension and verbal memory
D. nondominant temporal lobe	d. reading and writing
E. dominant temporal lobe	e. body schema and spatial attention
F. bilateral occipital lobe lesions	f. visual–spatial and constructional skills

3. Match each of the following aphasia types with its associated clinical characteristics:

A. Broca aphasia	a. impaired verbal expression
B. Wernicke aphasia	b. impaired auditory comprehension
C. anomia	c. impaired repetition
D. conduction aphasia	d. difficulty finding and retrieving lexicon

4. Match each of the following disorders with its associated dysfunction:

A. deep dyslexia	a. acquired illiteracy with impaired ability to read and write
B. surface alexia	b. pure alexia with word blindness with preserved ability to write
C. phonological alexia	c. semantic and visual errors in reading words
D. alexia with agraphia	d. reading by the recognition of words' meanings and by conversion of words to phonemes
E. alexia without agraphia	e. reading by grapheme-to-phoneme conversion, without directly recognizing words

5. Match each of the following apraxia types with its associated description:

A. ideomotor apraxia	a. failure to carry out a motor act in response to a verbal command
B. limb-kinetic apraxia	b. failure to use a real object
C. ideational apraxia	c. impaired skilled motor acts involving only one limb

6. Define three major categories of dementia causing conditions/diseases.

7. Match each of the following neurological conditions with the associated disease categories:

A. Alzheimer disease	a. systemic diseases associated with dementia
B. Pick disease	b. neurological diseases associated with dementia
C. Creutzfeldt–Jakob disease	c. degenerative brain diseases causing dementia
D. infections	
E. neoplasm	
F. normal pressure hydrocephalus	
G. Huntington chorea	
H. Parkinson disease	

8. Match each of the following dementing diseases with its associated pathophysiology:

A. Alzheimer disease	a. caused by an infectious agent, this rapidly progressive disease is marked by mood changes, dementia, seizures, and myoclonus.
B. Pick disease	b. a disease of frontal and temporal degeneration and includes Pick bodies
C. Creutzfeldt–Jakob disease	c. a disease marked by senile plaques and neurofibrillary tangles in the cerebral cortex, hippocampus, and nucleus basalis of Meynert

20

Diagnostic Techniques and Neurologic Concepts

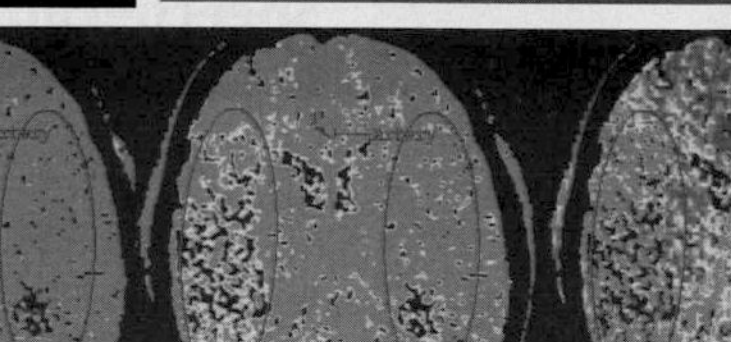

LEARNING OBJECTIVES

After studying this chapter, students should be able to:

- Understand the basics of brain imaging techniques
- Outline the diagnostic usefulness of each brain imaging technique
- Explain the sodium amytal infusion technique
- Explain the electromyography and its clinical significance
- Discuss the clinical value of electroencephalography in measuring seizures and altered consciousness
- Describe the physiology of sleep and explain associated patterns of brain activity
- Discuss the concept of the event-related evoked potential technique
- Describe the dichotic listening paradigm
- Discuss the neurolinguistic significance of corticography, subcortical electrode implants, and stereotaxic surgery
- Discuss myopathic, neuropathic, and seizure disorders
- Explain common patterns of inheritance and associated genetic disorders

A number of diagnostic techniques are available for the study of neurologically impaired patients, each based on a particular physical or biological mechanism. A thorough review of all these techniques is beyond the scope of this chapter; only the most relevant neurological concepts, and diagnostic techniques related to neurocognitive and neurolinguistic impairments are discussed.

BRAIN IMAGING**

Historical Background

The discovery of X-rays in 1895 by Wilhelm Conrad Roentgen, a German physicist, had an immediate and profound impact on the diagnosis of diseases and changed the practice of medicine so rapidly that Roentgen was awarded the Nobel Prize for Physics in 1901. Early neuroradiological diagnostic techniques such as skull films, **pneumoencephalography** and **cerebral angiography**, have been based on the use of X-rays. Skull X-rays were used mostly to detect skull fractures and displacement of bony and calcified structures (i.e., the pineal gland, the falx cerebri) in response to expansile processes (tumors, hematomas). Pneumoencephalography was performed by injecting air into the cerebrospinal spaces through a lumbar puncture (see Chapter 8) allowing the evaluation of pathological processes in the brain. Cerebral angiograph (discussed later in the chapter) is performed by obtaining high-speed X-ray imaging during the intravascular injection of contrast medium.

Developed in 1972 in England by Geoffrey Hounsfield, **computed tomography** (CT) has truly revolutionized the study of the brain. Introduced in the early 1980s as a clinical tool, **magnetic resonance imaging** (MRI) has further energized the diagnostic field, particularly in neuroradiology, and has replaced CT and other techniques in the evaluation of many disease conditions. The current growth in the number of MRI scanners makes it the most common of all imaging devices. Other techniques occasionally used in neuroradiology include nuclear medicine techniques, some of which are reviewed later in this chapter.

Key Terms:

Anisotropic media	**Isotropic media**
Blood oxygen level dependent	**Low density lesion**
Diffusion-weighted image	**Perfusion-weighted image**
High density lesion	**Pixel**
Hounsfield unit	**T1-weighted image**
	T2-weighted image

Cerebral Angiography

Cerebral angiography is usually performed via the transfemoral approach using the Seldinger technique (a method of needle insertion into a blood vessel). Catheters are advanced from the groin to the carotid or vertebral arteries. The risks inherent to angiography are the possibility of transient ischemic attacks or stroke, arterial injuries, and

**Jointly written with Lotfi Hacein-Bey, MD. Radiological Associates of Sacramento Medical Group Inc, CA.

BOX 20-1

Speech–Language Pathology in Medical Environment

Students working with human behaviors in medical settings not only require a functional knowledge of neuroscience and brain–behavior relationship, but they must also familiarize themselves with important neurological concepts. These clinical concepts include imaging techniques, neurosurgical procedures, electrodiagnostic tools, procedural issues involved with sodium amytal infusion, altered types of consciousness, neuropathies, infections, and the modes of genetic inheritance. A basic understanding of these concepts and procedures helps them become better clinicians by allowing the integration of their clinical knowledge with advances in medical fields, which is needed for presenting a broader and encompassing view of their field.

groin hematomas. Contrast medium is injected at a rate that varies inversely with the size of the vessel. Although modern nonionic contrast agents have become relatively safe, they are treated with their use limited to the necessary amount since they can cause seizures and have potential nephrotoxicity. Images are acquired by a powerful **X-ray** angiography equipment at a high rate (usually between 2 and 4 images per second), and for several seconds, so as to cover the arterial, capillary, and venous phases of contrast passage. Vascular structures are depicted as the radiopaque contrast agent outlines their margins. In the anterior (carotid) circulation, the anterior and middle cerebral arteries are visualized, while the posterior cerebral arteries are usually seen after the posterior (vertebrobasilar) circulation has been injected (Fig. 20-1).

Cerebral angiography remains the gold standard by which to evaluate the cerebral vasculature, primarily cerebral aneurysms, arteriovenous malformations (AVMs), fistulas, and hypervascular tumors. The explosion of neurointerventional techniques in the past two decades has resulted in major improvements in the catheter and device technology (coils, stents, embolic agents, clot-retrieving

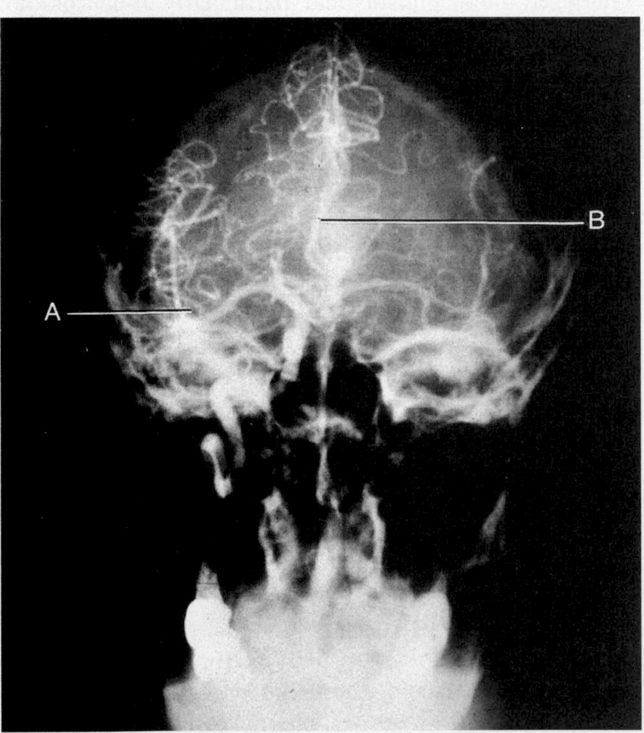

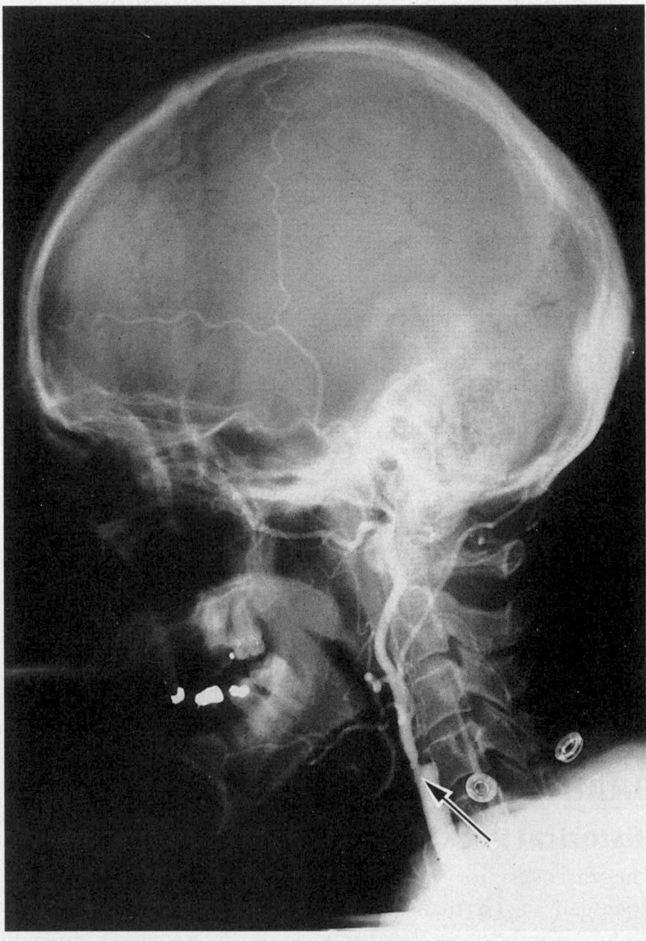

Figure 20-1 Angiographic illustration of major cortical arteries. Frontal (anteroposterior) view of middle (**A**) cerebral artery branches and anterior (**B**) cerebral artery branches. Lateral angiographic view of a left internal carotid artery thrombosis (*arrow*) with no filling beyond the carotid bifurcation point.

devices, thrombolytic drugs) used for the treatment of stroke and intracranial vascular lesions, that is, aneurysms and AVMs; also see Chapter 7.

Computed Tomography Techniques

Computed tomography (CT) technology is based on the use of highly collimated X-ray beams rotating around and traversing the patient and then collected by CT detectors. Each projection of an X-ray is made at a certain angle and consists of a certain number of individual X-ray photons. The emergent X-ray beam is expressed as a fraction of the original X-ray beam after it has been attenuated by the tissues traversed, therefore defining a "**linear attenuation coefficient**" or "**absorption value**" for each point of space. Slices of tissue are then reconstructed using complex mathematical methods, and the various tissues are displayed on an image within which various shades of gray represent the corresponding tissues.

CT remains either the examination of choice or the first-line test in many indications, including subarachnoid hemorrhage, trauma, and hydrocephalus. CT uses a narrow beam of X-ray photons that are emitted by a rotating X-ray tube; the thickness of the beam may be adjusted to produce axial slices of various thicknesses, usually 10, 5, or 3 mm. After having traversed the patient's head, the photon beam is "attenuated," that is, a number of photons are stopped by the tissues. The difference between the original and resulting beams is analyzed and displayed as a wide variety of shades of gray applied to various points in space represented in volume cell elements (voxels) to produce a two-dimensional (2D) picture (Fig. 20-2*A*), which contains a number of picture cell elements or "pixels." The higher the pixel number, the higher the resolution. The various shades of gray correspond to X-ray photon absorption coefficients, also called Hounsfield units. By definition, the gray scale ranges between the lowest Hounsfield unit, −1,000, which represents air, and the highest Hounsfield unit, +1,000, which represents dense bone; while water (represented by cerebrospinal fluid) appears dark on CT and has a value of 0 on the scale (Table 20-1). Pathological processes are usually labeled as either high- or low-density lesions. High-density intracranial lesions, which are especially significant to students in communicative disorders, are acute hemorrhages and calcified lesions. Important low-density lesions are cerebral chronic infarction, edema, and cystic lesions (Fig. 20-2*B*; Table 20-2). Tumors may be either high or low density.

Various radiopaque contrast agents can be used to better characterize pathologic processes and demonstrate certain vascular anatomy. Intravascular contrast agents may be injected intravenously (most commonly) or intra-arterially and localized in the intravascular space, which becomes more conspicuous because of the greater attenuation of X-rays by the contrast. Some pathologic conditions, that is, tumors and inflammatory processes show contrast enhancement as a result of a breakdown of the blood–brain barrier, allowing seepage of contrast from the intravascular compartment into the cerebral tissues. In some pathologic states, contrast enhancement occurs only during certain stages of the disease.

CT has been used extensively in neurolinguistics for the study of brain–behavior relationships. In an excellent description of CT applications, Gado et al. (1979) provided a comprehensive framework for relating brain anatomy on CT to language regions and Brodmann areas of interest. Naeser and Hayward (1987), Damasio (1998), and many other researchers have used CT to demonstrate anatomic correlations for classical aphasias. Alexander et al. (1987) used CT-based evidence to demonstrate the existence of subcortical aphasias.

Despite the disadvantages of using ionizing radiation, limited resolution, and poor differentiation between gray and white matter as well as an inability to diagnose an acute infarct, CT remains cost-effective compared to newer imaging techniques, especially MRI. For example, it is the preferred diagnostic tool in uncooperative patients because the image is not significantly degraded by motion artifacts. It can readily detect fresh (acute and subacute) hemorrhages and can identify bone fractures. The advent of 3D CT reconstructions allows clinicians to create images in multiple planes from volume rendering (VR).

CT Angiography

In the past decade, **CT angiography** (CTA) has gained acceptance for the noninvasive evaluation of extracranial and intracranial circulations. Clinical conditions that at present are routinely evaluated with CTA include carotid steno-occlusive disease, cerebral venous thrombosis, cerebral aneurysms, and acute stroke. Newer-generation CT machines allow the evaluation of large volumes of tissue, and therefore large vascular segments. Although cerebral angiography remains the gold standard to study the cerebral vasculature, comparative sensitivity and specificity rates for CTA are reported to be in the 98% to 99% range. CTA is obtained with a rapid intravenous injection of iodinated contrast medium, which localizes in high concentration in the arterial system. Fast imaging, referred to as "**dynamic CT scanning**," is obtained, and volume reconstructions are achieved with 2D and 3D postprocessing software. Multiplanar reconstruction is commonly used to display 2D reconstructions, and VR to display 3D reconstructions (Fig. 20-3).

CT Perfusion

CT perfusion (CTP) is now routinely performed to evaluate a variety of etiologies, including acute stroke, carotid steno-occlusive disease, certain brain tumors, and cerebral vasospasm following subarachnoid hemorrhage. The principles behind CTP rely on the assumption that (1) most of the brain tissue has a normal cerebral autoregulation for the maintenance of energy needs and that (2) contrast

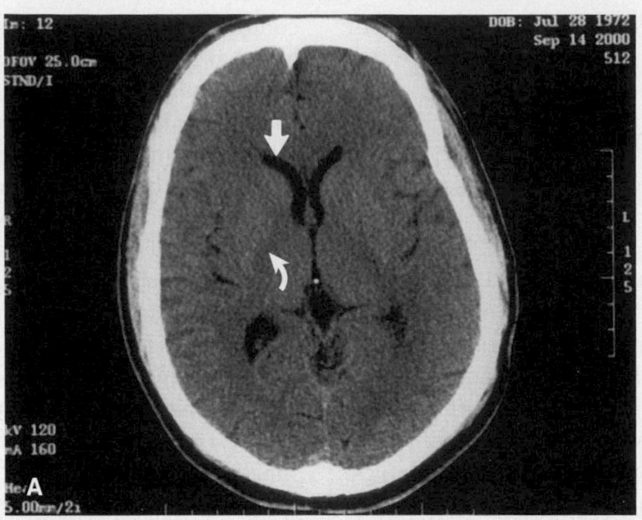

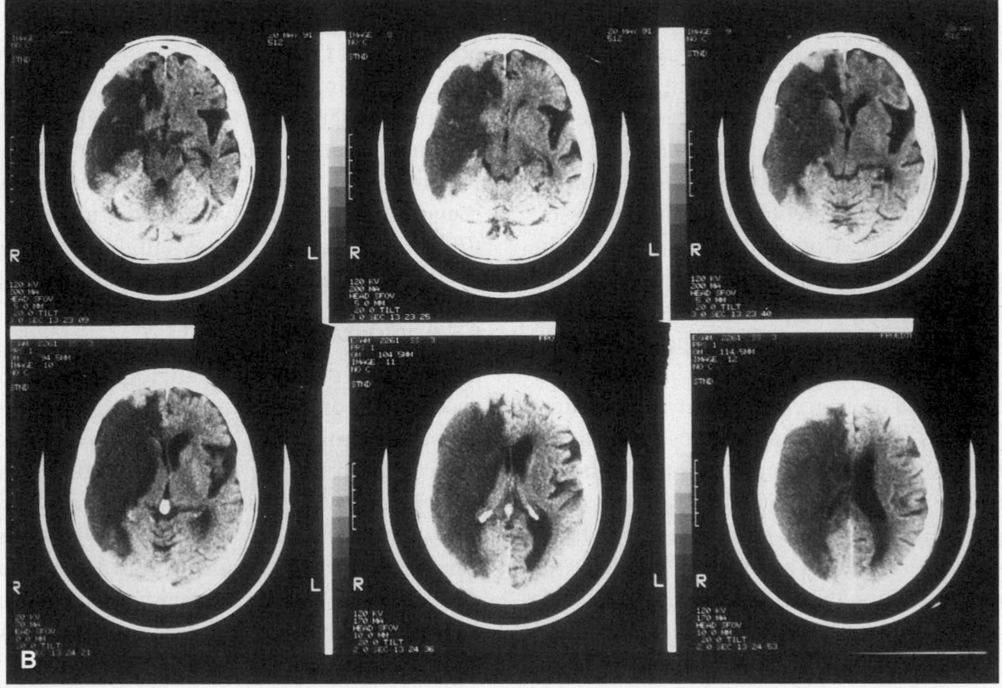

Figure 20-2 CT scans of a normal brain (A) with low density of the fluid-filled anterior horns of the lateral ventricle (*straight arrow*), adjacent brain parenchyma, and the basal ganglia (*curved arrow*). Series of CT scans of a massive infarct in the right hemisphere (B) involving the frontal, parietal, and occipital lobes.

material is limited to blood vessels, at least at first pass and in healthy cerebral parenchyma. CTP data analysis relies on the central volume principle, that is, the behavior of an iodinated contrast material bolus crossing the cerebral capillary networks, with subsequent modifications of contrast-enhancement profiles. CTP does not require any special equipment, only dedicated postprocessing software. Dynamic contrast-enhanced CTP uses an *intravascular* tracer instead of a *freely diffusible* tracer, and kinetic analysis and data acquisition methodology that is different from those of established methods of flow quantitation, that is, Xe-washout, Xe-CT, and positron-emission tomography (PET), which are all superior to CTP mainly because of the much quicker kinetics of iodinated contrast material compared with that of stable xenon-CT, and the limited volume coverage offered by CT. In practice, a rapid injection of contrast medium is made and rapid imaging is obtained within 40 seconds. A given volume of brain

Table 20-1

Pixel Attenuation Values

Hounsfield Unit Range	Appearance	Tissue Representation
High, 1–1,000	White	Bone and acute blood
Medium, 0	Gray to light gray	Chronic blood, brain (gray and white) substance
Low, –1 to –1,000	Light to dark black	Fat and air

(between 10 and 40 mm thickness) has to be selected, which limits the spatial resolution of CTP. Postprocessing allows for quality control (correction of motion, timing of contrast injection) and for the application of a deconvolution mathematical analysis (arterial and venous). This allows the calculation of the major perfusion parameters, which are mapped on anatomical images (Fig. 20-4): **cerebral blood volume** (CBV), **cerebral blood flow** (CBF), and **mean transit time** (MTT).

Magnetic Resonance Imaging Techniques

MRI contrast mechanisms are very different from those of CT. MRI relies on complex responses of living tissues to an applied magnetic field and exposure to radiofrequency (RF) waves. MRI does not use hazardous ionizing radiation, as do CT and conventional X-ray techniques. Rather, it creates images of structures in living brains or organs from the magnetic signal of the atomic nuclei of water, the hydrogen protons. Water is one of the main body components, though body tissues differ in their water concentrations. Hydrogen protons, with positive and negative areas, have north and south poles and act as spinning magnetic bars. In the absence of external interference, the magnetic activity of hydrogen protons is random so that overall they cancel each other out.

Table 20-2

Brain Structures Appearance on CT Images

Structure	Appearance
Acute blood and bone	Bright white
Subacute blood	Light gray
White and gray matter	Gray
Tumor	Gray to white
Fat	Light black
Air	Dark black

To obtain an MRI study, the body (e.g., the brain) is placed in an artificial external magnetic field, which causes the hydrogen protons of the tissue to align along a single vector. The strength of this strong external magnetic field commonly ranges from 0.3 to 5 T, which is about 100,000 times greater than the earth's average magnetic field of 50 μT, with most machines operating at 1.5 T. While the protons are aligned along a vector, a RF wave is emitted in continuous short bursts by an external RF-transmitting coil and excites the hydrogen protons. As a result, hydrogen protons realign themselves in various ways depending on their chemical environment and tissue type. When the external RF signal ends, protons return to their previous orientation along the main magnetic field by releasing the RF energy in the form of electromagnetic signal, which constitutes the basic image data.

This RF signal is collected by a receiving coil, and decomposed into the various components of the MRI image. Each point of the 3D space is therefore displayed on 2D or 3D pictures with various shades of gray according to the signal strength and the MR parameter studied. The protons have a variety of intrinsic characteristics, the most important being the T1 and T2 relaxation factors, the susceptibility, diffusibility, and flow characteristics. Because bone contains limited water, it produces fewer signals relative to the other cerebral structures (Fig. 20-5).

MRI relies on complex responses of living tissues to an applied magnetic field and exposed to RF waves. All molecules have natural motions within their environment as a result of naturally occurring rotation, vibration, and translation. Smaller molecules like water move faster than larger molecules like proteins. The major physical phenomena underlying clinically useful MRI involve the T1 and T2 relaxation times.

T1 is the "longitudinal" relaxation time and reflects the relationship between the frequency of the molecular motion and the Larmor frequency (also called the resonance frequency, dependent on the scanner's magnetic field strength). Therefore, T1 indicates the time required by a molecule to become fully magnetized after it is placed in the magnetic field; in practice, T1 represents the time required by the molecule to regain full magnetization after receiving a RF pulse. T2, on the other hand, is the "transverse" relaxation time. In practice, T2 is the time during which protons remain coherent in their motion, or "in-phase," after being exposed to an RF pulse. While the T2 signal decays because of interactions between protons, the T1 signal decays because of interactions between the protons and the surrounding magnetic environment.

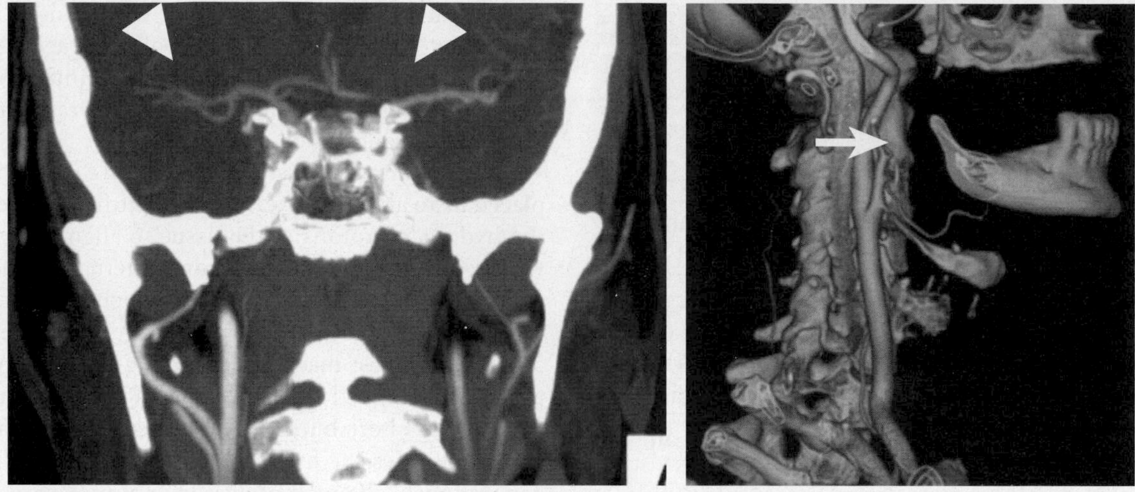

Figure 20-3 CT angiography image of a **left**, maximum intensity projection image shows intracranial circulation, and particularly both middle cerebral arteries (*small* arrows). **Right** 3D volume rendering of right carotid bifurcation (*arrow*) and its relations to the bony skeleton.

In order to obtain an image, the area to be studied, that is, the brain is submitted to a pulse sequence. Although a number of different pulse sequences are available, they all rely on acquiring multiple signals. The **spin-echo sequence** is the most commonly used, and has been refined throughout the years, with fast imaging techniques.

Clinically, T1-weighted images are good for depicting anatomical detail. They provide a better contrast between the gray and white matters based on the difference in fat concentration: white matter appears brighter than gray matter because of the presence of lipid-containing myelin. T1 image, though, is a poor indicator of water changes in tissue that are affected with edema and stroke; on a T1 sequence, edema would appear dark, fat appears bright, water appears dark, gray matter appears dark gray, and white matter appears light gray.

T2-weighted images, as well as fluid-attenuated inversion recovery (FLAIR), are sensitive to changes in water content and have proven to be a better diagnostic tool for the identification of edema and ischemia. On this sequence, the fat appears gray, water appears very bright, and gray matter is lighter than white matter (Fig. 20-6 and Table 20-3).

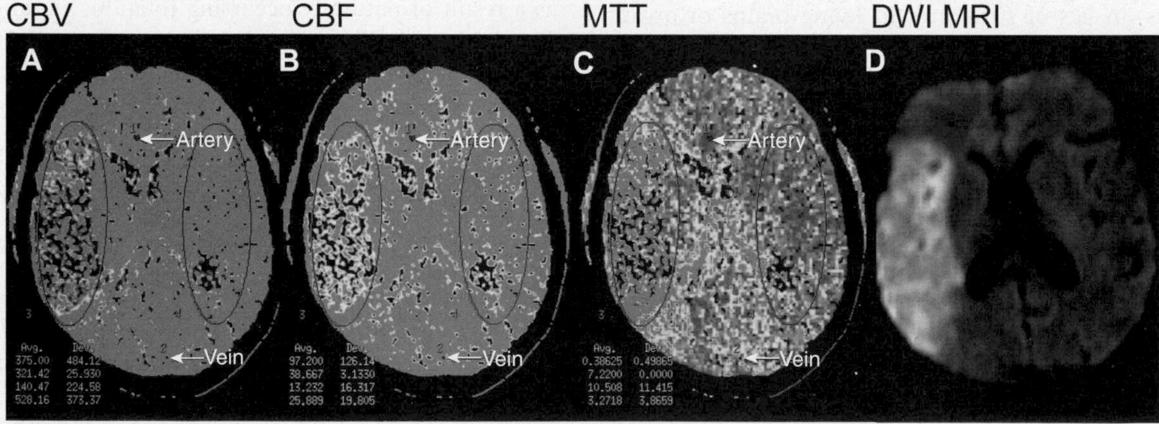

Figure 20-4 CT perfusion image of a patient with left hemiparesis with suspected right hemispheric stroke exhibiting a decreased cerebral blood volume (A) and cerebral blood flow (B), and increased mean transit time (C), diffusion-weighted MRI (D) in right MCA territory. These perfusion abnormalities match exactly the diffusion abnormality seen on MRI (D).

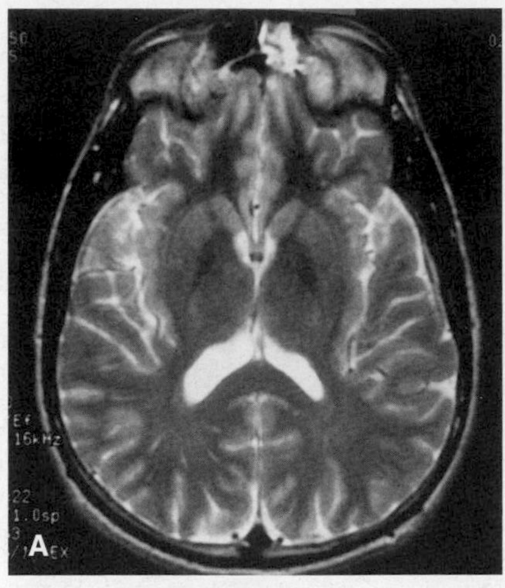

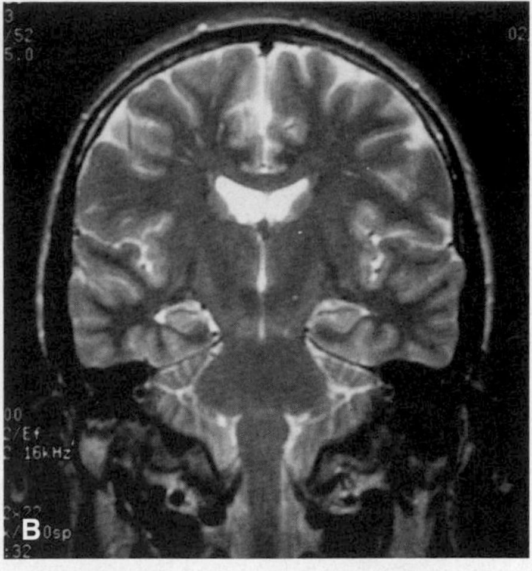

Figure 20-5 A. A normal T2-weighted (fast spin echo; FSE) axial MRI image of the brain with a small incidental left frontal sinus disease. B. A normal T2-weighted (FSE) coronal MRI image of the brain.

Fluid-Attenuated Inversion Recovery

The **fluid-attenuated inversion recovery** (FLAIR) sequence is a combination of T1 and T2, making CSF appear dark, while water in tissues (i.e., edema) appears bright. The FLAIR sequence involves subtraction of the CSF for clarity and is useful to demonstrate inflammatory lesions such as multiple sclerosis or infectious lesions, most tumors, edema, and subacute strokes (see Figs. 5-9 and 19-1*B*).

The **gradient-echo sequence**, also called the susceptibility sequence, is designed to detect metallic moieties, mostly iron from blood, and is used clinically to detect previous hemorrhage within the brain, in conditions such as cavernomas, capillary telangiectasias, amyloid angiopathy, and petechial transformation in stroke.

Diffusion-Weighted Imaging

Diffusion is a molecular property that refers to the random, uniform, and constant movements of water molecules in all directions (the Brownian motion principle); this is true of **isotropic** media, such as water and gases. However, the rate of water molecular movement in body tissues is related to cellular kinetic energy, which depends on thermal energy. Because molecular diffusion is not uniform (**anisotropic**) in body tissue because of barriers placed by tissue structures (cell membrane, axons, and vascular components), it is referred to as **apparent diffusion**. Diffusion-weighted (DW) MRI measures the variability of Brownian uniform water diffusion in terms of an apparent diffusion coefficient (ADC).

In case of an infarct, the affected area in the brain undergoes cellular swelling (cytotoxic edema), which impairs water diffusion and results in increased signal. As a diagnostic tool, the DWI MRI is extremely sensitive to even minute molecular motion, which makes it highly responsive to ischemic stroke, a neurologic condition of great importance to students of human behavior. In ischemia, the diffusion coefficient in affected tissue attenuates by 50% or so within 3 to 4 minutes of the onset of the infarct (Figs. 20-7 and 20-8*A*).

The loss of blood supply in ischemic stroke contributes to an increased retention of intracellular water volume in brain tissue secondary to cytotoxic edema, resulting in restricted diffusion of water and leading to hyperintensity on DWI studies. This diminished diffusion results in a bright appearance of the diseased area so that an infarct can be identified within 15 to 30 minutes from the onset, a great improvement over standard T1- and T2-weighted MRI studies (4 to 6 hours) and CT scans (24 to 48 hours). DWI also readily differentiates subacute lesions (old infarcts, vasogenic infarcts, and deep white matter pathologies, dilated ventricular spaces, some neoplasms, and demyelination), which do not become hyperintense (bright), as they do with acute stroke.

The underlying mechanism in DWI also could be related to energy failure, with a loss of Na+/K+ pump activity and reduction of extracellular volume. With its sensitivity to molecular motion, DWI has been accepted by neuroradiologists and neurologists as an accurate method for detecting acute stroke within minutes of onset; it is also being evaluated in a variety of other intracranial disease processes.

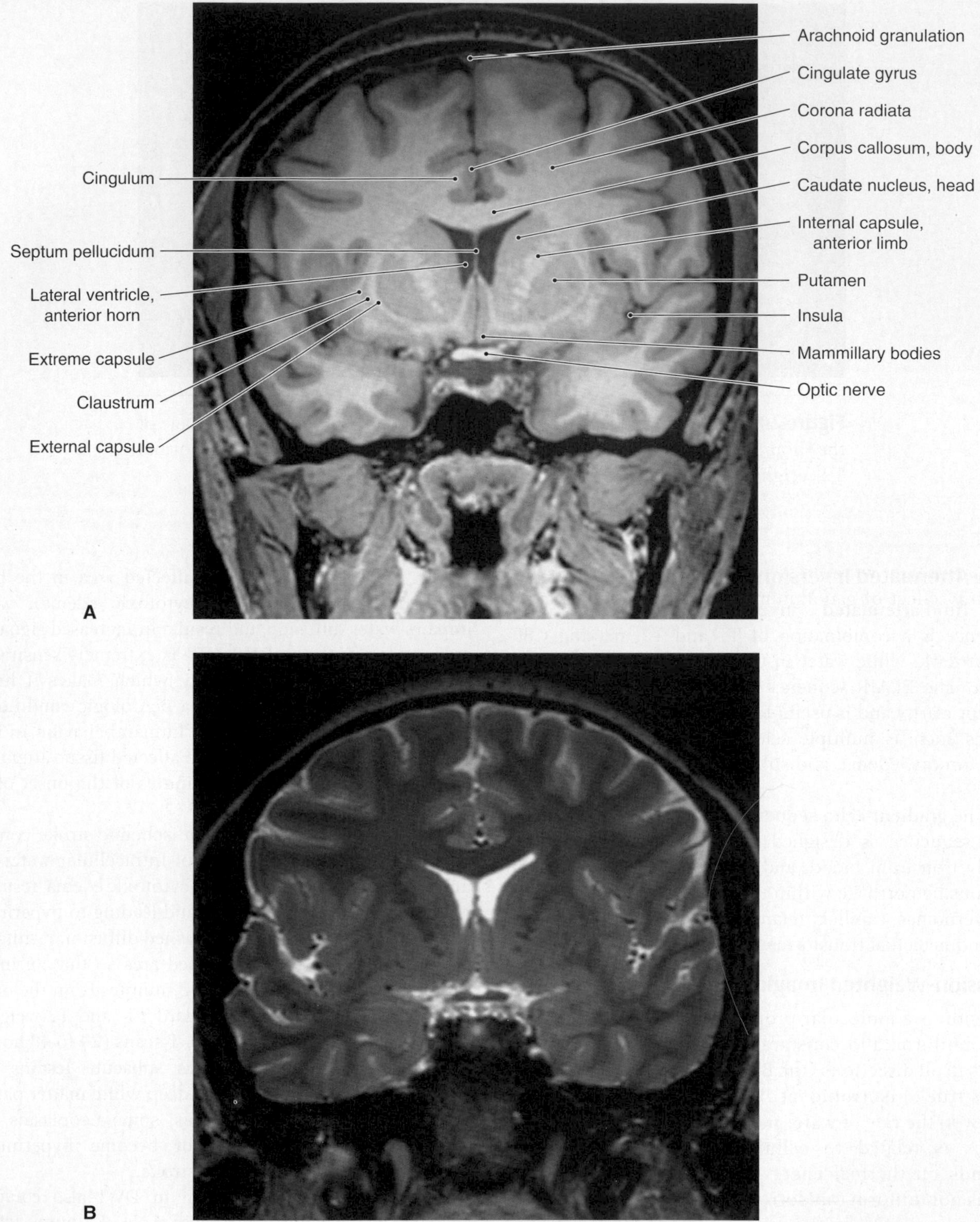

Figure 20-6 Two normal coronal MRIs: T1 (A) and T2 (B).

Table 20-3

Views of Normal and Pathologic Structures on T1- and T2-Weighted MRI Studies

State of Health	Structure	T1	T2
Normal	Bone	Black (+)	Black (+)
	Gray matter	Gray (dark)	Gray
	White matter	Gray	Gray (dark)
	Cerebrospinal fluid	Black (+)	White
Pathologic	Infarct (acute and subacute)	Gray (dark)	Gray to white
	Ischemia (acute and subacute)	Gray (dark)	Gray to white
	Tumor	Gray (dark)	Gray to white
	Edema	Gray (dark)	Gray to white

Perfusion-Weighted Imaging

Perfusion-Weighted Imaging (PWI) is sensitive to microscopic levels of blood flow. The most commonly used MR perfusion method is the contrast-enhanced rCBV (relative CBV) technique, which relies on the T2-shortening susceptibility effect of gadolinium contrast medium. Again, the susceptibility effect refers to loss of MR signal due to distortion of the local magnetic field by the paramagnetic contrast agent. The CBF can be inferred from the rCBV measurements, provided that the transit time of the contrast agent, CBF, is known.

More recently, an alternative noninvasive method of perfusion imaging has emerged called the **arterial spin-labeling** (ASL) technique. ASL allows the direct measurement of CBF by using the signal of water molecules in arterial blood as a natural tracer. Protons from arterial blood are "magnetically' labeled by using saturation pulses, and function as diffusible tracers. Perfusion MRI has become an established diagnostic tool in the evaluation of incipient or acute stroke and is sensitive to ischemia within minutes of onset (Fig. 20.8C–E). Perfusion MRI is also useful to assess blood flow and angiogenesis in brain tumors, and to distinguish tumor recurrence from post-treatment radiation necrosis.

Functional MRI

Functional MRI (fMRI) measures the effects of blood oxygen level dependent (BOLD), which represent the differential activity of hemoglobin and deoxyhemoglobin in the magnetic environment of the MRI machine. Any eloquent part of the brain that participates in a specific linguistic or sensorimotor task exhibits greater neuronal activity in the corresponding brain region, which initiates greater oxygen consumption, subsequently causing increased amounts of released deoxygenated hemoglobin (deoxyhemoglobin) in the surrounding veins. Deoxyhemoglobin is highly paramagnetic and generates a signal that triggers a greater redistribution of blood to the target area. However, the

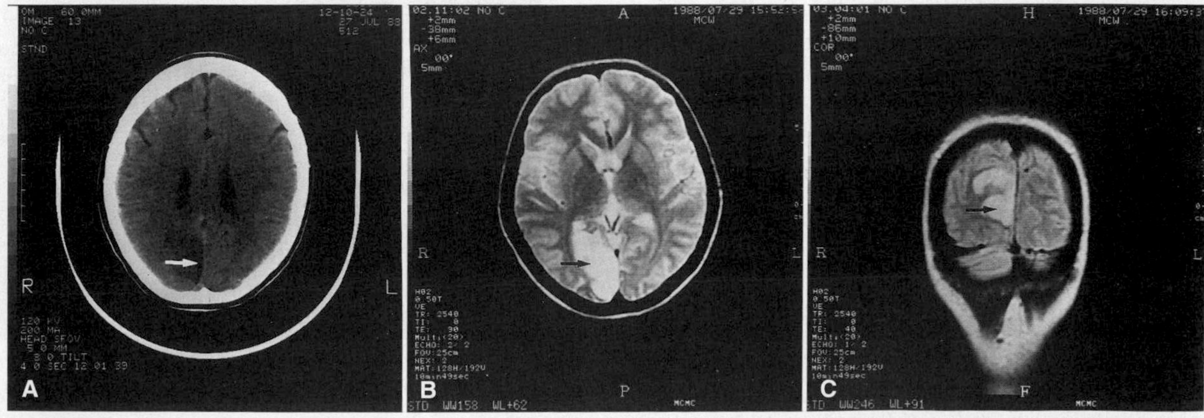

Figure 20-7 Three views of a massive right occipital infarct in a single patient. A. CT image. B. axial MRI. C. Coronal MRI study.

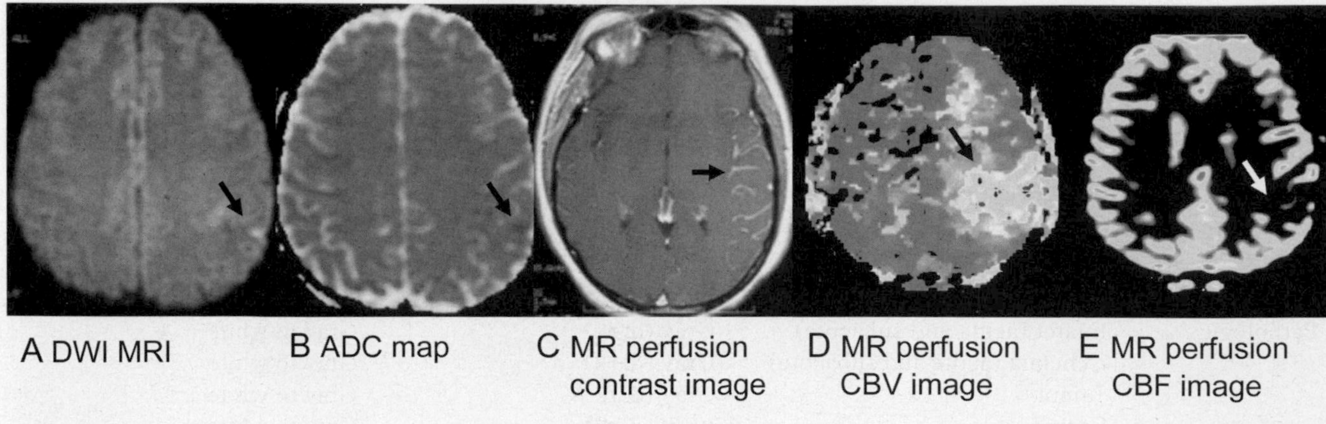

Figure 20-8 MRI showing diffusion-perfusion mismatch in stroke patient. **A.** Diffusion-weighted MRI image with a hypertense area of abnormal diffusion in the left motor cortical region. **B.** Apparent diffusion coefficient image with an area of abnormal diffusion (*dark*) consistent with an acute ischemic lesion in the left frontal posterior region. **C.** Contrast-enhanced MRI perfusion image with a contrast stagnation in the left middle cerebral artery territory. **D.** Cerebral blood volume MRI perfusion image with a decreased blood volume in the area of injury. **E.** Cerebral blood flow MR perfusion image with decreased perfusion in the entire left hemisphere, an excellent example of a diffusion–perfusion mismatch in which the area of perfusion deficit is larger than the area of injury seen on diffusion imaging.

stipulation is that there is a lag of 3 to 6 seconds before blood flows to the target area. The time gap between the presence of deoxygenated and the return of oxygenated hemoglobin is related to the BOLD effect. Therefore, and importantly, fMRI does not directly reflect neuronal activity, but rather the flow changes which are induced by it.

The BOLD-fMRI research paradigm involves several periods of rest alternated with periods of activation. A series of images of the brain region of interest are taken while the patient rests. A second set of images are taken while the patient performs a controlled sensorimotor or linguistic task. In general, 30 images are acquired in a period of 90 seconds. The first 10 images (30 seconds) and the last 10 images (30 seconds) are used as the baseline; the middle 10 images (30 seconds) images are acquired when the patient is performing the specific task and engaging the eloquent brain. The baseline images are subtracted from the task images, and the activated cortical areas are considered to be related to specific functions (Figs. 20-9 and 20-10). Although BOLD is the primary method employed for fMRI, other methods are evaluated: arterial **spin labeling** (ASL), MRI signal weighting by CBF, and CBV.

As an important neurolinguistic technique for students of human behavior, fMRI is used to precisely map brain areas activated through specific stimuli, such as sensorimotor, visual, linguistic, and nonlinguistic tasks (Figs. 20-9 and 20-10). This has allowed researchers to observe the differences and/or progressive physiologic changes in activated brain regions. Altered blood flow patterns are associated with a variety of pathologic states in brain tissue. fMRI not only is important for the investigation of normal or basic function in vivo but

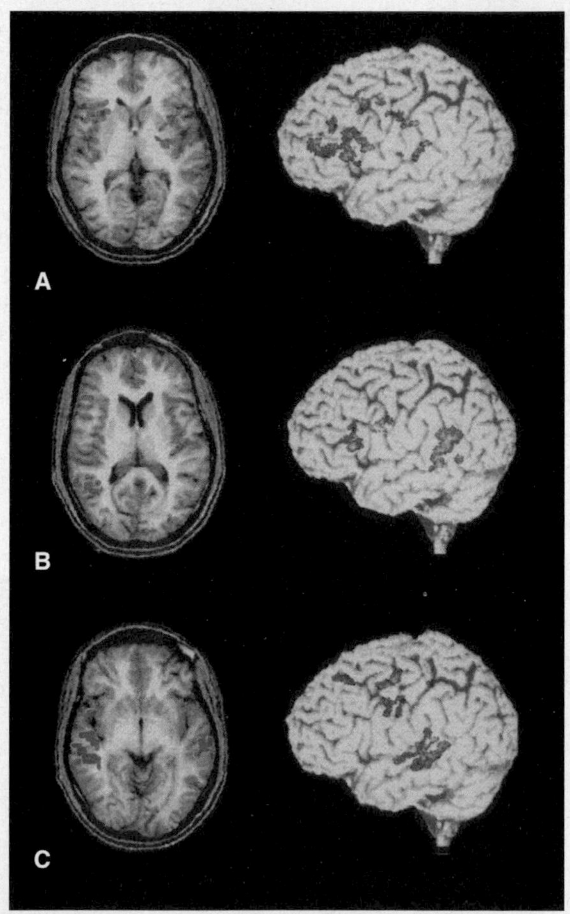

Figure 20-9 Anomalous cortical representation in a patient with demonstrated left hemispheric dominance on the Wada test. The fMRI images show bilateral cortical activation of the language areas during three tasks. **A.** Lexical generation. **B.** Silent sentence repetition. **C.** Listening.

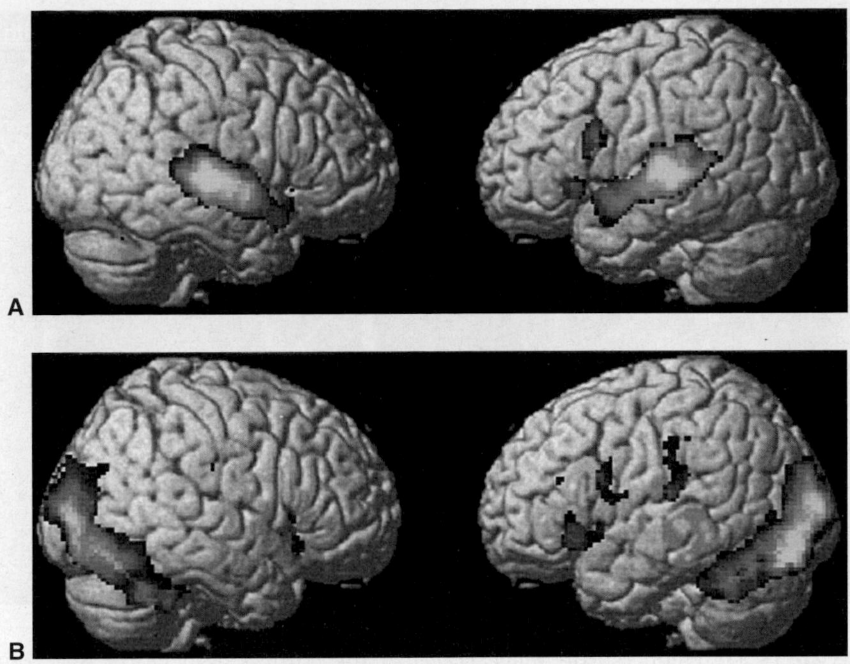

Figure 20-10 Functional MRI images with a bilateral cortical activation during a lexical decision task. **A.** The effect of contrasting lexical decisions when listening to real words and pseudo-words against null events. **B.** The cortical area activated during the lexical decision task on visually presented stimuli. The threshold of activation is significant at $p < 0.05$ (FWE [family wise error] corrected for multiple comparisons); activity is seen on the surface of the right and left hemispheres of the SPM2 single-subject template brain.

also has become a valuable source of information for guiding the treatment of pathologic conditions. The imaging technique helps clinicians monitor brain tumors, stroke, and degenerative or chronic central nervous system (CNS) disorders, such as seizures and multiple sclerosis. The localization of the sensorimotor cortex by fMRI has proved to be extremely useful in the preoperative planning of brain surgery for tumors, epilepsy, and other lesions, decreasing the risk of a neurologic deficit.

Diffusion Tensor Imaging

Diffusion tensor imaging (DTI), another recent development in MRI technology, evaluates the directionality of water molecular movements affected by tissue barriers in the body. This technique provides a way to identify normal and dysfunctioning parallel-running myelinated axonal tracts in the cortical white matter (Fig. 20-11). Molecular diffusion depends on the orientation of the white matter tracks and on the integrity of the myelin. The technique is based on the understanding that nerve fibers have a typical and standard microstructure that regulates the characteristic pattern of water-molecule diffusion. By including diffusion gradients of water molecules in at least six noncollinear directions for a uniform sampling, directionality of water movement can be calculated by eigenvectors (a mathematical value indicating directional movement). DTI involves an analysis of the magnitude and direction of water molecules and provides an averaged measure of water diffusion in one given orientation, called mean diffusivity (D'), and the degree of diffusion anisotropy (differential diffusional properties in different directions), which is also called fractional anisotropy (FA).

From the data collected via DTI, clinicians are able to generate color-coded maps of the diffusion anisotropy and direction of maximum diffusivity, which reflect properties of tissue microstructure. In general, water diffuses in the direction of the fiber orientation (parallel) more quickly than in other directions; this quality plays a role in clinical diagnosis. This technique is sensitive to subtle microstructural changes in white matter wiring in diseases such as multiple sclerosis, Alzheimer disease, aphasia, alexia, autism, and schizophrenia. This will also provide evidence to prove or disapprove Geschwind-connection theory. DTI is particularly useful in the evaluation of the anatomic correlates of disconnection syndromes (see Box 20-2). In its clinical applications, it has been suggested that a drop in

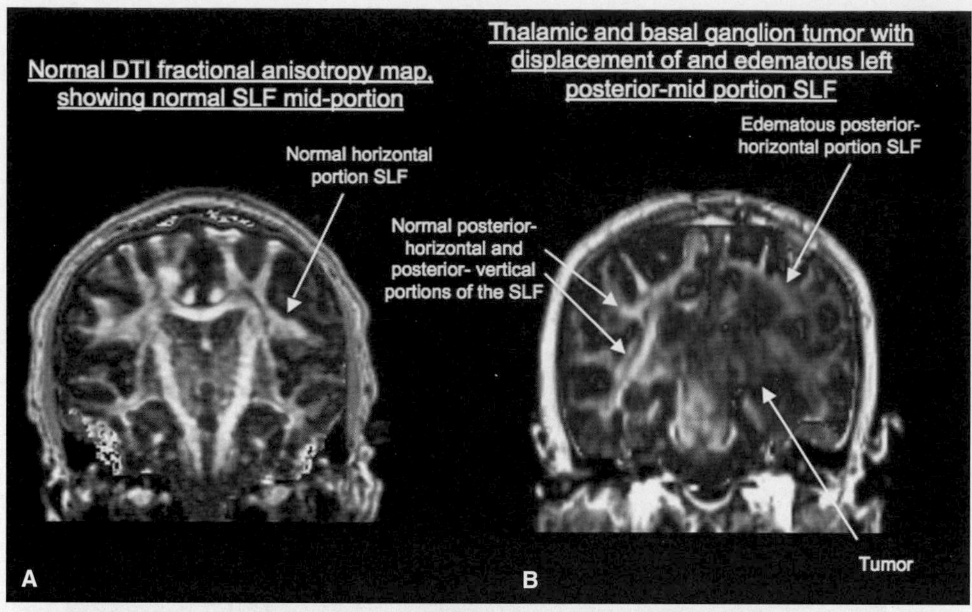

Figure 20-11 Diffusion tensor image (*DTI*) of the cortical association fiber bundle. **A.** A normal DTI fractional anisotropy map indicating a normal superior longitudinal fasciculus (*SLF*). **B.** A subcortical tumor with displacement of an edematous SLF.

FA reflects myelin disintegration and axonal disruption, whereas an increase in *D′* results from increased free water content and injury in structures that restrict water diffusion.

Magnetic Resonance Angiography/Venography

Blood flow is another phenomenon that can be utilized by MRI to generate information. The physical modifications linked to flow have been at the origin of vascular imaging, which can target the arterial system (**magnetic resonance angiography**—MRA) or the venous system (**magnetic resonance venography**—MRV). All flow imaging techniques are based on (1) the suppression of background signal represented by stationary tissues, and (2) the postprocessing of data to reconstruct maximum intensity projection (MIP) and 3D images (Fig. 20-12).

The major techniques used for flow imaging are time-of-flight (TOF) imaging, phase contrast (PC) imaging, fresh blood imaging, and contrast-enhanced MRA. While the first three techniques use the spontaneous contrast of flowing blood, the latter uses an intravenous bolus of contrast medium (gadolinium) coupled with a dynamic gradient-echo MRI technique; finer contrast spatial resolution comes at the cost of the use of contrast medium, which has potential toxicity in patients with renal insufficiency.

MRA is routinely used for the workup of patients with carotid, vertebrobasilar, or intracranial atheromatous disease, either preventively or after a stroke. MRA is also routinely used in the screening and follow-up of patients with intracranial aneurysms, and for the diagnostic workup of patients with AVMs.

MRV is usually obtained with either TOF or PC technique. MRV allows the imaging of intracranial dural sinuses and veins and is most commonly used when dural sinus thrombosis is suspected. It is also useful to study large veins in proximity to brain tumors prior to surgery.

Magnetic Resonance Spectroscopy

Magnetic Resonance Spectroscopy (MRS) provides a measure of brain chemistry. The most common nuclei that are used are ^{1}H (proton), ^{23}Na (sodium), and ^{31}P (phosphorus). Proton spectroscopy is easier to perform and provides much higher signal to noise than either sodium or phosphorus. Unlike for MRI, where the total signal from all the protons in each voxel is used to make the image, for MRS, the fat and water peaks are eliminated by using suppression techniques. These suppression techniques are generally used with a "STEAM" (STimulated Echo Acquisition Mode) or "PRESS" (Point RESolved Spectroscopy) pulse sequence acquisition. A Fourier transform is then applied to the data to separate the signal into individual frequencies. Protons in different molecules resonate at slightly different frequencies because the local electron cloud affects the magnetic field experienced by the proton. Proton MRS can be performed within 10 to 15 minutes and can be added on to conventional MRI protocols. It can be used to serially monitor biochemical changes in tumors, stroke, epilepsy, metabolic disorders, infections, and neurodegenerative diseases like AD.

BOX 20-2

Clinically Important Points of Neuroimaging

- Despite advances in imaging, cerebral angiography remains the gold standard for evaluating the cerebral vasculature, and particularly cerebral aneurysms, arteriovenous malformations and fistulas, and hypervascular tumors.
- Computed tomography (CT) remains the first-line test in many clinical conditions including subarachnoid hemorrhage, trauma, and hydrocephalus. Easy availability and low cost make CT a desired diagnostic technique. Furthermore, its acute sensitivity to hemorrhage in the brain has made it essential for the determination of eligibility of acute stroke patients for thrombolytics like tPA. Exposure to harmful ionizing radiation and indefectibility of an acute infarct remain two major drawbacks of CT imaging.
- The distinction between T1 and T2 sequences in MRIs is extremely important to students in human behaviors as they both provide two different clinically important pieces of information about the brain. T1-weighted image provides a better anatomical contrast between the gray and white matters based on the difference in fat concentration but it is a poor indicator of edema and stroke. With a heightened sensitivity to water-molecule changes in brain tissues, the T2-weighted sequence serves as a better diagnostic tool for the identification of edema and ischemia.
- With diffusion-based and perfusion-based advances in MRI, the time needed to detect ischemic pathology has significantly decreased. When cytotoxic edema is present, the movement of water molecules is restricted in ischemic tissue. Thus, a diffusion-weighted MRI can identify an infarct within 15 to 30 minutes from the onset, a great improvement over standard T1- and T2-weighted MRI studies (4 to 6 hours) and CT scans (36 to 48 hours). This diagnostic period is substantially reduced in the perfusion-based MRI, which is extremely sensitive to an acute or incipient stroke and can detect ischemia within minutes of its onset.
- Functional MRI (fMRI) relies on blood oxygen level differences between active and inactive brain tissue. In order to exhibit greater neuronal activity, active and eloquent brain tissue requires greater oxygen consumption, and releases increased amounts of released deoxygenated hemoglobin (deoxyhemoglobin) in the surrounding veins. This increase in oxygenated blood in the veins surrounding active cortex is measured and amplified to generate fMRI signal. Therefore, fMRI does not directly reflect neuronal activity, but rather the flow changes that it induces.
- With sensitivity to the directionality of water molecular movements in the myelinated white matter tracks, diffusion tensor imaging is a tool for evaluating the integrity of the association fiber bundles in the brain. This procedure will not only help demonstrate the disconnection theory in neurolinguistics but it also will shed light on to which extent the mental functions are controlled by the connections and the cortical centers, since the DTI technique is based on the understanding of nerve fibers that have a standard microstructure. Will any deviance from this typical format result in a behavioral pattern like stuttering or learning deficit? This might prove to be a tool of profound significance for research neurolinguistics.

Magnetoencephalography

Another, newer technique, magnetoencephalography (MEG) is performed by obtaining somatosensory event-related evoked potentials from the cortex in response to a specific task. Therefore, images obtained are plots of nerves' action potentials. These are co-registered and placed over the patient's MRI data to show the cortical representation. There is another technique, called magnetic source imaging, which is basically an MRI scan with a MEG machine within it. MEG and MRI data are obtained and merged automatically in those machines.

Radionuclide-Based Imaging Techniques

The underlying principle behind nuclear medicine techniques is the introduction into the body of radioactive agents, whose emissions are then detected and recorded by crystal scintillation cameras. In most cases, the emissions consist of gamma particles, whose amplitude is proportional to the intensity of the scintillation recorded by the camera.

^{133}Xenon Cerebral Blood Flow Measurement

Regional cerebral blood flow (rCBF) evaluation with radioisotopes was first reported in 1961 by Ingvar, who used ^{85}Kr (Krypton) to measure CBF in a surgically exposed brain. Subsequently, ^{133}Xe (Xenon) was selected as the preferred radioisotope as it was significantly more effective because (1) it is liposoluble, and therefore easily diffusible in the brain, (2) it is a gamma emitter and can be measured extracranially, and (3) it is safer because of a shorter half-life. Initially, ^{133}Xe was injected into the carotid artery. In 1967, Obrist developed a technique of inhalation of a gas. Using the inhalation technique, CBF measurements require knowledge of the arterial concentration of the isotope (measured in end-tidal air with the patient wearing a mask), and the ^{133}Xe concentration in the brain, measured by scintillation detectors placed on the skull. Obrist also developed a more simplified technique of intravenous ^{133}Xe administration.

This technique of CBF measurement is commonly referred to as the ^{133}Xe "washout" technique, as the isotope is gradually attenuated. Since blood flow and local metabolic activity are directly related under normal conditions of coupling of flow and metabolism, CBF measurements provide insights regarding which brain areas participate in various activities.

In a detailed study of specific brain function and blood flow by Lassen et al. (1978), observations of blood flow that were not uniform throughout the brain reaffirmed the conviction that there is functional localization in the brain, a belief held by classical neurologists. The study further demonstrated that there is greater blood flow to the prefrontal cortex, even during rest. Furthermore, the right nondominant hemisphere exhibited greater functional participation in speech than was previously thought, and the supplementary motor area was also important, primarily in dynamic motor activity.

More recently, improvements in CT technology have allowed measuring CBF with the "stable xenon CT" technique. The technique is based on the Fick principle, which states that the concentration of a freely diffusible, nonmetabolized gas can be measured in living tissue (i.e., the brain) as a function of time by measuring the differences in concentration of the gas in arterial and venous blood, provided that the distribution coefficient (blood–brain partition coefficient) of the gas is known. The blood–brain partition coefficient of ^{133}Xe was determined in 1978 by Kelcz. The inhalation technique allows the determination of arterial concentrations directly from end-tidal ^{133}Xe measurements within the inhalation mask using a thermoconductivity analyzer. Since xenon is radiodense, CT can measure directly its concentration within the brain, so that venous measurements are not needed. Therefore, with the ability to measure the concentration of xenon in the blood and brain, the time for which xenon has been administered and knowing the blood–brain partition coefficient for xenon, the CBF can be calculated, using a special formula (Kety–Schmidt formula).

Single Photon Emission Computed Tomography

Single Photon Emission Computed Tomography (SPECT) integrates two technologies: CT and a radioactive tracer. The tracer is a gamma-emitting radioisotope that localizes to tissues and organs. Radioisotopes typically used in SPECT to label tracers are ^{99m}Tc (technetium-99m), ^{123}I (iodine-123), ^{133}Xe (xenon-133), ^{201}Th (thallium-201), and ^{18}F (fluorine-18). Various radiopharmaceuticals can be labeled with these isotopes.

The information emitted by the gamma rays is received by a gamma camera and analyzed by a computer that translates it into 2D cross sections. These cross sections can be added back together to form a 3D image of the brain (Fig. 20-12). Bhatnagar et al. (1989, 1990) and Tikofsky and Hellman (1991) used SPECT to examine cognitive and language functions in neurosurgery and neurology patients.

Positron Emission Tomography

Positron emission tomography (PET) The most important elements involved in biological processes are carbon, nitrogen, and oxygen. These elements, which decay by the process of pure positron emission, could be artificially produced by a cyclotron in the late 1930s. When bombarded by an electron, a positron is annihilated, resulting in the emission of two coincident gamma particles of 511 Kev and at 180 degrees of each other. As a result, the study of human metabolism in vivo by measuring the decay of radioactive elements involved in biological and biochemical processes was not possible until the recent invention of PET. PET could only be realized when (1) inorganic scintillation detectors for the detection of gamma radiation, (2) electronic systems for coincidence measurements, and (3) computer capacity for data acquisition and image reconstruction became available, in the mid- to late 1980s (Figs. 20-13 and 20-14).

The radionuclides commonly employed in PET are the following short-lived radioactive elements: ^{18}F (with a half-life of about 2 hours), ^{11}C (with a half-life of 20 minutes), ^{13}N (with a half-life of 10 minutes), and ^{15}O (with a half-life of 2 minutes). Carbon, oxygen, nitrogen, and hydrogen are the elements of life and the building stones of nearly every molecule of biological importance. However, hydrogen has no radioactive isotope decaying with emission of radiation which can be detected outside the human body. For this reason, a fluorine isotope (^{18}F) is used as a replacement for a hydrogen atom in a molecule. Due to their short half-lives, other radionuclides have to be produced in house, preferably with a small, dedicated cyclotron, in a simple chemical form. When a complex molecule is needed, its synthesis requires help from organic and radiochemistry services.

Radioactive isotopes are tagged with a naturally occurring molecule, which is injected into the body, and the spatial distribution of radiation emission is measured and mapped out by the scanner.

Glucose metabolism is commonly evaluated by fluorodeoxyglucose (^{18}FDG) to study cognitive, language, speech functions, tumor metabolism, and epilepsy (Fig. 20-13). ^{18}FDG PET has been used to examine the physiology of brains in normal individuals and brain-damaged

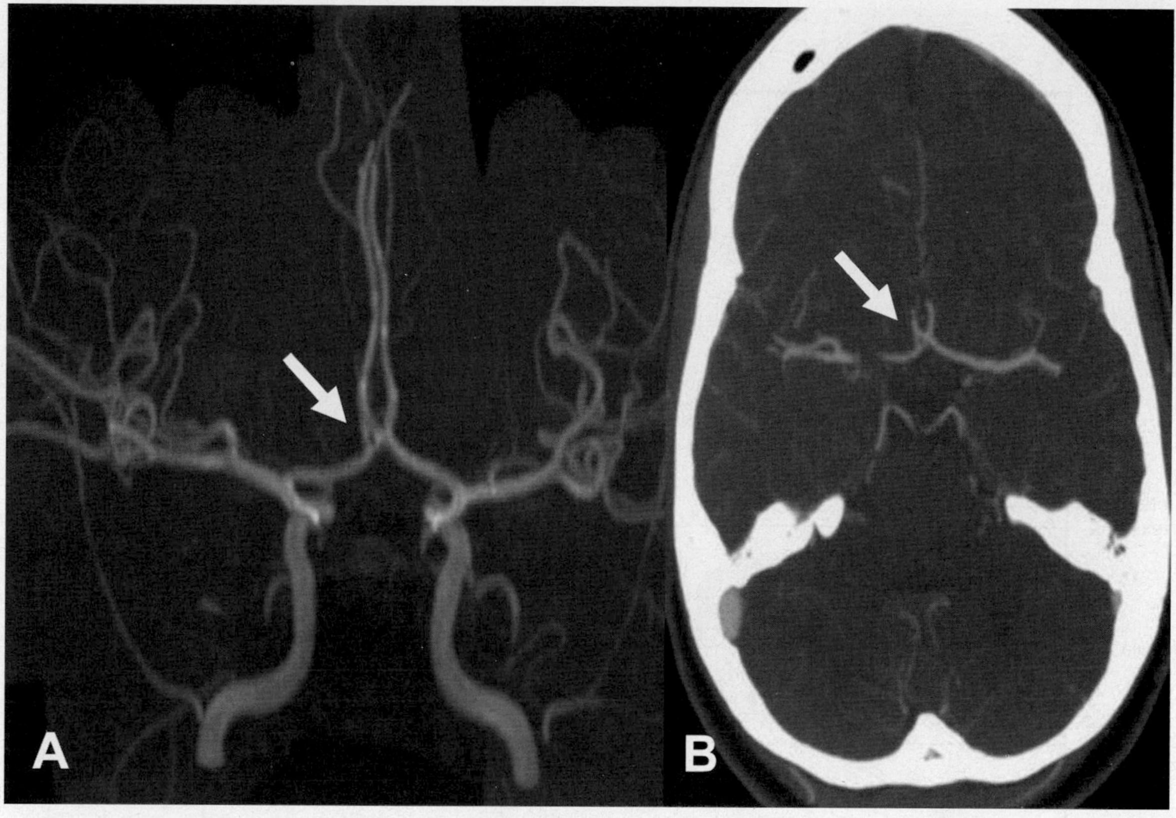

Figure 20-12 MRA of the brain (**A**) shows filling defect of the anterior communicating artery region suspicious for small aneurysm. CTA (**B**) confirms fenestration (duplication) of the anterior communicating artery region without associated aneurysm.

patients to determine the neuroanatomic correlates of different functions (Fig. 20-14). Studies of cellular glucose metabolism in aphasic patients have repudiated the belief that there is a strict localization of functions in the brain. Rather, these images demonstrated that focal brain pathology also affected the function of distant brain regions, commonly the prefrontal cortex, basal ganglia, and thalamus. For a better understanding of the application of PET to neuroanatomic pathologies in aphasic patients, consult these publications: Mazziotta et al. (1981, 1982), Metter (1987), Metter and Hanson (1985), and Metter et al. (1986).

PET is also used for detecting abnormal brain tissue, which causes seizures or psychiatric disorders, in which the metabolism of glucose is different from the rest of the brain. Such localization of abnormal brain tissue provides important diagnostic information before surgery.

PET is also used for identifying the limit and spread of tumors in the body and the brain to assist treatment planning and predict outcome. Because tumor cells are generally characterized by increased metabolism, the affected areas show increased cellular activity, which can be measured with ^{18}FDG.

rCBF may also be evaluated by ^{15}O-water PET, which is a sensitive method to measure regional cerebral activation secondary to specific task stimulation due to the high extraction of water in the brain.

Other radionuclides may be used with PET to study other functions: for example, ^{13}N may be used to study the metabolism of ammonia and ^{18}F-DOPA may be used to study Parkinson disease.

WADA TEST

The Wada test, also referred to as **sodium amytal infusion**, involves the intra-arterial carotid injection of sodium amobarbital during cerebral angiography to determine hemispheric dominance. Initially introduced by Juhn Wada in the early 1940s, the technique was developed to evaluate language dominance in patients with epilepsy and psychiatric conditions so that electroconvulsive therapy could be given to the hemisphere, which was not responsible for serving language (Box 20-3). With the advent of surgical management of epilepsy and intraoperative electrocorticography

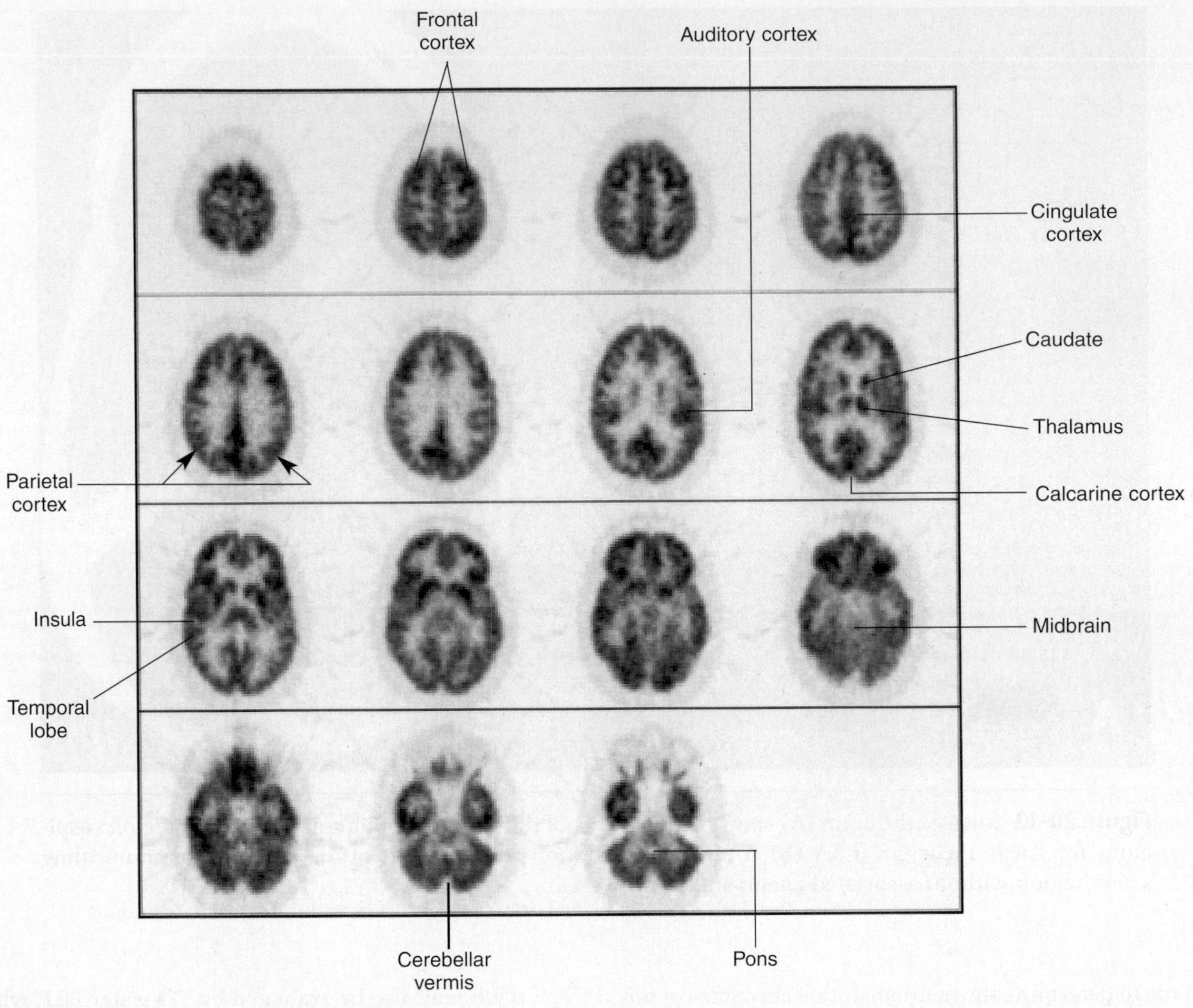

Figure 20-13 Positron emission tomography image of a normal brain.

undertaken at the Montreal Neurological Institute in 1940s, the Wada test became the standard tool for evaluating language dominance in patients with medically intractable epilepsy.

The intracarotid injection of sodium amobarbital induces a functional loss in the injected hemisphere which lasts 2 to 10 minutes. The underlying assumption of the test is that interruption of language function after sodium amytal infusion in either hemisphere should allow clinicians to identify the hemisphere that is dominant for language.

The Wada test starts with a cerebral angiogram, with a catheter placed in the femoral artery under local anesthesia and advanced into the carotid artery. The left carotid artery is usually the first studied, as most patients are left hemisphere dominant. First, an angiogram is obtained to determine the arterial blood supply to the hemisphere and the degree of collateral circulation, which could result in bihemispheric deactivation after the sodium amobarbital injection. Then a bolus of sodium amobarbital is injected over a 4-second period for maximum effectiveness; an average dose of 100 mg of amobarbital is used, diluted in 10 mL of saline solution. During slow drug infusion, patients are instructed to count backward from 10 to 1, and with their arms and fingers extended. Within seconds of the drug injection, the patient's contralateral arm becomes flaccid and drops suddenly and the counting stops, which confirms successful pharmacological anesthesia of the targeted hemisphere. Linguistic functions, such as ongoing counting and then confrontation naming, are also impaired if the injected hemisphere is dominant for language.

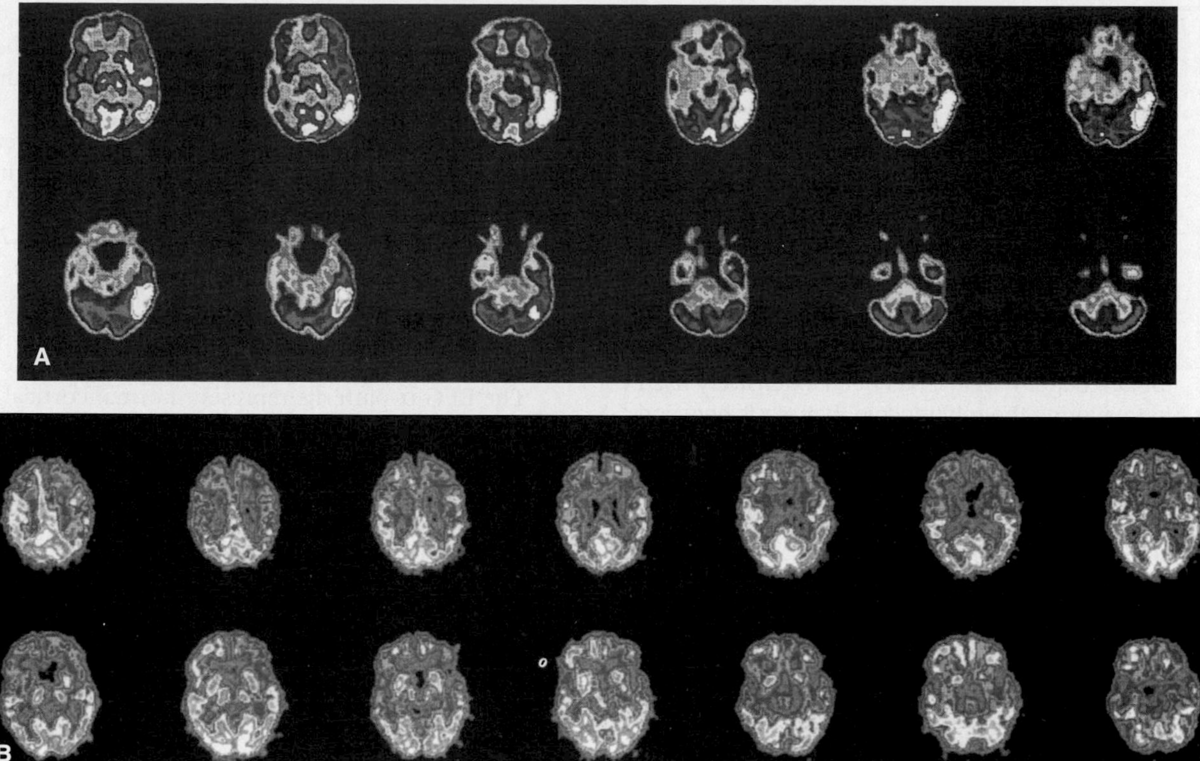

Figure 20-14 A. Positron emission tomography (PET) image exhibiting hyperactive metabolic activity in Wernicke area and a left inferior parietal lobule during a seizure. B. PET image indicating hypometabolism in the bifrontal and bitemporal regions in a patient diagnosed with Pick disease.

The Wada test has been extensively used for exploring the relationship between cerebral dominance and handedness. Do left-handed individuals have left cerebral dominance similar to right-handed individuals? Or do they have a right hemispheric or bilateral language and speech representation? When used to explore this relationship, the Wada test confirmed that most right-handed individuals have left hemispheric dominance for speech (Table 20-4); however, so do most left-handed individuals. This test further revealed that a significant number of left-handed individuals also exhibit right hemisphere language or dual hemisphere language representation (Wada and Rasmussen, 1960).

> *Key Terms :*
>
> **Brain-waves**
> **Cortical mapping**
> **Evoke potentials**
> **Polyphasic action potentials**
> **Dominant inheritance**
> **Recessive inheritance**
> **Sodium amobarbital infusion**
> **X-linked inheritance**

Recently, an effort was made to unravel the mental lexicon by examining the sequential unfolding of the processes of lexical access, retrieval, and production during the recovery of the left hemisphere from a complete drug-induced functional ablation with sodium amytal in neurosurgical patients (Bhatnagar, Barber, Mandybur, & Buckingham, 2005). It was noted that the access to the lexicon in all recovering neurosurgical subjects followed a consistently sequential pattern (Fig. 20-15). All the patients passed through the stages of fillers, perseveration, neologisms, and semantic paraphasia before producing the target lexicon; however, the duration of each lexical stage was different for each patient. The other point noted in the lexical restitution was that the linear recovery was marked with fluctuating brain functioning involving different levels of lexicon.

ELECTROENCEPHALOGRAPHY

The electroencephalogram (EEG) provides a graphic representation of the summated electrical activity in the brain cells. It measures potential differences between two

BOX 20-3

Wada Test

Sodium amytal infusion in the brain induces a transient functional anesthetization of the brain cells that can last from 2 to 10 minutes. The neurolinguistic assumption underlying the Wada test is that loss or altered language functions after the sodium amytal infusion will allow clinicians to identify the hemisphere that is or is not dominant for language. This test has been extensively used for exploring the relationship that exists between cerebral dominance and handedness. This is routinely undertaken on all the subjects that undergo cortical tissue removal for medically intractable epilepsy.

separated points on the scalp surface that represent brain-transmitted electrical potentials or brain waves of the cortex below, specifically of the vertical pyramidal cells. Spontaneous cortical surface activity is generated from the fluctuating voltage differences between the apical and the basal portion of the cortical dendrites. The greatest voltages are found in areas containing masses of dendrites.

EEG brain wave recordings are made by placing silver chloride metal electrodes (5 to 10 mm in diameter) at different points on the scalp using a standard 10/20 system of electrode placement (Fig. 20-16). Brain signals are simultaneously recorded from the frontal, parietal, occipital, and temporal scalp areas. Comparisons are made between corresponding areas of the brain hemispheres and among various areas within a single hemisphere for evaluating symmetry in wave patterns, amplitude and duration. In the 10/20 system, electrodes are labeled according to their locations (F = frontal, C = central, P = parietal, T = temporal, O = occipital) and the involved hemisphere (odd number for left, even number for right, and z for the midline).

Eight basic points corresponding to the frontal, parietal, occipital, and temporal lobes are used. In **bipolar** recordings, interconnecting electrodes are paired in the sagittal, transverse, and circular planes. The earlobes and mastoid processes are used as references for unipolar recordings.

The dominant electrical brain activity appears to cluster within a few frequency ranges. The different brain activities are represented by Greek letters and have a well-defined frequency range: α (8 to 12 Hz), β (12 to 30 Hz), θ (4 to 7 Hz), and δ (up to 4 Hz) (Table 20-5). There is no specific frequency for particular brain regions, although the α-frequency tends to predominate in the occipital area.

The EEG α-patterns represent normal cortical activity, predominantly in the posterior part of the brain. However, central and temporal regions may also have independent foci of α-rhythms. Eye opening and mental concentration usually suppress α-activity. The fast frequencies of β-rhythms are present in the central and frontal areas. β-Activity has relatively low voltage, usually not more than 20 μV, whereas θ- and δ-activities are not common patterns in normal adults but are seen in some normal children. The central brain areas may contain some θ-patterns, but they do not represent dominant EEG patterns. Brain potentials are measured in microvolts (μV), and the waves may vary from 25 to 300 μV. A seizure may display 1,000-μV discharge amplitudes. The frequencies are usually between 0.5 and 35 Hz (cycles per second).

In normal clinical conditions, the electrical patterns in homologous parasagittal areas are similar. In contrast, patterns in the two temporal areas are usually not synchronous. EEG is an excellent diagnostic procedure for seizures and measures abnormal brain wave patterns that are usually combinations of high-voltage spikes and/or sharp-wave discharges of varied frequencies. Focal discharge areas often display spike or sharp-wave reversal patterns (discussed with epilepsy). Similarly, asynchronized brain waves can be used to evaluate altered levels of consciousness, reduced responsiveness of the brain (discussed with sleep). However, in evaluation of seizures, problems arise in deciding when to perform the test. In some cases, such as grand mal seizures, it is not feasible to run an EEG when the patient is going through a seizure for two reasons: first, because of movement artifacts and second,

Table 20-4

Cerebral Dominance in Relation to Handedness, Based on Seizure Patients

Handedness	Total Cases	Left Hemisphere (%)	Right Hemisphere (%)	Bilateral (%)
Right	140	96	4	0
Left	122	70	15	15

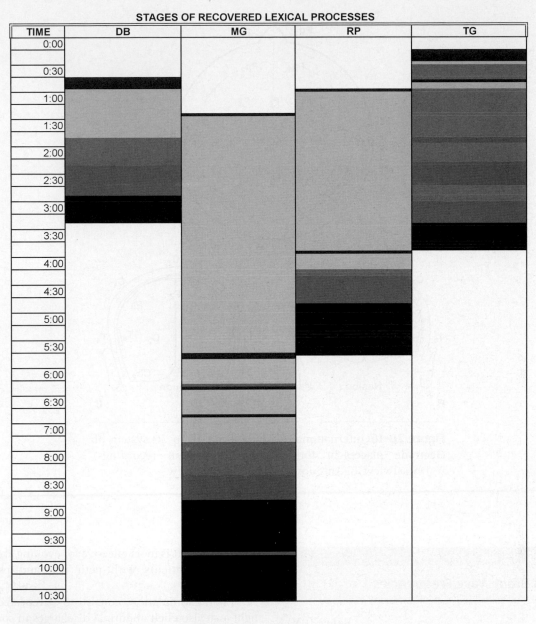

STAGES OF RECOVERED LEXICAL PROCESSES

TIME | DB | MG | RP | TG

0:00
0:30
1:00
1:30
2:00
2:30
3:00
3:30
4:00
4:30
5:00
5:30
6:00
6:30
7:00
8:00
8:30
9:00
9:30
10:00
10:30

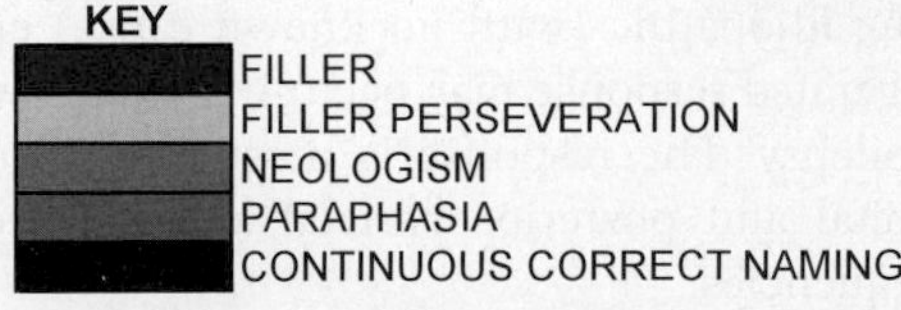

Figure 20-15. An illustration of sequential lexical recovery stages from an amytal-induced functional ablation of the brain in a right-handed subject with left cerebral dominance.

most patients have their seizures outside the hospitals. Initial routine EEG tests undertaken between seizures have been reported to demonstrate interictal epileptiform discharges (IEDs) in only 29% to 55% of patients. However, serial EEGs performed at various time periods have been reported to show IEDs in 80% to 90% patients. Specific techniques are used to evoke transient seizure activities for diagnostic reasons. Standard specific seizure-evoking methods are **hyperventilation**, **photic stimulation**, **sleep induction** and **sleep deprivation**.

Hyperventilation is used to activate the epileptic brain, which may be in a state of relative low excitability

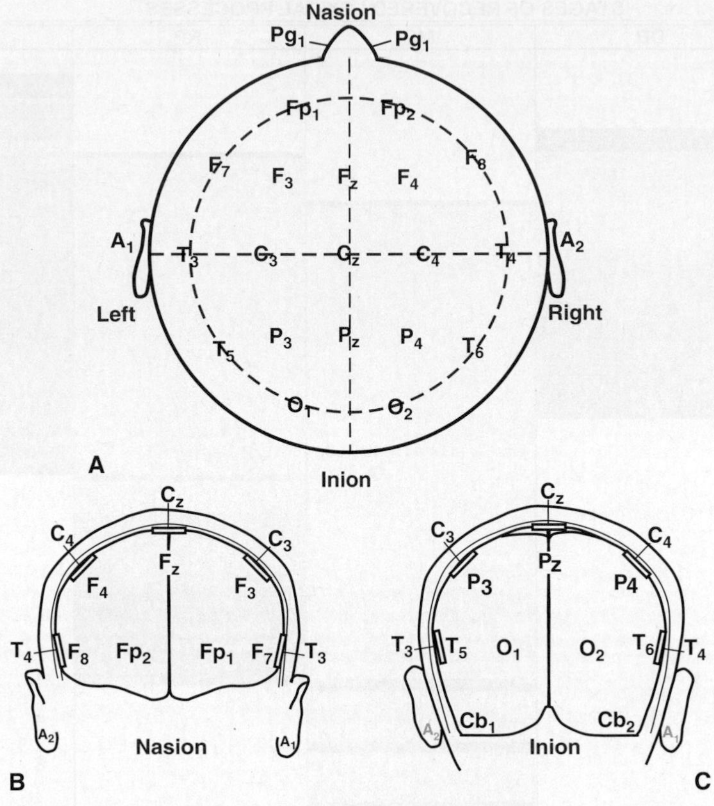

Figure 20-16 internationally standardized 10 to 20 system of electrode placement for electroencephalogram recordings. A. Dorsal view. B. Anterior view. C. Posterior view.

Table 20-5

Common Brain Wave Frequencies

Type	Range (μV)
Delta (δ: generalized brain region)	1–3
Dominant during dreamless deep sleep	
Theta (θ: generalized brain region)	4–7
Dominant during relaxed state of meditation	
Alpha (α: posterior cortex)	8–13
Dominant during deep and calm state with eyes closed	
Beta (β: anterior cortex)	>13
Dominant during fully awake and conscious state	

(quiescence). It is most effective for evoking abnormal discharges in patients with petit mal and psychomotor seizures.

Photic stimulation, consisting of repeated flashes of light, can also elicit abnormal discharges in some patients having idiopathic (with no known cause) epilepsies. An exaggerated response may occur in patients with a history of epilepsy. The response is most pronounced over the occipital and posterior parietal areas, especially in the α-frequencies.

Sleep is effective for activating discharges in all forms of epilepsy and most productive in psychomotor epilepsy. In addition, sleep deprivation has also been found to elicit paroxysmal activity in some patients having epilepsy.

EEG is also used to evaluate brain death, which refers to an irreversible loss of functions in the brain and brainstem (Box 20-4). Brain-death patients do not respond to external stimuli, cannot spontaneously breathe, and show no cranial nerve–mediated reflexes. The absence of their brain activity is marked by a flat line on **electroencephalogram**.

ELECTROMYOGRAPHY

Electromyography is the visual record of muscular electrical activity during spontaneous and/or voluntary movements. During contraction, muscle fibers generate action potentials that represent the transmembrane current of muscle fibers. This electrical activity of muscles can be recorded by placing a small electrode on the skin surface over the muscle or by a needle inserted into the muscle.

Electromyography is used to diagnose diseases of the nerves or muscles (muscular atrophy, myoneural junction disorders, and muscle diseases secondary to denervation) when clinical evidence is absent or equivocal or must be confirmed. An examination of the quality, speed, and magnitude of electrical impulses in muscles can help detect nerve or muscle damage (Fig. 20-17). It can also differentiate among muscle disease (myopathy), atrophy of spinal motor neurons (anterior horn cell disease), disorders of the nerves (neuropathy), interruption of the nerve supply (denervation), and neuromuscular (myoneural) problems.

Muscle pathologies are determined by comparisons made with normal patterns of muscle electrical activities. For example, there is no electrical activity in a normally functioning muscle during rest. In addition, the electrical potentials that result from the nerve irritation after electrode insertion do not last more than about a second in normal muscle tissues. This provides a point for the interpretation of pathologic patterns in muscles. In denervated (interrupted nerve) muscle fibers, for instance, there is initially spontaneous electrical activity, after which the insertional potentials can last a long time. Furthermore, denervation leads to high-frequency polyphasic discharges, fibrillations, and fasciculations.

In paralyzed and atrophied muscle, there is no spontaneous electrical activity. Low-amplitude, short-lasting motor unit potentials are usually seen in cases of muscle weakness owing to myopathy (muscular disease), involvement of the roots of the peripheral nerve fibers (neuropathy), or the pathology of anterior horn nerve cells (motor neuron disease). Fibrillation is the spontaneous action potential of a single muscle fiber, whereas fasciculation is the spontaneous discharge from an entire motor unit.

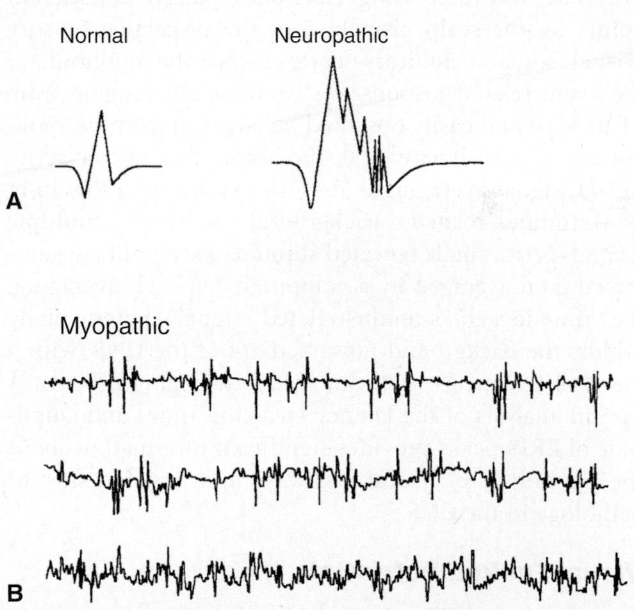

Figure 20-17 A. Normal motor action potentials have at least two phases. The phasic profile is altered in patients with neuropathic lesions and is characterized by high amplitude, long duration, and polyphasic motor unit action potentials. B. Myopathic lesions produce polyphasic motor action potentials with small amplitude and short duration.

BOX 20-4

Brain's Electrical Activity

Electrical activity in a normal brain is remarkably stable with balanced nerve membrane polarization and depolarization. However, an instability or volatility in brain's electrical activity causes epilepsy in which the waves of electrical activity are characterized by prolonged high-frequency neuronal discharges; these discharges represent rapid and excessive depolarizations of membrane potentials; subsequently, the electrical activity in one or more brain structures rises above a critical threshold. Seizures include sensory, motor, cognitive, and affective disorders that are the clinical manifestations of abnormal electrical neuronal discharges in the brain. Approximately 70% to 75% of initial seizures occur before age 20 and >30% of them occur before age 4 or 5. Seizures in small children associated with high fever are called febrile seizures, and in most cases they are not recurrent. The causative factors in 50% of seizure disorders are metabolic abnormalities, tumors, infarcts, infections, trauma, anoxia, perinatal insult, and physiologic disturbances. Among the remaining 50% of patients, there is no specific cause. Most types of the epilepsy can be controlled with medications. However, medically intractable epilepsy is treated with the surgical removal of the implicated brain tissues.

Patients with neuromuscular junction disorders may exhibit one of the two following patterns: progressively increasing motor unit action potentials with repetitive stimulation of the motor nerve (as in presynaptic impairment) or gradually decreased response of muscle action potential with repetitive nerve stimulation (as in postsynaptic myoneural junction disease).

Nerve conduction studies are used to identify disorders in the transmission of impulses to muscles. A peripheral nerve is stimulated, and the resultant electrical activity from the muscle is recorded. The latency of impulse, amplitude, speed, and direction of impulse conduction provide important clinical information. Measuring the amplitude of subsequent motor responses provides information about the number of muscle fibers activated, whereas recording nerve impulses at two points along the nerve helps determine the speed (velocity) of the nerve impulse and the time the impulse transmission takes. In denervating diseases, impulse transmission is slow.

EVENT-RELATED POTENTIALS

Event-related potentials (ERP) are the normal electrical signals of the CNS that instantly occur in response to specific and controlled sensory stimulation. Whether the sensory stimulus is visual, somatosensory, or auditory, the ERPs are recorded using electrodes placed at different points on the scalp, usually over the respective sensory (visual, somatic, auditory) cortex. Since the amplitude of the event-related responses is quite small, ranging from <1 to 5 μV and easily obscured by larger magnitude spontaneous electrical activity in the brain or myogenic activity, the signal averaging is used to extract the ERPs from non–stimulus-related background activity; multiple responses to a single repeated stimulus are amplified, summated, and averaged by a computer. Through averaging, the time-locked stimulus-related signal incrementally builds; the background noise activity of the CNS, with a mean of 0, cancels itself out in the averaging process. A careful analysis of the latency (reaction time) and amplitude of ERPs peaks provides significant information about the physiology of neural pathways and possible sites of pathology in the CNS.

Visual Evoked Potentials

The **visual evoked potential** (VEP) is used to evaluate electrical conduction along the optic nerve, optic tract, lateral geniculate body, optic radiations, and visual cortex. The eye is stimulated with flashes of light or black- or white-checked patterns, and electrical components of the visual response are recorded from scalp electrodes placed over the occipital area. The impulse transmission takes about 100 ms. Variations of reaction time, amplitudes, and wave patterns may occur in response to abnormalities at specific anatomic sites of electrical transmission. The slowed impulse latency in a VEP test is sensitive to the presence of a white matter lesion. The VEP is an important diagnostic test for identifying conditions like optic neuritis and multiple sclerosis in which the transmission of neural impulses is degraded.

Somatosensory Evoked Potentials

Somatosensory evoked potentials (SEPs) are elicited in the CNS through the electrical simulation of a peripheral nerve, such as the median nerve. The SEP wave pattern recorded from the scalp represents the functioning of the structures in the somatosensory pathway. Electric potentials that result from stimulation of the nerve are recorded from electrodes placed over the contralateral cortex. The intensity of the stimulation used is just above that needed to elicit a motor response from a muscle group innervated by the stimulated nerve. The reaction time gradually increases with distance from the primary sensory area. However, delayed latency or diminished amplitude of sensory evoked potentials indicates PNS and CNS diseases. The lesion may be in the nerves, nerve roots, or spinal cord. Clinical conditions in which SEPs have diagnostic value include multiple sclerosis, head injuries, brain death, and posterior column spinal cord lesions.

Auditory Evoked Potentials

Auditory evoked response testing provides electrophysiologic assessment of the auditory pathways which is important to students in human behaviors. Neural activity generated in response to the controlled acoustic stimuli presentation (clicks, tones, and speech sounds) is recorded from the scalp. Evoked response audiometry involves assessing auditory neural pathway function to estimate hearing thresholds in patients who are difficult to test. **Auditory evoked potentials** can also help identify the site of dysfunction in the auditory system.

Brainstem auditory evoked response (BAER) tests synchronous neural firings from the brainstem auditory pathway that occur within 10 ms of the stimulus onset. Five vertex positive wave forms represent the electrical signals produced in the auditory pathway (Fig. 20-18). Wave response classes appear to represent a specific anatomic point in the auditory pathway (Table 20-6). For example, wave I appears to arise from the peripheral and distal fibers of the vestibulocochlear nerve (CN VIII); wave II, from the proximal or brainstem portion of the vestibulocochlear nerve; wave III, from the first brainstem synapse, including the cochlear complex and trapezoid body; and waves IV and V, from the auditory pathway to the midbrain, including the lateral lemniscus and inferior colliculus. The additional wave patterns remain, anatomically and clinically, undetermined. The first two wave responses arise ipsilateral to the stimulus,

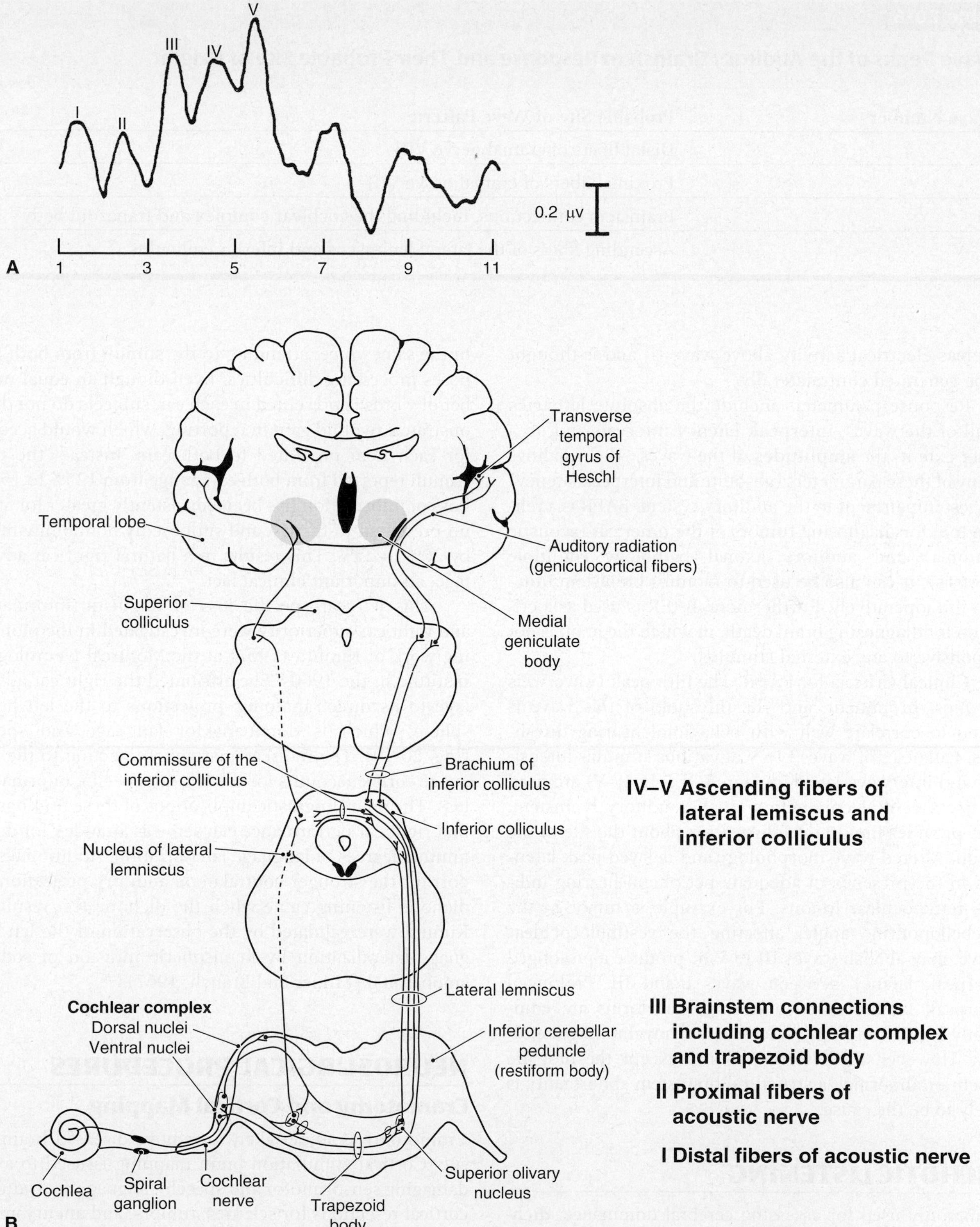

Figure 20-18 A. Normal brainstem auditory evoked responses within 10 ms from the onset of clicks. B. The relationship of the anatomic levels (*I–V*) of the auditory pathway to the brainstem response wave patterns.

Table 20-6

Wave Peaks of the Auditory Brainstem Response and Their Probable Site of Origin

Wave Number	Probable Site of Wave Pattern
I	Distal fibers of cranial nerve VIII
II	Proximal fibers of cranial nerve VIII
III	Brainstem connections, including the cochlear complex and trapezoid body
IV–V	Ascending fibers of the lateral lemniscus and inferior colliculus

whereas electrical activity above wave III and is thought to be generated contralaterally.

Response parameters include the **absolute latencies** of all of the waves, **interpeak latency intervals** and, to a lesser extent, the **amplitudes** of the waves. Abnormalities in any of these parameters (absolute and interpeak latency) suggest impairment in the auditory system. BAER is a reliable tool for diagnosing tumors of the inner ear (acoustic neuroma) and auditory axonal pathology (multiple sclerosis). It can also be used to monitor brainstem function intraoperatively. Furthermore, BAER is used as a criterion for diagnosing brain death, in which the brain is not responsive to any external stimulus.

Clinical Criteria for BAER. The fifth peak (wave V) is the most prominent, and the threshold of this wave is found to correlate well with behavioral hearing thresholds. Latencies of waves I to V at various stimulus intensities and interwave latencies (i.e., I–V, I–II, II–V) are used to assess central conduction in the auditory brainstem. This provides important information about the site of the lesion. Altered wave morphology and delayed peak latencies in the presence of adequate peripheral hearing indicate retrocochlear lesions. For example, a tumor in the cerebellopontine angle, affecting the vestibulocochlear nerve, may abolish waves III to V or produce a prolonged interpeak latency between waves I and III. Prolonged interpeak latencies and abnormal waveforms are commonly seen in multiple sclerosis, a demyelinating condition. However, if all wave patterns except the first are absent or abnormal, a structural brainstem abnormality is likely to be the cause.

DICHOTIC LISTENING

Commonly used for assessing cerebral dominance, **dichotic listening**, a noninvasive neuropsychologic tool, uses auditory stimuli. It involves presenting simultaneous but slightly different auditory stimuli to both ears. The attention factors are minimized by requiring patients to attend to both ears simultaneously and report the stimuli they perceive. When the linguistic material presented in both ears is digitized that means it is largely similar and spoken in the same voice; attending to the stimuli from both ears poses processing difficulties. Even though an equal number of words is presented in each ear, subjects do not demonstrate a twofold gain in reporting, which would account for each item presented to both ears. Instead, the total stimuli reported from both ears range from 125% to 150%. Loss of information has been consistently greater for stimuli presented to the left and supposedly nondominant ear by 20% to 25%. This results in a natural right ear advantage, an important clinical fact.

This left ear–specific loss of linguistic information and right ear superiority were investigated in the pioneering work of Kimura (1967) at the Montreal Neurological Institute in the 1960s. She attributed the right ear advantage to its direct anatomic projections to the left hemisphere, which is dominant for language and speech (Fig. 20-19). The indirect anatomic projection to the language cortex accounts for the left ear–specific information loss. The neurolinguistic implications of these findings are that right ear performance can serve as an index for determining degrees of language lateralization. Additional support for the stronger contralateral auditory projections in dichotic listening came when the dichotic test results of Kimura were validated by the observation of the left language lateralization by hemispheric infusion of sodium amobarbital (Milner and Branch, 1967).

NEUROSURGICAL PROCEDURES

Craniotomy and Cortical Mapping

Craniotomy is undertaken to remove diseased brain tissue. Cortical stimulation brain mapping is used to avoid damaging sensorimotor and speech–language areas during cortical resections for seizures, tumors, and aneurysms.

Focal external electric stimulation is based on observations by Fritsch and Hitzig (1870) and Bartholow (1874), who found that electric current externally applied to the exposed brain altered sensorimotor functions in animals and humans. After the safety and reliability of focal stimulation were established, stimulation mapping became a standard part of surgical treatment for medically intractable

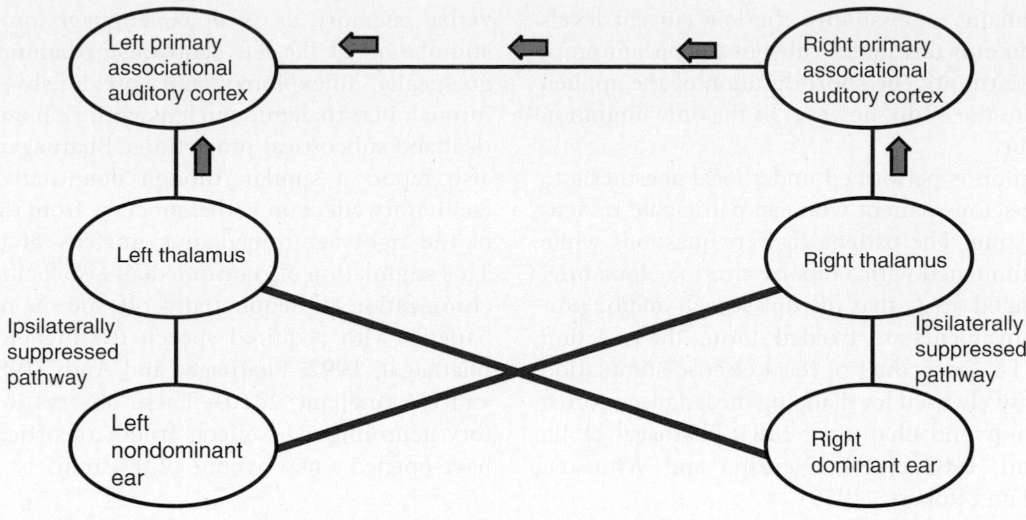

Figure 20-19 Ear projections to the auditory cortex during a dichotic listening task.

epilepsy and was used to identify the somatosensory cortex and map out the human brain involvement with memory and language at the Montreal Neurological Institute (Penfield and Roberts, 1959). Completed under local anesthesia while the patients remained awake, focal stimulation was used first to determine the stimulation threshold that produced after discharges and second to determine whether the diseased part of the brain was critical for language and sensorimotor functions (Andy and Bhatnagar, 1984; Bhatnagar et al., 2000, Ojemann et al., 1989).

Since many language functions are represented in the cortical tissue around the diseased part of the brain, the mapping of language in and around the area of pathology helps neurosurgeons determine whether it is safe to remove the diseased cortical tissues without any unacceptable loss, primarily of higher mental functions (speech, language, and memory) and secondarily of sensorimotor functions. This mapping also helps determine the size and extent of the tissue that can be safely resected. As a rule of thumb, no tissue resection is undertaken from the somatosensory area in the frontoparietotemporal cortex unless there is preexisting hemiplegia or the diseased tissue is not involved with language (Andy and Bhatnagar, 1991; Ojemann, 1983; Penfield and Roberts, 1959).

In the post-Penfield era, this technique was extensively used to treat patients with epilepsy and in surgical management of other conditions, such as tumors and AVMs. Focal stimulation acts like a reversible lesion of the brain, ranging from 4 to 8 seconds; its interruption lasts only for the duration of the applied current. Furthermore, the stimulation-induced interruption provides precise details about functional localization because the lesion is only 0.5 to 3 mm in diameter. The technique is not known to leave any lingering effect and/or postoperative aphasia. Carefully controlled stimulation parameters pose no safety concern to patients, cause no injury to the examined brain tissue, and produce no evidence of acute inflammation to the mapped region of the brain. Multiple samples of a single behavior from a single site allow for the necessary statistical analysis and can help determine whether the evoked linguistic errors are significant.

Interpretation of the physiologic effects of focal stimulation is based on the interference it produces during ongoing activity. For example, if stimulation at a cortical site disrupts ongoing naming or speaking, the cortical area in question is considered to be functional for the task (Fig. 20-20). If the stimulation does not block or alter the naming or speaking process, the stimulated area is not considered to be involved in the ongoing language activity. Although evoking distant effects of the applied

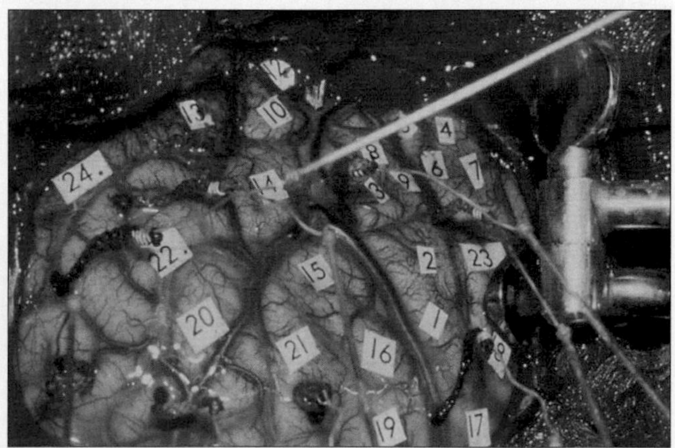

Figure 20-20 Exposed brain during electrocorticography. Numbered tickets, sites that were functionally mapped during intraoperative neurolinguistic testing. Many of these sites have been associated with language and memory functions.

stimulation remains a possibility, the low current levels (below sensorimotor threshold) rule out any distant propagation of the current. The short duration of the applied current trains to the brain, however, is the only limitation of the technique.

The operation is performed under local anesthesia to maintain a conscious patient who can participate in neurolinguistic testing. The patient answers questions while the cortex is stimulated with a bipolar electrode for a brief period. Stimulated areas that disrupt speech and/or produce motor movements are avoided during the resection of the lesion. The procedure of focal electric stimulation has been extensively used for mapping the language cortex in humans (Andy and Bhatnagar, 1983; Bhatnagar et al., 2000; Ojemann, 1983, 1989; Ojemann and Whitaker, 1978; Penfield and Roberts, 1959).

Subcortical Mapping

Stereotactic surgery is a method for identifying a precise nonvisualized deep brain structure by using 3D coordinates, which involves placing a discrete lesion at the selective subcortical location to manage involuntary movements and intractable pain. The subcortical brain structures are mapped by electrical stimulation for guidance while the patient is under local anesthesia. **Subcortical mapping** optimizes the beneficial results from the involvement of normal structures. Two examples of stereotactic surgery are a lesion or stimulation in the subthalamus or the ventrolateral nucleus of the thalamus that is used to treat Parkinsonian tremors and a lesion or stimulation in the globus pallidus that is used to treat parkinsonian tremor and rigidity.

Investigators have examined subcortical participation in speech, language, and verbal memory by stimulating discrete subcortical areas through depth electrodes. Ojemann (1983) noted facilitation of verbal recall via the application of stimulation parameters below the threshold for induced language disturbance during a left thalamotomy. He attributes this effect on the registration and recall of verbal stimuli to the thalamic evoked **alerting response mechanism**.

Stereotaxic procedures have given way to another advanced mode of treatment called **deep brain stimulation**, which involves a chronic electrode implant in deep thalamic nuclei and a stimulation programmer or pulse generator, similar to a pace maker, which not only controls the stimulation parameters but also regulates the consistency of the therapeutic stimulation. Without damaging the tissues, deep brain stimulation is known to remediate involuntary movements supposedly by blocking the brain signals that cause the abnormal symptoms. The electrode is connected to the stimulator through a wire that is placed below the skin. Bhatnagar et al. (1989, 2005) took advantage of this therapeutic paradigm for examining the role of subcortical reticular mechanism on speech and language. They noted a facilitatory effect on verbal memory as well as language processing from stimulation of the left centrum medianum, a neurolinguistically unexplored and previously unimplicated intralaminar thalamic nucleus with rich and diffuse cortical and subcortical projections. Bhatnagar et al. (1990) also report a similar, though quantitatively different, facilitatory effect on verbal memory from the stimulation of the right centromedianus nucleus of the thalamus. This stimulation of centromedian also facilitated the synchronization of sequentially off speech movements in patients with acquired speech dysfluencies (Andy and Bhatnagar, 1992; Bhatnagar and Andy, 1989; Bhatnagar and Buckingham, 2010). These observations of facilitatory neurolinguistic effects from subcortical stimulation have opened a new avenue of research.

Cordotomy

Cordotomy, a procedure used relatively infrequently, involves the sectioning of the lateral spinothalamic tract to relieve chronic pain; it is performed when medication proves ineffective. The procedure is performed under local anesthesia so that the patient can tell the surgeon when the pain is relieved and in which part of the body it is no longer felt. The ventrolateral spinothalamic tract of the cord is sectioned on the side opposite to the painful body part (see Chapter 11). The sectioning is performed three segments above the top segment level of pain. The spinal cord attachments of the dentate ligament are used as a reference point for sectioning the cord. They mark the plane between the overlying pyramidal tract and the underlying spinothalamic pain-conducting tract to be sectioned. The level of the sectioning is usually in the thoracic spinal cord for pain below the dermatomal nipple line. The cervical spinal cord is sectioned to eliminate pain in the upper extremities, shoulders, and neck.

Recently, stimulation of the cord using a chronically implanted electrode has also been used to relive intractable pain. In this procedure, an electrode is placed in the spinal canal over the cord, and it is stimulated through a battery-operated unit implanted subcutaneously in the infraclavicular fossa.

Vascular Surgery Procedures

Internal–External Carotid Anastomosis

A decrease in blood supply to the cortex and subcortical structures occurs when a blood vessel is occluded by either an embolus or a thrombosis with a local sclerotic plaque. Restoration of the blood supply in this case is performed by anastomosing the distal segment of the occluded internal carotid artery to the superficial branch of the external carotid artery. This surgery is performed through a craniotomy so that both blood vessels can be connected. This anastomotic surgery is used for the restoration of blood circulation only in selected patients since in some medical opinions, the clinical benefits of this procedure have been less than satisfactory.

Carotid Endarterectomy

Occlusive sclerotic plaques are usually found at the region of common carotid bifurcation. **Carotid endarterectomy** is a surgical procedure used to remove atherosclerotic plaque from the walls of the internal carotid artery. The plaque, formed by gradual accumulation of cholesterol, undissolved fatty, lipid-rich substances, cellular deposits and calcium elements, causes stroke by either impeding flow to the brain or by rupturing and releasing debris into the cerebral bloodstream. When this occurs, small particles of the plaque migrate upstream and occlude the smaller arteries within the brain. Endarterectomy is performed to physically remove the plaque to reduce the risk of subsequent stroke. The risk of stroke has been found to increase with increasing amount of plaque present within the artery measured as a percent narrowing (stenosis). Endarterectomy is indicated in symptomatic patients with 70% to 99% stenosis and in asymptomatic patients with more than 80% stenosis.

Carotid endarterectomy is performed with the patient under general anesthesia or partially awake. An incision is made in one of the skin folds of the neck to access the affected carotid artery. The common, internal, and external carotid arteries are controlled with vascular clamps. Blood flow to the brain is temporarily occluded and a longitudinal incision is made through the area of the plaque. Patients under general anesthesia are checked to ensure cerebral perfusion is adequate. Several methods can be employed, but if perfusion is low, a temporary silastic tube is placed to "shunt" blood from the common carotid artery to the internal carotid artery upstream from the area of the plaque. The plaque is then completely removed from the artery. The artery is then closed using an intervening patch to repair the incision. This patch technique helps to prevent renarrowing as the artery heals. The operation lasts approximately one and a half to two hours, does not involve much blood loss, and is typically well tolerated by even high-risk patients. Two main complications that can occur with endarterectomy are stroke and nerve injury. The periprocedural stroke risk is about 1% to 2% in asymptomatic patients and 3% to 5% in symptomatic patients. Permanent or temporary nerve injury can occur to the hypoglossal, marginal mandibular, and recurrent laryngeal nerves. Rarely, nerve injury can also occur to the glossopharyngeal, spinal accessory, and superior laryngeal nerves if dissection of the artery is more extensive due to anatomical concerns. Most nerve injury is temporary and resolves by 6 months postoperatively (see Chapter 7).

Aneurysm Clipping

Aneurysm is a bulging defect of the blood vessel wall that looks like a protruding nipple or balloon attached to the vessel. Aneurysms that hemorrhage or cause neurologic deficits and seizures require immediate attention. The medical management of an aneurysm involves lowering blood pressure to prevent bleeding; **aneurysm clipping** is used to obliterate the neck or attachment of the aneurysm to the blood vessels, thus disabling it. Aneurysms are also treated without opening the skull through coiling, which involves placing a platinum coil in the aneurysm that causes a blood clot to form, sealing off the aneurysm (see Chapter 7).

GENETIC INHERITANCE

The way in which an organism passes its physical attributes to its offspring is the subject of genetics. What we know about inheritance and genetic transmission can be traced to the late-19th-century work of Gregor Johann Mendel, who observed several patterns of inherited traits by examining the crossings of different-colored flowers and pea plants. In his work known as the Mendelian inheritance, Mendel examined the genotype and phenotype of genes and established two rues: law of segregation and law of independent assortment. The first law suggests that each sex chromosome gets an allele of genes and the second law suggests that the segregation of one trait (like height) does not affect the segregation of other trait (like eye color)

Genes regulate the formation, distribution, and growth of cells in an embryo. The blueprint for these processes is received from both parents at the time of conception. After passing through mitotic and meiotic divisions, each parental germ cell (oogonia and spermatogonia) contains 22 somatic chromosomes and one sex chromosome (see Chapter 4). At conception, cells from the two parents combine their genetic material to form a zygote that contains 44 (22 + 22) autosomal chromosomes and either 2 X chromosomes or 1 X and 1 Y chromosomes. The genes consist of 6 to 7 billion base pairs of DNA arranged linearly in 23 pairs of chromosomes. Each coiled chromosome contains tens of thousands of genes. One or more pairs of genes received from the parents regulate most physical traits, such as height, hair color, body shape, aptitude, and others.

Among these thousands of genes, everyone carries a few dysfunctional genes. Some diseases are caused by one faulty gene (**dominant inheritance**, only one mutant allele is required for expression of the phenotype), and some morbid conditions occur when a defective gene comes from both parents (**recessive inheritance**, both alleles must be mutant alleles to express the phenotype). There is no immunity against genetic illness, and large numbers of serious disorders are associated with chromosome abnormalities. Chromosomal errors occur primarily during the formation of germ cells, when meiotic processes that are supposed to reduce the chromosomes to the haploid number (23) produce a gamete cell with an extra or missing chromosome.

Most trisomies (three copies of a particular chromosome) cause severe developmental deficits and mental retardation (see Chapter 4). Three common trisomy syndromes are Down syndrome (trisomy 21), **Edward syndrome** (trisomy 18), and **Patau syndrome** (trisomy 13). Incidentally, most (75%) severe chromosomal malformations result in spontaneous abortion and >40% of infants born with abnormalities die. Errors of genetic inheritance also have implications for altered physiologic functions, such as metabolic, endocrine, and neurologic diseases.

Tracing the distribution of genes in the extended family is an important concept for understanding inheritance. Investigators use standard symbols to construct pedigrees. The pedigree charts are used in genetics to analyze inheritance and to show ancestral history (Fig. 20-21).

Mendel related his observations to the mathematical probability of inheritance. Most mathematical patterns of gene expression are calculated on the basis of gene penetration. However, if gene expression is not fully penetrated, the genetic traits may not follow the exact mathematical pattern. There are three common modes of genetic inheritance: **dominant**, **recessive**, and **X-linked**.

Dominant Inheritance

Even a single faulty gene can pass on a dominant autosomal genetic disease (Fig. 20-22). A child has a chance of receiving this kind of disease if he or she has one parent affected with the disorder. The defective gene dominates the gene from the other parent with which it is paired. In these cases, there is a 50% probability for each child to inherit the disease. At the same time, of course, there is a 50% chance that the child will not receive the faulty gene. Diseases inherited through dominant genes exhibit various degrees of symptoms, with severity ranging from mild to moderate, and most appear late in life. There are >2,000 known dominant autosomal disorders, but one of the most pertinent conditions to students in communicative disorders is **Huntington chorea**, a progressive degenerative disease that is characterized by movement disorders and cognitive impairments.

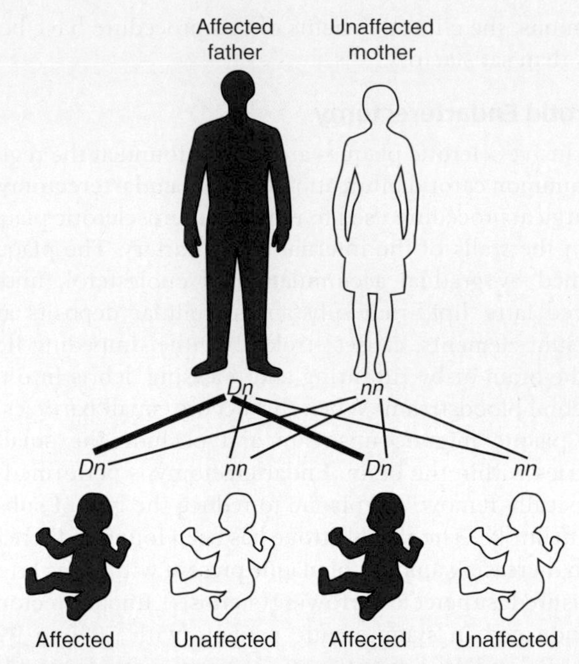

Figure 20-22 In simple dominant inheritance, one affected parent has a single faulty gene (*D*) that dominates its normal counterpart (*n*). Each child's chance of inheriting *D* or *n* from the affected parent is 50%.

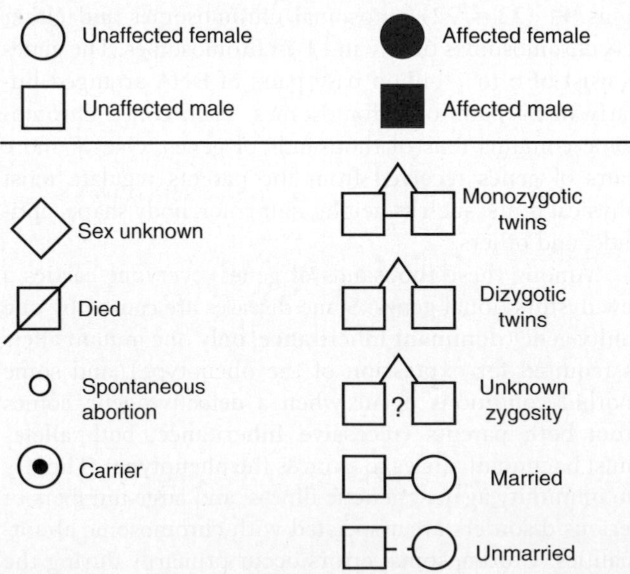

Figure 20-21 Symbols used when creating pedigree charts.

Recessive Inheritance

Recessive inheritance requires that both parents carry the faulty gene and transmit that gene to the child (Fig. 20-23). If one parent alone is a carrier of the dysfunctional gene, this gene is not likely to be harmful because it is dominated by the normal gene that is received from the other parent. With so many genes passing from parents, it is quite rare for both parents to be affected with and carry the same faulty gene. Even though there is a low probability of this, both parents occasionally do carry the same faulty gene, in which case the child is at risk for major birth defects. In such cases, each child has a 25% chance of inheriting the disease, a 25% chance of not inheriting the disease, and a 50% chance of receiving the faulty gene from one parent, which would make the child a carrier of the dysfunctional gene. The child's probability of getting an autosomal-recessive disorder is very high if the parents have common ancestors or are close relatives. Some well-known recessive disorders are **cystic fibrosis** and **Tay–Sachs disease**.

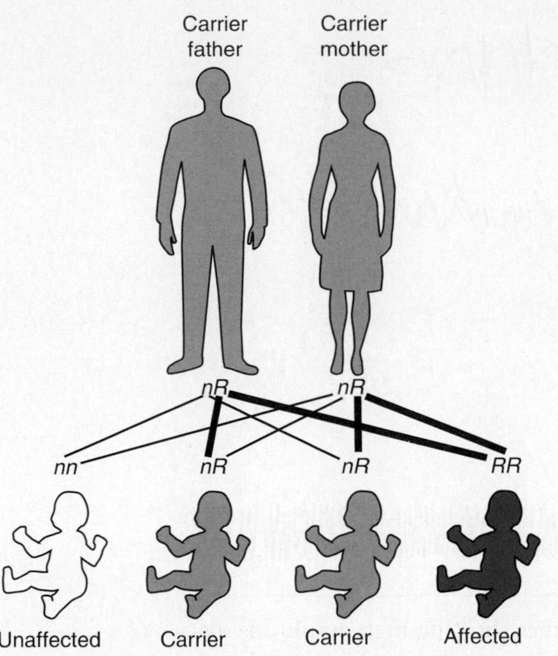

Figure 20-23 In simple recessive inheritance, both parents, usually unaffected, carry a normal gene (*n*) that takes precedence over its faulty counterpart (*R*). Each child has the following chances of inheritance: a 25% risk of inheriting two mutant *R* genes and thus having a serious birth defect; a 25% chance of inheriting two normal *n* genes and thus being an unaffected noncarrier; and a 50% chance of inheriting one *n* and one *R* gene and thus being an unaffected carrier.

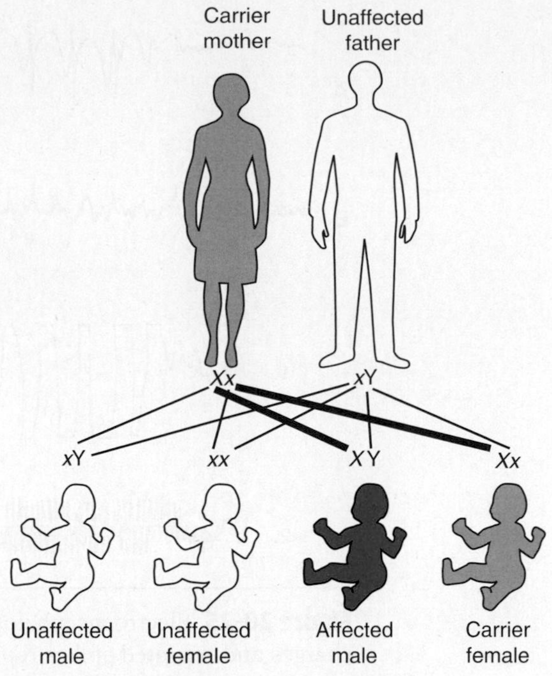

Figure 20-24 In X-linked inheritance, the unaffected, carrier mother has one faulty gene (*X*) and one normal gene (*x*), which are located on the X chromosome. The father has a normal *X* gene on the X chromosome and a normal Y chromosome. Each male child has the following chances of inheritance from his mother: a 50% risk of inheriting the faulty *X* gene and thus having the disorder and a 50% chance of inheriting the normal *x* gene and thus being normal and a noncarrier. Each female child has the following chances of inheritance from her mother: a 50% risk of inheriting one faulty *X* gene and thus being a normal carrier and a 50% chance of inheriting the normal *X* gene and thus being a normal noncarrier.

X-Linked Inheritance

Males and females carry different sex chromosomes; males have one X and one Y chromosome (XY), whereas females have two X chromosomes (XX). Consequently, a female has pairs of the genes found on the X chromosome, whereas a male cannot because he has only one X chromosome. If a fertilized egg receives an X chromosome from each of the parents, the child is a female; if the fertilized egg receives an X chromosome from its mother and a Y chromosome from its father, the child is a male.

X-linked inheritance involves the genes situated in the X chromosome. Generally, it is the mother who carries a faulty gene in one of her X chromosomes (Fig. 20-24). If a boy inherits a defective X-linked gene, he received it from his mother because the father passes only the Y chromosome on to a son. On the other hand, if a girl receives a faulty X chromosome from her mother, it will be dominated by the normal X chromosome from her father. Overall, each male child has a 50% risk of inheriting the faulty gene and accompanying disorder. Although each female has a 50% risk of inheriting the faulty gene, she will not exhibit the disease but would become a carrier like her mother. Obviously, no male-to-male transmission of a faulty X-linked gene occurs. Commonly known X-linked diseases are **color blindness**, **hemophilia** (blood clotting disorder), and **Duchenne muscular dystrophy**.

Key Terms:

Cataplexy	**Non–rapid-eye movement stages**
Cerebral death	**Oncogenes**
Coma	**Seizure**
Delirium	**Stupor**
Encephalopathy	**Tonic-clonic phases**
Epilepsy	
Neuropathy	

SPECIFIC NEUROLOGIC DISORDERS

Any alteration in neuronal functioning results in specific sensorimotor disturbances and/or diseases. Some of these disorders, listed here, might have briefly been discussed under the "Clinical Considerations" sections in different chapters:

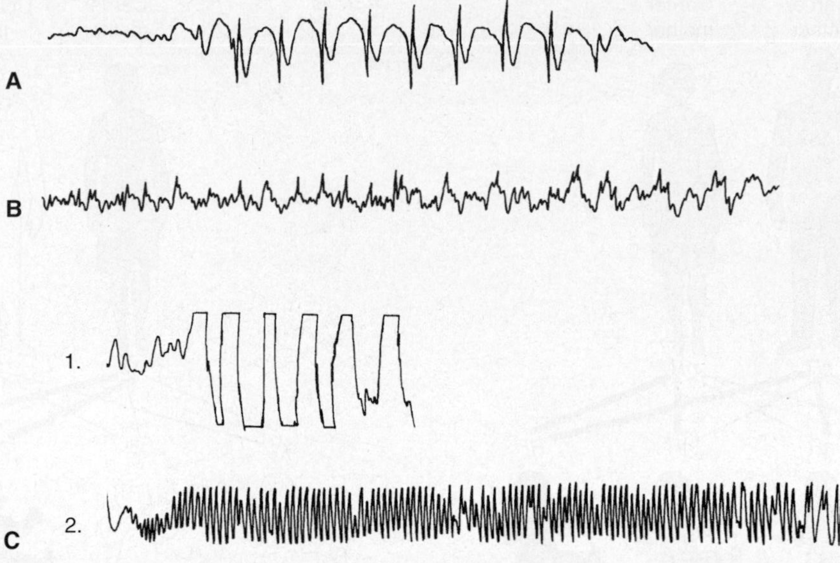

Figure 20-25 Electroencephalographic studies showing high-amplitude discharges and repeated spikes representing abnormal electrical activity during a seizure. A. Petit mal (absence) epilepsy in a 15-year-old boy. B. Psychomotor epilepsy. C. Grand mal (tonic–clonic) epilepsy with two frequency patterns.

Seizures and Epilepsy

Seizures are sensory, motor, cognitive, and affective disorders that are the clinical manifestations of abnormal electrical neuronal discharges in the brain (Fig. 20-25). Epilepsy refers to two or more (recurring) unprovoked seizures. Approximately 70% to 75% of initial seizures occur before age 20 and >30% of them occur before age 4 or 5. Seizures in small children associated with high fever are called **febrile seizures**, and in most cases they are not recurrent. The causative factors in 50% of seizure disorders are metabolic abnormalities, tumors, infarcts, infections, trauma, anoxia, perinatal insult, and physiologic disturbances. Among the remaining 50% of patients, no specific cause can be detected.

In a normal brain, electrical activity is remarkably stable, and nerve membrane polarization and depolarization are delicately balanced. However, in epilepsy, the brain's electrical activity becomes unstable and it is characterized by a prolonged high-frequency neuronal discharge, which represents rapid and excessive depolarization of membrane potentials (Fig. 20-25). The seizures occur when electrical activity in one or more brain structures rises above a critical threshold. Epileptic discharge can recruit neighboring and functionally related neuronal elements, and thus it replicates itself while spreading from one area to another, which is called Jacksonian march. During the course of frequently recurring epileptic discharges, some neurons remain quiescent (nonactive) for varying periods, representing excessive depolarization (fatigue) or hyperpolarization (inhibition).

Epileptic seizures are commonly divided into two types: **partial** (focal) and **generalized**. Partial seizures are further divided into **partial simple** and **partial complex**. Partial seizures can remain focal or can get secondarily generalized. Primary generalized seizures may be **petit mal** (brief absences) type, such as sudden and brief jerks (myoclonic seizures, marked by contraction and relaxation of muscles), or **grand mal (tonic–clonic)** type (Table 20-7). In the tonic phase the entire is rigid and stiff, while in the clonic phase the body has uncontrolled jerking movements.

Partial Simple Seizures

Partial focal (simple) seizures are usually caused by a single cortical or subcortical lesion. The symptoms are characterized by sudden onset of sensory and/or motor behaviors confined to a single body part, such as the leg, arm, or face, depending on the site of lesion. For example, a lesion in the motor cortex may generate the jerking of the opposite side arm. Involvement of the sensory cortex causes altered sensory perception, such as numbness or tingling. Spread of the abnormal discharge activity to adjacent cortical areas recruits other body parts into the seizure. The progressive recruitment of other body parts is called the **Jacksonian march** after the English neurologist who first described it. For example, a Jacksonian seizure may start in the foot and spread to the lower leg, thigh, abdomen, shoulder, and arm. A Jacksonian sensory spread may start as a tingling sensation in the thumb that spreads to the fingers, forearm, upper arm, and shoulder.

An aura is the first sign of a focal seizure and is usually characterized by a specific sensory experience that precedes the full-blown seizure. Auras are warnings of impending seizures that help to localize the site of origin of the seizures.

Table 20-7

Classification of Seizures

Partial seizures	**Partial simple**: rhythmic spike and/or slow-wave focal discharges with sensorimotor, visceral, and/or emotional symptoms
	Partial complex (psychomotor): abnormal electrical activity in amygdala, hippocampus, septum, mesodiencephalic, and association cortices with complex sensorimotor, visceral, and emotional symptoms
Generalized seizures	**Petit mal**: symmetrical 3-Hz spike and wave with brief episodes of automatisms
	Grand mal: high-voltage spike and wave activities with varied frequencies and duration, usually associated with loss of consciousness and tonic–clonic movements

Patients generally remember the aura of a simple focal seizure but do not remember the abnormal behavior (automatisms) at the onset of a temporal lobe seizure that emanates from the amygdala and hippocampus. In most cases of focal seizures, antiepileptic drugs (AEDs) are effective. However, in some cases, focal seizures do not respond to AEDs; such patients may need to be investigated and subsequently treated by surgical removal of the localized lesion and the surrounding brain tissue that may be responsible for seizure activity. The protocol of this surgical procedure involves determining the cerebral dominance through sodium amytal infusion and also provides opportunity for a functional mapping of the brain (see Fig. 20-20).

Partial Complex (Psychomotor) Seizures

Partial complex (psychomotor) seizures are very often the result of congenital and postnatal lesions of the medial temporal lobe structures consisting of the amygdala, hippocampus, and overlying temporal cortex. These types of seizures, occurring most frequently in young adults and older age groups, are characterized by recurring episodes of automatic, irrational behavior of which there usually is no memory. The individual is cognizant of neither the actions nor the consequences of them. In addition, the patient may have episodes of aggressive behavior. There are also notable cognitive deficits characterized by inattentiveness, unclear thinking, compulsive thoughts, sensory illusions, and apathy. These types of automatic behaviors occur in complex partial seizures because the discharge spreads to the adjoining cortical association areas thereby impairing the mechanisms of thought. The automatic actions represent programmed behaviors that are released from inhibition because they no longer are under direct control of the prefrontal associational cortex. In contrast, the premotor and primary sensorimotor cortices are spared. The emotional components of automatism related to mood, sexuality, and aggression are generated in the hypothalamus and integrated with the cortically programmed behaviors at the level of the diencephalon and brainstem.

Petit Mal (Absence) Seizures

Petit mal (absence) seizures occur in children aged 3 to 12, and they usually disappear after the third decade of life. These seizures involve a brief loss of awareness and are often associated with staring, chewing, blinking, and occasional myoclonic jerks. A dominant familial predisposition is evident. The electrical discharge is primarily thought to involve a reverberating circuit between the cortex, thalamus, and brainstem reticular formation. The EEG brain wave pattern consists of a slow wave with spikes usually appearing at 3 Hz. Drug therapy is effective in controlling this type of seizure.

Grand Mal (Tonic–Clonic) Seizures

Grand mal (tonic–clonic) seizures usually involve the cortex, basal ganglia, diencephalon, and brainstem reticular formation. Symptoms of grand mal seizures include loss of consciousness followed by tonic convulsions consisting of repeated hyperextension of the body (tonic–clonic convulsions) and breath-holding spells resulting in cyanosis and tongue biting (Table 20-8). The average length of a tonic–clonic seizure is 1 to 3 minutes. At the end of the seizure, the patient remains tired and listless for approximately 1 hour. During the seizure, the EEG reveals high-frequency spikes.

A hereditary predisposition is thought to be the underlying substrate for most patients having grand mal epilepsy. The precipitating factors consist of strong emotional stimuli, hyperventilation, drugs, alcohol, fever, infections, sleep deprivation, and physical stimuli such as loud noises and flashing lights. A grand mal seizure may last for several minutes before it stops completely. It is thought that two factors bring about the termination of these seizures: fatigue of the firing neurons and neuronal inhibition.

Drug Therapy for Epilepsy

Diphenylhydantoin (phenytoin, or Dilantin), **phenobarbital**, **valproate**, and **carbamazepine** (Tegretol) are the

Table 20-8

General Symptoms Associated with Tonic–Clonic Phases of Grand Mal Seizures

Tonic Phase	Clonic Phase
Unconsciousness	Alternate muscle relaxation
Failing to ground	Tongue biting
Spasticity in muscles	Salivation
Transient interruption of breathing	Turning blue

commonly used drugs for epilepsy. With these therapeutic drugs, there usually is a marked reduction of paroxysmal (sudden and sharp) discharge, and consequently the seizures are controlled. Drug combinations are often required, especially for some epilepsy syndromes made up of two or more seizure types. If appropriate drug therapy fails to control the seizures, the patients are investigated further and if it is feasible, the discharging brain tissue can be surgically removed, which opens opportunity for mapping the cognitive and linguistic functions of the epileptogenic tissue (Fig. 20-20).

Altered Consciousness and Sleep

Many neurological conditions are known to impair the consciousness, the external and internal awareness of self. More specifically, it is the awareness that individuals have about their external and internal environments that include their perceptions, thoughts, and memories. Consciousness is closely related to attention.

The disorders of consciousness can range from mild to profound depending on the degree and extent of injury to the bilateral cerebral cortex and the brainstem reticular formation. Some of the common states of altered consciousness are **acute confusional state**, **minimal consciousness**, **stupor**, and **coma** (Table 20-9). Common causes of altered consciousness are traumatic brain injury, oxygen deprivation to the brain, and anesthetics.

Acute confusional state, also known as **delirium**, is the least but fluctuating impaired level of consciousness. Characterized by confusion, psychomotor excitability distractibility, agitation, and disorientation, its additional behavioral attributes are slowed thinking, reduced processing, reduced information integration, and incoherent thinking subsequent to CNS dysfunctioning. Linguistically, this stage is marked by confused language, incomplete and inconsistent thoughts, lexical paraphasia, and semantically anomalous verbal output. The patient is not clear about time and space.

A state of minimal consciousness, which represents a deeper state of impaired consciousness, signals a functional and communicative paucity where the person can spontaneously undertake small movements (involving hand and eye) and are able to verbalize little and follow brief commands. Behaviorally, such patients are able to undertake short and brief communication, such as uttering a few words and answer yes/no questions.

Stupor is a level of significantly altered consciousness. Patients in stupor are generally unconscious but can be brought to a higher level of consciousness only through a strong stimulus, such as pain. Even after the state of consciousness is regained, the individual may not fully participate in any activity and may lapse back into stupor.

Table 20-9

Disorders of Altered Consciousness

Altered Consciousness Types	Clinical Characteristics
Confusion	Reduced responsiveness due to slow thinking, disorientation, and inattention
Acute confusional state (delirium)	Confusion, distractibility, agitation, disorientation, slowed thinking, reduced information processing and integration, and incoherent thinking, incomplete and inconsistent thoughts, and semantically anomalous verbal output
Minimum consciousness	A deeper state of impaired consciousness marked by paucity of spontaneous functional, physical, and communicative responsiveness
Stupor	A state of significantly impaired consciousness in which the patient can respond to only continuous painful stimuli
Coma	Representing the deepest state of impaired consciousness and with a general amnesia for the coma duration, the patient is unresponsive to even painful stimuli and with a general amnesia for the duration of the coma in comatos, the patient is completely noncommunicative and does not undergo a sleep/wake cycle.

Coma, the deepest state of impaired consciousness, is a profoundly decreased level of wakefulness in which the patient remains unresponsive to painful stimuli and cannot be awakened. There is general amnesia for the duration of the coma in patients who recover. Patients in this state are completely unresponsive, noncommunicative, and do not undergo a sleep–wake cycle.

Brain or cerebral death, an irreversible form of unconsciousness, is characterized by a completely nonfunctional cerebral cortex and the loss of reflexive brainstem functions. The patient is totally unresponsive to external stimuli, and the EEG is flat for at least 30 minutes. A related condition is persistent vegetative state, where the neocortex is nonfunctional with preserved brainstem reflexes—breathing and heartbeat control. Patients are incognizant of the environment, display no cognitive function, lack responsiveness to commands, but can breathe on their own, open their eyes reflexively, and follow sleep–wake cycle. Keeping such a person alive has become a bioethical issue that has been extensively debated, best illustrated by the legal proceedings for the right to die in the case involving Terri Schiavo, a 41-year-old brain-damaged woman in Florida.

As a diagnostic tool of cortical activity, the EEG is used to differentiate between altered states of consciousness such as stupor, coma, and brain death; EEG is also used to measure brain activity during **sleep**, which is another state of mind with different stages of self-consciousness. The cerebral cortex, which is active during periods of wakefulness, controls sensorimotor activity through a stream of impulses that diminish during sleep. The cortical activity in the awakened state is regulated by the projections of the reticular activating system (RAS), which is responsible for cortical activation and arousal and regulates the levels of consciousness. The RAS itself can be activated by any internal or external stimulus. Reduced activation of the RAS lowers consciousness and responsiveness to external and internal stimuli (see Chapter 18). Only a massive pathology of the cerebral cortex and/or thalamus bilaterally or of the reticular formation is associated with a profound loss of consciousness.

Sleep

Although an active state of mind, is different from wakefulness and is characterized by diminished responsiveness. It is an important physiologic state for replenishing body energy. Deprivation of sleep negatively affects the quality of cortical functions and has been associated with difficulty in reasoning, attending, self-monitoring, and maintaining concentration; it also makes individuals irritable and fatigued.

Normal sleep consists of two categories: **rapid-eye movement (REM)** and **non–rapid-eye movement (NREM)**. NREM sleep further consists of four stages (Fig. 20-26). The EEG correlates of sleep are measured by the increased degree of the dominance of two slow waves—θ and δ—which become more and more synchronized as one enters the cycle of sleep.

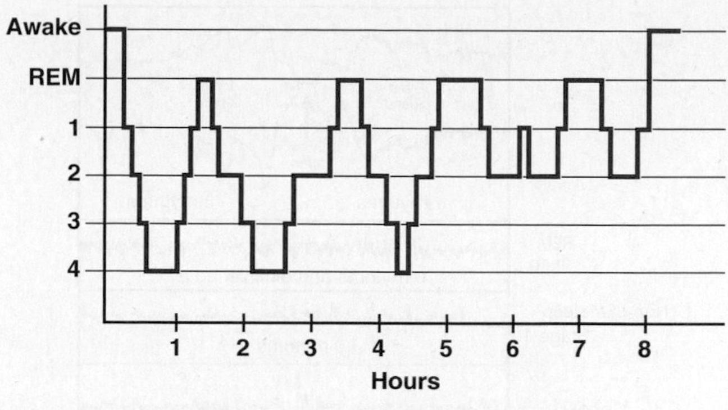

Figure 20-26 Graphic display of time spent in the stages of rapid-eye movement (*REM*) sleep.

One enters the REM and NREM stages many times during the sleep cycle. In the REM stage, the representative EEG pattern remains desynchronized, similar to the one seen in an awake stage (Box 20-5; Fig. 20-27). It is characterized by mixed electric wave frequencies, with θ- and decreased α-activity (1–2 cycles/second lower than waking). However, during the REM stage, there is substantial inhibition of sensory systems and the motor neurons in the spinal cord and brainstem. This immobilizes skeletal muscles except for the muscles of eye and diaphragm. On the one hand, the dominance of the parasympathetic system during REM slows down important body systems by lowering respiration, blood pressure, heartbeat, and body temperature. On the other hand, it increases gastric mobility. Disconnected from the external stimuli during this stage, the CNS becomes sensitive to internally

BOX 20-5

Important Clinical Points about Sleep

- Adequate sleep is needed for replenishing bodily and mental energies.
- Sleep deprivation affects our ability to optimally use cognitive processes, such as attention, memory, and thinking.
- Neural mechanism of sleep includes reticular ascending projections, pontine rapid-eye movement (REM) center, and the hypothalamus.
- With age, elderly subjects spend more time in non-REM (NREM) stages of 1 and 2 and have lesser deep slow-wave sleep cycles of NREM state 3 and 4.
- Sleepwalking, sleep talking, and sleep terror are known to occur during δ-sleep, which includes stages 3 and 4 of deep NREM.

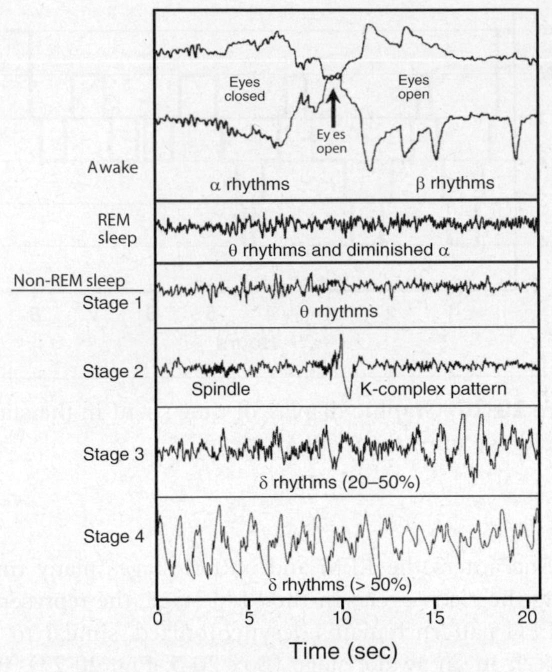

Figure 20-27 Graphic display of electroencephalographic rhythms during the rapid eye movement (*REM*) and non–REM sleep stages.

generated signals, as seen by the imagery experiences of dreams, which are accompanied by rapid movements of the eyes. Events like dreams, nightmare, erection, and bed-wetting, of which individuals may not retain any memory, are known to occur at this stage.

The rest of sleep time is spent in NREM sleep, which is marked by a greater synchronization of electroencephalographic rhythms. In NREM sleep, muscle tension is significantly reduced, and movement, though possible, is minimal. This movement is usually limited to the movements that change body position, if needed. The energy consumption of the body remains low because of the dominance of the parasympathetic system. In terms of electrical functioning, the slow EEG rhythms with large amplitude represent the synchronized neuronal activity at this stage.

During NREM sleep, a person progresses from stage 1 to stage 4; each of the stages is identified by a distinctive EEG pattern. For example, stage 1, also called quiet wakefulness, is characterized by low-amplitude θ-EEG activity replacing the high-frequency α-wave pattern. The individual is fully relaxed, with eyes closed and fleeting thoughts. In terms of EEG activity, this stage is hard to distinguish from the REM stage. NREM stage 2 is marked by the emergence of short sharp bursts of α-waves, known as high-amplitude sleep spindles (12- to 14-Hz wave pattern) and K complexes in the presence of background θ-activity; the person at this stage is easily awaken. NREM stage 3 is somewhat similar to stage 2, with 20% to 50% δ-activity and the sleeper in a state of extreme relaxation.

Representing the deepest level of sleep, stage 4 is dominated by >50% δ-electrical waves. The person at this stage is relaxed and difficult to awaken. Sleepwalking, sleep talking, and sleep terror are known to occur during δ-sleep, which includes stages 3 and 4. After progressing through these stages, one may reverse to different stages until reaching NREM stage 1 or REM level, completing the sleeping cycle. In a typical period of 7- to 8-hour sleep, an individual alternates from NREM to REM stage every 70 to 120 minutes. This cycle repeats three to five times during the entire sleep period.

Aging-related changes in sleep patterns involve a decrease time in the slow-wave stages of 3 and 4 of NREM and an increase time in stages 1 and 2. There are many sleep-related problems, such as disorders of initiating and maintaining sleep during normal sleeping periods, excessive daytime sleepiness, disorders of the sleep cycle, and dysfunctions associated with various stages of sleep. **Insomnia** (inability to initiate and maintain sleep during normal hours) is a common problem and is usually associated with such conditions as stress or emotional changes in life, most of which are temporary. **Hypersomnia**, or sleeping during normal waking hours, is caused by dysfunction of sleep. **Narcolepsy** is a common type of hypersomnia. In narcolepsy, which is inherited as an autosomal-recessive trait, a person exhibits uncontrollable napping during the day. Other symptoms are **cataplexy** (brief loss of muscle tone with sudden emotional bursts), vivid hallucinations, and sleep paralysis, in which the patient appears awake but cannot move the limbs. One of the causes of hypersomnia is **obstructive sleep apnea**, in which excessive relaxation of the pharyngeal muscle closes the upper airway during sleep. In apnea, the person may stop breathing and awake in panic.

Toxic Encephalopathies

Encephalopathy refers to CNS dysfunctions that primarily result from impaired cellular metabolism. As discussed in Chapter 7, the metabolic functioning of the CNS depends on a consistent availability of oxygen and glucose supplied by blood. Any interruption in this supply of glucose and oxygen to the brain can cause toxic or metabolic encephalopathy. The factors affecting brain metabolism can be intrinsic or extrinsic. Degenerative brain changes in **Parkinson**, **Huntington**, and **Alzheimer** diseases are intrinsic factors, whereas externally introduced toxic agents and co-agents are extrinsic factors.

The onset of toxic encephalopathy is usually gradual. Early signs include slowed cognitive processing, confusion, memory loss, impaired ability to communicate, difficulty finding words, depression, withdrawal, and indifference. In its advanced stages, these symptoms become more pronounced and include hallucinations, agitation, communicative breakdown, inattention, seizures, and coma.

Various conditions can alter the brain's metabolism and cause toxic encephalopathy. Persistent anoxia can severely affect the brain's oxygen supply. Both vascular and pulmonary diseases contribute to anoxia. Lasting anoxia to the medulla depresses respiration and can be fatal. A depleted supply of glucose, as seen in **hypoglycemia**, and excessive concentration of blood sugar, seen in **hyperglycemia**, directly affect brain functioning.

Blood lead levels >40 mg/100 mL cause lead poisoning, a condition common in children who live in old buildings with chipped lead paint. Manifestations of lead poisoning include hyperactivity, behavioral problems, psychomotor (lethargy) retardation, mental insufficiency, epilepsy, and neuropathy. Liver diseases and renal failure are the other causes of metabolic disturbances that lead to cognitive and sensorimotor functions and personality.

Malnutrition and alcohol dependency are two of the most common causes of **thiamine deficiency**, which can be seen in **Wernicke** and **Korsakoff encephalopathy**. However, in many instances, encephalopathic manifestations are reversible if they are treated early.

Myopathies

Myopathy is a collective term referring to a group of diverse muscle diseases caused by tissue degeneration, toxicity, and inflammatory changes. The primary manifestation is muscle weakness, although the muscles appear normal on clinical examination. Problems with speech and swallowing can also be found in the later stages. There are various types of muscular abnormalities. **Muscular dystrophy** is a hereditary myopathy marked by progressive weakness and atrophy. **Duchenne muscular dystrophy** is an X-linked myopathy transmitted to male children from their mothers, who never manifest the condition. **Oculopharyngeal** and **facial dystrophies** affect extrinsic ocular and facial muscles, causing dysarthria and severe problems with ocular movements.

Peripheral Neuropathies

Neuropathy is a disease of the peripheral nerves, interrupting the transmission of impulses from motor neurons to muscles. It can be inherited, idiopathic, or caused by trauma, toxicity, infection, or neoplastic growth. It can involve a single peripheral nerve (mononeuropathy) or several peripheral nerves (polyneuropathy). It may affect only sensory and/or motor functions (see Chapter 2); the symptom profile may be acute, chronic, or relapsing. Common peripheral mononeuropathies include neuropathy at the wrist (carpal tunnel syndrome), elbow, or knee. This syndrome results from the entrapment of the **median nerve** at the wrist level and is seen in people whose work activity regularly requires wrist movement.

Elbow neuropathy involves the **ulnar nerve**, which is susceptible to damage at the elbow. Initial symptoms of ulnar neuropathy are numbness and tingling at the area of nerve distribution. The nerve involved in knee neuropathy is the **peroneal**. It is especially susceptible to damage as it passes laterally around the fibula. Sitting with the legs crossed is often a cause of this neuropathy, and foot drop and sensory and motor disturbances characterize it.

Cranial neuropathies usually involve muscles of the eye, jaw, or face. Lesions of the fibers supplying the ocular nerves can affect movements of the eye and the parasympathetic functions of the iris. Lesions of the trigeminal nerve result in sensory symptoms in the face and motor problems for the mastication muscles. Damage to the facial nucleus and its nerve results in facial paralysis (Bell palsy), and associated visceral and parasympathetic disturbances.

Neoplastic Growth

A neoplasm (or tumor) is uncontrolled growth of body tissue and glia cells (see Chapter 5). The underlying cause may have to do with a faulty expression of **oncogenes** (proteins involved with cellular growth) and/or a loss of tumor-suppressor genes as well as the growth of new blood vessels (**angiogenesis**). A tumor can be primary or metastatic. Primary tumors arise from glia or meninges within the CNS. Metastatic, also known as secondary, tumors arise elsewhere in the body and spread to the brain. Most of the spreading tumors in the brain come from cancer of the breast or lung or from melanoma (malignant cells that contain melanin and are usually found in the skin). This spread from the remote sources occurs through the lymphatics or blood vessels.

Tumors are either malignant or benign. Malignant brain tumors grow to infiltrate the surrounding tissue, and are mostly fatal. These tumorous tissues are often multifocal and microscopically undifferentiated from the surrounding unaffected tissues. Malignancy is graded on a scale I to IV. Low-grade tumors are benign; high-grade tumors are malignant (see Chapter 5).

With the brain's unique ability to reorganize, patients with tumors present slowly developing and subtle clinical signs. Neoplastic growth in the brain primarily increases intracranial pressure, which slowly irritates and damages the surrounding brain tissues.

Most brain tumors originate from glia cells (gliomas) and include astrocytomas, ependymomas, and oligodendrogliomas. Other benign brain tumors are meningiomas, which arise from the dura mater; acoustic neuromas or vestibular schwannoma, which arise from the Schwann cell sheath of the nerve; and pituitary adenoma.

Tumors that initially involve the silent brain regions become symptomatic in later stages. Besides focal symptoms, common clinical symptoms of a brain tumor include progressive weakness, speech or visual loss, anomia, headache, impaired concentration, forgetfulness, double vision, altered cognitive ability, nausea, seizure-altered personality, and mental confusion. The most notable complications of a tumor are seizures and increased intracranial pressure with resulting complications of tissue herniations. Medical treatment of tumors involves surgical excision, chemotherapy, and/or radiation therapy (γ-knife). A modern gamma knife can deliver of over 200 beams of radiation with scalpel-like precision to tumors and lesions killing over 90% to 95% of all tumors.

Cerebral Infections

Various bacteria, viruses, and other organisms can cause infections in the CNS. Generally, the effect of an infection on the brain is diffuse and most commonly affects the meninges (meningitis) and cerebral cortex (encephalopathy). Infections can also be local, such as cerebral abscess, which occur in different parts of the brain. Some common infections are **viral infections**, **herpes simplex**, ***Escherichia coli***, **brain abscess**, **subdural empyema**, and **syphilis**.

SUMMARY

Students working with human behaviors in medical settings not only require a functional knowledge of neuroscience, but they must also familiarize themselves with imaging techniques and common neurological concepts and conditions. These concepts include the management of neurologic patients who are seen by professionals working primarily in medical settings (audiologists, speech–language pathologists, and psychologists). These concepts include imaging techniques, electrodiagnostic tools, procedural issues of sodium amytal infusion, and disorders of consciousness, physiology of speech, neuropathy, infections, and the modes of genetic inheritance. This chapter presented the pertinent neurosurgical procedures, along with their neurolinguistic implications, as well as a discussion of the modes of genetic inheritance and common neurologic diseases.

REVIEW QUESTIONS

1. Complete the following statements using the appropriate technical terms:
   A. ________ ________ is an excellent tool for evaluating the cerebral vasculature (________ ________, and ________ ________).
   B. The ________ procedure is used for relieving intractable pain by sectioning the lateral spinothalamic tract.
   C. As a treatment for Parkinson disease, the ________ ________ ________ involves a subcortical chronic electrode implant and the use of a stimulation programmer.
   D. ________ ________ involves the simultaneous presentation of largely identical words to both ears; the number of words recalled from each ear is used to measure cerebral dominance.
   E. In ________ ________, the faulty gene dominates the gene from the other parent with which it is paired and has a 50% probability of a trait inheritance.
   F. As a graphic representation of the brain's summated electrical activity, ________ reflects potential differences between two separated points on the scalp surface.
   G. ________ provides a visual record of muscular activity during spontaneous and/or voluntary movements.
   H. A________ ________ is undertaken to remove the CSF for a chemical analysis.
   I. As a peripheral nerve disease subsequent to trauma, toxicity, infection, or neoplasm, ________ slows the nerve impulses by interrupting their transmission.
   J. In________ ________, both parents carry and transmit the faulty gene, and the child has a 25% probability of inheriting the disease.
   K. Patients in________ can be brought to consciousness only through a painful stimulus.
   L. ________ refers to the brain dysfunctions that result from impaired cellular metabolism and vascular toxicity.
   M. ________ represents two or more incidences of (recurring) unprovoked seizures.
   N. ________ ________ ________ represents the normal CNS signals in response to specific and controlled sensory stimulations.
   O. ________ inheritance involves a faulty gene that is located on the mother's sex chromosome.
2. List the four major types of brain waves and their frequencies.
3. Name the preferred imaging technique for identifying subarachnoid hemorrhage, trauma, and hydrocephalus.
4. Name the imaging technique that measures responses of living tissues to an applied magnetic field and to radiofrequency waves.
5. List the major imaging technique that does not expose the patient to potentially harmful ionizing radiation.
6. Name the technique that measures electrical signals occurring in the CNS in response to specific and controlled sensory (visual, tactile, somatosensory, or auditory) stimulation.
7. Name the MRI technique that is extremely sensitive to even minute molecular motion and detects an ischemic stroke within 10 to 15 minutes.
8. Name the MRI technique that can immediately identify an eloquent part of the brain during participation in any linguistic or sensorimotor task based on the degree of oxygen consumption.
9. Name the MRI technique that provides functional (normal and abnormal) information about the cerebral white matter by measuring the directionality of water molecular movement in myelinated axonal tracts.

10. Name the MRI technique that measures brain chemistry.
11. Name the technique that uses intracarotid infusion of sodium amytal for measuring cerebral dominance.
12. Match each of the following MRI image types with its diagnostic efficacy:

    A. T1 sequence

    B. T2 sequence

    a. anatomical detail including gray and white matter

    b. water content to help identify tumors, infarcts and infections.
13. Match each of the following seizure types with associated function:

A. partial simple	a. a sudden onset of sensorimotor behaviors confined to a single body part from a single cortical or subcortical lesion
B. partial complex	b. also known as psychomotor, the recurring episodes of automatic, irrational and aggressive behavior with no memory secondary to medial temporal lobe lesions
C. petit mal	c. a brief loss of consciousness associated with staring, chewing, blinking, and occasional myoclonic jerks
D. grand mal	d. loss of consciousness with repeated hyperextension of the body (tonic–clonic convulsions) and breath-holding spells

14. Match each of the following techniques with the activities it measures:

A. electroencephalography	a. muscle activity and nerve conduction
B. electromyography	b. electrical brain activity in response to specific stimuli
C. sodium amytal infusion	c. brain's electrical potentials
D. evoked potentials	d. cerebral dominance
E. dichotic listening	e. CNS infections and intracerebral hemorrhages
F. lumbar puncture	f. ear superiority

15. What is the difference between coma and stupor?
16. What is the difference between coma and sleep?
17. Name the technique that is used to study brain–behavior relationship in case of surgical removal of epileptogenic brain tissue.
18. Describe the phasic profile of action potentials in patients with neuropathy (A) and myopathy (B).

Discussion of Review Questions

Chapter 1 Essential Neurological Concepts and Principles

1. Complete the following statements using the appropriate technical terms:

A. A left hemispheric lesion results in right hemiplegia and hemianesthesia.
B. In clinical orientation, the patient faces the clinician so that the patient's left and right corresponds to clinicians' right and left.
C. Brain's inherent capacity to reorganize when faced with injuries is known as neuroplasticity.
D. The decussation of sensory and motor fibers accounts for the contralaterality of sensorimotor organization in the brain.
E. Clinical symptoms are ipsilateral if they appear on the side of the body which is identical to the lesion side.
F. The topographical organization refers to the discreteness with which sensorimotor information is retained in the axonal pathways from the specialized peripheral receptors in the body to the brain.
G. Spasticity refers to a hypertonic state of muscle which is marked by increased tone.
H. As an example of muscle tone abnormality, rigidity refers to a constant resistance that is present throughout a passive limb movement.
I. The central part of the body which is made up of the head and trunk is known as the axial region. Appendicular, on the other hand, relates to the limbs, which are attached to the central body region.
J. The brainstem consists of three structures: midbrain, pons, and medulla.
K. Cerebral hemispheres, limbic lobe, and basal ganglia are derived from the telencephalon, which itself relates to the prosencephalon.
L. Tract/fasciculus is a collection of nerve fibers that have a common origin and termination.

2. Match each of the following functional categories with its examples:

A. general somatic afferent (GSA) (a)	a. pain and temperature
B. special somatic afferent (SSA) (d)	b. autonomic nervous system activity
C. general visceral afferent (GVA) (e)	c. limb movement involving skeletal muscles
D. special visceral afferent (SVA) (f)	d. audition
E. general somatic efferent (GSE) (c)	e. organ content
F. general visceral efferent (GVE) (b)	f. taste and smell
G. special visceral efferent (SVE) (g)	g. articulation, phonation, facial expression, and swallowing

3. Match the following lexical roots with their meanings. (see Appendix C for help)

A. kinesis (f)	a. paralysis
B. opsis (e)	b. old
C. phagein (d)	c. tongue
D. plege (a)	d. eat
E. prattein/praxis (h)	e. vision
F. presbys (b)	f. movement
G. taxis (g)	g. order
H. gloss (c)	h. act or action

4. Match the Brodmann area numbers for the following cortical regions:

A. primary motor cortex (c)	a. 41, 42
B. primary somatosensory area (b)	b. 3,1,2
C. primary visual cortex (d)	c. 4
D. primary auditory cortex (a)	d. 17

5. Provide the directional terms above and below the neuroaxial bend on the figures below:

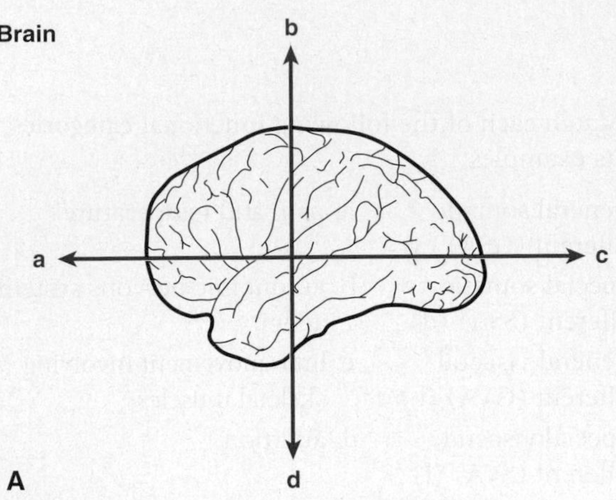

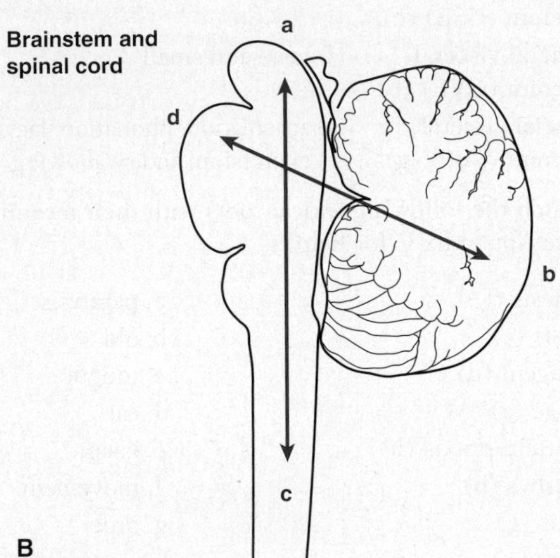

A. Above the neuroaxial bend (the brain):

a. Rostral
b. Dorsal
c. Caudal
d. Ventral

B. Below the neuraxial bend (the brainstem and spinal cord):

a. Rostral
b. Dorsal
c. Caudal
d. Ventral

6. Match each of the branches of neuroscience with its associated definition:

A. neurology (a)	a. nervous system and its diseases
B. neurosurgery (g)	b. structure and anatomy of the CNS
C. neuroanatomy (b)	c. imaging of brain structures in vivo
D. neuroradiology (c)	d. development of the CNS
E. neuroembryology (d)	e. chemical/physical processes of the CNS
F. neurophysiology (e)	f. pathologic changes in the CNS
G. neuropathology (f)	g. surgical removal of pathologic tissue from the nervous system

7. Match the following neurological conditions with the associated statement:

A. Huntington disease (d)	a. a degenerative disease of the aging brain associated with dementia
B. cerebral palsy (b)	b. a motor disorder caused by damage to the brain pre, post, or during birth
C. Parkinson disease (g)	c. an abnormality in the brain's electrical activity
D. Alzheimer disease (a)	d. a progressive and hereditary brain disease leading to chorea and dementia.
E. stroke (f)	e. a progressive demyelinating disease of the CNS
F. epilepsy (c)	f. a loss of function due to the interruption of blood circulation in the brain
G. multiple sclerosis (e)	g. a progressive disease of the brain characterized by tremor, reduced strength, and slow movements.

8. Provide two examples of reorganization in the adult brain as a reflection of cerebral plasticity.

- *establishment of the dominance for the projections from the stronger eye*
- *the reallocation of the committed cortical motor region after the amputation of a digit*

9. List six reasons why training in neuroscience helps you become a better SLP clinician.
   - *ability to understand the genesis of neurological conditions associated with communicative disorders*
   - *ability to appreciate the signs and symptoms associated with cortical and subcortical lesions*
   - *ability to interpret the scope of neuroimaging in the context of higher mental dysfunctions*
   - *ability to provide effective rehabilitation*
   - *ability to form a constructive working relationship with colleagues from a variety of disciplines (neurology, neurosurgery, radiology, pediatrics, and physiatry)*
   - *ability to present a broader view of the profession*
10. How does a stroke (cerebral vascular accident) affect cortical functions?
    - *On being deprived of oxygen in CVA, the brain cells die, affecting behaviors and skills.*
11. How does familiarity with clinical orientation help reading brain images?
    - *It helps you read neuroimages with precision as the patient's left and right brains are reversed.*
12. Name the principles that regulate brain functions dealing with connectivity, decision making, dominance, reorganization, and discreteness of sensorimotor representation.
    - *interconnectivity in the brain*
    - *centrality of the CNS*
    - *laterality of brain organization*
    - *plasticity in the brain*
    - *topographical organization*
13. Name three major structures of the brain.
    - *cerebrum*
    - *brainstem*
    - *cerebellum*
14. Name the brain region that contains six layered cortex and list its function.
    - *neocortex*
    - *higher mental functions and sensorimotor skills*
15. Name three major areas covered in a neurological examination.
    - *higher mental functions*
    - *sensory functions*
    - *motor functions*

Chapter 2 Gross Anatomy of the Central Nervous System

1. Complete the following statements using the appropriate technical terms:

A. Comprised of caudate nucleus, putamen, globus pallidus, claustrum, and amygdaloid nucleus, the basal ganglia are known to regulate cortically generated motor functions.

B. Consisting of cranial nerve nuclei, longitudinal fiber tracts, and the reticular formation, the brainstem connects the forebrain to the spinal cord.

C. The brainstem exits the cranium through the foramen magnum and connects with the spinal cord.

D. The cauda equina represents the spinal nerve roots that arise from the lumbosacral region and pass through the lumbar cistern before exiting the vertebral canal

E. The lower terminal point of the spinal cord is referred to as the conus medullaris.

F. Bordering medially the inferior horns of the lateral ventricles, the limbic structure of hippocampus is thought to be related to memory functions.

G. As the controller of the autonomic nervous system, the hypothalamus also regulates endocrinic functions, maintains body temperature, blood volume, food and water intake, body mass, reproduction, and the regulation of circadian rhythms.

H. The brain system that regulates emotional drive to visceral and vegetative functions such as instinctual reflexes, aggression, anxiety, and fear is the limbic system.

I. The meninges that protect the CNS consist of three layers of concentric fibrous tissue that include the dura mater, arachnoid membrane, and pia mater.

J. Also referred to as the craniosacral system, the parasympathetic system functions to conserve energy and regulates optimum visceral functions essential to survival.

K. A plexus is a network of interconnected nerves that originate from multiple segments of the spinal cord.

L. Also referred to as the thoracolumbar division of the ANS, the sympathetic system functions to expend energy in flight, fright or fight conditions.

M. Besides providing the organism with a three-dimensional orientation map that guides eye movements and head and body turning in response to bright light and directional sounds, the tectum also mediates visual reflexes.

N. The free borders of the tentorium cerebelli form an opening called the tentorial incisure, through which the brainstem exits the posterior cranial fossa.

O. Afferent axonal fibers carry sensory impulses toward the CNS, while the efferent fibers carry the commands away from the CNS.

P. The corpora quadrigemina that consist of the superior and inferior colliculi serve as the reflex centers for vision and audition.

Q. The peduncle is the bundle of fibers that connects the cerebellum with the brainstem.

2. Match each of the following structures with the associated vesicle:

A. pes pedunculi (c)	a. telencephalon
B. limbic system (a)	b. diencephalon
C. fourth ventricle (d)	c. mesencephalon
D. basal ganglia (a)	d. metencephalon
E. thalamus (b)	e. myelencephalon
F. substantia nigra (c)	
G. medulla (e)	
H. pons (d)	
I. cerebellum (d)	

3. Match each of the following cortical structures to the lobes in which they are located:

A. supramarginal gyrus (b)	a. frontal
B. angular gyrus (b)	b. parietal
C. calcarine sulcus (d)	c. temporal
D. olfactory sulcus (a)	d. occipital
E. uncus (c)	
F. parahippocampal gyrus (c)	
G. premotor cortex (a)	
H. amygdala (c)	
I. precentral gyrus (a)	
J. postcentral gyrus (b)	

4. Match each of the following cortical structures to the associated cortical surface:

A. central sulcus (a)	a. dorsal-lateral
B. lateral sulcus (a)	b. ventral
C. supramarginal gyrus (a)	c. midsagittal
D. angular gyrus (a)	
E. calcarine sulcus (c)	
F. olfactory sulcus (b)	
G. parahippocampal gyrus (c)	
H. collateral sulcus (b)	
I. orbital cortex (b)	
J. olfactory nerve (b)	
K. cingulate gyrus (c)	
L. corpus callosum (c)	

5. Match the major divisions of the brain with the corresponding ventricular spaces:

A. telencephalon (c)	a. cerebral aqueduct
B. diencephalon (d)	b. fourth ventricle
C. midbrain (a)	c. lateral ventricles
D. metencephalon (b)	d. third ventricle

6. List the number of spinal nerves that exit from the following spinal regions.

A. cervical (8)
B. thoracic (12)
C. lumbar (5)
D. sacral (5)

7. List the cranial nerves by name and in the order they exit the brainstem.

- *III oculomotor*
- *IV trochlear*
- *V trigeminal*
- *VI abducens*
- *VII facial*
- *VIII acoustic; vestibulocochlear*
- *IX glossopharyngeal*
- *X vagus*
- *XI accessory*
- *XII hypoglossal*

8. Match each of the following pathologies to the associated statement:

A. lesion in area 17 on the left (b)	a. incomprehension of spoken language
B. lesion in area 41 on the left (d)	b. right hemianopsia
C. lesion in area 22 on the left (a)	c. loss of executive function
D. prefrontal lobe white matter lesion (c)	d. auditory imperceptibility
E. cutting the corpus callosum (e)	e. separation of hemispheres

9. Match each of the dysfunctions to the associated lesion site:

A. hemiplegia (d)	a. postcentral gyrus
B. hemianesthesia (a)	b. cerebellum
C. impaired motivation and emotion (f)	c. ventricles and CSF
D. involuntary movements (h)	d. precentral gyrus
E. hydrocephalus (c)	e. hypothalamus
F. hormonal disorder (e)	f. limbic lobe
G. meningitis (g)	g. arachnoid–pia membranes
H. incoordination (b)	h. basal ganglia

10. Why should SLPs be concerned about traumatic injuries at the cervical spinal cord?

- *Damage to phrenic nerve in cervical region of the cord results in respiratory palsy.*

11. List two common herniations that occur after increased intracranial pressure in the brain.

- *uncal (temporal) herniation*
- *tonsilar (cerebellum) herniation*

12. Which system is responsible for expending energy in flight, fight, or fright conditions? Which system helps to restore energy when threats are gone?

- *sympathetic system for energy expenditure*
- *parasympathetic system for energy restoration*

13. List the primary and secondary brain vesicles along with their brain derivatives.
    - *prosencephalon (forebrain): telencephalon, diencephalon*
    - *mesencephalon (midbrain): mesencephalon*
    - *rhombencephalon (hindbrain): metencephalon, myelencephalon*
14. Name the three meninges in the order from external to inward.
    - *dura mater*
    - *arachnoid membrane*
    - *pia mater*
15. Name the three types of fiber bundles in the brain.
    - *projection fibers*
    - *association fibers*
    - *commissural fibers*
16. List three extensions of the meningeal layer of the dura mater.
    - *falx cerebri*
    - *tentorium cerebelli*
    - *falx cerebelli*
17. Name the location of the reticular cortical arousal system.
    - *brainstem*
18. Name the parts of the corpus callosum.
    - *rostrum*
    - *genu*
    - *body*
    - *splenium*

Chapter 3 Internal Anatomy of the Central Nervous System

1. Complete the following statements using the appropriate technical terms:

A. The cerebral aqueduct connects the third and fourth ventricles.
B. The inferior colliculus in the midbrain is concerned with the transmission of auditory signals to the medial geniculate body of the thalamus.
C. The lateral geniculate body of the thalamus relays visual information to the cortex.
D. The medial longitudinal fasciculus plays an important role in coordinated conjugate eye movements by integrating vestibular projections with ocular cranial nerve nuclei.
E. The decussation of motor fibers in the caudal most medulla accounts for contralateral motor organization in the brain.
F. The midbrain cell cluster in the red nucleus relays cerebellar output to the motor cortex as well as the spinal cord.
G. The dopaminergic nuclei, with inhibitory projections to the caudate and putamen, are located in the substantia nigra. Degeneration of these inhibitory nuclei is associated with Parkinson disease.
H. The subthalamic nucleus, a basal ganglia nucleus located between the internal capsule and the substantia nigra, is involved with hemiballism.
I. The superior colliculus, a midbrain structure, regulates visual reflexes such as ocular accommodation and coordinated head and eye movements.
J. Located above the internal capsule, fanned sensorimotor fibers are known as the corona radiata.
K. The fornix provides a two-way connection between the hypothalamic mammillary bodies and hippocampus.
L. The medial lemniscus, containing the sensory fibers that mediate proprioception and discriminative touch, projects to the ipsilateral sensory cortex.
M. The corpus callosum forms the roof of the lateral ventricles, whereas their floor is formed by the caudate and the thalamus.

2. List two structures whose varying shapes help identify the neuraxial levels in the brain.
    - motor fiber shape
    - ventricular cavity shape
3. List the internal medullary constructs that are associated with the following concepts:

A. contralateral motor organization
- *decussation*

B. condensed motor fibers
- pyramida*l*
- *corticospinal tract*

C. crossed motor fibers
- lateral *corticospinal* tract

4. List at least three structures in the medulla that are associated with the transmission of somatic sensation.
    - *fasciculi of gracilis and cuneatus*
    - *internal arcuate fibers*
    - *medial lemniscus*
5. What ventricular cavity is located dorsal to the pons and what pontine region is located beneath this ventricle?
    - *fourth ventricle*
    - *tegmentum of the pons*
6. List the pontine structures that are related with the following concepts:

A. descending motor fibers
- *diffuse corticospinal fibers*

B. somatic sensation
- *medial lemniscus*

C. projections to the cerebellum
- *middle cerebellar peduncle (brachium pontis)*

D. auditory transmission

- *lateral lemniscus*

7. What structure differentiates the tectal and tegmental regions in the midbrain?

- *cerebral aqueduct*

8. Name the internal structures of the midbrain that are associated with the clinical concepts of

A. dopamine-secreting cells

- *substantia nigra*

B. mediation of visual reflexes

- *superior colliculi*

C. relay nuclei for the auditory information

- *inferior colliculi*

D. cerebellar projections to the motor cortex

- *superior cerebellar peduncle (brachium conjunctivum)*

9. List the structures that are present on a coronal section at the caudate-head level and are related to the following constructs:

A. interhemispheric fibers

- *corpus callosum, genu*

B. separation of the lateral ventricles

- *septum pellucidum*

C. Huntington chorea

- *caudate nucleus, head*

D. concentrated descending sensorimotor fibers.

- *internal capsule*

10. A lesion in the right caudal medulla involving the corticospinal fibers is likely to result in a sensorimotor loss on what half of the body?

- *left hemiplegia*

11. Will a lesion at internal capsule level result in language disorders? Why or why not?

- *no*
- *language is a neocortical function*

12. What half of the body is involved with the loss of proprioception and discriminative touch subsequent to a cervical spinal lesion?

- *ipsilateral half of the body*

13. List three fiber tracts that connect brainstem with the cerebellum.

- *inferior cerebellar peduncle*
- *middle cerebellar peduncle*
- *superior cerebellar peduncle*

14. Name the tract that coordinates ocular movements and integrates it with vestibular input.

- *medial longitudinal fasciculus*

15. A lesion in the right medulla involving the medial lemniscus fibers is likely to result in a loss of discriminative touch on what half of the body?

- *left side of the body*

16. What are the three parts of the internal capsule?

- *genu*
- *anterior limb*
- *posterior limb*

17. Order the structures starting medial to laterally from the third ventricle: thalamus, claustrum, external capsule, globus pallidus, internal capsule, insula.

- *thalamus*
- *globus pallidus*
- *internal capsule*
- *external capsule*
- *claustrum*
- *insula*

Chapter 4 Development of the Nervous System

1. Complete the following statements using the appropriate technical terms:

A. The haploid normal gamete, or sex cell, contains 23 chromosomes: either 23, Y or 23, X. It is only the male gamete that has either an X or a Y chromosome.
B. Disjunction represents the normal separation of pairs of chromosomes.
C. The embryo refers to the developing human organism from conception until the end of the eighth week, whereas the developmental period from two months to the birth is the fetal stage.
D. Gametogenesis refers to the formation of the male and female gametes, the spermatozoa and the ova, respectively.
E. Sex cells or gametes are formed by a type of cell division called meiosis, which is characterized by reduction of chromosomes to half the usual number.
F. The other type of cellular division is mitosis in which the daughter cell contains the number of chromosomes that is equal to the mother cell.
G. Neural plate is the neuroectodermal region of the early embryo's dorsal surface that later develops into the nervous system.
H. Nondisjunction refers to a failure of one or more pairs of chromosomes to separate, which is one of the common causes of abnormal gametes.
I. The disturbed growth process in malformed babies is teratogenesis.

J. Attention–deficit/hyperactive disorder is a common cause of developmental disability with profound implications for cognitive and educational abilities.

K. A trisomy involving the chromosome 21 results in Down syndrome, which is characterized by mental retardation and physical abnormalities.

L. One of the original two germ layers is the epiblast.

M. Fragile-X syndrome is an X-linked recessive syndrome characterized by mental retardation, atypical facial appearance, and abnormally large testicles.

N. As an embryonic forebrain syndrome with poorly developed midline structures, holoprosencephaly is characterized by fused eyes, a single nasal chamber, a single ventricle, and underdeveloped corpus callosum.

O. Myelination refers to the development of myelin before and after the birth.

P. The neural crest is the structure that gives rise to the peripheral nervous system.

Q. The neural plate is the forerunner of the central nervous system.

R. Trilaminar embryo refers to the development of three germ layers.

S. Trisomy involves the presence of an extra chromosome.

T. The anterior and posterior pores of the neural tube, respectively, close on the 25th and 27th day, otherwise serious birth defects result.

U. Except for some later developing cells in the cerebellum and possibly in hippocampus, the full complement of neurons is in place by week 25 of gestation and no cells develop after the birth.

2. By which gestation week does the human embryo have three primary brain vesicles?
   - *third gestation week*
3. True or false? Normally developing humans have 46 somatic chromosomes.
   - *true*
4. True or false? There are 24 types of human chromosomes; 22 autosomes, and one X and one Y chromosome.
   - *true*
5. Name the structure that is the forerunner of the nervous system.
   - *the neural plate*
6. True or false? The neural tube develops into the brain and the spinal cord.
   - *true*
7. Name the period duration, in which the CNS is most susceptible to major congenital defects:
   - *during weeks 3 to 16 of development*
8. Match the following disorders with their associated statements:

A. anencephaly (d)	a. failure of the brain to form two hemispheres
B. holoprosencephaly (a)	b. developmental failure of the gyri/sulci formation
C. lissencephaly (b)	c. miniature brain and small skull cap with normal face size
D. microcephaly (c)	d. congenital absence of the cranial vault with missing or reduced forebrain
E. Arnold–-Chiari syndrome (e)	e. Cerebellar protrusion into the vertebral cavity

9. List three common trisomies naming the involved chromosome number.
   - *trisomy 21, Down syndrome*
   - *trisomy 18, Edwards syndrome*
   - *trisomy 13, Patau syndrome*
10. List four common forebrain malformations.
    - *anencephaly*
    - *lissencephaly*
    - *microcephaly*
    - *cranium bifidum*
11. List two structural malformations that are associated with the Arnold–Chiari malformation.
    - *hydrocephalus*
    - *syringomyelia*
12. Name the single most important difference between oogenesis and spermatogenesis.
    - ***As part of the first meiotic division, the suspended prophase is not completed until after puberty in females making their eggs vulnerable to bodily and environmental toxicity.***
13. List four common developmental disorders.
    - *mental retardation*
    - *Down syndrome*
    - *childhood autism*
    - *attention-deficit/hyperactivity disorder (ADHD)*
14. What percent of infant deaths occurring during the first year of life are related to CNS malformations?
    - *40 percent*

Chapter 5 Nerve Cell Physiology

1. Complete the following statements using the appropriate technical terms:

A. A cellular depolarization from a resting membrane potential to a less negative state by 10 to 15 mV results in the generation of an action potential.
B. Besides reacting to brain injuries by proliferating in size (hypertrophy) and numbers (hyperplasia), the astrocytes also contribute to the blood–brain barrier, the first line of defense for the brain from harmful substances.
C. The microglia cells contribute to the natural recovery process by ingesting and removing the cellular debris.
D. Two types of degenerative changes follow an axonal sectioning: in axonal reaction, the retrograde degenerative changes extend to the cell body, while Wallerian degeneration involves the axonal region detached from the cell body.
E. Acetylcholine, dopamine, norepinephrine, serotonin, glutamate, and gamma-aminobutyricacid (GABA) are the small molecule neurotransmitters; they are known to have short-lasting effects, in contrast to long-lasting effects on postsynaptic nerve cells by large molecule neurotransmitters.
F. The myelin sheath, a multilayered lipid material, not only protects the nerve fibers by insulating them but it also regulates the speed of nerve impulses.
G. Abnormalities of the cellular cytoskeletal (microtubules, neurofilaments, and microfilaments) structures in the form of tangles and, subsequently, the reduced intracellular protein transfer has been associated with the Alzheimer disease.
H. The dendrites are the short cytoplasmic extensions that transmit information to the cell body from other cells via synaptic sites; the axons are efferent structures that transmit information away from the cell body to other neurons or target organs.
I. The condition in which antibodies attack the body's own normal tissues is called an autoimmune disease.
J. Chromatolysis refers to cellular changes marked by swelling, dissolution of cellular organelles (specifically Nissl bodies), and shifting of the nucleus peripherally in soma in response to an injury.
K. Microphagic cells that ingest cellular debris are called phagocytes.
L. The Schwann cells form myelin around the axons in the peripheral nervous system.
M. The point of contact between two neurons is called a synapse.

2. How does myelin loss in the CNS lead to neurological symptoms?

- *Demyelination affects the speed and efficiency of saltatory impulse transmission; thus, the sensorimotor functions are slowed.*

3. How does the blocking of postsynaptic receptor sites lead to neurological symptoms as seen in myasthenia gravis?

- ***The binding of antibodies with the acetylcholine receptor sites results in the underactivity of acetylcholine, the transmitter that is involved in myasthenia gravis.***

4. Match each of the following functions with its associated glia type:

A. Support for primary brain cells (e)	a. astrocytes
B. Seal cavity and form scar (a)	b. oligodendrocytes
C. Remove the debris by digesting them (c)	c. microglia
D. Myelin formation in the CNS (b)	d. Schwann cells
E. Contribute to blood–brain barrier (a)	e. Glia cells
F. Myelin formation in the PNS (d)	

5. Match each of the following neurotransmitters with its associated function:

A. acetylcholine (a)	a. voluntary movements
B. dopamine (b)	b. Parkinson disease
C. norepinephrine (c)	c. sleep, attention, and moods
D. GABA (d)	d. Huntington chorea

6. Name the roles of growth cone and chemical affinity in the synapse development.

- *promote axonal growth through tissue density to connect with functionally related target cells*

7. What is the difference between cellular apoptosis and necrosis?

- ***In necrosis, the cells die from an abnormal process such as stroke, tumor, or trauma; apoptosis is a programmed cell death due to the activation of an intrinsic program.***

8. What is the saltatory nerve conduction?

- *The action current jumps from one node to the next node in myelinated fibers.*

9. List three common malignant types of brain tumors.

- *astrocytoma*
- *oligodendroglioma*
- *ependymoma*

10. List four slow-growing tumors of the brain.
 - *meningioma*
 - *acoustic neuroma*
 - *vestibular schwannoma*
 - *pituitary adenoma*

Chapter 6 Diencephalon: Thalamus and Associated Structures

1. Complete the following statements using the appropriate technical terms:

A. The diencephalon is composed of four parts: thalamus, epithalamus, subthalamus, and hypothalamus.
B. As a sensorimotor integrator, the thalamus is the gateway for projecting sensorimotor information to the forebrain.
C. As the regulator of the autonomic nervous system, the hypothalamus also mediates endocrine functions, fat metabolism, and the metabolic states including the functions like body temperature, water balance, and sugar presence in the blood.
D. With projections to the prefrontal cortex and limbic structures, the dorsal lateral nucleus of the thalamus is known to integrate visceral information with affect, emotions, thought processes, personality, and judgment.
E. Caused by chronic alcoholism, Wernicke–Korsakoff syndrome is characterized by amnesia, disorientation, delirium, confabulations, and hallucinations.
F. In lowered pain threshold, a commonly seen symptom after thalamic lesion, patients become hypersensitive to the sensations of touch, pain, and temperature on the contralateral half of the body.

2. Name the thalamic nuclei that are marked with letters in the figure (Exercise Fig. 6-1 given below):

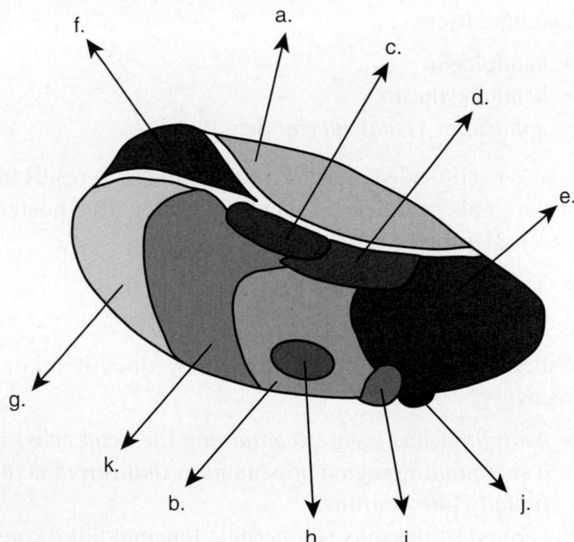

A.
 - *dorsal medial*

B.
 - *ventral posterior lateral*

C.
 - *lateral dorsal*

D.
 - *lateral posterior*

E.
 - *pulvinar*

F.
 - *anterior nucleus*

G.
 - *ventral anterior*

H.
 - *ventral posterior medial*

I.
 - *lateral geniculate body*

J.
 - *medial geniculate body*

K.
 - *Ventral lateral*

3. Match each of the following thalamic nuclei with its associated area of projection in the brain:

A. ventral lateral (g)	a. transverse gyri of Heschl
B. ventral anterior (b)	b. premotor cortex
C. pulvinar (e)	c. cingulate gyrus
D. dorsal medial (d)	d. prefrontal cortex
E. anterior nucleus (c)	e. inferior parietal lobule
F. lateral geniculate (f)	f. calcarine cortex
G. medial geniculate (a)	g. precentral gyrus

4. List three characteristics of the thalamic syndrome.:
 - *Nonlocalized pain sensation;*
 - *Contra lateral hemiplegia;*
 - *Contralateral hemianesthesia.*

5. List three symptoms of the hypothalamic syndrome.:
 - *Autonomic dysfunctions;*
 - *Hormonal abnormality*
 - *Impaired visceral functions like body temperature, water and food intake, sugar metabolism, and sexual behavior.*

6. What thalamic structures and pathway are affected in Wernicke--Korsakoff syndrome?
 - *Dorsal medial nucleus;*
 - *Mammillothalamic tract.*

7. Which thalamic nucleus mediates afferents from the medial lemniscus to the cerebral cortex?
 - *Ventral posterior lateral nucleus.*

8. Which thalamic nucleus is dedicated to mediating trigeminal projections to the cerebral cortex?
 - *Ventral posterior medial nucleus.*

9. A patient presenting with altered (increased or decreased) thresholds for the sensations of touch, pain, and temperature on the contralateral half of the body is likely to have what syndrome?

   - *thalamic syndrome*

10. What thalamic nucleus is reciprocally connected with the language cortex in the inferior parietal lobule?

    - *pulvinar*

Chapter 7 Cerebrovascular System

1. Complete the following statements using the appropriate technical terms:

A. Anastomosis marks a natural link between two blood vessels.
B. The development of collateral circulation to an ischemic tissue plays an important role in the natural recovery.
C. Subsequent to a congenital weakness in the arterial wall, aneurysm results in a localized dilation of an artery.
D. A transient ischemic attack results in temporary focal neurological symptoms that can last up to 30 minutes.
E. The vascular volume that is needed for the optimal brain functioning is approximately 50 to 60 mL per minute per 100 g of brain tissue.
F. The anticoagulant drugs are used to reduce or prevent intravascular clotting in the brain.
G. Representing the selective permeability of the blood vessels in the brain, the blood–brain barrier restricts the movement of harmful substances from the bloodstream to the brain tissue.
H. In hemorrhagic pathology, the blood leaks from a ruptured artery and increases pressure in the brain by occupying an intracranial space.
I. In hypertension, the sustained presence of elevated arterial blood pressure can cause damage to the heart and the brain.
J. Thrombolytic drug like tPA (tissue plasminogen activator) restores blood circulation by dissolving the clot.
K. Three cortical (middle, anterior, posterior) arteries originate from the circle of Wills.
L. Arteriovenous malformation is a congenital condition in which the arterial blood shunts to the veins, bypassing the underlying cortical tissue.
M. In embolism, a clump detached from the atherosclerotic plaque flows in the bloodstream and blocks a smaller and distal artery.
N. A thrombosis refers to a localized clot that blocks the lumen of a blood vessel.
O. Atherosclerosis is the process of narrowing of the arterial lumen owing to accumulation of fatty substances (cholesterol and triglycerides) and lipids along the intimal walls of the blood vessels.
P. By joining the circle of Willis at the base of the brain, the carotid and vertebrobasilar systems form a major anastomotic point.
Q. As an indicator of generalized hypoperfusion cellular death in the area peripheral to the primary distribution zones for the three cerebral arteries is the watershed infarct.
R. Subdural pathologies are located beneath the dura mater.
S. Extradural vascular pathologies are located external to the dura mater.
T. In stroke, an interruption of blood supply kills brain cells by affecting the oxygen supply.

2. Match each of the following cortical arteries with the brain region it supplies:

A. Anterior cerebral artery (c)	a. occipital lobe
B. Posterior cerebral artery (a)	b. lateral cortical surface
C. Middle cerebral artery (b)	c. midsagittal and ventral frontal surface

3. List three clinical symptoms that are likely to result from a CVA involving the anterior cerebral artery.

   - *impaired abstract reasoning*
   - *weakness in the lower leg*
   - *sensory loss in the lower leg*

4. List three clinical symptoms that are likely to result from a cerebral vascular accident involving the middle cerebral artery.

   - *hemiplegia*
   - *hemianesthesia*
   - *aphasia or visual special deficit*

5. List two clinical symptoms that are likely to result from a cerebral vascular accident involving the posterior cerebral artery.

   - *homonymous hemianopsia*
   - *visual agnosia*

6. What is ischemic penumbra? How does it relate to recovery?

   - *An infarct has a core (containing the dead cells) and a surrounding region of penumbra that contains functionally idle neurons.*
   - *Penumbra neurons can become functional if a consistent collateral circulation is operative within the critical time of 6–8 hours.*

7. Define stroke.
   - *brain cell death because of blood flow interruption in the brain*
8. Why is the blood–brain barrier important for the brain?
   - *As a unique property of the brain arteries, it prevents the flow of noxious substances in the blood to the brain.*
9. Name the mechanism that maintains a stable blood flow to the brain.
   - *autoregulation*
10. List two goals of the medical management of a cerebral vascular accident.
    - *restoring blood circulation to the brain*
    - *preventing another stroke*

Chapter 8 Ventricles and Cerebrospinal Fluid

1. Complete the following statements using the appropriate technical terms:

A. At the collateral trigone, the ventricular body enlarges before diverging into the posterior and inferior horns.
B. A blockage of the draining passage through which CSF reaches the subarachnoid space causes noncommunicating type of hydrocephalus.
C. A pressure difference between the sinus system and ventricular cavity regulates normal CSF drainage through the arachnoid granulations into the superior sagittal sinus.
D. If the sinus pressure exceeds ventricular pressure, the arachnoid villi close, causing an increased intracranial pressure in the brain.
E. The choroid plexus covered with ependymal cells secretes CSF through a passive diffusion from the blood.
F. Hydrocephalus is an accumulation of cerebrospinal fluid in the brain ventricles secondary to its impaired absorption in the sinus system.
G. A lumbar puncture is a diagnostic procedure that involves removing CSF from the lower lumbar section of the vertebral canal for chemical analysis.
H. Spinal anesthesia involves the injection of an anesthetic drug into the lumbar spinal subarachnoid space to suppress the sensation from the lower body.
I. The ventricles are the sites for the secretion and storage of CSF.
J. The common midbrain site associated with obstructive hydrocephalus and the enlargement of the lateral ventricles is the cerebral aqueduct.

2. Match the type of hydrocephalus with its associated description:

A. Communicating (a)	a. impaired CSF drainage into the superior sagittal sinus
B. Obstructive (Noncommunicating) (c)	b. large ventricular cavities subsequent to brain atrophy
C. Normal pressure hydrocephalus (d)	c. blocked access of the CSF to the subarachnoid space
D. Hydrocephalus ex vacuo (b)	d. hydrocephalus with impaired gait, frequent urination, and dementia

3. What is the major complication of increased intracranial pressure in the brain?
   - *brain tissue herniation*
4. Name the spinal site used for lumbar puncture.
   - *L3–L4*
5. Name two clinical functions of the lumbar puncture.
   - *removal of the CSF for a chemical analysis*
   - *administration of anesthetics for a spinal block*
6. Name the foramina that are associated with the following functions.

A. Connecting lateral ventricles to the third ventricle
   - *intraventricular foramen*

B. Connecting the third ventricle to the fourth ventricle
   - *cerebral aqueduct*

C. Discharging CSF from the fourth ventricle to the subarachnoid space
   - *foramen of Luschka and foramina of Magendie.*

7. Which of the ventricles in the brain has cavities in both hemispheres?
   - *the lateral ventricle*
8. How does a cerebral aqueduct stenosis contribute to hydrocephalus?
   - *enlarges lateral and third ventricles by blocking CSF flow to the fourth ventricle*
9. Name the structure that drains CSF into the superior sagittal sinus.
   - *arachnoid granulations*

Chapter 9 Auditory System

1. Complete the following statements using the appropriate technical terms:

A. The endolymph-filled cavities of saccule, utricle, semicircular ducts, and the scala media form the membranous labyrinth.
B. Located in the middle ear, the tensor tympani and stapedius muscles reflexively protect the auditory mechanism from damage by controlling ossicular motion.
C. The stapedius muscle, controlled by the facial nerve (CN VII), restricts stapes movement. The tensor tympani muscle, controlled by the trigeminal nerve (CN V), participates in restricting ossicular movements.
D. The retrocochlear auditory system includes the signals from hair cells in the organ of Corti to the brainstem cochlear nuclear complex.
E. The superior olivary nucleus is the first structure to receive auditory inputs from both (the ipsilateral and the contralateral) cochlear nuclei.
F. The lateral lemniscus contains the brainstem auditory fibers that originate from the superior olivary nucleus and project to the inferior colliculus.
G. A lesion above the cochlear nuclear complex is not likely to cause a profound hearing loss in either of the ears because of multiple crossing of the fibers.
H. The transverse Heschl gyri are the site of the primary auditory cortex.
I. Medial geniculate body mediates auditory information from the thalamus to the primary auditory cortex.
J. The labyrinthine artery that supplies blood to the inner ear and cochlear complex is a branch of the anterior inferior cerebellar artery, which originates from the basilar artery.
K. The primary auditory cortex is not absolutely essential for frequency discrimination; rather, it screens properties that are important in auditory discriminations.
L. In most right-handed individuals, the temporal planum is larger in the left brain and this in humans has been related to the cerebral dominance.

2. List two functions of the superior olivary nucleus.

- *receives projections from both ears*
- *first neuroaxial site to localize the sound source*

3. Match each of the following clinical concepts with its associated statement:

A. conductive hearing loss (d)	a. with a tuning fork placed on the vertex, subject reports in which ear the tone was perceived better
B. sensorineural hearing loss(c)	b. with a tuning fork pressed against the mastoid process, subject hears by bone conduction
C. Rinne test (b)	c. pathologies of hair cells in the cochlea
D. Weber test (a)	d. impaired sound transmission in the middle ear

4. Match each of the following structures with its associated vascular sources:

A. hair cells in the cochlea and three semicircular canals (c)	a. middle cerebral artery
B. lateral lemniscus (b)	b. pontine branches
C. inferior colliculus (e)	c. labyrinthine artery
D. medial geniculate body (d)	d. thalamogeniculate artery
E. primary auditory cortex (a)	e. superior cerebellar artery

5. Order these auditory relay nuclei (superior olivary nucleus, cochlear nuclear complex, 8th cranial nerve, lateral lemniscus, inferior colliculus, primary auditory cortex, medial geniculate body, auditory radiation fibers) in a hierarchic sequence reflecting the transmission of the ascending auditory information from the ear to the cortex:

1. 8th cranial nerve
2. cochlear nuclear complex
3. superior olivary nucleus
4. lateral lemniscus
5. inferior colliculus
6. medial geniculate body
7. auditory radiation fibers
8. primary auditory cortex

Chapter 10 Vestibular System

1. Complete the following statements using the appropriate technical terms:

A. Dynamic equilibrium regulates the maintenance of body and head positions during rotational and angular acceleration and deceleration.
B. Inertia represents a tendency of fluid to oppose any movement from a rest position.
C. Nystagmus is the oscillating movements of the eye, which is caused by dysfunctioning of the vestibular mechanism.
D. The dysfunction of the medial longitudinal fasciculus, which integrates the vestibular input with the coordinated eye movement, leads to double vision.
E. Characterized by vertigo, nausea, vomiting, tinnitus, and progressive but fluctuating sensory hearing loss, the Ménière disease is associated with increased endolymphatic pressure in the inner ear.
F. Static equilibrium regulates straight-line (linear) movements of the head in space and both head and body position during rest.
G. As a disorder of the vestibular system, vertigo refers to a sensation of self-rotation or the spinning of the space around.
H. The vestibular system regulates the position of the head and neck in space besides monitoring upright posture reflexes.

2. A 28-year-old woman was seen for a complaint of dizziness, nausea, and vomiting. On examination, she exhibited a tendency of falling to the right, left nystagmus, and deafness in the right ear, analgesia on the left body, hoarseness, and swallowing difficulty. Name the side and location of the lesion.
   - *right*
   - *cerebellopontine angle*
3. Professionals participating in which two activities do not exhibit reflexive rotational nystagmus?
   - *ballet dancers*
   - *figure skaters*
4. Provide three cardinal clinical symptoms that are associated with the Ménière disease:
   - *vertigo*
   - *tinnitus*
   - *progressive but fluctuating sensory hearing loss*
5. Name the purpose of irrigating the external auditory canal with warm and cold water.
   - ***To evaluate the integrity of the vestibular system. The thermal stimulation causes the hair cells in the ampulla of the vestibular apparatus to deflect, resulting in a nystagmatic eye movement, a normal response.***

Chapter 11 Somatosensory System

1. Complete the following statements using the appropriate technical terms:

A. Anesthesia refers to sensation loss that results either from a neurological disconnection/dysfunction or through a drug-induced suppression of nerve activity.
B. In graphesthesia, the patient's tactile recognition is tested by writing letters and drawing shapes on the skin surface.
C. Kinesthesia represents an internal awareness of the range and direction of the movement, whereas proprioception is the inner awareness of the limb position.
D. In stereognosis, one uses the discriminative ability to identify the shape, size, and texture of the object through tactile sensation.
E. Analgesia is the state in which painful stimuli are no longer perceived as being hurtful.
F. Epicritic sensation includes discriminative touch and proprioceptive awareness.
G. A sensation of pain in the area of a nerve distribution is an example of neuralgia.
H. Protopathic system includes the sensation of pain, temperature, and/or nonlocalized sense of touch.
I. Chordotomy is a surgical procedure that involves sectioning of the lateral spinothalamic tract to relieve medically intractable pain.
J. Patients' inability to perceive sensation from delineated body areas allows neurologists to identify the involved dermatomes with the spinal cord damage.

2. Match the following clinical concepts with associated statements:

A. referred pain (b)	a. pain sensation from an amputated limb
B. phantom pain (a)	b. source of pain being different than sensed
C. trigeminal pain (e)	c. evaluation of proprioception
D. carpal tunnel syndrome (d)	d. nerve entrapment syndrome
E. Romberg test (c)	e. neuralgia with trigger point

3. Name the etiology that is often associated with bilateral loss of pain and temperature, usually in the upper extremities.
   - *syringomyelia*
4. Name the spinal syndrome that is characterized by ipsilateral sensory (proprioception) loss and paralysis as well as contralateral loss of pain and temperature.
   - *spinal hemisection (Brown-Séquard syndrome)*
5. Match each of the following sensation types with its associated spinal tract:

A. thermal sensitivity (a)	a. lateral spinothalamic tract
B. crude/diffuse touch (b)	b. anterior spinothalamic tract
C. pain sensation (a)	c. spinocerebellar tracts
D. unconscious proprioception (c)	d. dorsal column–medial
E. vibratory sense (d)	
F. position sense (d)	
G. two-point discrimination (d)	

6. A person who tends to fall with eyes closed is lacking what kind of information?
   - *proprioception*

Chapter 12 Visual System

1. Complete the following statements using the appropriate technical terms:

A. An irregular curvature of the lens and/or the cornea causes a focusing disorder, in which vertical and horizontal rays focus at two different retinal points; this leads to astigmatism.
B. In binocular vision, the visual field area is simultaneously processed in both eyes.
C. The retinal point at which light rays converge for focusing is called the focal point. The focal length is the distance between the lens and this retinal focal point.
D. The parasympathetically mediated response that the lens undergoes to keep a near object in focus is the accommodation reflex.
E. The optic disk is the area through which the optic nerve (CN II) exits and arteries enter the eyeball; with no presence of photoreceptors at this point, it is also called the blind spot.
F. Change in diameter of the pupils in response to a projected light is called the light reflex, which is mediated by the visceral fibers of the oculomotor nerve (CN II).
G. The eye ball contains two types of fluids: aqueous humor, a substance similar to CSF that is produced and drained in the posterior chamber of the anterior ocular cavity, and vitreous humor in the posterior cavity that prevents the eyeball from collapsing.
H. On exposure to light, the parasympathetic constriction of the circular fibers narrows the aperture of the pupil, a condition called miosis; on the other hand in darkness, the sympathetic constriction of the radial (dilator) fibers of the iris results in pupil dilation, a condition called mydriasis.
I. Myopia is an optical condition in which the divergent light rays from a near (less than 20 ft away) object focus on the retina.
J. Hyperopia is an optical condition in which only the convergent rays from a far object focus on the retina.
K. Visual field is the entire external area that is perceived in one eye.
L. Containing only the cones, the fovea is the retinal site responsible for sharp vision and color vision.
M. Visual acuity represents one's ability to resolve the perceptual detains, and it is measured using a Snellen chart.
N. As an eye disease and a common cause of blindness, glaucoma is marked by increased intraocular pressure and subsequent atrophy of the optic nerve.

2. Match the following conditions with corresponding description:

A. Myopia (g)	a. sympathetic constriction of radial fibers in dark
B. Hypermetropia (f)	b. parasympathetic constriction of circular fibers in response to light
C. Astigmatism (d)	c. autonomic regulation of lens refractive power
D. Emmetropia (e)	d. different refractivity at different retinal points due to unequal refractive surfaces
E. Lens accommodation (c)	e. adequately refracted image on the retina
F. Pupil constriction (b)	f. focusing of near object behind the retina
G. Pupil dilation (a)	g. focusing of converging rays from a far object in front of the retina

3. Name each quarter and the side of the visual fields for each eye:

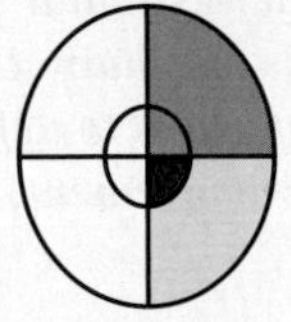
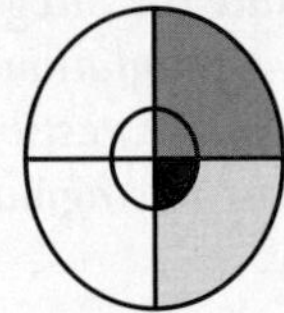

- *Left Eye:*
  - ***left upper nasal visual field quadrant***
  - ***left lower nasal visual field quadrant***
  - ***left upper temporal visual field quadrant***
  - ***left lower temporal visual field quadrant***
- *Right Eye:*
  - ***right upper nasal visual field quadrant***
  - ***right lower nasal visual field quadrant***
  - ***right upper temporal visual field quadrant***
  - ***right lower temporal visual field quadrant***

4. Name each of the visual field defects illustrated in the figure:

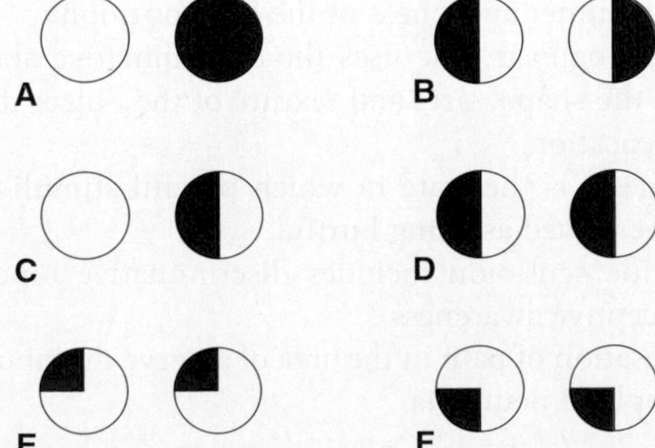

A. right monocular blindness
B. bitemporal hemianopsia
C. right nasal hemianopsia
D. left homonymous hemianopsia
E. left homonymous superior quadrantanopsia
F. left homonymous inferior quadrantanopsia

5. Match each of the following structures to its associated statement:

A. sclera (b)	a. drains aqueous humor into the venous system
B. canal of Schlemm (a)	b. outer tissue layer covering the eyeball
C. rods (j)	c. transparent covering of the anterior eye chamber
D. cornea (c)	d. containing melanocytes to make the eyeball opaque to stray light
E. choroid (d)	e. regulation of the pupil size to control the light amount entering the eye
F. iris (e)	f. smooth muscle fibers that reduce tension on the lens
G. lens (g)	g. transparent structure that refracts light rays on retina
H. ciliary body (f)	h. corresponds to the central retinal field
I. macula lutea (h)	i. photoreceptors for visual acuity and color vision
J. cones (i)	j. photoreceptors mediating night vision

6. What type of visual deficit results after a lesion affecting the Meyer's loop?
   - *homonymous upper quadrantanopsia*
7. What visual deficit results from a lesion in the dorsal/superior geniculocalcarine fibers?
   - *homonymous lower quadrantanopsia*
8. List the light conditions in which rods and cones are, respectively, operational.
   - *dark and twilight*
   - *daylight*

Chapter 13 Motor System 1: Spinal Cord

1. Complete the following statements using the appropriate technical terms:

A. The atrophy is the wasting away of muscle tissue secondary to damage to the lower motor neurons and/or subsequent loss of nerve supply (denervation).
B. The crossed extension reflex involves the withdrawal of a limb in response to painful stimuli with the simultaneous extension of the limb on the opposite side.
C. Located in specialized intrafusal fibers of skeletal muscle, the muscle spindles are sensitive to changes in muscle length.
D. The myoneural junction is the area of synaptic connection between an axon terminal and single skeletal muscle fiber, and it is also the site in which the acetylcholine is released.
E. Using selective inhibitory and excitatory circuits, reciprocal inhibition ensures that when one muscle is contracting, its paired (agonist) muscle is relaxed.
F. A stretch reflex refers to skeletal muscle contraction resulting from passive or active stretching of the same muscle.
G. Withdrawal of a limb by the flexions of multiple joints in response to a painful stimulus is a withdrawal reflex.
H. The skeletal muscles are under voluntary control.
I. As part of the LMN syndrome, hyporeflexia is marked by reduced or absent reflexes in a hypotonic muscle.
J. The degeneration of lateral and posterior spinal columns secondary to vitamin B_{12} deficiency (pernicious anemia) is known as subacute combined degeneration of spinal cord.
K. As part of the UMN syndrome, hyperreflexia is characterized by brisk reflexes in addition to increased muscle tone.

2. Name the parts of a motor unit.
   - *motor neuron*
   - *efferent fiber (axon)*
   - *myoneural junction*
   - *innervated muscle*
3. List five clinical characteristics of LMN syndrome.
   - *flaccid tone*
   - *paralysis*
   - *twitchings*
   - *atrophy*
   - *reduced reflexes*
4. List the location of the spinal motor neuron innervating the following muscles of respiration.

A. diaphragm (C3-C5, predominantly C4)
B. internal and external intercostals (T1-T12)
C. abdominal muscles (T6–T12)

5. Match each of the following clinical concepts with its associated information:

A. complete spinal transection (f)	a. degenerating alpha motor neurons
B. spinal hemisection (e)	b. denervated unused muscle fibers
C. syringomyelia (d)	c. bilateral spinal (dorsal column and corticospinal tract) degeneration due to pernicious anemia
D. subacute combined degeneration (c)	d. interrupted crossing of the pain and temperature fibers in the anterior commissure
E. muscle atrophy (b)	e. loss of sensorimotor functions ipsilaterally and pain and temperature contralaterally
F. fasciculation (a)	f. total bilateral loss of sensorimotor functions below the lesion site

Chapter 14 Motor System 2: Cerebellum

1. Complete the following statements using the appropriate technical terms:

A. Asthenia is the muscle weakness caused by cerebellar dysfunctioning.
B. Ataxia is the impaired ability to coordinate muscular activity during voluntary movement subsequent to a cerebellar pathology.
C. Dysarthria is a disorder of motor speech that results from central or peripheral disturbances and affects motor control of the articulators.
D. Asynergia is the decomposed motor activity marked with the loss of speed and skill in a movement.
E. As an error in the judgment of a movement's range and distance to the target, dysmetria is another cerebellar motor disorder.
F. The intention tremor is the jerky motor action present during the performance of a movement subsequent to a cerebellar pathology.
G. Hypotonia represents a reduced tone and lessened resistance to passive movement.
H. As a disorder of impaired motor tone adjustment and the loss of rapid and precise corrective response, rebounding refers to an inability to predict, stop, or dampen a movement.

2. Match each of the following statements with its associated neurological condition:

A. incoordination of muscular activity (a)	a. ataxia
B. Impaired control of distance and speed (b)	b. dysmetria
C. Impaired ability for controlling alternating movements (d)	c. asthenia
D. muscle weakness (c)	d. dysdiadochokinesia
E. Inability to dampen accessory movements during voluntary movement (f)	e. rebounding
F. Impaired ability to predict and stop movements (e)	f. intention tremor

3. A lateralized cerebellar lesion is likely to cause motor dysfunctions marked by intention tremor, ataxia, asynergia, and dysdiodochokinesia; these dysfunctions would affect which half (ipsi- or contra-) of the body?
   - *body ipsilateral to the lesion site*
4. Name the most recently developed cerebellar lobe and describe its function.
   - *neocerebellum*
   - *skilled movements*
5. What part of the cerebellum is likely to cause truncal ataxia, unsteadiness, and postural abnormality?
   - *midline cerebellar lesion including the flocculonodular lobe*
6. List four clinical signs of cerebellar pathology.
   - *ataxia*
   - *asynergia*
   - *intention tremor*
   - *rebounding dysdiadochokinesia*
7. Name the common cerebellar degenerative disease.
   - *Friedreich ataxia*
8. Why is it that a person with cerebellar lesion demonstrates unsteadiness and arm drifting even with the eyes open?
   - *The vision cannot compensate for a cerebellar abnormality.*

Chapter 15 Motor System 3: Basal Ganglia

1. Complete the following statements using the appropriate technical terms:

A. Akinesia refers to a loss of motor power of voluntary movements secondary to basal ganglia pathology.
B. Athetosis is the slow writhing (undergoing constant flexion and extension) movements of the limb.
C. Hemiballism refers to the acquired wild flinging movements involving one side of the body secondary to a lesion in the subthalamic nucleus.
D. Located within the white matter of the brain, the basal ganglia include a group of nuclei that refine the cortically generated motor movements.
E. As a clinical symptom of Parkinson disease, bradykinesia marks the slowness in the initiation of voluntary motor movements.
F. The chorea refers to irregular, spasmodic, involuntary movements of the limbs or facial muscles, which are commonly seen in patients with Huntington disease.
G. Emerging subsequent to lesions in the brainstem reticular formation above the vestibular nucleus, the decerebrate rigidity is marked by the sustained stiffness in the extensor limb muscles.
H. Developing as a complication of neuroleptic medications, the tardive dyskinesia is marked by involuntary and deforming movements involving the facial muscles.
I. Tremor, a repetitive movement secondary to alternate contraction of opposing muscles, is associated with pathologies of the basal ganglia circuitry.
J. The cogwheel rigidity is marked by stiffness and tremor so that the muscle responds with intermittent spasms (ratchety feeling) to a constant limb bending.
K. Dyskinesia stands for the inability to perform a voluntary movement because of the presence of abnormal and involuntary movements in basal ganglia diseases.

2. List four major basal ganglia nuclei.
   - *caudate nucleus*
   - *globus pallidus*
   - *putamen*
   - *subthalamic nucleus*
3. Name the midbrain structure with the dopaminergic projections to the striatum.
   - *substantia nigra*
4. Match each of the following diseases with associated description:

A. Huntington chorea (b)	a. tremor in young age after streptococcal infection and rheumatic fever
B. Parkinson disease (e)	b. disease of gene mutation marked with chorea and dementia
C. Wilson disease (d)	c. degenerative disease initially marked with balance disorders, loss of ocular movement, dysarthria, and dysphagia
D. progressive supranuclear palsy (c)	d. progressive motor disease with dysarthria and dementia secondary to impaired copper metabolism
E. Sydenham chorea (a)	e. motor disorder marked with tremor and rigidity subsequent to dopaminergic cell loss

5. Match each of the following definitions with its associated statement:

A. sudden and forceful movements (c)	a. athetosis
B. pill-rolling movements of fingers during rest (e)	b. chorea
C. rhythmic, quick, involuntary movements of proximal muscles (b)	c. ballism
D. difficulty in performing voluntary movements (d)	d. dyskinesia
E. slow twisting movements in the muscles of the upper extremities (a)	e. tremor

6. Loss of which neurotransmitter is associated with Parkinson disease?
   - *dopamine*
7. What structure and neurotransmitter are implicated with Huntington chorea?
   - *caudate nucleus*
   - *GABA*
8. What basal ganglia structure is associated with hemiballism?
   - *subthalamic nucleus*
9. What structure first receives net summative basal ganglia output from the globus pallidus?
   - *ventral lateral thalamus*
10. The presence of the Kayser–Fleischer ring at the edge of the cornea is suggestive of what disease?
    - *Wilson disease*
11. Name four signs of basal ganglia dysfunction.
    - *tremor*
    - *athetosis*
    - *chorea*
    - *hemiballism*
12. What mental disorder has been associated with increased dopaminergic projections to the forebrain?
    - *schizophrenia*

Chapter 16 Motor System 4: Motor Cortex

1. Complete the following statements using the appropriate technical terms:

A. Dorsal flexion of the great toe and fanning of other toes on the stroking of the sole are indicative of pyramidal tract pathology, and is called the Babinski reflex.
B. Homunculus is the representation of the body in the sensorimotor cortex.
C. The decussation of the descending and ascending fiber tracts accounts for the contralateral sensorimotor organization in the brain.
D. The upper motor neurons include the motor cells in the primary motor cortex and their descending axonal fibers.
E. The motor neural fibers that travel in the pyramidal tract arise from three cortical regions: primary motor cortex, premotor cortex, and sensory cortex.
F. Interruption of the descending corticospinal tract results in contralateral spastic hemiplegia.
G. Bilateral involvement of the corticobulbar fibers results in pseudobulbar palsy, which has a profound impact on motor speech and facial expression.
H. The primary motor cortex is located in the precentral gyrus, the Brodmann area 4.
I. Efferents from the motor cortex travel descend in two tracts: corticospinal and corticonuclear.

2. List two clinical signs of alternating hemiplegia.
   - *cranial nerve impairments ipsilateral to the site of lesion*
   - *motor control loss on the side opposite to the lesion*
3. What motor function that is important to SLPs is profoundly affected in pseudobulbar palsy?
   - *motor speech*
4. Match each of the following conditions with its associated lesion site:

A. muscle atrophy and flaccidity (a)	a. LMN
B. loss of stretch reflex (a)	b. UMN
C. spasticity and hypertonia (b)	c. cerebellum
D. fasciculation (a)	d. basal ganglia
E. positive Babinski sign (b)	
F. ataxia and asynergia (c)	
G. tremor and chorea (d)	
H. spastic hemiplegia (b)	

5. Name four clinical signs of UMN syndrome.
   - *spastic muscle tone*
   - *increased reflexes*
   - *Babinski sign*
   - *hemiplegia*
6. Why does a lesion at the internal capsule cause greater motor deficits than in the primary motor cortex?
   - *The internal capsule contains concentrated motor fibers as they descend from the entire motor and premotor cortices.*
   - *The motor cortex lesions result in deficits restricted to selected body regions.*
7. Is the presence of the Babinski sign in children considered abnormal?
   - *No, because the corticospinal tract is not yet fully developed and myelinated.*
8. Name the descending motor pathway that innervates cranial nerve nuclei.
   - *corticonuclear fibers*
9. From what layer of the cerebral cortex do the descending motor fibers originate?
   - *the fifth layer of the cerebral cortex*
10. Name the muscle spasticity in which initially there is resistance to any muscle stretch, which suddenly discontinues.
    - *clasp-knife spasticity*
11. Name the lesion site that is associated with clasp-knife reflex.
    - *descending corticospinal pathway lesion*

Chapter 17 Cranial Nerves Synopsis

1. Complete the following statements using the appropriate technical terms:

A. A lesion that interrupts olfactory fibers causes anosmia, in which the ability to smell is partly or fully impaired.
B. Diplopia is an optical condition in which an object is seen as being two.
C. In ophthalmoplegia, the internal and/or external ocular muscles are paralyzed.
D. Bilateral involvement of the corticonuclear fibers results in pseudobulbar palsy.
E. Denervated muscles become hypotonic and paralyzed, which eventually atrophy.
F. Bell palsy refers to the paralysis of the face subsequent to a unilateral involvement of the facial nerve or nucleus.
G. In light reflex, the pupils react to light by constricting, whereas in accommodation reflex the lens undergoes refractive changes in order to keep a moving object in focus.
H. In neuralgia, one experiences pain sensation along the course of the nerve.
I. The pseudobulbar palsy causes severe motor speech disorder because it has an impact on both the unilaterally and/or bilaterally innervated speech muscles.
J. Often confused with coma, the patients with locked-in syndrome are quadriplegic and can only communicate using the preserved vertical eye movement.
K. Often caused by the virus induced dysfunctioning of the 7th cranial nerve, Bell palsy results in paralysis involving one-half of the face.
L. Strabismus results in selected double vision subsequent to errors in improperly focused visual axes in misaligned eyes.

2. Match each of the following classification types with its associated function:

A. GSA (a)	a. pain and temperature
B. GSE (c)	b. vision and audition
C. SSA (b)	c. eye movements
D. SVA (e)	d. speech, phonation, and swallowing
E. SVE/BE (d)	e. taste and smell
F. GVA (f)	f. organ content
G. GVE (g)	g. autonomic activities

3. Match each of the following branchial arches with its associated motor cranial nerve:

A. first (d)	a. glossopharyngeal nerve
B. second (c)	b. vagus nerve
C. third (a)	c. facial nerve
D. fourth and sixth (b)	d. trigeminal nerve

4. A 45-year-old woman experiences decreased hearing in the right ear, the entire right side of her face is paralyzed, and she has no reflex to touch in the cornea of the right eye. What cranial nerves are suspected to be damaged?
   - *decreased hearing—acoustic portion of the vestibulocochlear nerve (CN VIII)*
   - *right-sided facial paralysis—facial nerve (CN VII)*
   - *loss of corneal reflex— trigeminal nerve (CN V)*

5. Clinical symptoms displayed by a stroke patient included left ptosis, pupil unresponsiveness to light with dilated left pupil, and laterally deviated left eye. Name the cranial nerve that is involved in this case.
   - *ptosis—oculomotor nerve (CN III)*
   - *loss of light reflex, dilated pupil—optic (CN II) and/or oculomotor nerve (CN III)*
   - *lateral fixation of the eye—oculomotor nerve (CN III)*
6. Which cranial nerve is involved in Tic douloureux?
   - *trigeminal nerve (CN V)*
7. What cranial nerve is involved with Bell palsy?
   - *facial nerve (CN VII)*
8. Why is pseudobulbar palsy so detrimental to speech and other facial functions?
   - *It affects speech muscles on both sides of the face.*
9. What cranial nerves provide the afferent and efferent paths for the pupillary light reflex?
   - *afferent arch—optic nerve (CN II)*
   - *efferent arch—oculomotor nerve (CN III)*
10. A lesion at what neuraxial region might produce right facial symptoms and left hemiplegia?
    - *right pontine lesion*
11. What communication mode can be used with a patient who has locked-in syndrome?
    - *scanning and ocular movement tracker*
12. Involvement of what primary cranial nerve is associated with abnormal phonation, resonance, and dysphagia?
    - *vagus nerve (CN X)*
13. In case of left hypoglossal nerve dysfunction, the weakened half of the tongue will deviate to which side on protrusion?
    - *left side*
14. A left lower motor neuron lesion involving the vagus and trigeminal nerves lowers the ipsilateral palate. Will this result in the deviation of the uvula toward the right (normal) or the left (paralyzed) side of the palate?
    - *right (normal) side*
15. How many cranial nerves are involved with ocular movements?
    - *three nerves (trochlear (CN IV), oculomotor (CN III), and abducens (CN VI)*

Chapter 18 Axial–Limbic Brain: Autonomic Nervous System, Limbic System, Hypothalamus, and Reticular Formation

1. Complete the following statements using the appropriate technical terms:

A. The activation and regulation of cortical arousal are perhaps the best known functions of the reticular formation.

B. As a subdivision of the nervous system, the autonomic nervous system regulates the activities of the heart, blood vessels, and lungs.

C. Resulting from a hypothalamic lesion, adipsia is marked by the absence of thirst.

D. Amnesia represents a long-term memory disturbance which is marked by impaired recall of past memories and failure to remember new details.

E. Dysphagia is an impaired ability to swallow.

F. In asphyxia, a reduced exchange of oxygen and carbon dioxide causes the brain cells to die secondary to anoxia.

G. As part of the three-layered cortex, the hippocampus is related to the registration and consolidation of memory.

H. Functionally related to the limbic system, the hypothalamus regulates visceral, somatic, and metabolic systems.

I. Associated with the bitemporal pathology, the Klüver–Bucy syndrome is marked by psychic blindness, increased oral tendency, and abnormal sexual behavior.

J. Representing a natural rhythm, the circadian rhythm occurs once each 24 hours.

K. As part of the limbic lobe, the cingulate gyrus has been linked with anxiety and obsessive behaviors.

L. Consisting of multiple polysynaptic descending and ascending connections, the reticular formation not only controls autonomic functions (e.g., respiration, blood pressure, and thermoregulation), but also regulates behavioral states such as alertness, cortical arousal, and sleep.

M. The antidiuretic hormone named vasopressin causes water retention in the body.

N. A complex neuronal circuitry in the mammalian forebrain involving the hippocampus, fornix, mammillary body, anterior thalamic nuclei, cingulate gyrus, and parahippocampal, the Papez circuit is dedicated to experiences of and responses to emotion.

2. Match each of the following structures with its associated function:

A. sympathetic system (b) — a. control of the heart, lungs, blood vessels, and the organs of the digestive, reproductive, and urogenital systems

B. parasympathetic systems (c) — b. energy expenditure during fight and flight experience

C. hypothalamus (d) — c. energy restoration

D. limbic lobe (e) — d. regulation of autonomic and endocrinic function

E. reticular formation (f) — e. control of motivation, moods, and emotional drive

F. autonomic nervous system (a) — f. maintenance of cortical arousal and brainstem-mediated visceral activities

3. Name the core structures of the limbic lobe.
   - ***amygdala***
   - ***hippocampus***
   - ***cingulate gyrus***
   - ***septum***

4. Name three primary functions of the limbic lobe.
   - ***emotional experiences***
   - ***motivational drives***
   - ***instinctual reflexes (feeding, mating, aggression, and flight)***

5. Which part of the axial–limbic brain has dedicated circuitries for the water intake, food intake, body temperature, and endocrinic secretion?
   - ***hypothalamus***

6. Match each of the hormones with its associated dysfunction:

A. growth hormone (a) — a. dwarfism/gigantism

B. thyroid-stimulating hormone (d) — b. reduced milk secretion

C. gonadotropic hormone (c) — c. impaired sexual function

D. adrenocorticotropic hormone (e) — d. low body development, low metabolism, and slow mental activity

E. prolactin (b) — e. impaired glucose synthesis

7. Which structure of the axial–limbic brain regulates cortical arousal, cardiovascular activity, respiration, swallowing, vomiting, and coughing?
   - ***reticular formation***

8. Why is it that a lesion in the brainstem is so damaging?
   - ***because of its regulation of cardiovascular and respiratory activities***

9. Match each of the activities by matching it with the associated autonomic system:

A. decreased lacrimal secretion (b) — a. sympathetic system

B. decreased intestinal secretion (a) — b. parasympathetic system

C. decreased gastric secretion (a)

D. reduced digestive tract activity (a)

E. increased lacrimal secretion (b)

F. increased intestinal secretion (b)

G. increased sweat secretion (a)

H. pupil constriction (b)

10. Match the following pathways with the structures it connects:

A. fornix (b) — a. hypothalamus and the midbrain (tegmental) region

B. mammillothalamic tract (c) — b. hypothalamus (mammillary bodies) with the hippocampus

C. stria medullaris (d) — c. hypothalamus (mammillary body) to the thalamus

D. stria terminalis (e) — d. septum with habenula thalamic nucleus

E. medial forebrain bundle (a) — e. hypothalamus and amygdala

11. At what area of the neuraxis are the autonomic respiratory centers located?
    - ***brainstem***

12. Which reticular nucleus with role in respiration receives projections from the chemoreceptors of the carotid body?
    - ***nucleus solitarius***
    - ***Its compression in case of increased intracranial pressure or herniation can cause death.***

Chapter 19 Cerebral Cortex: Higher Mental Functions

1. Complete the following statements using the appropriate technical terms:

A. As a common accompaniment of aphasia, acalculia is an acquired inability to perform simple mathematical problems.

B. A common accompaniment of aphasia, agraphia is an acquired inability to express through writing.
C. Impaired ability to read and comprehend written information secondary to brain damage is called alexia.
D. As a common accompaniment of aphasia, apraxia is the impaired ability to perform skilled movements on command.
E. Dementia is a progressive and persistent loss of cognitive functions, which are mostly caused by degenerative brain diseases.
F. A disorder of motor speech that results from central and/or peripheral lesions and affects muscular control of the articulators is dysarthria.
G. Neologisms are the new words or phrases of the patient's own making often seen in acute aphasia mostly by patients with Wernicke aphasia.
H. An inappropriate selection of related or unrelated words by subjects with aphasia is an example of paraphasia.
I. Agnosia is a disorder of recognition, which can involve one or multiple modalities (visual, auditory, or tactile).
J. Prosopagnosia is the failure to recognize familiar faces.
K. Anosognosia is a nondominant parietal symptoms in which the patients tend to deny the presence of paralysis.
L. The cerebral dominance may have a structural basis, which relates to the size of the planum temporale.
M. The Wada test involves carotid infusion of sodium amytal, and it is used to assess the cerebral dominance.
N. Related to traumatic brain injuries, contusion refers to a bruising of the brain marked by torn brain tissues; on the other hand, there is no visible bruising of the brain in concussion.

2. Match each of the following brain regions with its associated function:

A. superior parietal lobule (f)	a. visual agnosia
B. nondominant inferior parietal lobe (e)	b. musical function and nonverbal memory
C. dominant inferior parietal lobe (d)	c. language comprehension and verbal memory
D. nondominant temporal lobe (b)	d. reading and writing
E. dominant temporal lobe (c)	e. body schema and spatial attention
F. bilateral occipital lobe lesions (a)	f. visual–spatial and constructional skills

3. Match each of the following aphasia types with its associated clinical characteristics:

A. Broca aphasia (a)	a. impaired verbal expression
B. Wernicke aphasia (b)	b. impaired auditory comprehension
C. anomia (d)	c. impaired repetition
D. conduction aphasia (c)	d. difficulty finding and retrieving lexicon

4. Match each of the following disorders with its associated dysfunction:

A. deep dyslexia (c)	a. acquired illiteracy with impaired ability to read and write
B. surface alexia (e)	b. pure alexia with word blindness with preserved ability to write
C. phonological alexia (d)	c. semantic and visual errors in reading words
D. alexia with agraphia (a)	d. reading by the recognition of words' meanings and by conversion of words to phonemes
E. alexia without agraphia (b)	e. reading by grapheme-to-phoneme conversion, without directly recognizing words

5. Match each of the following apraxia types with its associated description:

A. ideomotor apraxia (a)	a. failure to carry out a motor act in response to a verbal command
B. limb kinetic apraxia (c)	b. failure to use a real object
C. ideational apraxia (b)	c. impaired skilled motor acts involving only one limb

6. Define three major categories of dementia causing conditions/diseases.
   - ***systemic diseases***
   - ***neurological diseases***
   - ***degenerative diseases***

7. Match each of the following neurological conditions with the associated disease categories:

A. Alzheimer disease (c)	a. systemic diseases associated with dementia
B. Pick disease (c)	b. neurological diseases associated with dementia
C. Creutzfeldt–Jakob disease (c)	c. degenerative brain diseases causing dementia
D. infections (a)	
E. neoplasm (a)	
F. normal pressure hydrocephalus (b)	
G. Huntington chorea (b)	
H. Parkinson disease (b)	

8. Match each of the following dementing diseases with its associated pathophysiology:

A. Alzheimer disease (c)	a. caused by an infectious agent, this rapidly progressive disease is marked by mood changes, dementia, seizures, and myoclonus
B. Pick disease (b)	b. a disease of frontal and temporal degeneration and includes Pick bodies
C. Creutzfeldt–Jakob disease (a)	c. a disease marked by senile plaques and neurofibrillary tangles in the cerebral cortex, hippocampus, and nucleus basalis of Meynert

Chapter 20 Diagnostic Techniques and Neurologic Concepts

1. Complete the following statements using the appropriate technical terms:

A. Cerebral angiography is an excellent tool for evaluating the cerebral vasculature (vasculitis, aneurysm, and arteriovenous malformation).
B. The cordotomy procedure is used for relieving intractable pain by sectioning the lateral spinothalamic tract.
C. As a treatment for Parkinson disease, deep brain stimulation involves a subcortical chronic electrode implant and the use of a stimulation programmer.
D. Dichotic listening involves the simultaneous presentation of largely identical words to both ears; the number of words recalled from each ear is used to measure cerebral dominance.
E. In dominant inheritance, the faulty gene dominates the gene from the other parent with which it is paired and has a 50% probability of a trait inheritance.
F. As a graphic representation of the brain's summated electrical activity, electroencephalography reflects potential differences between two separated points on the scalp surface.
G. Electromyography provides a visual record of muscular activity during spontaneous and/or voluntary movements.
H. A lumbar puncture is undertaken to remove the CSF for a chemical analysis.
I. As a peripheral nerve disease subsequent to trauma, toxicity, infection, or neoplasm, neuropathy slows the nerve impulses by interrupting their transmission.
J. In recessive inheritance, both parents carry and transmit the faulty gene, and the child has a 25% probability of inheriting the disease.
K. Patients in stupor can be brought to consciousness only through a painful stimulus.
L. Encephalopathy refers to the brain dysfunctions that result from impaired cellular metabolism and vascular toxicity.
M. Epilepsy represents two or more incidences of (recurring) unprovoked seizures.
N. Event-evoked potential represents the normal CNS signals in response to specific and controlled sensory stimulations.
O. X-linked inheritance involves a faulty gene that is located on the mother's sex chromosome.

2. List the four major types of brain waves and their frequencies.
   - ***delta-rhythm (1–3)***
   - ***theta-rhythm (4–7)***
   - ***alpha-rhythm (8–13)***
   - ***beta-rhythm (greater than 13)***
3. Name the preferred imaging technique for identifying subarachnoid hemorrhage, trauma, and hydrocephalus.
   - ***CT scan***
4. Name the imaging technique that measures responses of living tissues to an applied magnetic field and to radiofrequency waves.
   - ***magnetic resonance imaging***
5. List the major imaging technique that does not expose the patient to potentially harmful ionizing radiation.
   - **magnetic *resonance***
6. Name the technique that measures electrical signals occurring in the CNS in response to specific and controlled sensory (visual, tactile, somatosensory, or auditory) stimulation.
   - **event-evoked *potential***
7. Name the MRI technique that is extremely sensitive to even minute molecular motion and detects an ischemic stroke within 10 to 15 minutes.
   - **diffusion-weighted MRI**
8. Name the MRI technique that can immediately identify an eloquent part of the brain during participation in any linguistic or sensorimotor task based on the degree of oxygen consumption.
   - **functional MRI**
9. Name the MRI technique that provides functional (normal and abnormal) information about the cerebral white matter by measuring the directionality of water molecular movement in myelinated axonal tracts.
   - **diffusion tensor imaging**
10. Name the MRI technique that measures brain chemistry.
    - **magnetic resonance spectrography**
11. Name the technique that uses intracarotid infusion of sodium amytal for measuring cerebral dominance.
    - **Wada test.**
12. Match the following MRI image types with its diagnostic efficacy:

A. T1 sequence (a)	a. anatomical detail including gray and white matter.
B. T2 sequence (b)	b. water content to help identify tumors, infarcts and infections

13. Match each of the following seizure types with associated function:

A. partial simple (a)	a. a sudden onset of sensorimotor behaviors confined to a single body part from a single cortical or subcortical lesion
B. partial complex (b)	b. also known as psychomotor, the recurring episodes of automatic, irrational, and aggressive behavior with no memory secondary to medial temporal lobe lesions
C. petit mal (c)	c. a brief loss of consciousness associated with staring, chewing, blinking, and occasional myoclonic jerks
D. grand mal (d)	d. loss of consciousness with repeated hyperextension of the body (tonic–clonic convulsions) and breath-holding spells

14. Match each of the following techniques with the activities it measures:

A. electroencephalography (c)	a. muscle activity and nerve conduction
B. electromyography (a)	b. electrical brain activity in response to specific stimuli
C. sodium amytal infusion (d)	c. brain's electrical potentials
D. evoked potentials (b)	d. cerebral dominance
E. dichotic listening (f)	e. CNS infections and intracerebral hemorrhages
F. lumbar puncture (e)	f. ear superiority

15. What is the difference between coma and stupor?
    - *A patient can be aroused from the stage of unresponsiveness in stupor using a painful stimulus, which is not the case with coma, the deepest level of altered consciousness.*
16. What is the difference between coma and sleep?
    - *Coma is a nonsleep form of consciousness loss and there is no neural activity. Sleep is associated with increased brain activity.*
17. Name the technique that is used to study brain–behavior relationship in case of surgical removal of epileptogenic brain tissue.
    - *brain mapping through cortical stimulation*
18. Describe the phasic profile of action potentials in patients with neuropathy (A) and myopathy (B):
    - *A. high amplitude, long duration, polyphasic action potentials*
    - *B. small amplitude, short duration, polyphasic action potentials*

Discussion of Case Studies

Chapter 1 Essential Neurological Concepts and Principles

Case Studies For Problem Solving

Case (1-1) Discussion: The tumor is indeed in the right hemisphere. In clinical orientation, which is opposite of anatomic orientation, the patient's right and left, respectively, are the examiner's left and right. This clinical orientation applies to images in CT, PET, and MRI studies.

Case (1-2) Discussion: It is a hypothalamic syndrome. The hypothalamus, located below the thalamus, serves autonomic, visceral, and endocrine functions, including sexual drive, appetite, sleep–wake cycle, and body heat regulation.

Case (1-3) Discussion: This patient is likely to exhibit impaired motor control (Brodmann area 4); altered somatic sensation (Brodmann areas 3, 1, and 2); cognitive disorders and personality changes (Brodmann areas 10 and 11); and aggression and agitation (Brodmann area 38) owing to involvement of the amygdala and surrounding region.

Case (1-4) Discussion: Language is laterally located in the neocortex. This involves Brodmann areas 44 and 45 (expressive language cortex), 22 (receptive language cortex), and 39 and 40 (angular and supramarginal gyrus for reading and writing). The SLP needed to view the full extent of the lesion either on the leftmost parasagittal MRI slices or on an axial view of the brain.

Case (1-5) Discussion: Two pieces of information are missing here: first, detailed information about cognitive impairment that might have also included communicative deficiencies and, second, no information is provided about the nature and cause of speech unintelligibility. An SLP involvement would have revealed more information about these two aspects of communication and their treatments. This patient's speech problem was related to the involvement of multiple cranial nerves.

Chapter 2 Gross Anatomy of the Central Nervous System

Case studies for problem solving

Case (2-1) Discussion: The involvement of the frontoparietotemporal tissue accounts for all of the reported symptoms:

- Time-related confusion is characteristic of parietal involvement.
- Expressive aphasia reflects the involvement of the anterior language area, and the altered personality results from the involvement of the prefrontal projections.
- Right-sided paralysis and a positive Babinski sign indicate involvement of the motor and surrounding cortex.
- Progressive nature of the deficit rules out a cerebrovascular accident.

Case (2-2) Discussion: The tumor in the cauda equina region affected sacral motor control. The spinal nerves from the sacral region (S3–S5) innervate the bladder and anal sphincters (Fig. 2-34). Interruption of these sacral nerves affected bowel and bladder functions; incontinence issues are common after the involovement of the sacral roots.

Spinal cord injuries can also cause symptoms of urgency, but the bladder emptying is mostly incomplete. This is further compounded by immobility.

A temporal–parietal tumor affecting the language and cognitive cortex accounted for his cognitive and linguistic deficits.

Case (2-3) Discussion: This bilaterally located tumor had affected the inferior frontal cortex.

- The inferior frontal cortex (Brodmann areas 10 to 12) deals with personality and regulates executive–cognitive functions, such as reasoning, abstract thinking, self-monitoring, decision making, planning, and pragmatic behaviors.
- The reported behavioral deficits (altered personality, profanity, inactivity, and inappropriate behavior) implicate the orbitofrontal region.
- The tumor had also compressed the olfactory bulb and its tract, which accounts for the loss of the sensation of smell.

Case (2-4) Discussion: Massa intermedia, also called interthalamic adhesion, is present in only 70% to 80% of the human brains; it, however, is not related to any known neurologic (linguistic or cognitive) deficit.

Case (2-5) Discussion: The observed symptoms indicate that three cranial nerves were affected:

- Facial cranial nucleus/nerve: related to the paralysis of the right face and contributed to dysarthria
- Hypoglossal nerve: involved with the paralysis of the tongue and contributed to dysarthria
- Vagus nerve: contributed to the vocal cord paralysis and to the aphonia, diplophonia, and breathiness
- All three nerves: contributed to the articulatory precision causing speech to be unintelligible

Case (2-6) Discussion: The lateral ventricles are connected to the third ventricles through the interventricular foramina of Monro. The CSF from the third ventricle drains into the fourth ventricle through the cerebral aqueduct. A block involving the cerebral aqueduct in the midbrain region had resulted in an obstructive type of hydrocephalus.

Case (2-7) Discussion: This neurolinguistic symptomatology (fluently spoken, asemantic verbal output with anomia and impaired comprehension) indicates Wernicke aphasia. This type of aphasia is associated with damage to the posterosuperior temporal region and the inferior parietal lobule in the dominant hemisphere, which, in this case, includes the left supramarginal and angular gyri.

Chapter 5 Nerve Cell Physiology

Case studies for problem solving

Case (5-1) Discussion: In myasthenia gravis, the problem lies at the myoneural junction; the motor end plate is damaged by antibodies, which work against acetylcholine receptors; this leads to restrict muscle contraction and causes muscles to easily fatigue. Because normal-appearing muscles fatigue with persistent motor tasks, the stress testing is used to confirm this condition. The muscle fatigue has a generalized effect on all motor speech processes. See any textbook on motor speech disorders for the effect of this condition on speech. An administration of anticholinesterase drugs causes an increase in muscle strength by slowing the enzymatic destruction of acetylcholine at the myoneural junction.

Case (5-2) Discussion: This is a case of demyelinating disease. A history of neurologic symptoms with reoccurrence of symptoms marks the clinical pattern of exacerbations and remissions. Multiple but random and separated hyperintense patches (plaques) of demyelination suggest this to be a case of multiple sclerosis. While the moderate speech and swallowing problems emerge in the advanced stages of the disease, they can have subtle effects on complex coarticulator patterns even in the early stages.

Case (5-3) Discussion: This is a case of myasthenia gravis. In myasthenia gravis, elevated serum antibodies destroy the postsynaptic acetylcholine receptors of the myoneural junction. Thus, the acetylcholine released in the synaptic cleft is not quantitatively adequate to activate the muscle.

The muscle weakness is characterized by progressive fatigue and speech unintelligibility. Drug testing involves neostigmine administration, which inhibits the enzyme that degrades acetylcholine in the synapse, thereby increasing the amount of acetylcholine for muscle function, which contributes to an improved physical performance.

Case (5-4) Discussion: Guillain–Barré syndrome is a neuropathy of inflammatory demyelination involving the peripheral nervous system. Usually triggered by an acute infection, it involves the progression of weakness from the legs to the upper limbs but with intact sensations of pain, touch, and temperature. The recovery phase spontaneously begins in 2 to 3 weeks after the onset.

Chapter 6 Diencephalon: Thalamus and Associated Structures

Case studies for problem solving

Case (6-1) Discussion: A cerebrovascular accident in this patient affected the posterior region of the left thalamus and part of the internal capsule carrying descending motor fibers; this results in the following:

- Weakness in the arm and speech muscles subsequent to the interruption of adjacent motor fibers in the internal capsule
- Severe pain sensation resulted from the overreaction of the primitive pain mechanism of the thalamus secondary to the lesion
- Emotional instability, usually seen after a thalamic lesion
- Anomia subsequent to the involvement of the thalamocortical (parietal lobe) projections, which is a common constituent of the thalamic syndrome

Case (6-2) Discussion: This area is the site of part of the pulvinar and the geniculate bodies. The involvement of the geniculate bodies (LGB and MGB) appears to be implicated in this case. The involvement of the LGB resulted in the loss of the left visual fields for both eyes, also called left hemianopsia. The involvement of the adjacent MGB contributed to central auditory processing deficits, marked by a normal hearing threshold but impaired processing and reduced ability to identify the direction of sound.

Case (6-3) Discussion: The ventral posterior medial nucleus is involved with the facial sensation. It receives trigeminal afferents mediating pain, touch, and temperature from the face and projects to the lower third of the postcentral gyrus region, the primary sensory cortex. Impaired articulatory precision underlying distorted speech was related to disrupted proprioceptive afferents.

Case (6-4) Discussion: The primary motor cortex (Brodmann area 4) receives projections from the ventrolateral nucleus of the thalamus; this nucleus channels basal ganglia and cerebellar input to the motor cortex.

Chapter 7 Cerebrovascular System

Case studies for problem solving

Case (7-1) Discussion: A stroke involving the anterior branches of the left middle cerebral artery affected the motor cortex and Broca area (Brodmann areas 44 and 45), which resulted in right hemiplegia and expressive aphasia type with spared auditory comprehension.

Case (7-2) Discussion: A stroke in the posterior branches of the left MCA affected the temporal cortex, including the classical Wernicke area (Brodmann area 22), which impaired comprehension and meaningful expression in this patient. The temporal lesion also affected the geniculocalcarine visual radiation fibers. Intact sensorimotor function was related to the spared ascending branches of the MCA.

Case (7-3) Discussion: The stroke involving the left occipital lobe accounts for the focal symptom of right homonymous hemianopsia. The sudden emergence of the symptom implies a vascular cause (gradual appearance of the symptoms indicates a tumor or other progressive pathologies). The stroke affected the left PCA, which supplies blood to the visual cortex in the left occipital lobe (Figs. 7-3 and 7-4). The infarct was visualized only on a repeat CT because it takes nearly 36 hours for infarcts to show on CT.

Case (7-4) Discussion: Small lateral arterial branches of the basilar artery supply the pons and part of the medulla. The lateral medulla, which contains sensorimotor fibers, is supplied by the posterior inferior cerebellar artery, another branch of the vertebral artery.

A pontomedullary stroke involving the branches of the vestibular artery affected the trigeminal (CN V), facial (CN VII), and vestibulocochlear (CN VIII) nerves, as well as rootlets of the vagus (CN X) nerve. Effects on the facial (CN VII) and trigeminal (CN V) nerve fibers along with the rootlets of the vagus (CN X) nerve resulted in facial motor weakness, loss of sensation from the face, palatal paralysis, and swallowing difficulty. The involvement of vestibular and cochlear nuclei resulted in impaired equilibrium with a tendency to fall to the left and deafness in the left ear.

The interruption of the descending pyramidal (corticospinal) fibers above the point of decussation produced contralateral paralysis in the right arm and leg. The implicated cranial nerve fibers already had crossed, so there was left (ipsilateral) facial paralysis. This clinical picture is called alternating or crossed hemiplegia, which is a classical lateral medullary syndrome (see Chapter 16).

Case (7-5) Discussion: Vascular involvement of the lenticulostriate on the left affected the long sensory and motor projections fibers, which resulted in right-sided paralysis and hemianesthesia. The involvement of the corticobulbar system also affected the cranial motor nuclei of facial (CN VII), hypoglossal (CN XII), and vagus (CN X) nerves, which had contributed to his dysarthria and swallowing disorder. He could control the upper face, because it is known to have projections from both motor cortices.

Case (7-6) Discussion: This neurolinguistic symptomatology (fluently articulated but asemantic verbal output with anomia, impaired comprehension for both spoken and written language, and euphoria) is indicative of Wernicke aphasia. This aphasia type is associated with damage to the posterior superior temporal region (Brodmann area 22) and the inferior parietal lobule (Brodmann areas 39 and 40) in the dominant hemisphere. This infarct resulted in Wernicke-type aphasia.

Chapter 8 Ventricles and Cerebrospinal Fluid

Case studies for problem solving

(Case 8-1) Discussion: This is a case of an obstructive (noncommunicating) type of hydrocephalus, because the CSF did not have access to the subarachnoid space. The block occurred in the midbrain where the ventricular cavity is very narrow. There was tumor at the lower end of the third ventricle. The reported generalized symptoms are typical of hydrocephalus and did not point to a localized lesion.

Case (8-2) Discussion: This is a typical case of normal pressure hydrocephalus, which is characterized by urinary incontinence, unsteady gait, impaired equilibrium, urinary incontinence, and impaired cognition. The prefrontal symptoms result from pressure to the prefrontal cortex. Meningitis, subarachnoid hemorrhage, and trauma are the common causes of this condition. Impaired gait pattern is marked by wide-based stance and walking.

Chapter 9 Auditory System

Case studies for problem solving

Case (9-1) Discussion: The cochlear and vestibular branches of the vestibulocochlear nerve (CN VIII) enter the brainstem at the junction of the medulla and pons. Occlusion in the posterior inferior cerebellar artery resulted in a pontomedullary infarct that, in this case, affected the second-order (vestibular and cochlear) nuclei of CN VIII, the descending tract of the trigeminal nerve (CN V), lateral spinothalamic tract, and motor nucleus of the vagus nerve (CN X). The involvement of the left cochlear nuclear complex affected the hearing threshold in the left ear. Damage to the left vestibular nucleus accounted for her falling to the left. The involvement of the trigeminal system resulted in analgesia and thermal anesthesia on the left side of the face. The interruption of the crossed fibers of the lateral spinothalamic tract resulted in the loss of pain and temperature sensations from the right side of the body (see Chapter 11). The involvement of the adjacent vagus nerve (CN X) nucleus and fibers resulted in swallowing difficulty.

Case (9-2) Discussion: A Schwann cell tumor (schwannoma) at the cerebellopontine angle compressed both branches of vestibulocochlear (CN VIII) nerve roots. This resulted in right ear hearing loss and a right-sided equilibrium problem. The tumor also compressed the facial cranial nerve (CN VII) root, causing facial paralysis secondary to facial nerve (CN VII) injury. Unsteadiness while walking resulted from the involvement of the vestibular nerve.

Case (9-3) Discussion: The labyrinthine (internal auditory), a branch of the AICA, supplies blood to the inner ear, which includes the cochlea, spiral ganglion cells, and the vestibular apparatus. The occlusion of the labyrinthine artery in this case affected the cochlear mechanism (hearing loss) and the vestibular apparatus (disequilibrium).

Case (9-4) Discussion: This is a case of a central auditory processing deficit, in which the patient has performed well on traditional diagnostic tests but continues to have difficulty in processing linguistic signals. Bilateral involvement of the MGB has restricted the patient's ability to screen auditory information and regulate the speed of information processing as well as a mild sensorineural loss. The attenuated integration of attention might have also been involved in abnormal linguistic processing. The involvement of the LGB affected visual processing. The cerebellar hyperintensity contributed to disequilibrium.

Chapter 10 Vestibular System

Case studies for problem solving

Case (10-1) Discussion: The infarct in the left dorsal lateral medullopontine region affected the following structures:

- Vestibular nuclear complex, which was confirmed by the absence of nystagmus on caloric testing of the left ear.
- Vestibular projections to the cervico-spinal cord, which regulates head posture. Interruption of these fibers caused the head to tilt to the left.
- Interruption of the vestibulospinal projections to the extensor muscles of the limbs on the ipsilateral side. Consequently, the patient was falling to the left.
- Vestibular nucleus, which caused the sensation of vertigo.
- Vestibulocochlear (CN VIII) nucleus and possibly nerve afferents; this impaired hearing in the left ear.
- Crossing auditory pathway; this could have also impaired hearing in the right ear.
- Spinal nucleus of the trigeminal tract within the infarct region, which contributed to the mediation of pain and temperature from the left side of the face.

Case (10-2) Discussion: This is a case of minor stroke involving a small brainstem artery. The presence of sudden hearing impairment, unsteadiness, dizziness, and gait ataxia implicates ischemia in the territory of the AICA. This artery, which supplies blood to the inferior cerebellum, also gives off the labyrinthine artery, which supplies the membranous labyrinth (organ of Corti and semicircular canals), spiral ganglion, and vestibular ganglion.

Case (10-3) Discussion: This is a case of Ménière disease, in which excessive fluid accumulation or possibly rupture involving the membranous labyrinth causes fluctuating deafness, vertigo attacks, unsteadiness, and tinnitus. The repeated and periodic attacks of hearing impairment and dizziness are also associated with vomiting and nausea.

Case (10-4) Discussion: Cranial nerve dysfunctions are the best lesion localizers, which indicate the involvement of the cochlear–vestibular and vagus nerve on the pons and medulla on the right.

Chapter 11 Somatosensory System

Case studies for problem solving

Case (11-1) Discussion: There are three sensorimotor signs of spinal hemisection (Brown–Séquard syndrome, Fig. 11-11): (1) spastic paralysis on the side ipsilateral to the lesion; (2) ipsilateral loss of proprioception, kinesthetic sense, and discriminative touch below the level of the lesion; and (3) contralateral loss of pain and temperature below the level of the lesion.

- The descending corticospinal fibers cross the midline in the caudal medulla; thus, the T12 lesion caused flaccid paralysis in the limbs ipsilateral to the lesion site. Gradually within 3 weeks, the limb became spastic with a positive Babinski sign. These symptoms of the corticospinal tract lesion indicate the damage is to the upper motor neuron (see Chapter 14).
- The dorsal column fibers ipsilaterally ascend in the spinal cord and cross the midline in the caudal medulla; thus, the T12 lesion resulted in the loss of proprioception and discriminative touch on the side of the body ipsilateral to the lesion.

The fibers mediating pain and temperature cross to the opposite side at every spinal level in the spinal central gray region before forming the lateral spinothalamic tract. Thus, the T12 lesion blocked the transmission of pain and temperature from the contralateral (left side) body below the lesion site.

Case (11-2) Discussion: Formation of the syringomyelic cavity in the spinal cord from C6 to T1 affected the following structures:

- Crossing of pain and temperature fibers from the arm and hand regions; consequently, the patient did not have sensation of noxious stimuli in the arms and hands; this confirmed that the cavity was the cause of burn marks on the hands.
- Nearby α-motor neurons in the gray matter of the anterior horns; thus, the weakness and muscle wasting observed in his hands.

Case (11-3) Discussion: These dissociated (left and right sided) symptoms suggest the involvement of the vagus (CN X), facial (CN VII), and spinal trigeminal tracts/nuclei and the fibers of the lateral spinothalamic tract fibers. Only a right pontomedullary location of the lesion could affect these nerves and produce right facial and pharyngeal involvement. This lesion also affected the crossed ascending fibers of the lateral spinothalamic tract, which transmitted pain and temperature information from the left half of the body.

Case (11-4) Discussion: This is a case of trigeminal neuralgia, which is characterized by episodes of intense (sudden and stabbing) pain. The pain was initiated by touching a trigger zone in the mouth, which in this case was around the alveolar region. This condition of evoked pain caused the patient to refrain from speaking and eating.

Case (11-5) Discussion: As per rules of lesion localization (see Box 1-3), the ascending (sensory) and descending (motor) fibers are present throughout the neuraxis and, therefore, are susceptible to interruption at multiple levels. The cranial nerves, however, can be affected by a lesion located exclusively in the brainstem. Thus, the loss of facial sensation and the absent corneal reflex (afferent pathway = trigeminal [CN V] nerve; efferent pathway = facial [CN VII] nerve) indicate that the lesion site is in the brainstem.

Case (11-6) Discussion: This is a case of minor stroke involving the small parietal branches of the middle cerebral artery in the area of the superior parietal lobule (Brodmann areas 5 and 7). This parietal lobule serves cortical sensory integration and visual–spatial functions. Cortical sensory integration serves functions like recognition of information written on the skin and tactile identification of objects. Reading maps, identifying locations, following directions, drawing, and copying are examples of visual integration functions.

Chapter 12 Visual System

Case studies for problem solving

Case (12-1) Discussion: The tumor involved the pituitary gland region of the hypothalamus. The tumor compressed the retinogeniculate fibers from both nasal retinas at the optic chiasm. This resulted in a bitemporal hemianopia.

Case (12-2) Discussion: The left temporal and lower parietal lesion also resulted in severe comprehension deficit and moderate reading and writing problem; this aphasic syndrome is called Wernicke aphasia. The subcortical extension of the temporal lesion affected the left geniculocalcarine visual radiation fibers. These ventral fibers of the tract (passing through the loop of Meyer) carried information from the lower retinal quadrants, representing the upper quadrants of the visual field.

Case (12-3) Discussion: The larger left pupil dilation can result from either a right sympathetic or a left parasympathetic lesion. Clinically, the deciding point is the context in which the asymmetry is noticed: dark or light. The presence of pupillary asymmetry in the dark implies that the sympathetic system did not function well for the smaller (right) pupil. Thus, the patient had a right sympathetic lesion. However, if this pupillary asymmetry had been present in the light, it would have indicated a left parasympathetic disruption, which is responsible for constriction of the pupil.

Case (12-4) Discussion: The lesion involved the right temporal–parietal region. This is a case of left homonymous hemianopia, which refers to blindness in the left half of the visual fields for both eyes. Lesions anywhere from the LGB to the calcarine cortex can produce this type of visual field loss. In this case, a stroke involving the deeper temporal–parietal cortex not only interrupted the visual radiation fibers but also produced temporal and spacial deficits that include inattention and constructional deficit.

Case (12-5) Discussion: This is a case of monocular blindness secondary to the prechiasmatic involvement of the afferent fibers of the optic nerve. This interruption of the fibers had also affected the direct light reflex unilaterally, since the lesion blocked the afferent fibers. However, the presence of consensual reflex in the affected eye indicated the intact efferent oculomotor fibers from the midbrain.

Case (12-6) Discussion: Pupillary muscles receive both sympathetic and parasympathetic projections. Sympathetic projections travel to the radial (dilator) muscles through the superior cervical ganglion, whereas the parasympathetic projections innervate the circular (constrictor) muscles of the iris through the Edinger–Westphal nucleus and the oculomotor (CN III) nerve. This pupillary construction was a normal parasympathetic response to light exposure and was caused by the contraction of the circular fiber of the iris.

Chapter 13 Motor System 1: Spinal Cord

Case studies for problem solving

Case (13-1) Discussion: This is a case of a spinal tumor. The mass in this case had affected spinal LMNs from L2–S1 in the cauda equina and thereby caused weakness of the leg muscles (see the myotomal distribution in Fig. 2-34)

Case (13-2) Discussion: This is an example of Brown–Séquard syndrome (spinal hemisection) and is characterized by three signs:

- Paralysis on the side of the lesion
- Loss of position sense on the side of the lesion
- Impaired sensation of pain and temperature on the side opposite to the lesion

Flaccid paralysis followed by spastic paralysis indicates spinal shock secondary to a UMN lesion, which was confirmed by the positive Babinski sign in the left foot. The loss of position sense and discriminative touch from the left toes and leg indicates the involvement of the right dorsal column–medial lemniscal fibers; the loss of pain from the right leg suggests interruption of the left spinothalamic pathway mediating pain and temperature sensation from the right side of the body, this pathway crosses in the spinal cord at the level of entry.

Case (13-3) Discussion: A complete midthoracic transection of the cord affected the motor control of the lower limbs. The absence of muscle reflexes for a few days immediately after the injury is called spinal shock. The return of hyperactive reflexes and spasticity, indicating a UMN lesion, reflects the loss of descending inhibitory influences. In UMN involvement, Babinski sign is also expected. The loss of consciousness in this case was attributed to a cortical concussion, which is not related to a spinal cord injury.

Case (13-4) Discussion: The location of the tumor within the spinal central gray matter had affected the following structures:

- The tumor blocked the crossing fibers of the tract that carried the sensation of pain and temperature. Subsequently, this resulted in a bilateral loss of pain and temperature from both lower extremities.
- The tumor also encroached on the adjacent LMN tracts and neurons bilaterally, affecting lower limb muscle strength.
- A lumbar involvement is usually associated with bowel and bladder functions (see Fig. 2-34).

Case (13-5) Discussion: A lesion anywhere in the neuraxis is likely to affect the descending corticospinal fibers and ascending sensory fibers. However, a lesion only at the cervical spinal cord level is likely to interrupt the phrenic nerve fibers that innervate the diaphragm, the primary muscle of inspiration. In this case, the phrenic nerve injury had caused respiratory paralysis with marked difficulty in inhalation. A right cervical lesion also caused ipsilateral paralysis (subsequent to the interruption of the crossed fibers of the corticospinal tract) and ipsilateral loss of discriminative sensation (subsequent to the involvement of the uncrossed ascending fibers of the dorsal lemniscal system).

Chapter 14 Motor System 2: Cerebellum

Case studies for problem solving

Case (14-1) Discussion: The suspected Friedreich degenerative changes in the spinal cord had the following effects:

- Involvement of the corticospinal tract fibers resulted not only in weakness but also in the appearance of other pyramidal signs: loss of delicate movements and release of primitive reflexes.
- Damage to the spinocerebellar fibers prevented the transmission of unconscious proprioception to the cerebellum, which resulted in incoordination and unsteadiness.
- Damage to the fasciculus gracilis resulted in loss of discriminative sensation from the legs.

Case (14-2) Discussion: The gradual progression of the symptoms indicated a neoplastic (tumor) growth. The presence of a mass affected all cerebellar functions, including coordination, equilibrium, and motor speech.

Case (14-3) Discussion: Cerebellar cells are highly susceptible to alcohol toxicity. This case represents the degenerative effects of a long-term alcohol-induced toxicity, which had affected the following:

- Lateral cerebellar region that resulted in ataxic dysarthria subsequent to the incoordination of the articulators.
- Midline (vermian) structure, which contributed to the unsteady gait and impaired balance.
- Frontal lobe involvement that accounted for her personality changes; disorientation, confusion, and amnesia could have been related to nutritional deficiency as a result of persistent alcohol use.

Chapter 15 Motor System 3: Basal Ganglia

Case studies for problem solving

Case (15-1) Discussion: The subthalamic nucleus renders facilitatory influence on the intrinsically inhibitory globus pallidus. The irritative infarct impaired the smooth flow of facilitating impulses to the globus pallidus and inhibitory BG projections to the motor cortex, which resulted in hemiballism in the limbs contralateral to the lesion site.

Case (15-2) Discussion: This is a case of Parkinson disease, the most commonly known BG disease, which results from a degeneration of the dopaminergic neurons in the substantia nigra. Its symptoms include tremor at rest, cogwheel muscular rigidity, bradykinesia (slowed execution of body movements), akinesia (slow beginning or inability to initiate a movement), shuffling gate, expressionless face, flexed posture, and dysarthria. The muscle rigidity in Parkinson disease is commonly treated with L-dopa, a dopamine-replacement drug.

Case (15-3) Discussion: This is a case of HD, which is characterized by four clinical characteristics: heredity, onset in early adult age, chorea, and cognitive deficits (dementia). Personality changes and mood disorders, including depression, are also present. This neurologic condition, an autosomal-dominant disease, is associated with degenerative changes in the corpus striatum (putamen and caudate nucleus) followed by changes in other cortical areas.

Case (15-4) Discussion: This seems to a case of Wilson disease, which is marked by the retention of copper in the body. In normal conditions, the liver releases absorbed copper into the bile, which helps with digestion. The damaged liver in Wilson disease, however, frees copper into the bloodstream, which carries it to different organs in the body, damaging the kidneys, brain, and eyes. Copper accumulation around the cornea (Kayser–Fleischer ring) supports the diagnosis of Wilson disease. Basal ganglia degeneration affects the motor speech processes (hyperkinetic dysarthria) and produces tremor, rigidity, ataxia, and choreic movements. This pathophysiology has implications for language functions and eventually leads to dementia.

Case (15-5) Discussion: The "relapsing and remitting" pattern of sensorimotor impairment is largely exhibited by patients diagnosed with multiple sclerosis. Stroke patients usually display the most dramatic recovery within 2 to 4 weeks after the onset of the injury. The presence of the "Kayser–Fleischer" ring in the cornea is a clinical indicator of Wilson disease, which is marked by an abnormal accumulation of copper in the brain, kidney, and liver.

"Contre coup" is an injury pattern in traumatic brain injury in which the lesion occurs at the point that is opposite to the point of the blow. The peripheral demyelination refers to Guillain–Barré syndrome, which typifies an ascending pattern of sensorimotor deficit, and this symptomatology does not last more than 4 to 6 weeks.

The person with bacterial infection of the meninges is suspected to have meningitis. The myoneural motor condition refers to myasthenia gravis, an autoimmune disorder in which the patients do better after rest. A reduced caudate head with dementia and dysarthria is an indicator of Huntington chorea, a condition of dominant inheritance. The elderly patient with gait and balance problems and a lost control on eye movement is likely to have progressive supranuclear palsy.

Chapter 16 Motor System 4: Motor Cortex

Case studies for problem solving

Case (16-1) Discussion: The right internal capsule lesion interrupted the following structures:

- Interruption of the corticospinal tract fibers caused the left spastic hemiplegia.
- The affected portion of the corticobulbar fibers supplied the motor nucleus of the facial (CN VII) nerve (loss of delicate motor control for left lower facial muscles), hypoglossal (CN XII) nerve (imprecise speech), and vagus (CN X) nerve (weak voice). There was a differential effect of the lesion on the muscles of the larynx, lower face, and tongue. The effect was minimal on phonation because of the bilateral innervation of the nucleus ambiguus (vagus nerve nucleus), but maximal on articulation because of the profound impact on the facial (CN VII) and hypoglossal (CN X) nuclei because of unilateral innervation (see Chapter 17).
- Interruption in the thalamocortical (medial lemniscus) projections resulted in loss of proprioceptive and discriminative touch on the left half of the body.
- Damage to the thalamocortical projections accounted for the left-sided loss of pain and temperature sensation.

Case (16-2) Discussion: This is a case of crossed clinical findings suggestive of a brainstem process. The ventrolateral pontine infarct on the right side in the pons affected the following structures:

- Damaged facial (CN VII) nucleus and nerve caused the paralysis of the right half of the patient's face (LMN syndrome).
- Damaged trigeminal (CN V) motor nucleus caused the weakness of the right masticator muscles (LMN symptom).
- Damaged chief sensory nucleus and spinal trigeminal nucleus affected pain and touch sensation from the right half of the face.
- Interruption of the uncrossed descending corticospinal fibers resulted in paralysis of the left side of the body, and this was also associated with the Babinski sign.

Case (16-3) Discussion: This case may look similar to that of patient one, but patient three has a different lesion site. A cortical lesion had affected the following structures and their functions:

- Damaged corticospinal fibers in Brodmann area 4 caused the right (UMN) spastic hemiplegia.
- Affected corticobulbar fibers supplied the motor nucleus of the facial nerve (loss of motor control for right lower facial muscles) and hypoglossal nerve (imprecise speech), resulting in attenuated cranial nerve functions marked with facial and lingual paralysis and dysarthria. The effect on the upper facial muscles was minimal because the upper facial muscles receive bilateral cortical projections (see Chapter 17).
- Partial involvement of the somatosensory cortex resulted in the loss of pain, touch, and temperature.
- The involvement of the Brodmann area 44 (anterior association language cortex) resulted in nonfluent and effortful verbal output.

Case (16-4) Discussion: This is a brainstem syndrome associated with a right medullary lesion that had affected the following structures:

- Paralysis of the left hypoglossal (CN XII) nerve contributed to the speech unintelligibility.
- Involvement of the pharyngeal branches of the vagus (CN X) nerve resulted in the paralysis of the pharyngeal muscles, contributing to dysphagia.
- Involvement of the descending trigeminal (CN V) nucleus contributed to the facial anesthesia.
- Interruption of the ascending fibers of the lateral spinothalamic tract resulted in the loss of pain and temperature on the right half of the body.
- Involvement of the uncrossed descending motor fibers (pyramidal tract) contributed to the right hemiplegia.

Chapter 17 Cranial Nerves Synopsis

Case studies for problem solving

Case (17-1) Discussion: The motor functions of face and mandible (masticator) are mediated, respectively, by the facial (CN VII) and the trigeminal (CN V) nerves. Deglutition involves the pharyngeal plexus of the glossopharyngeal (CN IX) and vagus (CN X) nerves, and the tongue is controlled by the hypoglossal nerve (CN XII). In this case, the lacunar lesions impaired voluntary control of the connected muscles by injuring the corticobulbar pathway descending from the cortex to the nuclei of selected cranial nerve nuclei. As an example of the UMN lesion, this clinical condition, also known as the pseudobulbar palsy, is associated with bilateral cortical lesions. The term pseudobulbar implies that the problem is not in the medulla and does not affect the LMNs; rather it involves the bilateral corticobulbar pathways to the brainstem. Another term used to refer to a UMN lesion is supranuclear paralysis (injury above or rostral to the cranial nerve motor nuclei of the brainstem), owing to bilateral involvement of corticobulbar or corticonuclear pathways.

When the patient attempts to move his facial muscles, the muscles respond poorly, but they respond strongly to an emotional stimulus, which is not under direct control of the cerebral cortex. The pathways that are functional during an emotional response are not as well understood as the direct pathways controlling voluntary actions. The pathways involved with emotions are known to escape injury from lacunar strokes and cortical lesions in typical locations. When the cranial nerve nuclei are activated through the indirect and spared pathway known to mediate emotions, the facial response is actually exaggerated; the patient's face may assume an expressive mask, with forceful contraction of the muscles that otherwise appeared to be weak when he was asked to show his teeth or perform a voluntary smile. An emotional smile, in contrast, resulted in an exaggerated emotional expression accompanied by sobbing. It is important to avoid emotional stimulation when the patient is eating to minimize the risk of aspirating food or saliva.

Slow gait with hyperactive muscle stretch reflexes (deep tendon reflexes) and extensor plantar responses (Babinski signs) imply UMN symptoms. This means that the nerves of the LMNs directly supplying the muscles have not been damaged, but the descending corticospinal motor pathways from the brain have been damaged. The resulting spastic weakness with impaired voluntary control but uninhibited reflex activity (e.g., the hyperactive knee-jerk and ankle reflexes) is characteristic of UMN syndrome (see Chapter 14).

In pseudobulbar palsy, the reflex activities of laughing and crying are not just intact but are actually overactive or exaggerated for the same reason that hyperactive muscle stretch reflexes occur. The reflexes are normally modulated, or somewhat inhibited, by the activity in the intact corticonuclear or corticospinal pathways (corticonuclear or corticobulbar for the display of emotion in the face; corticospinal for the stretch reflexes in the limbs). When that inhibition is removed as the result of a lesion, the responses are uncontrolled, or hyperactive. The signs of cognitive impairment in this patient also resulted from multiple cortical infarcts.

Case (17-2) Discussion: The pontine tegmental lesion in this case affected four cranial nerves (abducens [CN VI], trigeminal [CN V], facial [CN VII], and vestibulocochlear [CN VIII]), which caused adduction of the left eye (impaired abducens function with paralyzed lateral rectus muscle), analgesia and anesthesia on the left face (trigeminal [CN V] interruption), paresis in the jaw (trigeminal [CN V] motor nerve involvement), left facial paralysis (facial [CN VII]), and hearing loss (vestibulocochlear [CN VIII]). The typical location of the lesion did not affect the descending corticospinal fibers, so limb motor functions were spared.

Case (17-3) Discussion: This patient exhibits the involvement of three cranial nerves: glossopharyngeal nerve (IX) with absent gag reflex and loss of palatal sensation; vagus nerve (X) with altered phonation, breathiness, diplophonia, dysphagia, and palatal immobility; and spinal accessory nerve (XI) with impaired shoulder elevation and lateral head rotation. The common binding factor involving these three nerves is that they exit the cranium through the jugular foramen (See Figure 17-5); a tumor adjacent to the jugular foramen is likely to have affected these nerves and impaired their functions.

Case (17-4) Discussion: A left pontine-medullary lesion resulted in alternating sensorimotor symptoms that included the following:

- The effects on the facial nerve (CN VII) and trigeminal nerve (CN V) fibers, along with the rootlets of the vagus nerve (CN X), were facial motor disturbance, loss of sensation from the face, palatal paralysis, and swallowing difficulty.
- Involvement of the vestibular nuclei resulted in the equilibrium problem.
- Interruption of the long descending pyramidal (corticospinal) fibers above the point of decussation produced paralysis in the right arm and leg.

Case (17-5) Discussion: This is another case of alternating hemiplegia in which a medullary lesion resulted in cranial nerve (LMN) symptoms on the ipsilateral side and hemiplegia (UMN) and hemianesthesia on the body contralateral to the lesion site. The lesion not only affected the cranial nerve projections but also interrupted long ascending and descending fibers:

- The ocular adduction (impaired ability to the move eye laterally) implies paralysis of the lateral rectus muscle subsequent to abducens nerve (CN VI) involvement; this nerve exists medially from the pontomedullary junction.
- Facial paralysis, imprecise articulation, and subsequent drooling of saliva resulted from the involvement of the facial nerve (CN VII), which exits laterally at the pontomedullary junction.
- The decreased pain and temperature sensation on the face was the result of interrupted fibers of the trigeminal nerve, which exits from the pontine tegmentum.
- Hypoglossal nerve (CN XII) and vagus nerve (CN X) involvement resulted in the paralysis of the right half of the tongue and caused speech to be poorly articulated and breathy; it also contributed to dysphagia. Hearing impairment (sensorineural type) indicated the involvement of the vestibulocochlear nerve (CN VIII), which is located lateral to the facial nerve at the pontomedullary junction. The presence of right hemiplegia and anesthesia resulted from the interruption of long ascending and descending projection fibers.

Case (17-6) Discussion: This is a case of trigeminal neuralgia, which is characterized by episodes of intense (sudden and stabbing) pain (see Chapter 11). The cause of neuralgia is not fully known. However, inflammation of the trigeminal ganglion and pressure caused by an arterial loop against the trigeminal nerve (CN V) are commonly implicated. The pain was initiated by touching a trigger zone, which for this patient was in the upper lip area. This evoked pain that caused her to refrain from speaking and eating.

Case (17-7) Discussion: This unilateral facial palsy is a case of Bell palsy, which could be caused by an idiopathic involvement of the facial nerve (CN VII). With no other sensorimotor (hemiplegia or hemianesthesia) symptoms and no higher mental function disorders (aphasia and amnesia), this is a case of focal pathology, most likely a viral infection, one of the most common causes of facial palsy. In this case, the inability to close the eye has serious implications, because a constantly exposed cornea leads to dryness and, if untreated, can lead to corneal ulceration, which may eventually damage the eye.

Case (17-8) Discussion: The motor nuclei for the vagus (CN X), hypoglossal (CN XII), and glossopharyngeal (CN IX) nerves are located in the upper medial medulla. A localized medullary stroke had selectively affected the nucleus ambiguus, which is shared by the glossopharyngeal (CN IX) and vagus nerve (CN X) (altered phonation and dysphagia). This also affected the hypoglossal nucleus, which resulted in lingual paralysis and further contributed to the dysarthria.

Case (17-9) Discussion: UMN signs produced by a lesion anywhere above the decussation of the pyramids in the caudal medulla manifest on the opposite side of the body. Therefore, a mass at the level of the pons and rostral medulla on the left can account for right-sided hemiparesis. Cerebellar signs of unsteadiness appear on the same side as the lesion, and injury to the left cerebellar hemisphere accounts for falling to the left, the side of the lesion. Therefore, a single site of lesion can account for both of these clinical abnormalities. The decreased sensation on the face can be explained by partial injury to the trigeminal (CN V) nerve on the left, with pain perception more affected than perception of touch. It may also be explained by injury to the sensory pathway for pain and temperature inside the brainstem on the left, because fibers mediating pain and temperature sensation (known as the descending or spinal tract of the trigeminal nerve) enter the brainstem at the midpons as part of the trigeminal nerve (CN V), then descend through the caudal pons and medulla as far as the high cervical spinal cord before synapsing and sending second-order sensory neurons across the midline to ascend to the thalamus on the right. The fibers mediating touch do not follow this descending course. They synapse, and the second-order axons cross at the level of entry in the midpons.

Absence of the corneal reflex can be explained by the loss of pain sensation on the cornea. The weakness of eye closure is also relevant to loss of the reflex, but without the sensory loss, some response of eye closure to touching the cornea with a wisp of cotton is likely, and the patient would feel the irritation of the stimulus.

The weakness of the face affects all components. When there is UMN facial weakness, the functions of forehead muscles are usually intact because they are controlled by both ipsilateral and contralateral descending motor pathways. Therefore, in this case, the weakness appears to be of the LMN variety (involvement of the nerve itself). This is consistent with the mass on the left at the level of the lateral recess of the medulla, where the facial and vestibulocochlear nerves enter the brainstem. The loss of hearing is the sensorineural type, affecting both air and bone conduction. Therefore, it is likely to originate in the nerve and is not consistent with middle ear disease, in which bone conduction is preserved.

The slow development of symptoms is consistent with tumor growth. Usually, a tumor in the cerebellopontine angle develops on the vestibular division of the vestibulocochlear nerve (CN VIII) from nerve sheath cells. The tumor is often called an **acoustic neuroma**, but better names for it are schwannoma (or Schwann cell tumor) and neurolemma.

It is necessary to remove a schwannoma surgically to prevent further compression of vital structures of the medulla. Because the expanding tumor tends to surround the facial nerve (CN VII), facial weakness, if present, is usually mild before surgery. It may not be possible to preserve the nerve during the operation, however, because it is engulfed in tumor, and the face may be paralyzed postoperatively. Similarly, hearing is usually not restored, and because the tumor most often develops on the vestibular division of the nerve, caloric testing (irrigating the ear canal with warm or cold water) gives no response—that is, there is no vertigo or nystagmus when the test is performed on the damaged side. This is true before the operation as well, if the test is performed during the diagnostic workup.

Chapter 18 Axial–Limbic Brain: Autonomic Nervous System, Limbic System, Hypothalamus, and Reticular Formation

Case studies for problem solving

Case (18-1) Discussion: With the tumor compressing the sacral cord, all afferent and efferent impulses of the spinal reflex to the bladder were interrupted. With the loss of motor control, the bladder became flaccid. Once the bladder was full, the urine dripped out gradually.

Case (18-2) Discussion: Horner syndrome results from a lesion of the sympathetic pathways to the eye and forehead. Clinical characteristics are miotic (constricted) pupil, ptosis of the upper eyelid, and inability to sweat on the forehead. Pupil constriction (miosis) is regulated by parasympathetic impulses, whereas pupil dilation (mydriasis) is controlled by sympathetic impulses. Sympathetic impulses originate in the ipsilateral hypothalamus and descend to the motor neurons in the

T1–T2 segments. Preganglionic neuron projections travel to the superior sympathetic cervical ganglion, which projects to the smooth dilator muscle of the iris. Damage to the superior cervical ganglia affected the sympathetic projections, resulting in unopposed actions of the parasympathetic system. This caused the pupil constriction and contributed to the inability to sweat.

Case (18-3) Discussion: Hypothalamic damage usually causes an imbalance in food and water intake and temperature control as well as a decrease in sexual drive. Weight loss is seen commonly in patients with anorexia. A vasopressin (antidiuretic hormone) deficiency causes excessive thirst and accompanying increased urinary output. Alterations in gonadotropic hormones lead to changes in the cycle of menses. Furthermore, hypothalamic damage causes a disturbance in temperature control.

Case (18-4) Discussion: Abnormal electric discharges of the temporal lobe stimulated the hippocampus and amygdala, resulting in automatic behaviors for which there was loss of conscious control. The involvement of association cortices during his seizures impaired his memory.

Case (18-5) Discussion: The laceration and concussion of the prefrontal lobe account for his personality changes, lack of hygiene, and cognitive deficits. The temporarily impaired functioning of the brainstem reticular formation was related to his loss of consciousness. The retrograde amnesia preceding the accident is typical of the traumatic brain injuries, which may largely relate to the structural damage to the hippocampus and/or its axonal connections to the neocortex.

Case (18-6) Discussion: It is a hypothalamic syndrome. The hypothalamus serves autonomic, visceral, and endocrine functions, including sexual drive, appetite, sleep–wake cycle, and body heat production. Impaired ANS control of the oral glands resulted in excessive saliva secretion (see Chapter 17).

Case (18-7) Discussion: Functionally related and adjacently located structures of the limbic lobes are involved with the reported behavioral symptoms of agitation and aggression (limbic lobe) and memory impairment (hippocampal formation).

Chapter 19 Cerebral Cortex: Higher Mental Functions

Case studies for problem solving

Case (19-1) Discussion: This collection of neurolinguistic symptoms (impaired auditory comprehension, paraphasic substitutions, and jargon utterances) indicates Wernicke (fluent) aphasia in its acute stage. Since the symptoms emerged suddenly, this syndrome likely resulted from an embolism that traveled into the middle cerebral artery and selectively occluded the inferior branches.

Case (19-2) Discussion: This is a case of pure alexia without agraphia, secondary to an infarction in the territory of the the left posterior cerebral artery, which had further involved the splenium of the corpus callosum, as evident in the MRI study. According to the disconnection theory of pure alexia, the callosal lesion prevents visual information processed in the intact right occipital lobe from reaching left hemisphere language centers for reading and color naming.

Case (19-3) Discussion: This is a case of ataxic dysarthria subsequent to a lateral medullary lesion; the cause of the infarct was occlusion of the left vertebral artery, which gives off the branch called posterior inferior cerebellar artery. The lateral medullary lesion (Wallenberg syndrome) affects the trigeminal spinal tract nucleus, nucleus ambiguus, and lateral spinothalamic tract containing spinothalamic fibers from the contralateral half of the body. It causes a dissociated loss of pinprick and temperature sensation from the ipsilateral face (trigeminal [CN V] nerve) and the contralateral side of the body (spinothalamic tract fibers). The involvement of the nucleus ambiguus (vagus [CN X] nerve) contributed to swallowing difficulty. Many patients with this syndrome, depending on the lesion size, show involvement of the inferior cerebellar peduncle and/or have a cerebellar infarction. The involvement of the inferior cerebellar peduncle in this case likely contributed to the dysarthric speech.

Case (19-4) Discussion: This is a case of primary progressive aphasia (nonfluent type). The primary progressive aphasia has apparent focal aphasic deficits that gradually progress over years. Some patients fail to show memory loss or other cognitive deficits for years after onset; the patient cannot think of names or understand the meaning of words. The nonfluent aphasia in dementia usually indicates pathology other than typical AD, whereas the pathology of semantic dementia and fluent progressive aphasia is more variable.

Case (19-5) Discussion: The left inferior parietal lobe is involved in multiple cognitive functions including language, praxis, constructions, and even memory. The "dementia" was in actuality due to a focal lesion in this case, and she improved after blood flow was restored via carotid surgery.

Case (19-6) Discussion: Vascular dementia is often cited as the second most common cause of dementia, after Alzheimer disease, though many cases actually involve a mixture of vascular and neurodegenerative pathology. This patient appeared to have a vascular dementia induced by three large infarctions.

Glossary

Abdominal muscles: Group of muscles innervated by the nerves originating from the T6–T12 spinal segments that regulate forced expiration.

Abdominal reflex: Contraction of the abdominal wall and retraction of the umbilicus towards the stimulus on stroking the skin over the abdominal quadrant. Absence of this reflex is associated with pyramidal tract lesions (upper motor neuron).

Abducens nerve: Cranial nerve VI, regulating the lateral rectus muscle, is responsible for moving eyeball outward laterally. The nerve involvement causes the eye to deviate to the middle (medial strabismus).

Abduction: Movement of the limb away from the central body axis.

Abscess: Localized accumulation of pus from liquefied tissue that is associated with swelling.

Absence (petit mal) seizures: Sudden and recurrent attacks of impaired consciousness, which are characterized by staring, blinking, and twitching of cranial muscles. The associated EEG pattern shows an abrupt onset of a 3 second spike.

Absolute refractive period: Cellular state immediately following the action potential in which no other action potential can be initiated by the cell.

Abulia: Impaired ability to take a decision and perform voluntary actions along with reduced speech output, usually associated with bilateral prefrontal lobe pathologies.

Acalculia: Impaired acquired ability, acquired after brain damage, to perform simple arithmetic calculation.

Accommodation: Parasympathetic visual response that the lens undergoes to keep a near object in focus.

Acetylcholine (ACh): Neurotransmitter released by cholinergic neurons and widely distributed in body tissues. It primarily regulates some brain activity and most of the muscular activity of the peripheral nervous system.

Acetylcholinesterase: Enzyme that breaks the neurotransmitter acetylcholine into choline and acetate, contributing to the termination of the postsynaptic current and signal. Much of the choline released by hydrolysis is recaptured by the presynaptic terminal.

Acoustic nerve: Part of the vestibulocochlear (CN VIII) nerve that serves audition.

Acoustic neuroma: Occurring usually on one side of the brainstem, this slow-growing benign tumor affects hearing and possibly also the ability to balance.

Acromegaly: Condition characterized by thickened bones and tissue and caused by oversecretion of human growth (hGH) hormone during adulthood.

Action potential: Electrical impulse representing a transient fluctuation in membrane potentials, which are propagated along axonal process to activate postsynaptic terminals.

Acuity: Measurement of perceptual clarity usually of auditory and visual stimuli.

Acute: Short-term physiologic effects emerging immediately after pathophysiology and requiring immediate medical attention.

Acute confusional state: Fluctuating level of altered consciousness marked by confusion, distractibility, disordered thinking, fluctuating attention, reduced memory, impaired perception, and agitation keep largely by toxicity in the brain; also known as delirium.

Adaptation: Gradually diminishing sensitivity of receptors to continued stimulation.

Adduction: Limb movement towards the midline/central body axis; it is opposite to abduction.

Adenohypophysis: Anterior lobe of the pituitary gland.

Adipsia: Condition marked by the lack of thirst or desire to take water.

Adrenal cortex: Outer portion of the adrenal gland, which releases cortisol on stimulation by pituitary gland.

Adrenal gland: Located superior to each of the kidneys. It contains cells that on sympathetic stimulation secrete epinephrine and norepinephrine.

Adrenergic: Neurons responsible for synthesizing and releasing epinephrine (adrenaline) and norepinephrine (noradrenaline).

Adrenocorticotropin: Hormone that stimulates growth of the adrenal (suprarenal) cortex and regulates the secretion of its hormones.

Afferent: Axonal bundles mediating bodily perceived sensations of pain, touch, and temperature toward the central nervous system.

Agnosia: Acquired impairment in recognizing objects while the primary modalities of sensation (touch, vision, and hearing) are normal.

Agraphia: Acquired impaired ability after brain damage to express through writing.

AIDS (acquired immunodeficiency syndrome): Disorder of the immune system owing to infection with the human immunodeficiency virus (HIV-1) in which the antibodies attack the body's own immune system.

AIDS dementia complex: Progressive cognitive (dementia) syndrome occurring after chronic HIV-1 encephalitis.

Akinesia: Slow initiation or loss of power of voluntary movements seen in patients with basal ganglia pathology.

Akinetic mutism: State of altered consciousness in which the patient appears intermittently alert but is unresponsive despite intact motor skills.

Alar lamina: Alar plate zone of the embryonic neural tube dorsal to the sulcus limitans. Dorsal gray columns of the spinal cord and sensory centers of the brain develop from this region.

Albinism: Genetically recessive condition involving partial or total lack of pigment in the skin, hair, and eyes due to the abnormalities of melanin production.

Alexia: Impaired acquired ability after brain damage to comprehend written information.

Alkalosis: Condition resulting from an increased acid (pH) level in body fluid.

Alleles: Genes at corresponding positions (loci) in a chromosome pair.

α-motor neuron: Largest and rapidly conducting spinal motor neuron, which controls the activity of skeletal muscle fibers.

alpha (α)-wave (α-rhythm): Brain wave with a frequency between 8 and 13 Hz that is present in the posterior brain region and represents the awakened and relaxed state of the brain with the eyes closed.

Alternating hemiplegia: Brainstem lesion characterized by cranial nerve impairments on the side ipsilateral to the lesion with motor and sensory loss on the opposite side.

Alzheimer disease: Chronic degenerative condition in the aging brain characterized by irreversible failing of memory, disorientation, impaired judgment, and disorders of language and cognition.

Amnesia: Impaired ability to remember. Forgetting information preceding cortical injury is retrograde amnesia, whereas the inability to learn newer information after injury is anterograde amnesia.

Ampulla: Sac-like canal dilation containing sensory receptors.

Amygdala: Almond-shaped medial limbic structure associated with visceral and vegetative activities needed for self-preservation, such as mating, fighting, and eating. Also controls autonomic responses to stress. It is reciprocally connected to the hypothalamus, hippocampus, and thalamus. Functionally, it is concerned with emotional responses.

Amyotrophic: Pertaining to muscular atrophy, as in amyotrophic lateral sclerosis.

Amyotrophic lateral sclerosis (ALS; Lou Gehrig disease): Progressive degenerative condition of spinal and cortical motor neurons characterized by progressive weakness and muscular atrophy.

Anabolism: Building of energy and cellular metabolic substances that are needed for the body.

Analgesia: Neurologic state in which painful stimuli are no longer perceived as being uncomfortable and painful.

Analgesics: Substances that relieve the sensation of pain.

Anaphase: Third stage in cell division.

Anastomosis: Natural connectivity involving two or more blood vessels that contributes to collateral circulation (reperfusion) for promoting natural recovery.

Anencephaly: Birth defect in which the forebrain and/or midbrain are diminished in size or are missing; it is caused by the defective fusion of the neural tube during embryologic development.

Anesthesia: Loss of touch and pain sensation either from a cortical lesion or from a drug-induced state of suppressed sensation.

Aneuploid: Having an extra chromosome.

Aneurysm: Localized, balloon-like dilation of a blood vessel caused by a weakened arterial wall or congenital defect.

Aneurysm clipping: Surgical treatment involving the use of a clip to obliterate the neck of an aneurysm.

Angiogenesis: Development of newer blood vessels, which can also promote abnormal cancerous tissue growth.

Angiography: X-ray technique that involves injection of radiopaque substance for examining the structural architecture of blood vessels.

Angioplasticity: Surgical procedure used to open blood vessels by using a dilated balloon and/or by placing a stent.

Angular gyrus: Neurolinguistically important and highly developed parietotemporal convolution in human brain, which is implicated with the reading function.

Anhidrosis: Autonomic disorder marked by reduced or absent sweating.

Annulospiral nerve endings: Specialized receptors that mediate muscle stretch.

Anomia: Impaired ability to name objects and find words acquired after brain injury.

Anorexia nervosa: Chronic psychological condition characterized by self-induced weight loss and distorted body image resulting from a loss of appetite.

Anosmia: Loss of the ability to smell.

Anosognosia: Failure to recognize one's own disease, a usual parietal syndrome.

Anoxia: Condition of oxygen deficiency in brain tissue.

Ansa lenticularis: Containing efferents from the globus pallidus to the thalamus, this motor pathway curves around the internal capsule to reach the ventral lateral thalamic nucleus.

Antagonist: One of the paired muscles that acts in opposition to the mover (agonist) muscle of the joint during a movement.

Anterior cerebral artery: Supplies blood to the medial surface of the frontal lobe and part of the parietal lobe, in addition to the anterior four-fifths of the corpus callosum.

Anterior commissure: Known to mediate olfaction, a smaller commissural fiber bundle that crosses the midline of the brain near the anterior limit of the third ventricle and interconnects the olfactory bulbs.

Anterior corticospinal tract: Descending motor fibers that do not cross the midline in the medulla oblongata.

Anterior horn: Ventral spinal gray region containing motor (final common pathway) nuclei.

Anterior lobe: Cerebellar region that is responsible for muscle tone and equilibrium during locomotion.

Anterior medullary velum: Thin white matter layer that forms the roof of the fourth ventricle.

Anterior nucleus: Thalamic nucleus mediating hypothalamic (mammillary body) projections to the cingulate gyrus of the limbic cortex. It participates in the regulation of visceral and emotional functions.

Anterior perforated substance: Region at the base of the brain near the optic chiasm through which the penetrating branches of the anterior and middle cerebral arteries enter to vascularize the deep subcortical structures.

Anterior (ventral) root: Collection of motor (efferent) fibers, emerging from the anterior aspect of the spinal cord and extending laterally to join a posterior root to form a spinal nerve.

Anterior spinothalamic tract: Axonal bundle mediating diffuse touch sensation to the thalamus.

Anterograde reaction: See WALLERIAN DEGENERATION.

Anterograde transmission: Forward flow of information from the soma (cell body) to the synapse.

Anterolateral spinothalamic system: Includes the spinal axonal bundle of fibers that mediate pain, touch, and temperature to the brain.

Antibody: Defensive substance produced in response to a specific antigen in the body.

Anticoagulant: Drugs that are used to prevent the clotting of blood. Warfarin (Coumadin) is a common anticoagulant drug.

Antidiuretic hormone (ADH): Hormone produced by neurosecretory hypothalamic cells that stimulates water reabsorption from the kidney, reduces urine output, and causes vasoconstriction of arterioles (vasopressin).

Antiepileptic drugs: Anticonvulsant medications used either to prevent or to treat seizure disorders.

Antigen: Foreign substances in the body whose contact with cells triggers a response from the body's immune system.

Aphagia: Impaired ability to swallow subsequent to brain injuries.

Aphasia: Impaired ability to process language, resulting from brain damage.

Apraxia: Impaired ability to execute skilled motor acts on commands, which is not caused by muscle paralysis, incoordination, or incomprehension.

Aqueduct: Narrow canal within the brainstem that connects the third and fourth ventricles.

Aqueous humor: Watery substance, similar to cerebrospinal fluid, that is continuously produced and drained in the posterior chamber of the anterior ocular cavity.

Arachnoid: Middle meningeal layer that protects the central nervous system by covering it and forms the subarachnoid space for the cerebrospinal fluid.

Arachnoid granulations: See ARACHNOID VILLE.

Arachnoid trabeculae: Fibrous tissue that maintains the subarachnoid space by serving as a ridge between the membranes of the arachnoid and the pia mater.

Arachnoid villi (granulations): Worm-like tufted structures that drain cerebrospinal fluid from the subarachnoid space into the superior sagittal sinus.

Archicerebellum: Oldest part of the cerebellum. Includes the flocculus and nodulus and is related to equilibrium.

Arcuate fasciculus: Fibers of the superior longitudinal fasciculus known to connect the association cortices of Broca area with Wernicke area.

Argyll Robertson pupil: Impaired pupillary reaction to light while the near vision reflex is preserved. Commonly seen with degenerative brain diseases such as Alzheimer, encephalopathy, and diabetes.

Arnold–Chiari malformation: Developmental malformation marked by a downward herniation of the medulla and cerebellum in the vertebral canal of the cervical region; it is often associated with spinal bifida and hydrocephaly.

Arteriosclerosis: Narrowing of arterial lumen owing to accumulation of lipids, fatty substances, and cholesterol along intimal walls of blood vessels; it is also called atherosclerosis.

Arteriovenous malformation: Congenital condition in which tangled and twisted arteries and veins are interconnected in a localized area, where the arterial blood shunts to the veins, bypassing the cortical tissue.

Artery: Vessel carrying blood from the heart to body parts.

Asphyxia: Brain cell anoxia secondary to a reduction in the regular exchange of oxygen and carbon dioxide.

Aspiration: Inhalation of water or food into the bronchial tree.

Association (secondary) cortex: Functionally uncommitted regions of the cerebral cortex at birth that later assume integration of multimodality information and include the parietal–temporal–occipital association cortex and prefrontal association cortex.

Association fibers: Short and long fibers that interconnect different regions within a cerebral hemisphere.

Astereognosis: Impaired ability to identify the shape, size, and texture of an object through touch; this is associated with a superior parietal lobule lesion.

Asthenia: Muscle weakness caused by cerebellar dysfunctioning.

Astigmatism: Focusing disorder in which vertical and horizontal rays focus at two different points on the retina. Results from irregular lens and/or cornea curvature.

Astrocytes: Neuroglia cells that support nerve cells and contribute to blood–brain barrier.

Asynergia: Impaired ability to coordinate different muscles in the performance of a skilled movement.

Ataxia: Lack of coordination in sequential voluntary muscular activities, resulting from cerebellar pathology.

Ataxic dysarthria: Acquired motor speech disorder subsequent to cerebellar pathology. Characterized by imprecise speech, articulatory breakdowns, and impaired stress applications.

Atheroma: Lipid deposit that compromises vascular supply to the brain by narrowing arterial wall as part of the atherosclerosis.

Atherosclerosis: Process of narrowing of the arterial lumen owing to accumulation of fatty substances (cholesterol and triglycerides) and lipids along the intimal walls of the medianum and larger blood vessels. The formation of an atherosclerotic plaque that decreases the size of the arterial lumen and is a common cause of hypertension and other vascular disorders.

Atherosclerotic plaque: Lesion causing plaque resulting from accumulated fatty substances involving the tunica media of an artery and leading to obstruction.

Athetosis: Involuntary, slow writhing movements of limbs subsequent to basal ganglia pathology.

Atrophy: Wasting away of muscle tissue, including reduction in muscle fiber diameter (weakening of the force of contraction owing to disuse atrophy) or disintegration of muscle fibers (denervation atrophy).

Atrophy of denervation (fiber wasting): Severely reduced muscle mass with loss of muscle fibers, resulting from prolonged loss (6 months or more) of lower motor neuron innervation of these fibers.

Atrophy of disuse: Reduction in muscle body mass without loss of muscle fibers (cells) caused by decreased muscular activity.

Attenuation reflex: Reflexive contraction of the middle ear muscles causing a decrease in auditory sensitivity.

Audiometry: Assessment of hearing sensitivity for a range of pure tones using the decibel (dBSPL) scale.

Auditory association (secondary) cortex: Brain region located around the primary auditory cortex, responsible for the elaboration of auditory information.

Auditory brainstem response (ABR): See BRAINSTEM AUDITORY-EVOKED POTENTIALS

Auditory reflexes: Protective simultaneous head and eye movements in response to loud auditory stimuli.

Auditory system: Neuroanatomic system, beginning in the inner ear, passing through the brainstem, thalamus (medial geniculate body), and terminating in the auditory cortex. Responsible for auditory perception.

Autoimmunity: Condition in which antibodies attack the body's own normal tissues.

Autonomic dysfunctions: Neurologic disorders involving pupil dilation/constriction, sexual activity, perspiration, thirst, hunger, urination, and gastric function.

Autonomic ganglia: Group of nuclei located in the peripheral nervous system that mediate impulses from the central nervous system to various visceral organs, cardiac muscles, smooth muscles, and glands.

Autonomic nervous system: Division of the peripheral nervous system with sympathetic and parasympathetic fibers. Works subconsciously and innervates blood vessels, internal organs, and glands.

Autoregulation: Autocerebral mechanism for regulating blood flow to the brain.

Autosomal: Related to chromosomes other than sex chromosomes.

Autosomal dominance: Genetic expression mode in which a dysfunctional allele possessed by one parent dominates the second allele from the other parent. Each offspring has a 50% probability of inheriting this dysfunctional gene and the disorder.

Axial muscles: Muscles associated with the central part of the body that regulate movements of the trunk.

Axon: Neuronal process capable of conducting neuronal impulses to other cell bodies.

Axon collaterals: Small branching processes attached to the main body of the axon.

Axon hillock: Dilated site of an axon where it joins the cell.

Axonal (retrograde) reaction: Retrograde chromatolytic changes in the soma marked by disintegration of the granules of the Nissl bodies after damage to an axon.

Axonal regeneration: Reconstitution of an injured axon. It is the most prevalent in the peripheral nervous system.

Babinski reflex: Dorsal flexion of the great toe and fanning of other toes being stroked on the sole of the foot. Presence of this response indicates pyramidal tract (upper motor neuron) pathology in adults.

Balint syndrome: Visual syndrome marked by inability to project voluntary gaze to certain points despite intact eye movements, which is associated with the bilateral parietooccipital lesions.

Ballism: Violent flinging movements usually involving one side of the body that are usually associated with a lesion of the contralateral subthalamic nucleus.

Bárány caloric test: Undertaken to evaluate vestibular functioning in cases of inner ear disease using the injection of water of different temperatures into the auditory canal. Cold water produces rotatory nystagmus toward the opposite direction, whereas warm fluid triggers nystagmus toward the injected (ipsilateral) side.

Basal ganglia: Group of subcortical nuclei (caudate, globus pallidus, and putamen) located within the white matter in each cerebral hemisphere. They play an important role in movement regulation.

Basis pedunculi: Also called pes peduncle or crus cerebri, it includes descending motor fibers in the midbrain on each side.

Bell palsy: Paralysis involving one side of the face in which weakened muscles are pulled toward unaffected side.

Benedikt syndrome: Midbrain cranial nerve syndrome marked by unilateral oculomotor paralysis with contralateral hemiplegia (corticospinal tract) and tremor (red nucleus).

Betz cells: Large motor (pyramidal) cells located in the primary motor cortex.

Bilaminar embryo: Human embryo in the second week of gestation, which consists of epiblast and the hypoblast.

Bilateral innervation: Mostly refers to cranial nerve motor nuclei that receive motor commands from both motor cortices, where each pyramidal tract provides both ipsilateral (minor) and contralateral (stronger) efferent fibers.

Binocular vision: Visual field area that is simultaneously processed in both eyes.

Biopsy: Removal of tissue from the living body usually for microscopic examination.

Biorhythms: Circadian (with a cycle of 24 hour) biologic rhythms regulating body homeostasis such as the sleep–wake cycle.

Bitemporal hemianopia: Loss of temporal visual fields for both eyes.

Blast: Immature cell.

Blastocyst: Stage in the first week of human development.

Blastomere: Cell resulting from cleavage of a fertilized ovum.

Blind spot: Retinal area, that contains no photoreceptors, located 15° medial to the visual axis and representing the optic disk through which optic nerve (cranial nerve II) fibers exit the retina.

Blood–brain barrier: Structural property of the CNS vessels formed by the endothelial cells that restricts (impermeability) the passage of most substances (many harmful) to the brain.

Blood pressure: Measurement of the force exerted by blood against the walls of blood vessels during ventricular systole (contraction of the heart, by which the blood is sent through the aorta for systemic circulation).

Bony labyrinth: Represents a series of cavities in the petrous portion of the temporal bone that contain the cochlea, semicircular canals, and vestibule.

Brachial plexus: Network of spinal nerve fibers exiting the ventral rami of the C5–T1 nerves that supply the upper limbs.

Brachium: Armlike fiber bundle. The brachium of the inferior colliculus is an auditory fiber bundle that connects the inferior colliculus to the thalamus. The brachium of the superior colliculus mediates visual information and bypasses the lateral geniculate body of the thalamus on its way to the pretectal region in midbrain.

Brachium conjunctivum: See Superior cerebellar peduncle.

Brachium pontis: See Middle cerebellar peduncle.

Bradykinesia: Slowness in the initiation of voluntary motor movements.

Brain waves: Electrical activity produced as a result of action potentials of brain cells

Brainstem: Stem part of the brain, which consists of midbrain, pons, and medulla.

Brainstem auditory-evoked potentials: Technique used for measuring brainstem neuronal responses to controlled auditory stimuli.

Branchial arches: Five pairs of arched embryologic structures that develop into laryngeal, pharyngeal, and facial muscles. These are remnants of arches in lower vertebrates that give rise to muscles for specialized functions like articulation, phonation, and swallowing in the humans.

Broad-based gait: Walking pattern characterized by placing the feet far apart. This gait pattern often results from cerebellar injury.

Broca aphasia: Type of aphasia associated with a lesion in the lower premotor cortex (Broca area or anterior language cortex), and it is characterized by impaired verbal output.

Brodmann areas: Approximately 50 or so brain areas identified and mapped by Brodmann on the basis of their cellular cytoarchitectonics.

Brownian motion: Physical property of water molecules, which refers to their constant motion and random movements in all directions.

Brown-Séquard syndrome: Hemi-spinal cord lesion resulting in spastic paralysis and proprioceptive loss in the body ipsilateral to the lesion and pain and temperature loss occurring contralateral.

Bulbar lesion: Lesions mostly related to the medulla that disrupts cranial nerve functions.

Bulbar palsy: Facial, lingual, and pharyngeal paralysis secondary to the involvement of the motor nuclei in the medulla, which has a profound impact on motor speech and swallowing.

Calcarine fissure: Located on the midsagittal surface of the occipital lobe, it separates the primary visual cortex into lower and upper opercula.

Callosal sulcus: Midsagittally located sulcus that separates the corpus callosum and cingulate gyrus.

Caloric stimulation test: Test of vestibular function that involves irrigating the external auditory canal to evaluate the functioning of the labyrinth. See Bárány caloric test.

Canal of Schlemm: Venous duct of the eye that drains the aqueous humor from anterior chamber of the eyeball. Its impaired drainage results in glaucoma.

Capillary: Terminal branches of arteries that supply blood to the brain.

Carbamazepine (Tegretol): An antiepileptic drug.

Cardiac muscle: Striated muscle fibers (cells) that form the wall of the heart. Stimulated by an intrinsic conduction system and autonomic motor neurons.

Cardiac output (CO): The measured volume of blood pumped from one ventricle of the heart in 1 minute, sending about 5.2 L/min.

Carotid endarterectomy: Surgical procedure to remove occlusive sclerotic plaques through an incision in the internal carotid artery.

Carotid sinus: A dilated region of the internal carotid artery containing receptors of the vagus (CNX) nerve that monitor blood flow and pressure.

Carotid vascular system: System formed by the internal carotid artery that supplies blood to the brain by dividing into the middle and anterior cerebral arteries.

Carpal tunnel syndrome: Pain and paresthesia of the hand caused by an entrapment of the median nerve.

Catabolism: Metabolic breakdown of complex substances into simpler substances, such as food digestion and oxidation of nutrient molecules for energy.

Cataract: Age-induced formation of nontransparent fibrous protein that affects vision by clouding the lens.

Catastrophic reaction: Uncontrollable emotional behaviors and psychological reactions that generally result from traumatic experiences and shocking accidents. These behaviors are characterized by crying, screaming, and depression.

Catecholamine: Group of neurotransmitters that includes epinephrine, norepinephrine, and dopamine.

Cauda equina: Bundle of spinal nerve roots that arise from the lumbosacral region and run through the lumbar cistern before exiting the vertebral canal.

Caudal: Toward back of brain or tail of the spinal cord.

Central (penetrating) arteries: Smaller arteries that supply blood to the subcortical structures.

Central canal: Narrow duct connecting the fourth ventricle with the lumbar cistern.

Central gray: Reticular core of nuclei around the cerebral aqueduct.

Central nervous system: Consisting of the brain and spinal cord. The CNS integrates all incoming and outgoing information and generates appropriate responses.

Central sulcus: Obliquely descending sulcus on the lateral surface of brain, marking the boundary between the frontal and parietal lobes.

Central visual pathways: Visual pathway from the retina to the primary visual cortex in the occipital lobe.

Cerebellar peduncles: Three pairs of fiber tracts that connect the cerebellum with the brainstem.

Cerebellar signs: Mostly ipsilateral symptoms of asynergia, ataxia, and/or action tremor.

Cerebral aqueduct (iter): Narrow ventricular passage in the midbrain that connects the third and fourth ventricles. Also called the aqueduct of Sylvius.

Cerebral cortex: Sheet of six-layered gray matter that covers the cerebral hemispheres.

Cerebral dominance: Brain's lateralized ability to exercise greater influence on a function. Usually refers to left hemispheric superiority for processing language.

Cerebral hemispheres: Bilaterally located parts of the cerebrum connected by the corpus callosum. Each hemisphere is made up of the cerebral cortex and deep-lying structures (basal ganglia, thalamus. and limbic structures).

Cerebral palsy: Group of motor disorders, characterized by muscle paralysis, weakness, and incoordination, caused by damage to motor areas of the brain during fetal life, birth, or infancy.

Cerebral veins: Venous network that collects circulated blood from the cortical and subcortical arteries and empties it into the sinus system.

Cerebrospinal fluid: Clear fluid produced in ventricular cavity that protects the CNS by forming a cushion in the subarachnoid space around the brain and spinal cord.

Cerebrovascular accident (CVA; stroke): Interruption of the blood supply to brain tissue resulting in neurologic symptoms.

Cerebrum: The cerebral hemispheres connected by the corpus callosum.

Chemotherapy: Chemical treatment of a disease, usually cancer.

Chief sensory nucleus: As the primary trigeminal nucleus in the pons, it mediates fine discriminative touch from the face, head, and neck.

Cholesterol: Fatlike substance abundantly found in food rich in animal fat and biles. Circulates in the blood plasma in various densities and plays a role in the pathogenesis of atheroma. There are two types: high-density lipoproteins (the good cholesterol) and low-density lipoproteins (the bad cholesterol).

Cholinergic: Pertaining to the cell that secrete acetylcholine in the nervous system and in body tissues.

Chorea: Rhythmic involuntary movements predominantly of distal extremities and muscles of the face, neck, tongue, and pharynx. Neostriatum is the suspected site of lesion.

Chorion: Fetal membrane enclosing the embryo. It also forms part of the placenta and is highly active and functional.

Choroid: Middle vascular coat of the eyeball that is the source of vascular supply to the sclera and outer retina.

Choroid plexus: Invaginated in the ventricles, the Pia–capillary network responsible for secreting the cerebrospinal fluid.

Chromatolysis: Cellular changes marked by swelling, dissolution of cellular organelles (specifically Nissl bodies), and shifting of the nucleus from its central position to the periphery in response to injury.

Chromosomal nondisjunction: Error in the separation of homologous chromosomes during anaphase of gametogenesis.

Chromosome: One of 46 small, dark-staining strands of condensed chromatin (DNA) located within the nucleus of a human diploid (2n) cell during cell division.

Chronic symptoms: Clinical symptoms developing and persisting over months to years.

Ciliary body: Parasympathetically regulated ocular muscles controlling lens shape and thus its refractive power.

Ciliary ganglion: Parasympathetic ganglion of the oculomotor nerve (CN III) responsible for regulating the ciliary muscle (for lens accommodation) and the sphincter muscle of the iris (for papillary constriction) with its postganglionic fibers.

Ciliary muscle: Muscle that regulates the refractive power of the lens in visual accommodation.

Cingulate gyrus: Limbic–cortical structure that serves emotional, somatic, and autonomic functions.

Cingulum: Association of limbic fiber bundle located under the cingulate gyrus that connects the medial, frontal, and parietal cortices with the temporal cortex.

Circadian rhythm: Biological rhythm based on a 24-hour cycle and controlled by the internal clock mechanism.

Circle of Willis: Arterial circle at the base of the brain that forms a major anastomotic point by connecting the carotid system with the vertebrobasilar system.

Clasp-knife spasticity: Increased resistance by the extensor muscles that gives way suddenly to an extension of continued pressure. This rigidity is the result of an exaggeration of the stretch reflex and is seen in spastic hemiplegia (upper motor neuron syndrome).

Claustrum: Subcortically located gray structure which is a part of the basal ganglia.***

Cleavage: Progressive mitotic division of the fertilized ovum.

Climbing fibers: Cerebellar afferent fibers (olivocerebellar projections) that directly activate Purkinje cells.

Coagulation: Process of blood clot formation.

Cochlea: Fluid-filled and spirally coiled structure that contains the organ of Corti, the sensory end organ of hearing.

Coelom: Body cavity containing the visceral organs, such as the heart, lungs, and intestines.

Cogwheel rigidity: Rhythmic interruption of resistance in a hypertonic muscle during passive manipulation, a clinical characteristics of Parkinson disease.

Colic: Painful spasmodic movement in any hollow internal tube mostly involving the abdomen.

Collateral circulation: Provision of an alternate blood flow via an anastomosis to a brain region that has lost its blood supply.

Collateral trigone: Wider posterior ventricular region from which the lateral ventricles diverge into temporal and occipital horns.

Color blindness: X-linked genetic condition in which perception of one or more colors is impaired.

Coma: State of profound unconsciousness in which the patient does not respond to sensory stimuli. It is usually seen in patients with TBI and with cerebral toxicity.

Commissural fibers: Association fibers that travel across the midline and connect the cerebral hemispheres.

Commissurotomy: surgical procedure that separates both hemispheres by dividing the corpus callosum, mostly undertaken to control the spread of epilepsy from one affected hemisphere to the other intact one.

Computerized tomography (CT): X-ray brain-imaging technique that provides cross-sectional images of the live brain and body in different planes.

Concave lens: Lens type used for correcting the refractive error in myopia (nearsightedness) by enlarging the focal length for the far vision.

Conceptus: Developing human along with its membranes. Term can be applied to any developmental stage from zygote through birth.

Concussion: Brain injury associated with a brief loss of consciousness in absence of any visible structural damage of cortical tissue.

Conduction aphasia: Type of aphasia associated with arcuate fasciculus lesion and characterized by disproportionately impaired verbal repetition with near-normal comprehension and comparatively good verbal expression.

Conductive hearing loss: Hearing loss that results from an interrupted transmission of sound through the outer or middle ear to the cochlea.

Cones: Retinal cells responsible for the highest visual acuity and color discrimination.

Confused language: Linguistically vague use of language indicating cognitive impairment as a result of brain damage. It is marked by slowed thinking, limited processing, and reduced integration of information mostly involving the right nondominant hemisphere or as a result of impaired consciousness.

Conjugate eye movements: Simultaneous movement of the eyes in the same direction, which is important for focusing and reading. In disconjugate movements, both eyes do not move together to one direction, resulting in strabismus and double vision.

Consciousness: State of wakefulness with intact feedback between the cerebral cortex and reticular activating system in which an individual is fully aware, and oriented.

Consensual response: Pupillary contraction in one eye in response to light exposure in the other eye.

Contralateral: The side opposite to the location of a lesion, to the location of a stimulus source, or to the location of a cortical motor control area.

Contusion: Injury characterized by a bruise and tissue damage under unbroken skin.

Conus medullaris: Terminal point of the spinal cord.

Convex lens: Lens type with an elevated surface used to correct refractive errors by shortening the focal length in hyperopia (farsightedness).

Convolution: Elevations forming the surface of the cerebral hemispheres, also called gyrus (pl. gyri).

Cordotomy: Surgical procedure used for sectioning a spinal tract usually for an intractable pain.

Cornea: Nonvascular, transparent outermost fibrous coat of the eye through which the iris can be seen.

Corona radiata: Crown-shaped, fanned sensorimotor fibers located above the internal capsule.

Coronal: Vertical section dividing the brain into front and back.

Coronary artery disease (CAD): Condition in which atherosclerotic plaque narrows the coronary arteries, reducing the blood flow to the heart muscles.

Corpora quadrigemina: Four egg-shaped structures (inferior and superior colliculi) in the dorsal midbrain (Tectum) that serve as reflex centers for vision and audition.

Corpus callosum: Largest bundle of axonal fibers that interconnects the cortex of the cerebral hemispheres, which consists of four parts: rostrum, genu, body, and splenium.

Corpus striatum: See STRIATUM.

Cortex: Six-layered collection of nerve cells that forms the external surface of the brain.

Cortical blindness: Neurologic syndrome characterized by blindness for shapes and patterns with preserved ability to distinguish light from dark, which is usually associated with bilateral damage to the visual cortex.

Corticobulbar fibers: See CORTICONUCLEAR FIBERS.

Corticonuclear fibers: Short axonal projections descending from the motor cortex and synapsing on the brainstem motor cranial nerve nuclei. This tract serves motor speech functions by innervating the musculature of the face, tongue, and jaws.

Corticospinal fibers: Long axonal projections fibers, also called pyramidal fibers, originating in the motor cortex and descending to terminate on spinal motor nuclei. This tract regulates the motor control of skeletal muscles.

Cortisol: Steroid hormone released by the adrenal cortex that inhibits the immune system and mobilizes energy.

Cranial nerves: The 12 pairs of nerves in the peripheral nervous system that innervate buccofacial muscles and mediate sensations of vision, smell, and touch from face.

Craniosacral outflow: Parasympathetic preganglionic neurons with their cell bodies located in the brainstem and in the lateral gray matter of the sacral portion of the spinal cord.

Craniosacral system: Parasympathetic division of the autonomic nervous system with preganglionic cell bodies located in the brainstem and in the lateral gray matter of the sacral portion of the spinal cord. Concerned with conserving bodily energy.

Craniotomy: Surgical procedure used to open the skull for removing pathologic tissue from the brain.

Cranium: Skeleton of the skull that protects the brain.

Cranium bifidum: Embryologic malformation marked by absence of cranial bone fusion leading to herniation of the meninges and cortex.

Cremasteric reflex: Retraction of the scrotum and testicle on stroking the skin of the inner thigh. Absence of this reflex indicates a pyramidal tract lesion (upper motor neuron).

Creutzfeldt–Jakob disease: Neurologic disorder marked by an ataxia, abnormalities of gait and speech, mood changes, cognitive impairments, seizures, and myoclonus. Caused by an infectious agent, such as the spongiform encephalopathies of animals.

Cristae: Vestibular sensory hair cells embedded in a gelatinous mass that project into the ampulla of each of the three semicircular canals.

Critical period: Important developmental period when stimulation and environmental input are capable of modifying the neuronal circuitry in the brain. This period may have different durations for different brain regions and different functions.

Crossed extension reflex: Withdrawal of a limb in response to painful stimuli with the extension of opposite side lower extremities.

Crossed hemiplegia: See ALTERNATING HEMIPLEGIA

Crus cerebri (pes pedunculi): Cortical pyramidal fiber tracts passing through the brainstem on their way to the lower motor neurons in the brainstem and spinal cord.

CT: See COMPUTERIZED TOMOGRAPHY.

CT angiography: Incorporating CT method and traditional angiography, it acquires multiple sectional images of the arteries and veins to reconstruct a three-dimensional view of vascular pathologies.

Cuneocerebellar tract: Spinal fibers mediating unconscious proprioception from the distal upper limbs to the cerebellum.

Cuneus: Occipital lobe region on midsagittal surface.

Cupula: Mass of gelatinous material covering the hair cells of a crista in the ampulla of a semicircular canal that are stimulated when the head moves.

Cutaneous: General sensation from skin.

Cystic cavity: Fluid-filled space outlined by astrocytes in large cortical lesions.

Cytoarchitectonism: Related to the structure, organization, and arrangement of nerve cells in the brain; cytoarchitectural map of brain areas is based on their cellular composition. Numbered Brodmann areas form the most widely used cytoarchitectural map of the brain.

Cytokine: Secreted by various cells, these molecular-weight proteins regulate the intensity and duration of immune response.

Cytoplasm: Substances present within the cellular plasma but external to the nucleus.

Dark adaptation: Physiological process of the retina becoming sensitive to light in dim and dark conditions.

Decerebrate rigidity: Sustained contractions of the extensor muscles that result from lesions in the brainstem reticular formation above the vestibular nucleus.

Decibel (dB): Unit used to measure sound intensity (loudness) in audiological examinations by calculating the ratio between two sound pressures.

Decussation: Crossing over of the midline by the sensorimotor fibers, which is illustrated by the decussation of the pyramidal tract and dorsal-column lemniscal fibers in the caudal medulla.

Deep cerebellar nuclei: Nuclei embedded within the cerebellar medullary region, including the dentate, emboliform, globose, and fastigial nuclei.

Deglutition (swallowing): Reflexive action instigated by the sensory and motor components of multiple cranial nerves along with the reticular participation.

Déjà vu: Sensation of having experienced a feeling or been in a place before.

Delirium: Altered state of consciousness of sudden onset that consists of fluctuating attention, confusion, distractibility, disorientation, disordered thinking, impaired memory, and agitation. Underlying causes include toxicity, structural damage, and metabolic disorders.

Dementia: Acquired progressive impairment of cognitive functions and altered personality subsequent to degenerative brain diseases. It is characterized by failing memory, disorientation, and impaired judgment.

Demyelination: Degenerative condition involving the insulating myelin sheath around the axon commonly seen in multiple sclerosis.

Dendrites: Cellular processes that receive impulses from other cells.

Denervation: Loss of nerve supply to muscles.

Dentate nucleus: Largest of the cerebellar nuclei, which is Involved with limb coordination.

Denticulate ligaments: Fibrous ligaments attaching the spinal cord to surrounding dura mater.

Depolarization: Changes in membrane potentials in which the cellular interior changes from negative (resting potential) to positive.

Depression: An altered mental state characterized by feelings of sadness, despair, low self-esteem, and compulsive thoughts. Subjects also exhibit reduced motor activity, and social withdrawal. Altered functions include loss of appetite, diminished libido, and loss of interest in things considered to be significant before.

Dermatome: Cutaneous body region receiving most of its sensory innervation from one dorsal root ganglion, brainstem segment, or spinal nerve.

Diabetes insipidus: Condition of excessive thirst and urination caused by inadequate secretion of the antidiuretic hormone.

Diabetes mellitus: Disease in which glucose is not adequately oxidized in the body tissue because of insufficient insulin.

Diadochokinesia: Ability to make rapid alternating movements of the limbs.

diaphragm: Primary muscle of inspiration. Also forms a partition between the abdominal and the thoracic cavities.

Dichotic listening: Neurolinguistic testing tool used for evaluating cerebral dominance. It involves simultaneous presentation of auditory stimuli to both ears requiring the subject to report the words, which generally favors the right ear.

Diencephalon: Inner part of the brain that is located beneath the cerebral hemispheres and includes the thalamus and hypothalamus.

Diffusion: Temperature-based movement of molecules from a region of high concentration to an area of low concentration, resulting in a balanced distribution of water molecules in all directions (Brownian motion principle). Equal molecular spread is particularly true in isotropic (water and gases) media.

Diffusion tensor imaging: MRI technique that evaluates the pathology of the white matter in the CNS by measuring movement and directionality of water molecules in the axonal tract.

Diffusion-weighted imaging: Measures the diffusion of water in tissues (apparent diffusion, based on Brownian motion) for constructing an image.

Diopter: Unit used for measuring the refractive power of the eye, which is reciprocally related to the focal distance.

Diplopia: Pathologic condition of double vision by which a single object is seen as being two objects.

Disconnection syndrome: Important neurolinguistic syndrome in which two major functional centers are disconnected from each other rather than damaged directly; thus, the central functions are preserved but the inability to execute a function is secondary to the pathway interruption.

Disjunction: Separation of bivalent chromosomes during anaphase.

Diuresis: Excessive secretion and output of urine. Commonly seen in diabetes mellitus.

Diurnal: Repeating once each 24 hours or a rhythm with a cycle of 24 hours.

DNA (deoxyribonucleic acid): Double-stranded molecular structure containing an organism's genetic information.

Dominant inheritance: Genetic expression mode in which a dysfunctional allele possessed by a parent dominates the second allele from the other parent. Each offspring has a 50% probability of inheriting this dysfunctional gene and the disorder.

Dopamine: One of the inhibitory neurotransmitters secreted by neurons in the brainstem. Its increased and decreased secretion is associated with schizophrenia and Parkinsonism, respectively.

Dorsal: Toward the superior surface of the brain.

Dorsal lemniscal column: Ascending medial lemniscal spinal system fibers mediating postural position sense, fine discriminative touch, and vibration.

Dorsal horn: Region of the spinal cord containing sensory cell bodies.

Dorsal motor nucleus: As a part of the vagus nuclear complex, this nucleus provides preganglionic parasympathetic projections to glands in oral–pharyngeal area.

Dorsal spinocerebellar tract: Spinal projections to the cerebellum mediating unconscious proprioception from the distal lower limbs.

Down syndrome (DS, trisomy 21): Inherited defect characterized by mental retardation, small skull flattened from front to back, short and flat nose, short fingers, and a widened space between the first two digits. Results from an extra copy of chromosome 21.

Dressing apraxia: Failure to dress the left half of the body owing to impaired spatial perception of a garment in relation to the body. Part of right parietal lobe syndrome.

Duchenne muscular dystrophy: Disease of muscular atrophy transmitted through X-linked inheritance.

Dura mater: Outermost and the toughest layer of the three meninges.

Dural sinuses: Network of dura-covered passages for blood in and around the brain.

Dynamic equilibrium: Ability to maintain balance during side-to-side and straight body movements.

Dysarthria: Disorders of motor speech that result from central or peripheral disturbances and affecting muscular control for the articulators.

Dysdiadochokinesia: Impaired ability to undertake rapidly alternating movements subsequent to cerebellar pathologies.

Dyskinesia: movement disorder in which the ability to perform voluntary movements is impaired by the presence of involuntary movements.

Dyslexia: Acquired impaired ability to read and comprehend written information subsequent to brain damage.

Dysmetria: Error in the judgment of a movement's range and distance to the target, which is associated with cerebellar lesions.

Dysphagia: Difficulty in swallowing.

Dystonia: Series of abnormally sustained postures and slow jerky movements mostly involving the trunk, neck, and proximal limbs.

Ectoderm: Outermost cellular layer of the three-layered embryo.

Edinger–Westphal nucleus: Visceral nucleus of the oculomotor nerve (cranial nerve III), which regulates ciliary muscles (lens accommodation) and iris muscle (papillary light reflex).

Edward syndrome: A trisomy of the 18th chromosome characterized by mental retardation, malformed ears, small mandible, cardiac defects, and short sternum.

Efferent: Axonal fibers that mediate nerve impulses away from the central nervous system and cell body.

Electroencephalography: Technique that records normal and abnormal electrical activity from the brain. It is primarily used to evaluate abnormal electric discharges in seizure disorders.

Electromyography: Visual record of muscle electrical activity during rest and spontaneous movements. It is used to determine causes of muscular weakness, paralysis, and involuntary twitching.

Emboliform nucleus: Located in the white substance of the cerebellum, this nucleus is involved with the processing of afferents from the spinal cord before sending the efferents to the motor cortex.

Embolism: Blocking of a smaller artery by a sclerotic tissue (embolus), which is detached from atherosclerotic plaque.

Embryoblast: Inner cell mass that gives rise to the embryo.

Embryonic (or animal) pole: Region of the blastocyst with inner cell mass; the opposite pole is abembryonic (vegetal) pole.

Emmetropia: Normal vision in which light rays from near and distant objects converge on the retina.

Encapsulated endings: Ovoid fluid-filled receptors with multiple layers that are highly sensitive to deformation but also highly adapting.

Encephalitis: Condition of brain inflammation, which is caused by viral or bacterial infection and is characterized by fever, stiff neck, and headache.

Encephalopathy: Dysfunction of the brain because of degenerative or structural changes in the brain.

Endarterectomy (carotid): Surgical procedure used for removing arterial plaque formed by an atheroma deposit along with the diseased arterial lining of the walls in the carotid artery. Performed if the artery is >70% blocked.

Endoderm: Innermost of the three primary germ layers.

Endolymph: Extracellular fluid that fills the semicircular canals, utricle, and saccule.

Endoneurium: Layer of connective tissue that wraps around axons in the peripheral nervous system.

Endorphins: One of the peptides in the brain that is concerned with pain and has similar effects as morphine.

Endothelial cells: Layer of cells lining the blood vessels.

Enkephalin: Neurotransmitter with projections in the basal ganglia and associated structures participating in controlling pain.

Enteric nervous system: Part of the autonomic nervous system regulating intestinal activity.

Ependymal cells: Layer of cells that lines the interior surface of the ventricular cavity and the central canal.

Epiblast: Embryonic germ layer on the dorsal aspect of the bilaminar disk that gives rise to ectoderm, neuroectoderm, and mesoderm.

Epicritic: Fine discriminative touch that includes two-point touch, stereognosis, and graphesthesia.

Epidural space: Potential space between the dura mater and the bone; this space is apparent in pathologic conditions.

Epilepsy: Sensory, motor, cognitive, and affective disorder with some altered consciousness that results from abnormal electric discharges in the brain.

Epinephrine (adrenaline): Important reticular formation catecholamine neurotransmitter that is synthesized from norepinephrine.

Epineurium: Connective tissue sheath that surrounds a nerve in the peripheral nervous system.

Epithalamus: Part of the thalamus consisting of posteriorly located pineal gland and habenular nucleus.

Equilibrium: State of body balance in space. Dynamic equilibrium maintains balance when moving. Static equilibrium maintains balance in a relatively stationary (nonmovement) state.

Estrogen: Female sex hormones that promote development of sex characteristics.

Etiology: Study of the causes of a disease.

Euploid: Exact multiple of haploid number of chromosomes.

Eustachian tube: Duct that connects the middle ear with the nasopharynx; it equalizes air pressure on both sides of tympanic membrane (eardrum).

Event-related potentials: Recording of brain electrical activity evoked in response to a controlled somatic, visual, or auditory stimulus.

Excitatory postsynaptic potential: Impulses that activate the postsynaptic cell to generate an action potential.

Expanded tip endings (receptors with): Receptors with expanded tips. Slow-transmitting and moderately adapting mechanoreceptors.

Expiration: Physiologic process of expelling air from the lungs. Also called exhalation.

Extension: Movement that straightens a limb.

Extensor: Muscle that causes limb extension by contraction.

External capsule: Slender white fiber bundle located immediately lateral to the putamen.

Extracellular fluid (ECF): Fluid outside body cells, similar to interstitial fluid.

Extradural: Referring to the location of pathology external to the dura mater.

Extraembryonic: Derived from a trophoblast.

Extrafusal fibers: Contractile muscle fibers that make up the bulk of a skeletal muscle.

Extrapyramidal pathways: Motor tract fibers that convey motor information from the brain down to the spinal cord and originate from the basal ganglia subthalamic nucleus, and substantia nigra.

Facial nerve: Cranial nerve VII, which is responsible for controlling all the muscles of facial expression, taste from the anterior two-thirds of the tongue, and secretory regulation of glands.

Falx cerebelli: Triangular-shaped vertical extension from tentorial cerebelli that separates the cerebellar hemispheres.

Falx cerebri: Large, sickle-shaped extension of dura between the cerebral hemispheres.

Far point: Point from which light rays originate.

Fasciculation: Involuntary contractions of groups (fasciculi) of muscle fibers from hyperexcitability of motor units.

Fasciculus (fasciculi): Bundle of nerve fibers that originate from a common source, terminate at a common point, and mediate a common function.

Fasciculus cuneatus: Sensory fibers carrying sensations of fine discriminative touch from the upper half of the body.

Fasciculus gracilis: Fibers carrying sensations of fine discriminative touch from the lower body.

Fastigial nucleus: Cerebellar nucleus connected to the vestibular system, which plays a role in equilibrium.

Febrile seizure: Seizure activity, lasting less than a few minutes that is associated with fever and is commonly seen in infants.

Fertilization: Penetration of a secondary oocyte by a sperm cell, resulting in a gamete.

Fetal alcohol syndrome (FAS): Refers to the effects of intrauterine exposure to alcohol on a fetus, resulting in retarded growth and limited cognitive skills subsequent to a reduced oxygen supply to the brain.

Fetus: Developing organism in utero from the beginning of the third month to birth.

Fibrillation: Spontaneous twitch of individual muscle fibers.

Fields of Forel (H fields): Prerubral region through which various basal ganglia projections pass before terminating in the thalamus.

Filum terminale: Fibrous extension of the spinal cord attached to the coccyx.

Fissure: Groove region bordering the gyri on the brain surface, also called sulcus (pl. sulci).

Flaccid: Weakened muscle with less than normal tone, which is a lower motor neuron symptom.

Flexion: Muscle movement that bends a limb.

Flexor: Muscle that contracts to cause flexion.

Flocculi (flocculonodular lobe): Oldest portion of the cerebellum that has a role in equilibrium.

Focal length: Distance between the lens and the point where light rays converge to form a focused image on the retina.

Focal point: Retinal point at which light rays converge for focusing.

Foramen: Opening or aperture.

Foramen magnum: Opening in the base of the skull through which the caudal end of the brainstem exits to connect with the spinal cord.

Foramen of Magendie: Medial aperture that releases cerebrospinal fluid from the fourth ventricle to the subarachnoid space.

Foramina of Luschka: Two laterally located apertures that release cerebrospinal fluid from the fourth ventricle to the subarachnoid space.

Forebrain: Brain (telencephalon and diencephalon) region that is derived from the rostral embryonic brain.

Fornix: Bundle of fibers that mediates two-way connections among the hypothalamus, septum, and hippocampus. Important in visceral functions.

Fourth ventricle: Cerebrospinal fluid–filled cavity lying between the cerebellum and the medulla oblongata and pons.

Fovea: Dipped area in the macula lutea. Site of central fixation, which is responsible for sharp vision.

Fragile X syndrome: X-linked recessive syndrome characterized by mental retardation, atypical facial features (long and narrow face with large ears, a prominent mandibular symphysis, and a high-arched palate), and macroorchidism (abnormally large testes).

Free nerve endings: Small and slowly conducting mechanoreceptors, which mediate pain and temperature.

Friedreich ataxia: Genetic condition of an autosomal-recessive trait, which involves the degeneration of the spinocerebellar tract and is characterized by skeletal deformations, limb weakness, and loss of vibration and position sense.

Frontal lobe syndrome (pseudopsychopathic behavior): Disorder of executive functions characterized by impairments of cognitive functions (attention, memory, reasoning, thinking, planning, self-monitoring, and purposeful activity) and decision making.

Frontotemporal dementia: Degenerative condition of the frontal and temporal lobes that results in personality changes, behavioral symptoms, and cognitive impairments. Also called Pick disease.

Functional MRI: Neuroimaging technique that measures cortical neuronal activity (increased blood flow to the cortical area) in response to specific somatosensory or linguistic tasks.

Functional plasticity: Capability of the brain to reorganize functionally after undergoing a pathologic condition.

GABAergic neurons: Inhibitory neurotransmitter neurons in the basal ganglia. Its deficiency leads to Huntington chorea.

Gag reflex: Brainstem-mediated reflex: from the glossopharyngeal nerve (cranial nerve IX) and vagus nerve (cranial nerve X): involving vomiting involuntarily, which is triggered by a touch on the posterior one-third of the tongue, the pharynx, or the soft palate.

γ-aminobutyric acid (GABA): Major inhibitory neurotransmitter of the brain synthesized from glutamate. Its deficiency in the striatum is implicated with Huntington chorea.

γ-motor neurons: Slow-conducting, small spinal motor neurons that supply intrafusal muscle fibers.

Gametes: Mature male and female sex cells containing haploid number of chromosomes.

Gametogenesis: Process through which mature male and female sex cells develop to fertilize.

Ganglion (pl. ganglia): Cluster of cell bodies in the peripheral nervous system.

Gene expression: Process that converts gene-coded information into the operating of a cell and structure.

Gene mutation: Any spontaneous heritable changes in the sequencing of DNA elements.

General functions: Touch, pain, and temperature information processed by general receptors.

General visceral efferent (GVE) fibers: Axonal fibers mediating autonomic commands to visceral structures.

Generalized seizure: Extensive and synchronized electrical activity in nerve cells that spreads to the entire brain.

Genes: Units of heredity located at a fixed position on a particular chromosome.

Genetics: Discipline concerned with the modes and consequences of hereditary transmission of human traits.

Geniculate bodies: Thalamic relay nuclei related to vision (lateral geniculate body) and audition (medial geniculate body).

Geniculocalcarine fibers (optic radiations): Visual fibers radiating from the geniculate body to the primary visual cortex in the occipital lobe.

Genome: Complete DNA sequence containing entire genetic information of an individual or a species.

Genotype: Genetic makeup of an individual.

Genu: Angular rostral region of the corpus callosum.

Glaucoma: Eye disease characterized by increased intraocular pressure in the anterior cavity caused by poor absorption of aqueous humor. If not treated causes optic nerve atrophy and blindness.

Glia cells: Association cells (astroglia, microglia, and oligodendroglia) in the nervous system that serve as supportive connective tissue.

Global aphasia: Aphasia characterized by profound impairment of language functions across all modalities.

Globose nucleus: Cerebellar nucleus participating in the coordination of skilled movements.

Globus pallidus: Part of the basal ganglia involved with motor activity.

Glossopharyngeal nerve: Cranial nerve IX, which has sensorimotor functions involving the oral and pharyngeal cavities.

Golgi complex: Microscopic organelle in the cytoplasm of cells responsible for processing, sorting, packaging, and delivering proteins and lipids to the plasma membrane.

Golgi tendon organ: Specialized receptive endings sensitive to muscle tension and interdigitated among the extrafusal muscle fibers in muscle tendons.

Gonadotropic: Hormones secreted in the anterior pituitary gland (adenohypophysis) that affect differential growth and function of sex gland cells.

Grand mal (tonic–clonic) seizure: Seizure disorder characterized by loss of consciousness and tonic convulsions, electric discharges originating from the cortex, basal ganglia, brainstem and/or reticular formation, repeated hyperextension of the body, and breath-holding spells resulting in cyanosis (skin discoloration owing deficient oxygenation of the blood).

Graphesthesia: Discriminative sensory ability used to recognize the outline of letters, words, or symbols written on the skin surface.

Gray matter: Term used for the collection of cell bodies in the central nervous system.

gray ramus communicans: Short nerve containing postganglionic sympathetic fibers that extend by way of the gray ramus to a spinal nerve and then to the periphery to supply smooth muscle in the blood vessels, arrector pili muscles, and sweat glands.

Guillain-Barré syndrome: Autoimmune demyelinating polyneuropathy (AIDP) affecting the PNS marked by an ascending pattern of weakness beginning in the feet and migrating towards the trunk.

Gyrus: Elevated cortical regions between sulci and fissures.

Haploid: Half of the normal number of chromosomes, which is the case with gametes.

Hearing level (HL): Individual threshold sensitivity to pure tone stimuli.

Hearing tests: Pure tone stimuli used to evaluate hearing thresholds.

Helicotrema: End region of the cochlea that connects the scala vestibuli to the scala tympani.

Hematoma: Accumulated mass of extravasated blood, usually located in a potential space like subdural or extradural.

Hemianesthesia: Loss of pain and touch sensation on one side of the body.

Hemianopsia: Loss of vision in half of the visual fields.

Hemiballism: Violent swinging movements on one side of the body associated with damage hemiparesis: Mild weakness of one side of the body to the subthalamic nucleus.

Hemiplegia: Paralysis of one side of the body involving both the upper and the lower limbs.

Hemophilia: Hereditary blood disorder characterized by deficient production of blood clotting factors and resulting in excessive bleeding.

Hemorrhage: Discharging of blood from a ruptured artery.

Hepatolenticular degeneration (Wilson disease): Disease resulting from degenerative changes in the basal ganglia and liver owing to a metabolic disorder. Clinically characterized by dysarthria and involuntary movement.

Herpes Zoster: Viral infection (herpesvirus), which is characterized by an eruption on one side of the body along the course of a nerve due to inflammation of ganglia and nerve roots.

Heschl gyri (gyri of Heschl): Refers to short and oblique convolutions in the lateral sulcus that form the primary auditory cortex.

High-altitude sickness: Condition characterized by headache, fatigue, insomnia, shortness of breath, nausea, and dizziness caused by decreased atmospheric levels of oxygen at high altitude.

High blood pressure (hypertension): Defined as a systolic pressure above 140 mm Hg or a diastolic pressure above 90 mm Hg, the elevated blood pressure is a common cause of vascular diseases including stroke.

Hippocampal gyrus: Long convolution that overlies the hippocampus and covers the medial ventral surface of the temporal lobe.

Hippocampus (hippocampal formation): Limbic structure bordering the lateral ventricle inferior horns in the temporal lobe. Thought to be related to the consolidation of memory.

Histology: Microscopic study of tissue structures.

Homeostasis: Optimal state of bodily equilibrium involving the chemical composition of fluids and tissues that is conductive to normal body functioning.

Homologous chromosomes: Two chromosomes that belong to a pair.

Homonymous hemianopia: Loss of vision in same visual fields for both eyes.

Homonymous left inferior quadrantanopsia: Blindness involving the left inferior quarters of the visual field in both eyes.

Homonymous left superior quadrantanopsia: Blindness involving the left superior quarters of the visual field in both eyes.

Homozygous: Possessing a pair of similar alleles on homologous chromosomes for a particular gene.

Homunculus: Representation of the body in the sensorimotor cortex.

Hormones: Chemical substances that originate in an organ and regulate important body activities.

Horner syndrome: Neurologic condition characterized by ptosis (unilateral eyelid dropping), miosis (pupil contraction), and anhidrosis (diminished perspiration) on the ipsilateral side of the forehead. Associated with a lesion of the cervical sympathetic chain or its central projections.

Human growth hormone (hGH): Hormone secreted by the anterior pituitary gland that stimulates growth of body tissues, especially skeletal and muscular.

Huntington chorea: Progressive degenerative condition of dominant inheritance characterized by involuntary movements, cognitive deficits, and dysarthric speech.

Hydrocele: Fluid-containing sac or tumor.

Hydrocephalus: Accumulation of cerebrospinal fluid in the brain ventricles secondary to its impaired absorption.

Hypalgesia: Increased threshold for pain resulting in a decreased sensitivity to pain.

Hyperacusia: Abnormal hearing sensitivity where normal sounds seem very loud.

Hyperalgesia: Decreased threshold for pain marked by increased response to painful stimuli.

Hypercholesterolemia: Excessive amount of cholesterol in the blood.

Hyperglycemia: Metabolic condition, marked by abnormally high blood glucose concentration, associated with frequent urination, increased thirst, and neurological conditions.

Hypermetropia (hyperopia): Optical condition in which light rays focus behind the retina, also called farsightedness.

Hyperparathyroidism: Increased level of parathyroid hormone secretion.

Hyperplasia: Increase in cell number due to an injury.

Hyperpolarization: Increased internal negativity across a cell membrane causing changes in voltage.

Hypersecretion: Overactivity of glands resulting in excessive secretion.

Hypersomnia: Excessive sleep, usually during normal waking hours.

Hypertrophy: Increase in the size of cells or organs.

Hypoblast: Embryonic germ layer on ventral aspect of the bilaminar disk that gives rise to endoderm.

Hypoglossal nerve: Cranial nerve XII, which controls tongue movements.

Hypoglycemia: Metabolic condition of lower blood sugar level is a common cause of neurological and autonomic dysfunctions including sweating, trembling, anxiety, dizziness, confusion, and fatigue.

Hypokinesia: Slow or limited movements.

Hypokinetic dysarthria: Type of dysarthric speech characterized by limited and slow movement. Associated with Parkinson disease.

Hyponatremia: Low level of serum sodium.

Hypophysis: Consisting of two (anterior and posterior) lobes, the pituitary gland controls the hormonal secretion.

Hyporeflexia: Diminished or reduced strength of a reflexive response of a skeletal muscle that results from pathology of the lower motor neuron or reduced lower motor neuron excitability.

Hypothalamus: Diencephalic structure, located beneath the thalamus, that secretes hormones and regulates feeding, fighting, and sexual behavior.

Hypothermia: Lowering of body temperature <35°C (95°F). In medical management, it involves a deliberate cooling of the body to slow down metabolism and reduce the oxygen needs of tissues.

Hypotonia: Muscle with reduced tone and lessened resistance to passive movement.

Hypoxemia: Low oxygen level in the arterial blood.

Hypoxia: Lower than normal level of oxygen in body tissues.

Ideomotor apraxia: Inability to carry on skilled purposeful movements to a verbal command secondary to a disconnection between motor and ideational centers.

Idiopathic: Emergence of a disease without an apparent cause.

Immunity: Body's natural power to resist the attack of disease or harmful agents.

Incus: Middle ear bone.

Inertia: Tendency of matter to resist change in motion (If matter is at rest, it remains at rest. If moving, it continues to move until acted on by an external force).

Infarct: Area of damaged tissues caused by insufficient or blocked blood supply.

Inferior cerebellar peduncle: Restiform body. One of the fiber bundles connecting the cerebellum with the brainstem. Mediates spinal and vestibular inputs to the cerebellar hemispheres.

Inferior colliculus: Midbrain structure involved with auditory reflexes and with the transmission of auditory signals to the medial geniculate body of the thalamus.

Inferior longitudinal fasciculus: Represents an intrahemispheric (corticocortical) association pathway connecting temporal lobe to the occipital lobe.

Inferior mesenteric ganglia: Prevertebral sympathetic nucleus.

Inferior olivary nucleus: Medullary structure that mediates spinal and vestibular afferents to the cerebellum.

Inflammation: Edematous response by tissue to an injury.

Infundibular stem: Stalk of the pituitary gland.

Inhibitory postsynaptic potentials: Impulses that inhibit the capacity of a postsynaptic cell to generate an action potential.

Insomnia: Inability to sleep during the night for no apparent reason.

Inspiration: Refers to the drawing of air into the lungs.

Instinctual reflexes: Protective stereotypical motor responses occurring in response to biologic needs.

Insula (isle of Reil): Triangular cortical brain area buried within the lateral sulcus.

Intensity: Amplitude of energy in sound waves that determines loudness.

Intention tremor: Rhythmic pill-rolling movements of fingers associated with cerebellar pathology, which are apparent during voluntary movements.

Intercostal muscles: Muscles located between the ribs.

Interhemispheric: Relating to a structure common to/located between both cerebral hemispheres.

Interhemispheric (longitudinal) fissure: Long vertical fissure that marks the medial boundary of the cerebral hemispheres.

Internal arcuate fibers: Crossing fibers of the dorsal lemniscal system at the medulla that form the medial lemniscus.

Internal capsule: Collection of concentrated ascending and descending fibers at the diencephalic level, which consist of three parts: the genu, internal, and external capsules.

Internal medullary lamina: Vertical layer of the white matter that divides the thalamus.

Interneurons: Spinal association neurons that interconnect other nerve cells and function to modify the lower motor neuron response via facilitation or inhibition.

Interpeduncular fossa: Area located on the inferior surface of the midbrain between the bilaterally located crus cerebri.

Interstitial fluid: Extracellular fluid that fills the spaces between the cells of tissues and regulates the internal environment of the body.

Interventricular foramen of Monro: Opening that connects the lateral ventricles in the forebrain with a single third ventricle in the midbrain.

Intracerebral: Referring to the location of pathology within the cerebrum.

Intracranial pressure: Pressure located within the cranium or skull, which is caused by space-occupying lesions in the brain.

Intrafusal fibers: Specialized skeletal muscle fibers contained in the encapsulated muscle stretch receptor, called a muscle spindle, that extend parallel to the extrafusal fibers. Innervated by small γ-motor neurons, their contraction modifies the responsiveness of the stretch receptor endings.

Intrahemispheric: Related to structures within one hemisphere.

Intralaminar centromedianum nucleus: Largest of the intralaminar nuclei in the thalamus and has extensive afferents and efferents to the brain and brainstem.

Ion: Electrically charged atoms

Ion selectivity: Membrane permeability restricted to only selected ions.

Ionic equilibrium: Electrical potential difference that regulates the ionic concentration gradient across the cell membrane.

Ipsilateral: The same side of the CNS with reference to a given point; it is best illustrated by the lesion and its effects being on the same side of the body.

Iris: Colored contractile fibers that regulate pupil size.

Ischemia: Reduced supply or unavailability of blood for tissue oxygenation owing to hemorrhagic stroke, stenosis, or thrombosis. It affects brain functions by causing cellular death.

Isocortex: See CEREBRAL CORTEX

Isthmus: Narrow passage or tissue strip connecting two larger parts.

Iter: See CEREBRAL AQUEDUCT.

Karyotype: Presentation of an individual's chromosomes arranged in a standard format according to their shapes and sizes.

Kayser–Fleisher ring: Circle formed by the deposition of copper in Descemet's membrane of the cornea, which is a common sign of Wilson disease.

Kinesthesia: Internal awareness of the range and direction of limb movements.

Klinefelter syndrome: Male chromosomal disorder in which the individual has an additional X chromosome (47, XXY); it is characterized by genital abnormalities and mental retardation.

Klüver–Bucy syndrome: Behavioral syndrome that results from bilateral ablation of the amygdala and surrounding temporal tissues; it is characterized by indiscriminate eating, oral exploration, fearlessness, loss of aggression, psychic blindness, and hypersexuality.

Korsakoff syndrome: Syndrome of amnesia, confusion, and memory impairment, which is caused by nutritional deficiency owing to chronic alcoholism. It is also called Korsakoff psychosis, which evolves from untreated Wernicke encephalopathy.

Labyrinth: Interconnecting and communicating bony and membranous ducts in the inner ear, including the semicircular ducts, vestibule, and cochlea.

Labyrinthine disease: Inner ear dysfunctions characterized by deafness, tinnitus, vertigo, nausea, and vomiting.

Labyrinthitis: Inflammatory condition of the inner ear clinically characterized by hearing impairment and vertigo.

Lacrimal: Related to tears.

Lacrimal gland: Secretory cells in the orbit responsible for the secretion of tears.

Lacunar stroke: Small multiple strokes in the thalamus and basal ganglia usually as a result of hypertension.

Lamina terminalis (lamina terminalis hypothalami): Thin plate derived from telencephalon. It is the rostral end of former neural tube. Develops into the anterior wall of the third ventricle of the cerebrum.

Lateral corticospinal tract: Represents the spinal location of the crossed fibers of the corticospinal tract.

Lateral (sylvian) fissure: Laterally located, a deep cortical fissure that separates the temporal lobe from the frontal and parietal lobes and serves as an important anatomical landmark.

Lateral geniculate body: Thalamic nucleus responsible for the transmission of visual information to the cortex.

Lateral lemniscus: Fibers projecting auditory impulses between the superior olivary nucleus and the inferior colliculus.

Lateral spinothalamic tract: Ascending fiber bundle that mediates the sensation of pain and temperature to the brain.

Lateral ventricle: Largest of the ventricular cavities in the cerebral hemispheres.

Laterality: Hemispheric superiority for serving language.

Lemniscus: Collection of nerve fibers carrying similar information.

Lens: Transparent organ constructed of proteins that refracts light rays on the retina.

Lenticular fasciculus: Fiber bundle that transmits basal ganglia projections from the globus pallidus to the thalamus.

Lenticular nucleus: General term for the globus pallidus and putamen.

Leptomeninges: General term for the pia and arachnoid membranes, which are infected in meningitis.

Levator palpebrae fissure: Extraocular muscle that is responsible for raising the upper eyelid.

Light reflex: Constriction of the pupil in response to light, a parasympathetic activity.

Limbic (visceral–emotional) brain: Mammalian portion of the brain responsible for motivation, emotional drive, and instinctual activities.

Limbic lobe: Phylogenetically an older part of the brain that regulates reproductive behavior, instinctual reflexes, and vegetative activities.

Limbic system: Visceral structures of the forebrain (dentate gyrus, amygdaloid body, septal nuclei, mammillary bodies, anterior thalamic nucleus, olfactory bulbs, and many bundles of myelinated axons) that regulate emotion and behavior.

Lissauer tract: Pain- and temperature-mediating fibers of the dorsolateral fasciculus that travel up or down a few segments of the spinal cord before penetrating the dorsal gray matter.

Locked-in syndrome: Often confused with coma, this condition of a bilateral basilar infarct results in quadriplegia, facial paralysis, and horizontal ophthalmoplegia; with consciousness and intact comprehension, the patient communicates only using vertical eye movements.

Locus ceruleus: Important reticular formation nucleus in the brainstem that produces norepinephrine and widely projects to different brain areas.

Lower motor neuron (LMN): Motor neurons of cranial nerves and spinal cord which send their axonal projections to the skeletal muscle; the loss of these neurons leads to weakness, twitching of muscle (fasciculation), and the atrophy of muscles.

Lower motor neuron syndrome: Neurological condition of clinical symptoms including flaccid paralysis, hyporeflexia, and muscular atrophy subsequent to a lesion involving spinal or cranial motor neurons and/or their axons.

Lumbar cistern: Enclosed space at the end of the cord containing the cerebrospinal fluid.

Lumbar plexus: Network of interwoven nerve fibers originating from T12–L4 and serving the abdomen, buttocks, and anterior thigh.

Lumbar puncture: Diagnostic procedure that involves removing the cerebrospinal fluid from the lower lumbar section of the vertebral canal for chemical and cellular analyses.

Luminosity curve: Visual representation of the spectral sensitivity of photoreceptors to light rays of various wavelengths.

Macrophage: Phagocytic cell that digests and removes cellular debris in the brain.

Macula: Specialized sensory structures in the vestibular apparatus that contribute to the maintenance of static equilibrium during linear acceleration and deceleration.

Macula lutea: Yellowish area in the posterior retina that contains cones and mediates color vision.

Magnetic resonance angiography (MRA): Used to evaluate the structural integrity of blood vessels. An important diagnostic tool for identifying arterial stenosis, aneurysm, and arteriovenous malformation.

Magnetic resonance imaging (MRI): Imaging technique that uses magnetic activity of the tissue to create clear images of the living brain and body.

Magnetic resonance spectroscopy: MRI application to evaluate the biochemical profile of nerve cells.

Malignant: Spreading and fast-growing tumor that causes death.

Malleus: Middle ear ossicle attached to the tympanic membrane.

Mammillary bodies: Two small, rounded hypothalamic structures posterior to the tuber cinereum that participate in related visceral and memory functions.

Massa intermedia: Crossing fibers that pass through the third ventricle and connect both thalami.

Maturation: Developmental processes through which a cell reaches its full functional potential.

Mechanoreceptors: Sensory receptor responsible for selective stimuli.

Medial forebrain bundle: Important limbic fiber bundle that interconnects the forebrain, limbic structures, hypothalamus, and the midbrain tegmentum and connects to dopaminergic, noradrenergic, and serotonic neurons.

Medial geniculate body: Thalamic nucleus responsible for transmitting auditory information to the primary auditory cortex.

Medial lemniscus pathways: Sensory pathways located in the dorsal third of the spinal cord and mediate epicritic proprioception, discriminative touch, two-point discrimination, pressure, and vibration sensation.

Medial longitudinal fasciculus: Brainstem fiber bundle that runs on each side of the midline in the brainstem beneath the fourth ventricle. It interconnects ocular cranial nerve nuclei with vestibular projections and plays an important role in coordinated head, eye, and body movements.

Medial strabismus: An optical condition in which the eyes do not concurrently point to the same object; this results in diplopia subsequent to the absence of parallelism of the visual axes due to the medial adduction of one paralyzed eye.

Median nerve: Originating from the brachial plexus, it supplies most of the forearm muscles. Esthesiometer-Instrument that is used for determining the discriminative touch sensitivity by touching two points.

Medulla oblongata: Most inferior part of the brainstem.

Medullary respiratory center: Reticular nuclear network in the medulla; that regulates the depth and cyclic nature of breathing.

Medullary reticulospinal tract: Located within the medulla. Projects to the spinal motor neurons and regulates muscle tone.

Meiosis: Cell division process that occurs during the formation of sex cells in which the number of chromosomes is halved.

Meissner corpuscles: Sensory receptors with encapsulated endings mediating the sensation of deep and discriminative touch.

Melanocytes: Pigment-producing cells in the choroid of the eyeball, which increase the clarity of visual perception by absorbing stray light elements.

Membrane: Thin sheet of tissue serving as a covering or as the lining of a cavity.

Membrane potentials: Electric voltages across a cell membrane.

Membranous labyrinth: Arrangement of endolymph-filled cavities that include scalae media of the cochlear duct and the vestibular labyrinth and contain receptive hair cells.

Ménière disease: Chronic condition of the membranous labyrinth. Marked by edema due to an increase in endolymphatic pressure. Characterized by progressive hearing loss, vertigo, and tinnitus.

Meninges: Three protective membranes (dura, arachnoid, and pia) that cover the central nervous system.

Meningitis: Bacterial or viral infection of the central nervous system that causes inflammation in the meningeal membranes of the brain and spinal cord.

Merkel receptors: Receptors with expanded tips mediating touch and temperature.

mesencephalon (midbrain): Midbrain region derived from the vesicle of mesencephalon.

Mesoderm: Middle of the three primary germ layers.

Metabolism: Cellular biochemical activities that include analytical (catabolic) and synthetic (anabolic) reactions that generate energy.

Metaphase: Stage in mitotic cellular division.

Metastasis: Spread of disease from a location in one part of the body to another, as is in the migration of cancerous cells through lymphatics and blood vessels.

Metencephalon: Subdivision of rhombencephalon consisting of the pons and cerebellum.

Meyer loop: Optic fibers of the geniculocalcarine tract radiating through the anterior and lateral temporal lobe before reaching the occipital cortex. The involvement of these fibers results in upper quadrantanopsia.

Microcephaly: Embryologic malformation in which the brain and skull cap are small in comparison to the face, resulting in mental retardation.

Microglia: Small scavenger glia cells that digest and remove cellular debris from the CNS.

Microtubules: Represented as straight protein tubulin that contribute to the cellular skeleton and are responsible for axoplasmic transport.

Micturition: Urination.

Midbrain: Part of the brainstem between the pons and the diencephalon. Also called the mesencephalon.

Middle cerebellar peduncle: Brachium pontis. A bundle of fibers that connects the cerebellum with the basilar pons.

Middle cerebral artery: Large intracranial vessel supplying blood to the entire lateral surface of the brain and parts of the basal ganglia structures.

Middle ear: Air-filled cavity containing three bones (incus, stapes, and malleus) and two muscles (tensor veli palatine and levator veli palatine).

Midsagittal plane: Vertical plane through the midline of the brain or body, dividing it into equal left and right halves.

Millard–Gubler syndrome: Alternating type of hemiplegia marked with contralateral hemiplegia and ipsilateral facial and ocular paralysis.

Minimal confusion state: As a state of altered consciousness, it is marked by a functional and communicative paucity in which the patient retains the ability to undertake short and brief but purposeful communication.

Miosis: Condition of a permanently constricted pupillary aperture.

Mitochondria: Organelle of the cellular cytoplasm containing enzymes providing the principle energy source for the cell.

Mitosis: Cell division process in which the daughter cell receives the identical number and kinds of chromosomes.

Modiolus: Conical bony structure around which the cochlea is wrapped.

Monoamines: Subgroup of small molecular neurotransmitters derived from amino acids.

Monoplegia: Paralysis confined to one limb.

Monosomy: Absence of one chromosome from a homologous pair.

Morula: Tiny sphere of blastomeres.

Mossy fibers: Afferent fibers that include all sensory projections to the cerebellum, except olivocerebellar fibers.

Motion sickness: Vestibular syndrome characterized by the sensation of vertigo, dizziness, nausea, and vomiting. Present when an individual is in motion.

Motion tremor (intention tremor): Oscillatory movements caused by irregular muscle contraction in the case of cerebellar pathology. Present only during an action period as opposed to a resting condition.

Motor cortex: Cortical region containing large Betz cells and consisting of Brodmann area 4, it is involved with control and regulation of voluntary movements.

Motor end plate: Postsynaptic membrane at the neuromuscular junction.

Motor neuron: Located in the anterior horn of the spinal cord. Controls muscle cells and muscle contraction.

Motor unit: Forming a neuronal circuit consisting of an α–lower motor neuron, its axon, myoneural junctions, and innervated muscles. It acts as a unit in that if the lower motor neuron fires, all the muscle cells of the unit fire at the same time.

Movement disorders: Tremor and chronic types of involuntary disorders commonly seen after basal ganglia pathologies.

Multiple sclerosis: Disease of progressive degeneration of the neuronal myelin sheath from an autoimmune disorder in the central nervous system, causing impaired nerve conduction, paresthesia, and disorders of equilibrium, movement, sensation, and vision.

Multipolar cells: Neurons containing many dendrites and one axon.

Muscle spindles: Intramuscular encapsulated receptor apparatus in specialized skeletal (intrafusal) muscle fibers that are sensitive to changes in muscle length.

Muscle tone: Defined by a "steady state of contraction which resists a force in the direction of passive stretch" such as gravitational pull or pull of flexor force from the opposite side of a joint. This is based on normal levels of excitability of the muscle spindles.

Muscles of respiration: Include the diaphragm, abdomen, and intercostals that participate in inspiration and expiration and are controlled by spinal motor neurons.

Muscular dystrophy: Inherited disease of muscle degeneration, characterized by weakness and progressive atrophy of the skeletal muscle. See also DUCHENE'S

Muscular fibrillation: Often seen in tongue muscles, the twitching of a single or a few muscle fibers secondary to the denervation.

Mutation: A spontaneous change in a gene or chromosomal structure.

Myasthenia gravis: Autoimmune neuromuscular disorder that results from growth of antibodies to acetylcholine receptors.

Mydriasis: Dilation of the pupil.

Myelencephalon: Medulla oblongata derived from the myelencephalic division of the rhombencephalon.

Myelin: Sheath of lipid and cell membrane wrapped around an axon and contributes to the speed of impulse transmission.

Myoneural junction: Synapse of an α–lower motor neuron axon on a single skeletal muscle fiber.

Myopathy: Disease of muscles.

Myopia: Refraction error in which light rays converge in front of the retina. Also called nearsightedness.

Myotatic reflex: Reflexive muscle contraction in response to muscle stretch.

Myotome: Muscles innervated by the motor neurons of a single spinal segment.

Narcolepsy: Sleeping disorder characterized by recurring episodes of excessive sleeping in the day and disrupted nocturnal sleep. Frequently accompanied by cataplexy, sleep paralysis, and hallucinations.

Narcotics: Drugs with analgesic effects, which are also used for changing moods and behaviors.

Nasal hemianopsia: Loss of vision in the nasal field of one eye.

Nausea: Sensation of impending vomiting.

Necrosis: Island of dead tissues surrounded by normal areas of tissues.

Neocerebellum: Newer part of the cerebellum concerned with skilled movements such as speech.

Neocortex: Six-layered cerebral cortex found in mammals.

Neologisms: Unrecognizable new word formations of patient's own making found in the acute stages of Wernicke aphasia.

Neoplasm: New and pathologic growth of tissue that can be benign or malignant.

Neostriatum: General term for the basal ganglia referring to the caudate nucleus and putamen.

Nerve(s): One or more bundles of myelinated or unmyelinated fibers in the peripheral nervous system.

Nerve cell: Specialized cell of the nervous system that conducts electrical impulses.

Nerve conduction: Measure of impulse transmission between two points on a nerve for identifying peripheral nerve pathologies.

Nervous system: Collectively refers to the brain, spinal cord, nerves (cranial and spinal), and autonomic ganglia that maintain the vital functions of the body in response to internal and external stimuli.

Neural crest: Segmentally arranged neuroectodermal tissue that separates from the neural tube dorsally before it closes. It develops into elements of the peripheral nervous system and other specialized structures.

Neural plate: Thickened midline plate of neuroectoderm that develops into the neural tube, giving rise to the central nervous system.

Neural tube: Embryologic structure that results from the fusion of neural folds and develops into the brain and spinal cord.

Neuralgia: Pain sensation extending along the course of a nerve.

Neuraxis: Brain and spinal axis.

Neurilemma: Outermost covering of axons formed by Schwann cells in the peripheral nervous system.

Neuritis: Inflammation of nerves from structural irritation or infection.

Neuroblast: Immature cell before cell division.

Neuroembryology: Study of the embryologic origins and development of the nervous system from fertilization to the 8th gestational week of development.

Neurofibrillary tangles: Age-induced twisting of fibers in the soma of nerve cells, often associated with Alzheimer disease. These are also found in the brains of Down syndrome patients.

Neurofibrils: Small fibers within the cytoplasm serving as the channels for intracellular communication among the cytoplasmic organelles.

Neurofilaments: Important components of the cellular skeleton. Serve as channels for intracellular communication.

Neuroglia: Cells associated with the nervous system: including astrocytes, oligodendrocytes, microglia cells, ependymal cells, and neurolemmal (Schwann) cells: responsible for a variety of supportive functions. Also called glial cells.

Neuroleptic: Class of drugs (tranquilizers) used for treating psychoses.

Neuromuscular junction: Myoneural junction marked by the space between the neuron and the muscle.

Neurons: Nerve cell with a cell body and its processes that participate in impulse transmission.

Neuropathy: Nerve disease.

Neuropeptide: Naturally occurring amino acid chain in the nervous system modulating the response of or to a neurotransmitter.

Neurophil: Mature white blood cell that is formed by the myelopoietic tissue found in the bone marrow.

Neuroplasticity: See PLASTICITY

Neurotransmitter: One of a variety of molecules within axon terminals released into the synaptic cleft in response to a nerve impulse and affects the membrane potential of the postsynaptic neuron. Also called a transmitter substance.

Night blindness (nyctalopia): Inability to see at night after a normal period of dark adaptation.

Nissl bodies: Endoplasmic structures in neuronal cell bodies that participate in protein synthesis.

Nociceptors: Receptors sensitive to harmful stimuli such as pain.

Nodes of Ranvier: Intervening space between two internodes (segments) of myelin.

Nodulus: Part of the flocculonodular lobe of the cerebellum. Serves a role in equilibrium.

Nondisjunction: Failure of two homologous chromosomes or two chromatids to dissociate during meiosis. Results in one cell having an extra chromosome and the other cell missing a chromosome.

Non–rapid-eye movement sleep: Stage in sleep characterized by slow and large waves. Marked with some muscle tone and paucity of dreams.

Noradrenergic synapses: Nerve endings in which norepinephrine is released.

Norepinephrine: Catecholamine neurotransmitter (noradrenalin) released by neurons primarily in the pons and medulla. Cells that produce norepinephrine are called noradrenergic cells.

Normal pressure hydrocephalus: Large ventricles with impaired absorbing dynamics of the cerebrospinal fluid. Clinically characterized by dementia and gait disturbances it is seen in elderly patients.

Notochord: Primitive, solid, skeletal structure derived from specialized mesodermal cells. Retained in the intervertebral disk as the nucleus pulposus and lies ventral to the neural tube.

Nuclear bag fibers: Intrafusal sensory fibers mediating dynamic sensory responses of the spindles.

Nuclear chain fibers: Intrafusal sensory fibers mediating static responses of the muscle spindles.

Nucleolus: Located within the nucleus of a cell body, and it contains RNA needed for protein synthesis.

Nucleus: Control center of a nerve cell.

Nucleus ambiguous: Shared by vagus and glossopharyngeal nerves, this cranial motor nucleus controls the muscles of larynx and pharynx.

Nucleus cuneatus: Specialized nerve cells in the caudal region of the medulla oblongata responsible for mediating fine discriminative touch from the upper half of the body.

Nucleus dorsalis of Clarke: Second-order spinal neurons that mediate unconscious proprioception.

Nucleus gracilis: Specialized nerve cells in the caudal medullary region responsible for mediating fine discriminative touch from the lower half of the body.

Nucleus pulposus: Adult remnant of the notochord in the intervertebral disk.

Nystagmus: Oscillatory movement of eyeballs consisting of slow and fast components. Identified according to direction of fast component.

Oblique plane: Section passing through the body or organ at an angle.

Occipitotemporal/fusiform gyrus: Located at the basal surface of the temporal and occipital lobe, this gyrus contributes to the recognition of faces and objects.

Occlusive vascular disease: Vascular diseases characterized by arterial occlusion, such as thrombosis and embolism.

Octonia: Gelatinous mass that incorporates sensory hair cells covered by a thin layer of densely packed calcium carbonate crystals.

Ocular convergence: Directing both eyes to a common focal point for a clear visual perception.

Oculomotor nerve: CN III, which regulates the majority of the ocular muscles except lateral rectus and superior oblique.

Olfactory bulb: Bulb-shaped brain structure that receives input from the olfactory receptor neurons.

Olfactory cortex: Region of the cerebral cortex in the medial temporal lobe uncus, anterior parahippocampal gyrus, and amygdala that receives projections from the olfactory bulb.

Olfactory epithelium: Cellular sheet that lines the nasal passages and contains olfactory receptor neurons.

Olfactory nerve: Cranial nerve I, which mediates smell.

Olfactory receptor: Bipolar neuron with a cell body, lying in the mucous membrane of each nasal cavity, responsible for transducing odors into neural signals.

Olfactory tract: Axonal bundle extending from the olfactory bulb to the primary olfactory cortex in the temporal lobe.

Oligodendroglia cells: Glia cells that produce the myelin sheath around axons in the central nervous system.

Olivocerebellar fibers: Medullary projection to the cerebellum mediating spinal and vestibular afferents.

Oogenesis: Development formation of a female sex cell (ova).

Oogonia: Primordial cell from which an oocyte is derived.

Operculum: Portions of the frontal, parietal, and occipital lobes that cover the lateral (Sylvian) sulcus and the insula.

Ophthalmoplegia: Paralysis of the extrinsic or intrinsic eye muscles.

Opsin: Protein found in the rhodopsin of rods.

Optic chiasm: Structure in the visual pathway where part of the fibers from each optic nerve decussate to form the optic tract.

Optic disk (papilla): Area through which the optic nerve (CN II) exits and arteries enter the eyeball.

Optic nerve: CN II, consisting of a bundle of ganglion cell receptors that passes from the retina to the optic chiasm.

Optic radiation: Refers to a collection of axons coursing from the lateral geniculate body to the visual cortex.

Optic tectum: Structure used to describe the superior colliculus.

Optic tract: Collection of retinal ganglion cell axons extending from the optic chiasm to the brain and brainstem.

Optokinetic nystagmus: Abnormal rotary ocular movements activated by visual fixation or moving visual patterns.

Organ of Corti: Auditory receptor organ that contains hair cells and supporting cells and is located in the scala media.

Ossicles: Three small bones in the middle ear: malleus, incus, and stapes.

Otitis media: Infectious accumulation of serous fluid in the middle ear that, if untreated, causes conductive hearing loss.

Otolithic membrane: Gelatinous membrane lying over the hair cells of the saccule and utricle in the vestibular sac.

Oval window: Hole in the bony cochlea at which movement of the ossicles is transferred to movement of the fluids in the cochlea.

Oxidation: Chemical dissolution of nutrients for energy.

Oxytocin (Pitocin): Peptide hormone released from the posterior pituitary. Stimulates uterine contractions in a pregnant uterus for inducing delivery and ejection of milk from mammary glands of breasts.

Pacinian corpuscle: Mechanoreceptor in the skin sensitive to vibrations.

Paleocerebellum: Anterior lobe of the cerebellum, primarily concerned with equilibrium and partial adjustments in locomotion.

Pallidum: General term referring to the globus pallidus.

Palsy: Muscle paralysis or paresis.

Papez circuit: Considered as the neurologic base of emotional expression and pain control, it is located on the medial brain surface and consists of the hypothalamus, brain, hippocampus (mammillary bodies), anterior thalamic nucleus, cingulate gyrus, and parahippocampal gyrus.

Paralysis: Refers to a loss of voluntary control of the muscles. Spastic paralysis is associated with upper motor neuron syndrome, whereas flaccid paralysis is associated with lower motor neuron syndrome.

Paraphasia: Inappropriate selection of words and phonemes commonly seen in aphasia.

Paraplegia: Paralysis of both lower limbs and lower trunk.

Parasagittal plane: Vertical plane parallel to the midline that divides the body into unequal left and right parts.

Parasympathetic system: Division of the autonomic nervous system with nuclei in the cranial and sacral region concerned with the conservation of body energy.

Parenchyma: Functionally specialized cells of an organ.

Paresthesia: Abnormal sensation such as numbness, crawling, and itching.

Parkinson disease: Movement disorder of the basal ganglia characterized by resting tremor, muscular rigidity, and paucity of movements.

Paroxysmal discharges: Periodic occurrence of abnormal electrical discharges in the brain.

Pars compacta: Region of the substantia nigra with dopaminergic projections to the striatum.

Pars reticulata: Substantia nigra region receiving inhibitory striatal projections.

Partial epilepsy: Sudden onset of sensory and/or motor behavior confined to a single body part and a progressive recruitment of other body parts. Referred to as the Jacksonian march.

Patau syndrome: A trisomy disorder of chromosome 13, which is characterized by mental retardation, malformed ears, cleft lip/palate, and small mandible.

Peduncle: Bundle of fibers that connects the cerebellum and brainstem.

Peptide neurotransmitters: Large molecules consisting of two or more amino acids that can function as neurotransmitters or neuromodulators.

Perfusion MRI: Neuroimaging technique that maps out the function of the cerebral cortex by measuring microscopic blood flow levels in the cerebral capillaries.

Periaqueductal gray matter: Region surrounding the cerebral aqueduct in the midbrain.

Perilymph: Fluid contained in the bony labyrinth (scalae vestibuli and tympani) that protects the membranous labyrinth.

Peripheral nervous system (PNS): Part of the nervous system that includes all the cranial and spinal nerves.

Peripheral neuropathies: Diseased conditions of peripheral nerves, such as carpal tunnel.

Peristalsis: Wavelike contracting movements in a hollow structure that propel its contents.

Peritoneal cavity: Potential abdominal space between the layers of the parietal and visceral peritoneum.

Periventricular zone: Hypothalamic region that medially borders the third ventricle.

Permeability: Property of brain vessels that restricts the passage of selective fluids and noxious substances.

Pernicious anemia: Anemic state characterized by a progressive decrease in red blood corpuscles. It can be fatal if not treated.

Persistent vegetative state: Altered consciousness state in which patients are not aware of the environment and display no cognitive functions but can breathe on their own, and follow the sleep–wake cycle.

PET: See POSITRON-EMISSION TOMOGRAPHY.

Petit mal (absence) seizures: Minimally involved seizure type that is commonly found in people under age 20 and is marked by a staring spell.

Phagocyte: Macrophagic microglia cells that ingest cellular debris.

Phagocytosis: Process of digestion by cells referring to the removal of dead tissue by microglia cells.

Phantom pain: Sensation of pain originating from the area of an amputated limb.

Phenobarbital: Family of drugs commonly used in the treatment of epilepsy.

Phenytoin (diphenylhydantoin, Dilantin): Drugs used in the treatment of seizure activity.

Phonologic dyslexia: Impaired ability to convert grapheme to phoneme, resulting in poor reading ability, particularly for pronounceable pseudo-words.

Photopigment: Rhodopsin or a visual pigment that absorbs light and undergoes structural changes, leading to the generation of an action potential.

Photopsin: Visual pigment found in retinal cones.

Photoreceptors: Specialized retinal cells that transfer light energy into action potentials.

Pia mater: Innermost layer of the three meninges.

Pick disease: Dementia-causing disease of the frontotemporal degeneration marked by the presence of pathologic Pick bodies in the brain.

Pineal gland: A diencephalic calcified glandular structure, located between the two superior colliculi, is involved with sexual development and is also the site for the secretion of melatonin and serotonin.

Pituitary gland: Hypothalamic structure of hormone synthesis in the central nervous system that is divided into a large anterior lobe (adenohypophysis) and a small posterior lobe (neurohypophysis).

Planum temporale: Area on the superior temporal lobe surface to Heschl gyri. It is larger in the left temporal lobe and is associated with cerebral dominance.

Plaque: Abnormal patch of lipid deposition along the inner arterial wall. Also refers to demyelinated areas in multiple sclerosis.

Plasticity: Brain's capability of being reorganized in the face of an injury, a property that is most evident in developing young brains, particularly before 6 years of age.

Platelet-inhibiting drugs: Medications such as acetylsalicylic acid (aspirin), dipyridamole (Persantine), clopidogrel bisulfate (Plavix), and ticlopidine (Ticlid) are commonly used to prevent platelet aggregation; the platelets in the blood have a tendency to adhere to each other and hence form a plug to prevent oxygen circulation.

Plexus: Network formed by the interconnected nerves from multiple spinal segments.

Polar bodies: Two or three cells formed during the first and the second meiotic division of oocytes that consists of almost all nuclear materials. Do not develop further and are lost.

Polarization: Electrical resting state of a cell characterized by the polarity of ions inside and outside the cell.

Poliomyelitis: Acute viral disease of the lower motor neurons in the spinal cord and brainstem.

Polydipsia: Condition characterized by excessive fluid intake.

Polyuria: Condition characterized by excessive discharge of urine.

Pontine gaze center: Collection of brainstem nuclei that coordinate the movement of the eyes by controlling the ocular cranial nerves.

Pontine nuclei: Nuclei clusters that mediate cortical projections to the cerebellar cortex.

Pontocerebellar fibers: Fibers arising from nuclei of the basilar pons and crossing to project to the cerebellum via the middle cerebellar peduncle.

Portal system: Low-pressure vascular system that carries hypothalamic hormones to the anterior pituitary gland (adenohypophysis).

Positron-emission tomography (PET): Imaging technique that measures live real-time cellular metabolism using radioactive substances (isotopes).

Postcentral gyrus (somesthetic cortex or primary sensory cortex): Cortical region (Brodmann areas 3, 1, 2) behind the central sulcus that integrates sensory inputs from the body and provides sensory awareness.

Posterior cerebral artery: One of the three cortical arteries originating from the circle of Willis and supplying blood to the basal surface of the occipital and temporal lobes and the midsagittal surface of the occipital lobe.

Postganglionic fibers: Sympathetic and parasympathetic fibers with cell bodies in the cells of the automatic ganglia. Project to the cells in the target muscles.

Postganglionic neuron: Second visceral motor neuron in an autonomic pathway with its unmyelinated axon ending at cardiac muscle, smooth muscle, or a gland.

Postsynaptic neuron: Neuronal surface located on the distal side of a synapse.

precentral gyrus: Primary motor cortex (Brodmann area 4), located rostral to the central sulcus.

Precuneus: Parietal lobe region located in the midsagittal surface.

Prefrontal cortex: Recent addition to the frontal cortex and with connections to the dorsomedial thalamus, it serves cognitive and personality functions.

Preganglionic fibers: Sympathetic and parasympathetic fibers before synapsing on the additional autonomic ganglia.

Preganglionic neurons: Autonomic nervous system neurons, with cell bodies in the spinal cord and brainstem, that project to the secondary ganglion.

Premotor cortex: Area located anterior to the motor cortex that programs and regulates skilled movements.

Preoptic area: Anterior portion of the hypothalamus located above the optic chiasm.

Presbyacusis: Age-induced sensorineural hearing loss due to the degeneration of hair cells.

Presbyopia: Age-induced impairment in the lens ability to accommodate the eyes for seeing near objects.

Primary auditory cortex: Located on the superior surface of the first temporal gyrus and receiving auditory projections. It is involved with higher-order analysis of the acoustic stimuli essential for the perception of sound.

Primary motor area: Precentral gyrus region of the cerebral cortex that controls specific or groups of muscles.

Primary somatosensory area: Postcentral gyrus area of the parietal cortex responsible for somatic sensation from the body.

Principal (inferior) olivary nucleus: Nucleus that projects spinal, vestibular, and reticular information to the cerebellum.

Progressive bulbar palsy: Motor neuron disease characterized by a progressive degeneration of cranial nerve nuclei in the brainstem.

Progressive supranuclear palsy: Often confused with Parkinson's disease, this progressive neurological condition affects brainstem cells that regulate ocular movements, equilibrium, and facial expression; it affects ability to move eyes, maintain equilibrium, and manifest facial expressions.

Progressive symptoms: Symptoms that continue to get worse.

Projection fibers: Descending and ascending axonal bundles of fibers mediating sensory and motor functions.

Prolactin (PRL): Hormone that is secreted by the anterior pituitary gland and is responsible for initiating milk secretion by the mammary glands.

Proprioception: Internal awareness of position, posture, and movement.

Prosencephalon (forebrain): Embryonic part of the brain that develops into the cerebral hemispheres, basal ganglia, and limbic system.

Prosopagnosia: Acquired impairment in the ability to recognize familiar faces. A right parietal lobe symptom.

Protopathic: Primitive sensory system that includes pain, temperature, and crude touch.

Pseudobulbar palsy: Pathologic condition involving bilateral supranuclear paralysis of the speech muscles: has significant implications for spastic dysarthria.

Psychomotor (complex) seizures: Convulsive disorders secondary to lesions involving the medial temporal lobe structures (amygdala, hippocampus, and overlying temporal cortex). Characterized by recurring episodes of automatic, irrational behavior of which there usually is no memory.

Psychosis: Severe form of mental disorder characterized by a disorganization of thinking, personality, and behavior; the presence of delusions and hallucinations interfere with daily life.

Psychosomatic: Refers to bodily disorders thought to be caused entirely or partly by emotional disturbances.

Pterygopalatine ganglion: Parasympathetic postganglion of the facial nerve.

pulvinar: The posterior most thalamic nucleus.

Pupillary accommodation: Bilateral reflexive constrictive reaction of the pupil in response to bright light. As a parasympathetic activity, it involves the projection of light to the midbrain pretectal area and to the Edinger–Westphal (visceral) nucleus of the oculomotor cranial nerve, the ciliary ganglion, and the pupillary constrictor muscle fibers.

Pupillary light reflex: Direct change in diameter of the pupils in response to projected light. It is mediated by the visceral fibers of the oculomotor cranial nerve from the brainstem tectum region to the iris.

Pure tone audiometry: Audiologic assessment evaluating hearing thresholds to pure tone stimuli.

Pure word deafness: Aphasic syndrome characterized by the isolation of the language cortex from the primary auditory cortices as a result of a bilateral lesion in the temporal lobes.

Purkinje cells: Large cerebellar nerve cells.

Putamen: Anatomic structure of the neostriatum in basal ganglia.

Pyknosis: A necrotic stage marked by a reduction in size of a cell.

Pyramidal decussation: Crossing of motor fibers that takes place in the most caudal medulla and accounts for contralateral motor organization.

Pyramidal fibers: Descending corticospinal fibers mediating motor impulses to spinal motor neurons.

Pyramidal tract: The descending motor fibers of the corticospinal tract named because of their location in the medullary pyramids.

Pyriform cortex: Primary olfactory cortex located on the medial rostral region of the uncus and hippocampal gyrus.

Quadrantanopsia: Blindness involving one-quarter of the visual field.

Quadriplegia: Paralysis of all four limbs.

Raphe nucleus: Collection of seratonin containing reticular cells located along the midline in the brainstem that diffusely project to hypothalamus, septum, hippocampus, and cingulate gyrus, brainstem, cerebellum, and spinal cord.

Rapid-eye movement (REM) sleep: Sleep stage characterized by high-frequency and low-amplitude EEG waves, vivid dreams, and rapid-eye movements.

Recessive inheritance: Genetic mode of inheritance in which both parents have the same affected alleles. It results in 25% probability of inheriting the dysfunctional genes and the condition.

Reciprocal inhibition: A neuronal circuitry in which an action potential is excitatory to motor units in an agonistic skeletal muscle and is excitatory to an inhibitory interneuron that, in turn, reduces the excitability of motor units in the paired antagonistic muscles. This ensures that when one muscle is contracting, its paired muscle is relaxing.

Red nucleus: Midbrain cell cluster that relays cerebellar output to the motor cortex and spinal cord.

Referred pain: The sensation of pain from a visceral organ is sensed as originating from another body part. The visceral structures do not have separate afferent pathways; rather they synapse on the same neurons in the dorsal root ganglion that also receives somatic sensation from the superficial structures.

Reflex: Hard-wired stereotypical response to a specific stimulus. All reflexes, except the stretch reflex, involve at least three neurons: the afferent neuron, one or more interneurons, and one or more efferent neurons.

Refraction: Bending of light rays as they travel from one medium to another.

Refraction errors: Focusing deviations from the optimal fixation point of the retina. Myopia (nearsightedness) and hyperopia (far-sightedness) are two common types of focusing errors.

Regional cerebral blood flow (rCBF): Neuroradiologic technique that measures blood flow to functionally active brain areas by monitoring a radioactive tracer.

Reissner membrane: Cochlear membrane that separates the scala media from the scala vestibuli.

Renshaw cells: Inhibitory neurons in the spinal cord that are connected to and inhibited by the collaterals of adjacent motor neurons.

Respiration: Involves the transfer of gases among the atmosphere, blood, and body cells and is marked by inhalation and exhalation.

Respiratory center: Reticular neurons in the brainstem that regulate the rate and depth of respiration.

Restiform body: Medially located division of the inferior cerebellar peduncle composed of the primarily bidirectional vestibular and reticular fibers connecting with the cerebellum, particularly the nodulus and flocculus.

Resting membrane potential: Membrane potential of –70 mV. At this stage, the nerve cell is not generating action potentials.

Resting state: Denotes the polarized state when the cell with an internal environment of –70 mV.

Resting tremor: Involuntary motor activity during rest. Associated with Parkinson disease.

Reticular formation: Diffuse core of brainstem nuclei with parallel and serial projections that integrates the entire nervous system and is involved with cortical arousal and muscle preparedness.

Reticulocerebellar pathway: Descending fibers that originate in the brainstem and mediate reticular projections to the cerebellum.

Retina: Neural layer of the eye that contains photoreceptor cells: rods and cones.

Retinal (visual yellow): Light-absorbing molecule of rhodopsin in rods, an aldehyde of vitamin A.

Retrocochlear auditory mechanism: Fibers of the acoustic cranial nerve and projections to the cochlear nuclei in the brainstem.

Retrograde reaction (degeneration): Changes occurring in the proximal portion of a damaged axon.

Rhodopsin: Visual purple pigment found in the outer segments of rod cells.

Rhombencephalon (hindbrain): Caudalmost of the primary vesicles of the embryonic neural tube. Divides into metencephalon and myelencephalon.

Righting reflex: Normal postural pattern that controls the position of the neck and extremities in space.

Rigidity: Stiff state of muscles involving both agonist and antagonist muscles, which is present throughout resistance (plastic pipe phenomenon). Clasp knife is the transient increased resistance of extensors to passive muscle movement, which melts away with persisting resistance.

Rinne test: Tuning fork test used to detect a conductive hearing loss. The stem of a tuning fork (512 Hz) is first held against the mastoid process and the patient listens to the tuning fork by bone conduction. When the patient no longer hears through bone conduction, the tuning fork is held near the opening of the external auditory meatus to determine if the patient can hear by air conduction. A patient with a conductive hearing loss will not hear the tuning fork by air conduction (negative Rinne).

Rods: Retinal photoreceptors responsible for night vision.

Romberg sign: Evaluates equilibrium in the case of impaired proprioception from the lower extremities. The patient is asked to stand with the feet together and eyes closed. A patient with the loss of proprioception is likely to fall when the eyes are closed.

Rostral: Toward the front of the head.

Rotational sensation: Persistent sensation of motion commonly seen in case of labyrinthine dysfunctioning.

Round window: Opening between the middle and inner ear covered by the secondary tympanic membrane.

Rubrospinal tract: Group of axons involved with motor movements that descend from the red nucleus and terminate on the motor neurons in the spinal cord.

Ruffini endings: Moderately adapting subcutaneous receptors mediating tactile and temperature information.

Saccadic: Rapid corrective movements of both eyes that are needed to keep words in focus (on fovea), while reading a printed line.

Saccule: Membranous sac in the vestibule of the labyrinth.

Sacral plexus: Formed by interjoined nerves originating from several sacral spinal segments.

Sagittal: Vertical section dividing the brain into left and right halves.

Saltatory conduction: Propagation of an action potential along a myelinated axon where current jumps from one node to the next.

Satiety center: Group of hypothalamic nuclei that, when stimulated, bring about a reduction in desire to eat.

Saturated fat: Fatty acid that is commonly associated with heart diseases and is prevalent in triglycerides of animal products, such as meat, milk, milk products, and eggs.

Scala media: Endolymph-filled cochlear region lying between the scala vestibuli and the scala tympani.

Scala tympani: Perilymph-filled lowermost compartment of the cochlea, which is connected to the scala vestibuli through the helicotrema.

Scala vestibuli: Perilymph-filled uppermost compartment of the cochlea.

Scarpa ganglion: Bipolar vestibular ganglia projecting impulses from the hair cells in the semicircular canals to the brainstem vestibular nucleus complex.

Schwann cells: Glia cells that form myelin around the axons in the peripheral nervous system.

Scotoma: Area of lost vision within the visual field.

Scotopic vision: Night vision mediated by rod cells.

Seizure disorders: Sensory, motor, cognitive, and affective disorders resulting from abnormal electrical discharges in the brain.

Semicircular canals: Three circular ducts containing sensory organs suspended in endolymph for reflexive control of dynamic equilibrium.

Semiovale center: Mass of white matter located below the cerebral cortex.

sensorineural hearing loss: Hearing loss resulting from a dysfunctioning organ of Corti or cochlear nerve (CN VIII).

Sensory cortex: Postcentral gyrus area responsible for the perception of bodily experienced modalities of pain, touch, and temperature.

Septum pellucidum: Thin membrane located above the septal nuclei and anteriorly dividing the lateral ventricles.

Serotonergic: Cells that secrete serotonin, a vasoconstrictor neurotransmitter in the CNS that also inhibits gastric secretion and stimulates smooth muscle.

Serotonin: Important central nervous system neurotransmitter that plays a role in sleep and wakefulness.

Sex chromosomes: The X and Y chromosomes that determine the sex of an individual (XY for males, XX for females).

Single photon–emission computed tomography (SPECT): Imaging technique that measures cerebral blood flow using a radioactive substance.

Sinus: Hollow channel covered with dura in the brain that receives deoxygenated blood after circulation.

Skeletal muscles: Muscles that contain striated fibers that move bones around a joint.

Sleep: State of partial unconsciousness characterized by a low level of activity in the reticular activating system.

Sleep disorders: Irregularity in reaching, maintaining, and leaving a physiologic state of partial unconsciousness marked with inactivity of the voluntary muscles of the body.

Smooth muscle: Tissue located in the walls of hollow internal organs and innervated by autonomic motor neurons.

Sodium amytal infusion: Test involves the infusion of sodium amytal, a chemical used for inducing a transient anesthetization of the human brain; this is used for determining the dominant cerebral hemisphere.

Somatic: Relating to structures derived from a series of mesodermal somites, including skeletal muscles, bones, and dermis.

Somatic nervous system (SNS): Division of the peripheral nervous system consisting of somatic sensory (afferent) neurons and somatic motor (efferent) neurons.

Somatosensation: Bodily experienced modalities of pain, touch, and temperature.

Somatosensory-evoked potentials: Evoked electric responses of the central nervous system to specific sensory activity.

Somatostatin: Capable of inhibiting the release of the hormone somatotropin by the anterior lobe of the pituitary gland.

Somite: Segmental block-like mass of mesoderm on either side of the notochord. Gives rise to muscles, vertebral bodies, and skin.

Sound pressure: Amplitude of sound in pressure units relative to a reference pressure.

Spastic dysarthria: Impaired motor speech functions secondary to bilateral interruption of corticobulbar fibers. Characterized by articulatory imprecision, monopitch, and reduced stress.

Spastic hemiplegia: Paralysis of one side of the body after a lesion in the pyramidal tract.

Spasticity: Hypertonic state of muscles characterized by increased muscle tone.

Spermatogenesis: Development of a male sex cell (spermatozoon).

Spermatogonia: Male germ cell or gamete, undifferentiated and arising from the seminiferous tubule, dividing into two primary spermatocytes.

Spina bifida: Neurological condition resulting from a fusion failure of the dorsal–caudal part of the neural tube on the first few embryonic weeks. It includes several types of embryonic malformation marked by the opening of the vertebral column.

Spina bifida cystica: Embryologic failure of fusion involving one or more vertebral arches, which is associated with a meningeal cyst (meningocele) or a cyst containing both meninges and spinal cord (meningomyelocele).

Spina bifida occulta: Genetic spinal defect with no protrusion of the cord or its membrane.

Spinal accessory nerve: Cranial nerve XI, which is responsible for raising the shoulders and turning the head contralaterally.

Spinal anesthesia: Injection of liquid anesthetic into the lumbar spinal subarachnoid space to cause a temporary loss of sensation in the lower body extending up to the level of injection.

Spinal nerve: Nerve of the spinal cord that innervates the body.

Spinal plexuses: Network of interconnected spinal nerves.

Spinal preparation: Cutting the spinal cord not only separates the cord from the forebrain, but it also allows the examination of spinal reflexes independent of the inhibitory or facilitatory influence exerted by higher motor centers.

Spinal tap (lumbar puncture): Procedure used for extracting the cerebrospinal fluid for diagnostic purposes. The cerebrospinal fluid is removed from the subarachnoid space in the lumbar region.

Spinal trigeminal nucleus (tract): Second-order nucleus and descending fibers that mediate pain and temperature from the face.

Spinocerebellar system: Spinal projection to the cerebellum mediating unconscious proprioception from the lower and upper limbs.

Spinocerebellar tract: Fiber bundle that mediates unconscious proprioception to the cerebellum.

Spinothalamic pathway: Ascending bundle of fibers that mediates the sensation of pain, touch, and temperature from the spinal cord to the thalamus.

Stapedius: A muscle, controlled by the facial nerve (cranial nerve VII), in the middle ear that reflexively contracts to attenuate hearing sensitivity by restricting ossicular movement.

Stapes: Middle ear ossicle that is attached to the oval window.

Static equilibrium: Balancing during a stationary posture.

Static labyrinth: Maintenance of a balanced position of the head and body in space against gravity during rest and during straight-line head movements.

Stenosis: Narrowing of arteries.

Stereognosis: Identification of objects by tactual sensation of shape, texture, and size.

Stereotaxic (stereotactic): Precise method of localization for lesion placement in a deep-seated brain structure using three-dimensional space.

Strabismus: Optic disorder in which visual axes of both eyes are not directed toward the same object.

Stretch reflex: Skeletal muscle contraction resulting from passive or active stretching of the same muscle. It involves two-neuron reflex circuitry.

Stria vascularis: Lining the cochlea, this vascular epithelial membrane is the site for the secretion of endolymph in the membranous labyrinth.

Striate cortex: Primary visual cortex, or Brodmann area 17.

Striatum: General term for the basal ganglia nuclei of the putamen and caudate nucleus.

Stroke: Suddenly emerging neurologic deficits that result from vascular circulatory impairments of embolism, thrombosis, and hemorrhage.

Stupor: Altered state of unconsciousness and unresponsiveness from which a patient can be aroused transiently with strong and repeated stimulation.

Subacute combined spinal degeneration: Spinal degeneration as a result of vitamin B_{12} deficiency. Commonly seen in chronic alcoholics, it is characterized by impaired transmission of proprioception and kinesthesia.

Subacute symptoms: Clinical features that appear after the acute phase and are of moderate duration.

Subarachnoid space: Real space that is filled with cerebrospinal fluid and is located between the pia mater and the arachnoid membrane.

Subcallosal gyrus: Limbic structure located beneath the rostrum of the corpus callosum.

Subdural: Referring to the pathology location in a potential space below the dura and external to the arachnoid membrane.

Substance P: Inhibitory basal ganglia neurotransmitter that causes the suppression of dopaminergic activity in the substantia nigra.

Substantia gelatinosa: Neurons located in the dorsal spinal column that receive nociceptive information.

Substantia nigra: Contains many dopaminergic nuclei which project to and are inhibitory to the cells of the caudate and putamen. Degeneration of its neuron is associated with Parkinson disease.

Subthalamic nucleus: Located between the internal capsule and the substantia nigra, this biconvex basal ganglia nucleus is involved with the movement disorders of hemiballism.

Subthalamus: Refers to a subcortical region that includes the subthalamic nucleus, zona incerta, and field H of Forel.

Sulcus: Also called fissure, it includes the groove or furrow markings on the cortical surface.

Superior cerebellar peduncle: One of the three fiber bundles that connects the cerebellum with the brainstem and motor cortex; it is also called the brachium conjunctivum.

Superior colliculus: Midbrain structure related to visual reflexes, such as ocular accommodation and coordinated head and eye movements.

Superior longitudinal fasciculus: Large intrahemispheric association pathway that connects frontal to the occipital lobe with projections to the Wernicke area in the temporal lobe.

Superior olivary nucleus: Nucleus in the medullary tegmentum that is the first to receive projections from both cochleae and plays an important role in sound localization.

Superior salivatory nucleus: Visceral cranial nucleus that is responsible for autonomic secretion of glands in the mouth and face.

Supination: Movement that causes the palm to turn upward.

Supplementary motor cortex: Midsagitally located extension of the premotor cortex, which is involved with bilateral aspects of motor control and planning.

Supramarginal gyrus: Located in the inferior parietal lobule, it is a linguistically important parietal lobe structure.

Supraoptic nucleus: Hypothalamic nucleus.

Surface dyslexia: Acquired reading impairment marked by phonemically relating grapheme to phoneme with no access to meaning through the entire word directly.

Sydenham chorea: Involuntary choreic movements appearing in children several months after streptococcal infection and subsequent rheumatic fever. The choreic movements involve the distal limbs and emotionally labile behaviors.

Sympathetic chain: Series of interconnected ganglia located adjacent to the vertebral column.

Sympathetic system: Anatomically and functionally distinct division of the autonomic nervous system with axonal projections from the thoracic and lumbar spinal regions. Concerned with the expenditure of body energy and with the regulation of bodily responses in fight-or-flight situations.

Sympathetic trunk ganglion: Cell bodies of postganglionic sympathetic neurons located lateral to the vertebral column. The ganglia chain extends inferiorly through the neck, thorax, and abdomen to the coccyx on both sides of the vertebral column.

Symptom: Patient-described subjective clinical observation.

Synapse: Point of contact between two neurons where the neurotransmitter is released.

Synaptic cleft: Point of junction between nerve cells.

Syringomyelia: Developmental presence of a longitudinal cavity, mostly in the cervical spinal cord, clinically marked by pain, paresthesia, and analgesia of the hands.

Tactile: Related to the sense of touch.

Tardive dyskinesia: Involuntary slow and stereotypical movements of facial muscles that emerge as the side effect of psychotropic drugs, such as haloperidol.

Tay–Sachs disease: Disorder of autosomal-recessive inheritance resulting in fatal brain damage with deterioration of mental and physical functions, convulsions, and enlarged head. Common in eastern European Jews.

Tectospinal tract: Tract that originates from nuclei in the superior colliculi and terminates on the spinal motor neurons. Regulates head and neck movements.

Tectum: Region of the brainstem dorsal to the cerebral aqueduct in the midbrain that serves visual and auditory reflexes and provides a map of external space.

Tegmentum: Cellular region of the midbrain and pons below the cerebral aqueduct and fourth ventricle.

Telencephalon: Subdivision of the prosencephalon, which develops into the cortex of the cerebral hemispheres, basal ganglia (nuclei), and limbic lobe.

Temporal Planum: See PLANUM TEMPORALE.

Tendon: Nerve fiber that attaches a muscle to a bone.

Tendon organ: Proprioceptive receptors, sensitive to muscle tension and force of contraction, found chiefly near the junctions of tendons and muscles. Also called a Golgi tendon organ.

Tensor tympani: Muscle, regulated by the trigeminal nerve (CN V), in the middle ear that reflexively contracts to attenuate hearing sensitivity by restricting ossicular movement.

Tentorium cerebelli: Dural extension that covers the cerebellum and the floor of the cranium.

Teratogenesis: Study of abnormal development of an embryo that results in a deformed fetus.

Teratogen: Fetotoxic drug that causes the abnormal development of structures in the embryo.

Teratology: Concerned with the development of malformed babies.

Terminal bouton: Nerve end synaptic vesicles filled with neurotransmitters.

Testosterone: Male sex hormone produced by the testicle. Promotes the development of sperm and sexual characteristics.

Thalamus: Major diencephalic structure located on either side of the third ventricle and medial to the internal capsules. Plays an important role in sensorimotor integration and projection to the cortex.

Thermal anesthesia: Loss of temperature sensation.

Thermal hyperesthesia: Abnormally lower threshold of sensitivity to heat and cold.

Thermal hypoesthesia: Diminished sensitivity to heat and cold stimuli.

Thermoreceptors: Receptors with sensitivity to heat and cold.

Thiamine: Essential for growth, a vitamin that is present in milk and grain husks. Its deficiency is associated with beriberi and Wernicke–Korsakoff syndrome, characterized by progressive personality changes and amnesia.

Third ventricle: Space in the diencephalon filled with cerebrospinal fluid.

Thoracolumbar outflow: Sympathetic preganglionic neurons with cell bodies in the lateral gray columns of the thoracic segments and the first two or three spinal lumbar segments.

Threshold: Value of membrane potential at which the ionic current change flows into the membrane, causing the cellular interior to become positive.

Thrombolytic agent: Chemical agents that dissolve blood clots and restore circulation. Also included in this category is tissue plasminogen activator (t-PA).

Thrombosis: Formation of a localized clot that blocks the lumen of a blood vessel.

Thymus: Lymphoid structure that functions as an endocrine gland.

Tic: Spasmodic involuntary twitching of mostly facial muscles (blinking, nose-twitching, or grimacing) usually associated with a basal ganglia lesion.

Tic douloureux: See TRIGEMINAL NEURALGIA.

Tinnitus: Perception of a (ringing or hissing) sound in the absence of an environmental acoustic stimulus, which is usually associated with a loss of hearing subsequent to the lesion is in the inner ear.

Tissue plasminogen–activating agent (tPA): Drug used to restore blood circulation in acute cases of thromboembolic stroke by dissolving the atherosclerotic clot.

Tonotopic: Systemic organization of frequency distribution in the auditory cortex.

Torticollis: Dystonic and abnormally sustained posture of neck muscles subsequent to basal ganglia pathology, in which the head rotates to one side so that the chin points to the other side.

Tract: Bundle of nerve fibers in the central nervous system.

Tranquilizers: Drugs used to calm emotions without sedation.

Transcortical motor aphasia: Severely limited verbal skills with preserved repetition skills caused by a lesion that separates Broca area from the surrounding association cortex.

Transcortical sensory aphasia: Severely limited comprehension of spoken language and unabated repetition that results from the separation of Wernicke area from an adjacent association cortex.

Transient ischemic attack (TIA): Temporary cerebral dysfunction caused by transient disruption of the blood supply to the brain; it is marked by transient symptoms that clear within 30 to 60 minutes.

Trapezoid body: Crossing fibers of the auditory pathway that are located in the pons.

Tremor: Rhythmic pin-rolling movements of the fingers at rest, along with akinesia and rigidity that characterizes Parkinson disease. Intention tremor occurs during movement and results from cerebellar pathology.

Trichromatic vision: Based on intact processing of three basic colors subsequent to possessing independent and specialized cone pigments with sensitivity to corresponding wave-lengths.

Trigeminal nerve: CN V, which is responsible for sensation from the face, head, and mouth. Its motor fibers regulate the muscle of mastication.

Trigeminal neuralgia: Intense and stabbing pain involving one or more of the branches of the trigeminal nerve (CN V) that has a trigger zone. It is also called tic douloureux.

Triplegia: Paralysis of any three limbs-an upper and both lower extremities or both extremities on one side and one extremity on the other side.

Trisomy: Abnormal addition of an extra chromosome to a normal diploid chromosomal set.

Trochlear nerve: CN IV, which innervates the superior oblique muscle and participates in looking downward and outward.

Trophoblast: Outer cell mass differentiating into cytotrophoblast and syncytiotrophoblast.

Tumor: Uncontrolled neoplastic growth of tissue.

Tuning fork tests: See WEBER AND RINNE.

Turner syndrome: Chromosomal syndrome with 1 X and no Y chromosome (45 chromosomes), characterized by short stature, webbed neck, abnormal sexual development, and broad chest.

Tympanic membrane: Soft tissue covering that separates the external ear from the middle ear.

UMN syndrome: Neurological condition that is marked by contralateral muscle spasticity, hyperreflexia, paralysis, and Babinski sign. Emerges a few days after an injury to the descending corticospinal tract fibers.

Uncinate fasciculus: Intrahemispheric association fiber bundle that connects frontal and temporal lobes.

Uncus: Structure of the limbic system associated with the perception of smell.

Unipolar neuron: Neuron with a single process (neurite).

Upper motor neurons (UMNs): Cell bodies in the motor cortex and their descending axonal processes that synapse on the cranial and spinal motor neurons.

Utricle: Membranous dilation of the vestibular apparatus.

Vagus nerve: CN X, which controls phonation and swallowing in addition to regulating many autonomic nervous system functions.

Vascular: Related to blood circulation and blood vessels.

Vasoconstriction: Decreased diameter of a blood vessel.

Vasodilation: Increased diameter of a blood vessel, resulting in greater blood flow.

Vasomotor center: Neural network localized in the medulla that controls arterial blood pressure and pulse rate.

Vasopressin: Hypothalamic hormone transported to the posterior lobe of the pituitary gland and has an antidiuretic effect.

Vein: Vessel that transports circulated blood from the body to the heart.

Venous sinus system: Veins and sinuses responsible for draining blood and cerebrospinal fluid.

Ventral horn: Ventral region of the spinal cord that houses motor neurons.

Ventral root: Bundle of motor fibers that originates from the spinal ventral horns.

Ventral spinocerebellar tract: Pathway that mediates unconscious proprioception from the lower limbs to the cerebellum.

Ventricles: Interconnected brain cavities that produce, store, and circulate the cerebrospinal fluid.

Vermis: Midline structure of the cerebellum.

Vertebra: Segment of spinal bone.

Vertebral basilar system: Vascular network that serves the brainstem and occipital lobe.

Vertebral column: Spinal cord containing bony case that extends from the cranium to the coccyx.

Vertigo: Sensation of self rotation (subjective vertigo) or of the surrounding environment (objective vertigo), which is associated with inner ear pathologies..

Vesicle (brain): Subdivisions of the embryonic neural tube, each with a wall of neuroectoderm and a cavity.

Vestibular apparatus: Part of the inner ear responsible for detecting head motion.

Vestibular labyrinth: Membranous labyrinth concerned with the regulation of equilibration, which is located within the semicircular canals and vestibule.

Vestibular nerve: Division of cranial nerve VIII, which serves equilibrium and, indirectly, ocular movement.

Vestibular schwannoma: Benign tumor arising from the myelin-forming Schwann cells of the vestibular division of the eighth cranial nerve.

Vestibular system: Brain mechanism responsible for maintaining equilibrium.

Vestibule: Part of the inner ear, consisting of the utricle and saccule, which contain sensory organs needed to facilitate reflexive control of static equilibrium.

Vestibulocochlear nerve: CN VIII, serving audition and equilibrium.

Visceral: Vital organs of the body that have nonstriated muscles, such as the larynx, pharynx, trachea, and lungs. Innervated by the autonomic nervous system and relates to respiration, phonation, and digestion.

Visceral afferent system: General sensation from the inner visceral organs.

Visceral efferent system: Autonomic nervous system regulating glandular secretion and visceral structure functions.

Visceral functions: Activities of the muscles of respiration, digestion, swallowing, phonation, and speech.

Visceral muscles: Muscles of the heart, the spleen, the great vessels, and the digestive, respiratory, urogenital, endocrine, and speech systems, which are autonomically controlled.

Visual agnosia: Impaired ability to recognize objects and printed words.

Visual field: Area seen by both eyes when looking straight ahead.

Visual reflexes: Include pupillary constriction in response to light and lens accommodation for near vision.

Vitreous humor: Jellylike substance in the posterior cavity of the eye. Prevents the eyeball from collapsing and contributes to intraocular pressure.

Wada test: Procedure in which the cerebral cortex is transiently anesthetized with sodium amobarbital infusion for assessing its functions.

Wallenberg syndrome: Associated with an infarct of the lateral medulla, it causes ipsilateral facial anesthesia, ipsilateral swallowing and phonatory problems, and a contralateral loss of pain and temperature.

Wallerian (anterograde) degeneration: Structural changes in a distal portion of an axon after it is sectioned and disconnected from the cell body as a result of an injury.

Watershed area: Tertiary brain area located peripheral to the primary distribution areas for the anterior, posterior, and middle cerebral arteries. This area is highly susceptible to vascular insufficiency because of its vascular dependency on multiple arteries.

Watershed infarct: Cellular death in the distal vascular distribution area due to an insufffiency of blood involving major cortical arteries.

Weber test: Tuning fork test in which the stem of a tuning fork is placed on the midline of the forehead. Lateralization to the poorer-hearing ear suggests a conductive hearing loss. Lateralization to the better-hearing ear suggests a sensorineural hearing loss in the other ear.

Wernicke encephalopathy: Syndrome of nutritional deficiency largely found in chronic alcoholics and characterized by ocular motility (ophthalmology), nystagmus, gait disturbances, and mental confusion.

White matter: General term for the axonal bundles in the central nervous system.

William syndrome: Congenital disorder caused by a continuous gene deletion and marked by distinctive facial and structural features, cognitive impairments (mental retardation and attention deficits), and hypercalcemia (elevated blood calcium levels).

Wilson disease: Neurological disorder of copper metabolism that results in dysarthria and impaired cognition subsequent to liver cirrhosis and basal ganglia degeneration.

Withdrawal reflex: Reflexive movement causing the withdrawal of a limb by flexion at more than one joint in response to a painful stimulus on the skin surface.

X-linked inheritance: Genetic inheritance mode where diseases or traits are transmitted by a gene or genes on the X (sex) chromosome.

Zygote: Fertilized ovum (first stage in human development).

Figure and Table Credits

FIGURES

Chapter 1

Figure 1-4: Modified from Standring S, Gray H. Gray's Anatomy. 40th ed. Edinburgh: Churchill Livingstone/ Elsevier, 2008.

Figure 1-7: Reprinted with permission from Carpenter MB. Core Text of Neuroanatomy. 4th ed. Baltimore: Williams and Wilkins, 1991.

Figure 1-6, 1-8, 1-8: Reprinted with permission from Haines DE. Neuroanatomy: An Atlas of Structures, Sections, and Systems. 8th ed. Baltimore: Wolters Kluwer Health/ Lippincott Williams & Wilkins, 2012.

Figure 1-10: Image courtesy of Lotfi Hacein-Bey, MD, Radiological Associates of Sacramento Medical Group Inc, CA.

Figure 1-16: Reprinted with permission from Haines DE. Neuroanatomy: An Atlas of Structures, Sections, and Systems. 8th ed. Philadelphia: Wolters Kluwer Health/ Lippincott Williams & Wilkins, 2012.

Figure 1-17: Reprinted with permission from Oatis C. A. Kinesiology: The Mechanics and Pathomechanics of Human Movement. Philadelphia: Lippincott Williams & Wilkins, 2004.

Chapter 2

Figure 2-1 B: Modified from Guyton AC. Organ Physiology: Structure and Function of the Nervous System. Philadelphia: Saunders, 1976.

Figures 2-3, 2-5, 2-7, 2-8, 2-10, 2-11, 2-12 B, 2-15 A, 2-16 A, 2-24 C, 2-27 A, B, 2-29, 2-39, 2-40 B, 2-41, and 2-50: Reprinted with permission from Haines DE. Neuroanatomy: An Atlas of Structures, Sections, and Systems. 8th ed. Philadelphia: Wolters Kluwer Health/ Lippincott Williams & Wilkins, 2012.

Figures 2-6, 2-12 A, 2-13, 2-17, 2-19, 2-32 B, 2-36 A, B, and 2-38: Modified from Parent A, Carpenter MB. Carpenter's Human Neuroanatomy. 9th ed. Baltimore: Williams & Wilkins, 1996.

Figures 2-9, 2-17, 2-18, 2-20, 2-21, 2-41 B, 2-42, 2-46 A, 2-47 A, 2-48 A, B, and 2-49: Reprinted with permission from Parent A, Carpenter MB. Carpenter's Human Neuroanatomy. 9th ed. Baltimore: Williams & Wilkins, 1996.

Figures 2-28, 2-43, and 2-44: Modified from Mettler FA. Mettler's Neuroanatomy. 2nd ed. St. Louis: Mosby, 1948.

Figure 2-31 A: Courtesy of Duane E. Haines PhD, Department of Anatomy, University of Mississippi Medical Center, Jackson.

Figure 2-31 B: Reprinted with permission from Mettler FA. Mettler's Neuroanatomy. 2nd ed. St. Louis: Mosby, 1948; Parent A, Carpenter MB. Carpenter's Human Neuroanatomy. 9th ed. Baltimore: Williams & Wilkins, 1996.

Figure 2-33: Reprinted with permission from Snell R. Clinical Neuroanatomy. 7th ed. Philadelphia: Wolters Kluwer Health/Lippincott Williams & Wilkins, 2010.

Figure 2-35: Modified from Kingsley RE. Concise Test of Neuroscience. Baltimore: Williams & Wilkins, 1996.

Figures 2-39 A and 2-45 A: Modified from Heimer L. The Human Brain and Spinal Cord: Functional Neuroanatomy and Dissection Guide. New York: Springer-Verlag, 1983.

Figure 2-40 A: Reprinted with permission from Haines DE. Neuroanatomy: An Atlas of Structures, Sections, and Systems. 7th ed. Philadelphia: Wolters Kluwer Health/ Lippincott Williams & Wilkins, 2008.

Figure 2-45 B: Modified from House EL, Pansky B. A Functional Approach to Neuroanatomy. New York: McGraw-Hill, 1967.

Figure 2-51: Modified from Barr ML, Kiernan JA. The Human Nervous System: An Anatomical Viewpoint. 7th ed. Philadelphia: Lippincott Williams & Wilkins, 1998.

Chapter 3

Figures 3-2 to 3-5, 3-7, 3-9 to 3-19, and 3-21 to 3-25: Reprinted with permission from Haines DE. Neuroanatomy: An Atlas of Structures, Sections, and Systems. 8th ed. Philadelphia: Lippincott Williams & Wilkins, 2012.

MRIs (3-21 to 3-25): Courtesy of Lotfi Hacein-Bey, Sutter Neuroscience Institute, Sacramento, CA, USA.

Figures 3-6 and 3-20: Modified from Haines DE. Neuroanatomy: An Atlas of Structures, Sections, and Systems. 8th ed. Philadelphia: Lippincott Williams & Wilkins, 2012.

Figure 3-26: Courtesy of Haines DE, PhD, Department of Anatomy, University of Mississippi Medical Center, Jackson.

Chapter 4

Figure 4-1: Modified from Kelley DE, et al. Bailey's Textbook of Microscopic Anatomy. Williams & Wilkins, 1984.

Figures 4-2 to 4-13: Reprinted with permission from Sadler TW, Langman J. Langman's Medical Embryology. 11th ed. Philadelphia: Lippincott Williams & Wilkins, 2009.

Chapter 5

Figure 5-5: Modified from Marieb EN. Essentials of Human Anatomy and Physiology. 10th ed. San Francisco: Benjamin-Cummings, 2011.

Figure 5-6: Modified from Gilman S, Manter JT, Gatz AJ, Newman SW. Manter and Gatz's Essentials of Clinical Neuroanatomy and Neurophysiology. 10th ed. Philadelphia: F.A. Davis, 2003.

Figure 5-9: Courtesy of Lotfi Hacein-Bey, MD, Radiological Associates of Sacramento Medical Group Inc, CA.

Chapter 6

Figure 6-1: Modified from Haines DE. Neuroanatomy: An Atlas of Structures, Sections, and Systems. 8th ed. Philadelphia: Wolters Kluwer Health/Lippincott Williams & Wilkins, 2012.

Chapter 7

Figures 7-2 A, 7-3 A, 7-4 A, 7-13 A, 7-14 A, B: Reprinted with permission from Parent A, Carpenter MB. Carpenter's Human Neuroanatomy. 9th ed. Baltimore: Williams & Wilkins, 1996.

Figure 7-2 B: Modified from Haines DE. Neuroanatomy: An Atlas of Structures, Sections, and Systems. 8th ed. Philadelphia: Lippincott Williams & Wilkins, 2012.

Figure 7-11: Courtesy of Leighton Mark, MD, Department of Neuroradiology, Medical College of Wisconsin, Milwaukee.

Figures 7-8, 7-9, 7-10: Courtesy of Lotfi Hacein-Bey MD. Radiology Associate of Sacramento Medical Group Inc, CA.

Chapter 8

Figures 8-2 A and 8-5: Reprinted with permission from Parent A, Carpenter MB. Carpenter's Human Neuroanatomy. 9th ed. Baltimore: Williams & Wilkins, 1996.

Chapter 9

Figure 9-1: Modified from Lavine RA. Neurophysiology: The Fundamentals. Lexington: Collamore Press, 1983.

Figures 9-2 and 9-3: Reprinted with permission from Parent A, Carpenter MB. Carpenter's Human Neuroanatomy. 9th ed. Baltimore: Williams & Wilkins, 1996.

Figures 9-5 and 9-6: Modified from Parent A, Carpenter MB. Carpenter's Human Neuroanatomy. 9th ed. Baltimore: Williams & Wilkins, 1996.

Figures 9-7 (modified) and 9-8: Reprinted with permission from Haines DE. Neuroanatomy: An Atlas of Structures, Sections, and Systems. 8th ed. Philadelphia: Lippincott Williams & Wilkins, 2012.

Chapter 10

Figure 10-2 B: Based after Kandel ER, Schwartz JH, Jessell TM. Principles of Neural Science. 4th ed. New York: McGraw-Hill, 2000.

Figure 10-3 C: Modified from Curtis BA, Jacobson S, Marcus EM. An Introduction to the Neurosciences. Philadelphia: Saunders, 1972.

Figure 10-4: Modified from Parent A, Carpenter MB. Carpenter's Human Neuroanatomy. 9th ed. Baltimore: Williams & Wilkins, 1996.

Figure 10-6: Modified from House EL, Pansky B. A Functional Approach to Neuroanatomy. New York: McGraw-Hill, 1967.

Chapter 11

Figures 11-3, 11-5 A and 11-7 A: Modified from on teaching material distributed at University of Rochester, College of Medicine, Rochester, NY.

Figures 11-5 B, 11-6, 11-7 B, 11-8, and 11-10: Modified from Parent A, Carpenter MB. Carpenter's Human Neuroanatomy. 9th ed. Baltimore: Williams & Wilkins, 1996.

Figure 11-9 B: Modified from Crosby E. Correlative Anatomy of the Nervous System. New York: Macmillan, 1962.

Chapter 12

Figure 12-1: Modified from Carpenter MB. Core Text of Neuroanatomy. 4th ed. Baltimore: Williams & Wilkins, 1991.

Figures 12-7 A, 12-8 A, and 12-13: Modified from Parent A, Carpenter MB. Carpenter's Human Neuroanatomy. 9th ed. Baltimore: Williams & Wilkins, 1996.

Chapter 13

Figure 13-1: Reprinted with permission from Haines DE. Neuroanatomy: An Atlas of Structures, Sections, and Systems. 8th ed. Philadelphia: Lippincott Williams & Wilkins, 2012.

Figures 13-3 to 13-5, and 13-9: Modified from Parent A, Carpenter MB. Carpenter's Human Neuroanatomy. 9th ed. Baltimore: Williams & Wilkins, 1996.

Figure 13-7 A, B: Modified from Gardener E. Fundamentals of Neurology: A Physiological Approach. Philadelphia: Saunders, 1975.

Chapter 14

Figures 14-1 A, B, 14-2 A, 14-3, and 14-4: Modified from Parent A, Carpenter MB. Carpenter's Human Neuroanatomy. 9th ed. Baltimore: Williams & Wilkins, 1996.

Figure 14-5: Modified from Carpenter MB. Core Text of Neuroanatomy. 4th ed. Baltimore: Lippincott Williams & Wilkins, 1991.

Figure 14-6: Modified from Guyton AC, Hall JE. Textbook of Medical Physiology. 11th ed. Philadelphia: Elsevier Saunders, 2006.

Chapter 15

Figures 15-1, 15-2, and 15-7: Reprinted with permission from Haines DE. Neuroanatomy: An Atlas of Structures, Sections, and Systems. 8th ed. Philadelphia: Lippincott Williams & Wilkins, 2012.

Figure 15-4: Modified from Carpenter MB. Core Text of Neuroanatomy. 4th ed. Baltimore: Lippincott Williams & Wilkins, 1991.

Figure 15-8 A, B: Courtesy of Madhuri Behari, MD, Department of Neuroradiology, All India Institute of Medical Sciences, New Delhi.

Figure 15-9 A, B: Courtesy of Alexandru Barboi, MD. Department of Neurology, Medical College of Wisconsin, Milwaukee.

Chapter 16

Figure 16-1 A, B: Reprinted with permission from Haines, De. Neuroanatomy: An Atlas of Structures, Sections, and Systems, 8th ed. Philadelphia: Lippincott Williams & Wilkins, 2012.

Figure 16-2: Modified from Parent A, Carpenter MB. Carpenter's Human Neuroanatomy. 9th ed. Baltimore: Williams & Wilkins, 1996.

Chapter 17

Figure 17-1: Reprinted with permission from Mettler FA. Mettler's Neuroanatomy. 2nd ed. St. Louis: Mosby, 1948.

Figure 17-2: Modified from Moore KL, Persaud TVN. The Developing Human: Clinically Oriented Embryology. 8th ed. Philadelphia: Saunders, 2007.

Figures 17-3 and 17-4: Reprinted with permission from Parent A, Carpenter MB. Carpenter's Human Neuroanatomy. 9th ed. Baltimore: Williams & Wilkins, 1996.

Figures 17-9 A–C, 17-12, 17-17, and 17-21: Modified from Parent A, Carpenter MB. Carpenter's Human Neuroanatomy. 9th ed. Baltimore: Williams & Wilkins, 1996.

Figure 17-13B: Modified from Campbell WW. DeJong's Neurologic Examination, 6th Edition. Philadelphia: Lippincott Williams & Wilkins, 2005.

Figures 17-14, 17-15, 17-18, 17-19, 17-22 to 17-26, 17-30 to 17-32, and 17-34: Based on data from House EL, Pansky B. A Functional Approach to Neuroanatomy. New York: McGraw-Hill, 1967.

Figure 17-29: Modified from Van Allen MW, Rodnitzky RL. Pictorial Manual of Neurologic Tests. 2nd ed. Chicago: Yearbook Medical Publishers, 1981.

Chapter 18

Figures 18-6, 18-7, 18-8, 18-9, and 18-10: Reprinted with permission from Parent A, Carpenter MB. Carpenter's Human Neuroanatomy. 9th ed. Baltimore: Williams & Wilkins, 1996.

Figure 18-11: Modified from Carpenter MB. Core Text of Neuroanatomy. 4th ed. Baltimore: Lippincott Williams & Wilkins, 1991.

Chapter 20

Figures 20-1 and 20-2 B: Courtesy of Varun K. Saxena, MD, Center for Neurological Disorders, Milwaukee.

Figures 20-3, 20-4, 20-6, 20-8, and 20-12: Courtesy of Lotfi Hacein-Bey, MD, Department of Radiology, Sutter Neuroscience Institute, Sacramento, CA.

Figures 20-7 and 20-11. Courtesy of Leighton P. Mark, MD, Department of Neuroradiology, Medical College of Wisconsin, Milwaukee.

Figure 20-9: Reprinted with permission from Lehericy S, Cohen L, Bazin B, et al. Functional MR evaluation of temporal and frontal language dominance compared with the WADA test. Neurology 2000;54:1625–1633.

Figure 20-10: Courtesy of Stefan Heim, PhD, Simon B. Eickhoff, MD, Anja K. Ischebeck, PhD, et al. Institute of Medicine, Research Centre Juelich, Juelich, Germany.

Figure 20-13: Courtesy of John Mazziotta, MD, Reed Institute, UCLA Medical Center, Los Angeles.

Figure 20-14 A, B. Courtesy of Howard S. Kirshner, MD, Vanderbilt Medical Center, Nashville, TN.

Figure 20-15: Modified from Bhatnagar SC, Barber SA, Buckingham HA, Mandybur GT. On lexical organization in the human brain: Evidence from intracarotid sodium amytal injection. ACTA Neuropsychologica 2005;3:107–119.

Figure 20-18 B: Modified with permission from Parent A, Carpenter MB. Carpenter's Human Neuroanatomy. 9th ed. Baltimore: Williams & Wilkins, 1996.

Figure 20-19: Modified from Bhatnagar SC, Andy OJ, Korabic EW, Tikofsky RS. Effects of bilateral thalamic stimulation on dichotic verbal processing. J Neurolinguistics 1990;4:407–425.

Figures 20-22 to 20-24: Modified from Genetic Counseling [March of Dimes Birth Defects Foundation Booklet 9-0022]. White Plains, NY, 1984.

TABLES

Chapter 4

Table 4-2: Modified from Arey LB. Developmental Anatomy. Philadelphia: Saunders, 1966.

Table 4-4: Modified from Moore KL, Persaud TVN. The Developing Human: Clinically Oriented Embryology. 8th ed. Philadelphia: Saunders, 2007.

Table 4-5: Modified from Menkes JH. Textbook of Child Neurology. 5th ed. Baltimore: Williams & Wilkins, 1995.

Chapter 10

Table 10-3: Data from Wada J, Rasmussen T. Intracarotid injection of sodium Amytal for the lateralization of cerebral dominance. J Neurosurg 1960;17:266–282.

Chapter 16

Table 16-3: Based on Castro AJ. Neuroscience: an outline approach. St. Louis: Mosby, 2002.

Suggested Readings

GENERAL SOURCES

Adams RD, Victor M, Ropper AH. Principles of Neuroanatomy. 7th ed. New York: McGraw-Hill, 2001.

Angevine JB, Cotman CW. Principles of Neuroanatomy. New York: Oxford University Press, 1981.

Arey LB. Developmental Anatomy: A Textbook and Laboratory Manual of Embryology. 7th ed. Philadelphia: Saunders, 1974.

Bear MF, Connors BW, Paradiso MA. Neuroscience: Exploring the Brain. 3rd ed. Baltimore: Lippincott Williams & Wilkins, 2007.

Brodal P. The Central Nervous System: Structure and Function. 3rd ed. New York: Oxford University Press, 2004.

Brown AG. Nerve Cells and Nervous Systems: An Introduction to Neuroscience. 2nd ed. New York: Springer, 2001.

Carpenter MB. Core Text of Neuroanatomy. 4th ed. Baltimore: Lippincott Williams & Wilkins, 1991.

Crafts RC. A Textbook of Human Anatomy. 3rd ed. New York: Wiley, 1979.

Crosby EC, Humphrey T, Lauer EW. Correlative Anatomy of the Nervous System. New York: Macmillan, 1962.

Gelb DJ. Introduction to Clinical Neurology. 3rd ed. Boston: Butterworth-Heinemann, 2005.

Gilman S, Newman SW. Manter and Gatz's Essentials of Clinical Neuroanatomy and Neurophysiology. 10th ed. Philadelphia: Davis, 2003.

Guyton AC, Hall JE. Textbook of Medical Physiology. 12th ed. Philadelphia: Saunders, 2011.

Haines DE. Fundamental Neuroscience for Basic and Clinical Applications. 3rd ed. Philadelphia: Churchill Livingston/Elsevier, 2006.

Haines DE. Neuroanatomy: An Atlas of Structures, Sections, and Systems. 8th ed. Baltimore: Lippincott Williams & Wilkins, 2012.

Heimer L. The Human Brain and Spinal Cord: Functional Neuroanatomy and Dissection Guide. 2nd ed. New York: Springer-Verlag, 1995.

Heuttel SA, Song AW, McCarthy G. Functional Magnetic Resonance Imaging. 2nd ed. Sunderland: Sinauer, 2008.

Hickok G, Poeppel D. Towards a functional neuroanatomy of speech perception. Trends Cogn Sci 2000;4:131–138.

Kandel ER, Schwartz JH, Jessell TM. Principles of Neural Science. 4th ed. New York: McGraw-Hill, 2000.

Kaufman DM. Clinical Neurology for Psychiatrists. 6th ed. Philadelphia: Saunders, 2006.

Kiernan JA. Barr's the Human Nervous System: An Anatomical Viewpoint. 9th ed. Philadelphia: Lippincott Williams & Wilkins, 2008.

Marieb EN. Essentials of Human Anatomy and Physiology. 10th ed. San Francisco: Benjamin-Cummings, 2011.

Martini FH, Nash Judi, Bartholomew EF, Seiger C. Fundamentals of Anatomy and Physiology. 7th ed. San Francisco: Benjamin-Cummings, 2004.

Nadeau SE. Medical Neuroscience. Philadelphia: Saunders, 2004.

Nolte J. The Human Brain: An Introduction to Its Functional Anatomy. 6th ed. St. Louis: Mosby, 2008.

Parent A. Carpenter's Human Neuroanatomy. 9th ed. Baltimore: Lippincott Williams & Wilkins, 1996.

Rowland LP, Pedley TA. Merritt's Neurology. 12th ed. Philadelphia: Lippincott Williams & Wilkins, 2009.

Standring S. Gray's Anatomy: The Anatomical Basis of Clinical Practice. 40th ed. Edinburgh, UK and New York: Churchill Livingstone/Elsevier, 2008.

Tortora GJ, Derrickson BH. Principles of Anatomy and Physiology. 13th ed. New York: Wiley, 2011.

Victor M, Ropper AH, Samuels M. Principles of Neurology. 9th ed. New York: McGraw-Hill, 2009.

Weiner HL, Levitt LP, Rae-Grant A. Neurology. 8th ed. Philadelphia: Lippincott Williams & Wilkins, 2008.

Wiederholt WC. Neurology for Non-Neurologists. 4th ed. Philadelphia: Saunders, 1995.

CHAPTER 1

Aronson AE. Aronson's Neurosciences Pocket Lectures. San Diego: Singular Publishing Group, 2000.

Broca P. Sur la faculte du language artiule. Bulletin de la Societe d'Anthropologie. 1961;6:337–393.

Brodmann K. Vergleichende Lokalisation lehre der Grosshirnrinde in ihren Prinzipien dargestellt auf Grunddes Zellenbaues. Leipzig, Germany: Barth, 1909.

Castro AJ, Merchut MP, Neafsey EJ, Wurster RD. Neuroscience : An Outline Approach. St. Louis, Mosby: 2002.

Donoghue JP, Sanes JN. Organization of adult motor cortex representation patterns following neonatal forelimb nerve injury in rats. J Neurosci 1988;8:3221–3232.

Dougherty DD, Rauch SL, Rosenbaum JF. Essentials of Neuroimaging for Clinical Practice. Washington DC: American Psychiatric Publishing, 2003.

Draganski B, Gaser C, Busch V, et al. Neuroplasticity: Changes in grey matter induced by training. Nature 2004;427:311–312.

Gottlieb G. Individual Development and Evolution. New York: Oxford University Press, 1992.

Guiraud J, Besle J, Arnold L, et al. Evidence of a tonotopic organization of the auditory cortex in cochlear implant users. J Neurosci 2007;27:7838–7846.

Jenkins WM, Merzenich MM, Ochs MT, Allard T, Guk-Robles E. Functional Reorganization of Primary Somatosensory Cortex in Adult Owl Monkeys After Behaviorally Controlled Tactile Stimulation. San Francisco, California, 1990.

Kingsley RE. Concise Text of Neuroscience. 2nd ed. Philadelphia: Lippincott Williams & Wilkins, 1999.

Ramachandran VS. Secrets of the Mind [Motion Picture]. Boston: WGBH Boston Video, 2001.

Sadato N, Campbell G, Ibanez V, Deiber M, Hallett M. Complexity affects regional cerebral blood flow change during sequential finger movements. J Neurosci 1996;16(8):2691–2700.

Ward J. The Student's Guide to Cognitive Neuroscience. New York: Psychology Press, 2010.

Wernicke K. The symptom complex of aphasia. In: Church ED, ed. Modern Clinical Medicine: Diseases of the Nervous System. New York: Appleton Century Crofts, 1874.

CHAPTER 2

Sperry RW. Forebrain commissurotomy and conscious awareness. J Med Philos 1977;2:101.

Catani M. From hodology to function. Brain 2007;130:602–605.

CHAPTER 4

Bhatnagar KP, Smith TD. The human vemeronasal organ. III. Postnatal development from infancy to the ninth decade. J Anat 2001;199:289–302.

Brodal P. The Central Nervous System: Structure and Function, 4th ed. New York: Oxford University Press, 2010.

Hamilton WJ, Mossman HW. Hamilton, Boyd, and Mossman's Human Embryology: Prenatal Development of Form and Function. 4th ed. Cambridge: Helfer, 1972.

Kelly DE, Wood RL, Enders AC. Baily's Text book of Microscopic Anatomy. Baltimore: Lippincott Williams & Wilkins, 1984.

Lander ES, Linton LM, Birren, Nusbaum C, et al. (some 50 more authors). Initial sequencing and analysis of the human genome. Nature 2001;409:860–921.

Langman J, Shimada M, Rodier P. Floxuridine and its influence on postnatal cerebellar development. Pediatr Res 1972;6:758–764.

Luckasson R, et al. Mental Retardation, Definition, Classification, and Systems of Support. 10th ed. Washington: American Association on Mental Retardation, 2002.

Moore KL, Persaud TVN. The Developing Human: Clinically Oriented Embryology. 8th ed. Philadelphia: Saunders, 2007.

Sadler TW. Langman's Medical Embryology. 11th ed. Philadelphia: Lippincott Williams & Wilkins, 2010.

CHAPTER 5

Lecours AR. Myelogenetic correlates of development of speech and language. In: Lenneberg EH, Lenneberg E, eds. Foundation of Language Development, Vol. 1. New York: Academic, 1975.

Lenneberg EH. Biological Foundations of Language. New York: Wiley, 1967.

Yakovlev PI, Lecours AR. The myelogenetic cycles of regional maturation of the brain. In: Minkowski A, ed. Regional Development of the Brain in Early Life. Oxford: Blackwell, 1967.

CHAPTER 6

Alexander MP. Clinical anatomic correlations of aphasia following predominantly subcortical lesions. In: Boller F, Grafman J, eds. Handbook of Neuropsychology, Vol. 2. Amsterdam: Elsevier, 1989.

Andy OJ, Bhatnagar SC. Inhibitory effects of thalamic stimulation on acquired stuttering: Physiological evidence from four neurosurgical subjects. Brain Lang 1992;42:385–401.

Andy OJ, Bhatnagar SC. Thalamic-induced stuttering (surgical observations). J Speech Hear Res 1991;34:796–800.

Bhatnagar SC, Andy OJ. Alleviation of acquired stuttering from thalamic stimulation. J Neurol Neurosurg Psychiatry 1989;52:1182–1184.

Bhatnagar SC, Andy OJ, Korabic EW, et al. The effect of thalamic stimulation in processing of verbal stimuli in dichotic listening tasks: A case study. Brain Lang 1989;36:236–251.

Bhatnagar SC, Andy OJ, Korabic EW, Tikofsky RS. Effects of bilateral thalamic stimulation on dichotic verbal processing. J Neurolinguistics 1990;5:407–425.

Bhatnagar SC, Buckingham HW. Neurogenic stuttering: its reticular modulation. Cur Neurol Neurosci Rep 2010;10:491–498.

Bhatnagar SC, Mandybur GT. Effects of intralaminar thalamic stimulation on language functions. Brain Lang 2005;92:1–11.

Ojemann GA. Organization of short-term verbal memory in language areas of human cortex: Evidence from electrical stimulation. Brain Lang 1978;5:331–348.

Ojemann GA. Brain organization for language from the perspective of electrical stimulation mapping. Behav Brain Res 1983;6:189–230.

Ojemann GA, Fedio P, Van Buren JM. Anomia from pulvinar and subcortical parietal stimulation. Brain 1968;91:99–116.

Penfield W, Roberts L. Speech and Brain Mechanisms. Princeton: Princeton University, 2003.

CHAPTER 7

Brott TG, Hobson RW, Howard G, et al. Stenting versus endarterectomy for treatment of carotid-artery stenosis. N Engl J Med 2010;363:11–23.

Executive Committee for the Asymptomatic Carotid Atherosclerosis Study. Endarterectomy for asymptomatic carotid artery stenosis. JAMA 1995;273:1421–1428.

Mas J-L, Chatellier G, Beyssen B, et al. Endarterectomy versus stenting in patients with symptomatic severe carotid stenosis. N Engl J Med 2006;355:1660–1671

North American Symptomatic Carotid Endarterectomy Trial Collaborators. Beneficial effect of carotid endarterectomy in symptomatic patients with high-grade carotid stenosis. N Engl J Med 1991;325:445–453.

Saver, J.L. Time is Brain-Quantified. Stroke 2006, 37:263-266.

The SPACE Collaborative Group. 30 day results from the SPACE trial of stent-protected angioplasty versus carotid endarterectomy in symptomatic patients: a radomised non-inferiority trial. The Lancet 2006;368(9543):1239–1247.

CHAPTER 9

Bhatnagar SC, Andy OJ. Tonotypic cortical representation. Presented at the Annual Meeting of the Pavlovian Society of North America, Orlando Florida, 1988.

Bhatnagar SC, Andy OJ, Korabic EW, et al. The effect of thalamic stimulation in processing of verbal stimuli in dichotic listening tasks: A case study. Brain Lang 1989;36:236–251.

Bhatnager SC, Andy OJ, Korabic EW, Tikofsky RS. Effects of bilateral thalamic stimulation on dichotic verbal processing. J Neurolinguistics 1990;5:407–425.

Donoghue JP, Sanes JN. Organization of adult motor cortex representation patterns following neonatal forelimb nerve injury in rats. J Neurosci 1988;8:3221–3232.

Geschwind N, Levitsky W. Human brain: Left-right asymmetries in temporal speech region. Science 1968;161:186–187.

Kilgard MP, Merzenich MM. Plasticity of temporal information processing in the primary auditory cortex. Nature Neurosci 1998;1:727–731.

Kingsley RE. Concise Text of Neuroscience. 2nd ed. Philadelphia: Lippincott Williams & Wilkins, 1999.

Lesser R, Lueders H, Klem G, et al. Extraoperative cortical functional localization in patients with epilepsy. J Clin Neurophysiol 1987;4:27–53.

Moore JK, Linthicum FH. Auditory system. In: Paxinos G, Mai JK, eds. The Human Nervous System. San Diego: Elsevier Academic Press, 2004:1242–1279.

Worden, F G. Hearing and the neural detection of acoustic patterns. Behavioral Science 1971;16(1):20-30.

CHAPTER 14

Guyton AC, Hall JE. Textbook of Medical Physiology. 11th ed. Philadelphia: Saunders, 2006.

CHAPTER 15

Battig K, Rosvold HE, Mishkin M. Comparison of the effect of frontal and caudate lesions on delayed response and attention in monkeys. J Comp Physiol Psychol 1960;53:400–404.

Bhatnagar SC, Mandybur GT. Effects of intralaminar thalamic stimulation on language functions. Brain Lang 2005;92:1–11.

Bhatnagar SC, Mandybur GT. Electrical stimulation of brain and language. In: Brown K, ed. Encyclopedia of Language and Linguistics, Vol. 4. England: Elsevier, 2006:97–105.

Brunner RJ, Kornhuber HH, Seemuller E, et al. Basal ganglia participation in language pathology. Brain Lang 1982;16:281–299.

Levy R, Friedman HR, Davachi KL, Goldman-Rakic PS. Differential activation of the caudate nucleus in primates performing spatial and nonspatial working memory tasks. J Neurosci 1997;17.

Middleton FA, Trick PL. Basal ganglia output and cognition: Evidence from anatomical, behavioral, and clinical studies. Brain Cogn 2000;42:183–200.

Paxinos G, Mai JK, eds. The Human Nervous System. New York: Elsevier, 2004.

Parkinson J. An essay on the shaking palsy. London: Sherwood, Neely and Jones, 1817.

CHAPTER 18

Additional Sources:

Andy O, Bhatnagar S. Stuttering acquired from subcortical pathologies and its alleviation from thalamic perturbation. Brain Lang 1992;42:385–401.

Andy O, Bhatnagar S. Thalamic-induced stuttering (surgical observations). J Speech Hear Res 1991;34:796–800.

Benarroch, E.F. Respiratory Chemosensitivity: New insights and clinical implications. Neurology, 68, June 12, 2140-2143, 2007.

Bhatnagar S, Mandybur G, Silverman F, Buckingham H. Stimulation-evoked dysfluency during cortical mapping. Paper Presented at the Meeting of the International Academy of Aphasia. Boulder, 2001.

Bhatnagar SC, Mandybur GT. Electrical stimulation of brain and language. In: Brown K, ed. Encyclopedia of Language and Linguistics, Vol. 4. England: Elsevier, 2006:97–105.

Magoun HW. The Waking Brain. 2nd ed. Springfield: Thomas, 1963.

CHAPTER 19

Alexander MP, Benson DF. The aphasias and related disturbances. In: Joynt RJ, ed. Clinical Neurology, Vol. 1. Philadelphia: Lippincott Williams & Wilkins, 1998.

Benson DF. The third alexia. Arch Neurol 1977;34:327–331.

Benson DR, Sheremata WA, Bouchard R, et al. Conduction aphasia: A clinicopathological study. Arch Neurol 1973;28:339–346.

Bhatnagar SC, Mandybur GT, Buckingham HW, Andy OJ. Language representation in the human brain: Evidence from cortical mapping. Brain Lang 2000;74:238–259.

Bigio EH. Update on recent molecular and genetic advances in frontotemporal lobar degeneration. J Neuropathol Exp Neurol 2008;67:635–648.

Blumer D, Benson BF. Personality changes with frontal and temporal lesions. In: Benson DF, Blumer D, eds. Psychiatric Aspects of Neurologic Disease. New York: Grune & Stratton, 1975.

Damasio H, Damasio AR. The anatomical basis of conduction aphasia. Brain 1980;103:337–350.

Darley FL, Aronson AE, Brown JR. Motor Speech Disorders. Philadelphia: Saunders, 1975.

Déjérine J. Contribution a letude anotomo-pathologique et cliniques des differentes varietes de cicite verbale. Memories-Societe Biologie 1892;4:61–90.

Demonet JF, Chollet F, Ramsay S, et al. The anatomy of phonological and semantic processing in normal subjects. Brain 1992;115:1753–1768.

DeRenzi E, Motti F, Nichelli P. Imitating gestures: A quantitative approach to ideomotor apraxia. Arch Neurol 1980;37:6–10.

Duffy JR. Motor Speech Disorders: Substrates, Differential Diagnosis, and Management. 2nd ed. St. Louis: Elsevier Mosby, 2005.

Evans DA, Funkenstein HH, Albert MS, et al. Clinically diagnosed Alzheimer's disease: An epidemiologic study in a community population of older persons. JAMA 1989;262:2551–2556.

Gerstmann J. Zur Symptomatologie der Hirnlasionen im Bergangsgebiet der unteren Parietal und mittleren Occipitalwindung (das Syndrom: Fingeragnosie, Rechts-Links Strung, Agraphie, Akalkulie). Nervenartzt 1930:691–695. [Reprinted in Rittenberg DA, Hochberg FH, eds. Neurological Classics in Modern Translation. New York: Hafner, 1977.]

Geschwind N. The organization of language and the brain. Science 1970;170:940–944.

Geschwind N. The apraxias: Neural mechanisms of disorders of learned movement. Am Sci 1975;63:188–195.

Geschwind N, Levitsky W. Human brain: Left-right asymmetries in temporal speech region. Science 1968;161:186–187.

Geschwind N, Quadfasel F, Segarra J. Isolation of the speech area. Neuropsychologia 1968;6:327–340.

Goldman-Rakic PS. The prefrontal landscape: Implications of functional architecture for understanding human mentation and the central executive. Philos Trans R Soc Lond B Biol Sci 1996;351:1445–1453.

Gorno-Tempini ML, Dronkers NF, Rankin K, et al. Cognition and anatomy in three variants of primary progressive aphasia. Ann Neurol 2004;55:335–346.

Heilman KM, Meador KJ, Loring DW. Hemispheric asymmetries of limb-kinetic apraxia: A loss of deftness. Neurology 2000;55:523–526.

Heilman KM, Maher LM, Greenwald ML, Rothi L. Conceptual apraxia from lateralized lesions. Neurology 1997;49:457–464.

Hickok G, Poeppel D. Towards a functional neuroanatomy of speech perception. Trends Cogn Sci 2000;4:131–138.

Josephs KA. Frontotemporal dementia and related disorders: deciphering the enigma. Ann Neurol 2008;64:4–14.

Kirshner HS. Apraxia of speech: A linguistic enigma. A neurologist's perspective. Semin Speech Lang 1992;13:14–24.

Kirshner HS, ed. Handbook of Neurological Speech and Language Disorders. New York: Marcel Dekker, 1995.

Kirshner HS. Behavioral neurology. Practical Science of Mind and Brain. 2nd ed. Boston: Butterworth Heinemann (now Elsevier) 2002:1–474.

Kirshner HS. First Exposure Neurology. New York: McGraw Hill, 2007:1–429.

Kirshner HS, Tanridag O, Thurman L, Whetsell WO Jr. Progressive aphasia without dementia: two cases with focal spongiform degeneration. Ann Neurol 1987;22:527–532.

Kirshner HS, Casey PF, Henson J, Heinrich JJ. Behavioral features and lesion localization in Wernicke's aphasia. Aphasiology 1989;3:169–176.

Liepmann H. Apraxie. Ergbn der ges Med 1920;1:516–543. [Cited in Brown JW. Aphasia, Apraxia, and Agnosia. Springfield: Thomas, 1972.]

McIntosh RD, Schenk T. Two visual streams for perception an action: current trends. Neuropsychologia 2009;47:139–136.

Mesulam MM. Slowly progressive aphasia without generalized dementia. Ann Neurol 1982;11:592–598.

Mesulam MM, ed. Principles of Behavioral and Cognitive Neurology. 2nd ed. New York: Oxford University Press, 2000.

Mesulam MM. Primary progressive aphasia–a language-based dementia. N Engl J Med 2003;349:1535–1542.

Milner AD, Goodale MA. Two visual systems re-viewed. Neuropsychologia 2008;46:774–785.

Mohr JP, Pessin MS, Finklestein S, et al. Broca aphasia: Pathologic and clinical. Neurology 1978;28:311–324.

Naeser MA, Palumbo CL, Helm-Estabrooks N, Stiassny-Eder D, Albert ML. Severe nonfluency in aphasia: Role of the medial subcallosal fasciculus plus other white matter pathology in recovery of spontaneous language. Brain 1989;112:1–38.

Neary D, Snowden J. Fronto-temporal dementia: Nosology, neuropsychology, and neuropathology. Brain Cogn 1996;31:176–187.

Ochipa C, Rothi LJG, Heilman KM. Ideational apraxia: A deficit in tool selection and use. Ann Neurol 1989;25:190–193.

Ojemann G, Ojemann J, Lettich E, Berger M. Cortical language localization in left, dominant hemisphere. An electrical stimulation mapping investigation in 117 patients. J Neurosurg 1989;71:316–326.

Rasmussen T, Milner N. The role of early left brain injury on the lateralization of cerebral speech functions. Ann NY Acad Sci 1977;355–369.

Sacks O. The Man Who Mistook His Wife for a Hat and Other Clinical Tales. New York: Simon and Schuster, 1998.

Shallice T, Warrington EK. Auditory-verbal short-term memory impairment and conduction aphasia. Brain Lang 1977;4:479–491.

Wada J, Rasmussen T. Intracarotid injections of sodium amytal for the lateralization of cerebral speech dominance. Experimental and clinical Observations. J Neurosurg 1960;17:266–282.

CHAPTER 20

Alexander MP, Naeser MA, Palumbo CL. Correlations of subcortical CT lesion sites and aphasia profiles. Brain 1987;110:961–991.

Andy OJ, Bhatnagar SC. Right hemispheric language: Evidence from cortical stimulation. Brain Lang 1984;23:159–166.

Andy OJ, Bhatnagar SC. Thalamic-induced stuttering (surgical observations). J Speech Hear Res 1991;34:796–800.

Andy OJ, Bhatnagar SC. Inhibitory effects of thalamic stimulation on acquired stuttering: Physiological evidence from four neurosurgical subjects. Brain Lang 1992;42:385–401.

Bartholow R. Experimental investigations into functions of the human brain. Am J Med Sci 1874;67:305–315.

Bhatnagar SC, Andy OJ. Alleviation of acquired stuttering from thalamic stimulation. J Neurol Neurosurg Psychiatry 1989;52:1182–1184.

Bhatnagar SC, Buckingham HW. Neurogenic stuttering: Its reticular modulation. Curr Neurol Neurosci Rep 2010;10:491–498.

Bhatnagar SC, Mandybur GT. Effects of intralaminar thalamic stimulation on language functions. Brain Lang 2005;92:1–11.

Bhatnagar SC, Mandybur GT. Electrical stimulation of brain and language. In: Brown K, ed. Encyclopedia of Language and Linguistics, Vol. 4. England: Elsevier, 2006:97–105.

Bhatnagar SC, Andy OJ, Korabic EW, Tikofsky RS. Effects of bilateral thalamic stimulation on dichotic verbal processing. J Neurolinguistics 1990;5:407–425.

Bhatnagar SC, Barber SA, Mandybur GT, Buckingham HW. On lexical organization in the human brain: Evidence from intracarotid sodium amytal injection. Acta Neuropsychologica 2005;3:107–119.

Bhatnagar SC, Mandybur GT, Buckingham HW, Andy OJ. Language representation in the human brain: Evidence from cortical mapping. Brain Lang 2000;74:238–259.

Bhatnagar SC, Andy OJ, Korabic EW, et al. The effect of thalamic stimulation in processing of verbal stimuli in dichotic listening tasks: A case study. Brain Lang 1989;36:236–251.

Bruxton RB. Introduction to Functional Magnetic Resonance Imaging, Principles, and Techniques. Cambridge: Cambridge University Press, 2002.

Damasio H. Neuroanatomical correlates of the aphasias. In: Sarno MT, ed. Acquired Aphasia. 3rd ed. San Diego: Academic, 1998.

Dougherty DD, Rauch SL, Rosenbaum JF. Essentials of Neuroimaging for Clinical Practice. Washington: American Psychiatric Publishing, 2004.

Fritsch G, Hitzig E. Uber die elektrische erregbarkeit des Grosshirns. Archiv der Anatomische Physiolosische Weisenschaftliche Medizine 1870;37:300–332. [Translated into English and reprinted as: On the electrical excitability of the cerebrum. In: von Bonin G, ed. Some Papers on the Cerebral Cortex. Springfield, IL: Thomas, 1960:73–96.]

Gado M, Hanaway J, Frank R. Functional anatomy of the cerebral cortex by computed tomography. J Comput Assist Tomogr 1979;3:1–19.

Grossman CB. Magnetic Resonance Imaging and Computer Tomography of the Head and Spine. 2nd ed. Baltimore: Lippincott Williams & Wilkins, 1996.

Heilman KM, Meador KJ, Loring DW. Hemispheric asymmetries of limb-kinetic apraxia: A loss of deftness. Neurology 2000;55:523–526.

Kimura D. Functional asymmetry of the brain in dichotic listening. Cortex 1967;3:163–178.

Lassen NA, Ingvar DH, Skinhoj E. Brain function and blood flow. Sci Am 1978;239:62–71.

Lesser R, Hahn J, Lueders H, et al. The use of chronic subdural electrodes for cortical mapping of speech. Epilepsia 1981;22:240.

Lesser R, Lueders H, Klem G, et al. Extraoperative cortical functional localization in patients with epilepsy. J Clin Neurophysiol 1987;4:27–53.

Mazziotta JC, Phelps ME, Carson RE, Kuhl DE. Tomographic mapping of human cerebral metabolism: Sensory deprivation. Ann Neurol 1982;12:435–444.

Mazziotta JC, Phelps ME, Miller J, Kuhl DE. Tomographic mapping of human cerebral metabolism: Normal unstimulated state. Neurology 1981;31:503–506.

Metter EJ. Neuroanatomy and physiology of aphasia: Evidence from positron emission tomography. Aphasiology 1987;1:3–33.

Metter EJ, Hanson WR. Brain imaging as related to speech and language. In: Darby J, ed. Speech Evaluation in Neurology. New York: Grune & Stratton, 1985.

Metter EJ, Jackson C, Kempler D, et al. Glucose metabolic asymmetries in chronic Wernicke's, Broca's and conduction aphasias. Neurology 1986;36(suppl 1):317.

Milner B, Branch C. Experimental analysis of cerebral dominance in man. In: Millikan CH, Darley FL, eds. Brain Mechanism Underlying Speech and Language. New York: Grune & Stratton, 1967:177–184.

Naeser MA, Hayward RW. Lesion localization in aphasia with cranial computed tomography and the Boston diagnostic aphasia examination. Neurology 1987;28:545–551.

Ojemann GA. Brain organization for language from the perspective of electrical stimulation mapping. Behav Brain Res 1983;6:189–230.

Ojemann G, Whitaker H. The bilingual brain. Arch Neurol 1978a;35:409–412.

Ojemann G, Ojemann J, Lettich E, Berger M. Cortical language localization in left, dominant hemisphere. An electrical stimulation mapping investigation in 117 patients. J Neurosurg 1989;71:316–326.

Penfield W, Roberts L. Speech and Brain Mechanisms. Princeton: Princeton University, 1959.

Tikofsky RS, Heilman RS. Brain single photon emission computed tomography: New activation and intervention studies. Semin Nucl Med 1991;21:40–57.

Wada J, Rasmussen T. Intracarotid injection of sodium Amytal for the lateralization of cerebral dominance. J Neurosurg 1960;17:266–282.

Index

Note: Page numbers in *italics* refers to figures; those followed by b and t refer to boxes and tables, respectively.